Giovanni Mantovani (Ed)

Cachexia and Wasting: A Modern Approach

Giovanni Mantovani (Ed)

# Cachexia and Wasting: A Modern Approach

*Co-editors:*
Stefan D. Anker
Akio Inui
John E. Morley
Filippo Rossi Fanelli
Daniele Scevola
Michael W. Schuster
Shing-Shing Yeh

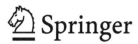 Springer

G. Mantovani (*Editor*)
Department of Medical Oncology
University of Cagliari,
Cagliari, Italy

*Co-editors*
S.D. Anker
Imperial College, NHLI, Department of Clinical
Cardiology, London, United Kingdom
Applied Cachexia Research, Department of Cardiology
Charité, Campus Virchow-Klinikum, Berlin, Germany

J.E. Morley
GRECC, VA Medical Center and Division of Geriatric
Medicine, Saint Louis University, St. Louis, MO, USA

D. Scevola
Department of Infectious Diseases, IRCCS S.Matteo
Polyclinic, University of Pavia, Pavia, Italy

S.-S. Yeh
Department of Medicine - Geriatrics
University of New York at Stony Brook
VAMC, Northport, NY USA

A. Inui
Kagoshima University
Graduate School of Medical and Dental Sciences
Department of Behavioral Medicine
Kagoshima, Japan

F. Rossi Fanelli
Department of Clinical Medicine, University of Rome,
La Sapienza, Rome, Italy

M.W. Schuster
Bone Marrow and Blood Stem Cell Transplantation
Program, Center for Lymphoma and Myeloma,
New York Presbyterian Hospital/Weill Medical Center,
New York, NY, USA

Library of Congress Control Number: 2006922659

ISBN-10 88-470-0471-3 Springer Milan Berlin Heidelberg New York
ISBN-13 978-88-470-0471-9 Springer Milan Berlin Heidelberg New York

Springer is a part of Springer Science+Business Media

springer.com
© Springer-Verlag Italia 2006
Printed in Italy

Cover design: Simona Colombo, Milan, Italy
Cover illustration: Roberto Serpe, Cagliari, Italy
Typesetting: Graphostudio, Milan, Italy
Printing and binding: Printer Trento, Trento, Italy

# Preface

Cachexia may well represent the devastating flip side of the tremendous achievements of modern medicine, as the incidence of cachexia is also a function of survival of chronic illness.

Many diseases – which rapidly led to death only a few years ago – are now better controlled by new therapies. Even if we cannot cure and eradicate these diseases, their natural history has significantly increased by months and years. Although these new therapeutic strategies represent a remarkable advantage over the previous standards of care, it is impossible to ignore the fact that many more patients are now facing the nutritional and metabolic consequences of prolonged immunological and hormonal challenges due to both the illness process itself and the aggressive therapies.

This book aims to conceptualise the fact that cachexia is a clinical syndrome that accompanies the course of several medical conditions such as cancer, heart failure, diabetes, chronic renal failure and chronic obstructive lung disease, as well as gastrointestinal and infection-related diseases (e.g. HIV infection and sepsis) and ageing. Cachexia is a complex syndrome with many possible scenarios, not just one disease. This is one reason why there is not yet a unified definition of cachexia.

From a pathophysiological standpoint, cachexia can be considered the result of a complex cascade of many different events, such as chronic inflammation and free radical generation, chronic hyperactivation of immune and many different endocrine systems causing dysregulation of appetite, hormone resistance syndromes, catabolism and impaired anabolism. In the past, inflammatory cytokines have received the most attention; today, for instance, the ubiquitin-proteasome system is at the centre of research attention. New treatments based on this research have not yet been proven to be effective, but we are optimistic that the near future will bring many positive developments.

It appears that the high prevalence of cachexia has not yet been matched by a similar rise in awareness of its clinical consequences among healthcare professionals around the world. Weight loss, muscle wasting, inflammation, asthenia and loss of appetite are important signs and symptoms of cachexia. They often go under-recognised in clinical practice. Interestingly, it seems that patients are more concerned than doctors about their nutritional status and related debilitating symptoms, such as fatigue and shortness of breath. Therefore, one of the aims of our book is to increase awareness. Only if cachexia is recognised can research efforts start and available treatments be used to improve the health status of our patients.

The past decade has seen rapid advances in knowledge of every aspect of cachexia, mainly in the pathophysiological mechanisms leading to the syndrome. The next decade – we believe – will bring an even better understanding of the processes leading to muscle and fat tissue wasting. But, particularly, it will bring the first successful therapies. An important aspect in these treatment development efforts will be the cooperation of physicians and scientists across specialties. A successful cachexia treatment in one disease area is also likely to work in another area. This is also a form of translational medicine.

Due to the enormous efforts of scientific societies, individual researchers and patient associations, and with the support of the pharmaceutical industry, a series of congresses, workshops, public conferences and seminars have been organised in the past 6 years, and the clinical consequences of cachexia are now receiving more attention from health-related professionals, the media, and even political institutions. It is now acknowledged that the cachexia syndrome is an extremely interesting biological phenomenon. Cachexia – in itself – is a relevant clinical event, particularly when considering its implications in terms of increased morbidity and mortality, and it is therefore also an important socio-economic issue.

In summary, cachexia is a complex syndrome/disease, which can be analysed from different perspectives, including, but not limited to, those of morphologists, epidemiologists, biochemists, biologists, physiologists, clinicians (oncologists, surgeons, cardiologists, nephrologists, pulmonologists, nutritionists, immunologists, etc.).

The primary purpose of this reference work is to share the knowledge on cachexia with researchers and scientists in this field. The text is mostly based on observations and studies performed by scientists over the past 15 years. We express our sincere appreciation and thanks to our many colleagues who provided us with unusually fine unpublished manuscripts to be included in this book.

We hope that this book will help facilitate understanding of the complex yet unequivocal clinical role of the cachexia syndrome. Cachexia is a worldwide inter-disciplinary problem. This makes it an exciting and very worthwhile area of research and clinical work.

*Giovanni Mantovani*
*Stefan D. Anker*
*Akio Inui*
*John E. Morley*
*Filippo Rossi Fanelli*
*Daniele Scevola*
*Michael W. Schuster*
*Shing-Shing Yeh*

# Contents

## 4. THE DIFFERENT FEATURES OF WASTING IN HUMANS

## 5. PATHOPHYSIOLOGY OF WASTING/CACHEXIA

## 6. MEDICAL CAUSES OF WASTING/CACHEXIA

## 7. CACHEXIA AND AGEING

# 10. TREATMENT OF CANCER CACHEXIA

## 11. TREATMENT OF CACHEXIA IN THE ELDERLY

## 12. A GLOBAL PERSPECTIVE FOR THE TREATMENT OF CACHEXIA

# List of Contributors

**Almendro V.**
Cancer Research Group,
Department of Biochemistry and Molecular
Biology, University of Barcelona,
Barcelona, Spain

**Anderson M.**
Clinical Hematology/Oncology, Centocor,
Malvern, PA, USA

**Anker S.D.**
Department of Clinical Cardiology,
National Heart and Lung Institute,
Imperial College School of Medicine,
London, United Kingdom and Department of
Cardiology, Division of Applied Cachexia Research,
Charité Medical School,
Berlin, Germany

**Argilés J.M.**
Cancer Research Group, Department
of Biochemistry and Molecular Biology,
University of Barcelona,
Barcelona, Spain

**Asakawa A.**
Department of Clinical Molecular Medicine,
Division of Diabetes,
Digestive and kidney Diseases,
Kobe University Graduate School of Medicine,
Kobe, Japan

**Astara G.**
Department of Medical Oncology,
University of Cagliari,
Cagliari, Italy

**Baldi M.**
Department of Internal Medicine,
Division of Endocrinology, University of Turin,
Turin, Italy

**Balducci L.**
H. Lee Moffitt Cancer Center & Research Institute,
Senior Adult Community Program,
Tampa, FL, USA

**Baracos V.E.**
Department of Oncology,
University of Alberta,
Edmonton, Canada

**Bonometto P.**
Department of Medical and Surgical Sciences,
Geriatrics Division, University of Padua,
Padua, Italy

**Bosaeus I.**
Clinical Nutrition, Göteborg University,
Sahlgrenska University Hospital,
Göteborg, Sweden

**Bossola M.**
Department of Surgery,
The Catholic University of Rome,
Rome, Italy

**Bowers C.Y.**
Department of Medicine,
Division of Endocrinology and Metabolism,
Tulane University Health Sciences Center,
New Orleans, LA, USA

**Bozzetti F.**
Department of Surgery, Hospital of Prato,
Prato, Italy

**Brivio F.**
Department of Surgical Sciences and Intensive
Therapy, Department of General Surgery,
Surgery Unit 3, University of Milano-Bicocca
at San Gerardo Hospital,
Monza, Italy

**Broglio F.**
Department of Internal Medicine,
Division of Endocrinology and Metabolism,
University of Turin,
Turin, Italy

**Busetto L.**
Department of Medical and Surgical Sciences,
Geriatrics Division,
University of Padua,
Padua, Italy

**Busquets S.**
Cancer Research Group,
Department of Biochemistry and Molecular
Biology, University of Barcelona,
Barcelona, Spain

**Cascino A.**
Department of Clinical Medicine,
University of Rome La Sapienza,
Rome, Italy

**Chang J.-K.**
Phoenix Pharmaceuticals Inc.,
Belmont, CA, USA

**Cinti S.**
Institute of Normal Human Morphology,
School of Medicine, Polytechnic
University of Marche,
Ancona, Italy

**Coin A.**
Department of Medical and Surgical Sciences,
Geriatrics Division,
University of Padua,
Padua, Italy

**Cova D.**
Onco-Geriatric Unit, Pio Albergo Trivulzio
Institute, Milan, Italy and Geropharmacological
Pharmacosurveillance Center,
Department of Pharmacology,
University of Milan,
Milan, Italy

**Dahele M.**
Department of Clinical and Surgical Sciences
(Surgery), The University of Edinburgh,
Royal Infirmary, Edinburgh,
United Kingdom

**de Witte M.**
Clinical Hematology/Oncology,
Centocor,
Malvern, PA, USA

**Destefanis S.**
Department of Internal Medicine,
Division of Endocrinology and Metabolism,
University of Turin,
Turin, Italy

**Di Matteo A.**
Department of Infectious Diseases,
University of Pavia, IRCCS Policlinico S. Matteo,
Pavia, Italy

**Doehner W.**
Applied Cachexia Research,
Department of Cardiology,
Charité Medical School,
Campus Virchow-Klinikum, Humboldt University,
Berlin, Germany

**Doglietto G.B.**
Department of Surgery,
The Catholic University of Rome,
Rome, Italy

**Enzi G.**
Department of Medical and Surgical Sciences,
Geriatrics Division,
University of Padua,
Padua, Italy

**Evans W. J.**
Department of Geriatrics, Nutrition,
Metabolism and Exercise Laboratory,
University of Arkansas for Medical Sciences,
Little Rock, AR, USA

**Faga A.**
Department of Surgery, Section of Plastic and
Reconstructive Surgery,
University of Pavia,
Pavia, Italy

**Fearon K.C.H.**
Department of Clinical and Surgical Sciences
(Surgery), The University of Edinburgh,
Royal Infirmary, Edinburgh,
United Kingdom

**Fumagalli L.A.**
Department of Surgical Sciences and Intensive
Therapy, Department of General Surgery,
Surgery Unit 3, University of Milano-Bicocca
at San Gerardo Hospital,
Monza, Italy

**Gardani G.**
Department of General Surgery,
Division of Oncology and Radiotherapy,
University of Milano-Bicocca at San Gerardo
Hospital,
Monza, Italy

**Ghigo E.**
Department of Internal Medicine,
Division of Endocrinology and Metabolism,
University of Turin,
Turin, Italy

**Gianotti L.**
Department of Internal Medicine,
Division of Endocrinology and Metabolism,
University of Turin,
Turin, Italy

**Giglio O.**
Department of Infectious Diseases,
University of Pavia,
IRCCS Policlinico S. Matteo,
Pavia, Italy

**Gilli G.**
Department of Oncology-Pathology,
Clinical Oncology Unit,
University Hospital of Ferrara,
Ferrara, Italy

**Giordano K.F.**
Department of Oncology, Mayo Clinic,
Rochester, MN, USA

**Giordano R.**
Department of Internal Medicine,
Division of Endocrinology, University of Turin,
Turin, Italy

**Goncalves C.G.**
Department of Surgery,
Surgical Metabolism and Nutrition Laboratory,
Neuroscience Programs, University Hospital,
Upstate Medical University,
Syracuse, NY, USA

**Gottero C.**
Department of Internal Medicine,
Division of Endocrinology and Metabolism,
University of Turin,
Turin, Italy

**Gramignano G.**
Department of Medical Oncology,
University of Cagliari,
Cagliari, Italy

**Hurley D.L.**
Department of Biochemistry,
Tulane University Health Sciences Center,
New Orleans, LA, USA

**Inelmen E.M.**
Department of Medical and Surgical Sciences,
Geriatrics Division,
University of Padua,
Padua, Italy

**Inui A.**
Kagoshima University
Graduate School of Medical
and Dental Sciences
Department of Behavioral Medicine
Kagoshima, Japan

**Jatoi A.**
Department of Oncology, Mayo Clinic,
Rochester, MN, USA

**Kalantar-Zadeh K.**
Los Angeles Biomedical Research Institute at
Harbor-UCLA Medical Center,
Division of Nephrology and Hypertension,
and David Geffen School of Medicine,
University of California Los Angeles,
Los Angeles, CA, USA

**Kopple J.D.**
Division of Public Health,
Nutrition and Epidemiology,
University of California Berkeley
School of Public Health,
Berkeley and UCLA School of Public Health,
Los Angeles, CA, USA

**Lambert C.P.**
Department of Geriatrics, Nutrition,
Metabolism and Exercise Laboratory,
University of Arkansas for Medical Sciences,
Little Rock, AR, USA

**Lanfranco F.**
Department of Internal Medicine,
Division of Endocrinology, University of Turin,
Turin, Italy

**Langhans W.**
Institute of Animal Sciences,
Physiology and Animal Husbandry,
Schwerzenbach, Switzerland

**Laviano A.**
Department of Clinical Medicine,
University of Rome La Sapienza,
Rome, Italy

**Lelli G.**
Department of Oncology-Pathology,
Clinical Oncology Unit,
University Hospital of Ferrara,
Ferrara, Italy

**Linse K.D.**
Institute for Cellular and Molecular Biology,
University of Texas,
Austin, TX, USA

**Lissoni P.**
Department of General Surgery,
Division of Oncology and Radiotherapy,
University of Milano-Bicocca at San Gerardo
Hospital, Monza, Italy

**López-Soriano F.J.**
Cancer Research Group,
Department of Biochemistry and Molecular
Biology, University of Barcelona,
Barcelona, Spain

**Lorusso V.**
Medical Oncology Unit, IRCCS Oncology Institute,
Bari, Italy

**Lucatello B.**
Department of Internal Medicine,
Division of Endocrinology and Metabolism,
University of Turin,
Turin, Italy

**Lucca A.**
Psychiatric Clinic, San Raffaele Hospital,
Milan, Italy

**Lundholm K.**
Department of Surgery, Göteborg University,

Sahlgrenska University Hospital,
Göteborg, Sweden

**Lusso M.R.**
Department of Medical Oncology,
University of Cagliari,
Cagliari, Italy

**Maccario M.**
Department of Internal Medicine,
Division of Endocrinology, University of Turin,
Turin, Italy

**Macciò A.**
Obstetrics and Ginecology Unit,
Sirai Hospital,
Carbonia, Italy

**Madeddu C.**
Department of Medical Oncology,
University of Cagliari,
Cagliari, Italy

**Maltoni M.**
Department of Hospice and Palliative Care,
City Hospital of Forlìmpopoli,
Forlì, Italy

**Mantovani G.**
Department of Medical Oncology,
University of Cagliari,
Cagliari, Italy

**Manzato E.**
Department of Medical and Surgical Sciences,
University of Padua,
Padua, Italy

**Massa E.**
Department of Medical Oncology,
University of Cagliari,
Cagliari, Italy

**Me E.**
Department of Internal Medicine,
Division of Endocrinology and Metabolism,
University of Turin,
Turin, Italy

**Meguid M.M.**
Department of Surgery, Surgical Metabolism and
Nutrition Laboratory, Neuroscience Programs,
University Hospital, Upstate Medical University,
Syracuse, NY, USA

**Merendino N.**
Department of Environmental Sciences,
University of Tuscia, Viterbo, Italy

**Millioni R.**
Department of Clinical and Experimental Medicine,
University of Padua,
Padua, Italy

**Moore-Carrasco R.**
Cancer Research Group,
Department of Biochemistry and Molecular
Biology, University of Barcelona,
Barcelona, Spain

**Morley J.E.**
GRECC, VA Medical Center and Division of
Geriatric Medicine, Saint Louis University,
St. Louis, MO, USA

**Muscaritoli M.**
Department of Clinical Medicine,
University of Rome La Sapienza,
Rome, Italy

**Nespoli A.**
Department of Surgical Sciences and Intensive
Therapy, Department of General Surgery, Surgery
Unit 3, University of Milano-Bicocca at San
Gerardo Hospital,
Monza, Italy

**Nguyen P.L.**
Department of Laboratory Medicine and Pathology,
Mayo Clinic,
Rochester, MN, USA

**Ohara T.**
Department of Clinical Molecular Medicine, Division
of Diabetes and Digestive and Kidney Diseases, Kobe
University Graduate School of Medicine,
Kobe, Japan

**Okano H.**
Department of Internal and Geriatric Medicine,
Kobe University,
Kobe, Japan

**Perboni S.**
Department of Medical Oncology,
University of Cagliari,
Cagliari, Italy

**Picu A.**
Department of Internal Medicine,
Division of Endocrinology, University of Turin,
Turin, Italy

**Pigozzo S.**
Department of Medical and Surgical Sciences,
Geriatrics Division, University of Padua,
Padua, Italy

**Plata-Salaman C.R.**
Global External Research & Development, Lilly
Research Laboratories, Lilly Corporate Center,
Indianapolis, IN, USA

**Preziosa I.**
Department of Clinical Medicine,
University of Rome La Sapienza,
Rome, Italy

**Prodam F.**
Department of Internal Medicine,
Division of Endocrinology and Metabolism,
University of Turin,
Turin, Italy

**QuBaiah O.**
GRECC, VA Medical Center and Division of
Geriatric Medicine, Saint Louis University,
St. Louis, MO, USA

**Ragazzoni F.**
Department of Internal Medicine,
Division of Endocrinology and Metabolism,
University of Turin,
Turin, Italy

**Ramos E.J.B.**
Department of Surgery,
Surgical Metabolism and Nutrition Laboratory,
Neuroscience Programs,
University Hospital, Upstate Medical University,
Syracuse, NY, USA

**Riganti F.**
Department of Internal Medicine,
Division of Endocrinology and Metabolism,
University of Turin,
Turin, Italy

**Robinson D.**
Clinical Hematology/Oncology, Centocor,
Malvern, PA, USA

**Romanato G.**
Department of Medical and Surgical Sciences,
University of Padua,
Padua, Italy

**Rossi Fanelli F.**
Department of Clinical Medicine,
University of Rome La Sapienza,
Rome, Italy

**Scapoli D.**
Department of Oncology-Pathology,
Clinical Oncology Unit,
University Hospital of Ferrara,
Ferrara, Italy

**Scevola D.**
Department of Infectious Diseases,
IRCCS S. Matteo Polyclinic, University of Pavia,
Pavia, Italy

**Scevola S.**
Department of Surgery, Section of Plastic Surgery,
IRCCS Maugeri Foundation, University of Pavia,
Pavia, Italy

**Schuster M.W.**
Bone Marrow and Blood Stem Cell Transplantation
Program, Center for Lymphoma and Myeloma,
New York Presbyterian Hospital/Weill Medical
Center, New York,
NY, USA

**Seardo M.A.**
Department of Internal Medicine,
Division of Endocrinology and Metabolism,
University of Turin,
Turin, Italy

**Sergi G.**
Department of Medical and Surgical Sciences,
Geriatrics Division, University of Padua,
Padua, Italy

**Serpe R.**
Department of Medical Oncology,
University of Cagliari,
Cagliari, Italy

**Silvestris N.**
Medical Oncology Unit,
Giorgio Porfiri Oncology Center,
Hospital of Latina,
Latina, Italy

**Skipworth R.J.E.**
Department of Clinical and Surgical Sciences
(Surgery), The University of Edinburgh, Royal
Infirmary, Edinburgh,
United Kingdom

**Smeraldi E.**
Psychiatric Clinic, San Raffaele Hospital,
Milan, Italy

**Strassburg S.**
Applied Cachexia Research,
Department of Cardiology, Charité, Campus
Virchow-Klinikum,
Berlin, Germany

**Strasser F.**
Department of Internal Medicine,
Section Oncology/Haematology,
Oncology and Palliative Medicine,
Cantonal Hospital,
St.Gallen, Switzerland

**Sullivan D.H.**
Department of Geriatrics, Nutrition,
Metabolism and Exercise Laboratory,
University of Arkansas for Medical Sciences and
Geriatric Research Education and Clinical Center,
Central Arkansas Veterans Healthcare System,
Little Rock, AR, USA

**Suzuki S.**
Department of Surgery, Surgical Metabolism
and Nutrition Laboratory,
Neuroscience Programs, University Hospital,
Upstate Medical University,
Syracuse, NY, USA

**Tassinari D.**
Department of Oncology,
Supportive and Palliative Care Unit,
City Hospital of Rimini,
Rimini, Italy

**Tassone F.**
Department of Internal Medicine,
Division of Endocrinology, University of Turin,
Turin, Italy

**Tessari P.**
Department of Clinical and Experimental Medicine,
Chair of Metabolism, University of Padua,
Padua, Italy

**Thomas D.R.**
Division of Geriatric Medicine,
Saint Louis University Health Sciences Center,
Saint Louis, MO, USA

**Tisdale M.J.**
Pharmaceutical Sciences Research Institute,
Aston University,
Birmingham, United Kingdom

**Tomassi G.**
Department of Environmental Sciences,
University of Tuscia,
Viterbo, Italy

**Uberti F.**
Department of Infectious Diseases,
IRCCS S.Matteo Polyclinic, University of Pavia,
Pavia, Italy

**Urbini B.**
Department of Oncology-Pathology,
Clinical Oncology Unit,
University Hospital of Ferrara,
Ferrara, Italy

**van der Lely A.J.**
Department of Internal Medicine,
Division of Endocrinology and Metabolism,
Erasmus University,
Rotterdam, The Netherlands

**Veldhuis J.D.**
Department of Internal Medicine,
Division of Endocrinology and Metabolism,
Mayo Medical and Graduate Schools,
Rochester, MN, USA

**Von Haehling S.**
Department of Clinical Cardiology,
National Heart and Lung Institute,
Imperial College School of Medicine,
London, United Kingdom

**von Roenn J.H.**
Department of Medicine,
Division of Hematology/Oncology,
The Feinberg School of Medicine of
Northwestern University and the Robert
H. Lurie Comprehensive Cancer Center,
Palliative Care and Home Hospice Program,
Northwestern Memorial Hospital,
Chicago, IL, USA

**Wouters E.F.M.**
Department of Respiratory Medicine,
University Hospital Maastricht,
Maastricht, The Netherlands

**Wu S.**
NMR Research Center, Emory University,
Atlanta, GA, USA

**Yeh S.-S.**
Department of Medicine - Geriatrics
University of New York at Stony Brook
VAMC, Northport, NY USA

# Index of Contributors

# Section 1
# Anatomy, Historical Perspective and Epidemiology

# Functional Anatomy of the 'Adipose Organ'

Saverio Cinti

## Introduction

White and brown adipose tissues have long been considered as two distinct and independent entities, underestimated by researchers.

White adipose tissue (WAT) has largely been ignored by researchers for many years. One major reason for this is its diffuse distribution and its apparently uninteresting localisation in the mammalian body, as if filling the interstitial spaces among the various organs like a connective tissue. WAT is distributed at the cutaneous (dermis), subcutaneous, perivisceral (mediastinal, retroperitoneal, intraperitoneal: omental, mesenteric, etc.) and intravisceral (parotid, bone marrow, parathyroid, pancreas) levels. When the cellular nature of this connective tissue was first unveiled, the functional interpretation came quickly and intuitively: given its high fat content (triglycerides), WAT had to be an energy depot for short or prolonged fasting periods; however, not being used in the physio-

logical daily routine, it could not be very important.

Its histological aspect (Fig. 1) was similarly uninspiring, consisting of spherical cells 70–90 μm in diameter with a thin rim of cytoplasm surrounding a single lipid droplet (triglycerides); scarce cytological tissue elements (macrophages, mast cells and fibroblasts); and unimpressive vascularity and innervation.

The description of mammalian brown adipose tissue (BAT) had a separate history. The term *adipose* is due to its high triglyceride content, whereas *brown* is due to its darker hue compared with white fat, a colour that is visible to the naked eye and stems from its different cellular and tissue anatomy: smaller (30–50 μm in diameter) and not properly spherical (polyhedral) cells with a rounded nucleus occasionally located in a central position.

The distinctive feature of BAT is the multilocular organisation of cytoplasmic triglycerides into

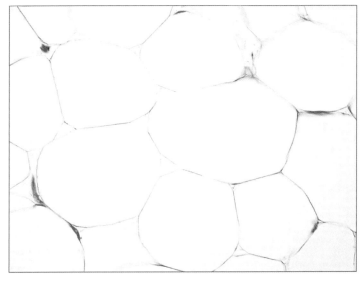

**Fig. 1.** Human subcutaneous white adipose tissue made up of unilocular adipocytes. Light microscopy 550x

multiple separate droplets that are easily seen at the light microscope (Fig. 2). The electron microscope shows large and cristae-rich mitochondria filling the cytoplasm (Fig. 3), another distinguishing characteristic from white fat. The histological features of BAT are also different: vessels are much more diffuse and the nerves appear to infiltrate the parenchyma, forming numerous neuro-adipocytic synaptic contacts. It is the high capillary density of this tissue and the large amount of mitochondria found in brown adipocytes that confer on BAT its brown colour. Despite a similar interstitial distribution, the mammalian BAT is easier to localise precisely compared with WAT, especially in smaller animals.

The function of BAT – heat production – and its large proportion in hibernating animals were described in the 1960s. This led to circumscription of the importance of this tissue, also because it was increasingly clear that its amount was negligible in large mammals, man included.

In the late 1970s, Stock's group in London revived the biomedical interest in BAT. In addressing the issues connected with human eating habits, especially in relation to the growing proportion of obese individuals in Western countries, these researchers – wondering why laboratory rats did not become obese – tried feeding them a diet similar to

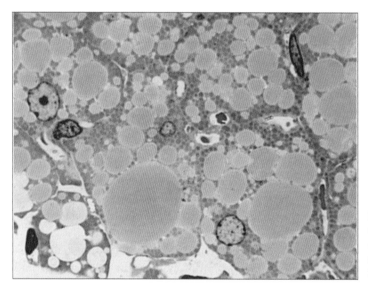

**Fig. 2.** Mouse brown adipose tissue composed of multilocular adipocytes. Note the dark dots in the cytoplasm corresponding to large mitochondria. Resin-embedded tissue. Light microscopy 1200x

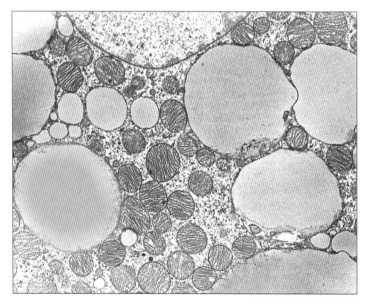

**Fig. 3.** Electron micrograph of the cytoplasm of a brown adipocyte. Note the large mitochondria rich in cristae. Transmission electron microscopy 10 000x

the one widely diffused in the West: the fat-rich, so-called cafeteria diet. Unexpectedly, although the rats did gain weight, they did not do so by the amount that had been forecast based on the calculation of the calories administered [1]. There therefore had to be a protective mechanism, whose enhancement could maybe help address human obesity and its complications (diabetes, hypertension, cardiovascular disease).

The significantly increased tissue function of BAT observed in rats fed the cafeteria diet prompted the hypothesis that the factor protecting against obesity could be the energy consumed by the tissue in response to food administration (diet-induced thermogenesis). Indeed, a very large amount of energy is theoretically dissipated through thermogenesis. It has been calculated that a gram of BAT can develop 300 Watts, i.e. 300 times the amount developed by all other mammalian cell types [2]; thus, 1 kg of BAT is capable of dispersing about 6200 kcal/day, corresponding to the energy requirements of an individual doing a heavy manual job (while most of us expend about one third of this energy). Therefore, a few hundred grams of fat tissue in our body can use the amount of energy required for the functioning of the whole body, and 50 g of BAT can use 10–15% of the whole energy turnover [2, 3].

In 1993, the hypothesis that BAT could be an anti-obesity factor received further support from experiments by the Boston group of Lowell and Flyer, who obtained genetically manipulated mice lacking BAT and reported that they became obese [4]. However, subsequent research on mice lacking the mitochondrial protein UCP1 – which is responsible for BAT's thermogenic activity and thus for its ability to disperse energy – showing that they were sensitive to cold (did not produce heat) but did not become obese [5], reopened the question of the role of BAT. In contrast, mice made to produce UCP1 ectopically in WAT were lean and resistant to obesity [6, 7].

## Functional Anatomy of White Adipose Tissue

Important discoveries in the 1990s rekindled the interest in white adipose tissue. In December 1994, the team of Friedman at New York Rockefeller University discovered the gene of obesity [8]; their subjects were mice, which in the 1950s had developed a spontaneous mutation resulting in hyperphagia, infertility and reduced activity of the sympathetic nervous system, and consequently in early, massive obesity (*ob/ob* mice) [9].

The alteration – detected on chromosome 6 – consisted of a C to T point mutation at codon 105, turning it into a stop codon and interrupting the synthesis of a 167 amino acid secretion protein, which was named leptin from the Greek *leptos* (thin) [8]. The mouse gene appears to be expressed solely in WAT and is 84% homologous to the human gene.

Within a few months, three groups demonstrated independently that leptin administration to obese mice corrected in a few weeks all the defects related to its absence, and that treated mice were then no longer distinguishable from lean controls [10–12]. The leptin receptor was discovered in 1995 [13]. Demonstration of at least five alternatively spliced forms [14], and reports that the functional form (i.e. the one activating intracellular signalling) appears to be prevalently expressed at the hypothalamic level and is mutated in mice phenotypically very similar to *ob/ob* mice (except for a proneness to develop diabetes, hence called *db/db*) [14, 15], came the following year.

These findings lent support to the hypothesis – advanced by Coleman in the 1970s based on parabiosis experiments [16] – that a circulating lipostatic factor must be implicated in maintaining body fat constant. By making the blood of lean and *ob/ob* mice circulate in parabiosis, Coleman noted that obese mice lost weight, benefiting from the lipostatic factor present in the bloodstream of lean mice. The same did not apply to *db/db* mice, since whereas *ob/ob* mice do not produce leptin, *db/db* ones do not produce its functional receptor.

The researchers' enthusiasm was dampened by a paper in which Maffei [17] reported in a large sample of patients an unexpected, close correlation between BMI (the body mass index obtained by calculating the ratio of weight in kg to the square of height in metres) and leptinaemia; as this entails that obese subjects have high values of leptinaemia and are thus prone to leptin resistance, they would be unaffected by the leptin treatment beneficial to *ob/ob* mice. Until now, rare cases of human genetic leptin deficiency have been discovered and successfully treated with leptin [18].

Flyer, noting that its administration restored plasma levels of thyroid, adrenal and gonadal hormones in fasting mice, hypothesised a prominent role for leptin in controlling the endocrine secretion in relation to food intake [19]. Accordingly, leptin functional receptors were identified in several peripheral organs [20], considerably broadening its role.

Further sites of leptin production were identified in placenta, mammary gland, stomach and salivary glands, further supporting the notion of a wider functional action of this protein (in vasculo-genesis, immune defence, food absorption) (see [21] for a review).

These reports revolutionised the concept of WAT, which finally came to be recognised as a real endocrine tissue capable of affecting the feeding behaviour of mammals.

Over time, other molecules were reported to be WAT secretion products (adipokines), and the relationship between their excessive secretion and the severe complications of obesity became increasingly apparent. Especially interesting was the correlation between secretion of tumour necrosis factor (TNF)-α, resistin and adiponectin and diabetes; between angiotensinogen and mineralocorticoid-releasing factors and arterial hypertension [21]; and between plasminogen activator inhibitor (PAI 1) and coagulation problems [22]. These data contributed to clarify the molecular mechanism underpinning the early clinical observation that androgenic obesity (i.e. central adiposity with a greater accumulation of visceral fat) carries more dangerous complications than gynoid obesity (peripheral adiposity with a greater accumulation of subcutaneous fat), because of the inhomogeneous secretion of adipokines across depots. An especially close relationship was described for adiponectin and diabetes.

## Functional Anatomy of Brown Adipose Tissue

In the 1990s, advances were also made in the study of brown adipose tissue. Especially following the studies by Stock et al. reported above, a rising number of laboratories began to focus on BAT, soon leading to the description of the main mechanisms of action of brown adipocytes.

An uncoupling protein (UCP1) expressed solely in brown adipocyte mitochondria was identified [23–25], as an atypical β-adrenergic receptor (β3-AR), which appeared to be prevalently expressed by adipose tissue [26, 27]. Therefore, brown adipocytes are activated by adrenergic stimulation of these receptors, leading to triglyceride lipolysis and new synthesis of UCP1. The fatty acids thus released are burnt by β oxidation, which gives rise to a hydrogenionic gradient between the two mitochondrial membranes. This gradient, commonly used by adenosinetriphosphatase to produce ATP, is abrogated by the abundance of UCP1 in the inner mitochondrial membrane, UCP1 being a protonophore [28].

All this allows for a fast and highly regulated transformation of the potential energy contained in triglycerides into heat, also accounting for brown adipocyte anatomy: given the enormous demand for oxidisable substrate (the lipid vacuoles), and that lipolysis can take place only on the surface of the vacuoles, a multilocular organisation is essential to increase the contact surface between lipids and hyaloplasm. Such ready substrate availability would be useless without a large number of mitochondria – which large size and abundance of cristae make very efficient – ready to carry out the oxidation process.

The presence of the protonophore UCP1 is thus the final step in a series of events beginning with the adrenergic stimulus and proceeding through lipolysis and fatty acid oxidation to the formation of an electrochemical gradient that is dissipated. These cells therefore represent a unique phenomenon in the mammalian organism because, unlike all the other cell types, which pursue optimal efficiency, they work via a loss of efficiency.

The enormous amount of heat produced requires a vascular bed capable of ensuring a large oxygen supply and the rapid transport of the heat from the tissue to the rest of the organism, not least to prevent the high temperature from damaging the tissue itself. This accounts for the impressive vascularity of BAT.

The obvious physiological stimulus capable of activating BAT is cold, and virtually all facultative non-shivering thermogenesis is to be ascribed to this tissue. As mentioned above, food intake is also capable of activating it [1], and several synthetic molecules, called specific β3-AR agonists, have been manufactured industrially. Pharmacological utilisation demonstrated their effectiveness in treating obesity and the consequent diabetes in both genetically and diet-induced rodent obesity [29, 30], whereas the drugs developed in the hope of treating human obesity gave disappointing results [31] commonly attributed to the scarce presence of BAT in adult humans.

For this reason, the work published in 1997 by Fleury et al. [32] has had the merit of rekindling the hope for a pharmacological intervention aimed at dissipating the excess energy accumulated by obese subjects. These researchers identified a new protein, homologous to UCP1 and also expressed in man, which they denominated UCP2, and demonstrated that UCP2 is not only expressed in BAT, but that it is widely distributed in all tissues and is thus well represented in adult human tissues [32].

Shortly after the publication of this paper, two different teams [33, 34] independently described a protein highly homologous to UCP1 and UCP2, hence designated UCP3. UCP3 is expressed in mice and human BAT and skeletal muscle. The enthusiasm generated by these findings was chilled by subsequent research showing the absence of any specific phenotype in transgenic mice lacking this protein [35, 36] and the absence of alternative non-shivering thermogenesis in cold-acclimatised transgenic mice lacking UCP1 [37]. Nonetheless, these studies opened new avenues of research in cell physiology, and the group of Lowell went on to discover the important role of UCP2 in pancreatic insulin secretion [38].

## The Adipose Organ

The new concept of an adipose organ was first proposed in the late 1990s.

### Anatomy

Using anatomical microdissection, our group demonstrated that not only is it possible to excise and isolate nearly the entire adipose content of mammalian organisms, but also that BAT is wholly found in fat depots that are often prevalently white. In other words, in adult rodents kept in standard feeding and environmental conditions there are no totally brown depots distinct from WAT depots, but a single organ articulated into several subcutaneous and visceral depots containing both tissues [39].

Rodents have two subcutaneous fat depots, one anterior and one posterior, lying in discrete

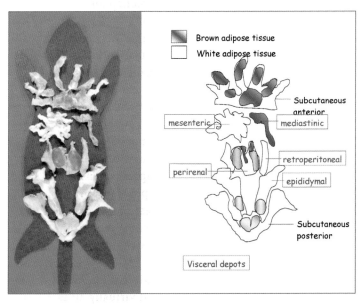

**Fig. 4.** Adipose organ of an adult C57/BL mouse maintained in standard conditions. The organ is made up of two subcutaneous and several visceral depots. The most representative visceral depots are shown. Kidneys and testes were dissected together with the depots. White areas made up of white adipose tissue and brown areas composed of brown adipose tissue are indicated by the scheme

anatomical locations (Fig. 4). The anterior depot is the more complex; it lies at the base of the fore-limbs and mainly occupies the dorsal body region between and under the scapulae, the axillary and proximal regions of the forelimbs, and the cervical area. The interscapular is the most conspicuous central portion of the depot (body) and extends laterally (lateral wings) and anteriorly (anterior wings). The body is made up of WAT in its superficial portion, and of BAT in its depth. The latter extends to the lateral wings and to the subscapular and axillary regions (all brown), which in turn are continuous with the region occupying the proximal portion of the forelimb and the lateral thoracic wall (both white). The anterior wings extend anteriorly between the superficial dorsal muscles and reach the base of the neck. In this area, the anterior wings are often white, whereas the more anterior region following the course of the neck nerve-vascular bundle is generally brown.

The posterior depot is located at the base of the hind legs. It is simpler, consisting of a single tissue band beginning from the dorsum at the lumbar level (dorso-lumbar portion), extending anteriorly in the inguino–crural region (inguinal portion) and further at the pubic level into the gluteal region (gluteal portion). At the pubic level this depot is continuous with the contralateral depot. The posterior depot is usually white.

The visceral depots are located in the thorax and abdomen. The former lie prevalently against the intercostal nerve-vascular bundles, the heart and the aorta. They are usually mixed, but in constant environmental and feeding conditions much depends on age and species.

The abdominal depots can be subdivided into retro- and intraperitoneal. The retroperitoneal depot *par excellence* has an elongated conical shape and lies in the paravertebral position, i.e. on the border between the spine and the posterior abdominal wall, and is generally white. The best known perirenal deposit is divided from the retroperitoneal by a peritoneal fold and can be dissected separately. It is generally mixed, with the brown component prevalently located at the level of the renal hilus.

The omental deposit is small in rodents and is made up of WAT, as is the mesenteric depot out-

lined by the two peritoneal leaflets holding the intestine against the posterior abdominal wall.

The perigonadal depot is consistently white and is simpler in males, where it is well circumscribed, enveloped and bound to the epididymis by the peritoneal leaflets. In females it surrounds the ovaries, uterus and bladder.

Thus, in adult mice and rats maintained in standard conditions, the BAT component is macroscopically visible in the sole anterior subcutaneous depot and in part of the thoracic and perirenal depots. However, light microscopic examination of WAT deposits shows the consistent presence of brown adipocytes, especially in the inguinal region of the anterior subcutaneous depot, in the periovarian region of the gonadal depot, and in the retroperitoneal region. It is important to stress that the amount of brown adipocytes found in the different depots is genetically determined, since in similar environmental and feeding conditions it is substantially species-related [40].

Subject age is also important in this respect. In a systematic study of the anterior subcutaneous depot in animals of different ages, we demonstrated that in ageing rats the BAT component undergoes a progressive substitution by WAT, albeit retaining a considerable size in older (2 years) animals [41, 42]. In general, the number of brown adipocytes tends to decrease with age in all depots.

Minor WAT depots are found in bone marrow, parotid, parathyroid and pancreas. Different amounts of mixed adipose tissue are found along the vasculo-nervous bundles of the limbs, and close to the superficial lymph nodes the adipose tissue is often brown.

## Vessels and Nerves

Each deposit is endowed with a well-organised vascular and nerve network. Whereas the former aspect is well explored and exhaustively described, studies addressing the specific innervation of each depot are few and scarcely informative.

The most widely investigated deposit is the anterior subcutaneous, which exhibits a dense vascularity and innervation [43]. Two anterior vessels reach the wings of the depot bilaterally from the axillary artery, accompanied by veins and nerves of different calibres. The thinner nerves are less myelinated and contain a larger number of noradrenergic fibres. The thicker and more myelinated nerves also contain fibres immunoreactive for neuropeptides that co-localise with noradrenaline in noradrenergic fibres (neuropeptide Y [NPY]) or that localise in sensitive fibres (or at least fibres immunoreactive for the neuropeptides that are commonly localised in sensitive fibres: substance P [SP] and calcitonin gene-related peptide [CGRP]). A peripheral cytotrophic and vasculotrophic action of the sensitive fibres containing these neuropeptides has been described [44]. Five nerves, prevalently made up of noradrenergic fibres, run bilaterally and symmetrically from the intercostal spaces into the body of the deposit. A large solitary vein (Sulzer's vein) ensures a conspicuous outflow from the depth of the BAT body and reaches the azygos vein via the intercostal space.

Immunohistochemical and ultrastructural studies from our and other laboratories have shown that the fibres innervate the vessels down to the more peripheral capillary ramifications and also branch directly into the parenchyma, giving rise to real, consistently noradrenergic, neuroadipocytic junctions [39]. The WAT component of the depot is similarly, but not quite as densely, vascularised and innervated.

Much less is known about the other depots. As a rule, all receive vessels from the main arterial and venous branches of the organs to which they are closest, and their innervation is very similar to the one described in the anterior subcutaneous depot; vessel and nerve density depend on the amount of BAT in the depot, greater vessel and nerve density being associated with greater amounts of BAT.

A recent immunohistochemical investigation by our group has demonstrated that the periaortic thoracic depot is also endowed with independent cholinergic parenchymal fibres of likely parasympathetic origin [45].

This pattern of vessel and nerve distribution is easily accounted for by the considerations made above on the physiology of brown and white adipocytes.

Whereas the high density of noradrenergic parenchymal fibres in the brown areas (BAT) obviously depends on the fact that the adrenergic stimulus is the trigger activating the molecular process of heat production, it is rather more difficult to explain the role of adrenergic fibres in WAT. White adipocytes express both β-ARs (including β3-AR) and α-receptors. The former are responsible for the lipolysis induced by the adrenergic stimulus [46], whereas α-receptors have the opposite effect. Their physiological role is thus still unclear.

Recent work prevalently conducted by the group of Lafontain and Valet points to a prominent role for α-ARs in the control of adipocyte precursor proliferation [47]. Indeed, stimulation of these receptors would induce adipocytic secretion of a protein, autotaxin, capable of promoting the proliferation and differentiation of new adipocytes by acting on lisophosphatidic acid (LPA) [48]. This is in line with previous work carried out by this group in collaboration with the team of Lowell, where transgenic mice expressing only α-AR in adipose tissue and fed a high-fat diet consistently developed small cell hyperplastic obesity [49].

According to a hypothesis recently advanced by Hodgson [50] based on anatomical studies of the distribution of adrenergic fibres, there would be two separate adipocyte populations, one prevalently expressing α-ARs and the other prevalently expressing β-ARs. Only the latter would be directly in contact with adrenergic parenchymal fibres. These two populations would respond differentially to the adrenergic stimulus: those expressing β-receptors would undergo prompt delipidisation, whereas those expressing α-receptor would remain intact to distribute paracrinely the fatty acids to delipidised cells.

If this hypothesis is correct, there would be two white adipocyte populations sharing functional tasks during hormone-driven lipolysis. This hypothesis is in line with the observation that during lipolysis due to acute adrenergic stimulation, only a fraction of adipocytes are delipidised, while the others are ostensibly unaffected. However, things seem to be rather more complicated, because a homogeneous delipidisation response by adipocytes has been described during chronic lipolytic stimulation [51]. Although a role for parasympathetic fibres in WAT lipolysis has also been hypothesised recently [52], unpublished immunohistochemical data from our laboratory do not lend support to this hypothesis.

## Development of the Adipose Organ

Developmental studies have mainly been conducted on small mammals on two depots considered representative: epididymal for WAT and the interscapular portion of the anterior subcutaneous depot for BAT.

### White Preadipocytes

The epididymal tissue is recognisable in the fetus in the last days of gestation. At this time, only the capillaries are morphologically visible, immersed in the extracellular matrix together with collagen fibres and undifferentiated cells. Postnatally, a profound rearrangement takes place (in rats and mice on days 4–6) marked microanatomically by areas well circumscribed by fibroblast-like cells and by numerous dilated capillaries. Among these vessels a rich cell population is observed, the vast majority of which is made up of preadipocytes at various stages of differentiation from cells barely showing the first signs of differentiation (glycogen and small triglyceride vacuoles) to unilocular cells similar to mature adipocytes in all but size (5–10 μm in diameter compared with the 70–80 μm of mature adipocytes) (Fig. 5).

It is important to note that the less differentiated cells are often found in the pericytic position (completely enveloped in a doubling of the basal capillary membrane). The extracellular matrix inside the area circumscribed by the fibroblast-like cells is very rich in collagen fibrils and is clearly different from the one surrounding it, where an amorphous matrix predominates. We designated these areas as *vasculo-adipocytic islands* and believe them to be the primary sites of adipocyte development in the epididymal depot. The preadipocytes developing in these areas are easily distinguished from the other cell elements (endothelial cells, fibroblasts, mast cells, macrophages) by their characteristic cytoplasm, which contains varying amounts of glycogen and

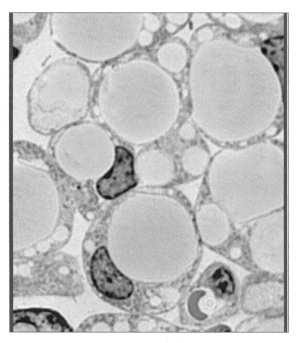

**Fig. 5.** White adipocyte precursor. This cell has a distinct morphology mainly due to early unilocular lipid accumulation, glycogen particles, pinocytotic vesicles, 'white' mitochondria and external lamina. Resin-embedded tissue. Light microscopy 1200×

lipids. Rough endoplasmic reticulum and Golgi apparatus are well represented when lipids are still scarce. Smooth endoplasmic reticulum is variable and is frequently associated with lipid vacuoles. Mitochondria are typically elongated with small, variously oriented cristae.

Vasculo-adipocytic islands are found in the first week of postnatal development, but preadipocytes are recognisable until postnatal weeks 3–6 in the epididymal depots of mice and rats (our unpublished data).

The study of subcutaneous adipose tissue in human fetuses has evidenced morphological developmental features very similar to those of mice and rats reported above. At present, it is impossible to say whether they are stem cells or cells genetically predisposed to differentiate into adipocytes, or to understand whether they originate from the vessels of the tissue itself or at distant sites like bone marrow.

## Brown Preadipocytes

In perinatal rat fetuses, the anterior subcutaneous depot contains exclusively brown adipocytes and is recognisable from day 15 of gestation. At the site where the anlage arises, few dilated capillaries are immersed in an extracellular matrix poor in cells and collagen fibrils and rich in amorphous substance. At this stage pericytes – which cannot be defined as 'pure' undifferentiated cells because of their characteristic mitochondria – are already recognisable. They are often numerous, large and rich in cristae (pretypical mitochondria), anticipating their differentiation into typical brown mitochondria. Another distinctive feature is the variable amount of glycogen (Fig. 6). Anlage cellularity, but not cell differentiation, increases on the following days.

Around day 18 of gestation, cell number and degree of differentiation augment greatly through the arising of further differentiation features of mitochondria, which become typical; the first lipid vacuoles also appear. Of note, lipid accumulation seems to be multilocular from the very first steps of differentiation.

Around day 20, mitochondria express the functional protein, and all the morphological features of mature brown adipocytes are detected at this time in most cells in the depot. In the first few postnatal weeks, elements at various stages of differentiation continue to be seen.

All such features of brown adipocytes are recognisable in subcutaneous BAT of human fetuses (our unpublished data).

Therefore, also in the case of BAT, stem cells cannot be identified based solely on morphological features; in fact, the most undifferentiated cells found in the pericytic position already exhibit minimal features of differentiation that allow them to be distinguished from 'pure' stem cells.

There thus seem to be two different types of precursor. Both appear to be programmed to form the organ's parenchyma independently of the animal's functional requirements; indeed, the complete absence of β1, 2 and 3 adrenergic receptors (which mediate thermogenic activity) does not prevent the arising of brown preadipocytes with a normal ultrastructure (our unpublished data), and the nearly complete absence of insulin receptor (which mediates liposynthesis) does not prevent the formation of either type of precursor in the adipose organ, even though they do not attain complete differentiation into mature adipocytes [53].

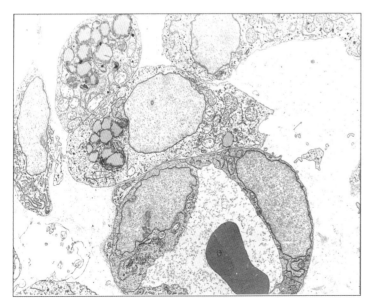

**Fig. 6.** Brown adipocyte precursor. This cell shows a distinct morphology mainly due to multilocular lipid accumulation, glycogen particles, pinocytotic vesicles, 'brown' mitochondria and external lamina. Transmission electron microscopy 7000x

## Adipose Organ Plasticity and Medical Implications

Different types of stimulation produce dramatic anatomical changes in the adipose organ, which is endowed with striking plastic properties. Given the considerations made above with regard to functional anatomy, it is easy to understand how nutritional stimuli or modifications in environmental temperature can bring about anatomo-functional modifications.

## Fasting

Fasting and food restriction produce organ modifications that vary based on their duration [39]. In the case of fasting, changes regard the sole white component via a focal tissue response. Indeed, areas can be observed where some adipocytes have shrunk and are surrounded by still apparently unaffected adipocytes. At extreme degrees of delipidisation, white adipocytes are elongated or star-shaped and are still easily distinguished from all other parenchymal cells, essentially due to the distinctive presence, on the surface of these slimming cells, of invaginations (described by some researchers as surface evaginations or villus-like structures) characterised by abundant pinocytotic vesicles. These invaginations arise early in the cell slimming process, because nearly unaffected cells (exhibiting prevalently unilocular lipid accumulations) show 'tails' of slimmed-down cytoplasm rich in invaginations. The tannic acid technique devised by Blanchette-Mackie and Scow [54] has made it possible to follow at the electron microscope the process of fatty acid migration during the slimming process by allowing electron-dense myelinic figures (corresponding to migrating free fatty acids) to be detected in the adipose tissue. These figures are found on the surface of lipid vacuoles; in the hyaloplasm; in direct contact with mitochondria and in close relation to the cytoplasmic invaginations rich in pinocytotic vesicles that are characteristic of this slimmed-down state; they are seen free in the interstitial space, in the cytoplasm of endothelial cells, and in vessel lumina. In practice, they are found at all the sites of fatty acid migration during lipolysis. Although they are not exclusively seen during the lipolytic process, they are significantly more numerous

during adipocyte delipidisation.

In conditions of protracted fasting, brown adipocytes with a complete lipid endowment can be observed side by side with slimmed-down adipocytes, easily recognised for the features described above [39]. We feel that this is the most convincing evidence that despite the organ's plasticity, a small component of either type of cells is consistently found in the organ. Indeed, in extreme fasting conditions a part of the energy contained in the organ's triglycerides is stored for the critical thermogenic requirements, obviously in brown adipocytes.

The fate of totally slimmed-down cells is unclear. According to some researchers they may undergo apoptosis. Still unpublished data from our laboratory seem to indicate that this is not the case: after protracted fasting, the retroperitoneal depot of three adult mice was completely delipidised, but careful electron microscopic examination (highly sensitive to signs of apoptosis) of about 500 delipidised cells/mouse showed no sign of apoptosis in any slimmed-down cell (Fig. 7).

## Warm Exposure

Warm exposure entails a reduction of the orthosympathetic stimulus, resulting in BAT inactivation. Morphologically, this corresponds to a transformation of brown fat cells into cells similar to white adipocytes. During this transformation, we have observed a reduced genic expression of UCP1 and increased genic expression of leptin [55]. This suggests that such morphological transformation is accompanied by a new functional situation, with adipocytes losing their thermogenic ability and acquiring the properties of white fat cells, including production of such an important hormone as leptin. This is in line with the observation that classic multilocular brown adipocytes subjected to adrenergic stimulation express UCP1 but not leptin [56, 55], whereas cold exposure and sympathetico-mimetic drugs reduce leptinaemia [57] and induce the transformation of white into brown adipocytes [58] (see below 'Transdifferentiation').

It is interesting to note that the energy required for basic metabolic activities is consider-

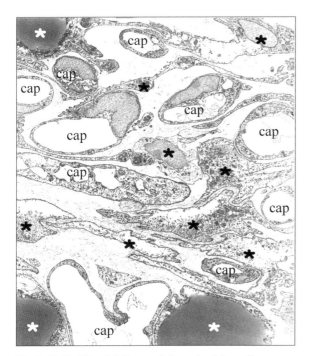

**Fig. 7.** Delipidised (slimmed-down) white adipocyte. Slimmed adipocytes (*asterisks*) show distinctive morphological features: external lamina, pinocytotic vesicles, cytoplasmic invaginations, cytoplasm rich in organelles including mitochondria, endoplasmic reticulum, Golgi complex and lipid droplets of variable size. Lipid droplet size depends on the stage of delipidisation. *Cap,* capillary. Transmission electron microscopy 5500x

ably reduced in animals maintained in thermoneutral conditions. Indeed, in an adult mouse subjected to prolonged fasting (48 h), the whole WAT shrinks almost to disappearance at around 10°C, whereas it is nearly unchanged if the animal is kept at 28°C [39].

## Cold Exposure

This condition involves the immediate activation of the orthosympathetic system, with the consequent, immediate functional activation of brown adipocytes via the innervation and the neuro-adipocytic junctions described above. In a matter of hours, activated adipocytes exercise their thermogenic function by synthesising new mitochondria and UCP1; in the course of a few days new cells develop, giving rise to a new tissue organisation characterised by an increased number of vessels and nerves [59, 60]. In the framework of the new concept of adipose organ, it is easy to understand that the arising of new brown cells involves not only some areas long considered as pure BAT, but the whole organ. It follows that its macroscopic appearance veers towards a brown aspect and that the microscopic features of the different depots progressively turn them into BAT (Fig. 8).

It is important to note that this process does not necessarily entail the arising of brown adipocytes in white depots – since, as mentioned above, brown cells may be present in the various depots (depending on age, strain, etc.; see above) – but rather an increase in their number [61, 62].

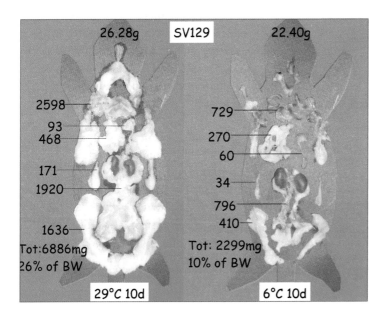

**Fig. 8.** Adipose organ of adult Sv129 mice maintained at 29°C or 6°C for 10 days. Note the evident reduction in organ size and the increase of brown areas corresponding to an increase in the brown component of the organ

Transmission electron microscopic (TEM) studies, which are very sensitive in detecting the different stages of cell development (see 'Development'), have shown that the adipose organ of adult mice and rats kept in thermoneutral conditions and fed a normal diet contains neither totally undifferentiated nor scarcely differentiated cells.

By contrast, in cold-exposed animals undifferentiated pericytes and brown preadipocytes (i.e. cells with minimal differentiation features that allow their morphological identification as cells committed to differentiate into brown adipocytes) arise both in BAT and in WAT. Preadipocytes may be found in the pericytic and/or perivascular position, suggesting that cold exposure induces the tissue conditions that lead to the arising of brown preadipocytes in all WAT and BAT areas of the organ. Therefore, irrespective of the existence of distinct white and brown cell precursors, their arising in different depots of adult animals clearly depends on microenvironmental tissue conditions. Cold exposure induces an increased activity of noradrenergic parenchymal fibres and simultaneous branching of nerve fibres both in WAT [63] and in BAT [43] areas. In turn, this induces an overall increase in noradrenaline tissue concentration followed by the development of brown cells in the various depots of the organ.

In contrast, development of white preadipocytes in the various areas appears to be triggered by different stimuli (see 'Positive Energy Balance: Overweight and Obsesity') directed at increasing the energy storage capacity.

## Transdifferentiation

Transdifferentiation is a biological phenomenon by which a differentiated cell turns phenotypically and functionally into a differentiated cell of another type without undergoing dedifferentiation [64]. We believe that brown and white adipocytes can transdifferentiate into one another in the adipose organ. We report some data providing evidence for physiological transdifferentiation of white into brown fat cells.

Since Ashwell's pioneering work (1984), it has been known that, after cold exposure, brown adipocytes expressing UCP1 arise in WAT areas of the adipose organ [61]. Our group has demonstrated that the precursors developing in the periovarian depot have ultrastructural and genic expression features typical of brown precursors [62]. A recent study of WAT tissue in different mice strains exposed to cold for varying periods of time has suggested that a significant number of multilocular adipocytes arise in a matter of days in visceral as well as subcutaneous WAT depots [65]. Analysis of the genic expression of these tissues after acute cold exposure (2 days) showed a significant increase in UCP1mRNA from baseline, suggesting that the new multilocular cells express UCP1mRNA.[1]

Interestingly, these cells do not express UCP1 protein (as demonstrated by immunohistochemical and Western blotting techniques), indicating that after 2 days of cold exposure a significant number of well-differentiated multilocular adipocytes express the UCP1 gene but not the protein. Considering that, in the course of fetal organ

---

[1]Whereas in the opinion of several researchers the presence of UCP1 is a brown adipocyte hallmark, in our view it is merely a cellular feature that subserves the main function of BAT; however, brown adipocytes do not consistently express it, and in some conditions in which they do not do so, they assume the appearance of white fat cells. For instance, in an animal maintained above its thermoneutral temperature (see 'Warm Exposure'), the BAT-activating adrenergic stimulus is off; brown adipocytes thus undergo a morphological transformation: they become unilocular and lose the typical mitochondrial features, thereby becoming similar to white adipocytes. This morphological transformation is accompanied by inhibition of UCP1 gene and by ob gene (leptin) activation [55]. The same process takes place in mice lacking all β-AR subtypes, demonstrating that this phenomenon is mediated by the β-adrenergic stimulus [66]. Although these data seem to be consistent with the concept that a brown adipocyte lacking UCP1 is a more or less typical white fat cell, this is denied by the fact that multilocular brown adipocytes quite different from white fat cells are found in the adipose organ of UCP1 knock-out mice (our unpublished data).

development, brown adipocyte precursors express UCP1 quite early with respect to the overall stage of cell differentiation, it seems reasonable also to hypothesise that the arising of the multilocular adipocytes in WAT depots after cold exposure is a phenomenon quite distinct from mere preadipocyte differentiation.

In the course of the same experiments, we also noted that the number of multilocular adipocytes increased further after a longer exposure to cold (10 days), and that, unlike those arising after acute exposure, these cells also expressed UCP1 protein. It thus appears that the continuous adrenergic stimulus prompted the multilocular cells already expressing UCP1mRNA to express also the protein and thus to acquire the functional thermogenic properties of brown adipocytes.

In transgenic animals not expressing β3-AR, the same experiments evidenced a nearly complete inhibition of this phenomenon, suggesting an important role for this receptor in its mediation. In addition, given that brown adipocyte precursors do not appear to express β3-AR, the hypothesis may be advanced that brown preadipocytes do not play a critical role in determining the presence of the new population of multilocular or brown adipocytes.

Immunohistochemical studies demonstrate that UCP1 protein is expressed by varying proportions of multilocular cells in the different depots. In this context, the most interesting observation, made in our laboratory in collaboration with the group of J.P. Giacobino (Geneva), was that in the subcutaneous depot of cold-exposed (6°C for 10 days) SV129 mice, about 35% of adipocytes were multilocular cells, 85% of which expressed UCP1. Also in this condition, then, the absence of β3-AR receptor significantly reduced the number of multilocular adipocytes (our unpublished data).

These findings seem to substantiate the hypothesis, advanced in a previous work by our group, that chronic (7 days) stimulation with the β3-AR agonist CL 316,243 could induce direct transformation of white into multilocular adipocytes, around 8% of which would express UCP1 [58]. Prolonged stimulation (7 more days) with the same drug induced a considerable increase in the proportion of UCP1-expressing cells (33%) without a concurrent increase in the number of multilocular cells (our unpublished data). This suggests that only a subpopulation of white adipocytes would be committed to this transformation, confirming that white-to-brown transdifferentiation passes through successive steps, beginning with the transformation of the lipid vacuole from unilocular into multilocular, followed by the expression of UCP1.

β3-AR receptor agonists administered to rats with genetic or diet-induced obesity are known to activate BAT, to induce the transdifferentiation of white into brown adipocytes [58], and to cure both their obesity and the consequent diabetes. Unfortunately, although some recent data indicate the presence of the receptor also in the human adipose organ [67], a drug inducing the same effects in man is still not available.

In a recent paper, Toseland [68] demonstrates that other drugs could be involved in the plastic modulation of the adipose organ, particularly the agonists of PPARγ – a nuclear receptor acting as a transcription factor and implicated in the process of development of fat cells [69, 70] – which induce the transformation of the adipose organ of treated dogs and rats into BAT.

## Molecular Mechanisms of Transdifferentiation

Energy expenditure via activation of the orthosympathetic system is essential for the energy balance; indeed, mice lacking all β receptors (1, 2 and 3), though not exhibiting changes in the amount of food intake or in motor activity, become precociously and massively obese [66]. These mice exhibit a complete and early transformation of BAT into WAT, in line with the observations that absence of BAT results in obesity and that ectopic UCP1 expression in WAT makes mice resistant to obesity. These data also agree with the finding that BAT activation and the white-to-brown transdifferentiation induced by administration of β3-AR agonists cure obesity. On the other hand, the mechanism by which mice lacking UCP1 fail to become obese is still obscure.

Since the white-to-brown transdifferentiation induced by the adrenergic stimulus appears to be difficult to harness for human therapeutic goals, recent works indicating possible alternatives to achieve transdifferentiation appear all the more interesting.

Transgenic mice lacking the RIIβ subunit (one of the subunits regulating AMPc-dependent proteinphosphokinase A, abundant in adipose tissues) overexpress RIα subunit, which involves increased sensitivity of proteinphosphokinase A to AMPc in WAT, and consequent UCP1 gene activation [71]. This entails a brown phenotype of abdominal fat and resistance to obesity.

Foxo2 is a gene for a transcription factor expressed exclusively in adipose tissue. Its overexpression in the adipose tissue of transgenic mice gives rise to an obesity-resistant and more insulin-sensitive lean phenotype. These mice show a transformation of white into brown adipocytes [72]. Interestingly, individuals with greater insulin resistance exhibit a reduction of FOXO2 (human foxo2) in subcutaneous abdominal fat accompanied by down-regulation of other genes of the brown adipocytic phenotype.

Expression of protein 4E-BP1, which is essential to regulate post-transcriptional protein synthesis, is high in WAT. In transgenic mice lacking 4E-BP1, brown adipocytes arise in WAT and the adipose organ shrinks in size [73]. This entails that 4E-BP1 protein regulates the post-transcriptional synthesis of some factor involved in the maintenance of the white phenotype in a portion of the adipose organ. The authors suggest that this factor may be PGC1 (peroxisome proliferator-activated receptor-gamma coactivator) – a recently described protein [70] acting as a co-factor of PPARγ (see above) in the transcriptional modulation of the adipocyte genome – and that it might be essential to induce transdifferentiation to a brown phenotype [74].

The recent demonstration that white adipocytes from human subcutaneous fat can turn into brown cells via PGC1 transfection [75] lends support to this hypothesis.

A final observation stemming from our collaboration with Kristiansen's group [76] is the demonstration of the important role of protein RB, both during development and in the transdifferentiation induced by the β3-AR agonist CL316,243, in inducing the two phenotypes. In particular, its expression would be responsible for the white phenotype and its inhibition would trigger white-to-brown transdifferentiation.

Promising metabolic routes to induce transdifferentiation have thus been opened downstream from β-ARs; we hope that they will provide fresh therapeutic options for human obesity and related diseases.

## Positive Energy Balance: Overweight and Obesity

When the energy balance is positive, the adipose organ prevalently undergoes an increment in its white component. White adipocytes become hypertrophic and subsequently hyperplastic (likely due to a close causal relationship). In fact, it has been suggested that adipocytes are unable to expand beyond a given maximum volume, or 'critical size', which is genetically determined and specific for each depot [77]. Adipocytes that have reached the critical size trigger an increase in cell number [78–80]. In a recent review, Hausman et al. [81], after considering the evidence for this theory, conclude that not only paracrine factors, but also circulating factors as well as neural influences may play a large role in regulating adipose tissue development and growth. They suggest that in the development of obesity, enlarged fat cells produce and release proliferative paracrine factors as internal controllers of preadipocyte proliferation, and that their proliferative response is modulated by neural inputs to fat tissue and/or serum factors. In any case, paracrine factors appear to play a pivotal role. Adipose tissue expresses numerous factors that could be implicated in the modulation of adipogenesis: IGF-1, TGF-α, TNF-α, macrophage colony-stimulating factor (MCSF), angiotensin II, autotaxin-lysophosphatidic acid (ATX-LPA), leptin, resistin, etc. [20].

Of note, in genetically obese *ob/ob* mice (lacking leptin) and in other types of genetic and diet-induced obesity, the fat mass is hypertrophic and hyperplastic, while in genetically obese *db/db* mice (lacking leptin receptor) the fat mass is increased only by a hypertrophic mechanism ([82] and our unpublished observations). Therefore, the presence of leptin receptor seems to be essential to induce hyperplasia. In the subcutaneous adipose tissue of a massively obese patient lacking leptin receptor [83], we recently observed that mean adipocyte volume was about half that usually seen in the same depot of patients with similar BMI due to 'primitive obesity'.

A recent study showed that obesity induced by a high-fat diet in mice is hypertrophic, while that induced by hypothalamic lesion due to administration of monosodium glutamate is hyperplastic [84].

A positive energy balance also affects the organ's brown component. The brown adipocytes of obese animals are generally similar to white cells. Prevalently unilocular cells are observed at the sites where brown adipocytes are normally found, but these cells often exhibit typical mitochondria distinct from the 'normal' organelles of white fat cells. They usually – though modestly – express UCP1 as well as the typical protein of white adipocytes: leptin [56]. Interestingly, the large amount of TNF-α found in obese mice induces an increased rate of apoptosis of brown fat cells [85].

Transgenic animals lacking β1, 2 and 3 receptors become massively obese eating the same amount of food as lean ones [66]. In such animals, brown adipocytes are identical to those found in the genetically obese (*ob/ob*) and *db/db* mice described above: they are unilocular and show leptin expression and modest UCP1 activity in mitochondria with the typical morphology. This is in line with the fact that obesity due to lack of leptin (*ob/ob*) or its receptor (*db/db*) is accompanied by reduced BAT adrenergic stimulation owing to the absence of the stimulus normally exerted by the hormone on hypothalamic orthosympathetic centres.

## The Human Adipose Organ

As in small mammals, the adult human adipose organ is made up of subcutaneous as well as visceral depots. In normal adult individuals it accounts for about 9–18% of body weight in men and 14–28% in women. Most of the organ is located subcutaneously; its distribution is sex-dependent,

the mammary and gluteo-femoral subcutaneous depots being more developed in women.

The visceral depots are very similar to those described in small mammals. In overweight or obese individuals, the abdominal visceral depots tend to grow in men and in post-menopausal women. This type of fat accumulation is dangerous for its association with the diseases secondary to overweight and obesity (diabetes, hypertension, myocardial infarct).

There are no histological differences between human and murine adipocytes, except for the larger size of the former. The maximum diameter measured in obese mice is ca. 140 μm (about 1.30 μg/cell in the epididymal depot), whereas in the subcutaneous depot of massively obese individuals the maximum diameter we measured is ca. 160 μm (about 1.95 μg/cell), a difference of 30–40%.

All the major molecules produced by murine fat cells (e.g. leptin, adiponectin, TNF-α, angiotensinogen, PAI 1, resistin, adipsin) are also produced by human adipocytes.

Human adipose tissue development entails a long phase of preadipocyte proliferation, which is complete at around 20 years of age. This is similar to rats and mice, where this phase is achieved by the second month of postnatal life [86].

Also in our species, regulation of the amount of fat tissue depends on the energy balance. If there is a positive balance, adult individuals exhibit an increase in adipocyte size, which, upon attainment of a critical size, will induce the development of new fat cells (see also 'Vessels and Nerves').

Indeed, the number of adipocytes, total fat mass and proportion of body fat correlate with age in both sexes, whereas adipocyte size does not appear to correlate with age, but with the amount of fat mass and its proportion of body weight in both sexes [87].

In massively obese individuals, the fat mass may quadruple to 60–70% of body weight [88, 89]. Recent works reporting a massive presence of macrophages in the adipose tissue of obese subjects hypothesise that many cytokines produced by adipose tissue and responsible for most of the adverse symptoms of obesity are in fact histiocytic in origin. The cause of this macrophage infiltration is unclear, but seems to be related to adipocyte size [90].

A negative energy balance induces a reduction in both fat mass and adipocyte size. The latter fact is important, because it results in improved cellular insulin sensitivity. Completely delipidised cells may be seen in the adipose tissue of individuals with a negative energy balance. Their morphology is very similar to that of the slimmed-down rat and mouse cells described above. In a TEM study of subcutaneous fat tissue from obese individuals administered a very low-calorie diet for 5 days, we detected severely slimmed-down adipocytes very similar to those observed in acutely fasted rats and mice. Interestingly, slimmed-down cells were side by side with unilocular adipocytes ostensibly not affected by the slimming process. The fate of completely slimmed-down cells is still unclear, and the hypothesis that they may undergo apoptosis is so far unsubstantiated.

Not all fat depots respond identically to a negative energy balance. Indeed, the gluteo-femoral subcutaneous tissue of adult pre-menopausal women is known to be much more resistant to the slimming process than abdominal subcutaneous fat, whereas both depots behave similarly in post-menopausal subjects. This seems to be due to a combination of increased lipoproteinlipase activity and reduced lipolytic activity in the former area.

The reduced lipolytic activity appears to stem from a relative preponderance of the antilipolytic activity of α2-ARs over that of lipolytic β-ARs [91]. In general, α2-ARs are more represented in human than murine adipose tissue. Transgenic mice with adipose tissue similar to human fat tissue have been obtained to mimic this situation in a murine model. These animals lack β3-ARs and express abundantly human α2-AR (β3-AR-deficient, human α2-expressing transgenic mice) [92]. In these animals obesity induced by a high-fat diet was exclusively of the hyperplastic type and the mice were not insulin-resistant. These data are in line with the important role of α2-AR in relation to the proliferative stimulus, and with the relationship between insulin sensitivity and adipocyte size.

Like the murine organ, the human adipose organ also contains BAT. Given its thermogenic function, animals with a small body volume and a larger relative body surface clearly have greater

thermogenic requirements; the greater heat dissipation occurring in these compared with larger animals (which have a smaller volume/surface ratio) results in greater heat dispersion; hence, also the smaller proportion of human vs murine BAT. For the same reason, human newborns exhibit a greater amount of BAT than adults. In the human newborn's adipose organ, BAT occupies the same sites as in the murine organ. In the adipose organ of adult humans, several studies have detected small amounts of BAT with the same morphological and functional characteristics as murine BAT [93]. An increase in BAT in cold-exposed human subjects has also been reported [94]. Considerable amounts of BAT, especially perirenal, have often been described in patients with pheochromocytoma (a tumour made up of endocrine cells secreting large amounts of adrenaline and noradrenaline) [95, 96].

It has recently been demonstrated that human preadipocytes from different depots stimulated in vitro with thiazolidinediones (drugs that act by stimulating the PPARγ transcription factor, which seems to have a large role in adipocyte differentiation) express UCP1 [97]. This suggests that human brown adipocyte development may be induced by drug treatment.

UCP1mRNA has been detected in the abdominal visceral depots of both lean and obese patients, though in significantly smaller amounts in the latter [98]. It is interesting to note that after dieting and consequent weight loss, UCP1mRNA levels remained lower than in lean subjects, suggesting a lesser genetic predisposition to energy dispersion in obese individuals [99]. This is in line with the observation that combined mutations of UCP1 and β3-AR induce additive effects on weight gain in human obesity [100].

Two recent papers stress the importance of the concept of the adipose organ in humans. In the first, in agreement with the experimental finding that transgenic mice lacking insulin receptor at the sole level of BAT are hyperglycaemic, a reduced 'brown' phenotype in human subcutaneous adipose tissue has been shown to predispose to diabetes [101]. In the second, in vitro transfection of PPARγ co-factor 1 (PGC1, see above) induced the transformation of human white adipocytes into fat cells capable of expressing UCP1, the molecular marker of brown adipocytes [75].

# Protein ZAG and Cachexia of the Adipose Organ

## Protein ZAG: A New Adipokine

A dramatic weight loss, entailing a reduction of the adipose organ by up to 85%, is a characteristic feature of tumour cachexia. Several factors are implicated in this process; one of them is possibly ZAG (zinc-α2-glycoprotein), a 43-kDa protein originally isolated in human plasma [102] and later described in several organs: breast, prostate, liver, lung and skin [103]. Overexpression of protein ZAG occurs in several malignant tumours and is thus used as a tumour marker.

The biological function of this protein is still largely unknown; its molecular identity with a lipid-mobilising factor isolated from MAC16 (a murine tumour inducing deep cachexia) and the urine of cachectic cancer patients has recently been reported [104].

Murine and human ZAG protein exhibit 59% homology of the amino acid sequence and 100% homology at the sites functionally involved in the action on lipid metabolism [105, 106]. Its administration to lean and obese animals induces a marked reduction in body fat, and a dose-dependent lipolytic activity has been demonstrated in vitro [107].

The specific β3-adrenoreceptor antagonist SR59230 reduces its lipolytic activity, suggesting that in rodents its action is mediated by β3-AR [108].

A recent study of its normal expression in adipose tissues in vivo and in vitro showed that protein ZAG is expressed in WAT and BAT in different murine depots as well as in human subcutaneous and visceral WAT. In particular, it has been detected in white adipocyte cytoplasm using immunohistochemical techniques. It is also found in the stroma-vascular fraction of adipose tissue [109].

Adipocytic overexpression of the protein in cachectic mice is consistent with a role for it in the local control of lipolysis. A recent paper reporting that protein ZAG stimulates adiponectin expression in adipocytes in vitro suggests that it may be a gene for body weight regulation.

# References

1. Rothwell NJ, Stock MJ (1979) A role for brown adipose tissue in diet-induced thermogenesis. Nature 281:31–35
2. Nedergaard J, Lindberg O (1982) The brown fat cell. Int Rev Cytol 74:187–284
3. Stock MJ (1989) Thermogenesis and brown fat: relevance to human obesity. Infusionstherapie 16:282–284
4. Lowell BB, S-Susulic V, Hamann A et al (1993) Development of obesity in transgenic mice after genetic ablation of brown adipose tissue. Nature 366:740–742
5. Enerback S, Jacobsson A, Simpson EM et al (1997) Mice lacking mitochondrial uncoupling protein are cold-sensitive but not obese. Nature 387:90–94
6. Kopecky J, Clarke G, Enerback S et al (1995) Expression of the mitochondrial uncoupling protein gene from the aP2 gene promoter prevents genetic obesity. J Clin Invest 96:2914–2923
7. Kopecky J, Hodny Z, Rossmeisl M et al (1996) Reduction of dietary obesity in aP2-Ucp transgenic mice: physiology and adipose tissue distribution.

Am J Physiol 270:E768–E775
8. Zhang YY, Proenca R, Maffei M et al (1994) Positional cloning of the mouse obese gene and its human homologue. Nature 372:425–432
9. Ingalls AM, Dichie MM, Snell GD (1950) Obese, a new mutation in the house mouse. J Hered 41:317–318
10. Campfield LA, Smith FJ, Guisez Y et al (1995) Recombinant mouse OB protein: evidence for a peripheral signal linking adiposity and central neural networks. Science 269:475–476
11. Halaas JL, Gajiwala KS, Maffei M et al (1995) Weight-reducing effects of the plasma protein encoded by the obese gene. Science 269:543–546
12. Pelleymounter MA, Cullen MJ, Baker MB et al (1995) Effects of the obese gene product on body weight regulation in ob/ob mice. Science 269:540–543
13. Tartaglia LA, Dembski M, Weng X et al (1995) Identification and expression cloning of a leptin receptor, OB-R. Cell 83:1263–1271
14. Lee GH, Proenca R, Montez JM et al (1996) Abnormal splicing of the leptin receptor in diabetic

mice. Nature 379:632–635

15. Ghilardi N, Ziegler S, Wiestner A et al (1996) Defective STAT signalling by the leptin receptor in diabetic mice. Proc Natl Acad Sci USA 93:6231–6235

16. Coleman DL (1978) Obese and diabetes: two mutant genes causing diabetes-obesity syndromes in mice. Diabetologia 14:141–148

17. Maffei M, Halaas J, Ravussin E et al (1995) Leptin levels in human and rodent: measurement of plasma leptin and ob RNA in obese and weight-reduced subjects. Nat Med 1:1155–1161

18. Farooqi IS, Jebb SA, Langmack G et al (1999) Effects of recombinant leptin therapy in a child with congenital leptin deficiency. N Engl J Med 341:879–884

19. Ahima RS, Prabakaran D, Mantzoros C et al (1996) Role of leptin in the neuroendocrine response to fasting. Nature 382:250–252

20. De Matteis R, Dashtipour K, Ognibene A, Cinti S (1998) Localization of leptin receptor splice variants in mouse peripheral tissues by immunohistochemistry. Proc Nutr Soc 57:441–448

21. Trayhurn P, Hoggard N, Rayner DV (2001) White adipose tissue as a secretory and endocrine organ: leptin and other secreted protein. In: Klaus S (ed) Adipose tissues. Landes Bioscience, Georgetown, pp 158–182

22. Ehrhart-Bornstein M, Lamounier-Zepter V, Schraven A et al (2003) Human adipocytes secrete mineralcorticoid-releasing factors. Proc Natl Acad Sci USA 100:14211–14216

23. Cannon B, Hedin A, Nedergaard J (1982) Exclusive occurrence of thermogenin antigen in brown adipose tissue. FEBS Lett 150:129–132

24. Klaus S, Casteilla L, Bouillaud F, Ricquier D (1991) The uncoupling protein UCP: a membranous mitochondrial ion carrier exclusively expressed in brown adipose tissue. Int J Biochem 23:791–801

25. Ricquier D, Casteilla L, Bouillaud F (1991) Molecular studies of the uncoupling protein. FASEB J 5:2237–2242

26. Zaagsma J, de VJ, Harms HH, Jansen JD (1995) The nature of adipocyte b-adrenoceptors. In: Pharmacology of adrenoceptors. MacMillan Press, London, pp 247–256

27. Emorine LJ, Marullo S, Briend-Sutren MM et al (1989) Molecular characterization of the human beta 3-adrenergic receptor. Science 245:1118–1121

28. Nicholls DG, Cunningham SA, Rial E (1986) The bioenergetic mechanisms of brown adipose tissue. In: Trayhurn P, Nicholls DG (eds) Brown Adipose Tissue. Edward Arnold, London, pp 52–85

29. Ghorbani M, Claus TH, Himms-Hagen J (1997) Hypertrophy of brown adipocytes in brown and white adipose tissues and reversal of diet-induced obesity in rats treated with a beta3-adrenoceptor agonist. Biochem Pharmacol 54:121–131

30. Ghorbani M, Himms-Hagen J (1997) Appearance of brown adipocytes in white adipose tissue during CL 316,243-induced reversal of obesity and diabetes in Zucker fa/fa rats. Int J Obesity 21:465–475

31. Buemann B, Toubro S, Astrup A (2000) Effects of the two beta-3-agonists, ZD7114 and ZD2079, on 24 hour energy expenditure and respiratory quotient in obese subjects. Int J Obesity 24:1553–1560

32. Fleury C, Neverova M, Collins S et al (1997) Uncoupling protein-2: a novel gene linked to obesity and hyperinsulinemia. Nat Genet 15:269–272

33. Boss O, Samec S, Paoloni-Giacobino A et al (1997) Uncoupling protein-3: a new member of the mitochondrial carrier family with tissue-specific expression. FEBS Lett 408:39–42

34. Vidal-Puig AJ, Solanes G, Grujic D et al (1997) UCP3: an uncoupling protein homologue expressed preferentially and abundantly in skeletal muscle and brown adipose tissue. Biochem Biophys Res Commun 235:79–82

35. Arsenijevic D, Onuma H, Pecquer C et al (2000) Disruption of the uncoupling protein-2 gene in mice reveals a role in immunity and reactive oxygen species production. Nat Genet 26:435–439

36. Vidal-Puig AJ, Grujic D, Zhang CY et al (2000) Energy metabolism in uncoupling protein 3 gene knock out mice. J Biol Chem 275:16258–16266

37. Golozoubova V, Hohtola E, Matthias A et al (2001) Only UCP1 can mediate adaptive nonshivering thermogenesis in the cold. FASEB J 15:2048–2050

38. Zhang CY, Baffy G, Perret P et al (2001) Uncoupling protein-2 negatively regulates insulin secretion and is a major link between obesity, beta cell dysfunction, and type 2 diabetes. Cell 105:745–755

39. Cinti S (1999) The adipose organ. Kurtis Ed, Milan

40. Guerra C, Koza RA, Yamashita H et al (1998) Emergence of brown adipocytes in white fat is under genetic control. Effects on body weight and adiposity. J Clin Invest 102:412–420

41. Sbarbati A, Morroni M, Zancanaro C, Cinti S (1991) Rat interscapular brown adipose tissue at different ages: a morphometric study. Int J Obesity 15:581–587

42. Morroni M, Barbatelli G, Zingaretti MC, Cinti S (1995) Immunohistochemical, ultrastructural and morphometric evidence for brown adipose tissue recruitment due to cold acclimation in old rats. Int J Obesity 19:126–131

43. De Matteis R, Ricquier D, Cinti S (1998) TH-, NPY-, SP-, and CRGP-immunoreactive nerves in interscapular brown adipose tissue of adult rats acclimated at different temperatures: an immunohistochemical study. J Neurocytol 27:877–886

44. Giordano A, Morroni M, Carle F et al (1998) Sensory nerves affect the recruitment and differentiation of rat periovarian brown adipocytes during cold acclimation. J Cell Sci 111:2587–2594

45. Giordano A, Frontini A, Castellucci M, Cinti S (2004) Presence and distribution of cholinergic nerves in rat mediastinal brown adipose tissue. J Histochem Cytochem 52:923–930

46. Murphy GJ, Kirkham DM, Cawthorne MA, Young P (1993) Correlation of beta 3-adrenoceptor-induced

activation of cyclic AMP-dependent protein kinase with activation of lipolysis in rat white adipocytes. Biochem Pharmacol 46:575–581

47. Bouloumie A, Planat V, Devedjian JC et al (1994) Alpha 2-adrenergic stimulation promotes preadipocyte proliferation. Involvement of mitogen-activated protein kinases. J Biol Chem 269:30254–30259

48. Valet P, Pages C, Jeanneton O et al (1998) Alpha 2-adrenergic receptor-mediated release of lysophosphatidic acid by adipocytes. A paracrine signal for preadipocyte growth. J Clin Invest 101:1431–1438

49. Valet P, Grujic D, Wade J et al (2000) Expression of human alpha 2-adrenergic receptors in adipose tissue of beta 3-adrenergic receptor-deficient mice promotes diet-induced obesity. J Biol Chem 275:34797–34802

50. Hodgson AJ, Wilkinson C, Abolhasan P, Llewellyn-Smith IJ (2001) Differential control of lipolysis by sympathetic nerves. Int J Obesity 25:27

51. Napolitano L, Gagne HT (1963) Lipid-depleted white adipose cells: an electron microscope study. Anat Rec 147:273–293

52. Kreier F, Fliers E, Voshol PJ et al (2002) Selective parasympathetic innervation of subcutaneous and intra-abdominal fat – functional implications. J Clin Invest 110:1243–1250

53. Kitamura T, Kitamura Y, Nakae J et al (2004) Mosaic analysis of insulin receptor function. J Clin Invest 113:209–219

54. Blanchette-Mackie EJ, Scow RO (1981) Lipolysis and lamellar structures in white adipose tissue of young rats: lipid movement in membranes. J Ultrastruct Res 77:295–318

55. Cancello R, Zingaretti MC, Sarzani R et al (1998) Leptin and UCP1 genes are reciprocally regulated in brown adipose tissue. Endocrinology 139:4747–4750

56. Cinti S, Frederich RC, Zingaretti MC et al (1997) Immunohistochemical localization of leptin and uncoupling protein in white and brown adipose tissue. Endocrinology 138:797–804

57. Rayner DV, Simon E, Duncan JS, Trayhurn P (1998) Hyperleptinaemia in mice induced by administration of the tyrosine hydroxylase inhibitor alpha-methyl-p-tyrosine. FEBS Lett 429:395–398

58. Himms-Hagen J, Melnyk A, Zingaretti MC et al (2000) Multilocular fat cells in WAT of CL-316243-treated rats derive directly from white adipocytes. Am J Physiol 279:C670–C681

59. Cannon B, Nedergaard J (2004) Brown adipose tissue: function and physiological significance. Physiol Rev 84:277–359

60. Lowell BB, Flier JS (1997) Brown adipose tissue, beta 3-adrenergic receptors, and obesity. Annu Rev Med 48:307–316

61. Young P, Arch JR, Ashwell M (1984) Brown adipose tissue in the parametrial fat pad of the mouse. FEBS Lett 167:10–14

62. Cousin B, Cinti S, Morroni M et al (1992) Occurrence of brown adipocytes in rat white adipo-

se tissue: molecular and morphological characterization. J Cell Sci 103:931–942

63. Giordano A, Morroni M, Santone G et al (1996) Tyrosine hydroxylase, neuropeptide Y, substance P, calcitonin gene-related peptide in nerves of rat periovarian adipose tissue: an immunohistochemical and ultrastructural investigation. J Neurocytol 25:125–136

64. Tosh D, Slack JMW (2002) How cells change their phenotype. Nat Rev Mol Cell Bio 3:187–194

65. Jimenez M, Barbatelli G, Allevi R et al (2003) Beta 3 adrenoceptor knockout in C57BL/6J mice depresses the occurrence of brown adipocytes in white fat. Eur J Biochem 270:699–705

66. Bachman ES, Dhillon H, Zhang CY et al (2002) BetaAR signalling required for diet-induced thermogenesis and obesity resistance. Science 297:843–845

67. De Matteis R, Arch JR, Petroni ML et al (2002) Immunohistochemical identification of the beta(3)-adrenoceptor in intact human adipocytes and ventricular myocardium: effect of obesity and treatment with ephedrine and caffeine. Int J Obesity 26:1442–1450

68. Toseland CDN, Campbell S, Francis I et al (2001) Comparison of adipose tissue changes following administration of rosiglitazone in the dog and rat. Diabet Obes Metab 3:163–170

69. Lowell BB (1999) PPARgamma: an essential regulator of adipogenesis and modulator of fat cell function. Cell 99:239–242

70. Spiegelman BM, Puigserver P, Wu Z (2000) Regulation of adipogenesis and energy balance by PPARgamma and PGC-1. Int J Obesity 24 (Suppl 4):S8–S10

71. Cummings DE, Brandon EP, Planas JV et al (1996) Genetically lean mice result from targeted disruption of the RII beta subunit of protein kinase A. Nature 382:622–626

72. Cederberg A, Gronning LM, Ahren B et al (2001) FOXC2 is a winged helix gene that counteracts obesity, hypertriglyceridemia, and diet-induced insulin resistance. Cell 106:563–573

73. Tsukiyama-Kohara K, Poulin F, Kohara M et al (2001) Adipose tissue reduction in mice lacking the translational inhibitor 4E-BP1. Nat Med 7:1128–1132

74. Wu Z, Puigserver P, Andersson U et al (1999) Mechanisms controlling mitochondrial biogenesis and respiration through the thermogenic coactivator PGC-1. Cell 98:115–124

75. Tiraby C, Tavernier G, Lefort C et al (2003) Acquirement of brown fat cell features by human white adipocytes. J Biol Chem 278:33370–33376

76. Hansen JB, Jorgensen C, Petersen RK et al (2004) Retinoblastoma protein functions as a molecular switch determining white versus brown adipocyte differentiation. Proc Natl Acad Sci USA 101:4112–4117

77. Di Girolamo M, Fine JB, Tagra K, Rossmanith R

(1998) Qualitative regional differences in adipose tissue growth and cellularity in male Wistar rats fed ad libitum. Am J Physiol 274:R1460-R1467

78. Lemonnier D (1972) Effect of age, sex, and site on the cellularity of the adipose tissue in mice rendered obese by a high fat diet. J Clin Invest 51:2907-2915

79. Faust IM, Johnson PR, Stern JS, Hirsh J (1978) Diet-induced adipocyte number increase in adult rats: a new model of obesity. Am J Physiol 235:E279-E286

80. Bjorntorp B (1991) Adipose tissue distribution and function. Int J Obesity 15:67-81

81. Hausman DB, Di Girolamo M, Bartness TJ et al (2001) The biology of white adipocyte proliferation. Obes Rev 2:239-254

82. Johnson PR, Hirsh J (1972) Cellularity of adipose depots in six strains of genetically obese mice. J Lipid Res 13:2-11

83. Clement K, Vaisse C, Lahlou N et al (1998) A mutation in the human leptin receptor gene causes obesity and pituitary dysfunction. Nature 392:398-401

84. Imai T, Jiang M, Chambon P et al (2001) Impaired adipogenesis and lipolysis in the mouse upon selective ablation of the retinoid X receptor alpha mediated by a tamoxifen-inducible chimeric Cre recombinase (Cre-ERT2) in adipocytes. Proc Natl Acad Sci USA 98:224-228

85. Nisoli E, Briscini L, Giordano A et al (2001) Tumor necrosis factor alpha mediates apoptosis of brown adipocytes and defective brown adipocyte function in obesity. Proc Natl Acad Sci USA 97:8033-8038

86. Hager A, Sjostrom L, Arvidsson B et al (1977) Body fat and adipose tissue cellularity in infants: a longitudinal study. Metabolism 26:607-614

87. Chumlea WC, Roche AF, Siervogel RM et al (1981) Adipocytes and adiposity in adults. Am J Clin Nutr 34:1798-1803

88. Prins JB, O'Rahilly S (1977) Regulation of adipose cell number in man. Clin Sci 92:3-11

89. Hausman DB, Di Girolamo M, Bartness TJ et al (2001) The biology of white adipocyte proliferation. Obes Rev 2:239-254

90. Xu H, Barnes GT, Yang Q et al (2003) Chronic inflammation in fat plays a crucial role in the development of obesity-related insulin resistance. J Clin Invest 112:1785-1788

91. Rebuffe-Scrive M, Enk L, Crona N et al (1985) Fat cell metabolism in different regions in women. Effect of menstrual cycle, pregnancy and lactation. J Clin Invest 75:1973-1976

92. Boucher J, Castan-Laurell I, Le Lay S et al (2002) Human alpha 2A-adrenergic receptor gene expressed in transgenic mouse adipose tissue under the control of its regulatory elements. J Mol Endocrinol 29:251-264

93. Kortelainen M-L, Pelletier G, Ricquier D, Bukowiecki LJ (1993) Immunohistochemical detection of human brown adipose tissue uncoupling protein in an autopsy series. J Histochem Cytochem 41:759-764

94. Huttunen P, Hirvonen J, Kinnula V (1981) The occurrence of brown adipose tissue in outdoor workers. Eur J Appl Physiol 46:339-345

95. Ricquier D, Néchad M, Mory G (1982) Ultrastructural and biochemical characterization of human brown adipose tissue in phaeochromocytoma. J Clin Endocrinol Metab 54:803-807

96. Lean MEJ, James WPT, Jennings G, Trayhurn P (1986) Brown adipose tissue in patients with phaeocromocytoma. Int J Obesity 10:219-227

97. Del Mar Gonzalez-Barroso M, Pecquer C, Gerlly C et al (2000) Transcriptional activation of the human ucp1 gene in a rodent cell line. Synergism of retinoids, isoproterenol, and thiazolidinedione is mediated by a multipartite response element. J Biol Chem 275:31722-31732

98. Oberkofler H, Dallinger G, Liu YM et al (1997) Uncoupling protein gene: quantification of expression levels in adipose tissues of obese and non-obese humans. J Lipid Res 38:2125-2133

99. Oberkofler H, Liu YM, Esterbauer H et al (1998) Uncoupling protein-2 gene: reduced mRNA expression in intraperitoneal adipose tissue of obese humans. Diabetologia 41:940-946

100. Clement K, Ruiz J, Cassare-Doulcier AM et al (1996) Additive effect of A—>G (-3826) variant of the uncoupling protein gene and the Trp64Arg mutation of the beta 3-adrenergic receptor gene on weight gain in morbid obesity. Int J Obesity 20:1062-1066

101. Guerra C, Navarro P, Valverde AM et al (2001) Brown adipose tissue-specific insulin receptor knockout shows diabetic phenotype without insulin resistance. J Clin Invest 108:1205-1213

102. Burgi W, Schmid K (1961) Preparation and properties of Zn-alpha 2-glycoprotein of normal human plasma. J Biol Chem 236:1066-1074

103. Tada T, Ohkubo I, Niwa M et al (1991) Immunohistochemical localization of Zn-alpha 2-glycoprotein in normal human tissues. J Histochem Cytochem 39:1221-1226

104. Todorov PT, McDevitt TM, Meyer DJ et al (1998) Purification and characterization of a tumor lipid-mobilizing factor. Cancer Res 58:2353-2358

105. Ueyama H, Naitoh H, Ohkubo I (1994) Structure and expression of rat and mouse mRNA for Zn-alpha 2-glycoprotein. J Biochem 116:677-681

106. Sanchez LM, Chirino AJ, Bjorkman P (1999) Crystal structure of human ZAG, a fat-depleting factor related to MHC molecules. Science 283:1914-1919

107. Hirai K, Hussey HJ, Barber MD et al (1998) Biological evolution of a lipid-mobilizing factor isolated from the urine of cancer patients. Cancer Res 58:2359-2365

108. Russell ST, Hirai K, Tisdale MJ (2002) Role of beta3-adrenergic receptors in the action of a tumour lipid mobilizing factor. Br J Cancer 86:424-428

109. Bing C, Bao Y, Jenkins J et al (2004) Zinc-alpha2-glycoprotein, a lipid mobilizing factor, is expressed in adipocytes and is up-regulated in mice with cancer cachexia. Proc Natl Acad Sci USA 101:2500-2505

# Body Silhouette and Body Fat Distribution

Angela Faga

## Introduction

Body silhouette is defined by skeleton framework, muscle masses and fat distribution. All these anatomical components are genetically fixed, related to growth hormones and sex hormones, and modified by extrinsic factors such as age, physical exercise, diet, constrictive garments, way of living and general health conditions.

As far as fat distribution is concerned, we recognise the subcutaneous and the central (visceral) fat.

## Central Fat

Fat is present, in a higher or lesser degree, in almost every anatomical compartment, inside parenchymatous organs, muscles and breasts and it is stored mainly in the omentum (intra-abdominal fat): this is the so-called 'central' fat and it is the most involved in metabolic variations, increasing in obesity and reducing in the case of weight loss. Intra-abdominal fat contributes to a significant degree, but not exclusively, to the increase of waist circumference and sagittal diameter [1], altering the normal ideal silhouette (Fig. 1a, b); even in normal non-obese subjects, it tends to increase in the elderly, owing to the redistribution of the adipose mass [2].

Besides the central fat, which is sensitive to weight variations, we recognise some anatomical districts where adipose fat pads are present, where volumes are constant irrespective of the degree of corpulence or even in the event of major weight loss. These are structures devoted to produce more protection in the regions of attrition and have been thoroughly described: around the kidneys, inside the joints, underneath the breasts

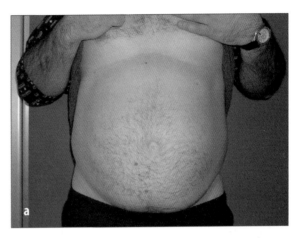

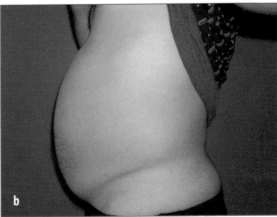

**Fig. 1.** Middle-aged man: typical silhouette from increased intra-abdominal fat. **a** Front view. **b** Side view

(Chassaignac retrommamary bursa), deep in the face (corpus adiposum buccae or bulla of Bichat, adipose body of the orbit, parapharyngeal adipose corpus), inside the hand (corpus adiposum palmare profundum [3]), and over the os pubis (mons Veneris). This fat has almost no influence on body silhouette and a few on face traits.

## Subcutaneous Fat

There are two distinctly different types of subcutaneous fat, separated by the fascia superficialis [4]: the superficial fat layer, which is distributed over almost the entire body, and the deep layer, located between the superficial and the deep fascia, which is found only in certain areas of the body [5, 6].

### Superficial Fat

The superficial fat (areolar fat) consistently lines the skin and follows the skin displacements. It can be considered a part of the skin, as it is responsible for the terminal vascularisation of the skin itself. Histologically it has a lobular pattern and a vertical orientation, being located within connective arches (retinacula cutis). Its mean dimensions are 0.5–1.0 cm per unit. It is firmly anchored both to the undersurface of the skin and to the fascia superficialis; these septa are able to adapt the adipocytes they contain only laterally: as fat hypertrophy increases, the tension within these fat pockets (their volume may increase a thousand fold) also increases, giving the skin the typical 'Chesterfield sofa' look (Fig. 2a, b). Adipocytes of the areolar layer are large, round, turgid, and piled together where small vessels pass directed towards the dermis [7]. Normally, it is approximately 1 cm thick and has a rather uniform distribution, although it tends to increase significantly with age on the upper abdomen, on the rear side of the body and on the buttocks [8], particularly in women. It is thinner in certain areas of the body (ankles and pretibial crest) and can reach several centimetres in cases of marked hypertrophy.

This fat is metabolically active and responds to weight loss, as its adipocytes are rich in beta 1 receptors, which are lipolytic and secrete lipase: thus, the superficial fat is responsible for the overall silhouette changes in size (but not in shape) according to changes in weight.

### Deep Layer Fat

The deep layer (lamellar fat) constitutes blocked reserve fat, easy to gain and difficult to lose, metabolised only when there is starvation. It has a laminar pattern and a horizontal orientation, and is arranged as fat pads (localised fat pads, LFP), surrounded by a fascia that is sometimes well identified as a specific capsule and sometimes indistinct from the fascias of the muscles, differently located according to sex, race and genetic

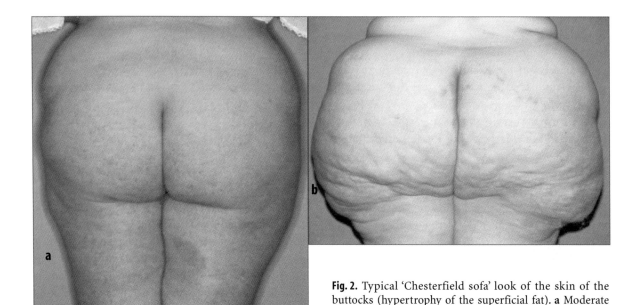

**Fig. 2.** Typical 'Chesterfield sofa' look of the skin of the buttocks (hypertrophy of the superficial fat). **a** Moderate grade. **b** Severe grade

characteristics. Fat pads appear at puberty or shortly thereafter and are the most responsible for the body silhouette. Larger vessels pass along connective trabeculas, destined to the superficial skin vascular net. Adipocytes in deep fat are smaller than in the areolar layer, and horizontally elongated [7]. Pad adipocytes are two to four times more receptive to glucose than other fat cells; they are also very rich in alpha 2 receptors, which block lipolysis and are stimulated by catecholamines.

Only surgery can modify the shape of the silhouette, through a direct approach to LFPs, both by dermolipectomy operations and, mainly, by different techniques of liposuction.

Different locations of fat pads have been described.

*Face* - Fat distribution in the face contributes to the face traits. A fat pad is observed around the buccal area (Fig. 3). It can be divided into three lobes: anterior, intermediate and posterior. Four extensions derive from the posterior lobe: buccal, pterygoid, pterygopalatine and temporal [9]. In the nose, an interdomal fat pad is present, varying in size from 1.2 × 2.4 mm to 3.6 × 5.2 mm [10]. Fat pads are also identified in the periorbital, nasolabial (Fig. 3), submental (Fig. 4) and temporal regions.

*Upper torso* - Three major fat pads are described: two even in the scapular regions, one odd in the interscapular area [7].

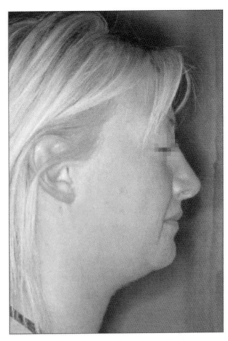

**Fig. 4.** Fat pad in the submental region of a young woman

*Chest* - Fusion of the superficial layer with the deep fascia on the ribs creates separate pockets responsible for the ripple effect (Fig. 5).

*Arms* - A posterior fat pad (subacromial) [11] and a deltoid fat pad have been described.

*Abdomen* - In the medial regions (supraumbilical, umbilical, infraumbilical), the fascia superficialis presents several layers separated by adipose tissue, while in the lateral regions localised adiposity is

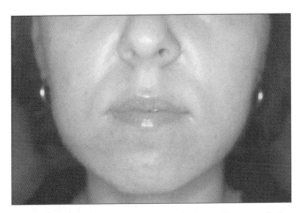

**Fig. 3.** Face of a young woman, with fat pads around the mouth and in the nasolabial regions

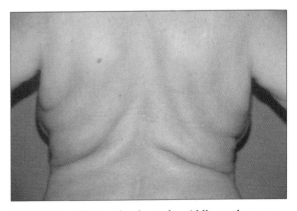

**Fig. 5.** Ripple effect on the chest of a middle-aged woman

very rare. A true LFP can be identified just in the lower half of the abdomen, limited between an ideal line that joins both iliac crests above the umbilicus and the superior border of the pubis (Fig. 6). The thicker zone of the abdomen corresponds to the projection of the rectus abdominalis muscle, where the large perforating vessels are situated.

*Hips* - An LFP may be found in the hips, limited by the 12th rib above, the muscles of the lumbar region posteriorly, the abdominal muscles anteriorly, and the iliac crest below.

*Gluteal region and flank* - The lumbo-gluteal adipose body (LGAB) has been identified in this area [12–14]. It is a symmetrical structure, shaped as a triangular pyramid, with a subcutaneous posterior base and an intermuscular anterior apex, which partially borders three regions: the inferior part of the lumbar region, the superior part of the gluteal region and the posterior part of the flank. It extends from the second lumbar to the second sacral vertebral body and between the anterior superior iliac spines, so corresponding to the lumbar trigone (Fig. 7). Inside the LGAB, two/three layers can be identified, separated by parallel fibrous septa: the more superficial layers are composed of smaller lobules, and the deeper layers of larger lobules.

*Buttocks* - Important LFPs in this region exist only in blacks, Brazilian mulatas, Asiatics and certain Slavic types. Owing to the adherence of the deep fascial layer to the underlying muscles, these fat pads do not tend to drop while standing (Fig. 8), sometimes giving the buttocks a particularly pleasant shape. Enormous buttock fat pads have been described in some African tribes.

*Pretrochanteric area* - This can be subdivided into four regions: the iliofemoral bulge, the middle femoral region, the anterior femoral region and the posterior extension, directed towards the infragluteal fold (Fig. 9). A large accumulation of fat in the iliofemoral area is typical among gynoid Caucasians.

*Thigh* - An LFP is present in both the upper and the lower third of the internal surface; the upper one

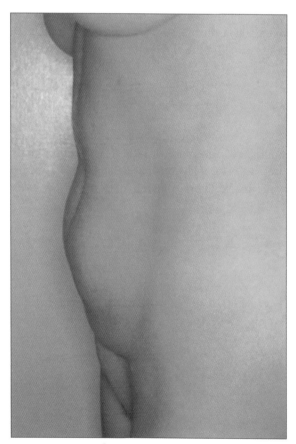

**Fig. 6.** Well-identified fat pad in the lower half of the abdomen in a thin young woman

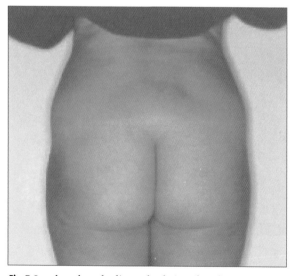

**Fig. 7.** Lumbo-gluteal adipose body in a female teenager

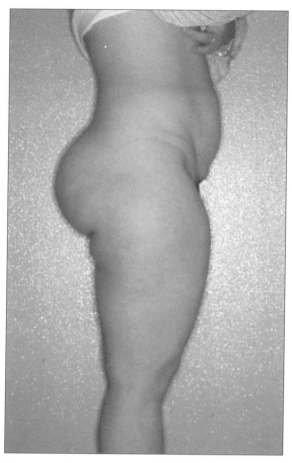

**Fig. 8.** Fat pads of the buttocks, with typical tendency to stay up

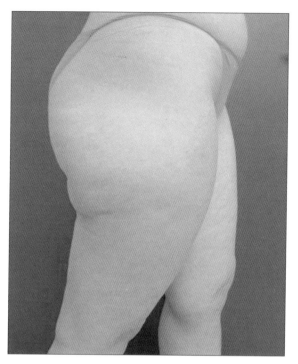

**Fig. 9.** Posterior extension of the pretrochanteric fat pad

extends from the inguinal crease to the middle third of the thigh and can reach dimensions large enough to impair a good deambulation. In the middle third the lamellar layer is almost absent (Fig. 10).

*Knees* - Between the inferior portion of the thigh and the superior portion of the leg there is a fat pad with an anteromedial extension, which curves inferiorly around the medial and inferior segment of the patella like a hook (infrapatellar fat pad) (Fig. 11).

*Legs* - An oval unilocular fat pad has been identified, vertically oriented from the lateral aspect of the ankle towards the head of the fibula: the lateral inframalleolar fat pad. The sural nerve and the short saphenous vein run over its external surface [15, 16] (Fig. 12).

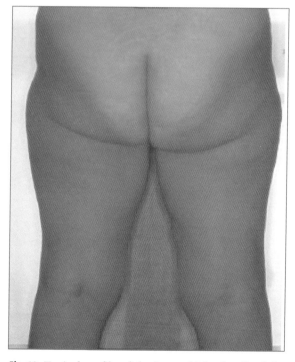

**Fig. 10.** Typical profile of the inner thighs: localised fat pads are present just in the upper and lower third

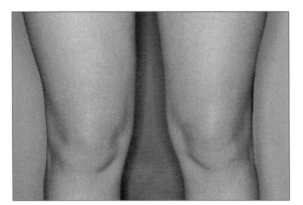

**Fig. 11.** Infrapatellar fat pads in a teenage girl

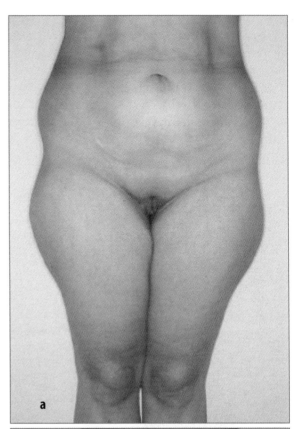

According to the sex (hormonal factors), we observe that the majority of LFPs in women and gynoid types are located around the pelvis and in the lower half of the body (rhizomelic silhouette), while in men and android morphotypes, LFPs are observed mostly in the trunk and the upper half of the body.

According to the ethnic origin, four types are described, depending on the prevalent distribution and thickness of the LFPs:

1. Latin, with a typical 'violin' shape (rolls on the hips and trochanteric fat) (Fig. 13a, b)

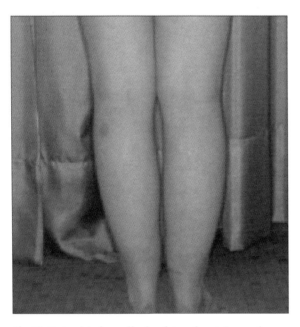

**Fig. 12.** Lateral inframalleolar fat pads, giving a clumsy aspect to the legs of a young woman

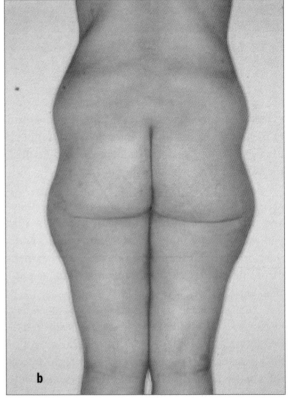

**Fig. 13.** Typical 'violin' shape. **a** Front view. **b** Back view

2. AngloSaxon and Nordic, with a typical 'life preserver' shape (hips and abdominal rolls), which resembles the 'Michelin man' shape in the fatter individuals.
3. Asiatic, with a typical 'kimono' shape (rolls mainly on the waist, chest, arms) (Fig. 14)
4. Black, where steatopygia is the most distinctive character (fat on the buttocks) (Fig. 15).

All the fat deposits described are composed of white adipocytes. Brown adipocytes are scattered among the white ones and constitute well-identified masses (as in the well-known buffalo hump on the back of the neck) only under pathological conditions (lipodystrophies).

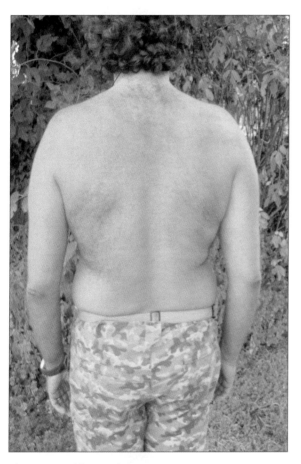

**Fig. 14.** Typical 'kimono' shape in a young man

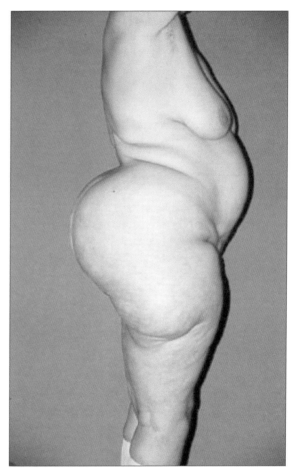

**Fig. 15.** Steatopygia in a middle-aged woman

# References

1. Harris TB, Visser M, Everhart J et al (2000) Waist circumference and sagittal diameter reflect total body fat better than visceral fat in older men and women. The Health, Aging and Body Composition Study. Ann NY Acad Sci 904:462–473
2. Schwartz RS, Shuman WP, Bradbury VL et al (1990) Body fat distribution in healthy young and older men. J Gerontol 45:M181-M185
3. Reidenbach MM, Schmidt HM (1993) Clinical anatomy of the fat body in the forearm and in the palm. Ann Anat 175:11–20
4. Testut L, Jacob O (1921) Traité d'anatomie topographique avec applications médico-chirurgicales. Paris, Doin
5. Illouz YG (1990) Study of subcutaneous fat. Aesth Plast Surg 14:165–177
6. Markman B, Barton FE Jr (1987) Anatomy of the subcutaneous tissue of the trunk and lower extremi-

ty. Plast Reconstr Surg 80:248–254

7. Avelar J (1989) Regional distribution and behaviour of the subcutaneous tissue concerning selection and indication for liposuction. Aesth Plast Surg 13:155–165

8. Murakami M, Arai S, Nagai Y et al (1997) Subcutaneous fat distribution of the abdomen and buttocks in Japanese women aged 20 to 58 years. Appl Human Sci 16:167–177

9. Zhang HM, Yan YP, Qi KM et al (2002) Anatomical structure of the buccal fatpad and its clinical adaptations. Plast Reconstr Surg 109:2509–2518

10. Copcu E, Metin K, Ozsunar Y et al (2004) The interdomal fat pad of the nose: a new anatomical structure. Surg Radiol Anat 26:14–18

11. Vahlensieck M, Wiggert E, Wagner U et al (1996) Subacromial fat pad. Surg Radiol Anat 18:33–36

12. Charpy M (1907) Le coussinet graisseux lombofessier. Bibliogr Anat Berger-levrault, Paris, pp 207–217

13. Giron JP, Sick H, Koritke JG (1981) Topography, structure and vascularization of the fat pad of the lumbar trigone (corpus adiposum trigoni lumbalis). Arch Anat Histol Embryol 64:173–182

14. Kahn JL, Wolfram-Gabel R (2004) The lumbo-gluteal adipose body. Surg Radiol Anat 26:319–324

15. Le Pasteur J (1994) Adipose pad of the external submalleolar fossa. Anatomy and value in liposuction of the lower limbs. Ann Chir Plast Esthet 39:377–383

16. Bremond-Gignac D, Copin H, Kohler C et al (2001) The lateral inframalleolar fat pad: a poorly recognized anatomical structure. Surg Radiol Anat 23:325–329

# Historic Views on Cachexia in Humans with Special Reference to Cardiac Cachexia

Wolfram Doehner

## Introduction

Extreme loss of body tissue in association with severe illness has been observed by physicians since ancient Greek times. The term 'cachexia' was the label for a 'signum mali ominis' in various, mostly fatal, diseases. Observing the chronicity of the course of a disease, cachexia was recognised as a severe complication indicating end-stage disease and poor quality of life. As modern treatment helps to prevent early death for an increasing number of chronic diseases, growing interest is focussed on chronic complications such as cachexia. Nevertheless, observation and clinical documentation of this condition go back as long as medical science itself. Pioneering studies on the reasons and mechanisms of cachexia were performed several decades ago. These studies provide fundamental insights and guidance towards a better understanding of cachexia.

In this review we present an historic overview of cachexia from the first anecdotal documentation to the beginning of its systematic investigation. The material reviewed is taken entirely from Western sources. We have concentrated on material that was published prior to the start of the online library *Medline* and is mainly based on the *Index Medicus*, which dates back as far as the nineteenth century (Fig. 1). Early thoughts and milestone studies on metabolic abnormalities leading to cachexia are presented.

Cardiac cachexia may serve as an example for cachexia secondary to chronic disease and has been focussed on for three reasons. First, especially in the field of cardiology, modern treatment options often prevent early death from acute events without completely erasing the source of the disease, such as surgical treatment in cases of some cancers. Second and following the former, chronic heart failure leading to cachexia may be

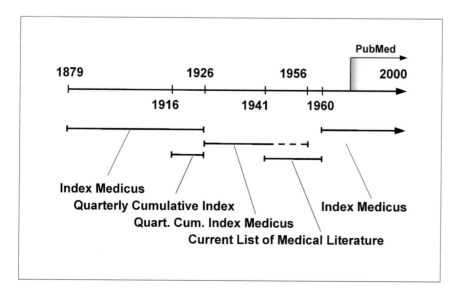

**Fig. 1.** The historic overview of cachexia is mainly based on material published in Index Medicus, which dates back as far as 1879

viewed as a rather isolated solitary origin for generalised deleterious and mal-adapting processes affecting global body functions. And third, the improved treatment of chronic heart failure and the gradual shift in the (patient) population towards elderly patients result in increasing numbers of patients with late-stage complications such as cachexia and hence a growing focus on this syndrome.

## Early Annotations

The earliest report on significant weight loss in relation to what can be diagnosed as chronic disease dates back 2400 years to classical Greece and the school of medicine of Hippocrates (about 460–377 BC) on the island of Cos. Observing an association between dropsy and cachexia, Hippocrates wrote that 'the flesh is consumed and becomes water, … the abdomen fills with water, the feet and legs swell, the shoulders, clavicles, chest and thighs melt away … This illness is fatal' [1]. Hippocrates also recognised the severity of this syndrome. The origin of the term 'cachexia' is also Greek: derived from the words *kakós* (i.e. bad) and *hexis* (i.e. condition or appearance). It was, however, established as a fixed term for a deleterious condition only many centuries later, as knowledge of the physiology of the severe weight loss and the association with underlying diseases did not exist in ancient Greece. Regardless of the lack of understanding of the underlying reasons, these passages in the Corpus Hippocraticum provide almost the only high-quality clinical records on cachexia for the next 1700 years.

It remains uncertain when the term 'cardiac cachexia' was first introduced into medical literature. Knowledge of the physiological function of the heart and the circulatory system was of course a prerequisite. In Greek times, this was completely unknown: in fact, the heart was debated as being the location for the intellect. In 1628 Harvey discovered the circulatory physiology and recognised the heart as the driving pump for the circular movement of the blood [2]. This finding replaced the then prevailing Galenic view of the heart generating and distributing *pneuma* and heat

throughout the body [3]. An anecdotal case of what most likely may have been cardiac cachexia was observed by Withering (1741–1799) in 1785. In his work 'An Account of the Foxglove and some of its Medical Uses with Practical Remarks on Dropsy and other Diseases' (an outstanding scientific contribution, which introduced digitalis into modern medicine), he observed '… his countenance was pale, his pulse quick and feeble, his body greatly emaciated, except his belly, which was very large' [4]. The earliest written documentation of the term 'cardiac cachexia' comes from the French physician Charles Mauriac. In his medical thesis, in 1860, he wrote of a 'commonly observed secondary phenomenon in patients affected with diseases of the heart … a peculiar state of cachexia which is… conventionally designated cardiac cachexia' [5]. Anorexia was known to accompany cardiac decompensation and the grave prognosis in those cases was well recognised. '… But other cases occur which are neither so frequent nor so well known; in these the exertion does not give rise to sudden death, but starts a slowly ingravescent asthenia from which there is no recovery' [6]. Similar observations were reported by others: 'Disease of the heart occasionally results in a certain picture of cachexia "Cachéxie cardiaque"' [7].

## The Missing Continuation

Apart from these few early reports, cachexia as a particular syndrome was not studied in much detail by clinical scientists for many years to come. If recorded, authors mostly did not extend their reports beyond the state of mere observation. However, potential mechanisms for this have not been explored in detail. Weakness and a reduced urge to eat were easily accepted as underlying mechanisms of weight loss. The lack of interest in this syndrome has to be viewed in the context and the background of the clinical setting in the nineteenth and the beginning of the twentieth centuries. Cachexia was of course known to physicians as a severe clinical condition indicating both grossly reduced quality of life and early death. It was, however, seen more in the broader context of diseases as an inevitable but unspecific consequence and serious complication in diseases such as tuberculosis, malignancies or uncontrolled metabolic disorders, for example, diabetes mellitus or thyrotoxicosis.

In comparison to those diseases, cardiac cachexia was a rather rare condition, simply because the vast majority of patients with heart failure would not reach the state of chronicity for cachexia to develop. No sufficient and practicable treatment to control fluid overload was available and heart failure patients – mostly with valve diseases following rheumatic fever or ischaemic heart disease – died early in the course of the disease in a state of acute decompensation. With the introduction of modern therapy it was possible to keep patients in a stable, compensated condition for longer time periods. Thus life with heart failure has been prolonged considerably, and consequently new aspects of the disease emerged with its extended duration, including a growing number of patients with cardiac cachexia. A shift in the perception of the disease occurred, which is also expressed by the gradual change from the term 'congestive heart failure' to the more commonly used term 'chronic heart failure' or 'chronic congestive heart failure' in today's literature.

## Pioneering Studies

The observation of major alterations in body composition that accompany chronic diseases has been attributed commonly to anorexia, i.e. reduced eating. Voluntary reduction of food intake was seen as a compensatory mechanism, to prevent the additional strain that a large meal with the resulting increase in splanchnic blood flow may impose [8]. 'The histories leave no doubt that anorexia is the chief cause of the malnutrition, with nausea and vomiting frequently acting as contributory factors' [9]. Although this view was widely accepted, quantitative data derived from controlled studies are rare. In a small study on decompensated heart failure patients with anorexia, a negative nitrogen and caloric balance was found, which became positive with recompensation and a voluntary increase in food intake [10]. The situation for patients might have been worsened by the fact that often the

caloric intake was further reduced by dietary restrictions imposed on patients with chronic disease by the physicians of that time. A restricted diet was widely accepted as beneficial for the 'senile' heart [11] and a variety of diets existed for that purpose. For example, the Karell diet [12] was very popular for several decades; however, the 800 ml milk and nothing else included in Karell's prescription was less than satisfactory.

Prospective studies on mechanisms of cachexia were very few in the first half of the twentieth century for the reasons given above. There was, however, pioneering work that provided the foundation for today's knowledge of the pathophysiology of the syndrome. Some of the current theories have their roots in the work that was done decades ago, such as, for instance, studies on hypoxia [13], subacute inflammation in heart failure [14] and upregulated sympathetic activation [15].

## Food Intake and Absorption

Several studies have shown a connection between cardiac congestion and impaired intestinal capacity for absorption of nutrients. As early as 1888, impairment of intestinal absorption was recorded in patients with congestive heart failure due to valvular defects. In this study, fat absorption was reduced by 18%, whereas nitrogen and carbohydrate absorption were only marginally impaired [16]. This is very similar to what was described by King et al. in two studies 108 years later [17, 18]. In 1938, an Italian group found increased steatorrhoea in 12 of 20 oedematous patients with heart failure [19].

In the early 1960s, several studies using [131]I-labelled fat administration gave further evidence of reduced fat absorption in congestive heart failure [20, 21]. The authors noted a correlation between severity of the congestion and the degree of steatorrhoea, as well as a reversion to normal fat absorption when compensation could be achieved. Those studies were based on the hypothesis that elevated venous pressure may cause congestive oedema of the intestinal wall, which was reported in 1943 [22]. Also abnormal protein absorption was reported for heart failure patients with the finding of protein-losing gastroenteropathy [23] contributing to reduced oncotic pressure and the production of cardiac oedema and impaired intestinal absorption of amino acids in oedematous patients [24].

## Tissue Metabolism

As early as the beginning of the nineteenth century, physicians noted an important factor in the wasting process that could not be explained by simple reduction of caloric intake. The meticulous observational skills of these physicians, were the basis for many discoveries at a time when today's technologies were not available.

In contrast to uncomplicated starvation, where the energy expenditure is decreased as compensation, an elevated metabolic rate was recognised. Several symptoms such as tachycardia, hyperpnoea, sweating and a rise in body temperature indicated an increase of the metabolic rate that was in sharp contrast to the reduced energy supply in these patients [25]. In 1916, the increase in the basal metabolic rate was directly documented [26, 27]. Increased metabolic demands of several specific tissues were discussed as one underlying reason for this finding. Decreased efficiency of the respiratory system due to reduced compliance [28] and capacity of the lungs, together with hyperventilation, result in higher energy demands of the respiratory muscles [29]. In the case of patients with congestive heart failure it was also suggested that the hypertrophic myocardium may contribute to the hypermetabolism in chronic heart failure [30, 31]. The combination of an increase in total energy consumption of the heart and reduced cardiac output [32] was viewed as diminished myocardial efficiency [33]. Enhanced tissue activities such as erythropoietic activity and hyperplasia of red bone marrow have also been demonstrated repeatedly [34, 35] and were also suggested to contribute to increased caloric turnover.

## Chronic Inflammation

In contrast to the increased metabolic demands of specific tissues, other abnormalities may produce a more generalised caloric effect. In this context, detailed studies revealed that high body tempera-

ture is a common finding in patients with chronic heart failure. In two large studies in the 1930s, most patients with heart failure were found to have at least mildly elevated body temperature.

In 1934, Cohn and Steel studied body temperature in 300 patients with cardiac disease by rectal measurement two or more times [14]: heart failure was diagnosed in 172 of these patients. In this study only 11% of the patients with heart failure had normal temperature, while 89% had some degree of pyrexia. This was often due to pneumonia or other infections. Other pathological situations, such as thrombosis, pulmonary or myocardial infarctions, rheumatic diseases and bacterial endocarditis were also diagnosed. Cohn and Steel also described a number of cases where the origin of the fever could not be established, mainly in those cases where temperature was only slightly elevated. In another study by Kinsey and White, only four out of 200 patients were free of fever [36]. Inflammatory immune activation may have been the cause of the fever.

Today, it may be hypothesised that bowel wall oedema causes bacterial translocation [37], which may explain the increased levels of endotoxin that are found in patients with congestive heart failure [38].

As early as 1934, Cohn and Steel discussed the possibility of a yet-unidentified pyrogen causing the higher temperature [14]. The accuracy and thoughtful interpretation of these old studies is stunning in the light of the more recent finding of mild but measurable immune activation in patients with chronic heart failure characterised by high levels of tumour necrosis factor-alpha and other pro-inflammatory cytokines [39, 40].

## Tissue Hypoxia

The observation of constant 'air hunger' brought attention to the role of reduced oxygen supply to the tissues. Cellular hypoxia became the focus of metabolic research at the beginning of the twentieth century. First blood gas analyses were reported as early as 1919 [13] and in 1923 it was observed that at high altitudes the study subjects involuntarily lost weight [41]. Evidence for reduced tissue oxygen supply came mostly from indirect observations such as increased erythropoietic activity and high lactate production. Increased lactate levels as a measure of an imbalance between aerobic and anaerobic metabolism were reported in the 1930s and repeatedly thereafter [42].

In 1958, Huckabee introduced the concept of 'excess lactate' production as a measure of tissue hypoxia [43]. It was estimated that in a chronic disease such as heart failure, 25–50% of the body's energy needs would be derived from anaerobic glycolysis [44]. In normal subjects, this study found that the anaerobic pathway would account for only 5% of the energy production during exercise. Those observations suggested that lack of oxygen at tissue level reduces energetic efficiency and also negatively affects protein biosynthesis, leading to the down-regulation of anabolic pathways and the increase of catabolic pathways.

Based on early observations of sweating, tachycardia, venoconstriction and systemic increased vascular resistance with reduced cutaneous and renal blood flow, an overactivity of the sympathetic nervous system was recognised. The finding of high norepinephrine levels in chronic heart failure patients by Chidsey, Harrison and Braunwald in 1962 supported this hypothesis [15]. The authors recognised this as a compensatory mechanism to improve cardiac performance.

## A Complex Picture Emerges

Many studies were carried out in the 1950s and 1960s aiming at investigating special aspects of metabolic malfunction and changes in body composition secondary to chronic diseases. The evidence emerging from these studies made it apparent that multiple mechanisms act in combination, forming a complex web of metabolic imbalance with catabolism dominating the anabolic drive, resulting in weight loss. A first attempt at a comprehensive overview of the complex pathophysiology of cachexia with special emphasis on cardiac cachexia was made by Pittman and Cohen in 1965 [45, 46] (Fig. 2). Their review of related studies addressed three main pathophysiological mechanisms of cardiac cachexia:

1. Dietary factors
2. Loss of potential nutrients
3. Abnormal metabolism of ingested food.

The findings of Pittman and Cohen may be summarised as follows: dietary factors, i.e. reduced supply of nutrients to the body, as discussed before, are generally accepted as a factor of primary importance in the genesis of cachexia. Many reasons for a reduced food intake in the setting of chronic disease have been discussed. Patients frequently complain of gastrointestinal problems and many reasons were identified: reduced gastric

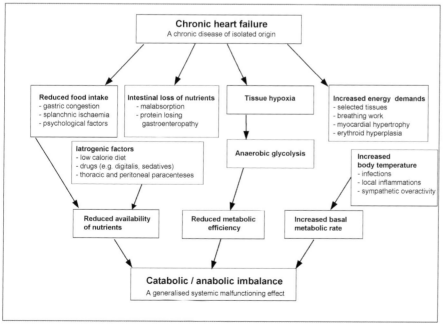

**Fig. 2.** Overview of the complex pathophysiology of cachexia with special emphasis on cardiac cachexia

motility, delayed gastric emptying, a reduced capacity due to hepatomegaly, ascitis, meteorism and pain due to distension or splanchnic angina. Psychological factors may also account for reduced eating, such as depression and fear of increased discomfort after a meal. In this context, a change in the pattern of eating was also shown. Instead of eating a full meal three times per day, patients start to eat small portions of food irregularly throughout the day. This 'nibbling' instead of 'gorging' has been suggested to affect the intermediate metabolism and make the calorie uptake less efficient [47, 48]. An excessive loss of potential nutrients due to impaired absorption or excessive excretion has been shown for fat as well as for protein and vitamins [49].

At the same time, an increased metabolic rate due to increased energetic demands of specific tissues and general calorie-consuming factors such as increased body temperature may further contribute to an unfavourable balance of the body energy metabolism. As a result, the catabolic drive may chronically dominate the anabolic pathways. The constant drain of the body's energy reserves may eventually lead to a pathological tissue degradation.

More than a century of studying the specific phenomenon of cachexia in patients with chronic heart failure has passed. The nineteenth century brought the medical term and the clinical recognition of cardiac cachexia; the twentieth century focussed on more sophisticated pathophysiological studies of this subject. With regard to therapeutic options, however, cachexia in chronic heart failure, as in many other diseases, is still a mostly unknown and unconquered territory. In 1964, Pittman and Cohen concluded: 'Besides the avoidance of … potentially harmful forms of therapy, the only known treatment of cardiac cachexia requires improvement in cardiac function' [45]. This may be extended reespectively to cachexia in general that occurs secondary to chronic diseases. We believe that the twenty-first century will see major improvements towards the development of therapy strategies aiming at reducing or even reversing cachexia in chronic diseases.

### Acknowledgements

I thank the staff of the libraries of the National Heart & Lung Institute, the Hammersmith Hospital, St Marie's Hospital, and the Imperial College South Kensington Campus for their support in the extensive literature search. Klaus Wojciechowski assisted substantially in the research of literature sources.

### Support

W.D. was supported by the 'Verein der Freunde und Förderer der Berliner Charité', Germany and the National Heart & Lung Institute, London, UK.

## References

1.  Katz AM, Katz PB (1962) Diseases of the heart in the works of Hippocrates. Br Heart J 24:257–264
2.  Harvey W (1889) On the movement of the heart and blood in animals. Willis TR, Bowie A (ed) George Bell and Sons, Covent Garden, London
3.  Katz AM (1997) Evolving concepts of heart failure: cooling furnace, malfunctioning pump, enlarging muscle. J Card Fail 3:319–334
4.  Aronson JK (1985) An account of the foxglove and its medical uses. University Press, London, pp 11–100
5.  Mauriac C (1860) Essai sur les maladies de cœur: de la mort subite dans l'insuffisance das valvules sigmoides de l'aorte. Leclerc, Paris
6.  Balfour GW (1888) The senile heart. Edinburgh Med J 33:681–688
7.  Kost P (1919) Kachexie und verwandte Krankheitsbilder. Ärztliche Rundschau 37:273–276
8.  Brandt JL, Castleman L, Ruskin HD et al (1955) The effect of oral protein and glucose feeding on splanchnic blood flow and oxygen utilisation in normal and cirrhotic subjects. J Clin Invest 34:1017–1025
9.  Payne SA, Peters JP (1932) The plasma proteins in relation to blood hydration. VIII. Serum proteins in heart disease. J Clin Invest 11:103–112
10. Jaenike JR, Waterhouse C (1958) The nature and distribution of cardiac disease edema. J Lab Clin Med 52:384–393
11. Schott T (1904) Diet in chronic heart disease. Lancet 2:138–141
12. Karell P (1866) De la cure de lait. Arch Gen de Med 2:513–533
13. Harrop GA (1919) The oxygen and carbon dioxide content of arterial and venous blood in normal individuals and in patients with anaemia and heart disease. J Exp Med 30:241-257
14. Cohn AE, Steel JM (1934) Unexplained fever in heart failure. J Clin Invest 13:853–868
15. Chidsey CA, Harrison DC, Braunwald E (1962) Aug-

mentation of the plasma norepinephrine response to exercise in patients with congestive heart failure. New Engl J Med 267:650–654

16. Grassmann X (1888) On the absorption of nutrients in cardiac patients [German]. Zeitschr F Klin Med 15:183–207

17. King D, Smith ML, Chapman TJ et al (1996) Fat malabsorption in elderly patients with cardiac cachexia. Age Ageing 25:144–149

18. King D, Smith ML, Lye M (1996) Gastro-intestinal protein loss in elderly patients with cardiac cachexia. Age Ageing 25:221–223

19. Bologna A, Castadoni A (1938) Osservazioni sulla funzione gastropancreatica nei cardiopazienti. Arch Ital Mal App Digest 7:215–254

20. Berkowitz D, Sklaroff D, Woldow A et al (1959) Blood absorptive patterns of isotopically labeled fat and fatty acid. Ann Intern Med 50:247–256

21. Hakkila J, Mäkelä TE, Halonen PI (1960) Absorption of I131triolein in congestive heart failure Am J Cardiol 5:295–299

22. Pollack AD, Gerber IE (1943) [No title available]. Arch Pathol 36:608

23. Davidson JD, Waldmann TA, Goodman DS, Gordon RS (1962) Protein losing gastroenteropathy in congestive heart failure. Lancet 1:892–893

24. Hardy JD, Schultz J (1952) Jejunal absorption of an amino acid mixture in normal and in hypoproteinemic subjects. J Appl Physiol 4:789–792

25. Silver S, Proto P, Crohn EB (1950) Hypermetabolic states without hyperthyroidism (non-thyroidism hypermetabolism). Arch Intern Med 85:479–482

26. Peabody FW, Meyer AL, DuBois EF (1916) Clinical calorimetry. VII. The basal metabolism of patients with cardiac and renal disease. Arch Intern Med 17:980–1009

27. Boothby WM, Willus FA (1925) The basal metabolic rate in cases of primary cardiac disease. Med Clin North Am 8:1171–1180

28. Christie RV, Meakins JC (1934) The intra-pleural pressure in congestive heart failure and its clinical significance. J Clin Invest 13:323–345

29. McKerrow CB, Otis AB (1956) Oxygen costs of hyperventilation. J Appl Physiol 9:375–379

30. Smith JA, Levine SA (1947) Aortic stenosis with elevated metabolic rate simulating hyperthyroidism. Arch Intern Med 80:265–270

31. Blain JM, Schafer H, Siegel AL, Bing RJ (1956) Studies on myocardial metabolism. IV Myocardial metabolism in congestive failure. Am J Med 20:820–833

32. Stead EA, Warren JV, Brannon ES (1948) Cardiac output in congestive heart failure. Am Heart J 35:529–541

33. Olson RE (1959) Myocardial metabolism in congestive heart failure. J Chron Dis 9:442–464

34. Shillingford JP (1950) The red bone marrow in heart failure. J Clin Path 3:24–39

35. Hedlund S (1953) Studies on erythropoiesis and total red cell volume in congestive heart failure. Acta Med Scand 146(Suppl 284):1–146

36. Kinsey D, White PD (1940) Fever in congestive heart failure. Arch Intern Med 65:163–170

37. Anker SD, Egerer KR, Volk HD et al (1997) Elevated soluble CD14 receptors and altered cytokines in chronic heart failure. Am J Cardiol 79:1426–1430

38. Niebauer J, Volk H-D, Kemp M et al (1999) Endotoxin and immune activation in chronic heart failure: a prospective cohort study. Lancet 353:1838–1842

39. Levine B, Kalman J, Mayer L et al (1990) Elevated circulating levels of tumour necrosis factor in severe chronic heart failure. N Engl J Med 323:236–241

40. Rauchhaus M, Doehner W, Francis DP et al (2000) Plasma cytokine concentrations and mortality in patients with chronic heart failure. Circulation 102:3060–3067

41. Barcroft J, Binger CA, Bock AV et al (1923) Observation upon the effect of high altitude on physiological processes of the human body carried out in the Peruvian Andes, chiefly at Cerroda Pasca. Philos Trans R Soc Lond B Biol Sci 211:351

42. Weiss S, Ellis LB (1935) Oxygen utilisation and lactic acid production in the extremities during rest and exercise in subjects with normal and in those with diseased cardiovascular systems. Arch Intern Med 55:665–680

43. Huckabee WE (1958) Relationships of pyruvate and lactate during anaerobic metabolism. I. Effects of infusion of pyruvate or glucose and of hyperventilation. J Clin Invest 37:244–254

44. Huckabee WE, Judson WE (1958) The role of anaerobic metabolism in the performance of mild muscular work. I. Relationship to oxygen consumption and cardiac output and the effect of congestive heart failure. J Clin Invest 37:1577–1592

45. Pittman JG, Cohen P (1964) The pathogenesis of cardiac cachexia. New Engl J Med 271:403–409; 453–560

46. Pittman JG, Cohen P (1965) Studies of intestinal absorption in chronic heart failure. Am J Gastroenterol 43:101–120

47. Cohn C, Joseph D (1960) Role of rate of ingestion of diet on regulation of intermediary metabolism ('meal eating' vs 'nibbling'). Metabolism 9:492–500

48. Gwuinup G, Roush W Byron R et al (1963) Effect of nibbling versus gorging on glucose tolerance. Lancet 2:165–167

49. Wenger J, Kirsner JB, Palmer WL (1957) Blood carotene in steatorrhea and in malabsorptive syndromes. Am J Med 22:373–380

# Epidemiology of Cachexia

Giovanni Mantovani, Clelia Madeddu

## Introduction

The interrelationships between clinical diseases and malnutrition have long been recognised. Malnutrition due to starvation, disease or injury is a very common phenomenon, even in current times. Our predecessors in medicine were more familiar with clinical malnutrition than we are, since observation and physical examination played a much greater role in diagnosis in the past. Century-old textbooks provide detailed descriptions of physical changes that occur with malnutrition. Classic studies document the complex adaptations that occur in response to starvation as well as the metabolic alterations associated with stress and trauma.

The rationale that effective treatment of malnutrition may have clinical benefit has led to renewed interest in applying the tools of clinical nutrition. As such, caregivers may need to reacquaint themselves with the topic of clinical nutrition while investigators continue to make advances in those fields that are relevant in the current health care environment [1].

Malnutrition means 'badly nourished' but it is more than a measure of what we eat, or fail to eat. Clinically, malnutrition is characterised by inadequate intake of protein, energy and micronutrients, and by frequent infections or disease. Although often an invisible phenomenon, malnutrition casts long shadows, affecting close to 800 million people – 20% of all people in the developing world (Fig. 1) [2].

Although the greatest number of people worldwide are affected by iron deficiency and anaemia, protein-energy malnutrition (PEM) has by far the most lethal consequences, accounting for almost half of all premature deaths from nutrition-related diseases. Also, although trends differ (for example, iodine-deficiency disorder is rapidly declining

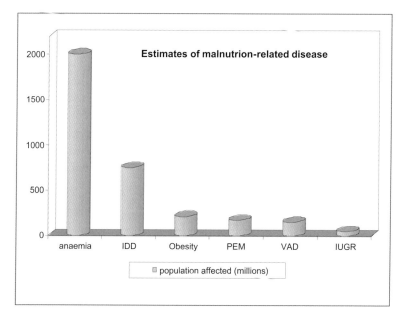

**Fig. 1.** Dimensions of malnutrition: casting long shadows of disability and death (Adapted from [2]). *IDD*, iodine-deficiency disorders; *PEM*, protein-energy manutrition; *VAD*, vitamin A deficiency; *IUGR*, intrauterine growth retardation

while obesity is rapidly increasing), the overall dimension of malnutrition gives serious cause for concern [2].

## The Spectrum of Malnutrition

Hunger and malnutrition remain among the most devastating problems facing the majority of the world's poor and needy, and continue to dominate the health of the world's poorest nations.

Nearly 30% of humanity – infants, children, adolescents, adults and older persons in the developing world – are currently suffering from one or more of the multiple forms of malnutrition. This remains a continuing travesty of the recognised fundamental human right to adequate food and nutrition, and freedom from hunger and malnutrition, particularly in a world that has both the resources and knowledge to end this catastrophe. The tragic consequences of malnutrition include death, disability, stunted mental and physical growth and as a result, retarded national socioeconomic development. Some 49% of the 10.7 million deaths each year among children aged under 5 in the developing world are associated with malnutrition. Iron-deficiency anaemia affects 2 billion people, especially women and children. Iodine deficiency is the greatest single preventable cause of brain damage and mental retardation worldwide: 740 million are affected. PEM affects 150 million children aged under 5. Intrauterine growth retardation affects 30 million per year (23.8% of all births). Vitamin A deficiency remains the single greatest preventable cause of needless childhood blindness, with 2.8 million children aged under 5 affected. At the same time, especially in rapidly industrialising and industrialised countries, a massive global epidemic of obesity is emerging in children, adolescents and adults, so that more than half the adult population is affected in some countries, with consequent increasing death rates from heart disease, hypertension, stroke and diabetes. Diet is also a major causative factor in the problems of post-menopausal women and in many types of cancer [2].

Other important nutrition issues affecting large population groups include:

- Only 35% of infants are exclusively breast-fed between 0 and 4 months of age
- Poor complementary feeding practices are very widespread – a major cause of childhood malnutrition
- Scurvy, beriberi and rickets occur in badly deprived and refugee populations
- Folate deficiency in women of child-bearing age and adolescent girls, causing three quarters of the cases of anaemia and neural tube defects
- Zinc deficiency in deprived populations, contributing to growth retardation, diarrhoea, immune deficiency, skin lesions
- Selenium deficiency, widespread in China and the Russian Federation, causing Keshan disease and Kashin-Beck disease.

## Protein-Energy Malnutrition

Protein-energy malnutrition is by far the most lethal form of malnutrition. Children are its most visible victims. Malnutrition, 'the silent emergency', is an accomplice in at least half of the 10.4 million child deaths each year. These young lives are prematurely, and needlessly, lost.

First recognised in the twentieth century, the full impact of PEM has been revealed only in recent decades. Infants and young children are most susceptible to PEM's characteristic growth impairment because of their high energy and protein needs and their vulnerability to infection. Globally, children who are poorly nourished suffer up to 160 days of illness each year. Malnutrition magnifies the effect of every disease. PEM affects every fourth child worldwide: 150 million (26.7%) are underweight while 182 million (32.5%) are stunted. Geographically, more than 70% of PEM children live in Asia, 26% in Africa and 4% in Latin America and the Caribbean. Their plight may well have begun even before birth with a malnourished mother [2].

## Clinical Relevance of Cachexia

Cachexia is one of the most visible and devastating consequences of human disease, seen in several chronic diseases, including cancer, acquired immunodeficiency syndrome (AIDS), thyrotoxicosis, chronic heart failure and rheumatoid arthritis. In malignant cancer and AIDS, cachexia is known to be a sign of very poor prognosis [3].

## Cancer Cachexia

Owing to the difficulties in clearly defining and diagnosing cancer anorexia, its prevalence is yet to be precisely assessed [4]. Based on different diagnostic tools, anorexia has been detected at the point of cancer diagnosis in 13–55% of patients [5]. Nevertheless, consistent evidence suggests that approximately 50% of cancer patients report abnormalities of eating behaviour at the time of first diagnosis [6] and prevalence in terminally ill cancer patients is even higher, at approximately 65% [7]. The incidence of weight loss upon diagnosis varies greatly according to the tumour site (Table 1) [8]. In less aggressive forms of Hodgkin's lymphoma, acute non-lymphocytic leukaemia, and in breast cancer, the frequency of weight loss is 30–40%. More aggressive forms of non-Hodgkin's lymphoma, colon cancer and other cancers are associated with a frequency of weight loss between 50 and 60% [9–11]. Patients with pancreatic or gastric cancer have the highest frequency of weight loss at over 80%. The onset of anorexia–cachexia significantly influences the clinical course of the disease, and most antitumour

**Table 1.** Incidence of weight loss in cancers of different sites. (Adapted from [8])

| Tumour site | Incidence of weight loss (%) |
| --- | --- |
| Pancreas | 83 |
| Gastric | 83 |
| Oesophagus | 79 |
| Head and neck | 72 |
| Colorectal | 55–60 |
| Lung | 50–66 |
| Prostate | 56 |
| Breast | 10–35 |
| General cancer population | 63 |

therapies actually exacerbate anorexia and worsen body weight loss. As a consequence, the higher prevalence and greater severity of anorexia–cachexia syndrome in advanced cancer patients is mostly due to iatrogenic causes. The presence of early satiety at any stage of the disease can significantly increase the risk of death by 30%. Similarly, the extent of body weight loss negatively influences survival not only per se, but also by delaying initiation and/or completion of aggressive antitumour therapy [12].

## Cachexia in Chronic Heart Failure

There is considerable disagreement as to the percentage of heart failure patients who develop cachexia and how this should be defined and measured. Carr et al. reported that up to 50% of patients with chronic heart failure suffered from some form of malnutrition [13]. Anker and Coats reported that up to 15% of patients attending their chronic heart failure clinic developed cachexia during the clinical course of the disease [14]. Roubenoff et al. observed that loss of more than 40% of lean body tissue would cause death [15]. Cardiac cachexia also occurs in childhood, related to malnutrition and/or malabsorption diseases such as kwashiorkor or marasmus [3].

## Cachexia and Infectious Diseases

Malnutrition, particularly that related to micronutrients (vitamins, trace minerals, essential amino acids, polyunsaturated fatty acids), is certainly one of the most easily preventable causes of death and disability. The 1995 World Health Organization (WHO) bulletin shows population-attributable risk for child deaths in 52 developing countries due to interaction between malnutrition and infectious disorders [16].

Malnutrition is a common complication of HIV infection and plays a significant and independent role in its morbidity and mortality. Malnutrition was one of the earliest complications of AIDS to be recognised and has been one of the most common initial AIDS-defining diagnoses to be reported to public health authorities [1]. The earliest studies of nutritional status in AIDS patients, performed between

1981 and 1983, were determined in hospitalised patients [17]. Weight loss to an average of 80% of ideal weight was found in this population. Evidence of protein deficiency was documented by demonstrating deficiencies in serum proteins (transferrin, albumin), haemoglobin, and by muscle wasting (midarm circumference). Several other studies also reported a high prevalence of severe weight loss in AIDS patients at the time of hospital admission.

The results of formal nutritional assessments in HIV infection, using high-precision techniques, were first reported in 1985 [18]. In a cross-sectional study, body cell mass as total body potassium content, fat content, and body water volumes (total body water, intracellular water and extracellular water), were measured in hospitalised, clinically ill AIDS patients and compared to results in normal controls. The AIDS patients averaged 82% of ideal body weight. However, the body cell mass was depleted disproportionately and was only 68% as compared to control. The magnitude of depletion of body cell mass was striking, since the body fat content was not severely depressed, at least in male subjects. The women studied had equivalent depletion of body cell mass as men, but were much more depleted of fat. This finding was confirmed in later studies performed in the USA and Africa [19, 20]. Other studies have concentrated on the body's protein status and have demonstrated that malnutrition is accompanied by depletion of nitrogen, which is directly related to protein content. Approximately one half of the weight difference between HIV-infected and control men could be ascribed to differences in skeletal muscle mass.

The cross-sectional studies described above have provided the field with a point of reference for over a decade. However, it is important to note that these studies were performed in the pre-zidovudine era, at which time the treatment of many complications of HIV disease was rudimentary. These reports document the natural history of untreated HIV infection and AIDS. While the findings may still reflect the nutritional consequences of HIV infection in much of the world, they may be less accurate in the USA, Europe and Australia. More recent studies have shown a relatively greater loss of fat than early studies, and lesser depletion of body cell mass [1].

Other studies have demonstrated that depletion of body cell mass may precede the progression to AIDS, suggesting that cause of the depletion may be related to the underlying HIV infection, rather than to an opportunistic infection [21]. Clinical stability is associated with nutritional stability [22].

Weight loss can be episodic and related to an acute event, often a specific disease complication [23].

Malnutrition in children is manifested as growth failure; a decrease in the rate of increase in linear height [24].

Most opportunistic infections and many lymphomas in AIDS patients are accompanied by cachexia. In such patients, weight loss is rapid (3–5 pounds per week or 5% per month). While the metabolic rate is extremely elevated, food intake is diminished. There is often extreme weakness and lethargy.

## Cachexia in Chronic Kidney Disease

Many reports indicate that in patients with advanced chronic kidney disease (CKD) and those on dialysis there is a high prevalence of PEM, up to 40% or more, and a strong association between malnutrition and greater morbidity and mortality [25]. CKD patients not only have a high prevalence of malnutrition, but also a higher occurrence rate of inflammatory processes. Many conditions leading to malnutrition and wasting may also cause inflammation. Oxidative stress may be a major underlying cause for both conditions [26]. Since both malnutrition and inflammation are strongly associated with each other and can change many nutritional measures and clinical outcomes in the same direction, and because the relative contributions of measures of these two conditions to each other and to poor outcomes in CKD patients are not yet well defined, the term 'malnutrition–inflammation complex syndrome' (MICS) has been suggested to denote the important contribution of both of these conditions to end-stage renal disease outcome [25]. The MICS may also be defined as the 'malnutrition–inflammation–cachexia syndrome' to indicate better the presence of the wasting syndrome pointed out recently. However, unlike cancer cachexia, the wasting syndrome in CKD usually does not lead to immediate death from the direct consequences of malnutrition, but acts over time to promote atherosclerotic cardiovascular disease [27].

# References

1. Kotler DP (1999) Nutrition and wasting in HIV infection. http://www.medscape.com/viewprogram/667

2. Anonymous (2000) Turning the tide of malnutrition: responding to the challenge of the 21st century. Geneva, World Health Organization, Document WHO/NHD/00.7

3. Anker S, Coats A (1999) Cardiac cachexia: a syndrome with impaired survival and immune and neuroendocrine activation. Chest 115:836–847

4. Laviano A, Meguid MM, Inui A et al (2005) Therapy insight: cancer anorexia-cachexia syndrome – when all you can eat is yourself. Nat Clin Pract Oncol 2:158–165

5. Geels P, Eisenhauer E, Bezjak A et al (2000) Palliative effects of chemotherapy: objective tumor response is associated with symptom improvement in patients with metastatic breast cancer. J Clin Oncol 18:2395–2405

6. Sutton LM, Demark-Wahnefried W, Clipp EC (2003) Management of terminal cancer in elderly patients. Lancet Oncol 4:149–157

7. Walsh D, Donnelly S, Rybicki L (2000) The symptom of advanced cancer: relationship to age, gender, and performance status in 1000 patients. Support Care Cancer 8:175–179

8. Laviano A, Meguid MM (1996) Nutritional issues in cancer management. Nutrition 12:358–371

9. Palesty JA, Dudrick SJ (2003) What we have learned about cachexia in gastrointestinal cancer. Dig Dis 21:198–213

10. Ruiz-Arguelles GJ, Gomez-Rangel JD, Ruiz-Delgado GJ et al (2004) Multiple myeloma in Mexico: a 20 year experience at a single institution. Arch Med Res 35:163–167

11. Thammakumpee K (2004) Clinical manifestation and survival of patients with non-small cell lung cancer. J Med Assoc Thai 87:503–507

12. Dewys WD, Begg C, Lavin PT et al (1980) Prognostic effect of weight loss prior to chemotherapy in cancer patients. Eastern Cooperative Oncology Group. Am J Med 69:491–497

13. Carr JG, Stevenson LW, Walden JA et al (1989) Prevalence and hemodynamic correlates of malnutrition in severe congestive heart failure secondary to ischemic or idiopathic dilated cardiomyopathy. Am J Cardiol 63:709–713

14. Anker SD, Coats AJS (1997) Syndrome of cardiac cachexia. In: Poole-Wilson PA, Colucci WS, Massie BM et al (eds) Heart failure: scientific principles and clinical practice. Churchill Livingstone, Edinburgh, pp 261–277

15. Roubenoff R, Kehayias JJ (1991) The meaning and measurement of lean body mass. Nutr Rev 49:163–175

16. Ambrus JL Sr, Ambrus JL Jr (2004) Nutrition and infectious diseases in developing countries and problems of acquired immunodeficiency syndrome. Exp Biol Med (Maywood) 229:464–472

17. Kotler DP, Gaetz HP, Klein EB et al (1984) Enteropathy associated with the acquired immunodeficiency syndrome. Ann Intern Med 101:421–428

18. Kotler DP, Wang J, Pierson RN (1985) Body composition studies in patients with the acquired immunodeficiency syndrome. Am J Clin Nutr 42:1255–1265

19. Grinspoon S, Corcoran C, Miller K et al (1997) Body composition and endocrine function in women with the acquired immunodeficiency syndrome. J Clin Endocrinol Metab 82:1332–1337

20. Kotler DP, Thea DM, Heo M et al (1999) Relative influences of race, sex, environment, and HIV infection upon body composition in adults. Am J Clin Nutr 69:432–439

21. Ott M, Lambke B, Fischer H et al (1993) Early changes of body composition in human immunodeficiency virus-infected patients: tetrapolar body impedance analysis indicates significant malnutrition. Am J Clin Nutr 57:15–19

22. Kotler DP, Tierney AR, Brenner SK et al (1990) Preservation of short-term energy balance in clinically stable patients with AIDS. Am J Clin Nutr 51:7–15

23. Macallan DC, Noble C, Baldwin C et al (1993) Prospective analysis of patterns of weight change in stage IV human immunodeficiency virus infection. Am J Clin Nutr 58:417–424

24. Arpadi SM, Wang J, Cuff PA et al (1996) Application of bioimpedance analysis for estimating body composition in prepubertal children infected with the human immunodeficiency virus type-1. J Pediatr 129:755–757

25. Kalantar-Zadeh K, Ikizler TA, Block G et al (2003) Malnutrition-inflammation complex syndrome in dialysis patients: causes and consequences. Am J Kidney Dis 42:864–881

26. Himmelfarb J, Stenvinkel P, Ikizler TA, Hakim RM (2002) The elephant in uremia: oxidant stress as a unifying concept of cardiovascular disease in uremia. Kidney Int 62:1524–1530

27. Stenvinkel P, Heimburger O, Lindholm B (2004) Wasting, but not malnutrition, predicts cardiovascular mortality in end-stage renal disease. Nephrol Dial Transplant 19:2181–2183

# Section 2
# Biochemistry, Physiology and 'Clinics' of Adipose Tissue

# Energy Values of Foods

Gianni Tomassi, Nicolò Merendino

## Energy Values of Foods

The human organism, like other higher animal organisms, derives the energy needed for its essential vital functions from the oxidation of organic substrates. In effect, the only form of energy that humans are able to utilise is the chemical energy contained in C-C or C-H bonds, while plants and vegetables can utilise solar energy in order to synthesise the complex molecules needed for their growth and survival [1].

Foods contain various amounts of organic oxidisable substrates that can be utilised to yield energy. The best substrates are the same as those present in the cells of the human organism, i.e. protein, carbohydrates and fats, since the cellular apparatus is equipped with enzymes and other necessary components for the metabolism of these compounds. However, even compounds that are not naturally present in cells, such as alcohol, may be utilised for energy production since they can be metabolised by existing, or inducible enzymes.

The energy value of foods is currently expressed in Kcalories* (Kcal) and in Kjoules** (Kj), the conversion factor being 4.184 to obtain Kjoules from Kcalories. This dual system emerged from a recommendation of the International Union of Nutritional Sciences to express the energy content of foods also in joules, since they represent a more scientifically correct unit to describe biological work, even though the use of calories is still predominant [2].

---

* 1 Kcalorie = amount of heat needed to raise the temperature of 1 l of water from 14.5 to 15.5° C (1 Kcal = 4.184 Kj).
** 1 Kjoule (1000 j), where j is the amount of energy expended when 1 kg is moved 1 m by a force of 1 Newton (1 Kj = 0.239 Kcal; 1 Mj = 1000 Kj)

## Physical Values

The energy values of a single food or nutrient can be directly measured by determining the amount of heat released upon its ignition and total combustion in a bomb calorimeter (Fig. 1). The values obtained with this direct measurement for different foods and nutrients are reported in Table 1 [3].

These values do not correspond to the amount of energy utilisable by the body, since they do not take into consideration the amount lost by digestive and metabolic processes, i.e. excretion in the faeces, sweat, and urine.

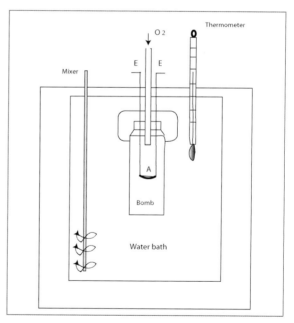

**Fig. 1.** 1 Schematic representation of a bomb calorimeter. A weighted portion of dried food, placed on a platinum plat (*A*), is ignited and burned by electrical wires (*electrodes E*) under oxygen pressure. From the increase of water temperature, it is possible to calculate how much heat has been released

**Table 1.** Physical energy values of common foods and nutrients (Data from [3])

| Food or nutrient | Kcal/g | KJ/g |
|---|---|---|
| Starch | 4.18 | 17.49 |
| Glycogen | 4.19 | 17.53 |
| Dextrins | 4.11 | 17.20 |
| Disaccharides | 3.95 | 16.53 |
| Monosaccharides | 3.74 | 15.65 |
| Glycerol | 4.31 | 18.03 |
| Butyric acid | 5.95 | 24.89 |
| Oleic acid | 9.41 | 39.37 |
| Stearic acid | 9.53 | 39.87 |
| Butter | 9.20 | 38.49 |
| Olive oil | 9.33 | 39.04 |
| Rapeseed oil | 9.49 | 39.71 |
| Peanuts oil | 9.47 | 39.62 |
| Beef tallow | 9.50 | 39.75 |
| Lard | 9.59 | 40.12 |
| Caseine | 5.86 | 24.52 |
| Gelatine | 5.25 | 21.97 |
| Ovoalbumine | 5.69 | 23.81 |
| Wheat Gluten | 5.95 | 24.89 |
| Ethanol | 7.11 | 29.75 |

## Physiological Values

To obtain physiological energy values from physical values, we have to know the digestibility coefficients

$$\frac{\text{energy intake–energy in faeces}}{\text{energy intake}} \times 100$$

for carbohydrates, fats, and proteins and the energy values of the final metabolic products.

For carbohydrates and fats, the final metabolic oxidation products are the same as those found in physical oxidation ($CO_2$ + $H_2O$), while for proteins the metabolic products that are eliminated in the urine (urea, creatinine, uric acid, and other nitrogenous compounds) still contain energy.

The energy content of the urine has been determined to be 1.25 Kcal/g ingested protein, which should to be subtracted from the physical value; the physiological energetic value for proteins is thus 4.40 Kcal/g (5.65 – 1.25 Kcal/g). Furthermore, if we consider the average values of the digestibility coefficients (97, 95, and 91%, respectively, for carbohydrates, fat, and proteins),

we obtain the corrected physiological energy values for the three energetic nutrients:

| | | |
|---|---|---|
| Carbohydrates | 4.1 x 0.97 = 4 | |
| Fats | 9.3 x 0.95 = 9 | |
| Proteins | 4.4 x 0.91 = 4 | |

These values represent the averaged energy values used for calculating the energy value of a food, when its chemical composition is known from food composition tables [4].

## History of the Energy Value of Foods

Most of the fundamental work on the energy value of foods was carried out by the pioneer scientists Rubner (in Germany) and his pupil Atwater (in USA) at the end of the nineteenth century.

Rubner measured the heats of combustion of a number of different proteins, fats, and carbohydrates in a bomb calorimeter and also studied the heat of combustion of urine passed by a dog, a man, a boy, and a baby. He realised that the heat of combustion of protein in a bomb calorimeter was greater than its caloric value in the body because the body oxidises proteins only to urea, creatinine, uric acid, and other nitrogenous end-products, all of which can be further oxidised [5].

Atwater, in a study of 46 persons, analysed urines and measured their heat of combustion. He found that for every gram of nitrogen in the urine there was unoxidised material sufficient to yield an average of 7.9 Kcalories, equivalent to 1.25 Kcalories per gram of protein in food, if the person is in nitrogen equilibrium [6].

Atwater also extensively studied the 'availability' of nutrients and distinguished between 'available' and 'digestible' nutrients. He regarded the faeces as having two parts: undigested and therefore unabsorbed food residues, and metabolic products of digestion, consisting of desquamated cells, bacteria, and substances in the digestive juices [7]. In other experiments, Atwater analysed the foods eaten in mixed diets and the faeces of human subjects. He then compared the data with reports in the literature on the availability of protein, fat, and carbohydrate in separate classes of food. The comparison gave very good agreement between the data and indicated average factors of 4.0, 8.9 (later rounded off to 9.0), and 4.0 for protein, fat, and carbohydrate, respectively. These factors, which Atwater intended only for use in calculating calories deriving from proteins, fats, and carbohydrates in mixed diets, came to be widely used for calculating the available energy value of individual foods. These factors also form the basis for the energy value of foods reported in the Food Composition Tables.

## Energy Values from the Food Composition Tables

These values represent the average calculations derived from the chemical composition of food, which can vary according to the sample and the method used, resulting in possible differences among the various tables applied by different countries. However, the differences are generally small and acceptable for evaluating the actual intake of food energy in a mixed diet.

For carbohydrates, a value of 3.75 Kcal/g, when expressed as monosaccharides (corresponding to the physical value), is used. In the case of disaccharides, because the molecular weight of a monosaccharide is higher than that of a disaccharide molecule, a factor of 1.05 is applied and the energy value is 3.75 x 1.05 = 3.94 Kcal/g. In the case of starch, the factor is 1.10 and the energy value is 4.125 Kcal/g [8].

Together, the monosaccharides + disaccharides + starch represent the available carbohydrates. Cellulose, hemicellulose, pectin, gums, and resistant starch* (collectively referred to as dietary

fibre or unavailable carbohydrates) are not considered to have energetic value. However, unavailable, unaltered carbohydrates reach the colon, where they can be fermented by the local microflora, which consist of several genera of anaerobic microorganisms. These utilise dietary fibre to produce pyruvic acid, an important metabolic intermediate from which short-chain fatty acids (SCFA), i.e. acetic, propionic, and butyric acids, and other gases are produced (Fig. 2) [9].

Since the SCFA, produced at an estimated average amount of 380 mmol/day, can be absorbed in the intestinal mucosa and metabolised to yield energy, an energetic value for dietary fibre of 1.5 Kcal/g can be calculated [10].

In practice, however, since dietary fibre reduces the absorption of other energetic nutrients and increases faecal mass, its contribution to the total energetic value of foods in a mixed diet is not considered. The same is true for organic acids, because of their presence in minimal amounts in foods and their low specific energy value (2 Kcal/g).

On the basis of the values reported in the Food Composition Tables, foods can be grouped into four main classes: (1) energy-dense foods, (2) high-energy foods, (3) moderate-energy foods, (4) low-energy foods. The first category comprises foods with energy values between 900 and 500 Kcal/100 g of edible part; the second category consists of foods with energy values between 500 and 300 Kcal/100 g; in the third category are foods with energy values between 300 and 100 Kcal/100 g; and in the fourth category are foods with energy values from 80 to 10 Kcal/100 g.

The most common foods in the four classes are listed in Table 2 [8].

## Energy Distribution Among Nutrients

The choice of foods according to their energy value represents the basis for building-up the energy-controlled dietary regimens that are required under different conditions, such as reduction of body weight (in overweight or obese patients), increased energy demand during recovery from illness or surgery, or high-level physical activity [11, 12].

---

* Resistant starch is the portion of starch that cannot be digested by human enzymatic activities or absorbed in the digestive tract. Generally it represents a small percentage of total starch (1–3%). The resistance to digestion can be due to physical inaccessibility (as in cereals and grain kernels that are whole or only partially minced) or to the absence of gelatinisation (green bananas, or uncooked potatoes) or to starch 'retrogradation' (as in bread, food cooked at elevated temperatures, corn flakes, or biscuits).

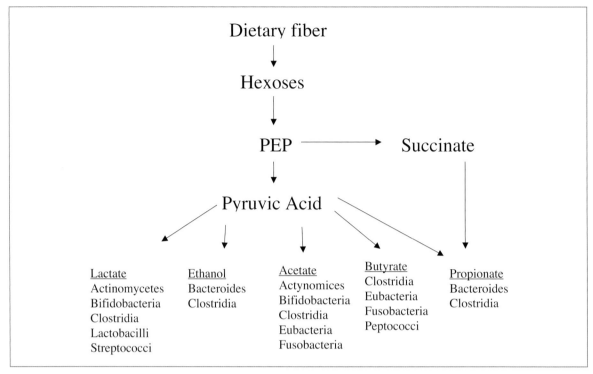

**Fig. 2.** Metabolic products of carbohydrate fermentation by colon microflora

**Table 2.** Distribution of foods according to the four energy categories[a]

| Foods | Kcal/100 g edible part |
|---|---|
| *Energy-dense foods* | |
| Oils and lard | 900 |
| Butter and margarines | 750 |
| Nuts | 650–700 |
| Chocolate | 550 |
| *High-energy foods* | |
| Biscuits, cakes, crackers | 400–450 |
| Salami | 350–450 |
| Cheeses | 300–450 |
| Sucrose | 400 |
| Milk creams | 350 |
| *Moderate-energy foods* | |
| Bread, pizza | 250–300 |
| Pasta, rice | 300–350 |
| Legumes (dried) | 300 |
| Meats | 120–200 |
| Fish | 100–150 |
| *Low-energy foods* | |
| Fresh fruits | 20–60 |
| Vegetables and fresh legumes | 10–40 |

[a]Values are referred to raw, uncooked weights (Data from [8])

However, in addition to the importance of controlling the total amount of dietary energy, food choices should be directed towards a balanced distribution of energy among nutrient sources. Epidemiological and experimental studies have led to the establishment of correct energy distribution among carbohydrates, fats, and protein, in order to prevent the onset of chronic diseases and to assure the maintenance of a good nutritional and health status. In this view, in the USA, more than 20 years ago, a Senate Select Committee stated that the energy distribution compatible with good health and that should be reached by the American population (dietary goals) should consist of 58% of energy from carbohydrates, 30% from fats, and 12% from proteins. Among carbohydrates, 15% of calories should derive from sugars and 40–50% from complex carbohydrates, while, among fats, 10% of calories should come from saturated fats and 20% from unsaturated fats [13].

Since then, many other studies have indicated more detailed distribution among dietary energy sources, with particular regard to the quality of carbohydrates and fats. For carbohydrates, there is now the tendency to ignore the previous distinction between simple and complex compounds (based on molecular weight) because physiological processes in the organism are not strictly dependent on the molecular complexity of the carbohydrate itself. In fact, the glycaemic index of foods (the response of glycaemia after carbohydrate ingestion) is influenced by factors other than the chemical nature of monosaccharides (glucose has a value of 138, while fructose has a value of 32, referred to the white bread = 100) and of starch (amylose, amylopectin, and resistant starch). These include cooking, other types of food processing, and the presence of other food components, such as fats and proteins, antinutrients, organic acids, dietary fibre. For example, among cereal products, cakes have a value of 87, cornflakes 119, spaghetti 59, and linguini 71; among potatoes, baked 121, boiled 80, and French fries 107 [14].

Therefore, the actual recommendation is consuming foods with a low glycaemic index value rather than excluding simple sugars from the diet. Nonetheless, control of the amount of energy from simple sugars is still recommended, with the value not to exceed 10–15% of total dietary energy [15].

For fats, taking into consideration their chemical nature and the relationship between fatty-acid composition and the risk of the onset of chronic diseases, such as cardiovascular diseases, diabetes, and cancer, the most recent scientific reports [16, 17] indicate the following distribution:

- Total fat energy: 25–35% of total calories
- Saturated fatty acids: up to 7% of calories
- Monounsaturated fatty acids: up to 20% of calories
- Polyunsaturated fatty acids: up to 7% of calories, of which not more than 5% from omega-6 fatty acids. For omega-3: up to 1g/day for linolenic acid and up to 1 g/day for eicosapentaenoic acid (EPA) + docosahexaenoic acid (DHA).

These indications refer to the optimal distribution of total diet and cannot be applied to a single food. It is only from a good selection of foods consumed in the total diet that a balanced energy profile can be reached at the end of the daily diet or also after a mixed meal.

# References

1. Passmore R, Eastwood MA (1986) Energy. In: Human nutrition and dietetics, 8th ed. Churchill, Livingston, pp 14–27
2. Anonymous (1972) Metric units, conversion factors and nomenclature. In: Nutritional and food sciences. Royal Society, London
3. Arienti G, Brighenti F, Fidanza F (1998) Ruoli e richieste di energia e nutrienti energetici. Gnocchi, Naples
4. Greenfield H (1992) Southgate DAT. Food composition data, production, management and use. Elsevier Applied Science, Amsterdam
5. Rubner M (1901) Der energiewert der Kost des Menschen. Z Biol 42:261
6. Atwater WO (1910) Principles of nutrition and nutritive value of foods. Fmrs Bull US Dep Agric 142
7. Atwater WO (1902) On the digestibility and availability of food materials. Conn (Storrs) Agric Exp Sta 1414 Ann Rep 1901
8. Carnovale E, Marletta L (2000) Tabelle di composizione degli alimenti. Istituto Nazionale di Ricerca per gli Alimenti e la Nutrizione, EDRA, Milan
9. Gentile MG (1996) Aggiornamenti in nutrizione clinica, 4. Il Pensiero Scientifico Editore, Rome
10. Brighenti F, Mariani-Costantini A, Cannella C, Tomassi G (1999) Carboidrati e fibra. In: Fondamenti di nutrizione umana. Il Pensiero Scientifico Editore, Rome, pp 197–222
11. Astrup A (1999) Dietary approaches to reducing body weight. Baillieres Best Pract Res Clin Endocrinol Metab 13:109–120
12. Drewnowski A (2000) Sensory control of energy density at different life stages. Proc Nutr Soc 59:239–244
13. Anonymous (1977) Senate dietary goals for the United States. Select Committe on Nutrition and Human Needs US, 1st and 2nd ed. US Government Printing office, Washington DC
14. Anonymous (1998) Carbohydrates in human nutrition. In: FAO, Food and nutrition, p 66
15. Anonymous (2002) Diet, nutrition and the prevention of chronic diseases. Report of the joint WHO/FAO expert consultation. Available at http://www.fao.org/documents/show_cdr.asp?url_file=/DOCREP/005/AC911E/AC911E00.HTM
16. Etherton P, Daniels S, Eckel R et al (2001) Summary of the scientific conference on dietary fatty acids and cardiovascular health. Circulation

103:1034–1039

17.  Anonymous (2001) Executive Summary of the Third Report of the National Cholesterol Education Program (NCEP). Expert Panel on Detection, Evaluation and Treatment of High Blood Cholesterol in Adults. JAMA 285:2486–2496

# Diet-Induced Thermogenesis

Gianni Tomassi, Nicolò Merendino

## Origin and Nutrient Determinants

Since the time of Lavoisier, it has been known that the ingestion of foods by animals and humans produces an increase in oxygen consumption. This increase in metabolic rate, originally called 'specific dynamic action' (SDA) is now widely referred to as the 'thermic effect' (TE) of food or 'diet-induced thermogenesis' (DIT) [1]. This effect starts generally 1 h after ingestion, reaches a maximum after 3 h later, and continues at this level for several hours [2]. The DIT is a component of the total energy expenditure, which includes energy expenditure required for performance of cellular and organ functions (basal metabolism [BM]), physical activity, and thermoregulation of body temperature. Supplementary energy is required for metabolic processes taking place during growth, pregnancy, and lactation [3]. In quantitative terms DIT represents about 10% of total energy expenditure (15%

together with cold-induced thermogenesis). BM accounts for about 60–75% of total energy expenditure, with the remaining due to physical activity (10–20% of total energy expenditure) (Fig. 1) [4].

There are two energetic aspects of the food intake effect: the first, and major one, is the obligatory expenditure in order to digest, absorb, distribute, and store the nutrients ingested; the second is the facultative expenditure inducing additional heat production by activation of brown adipose tissue (BAT) [5]. The amount of energy required for handling incoming food is related to the type and the quantity of carbohydrates, fats, and proteins ingested. Fat is the least 'expensive' in terms of DIT, since it requires relatively little hydrolysis and has a fairly direct pathway to storage tissue (3–4% of ingested calories). Protein is the most 'expensive' for DIT, requiring expenditures up to 30% of the inherent energy for processing, which includes removal of nitrogen, synthesis of urea, and gluconeogenesis (on average,

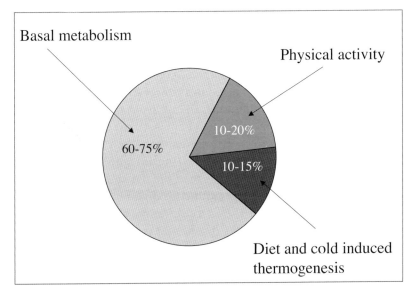

**Fig. 1.** Categories of energy expenditure

15–20% of ingested calories). Carbohydrate is intermediate with respect to DIT; it requires considerable metabolism when converted and stored as triglyceride and less when converted to glycogen (10–15% of ingested calories). Carbohydrate (and also fat) can also elicit increased heat production not related to the use of energy for nutrient digestion, transport, and storage.

## Physiological Regulation

Of the total energy expenditure for DIT, about one-third is ascribable to stimulation of BAT or to futile cycles to produce extra heat. Thus, DIT consists of adaptive thermogenesis together with thermogenesis induced by cold exposure. This adaptive thermogenesis, which responds to temperature and diet, is highly variable and is influenced by genetic makeup. It is regulated by brain activity throughout the sympathetic nervous system (SNS), an important efferent pathway.

β-Adrenergic receptors (βARS) transmit the thermogenetic signal to peripheral target tissue (brown fat, and possibly muscle and other tissues) and play an important role in diet-induced thermogenesis and therefore also in prevention of diet-induced obesity. Various components of the energy balance system in the brain have been identified and include the leptin receptor, melanocyte stimulating hormone (MSH), the melanocortin-4 receptor (MC4 receptor), neuropeptide Y (NPY), and agouti-related protein (AgRP) (Fig. 2) [6]. Alterations in DIT may be of great importance in controlling body weight and in promoting obesity, as indicated by the fact that most animal models of obesity (*ob/ob, db/db* and MC-4 receptor gene knock-out mice) have defects in adaptive thermogenesis.

The amount of DIT depends on the nutrient composition of the foods ingested and on the total amount of energy introduced. Higher energy requirements for subjects with higher physical activity or greater body dimensions correspond to higher energy expenditures in absolute values for digestion, absorption, and storage of ingested nutrients. Measurement of the energetic cost of DIT is not simple, since it is difficult to separate

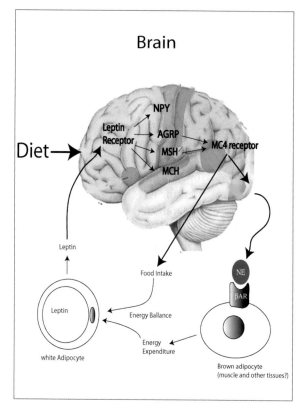

**Fig. 2.** Pathway for diet-induced thermogenesis. The brain receives signals from diet and adipose tissue. Neuronal circuits controlling energy expenditure are activated, which, in turn, increase sympathetic nerve activity. Brown adipose tissue is one effector of sympathetically driven thermogenesis. Other tissues, such as skeletal muscle, are also likely to be important effectors. *AgRP*, agouti-related protein; *MC4 receptor*, melanocortin 4 receptor; *MCH*, melanin-concentrating hormone; *MSH*, a-melanocyte-stimulating hormone; *NPY*, neuropeptide Y

the amount of energy expenditure above BM after a meal from the energetic cost due to physical activity related to sitting, eating, and digesting. In practical terms, DIT is determined by measuring the metabolism of subjects after a meal, without limiting small movements. The value so obtained represents the resting metabolic rate (RMR), which is higher than the BM since it includes the energy expenditure for digestion and metabolism and for the increase in muscle tone and small movements. From measurements made in the morning, afternoon, and evening, it is possible to obtain an average value of the RMR [7].

## Biochemical Mechanisms

Although the causes of DIT are not very clear, the mechanisms perhaps responsible for adaptive thermogenesis may be related to adenosine triphosphate (ATP) production and utilisation. In animal tissues, six different pathways for ATP production have been identified: two through anaerobic glycolysis of carbohydrates, one involving oxidative decarboxylation of carboxylic chetoacids, and three associated with electron transport to molecular oxygen. The energy required for ATP synthesis varies with the substrate considered, according to their different caloric value per 100 g, and to the yield in ATP per 100 g. The energy needed to produce 1 mol of ATP is therefore less for carbohydrates than for fats and proteins (Table 1).

Energy expenditure can be increased by increasing utilisation of ATP or by 'uncoupling' the tight relationship between fuel oxidation and biological work, allowing fuels to be oxidised in the absence of ATP consumption. ATP utilisation can be increased by physical activity and growth, or by processes referred to as 'futile cycles', in which ATP is consumed but net work is not performed. Examples of futile cycles include the synthesis and degradation of proteins, the pumping and leakage of ions across membranes, and esterification and lipolysis of fatty acids/triglycerides. Since the activity of these futile cycles is difficult to assess in intact organisms, it has been difficult to determinate their importance in adaptive thermogenesis. A clear example of uncoupling as a means of increasing energy expenditure is that brought about by uncoupling protein-1 (UCP1), a mitochondrial inner-membrane protein that leaks protons across the mitochondrial inner membrane. The energy that is stored in the mitochondrial proton electrochemical gradient is released [8] in form of heat and is not used to synthesise ATP. UCP-1 is expressed at very high levels in BAT, the primary function of which is to produce heat in response to cold exposure. Other homologues of UCP-1 (UCP-2, UCP-3, UCP-4, and UCP-5) have been found in other tissues, but they do not appear to play an important role in regulating whole-body energy expenditure. The reason for the lack of effect of UCP homologues is presently unclear [9]. UCP-2 is distributed in skeletal muscle, white and brown adipose tissue, the gastrointestinal tract, lung, and the spleen; and UCP-3 in skeletal muscle. Other actions of uncoupling proteins seem to be the regulation of insulin secretion and the protection of free-radical oxygen species [10]. Insulin plays a role in mediating DIT and insulin resistance, and may therefore be implicated in the defective thermogenesis observed in diabetes.

**Table 1.** Factors related to the energy available from ingested fats, carbohydrates and proteins. (Adapted from [4])

|  | Fats | Carbohydrates | Protein | Mixed diet |
|---|---|---|---|---|
| Digestibility (%) | 95 | 97 | 91 | 95 |
| Conversion to mol/100 g nutrient | 50.4 | 21.1 | 22.6 | 34.4 |
| Costs (Kcal/mol ATP) | 18.6 | 17.6 | 22.7 | 19 |
| Maximum percent Kcal converted to ATP | 40 | 40 | 32–34 | 40 |
| Diet-induced thermogenesis (% of ingested Kcal) | 3–4 | 10–15 | 15–30 | 10 |

*ATP,* adenosine triphosphate

## Non-nutrient Dietary Components

Non-nutrient substances, i.e. those other than carbohydrates, fats and proteins, are present as minor components of foods and may have an effect on DIT: examples of non-nutrient substances include caffeine, spices, and nicotine. A thermogenic stimulating effect has been found in green tea, attributed to its caffeine and catechin polyphenols content. Since the latter is capable of inhibiting the enzyme that degrades noradrenaline (catechol-o-methyl transferase) and caffeine inhibits transcellular phosphodiestcrases (enzymes that break down noradrenaline-induced cAMP), it has been proposed that the green-tea-stimulated thermogenesis is due to the relief of inhibition along the noradrenaline-cAMP axis [11]. Furthermore, an increase in energy expenditure has been observed in young and old women after caffeine ingestion, with the effect being greater in the former (15.4% vs 7.8%) [12]. Also, after caffeinated coffee consumption the thermogenic response was higher in lean subjects than in obese ones (7.6% vs 4.9%) [13].

Spices seem to show a stimulating effect on thermogenesis, as has been observed with red pepper and mustard [14]. In experiments in rats, nicotine significantly reduced body weight gain, but not food intake [15].

In general, the DIT produced by a mixed diet is lower than that resulting from consumption of single dietary components. It has been calculated that a mixed diet contributes to 10% of the total energy expenditure. The size of the effect also depends on the nutritional condition of the subject. For example, in malnourished children a test meal had a maximum DIT effect of 6%, while when the children were growing rapidly during nutritional rehabilitation the effect of the same meal was 23%; when recovery was complete, the value returned to 6% [16].

## References

1. Rothwell NJ, Stock MJ (1983) Diet-induced thermogenesis. Adv Nutr Res 5:201–220
2. Lanzola E, Turconi G (2001) Bisogni nutrizionali ed effetti farmacologici dei nutrienti in Farmacologia e Nutrizione. UTET, Torino, pp 1–14
3. Trayhurn P (1989) Thermogenesis and the energetics of pregnancy and lactation. Can J Physiol Pharmacol 67:370–375
4. Linder MC (1991) Energy metabolism, intake and expenditure. In: Nutritional biochemistry and metabolism with Clinical Applications, 2nd Edition. Elsevier, Amsterdam, pp 277–304
5. Rothwell NJ, Stock MJ (1997) A role for brown adipose tissue in diet induced thermogenesis. Obes Res 5:650–656
6. Lowell BB and Bachman ES (2003) b-Adrenergic receptors, diet-induced thermogenesis and obesity. J Biol Chem 278:29385–29388
7. Anonymous (1985) FAO/WHO/UNU Energy and protein requirements. Technical Report series n. 724, WHO, Geneva
8. Del Mar Gonzalez-Barroso M, Ricquier D, Cassard-Doulcier AM (2000) The human uncoupling protein-1 gene (UCP1): present status and perspectives in obesity research. Obes Rev 1:61–72
9. Erlanson-Albertsson C (2003) The role of uncoupling proteins in the regulation of metabolism. Acta Physiol Scand 178:405–412
10. Ferrannini E, Galvan AQ, Gastaldelli A et al (1999) Insulin: new roles for an ancient hormone. Eur J Clin Invest 29:842–852
11. Dulloo AG, Seydoux J, Girardier L et al (2000) Green tea and thermogenesis: interactions between catechin-polyphenols, caffeine and sympathetic activity. Int J Obes Relat Metab Disord 24:252–258
12. Arciero PJ, Bougopoulos CL, Mindi BC, Benowitz NL (2000) Influence of age on thermic response to caffeine in women. Metabolism 49:101–107
13. Bracco D, Ferrara JM, Arnaud MJ et al (1995) Effects of caffeine on energy metabolism heart rate and methylxanthine metabolism in lean and obese women. Am J Phys 269:E671-E678
14. Henry CJ, Emery B (1986) Effect of spiced food on metabolic rate. Hum Nutr Clin Nutr 40:165–168
15. Wellman PJ, Marmon HM, Reich S, Ruddle J (1986) Effects of nicotine on body weight, food intake and brown adipose tissue thermogenesis. Pharmacol Biochim Behav 24:1605–1609
16. Brooke OG, Ashworth A (1972) The influence of malnutrition on the postprandial metabolic rate and respiratory quotient. Br J Nutr 27:407–415

# SECTION 3
# ASSESSMENT OF NUTRITIONAL STATUS

# Biochemical Parameters of Nutrition

Emine M. Inelmen, Giuseppe Sergi

## Introduction

Nutrition is an important factor in the aetiology and management of several major causes of death and disability. The nutritional status of a person is the result of a balance between the intake and the requirement of nutrients. Optimal nutritional status is achieved when sufficient nutrients are consumed to support day-to-day body needs. This status promotes growth and development, maintains general health, support activities of daily living, and assists in protection from diseases. Several variables can influence the intake of food: economical, emotional, developmental and cultural factors, dietary patterns, unbalanced self-imposed diets, anorexia, bulimia, etc. The intake of food also varies in relation to many physiological situations, such as growth, pregnancy, breast-feeding and physical activity. Dysphagia, dyspepsia, malabsorption, loss of nutrients (vomit, diarrhoea, wounds, fistulas, drainage, etc.), alterations in metabolic and nutritional requirements, and drug interactions can be present in different pathological situations.

Malnutrition can be the result of nutrition in excess or in defect. Hyper-nutrition or hypo-nutrition could be more appropriate terms. There are many definitions of the term malnutrition, which vary significantly; this is one of the reasons for the heterogeneity in the epidemiological and clinical data [1]. Hypo-nutrition or under-nutrition occurs when nutritional reserves are depleted and/or when nutrient intake is inadequate to meet day-to-day needs. It has been defined as a nutritional disorder status resulting from reduced nutrient intake or impaired metabolism [2]. It is used to describe a broad spectrum of clinical conditions ranging from mild to very severe. The state of impending under-nutrition, or increased nutritional risk, has also been included under the umbrella of 'under-nutrition' [3, 4]. The vulnerable groups for under-nutrition are infants, children, pregnant women, low-income families, hospitalised patients, cancer patients and ageing adults.

Aetiologically, malnutrition should be regarded as a geriatric syndrome, because of the multiple factors, disease- and age-related risk factors, that disturb the balance between nutritional need and intake [5]. Malnutrition or nutritional deficiency is defined as a continuum starting with inadequate food intake, followed by decreased anthropometrical and biochemical values. The diagnosis of malnutrition is generally based on objective measurements of nutritional status, including assessments of oral energy intake, weight loss, anthropometric data, cell-mediated immunity, biochemical parameters and body composition analysis [6]. Although these indicators are epidemiologically useful, there is no gold standard; thus, nutritional evaluation tends to be overlooked [7–9]. Body weight, for example, can be inaccurate if oedema, ascites or fluid balance derangements are present, resulting in falsely high body mass index [10]. Hence, attention should be turned to combinations of different measurements to increase sensitivity and specificity [11]. Well-known clinical problems such as dehydration and dysphagia are highly prevalent in patients suffering from malnutrition, and initial screening should address these problems as well [12, 13].

## Nutritional Assessment in the Elderly

The percentage of elderly persons is rising in most countries around the world [14]. Ideally, people should survive to an advanced age, keeping their vigour and functional independence, and morbidity and disability should be confined to a relatively short period before death [15, 16]. Hence, a major challenge today is how we can improve overall health and quality of life at older ages; if the average age of onset of ill health remains unchanged, an increased life span would mean for an individual more years of ill health before death [17]. In fact, in an ageing population there are increased chronic disabilities and diseases [18], which are linked with loss of autonomy and health risks [14]. So, it is important to study the factors that modulate ageing; among these factors nutrition seems to have a very important role in health status and quality of life of elderly people [19]. Although the available surveys show that healthy elderly people generally have a good nutritional status, there is no doubt that the older population is at risk of malnutrition [20], and that the nutritional needs and problems of this group differ from those of their younger cohorts.

Physical activity decreases with age and results in an overall lower caloric intake [21]. Furthermore, elderly persons may change their eating habits because of health, social, or financial reasons [22]. Almost half of the elderly population is likely to experience olfactory dysfunction [23]. It is widely assumed that taste and smell dysfunction adversely influence food intake, nutrition status, and the occurrence of certain chronic diseases, confirmed by Schiffman [24]. The loss of sight and hearing, or the presence of osteoarthritis affecting mobility, may decrease the elderly person's ability to purchase and prepare food [25].

Nutritional assessment allows us to specify the nutritional needs and body reserves, as well as the metabolic and immunological functions; it is aimed at defining if the patient is well nourished, slightly or severely malnourished and if the aetiologies of the existing malnutrition will disappear, increase or decrease [26]. It consists of many different tests: clinical, biochemical and anthropometric [9]. However, objective markers of nutritional assessment often do not reflect physiological, physical, cognitive and emotional function [9]. Moreover, nutritional assessment using objective markers is less reliable in the older subject because metabolic changes, among others, affect some of the routine biochemical tests results, and the refer-

ence values of the anthropometric measures are not always age-adjusted [9]. Anyway, when malnutrition has been estimated using a combination of at least one anthropometrical and one biochemical variable, the sensitivity increases [27, 28].

The essential part of nutritional assessment in the elderly is an accurate medical history and a clinical evaluation. The medical history has to evaluate particularly the dietary intake (the techniques are given below). It is important to look for the presence of acute or chronic diseases, infections, trauma or stress in order to evaluate an increase of dietary requirements of the patient. Obtaining an accurate medical history from an older person can be challenging. Memory loss, cognitive decline and their consequences can limit its accuracy. Obtaining pertinent data from the caregiver and from medical records is often necessary. The aim of the clinical evaluation is also to identify the signs of malnutrition, which are given in Table 1.

Another essential part of the nutritional assessment is the measurement of anthropometrical parameters. These parameters are simple and not invasive: a meter and a plicometer allow the necessary information to be obtained for an adequate nutritional evaluation.

The biochemical parameters available for the nutritional situation have increased recently. Unfortunately, most of these indexes are expensive and not available in all laboratories. Besides, the results can often be influenced by factors that are independent from the nutritional condition of the patient. Hence, the basal parameters are still now essential for the nutritional status of a person.

Therefore, nutritional assessment becomes crucial in the elderly population as progressive undernutrition occurs, often without being diagnosed.

## Dietary Intake

There are several difficulties in selecting a sample of elderly people for a nutritional study. Some authors [29] suggest the selection of 'healthy' elderly. Even if it is possible to obtain an almost homogeneous group, this is not a 'real' sample of an elderly population, which is, on the contrary, characterised by a high heterogeneity of subjects:

**Table 1.** Clinical signs in malnutrition

| | |
|---|---|
| Hair | Thinness, sparseness, easy pluckability |
| Face | Diffuse depigmentation, nasolabial seborrhea |
| Eyes | Conjunctival xerosis, corneal xerosis, keratomalacia, blepharitis |
| Lips | Angular stomatitis, angular, scars, cheilosis |
| Tongue | Magenta tongue, glossitis |
| Gums | Spongy, bleeding |
| Glands | Thyroid enlarged, parotid enlarged |
| Skin | Xerosis, follicular hyperkeratosis, petechiae, ecchymoses, dermatosis |
| Nails | Koilonychia |
| Subcutaneous tissue | Oedema |
| Muscular and skeletral systems | Muscle wasting, osteomalacia |
| Internal systems | Hepatomegaly, listless, apathetic, mental confusion, irritability, sensory loss, motor weakness, loss of balance |
| Cardiovascular | Cardiac enlargement, tachicardia |

self-sufficient, not self-sufficient and institutionalised [30]. Besides, nutritional examination in a selected healthy elderly population would not show variations in dietary patterns; in fact, they try to maintain the food habits because of a reduction of the adaptation capacity with age [31]. Elderly people's associations with food are more emotional than those of younger adults; for some, food intake is the main event in the course of the day, often providing the only possibility of social contact [31]. The elderly have repeatedly been told that good food means good health [31]. So, the elderly may eat simply because they know they have to, even if they do not feel like eating, or they may eat because the food is delivered and throwing it away would be wasteful [32].

Another question is the continuing debate about the use of reference parameters in nutritional studies in the elderly. In fact, the value of dietary intake data as an indicator of health status in an elderly population is debatable [32]. In a population with an increased number of physical and mental disabilities like the elderly, dietary assessment methods might be adapted or different methodologies might be developed [19]. An independent measure of the reliability of reported energy can be obtained by calculating the ratio of energy intake to the resting metabolic rate (RMR) [33].

In spite of their limitations, dietary surveys are the main tool for assessing nutritional habits, establishing food policies, and creating awareness of nutritional needs [31]. Although biochemical tests have been widely accepted as an objective assessment of nutritional status, especially of marginal states, malnutrition and suboptimal nutrition can be adequately understood only in the light of dietary data on food consumption, meal patterns and methods of preparation [31]. Any method used for dietary surveys in the adult population can, theoretically, be used for surveys in the elderly [31].

## Survey Techniques for Assessment of Food Intake

### Dietary Records and Diaries

The most widely used technique for the assessment of food intake is keeping a record of food consumption [31]. Ideally, food should be weighed before and after preparation, records kept during the meal, and leftovers weighed again [31]. This technique produces data that can be expressed in quantitative terms, be converted into nutrients, and serve as the basis of clinical and biochemical research [31]. Investigators working with the elderly prefer the record system even if the food intake can be influenced by this process to such a degree that the subject's original food pattern can be changed. It is better to record dietary intake over a period of three non-consecutive days with a ratio of 5/2 between working days and holidays [34].

## Diet Histories

Several models of diet histories have been developed, but the most common are the 24-h diet recall and the modified dietary history.

The 24-h diet recall is characterised by the evaluation of the quantity and quality of the food consumed in 24 hours before the interview. It is a simple method and is particularly indicated for wide samples [34] but requires a highly skilled interviewer.

The modified dietary history is a classic method for evaluating the 'usual diet', that is the diet for at least 6–12 months before the interview. This method was validated in the elderly with the record for 3 days, in which the participant is asked to note all the foods and beverages consumed daily; illiterate or handicapped subjects are helped by a relative or a friend [35]. A sufficient concordance between the two methods emerged from the studies in the Italian population, even if the modified dietary history overestimated the intakes [36].

## Food-Frequency Lists

As in the diet history, the food-frequency method uses an interview, but the questions refer only to items previously listed and do not require active recall. The food-frequency checklists are simple to administer; they identify usual food intake rather than food consumption for specific periods, eliminating the variance associated with an individual's day-to-day changes in eating [37]. Food-frequency lists indicate only food patterns and can distinguish adequate from inadequate diets.

## Mini Nutritional Assessment (MNA)

The Mini Nutritional Assessment (MNA) is a rapidly administered, simple tool for evaluating the nutritional status of older persons. It consists of 18 items [38] and can be administered by a healthcare professional in less than 15 minutes. It involves a general assessment of health, a dietary assessment, anthropometric measurements, and a subjective self-assessment by the patient (Table 2). The results of the MNA test classify the patient as well nourished, at risk for malnutrition, or malnourished. The MNA test was shown to be 92–98% accurate. It is a simple, non-invasive, well-validated screening tool for malnutrition in elderly persons.

## Dietary Requirements for the Elderly

Nutrition may act in different ways: first, lifestyle and nutritional habits of adulthood may contribute to the age-related loss of tissue function; second, chronic degenerative diseases, such as atherosclerosis and cancer, appear to be influenced by nutrition; finally, since elderly people eat less, the intake of some nutrients may fall below the recommended dietary allowances (RDA) [39]. But, until now, most of the nutritional recommendations for the elderly have been derived by extrapolation from data of younger adults [32, 39]. The controversial point is the choice of two-thirds of the RDA as a cut-off value for determining insufficient intake [32]. This could be incorrect because the chronic disease widespread in geriatrics might interfere with the dietary intake for groups of elderly subjects [40].

The US RDA for the elderly are set for people aged over 51 years (with a reference body weight of 65 and 77 kg and a reference height of 160 and 173 cm for women and men, respectively) [39]. Other countries have established their RDA for subjects over 60 years of age: the French RDA are set for people aged over 65 years (with a reference body weight of 60 and 70 kg for women and men, respectively) [39]. In Bulgaria, the RDA are set for subjects over 90 years of age [41].

In Italy, the recommended nutrient levels (LARN) [42] are valid for a population up to 60 years old, while all the elderly are placed in a unique 'geriatric' group of age over 60. In a recent study of the Italian population aged 70–75 years, the authors [35] showed that in both genders energy and macro-nutrient mean values were similar to LARN

**Table 2.** The Mini Nutritional Assessment (MNA) questionnaire. (Modified from [38])

*Anthropometric assessment*

1. BMI (weight/height2)
   0 = BMI > 10
   1 = 21 ≤ BMI ≤ 23
   2 = BMI > 23

2. Mid Arm Circumference (MAC, cm)
   0.0 = MAC < 21
   0.5 = 21 ≤ MAC ≤ 22
   1.0 = MAC > 22

3. Calf Circumference (CC, cm)
   0 = CC < 31
   1 = CC ≥ 31

4. Weight loss during last 3 months
   0 = weight loss > 3 kg
   1 = does not know
   2 = weight loss between 1 and 3 kg
   3 = no weight loss

*Global evaluation*

5. Does the patient live independently
   in contrast to a nursing home?
   0 = no
   1 = yes

6. Does the patient take more than
   3 prescription drugs per day?
   0 = yes
   1 = no

7. In the past 3 months, has the patient suffered
   from psychological stress or acute disease?
   0 = yes
   1 = no

8. Mobility
   0 = bed or chair bound
   1 = able to get out of bed/chair but does not go out
   2 = goes out

9. Neuropsychological problems
   0 = severe dementia or depression
   1 = mild dementia
   2 = no psychological problems

10. Pressure sores or skin ulcers
    0 = yes
    1 = no

*Dietetic assessment*

11. How many full meals does the patient eat daily?
    0 = 1 meal
    1 = 2 meals
    2 = 3 meals

12. Does he consume
    At least one serving of dairy products per day
    (yes/no)
    Two or more servings of beans or eggs per week
    (yes/no)
    Meat, fish or poultry every day (yes/no)
    0 = if 0 or 1 yes
    1 = if 2 yes
    2 = if 3 yes

13. Does he consume two or more servings
    of fruits or vegetables per day?
    0 = no
    1 = yes

14. Has the patient food intake declined over the past
    3 months due to a loss of appetite, digestive
    problems, chewing or swallowing difficulties?
    0 = severe loss of appetite
    1 = moderate loss of appetite
    2 = severe loss of appetite

15. How many cups/glasses of beverages does
    the patient consume per day?
    0.0 = less than 3 glasses
    0.5 = 3 to 5 glasses
    1.0 = more than 5 glasses

16. Mode of feeding
    0 = fed requires assistance
    1 = self-fed with some difficulties
    2 = self-fed without any problem

*Subjective assessment*

17. Does the patient consider to have any
    nutritional problems?
    0 = major malnutrition
    1 = does not know or moderata malnutrition
    2 = no nutritional problem

18. In comparison with other people of the same age, how
    would the patient consider his/her health status?
    0.0 = not as good
    0.5 = does not know
    1.0 = as good
    2.0 = better

Score: well-nourished, ≥ 24 points; at risk of malnutrition,
17 to 23.5 points; undernutrition, < 17 points

[42]; these authors [35] suggested that LARN [42] could be used for people up to 75 years of age. According to LARN [42], 40% of men and 54% of women had an insufficient caloric intake. According to the authors [35], however, this fact did not indicate that they presented intakes below the recommended values; in fact, the recommended values of LARN [42] are reported to the average behaviour of the whole elderly population. So, it is necessary to know exactly the nutritional levels recommended for the elderly, in each decade of advanced age [43] and for different elderly populations [35].

## Energy

Energy requirements are defined by energy expenditure composed of RMR, physical activity and diet-induced thermogenesis [39]. With ageing there is a reduction in energy requirements related to a reduction in metabolic rate (due to the loss of lean body mass and the reduction of protein turnover) and to a diminution of physical activity [44]. However, some authors have stressed that the energy requirements to remain active are the same for the elderly as for younger adults; walking, however, seems to require more energy in the elderly due to the loss of balance (diminution of neuromuscular coordination) [45, 46].

The RDA for energy for the elderly (2300 kcal [9600 MJ] per day in males and 1900 kcal [8000 MJ] in females or 30 kcal/kg [125 MJ] for both males and females) are lower than those for younger adults [39]. These RDA assume light-to-moderate activity (1.5 times the RMR) in the elderly [39]. According to the updated LARN [47] for energy for the elderly, the requirements are defined taking into account the energy expenditure and not the dietary energetic intake, as in 1987 [42]. Physical activity, however, in healthy elderly people is very variable [48] and energy intakes are under-reported [48, 49]. When energy intake is below 1500 kcal/day, it becomes difficult to cover the micronutrient requirements [39]. As the age-related reduction of energy has to be re-examined, it is, therefore, difficult to make general recommendations for energy requirements for the elderly [39]. In Italy, it has been suggested that, without physical activity, the recommended

caloric intake is about 1900–2250 for males and 1600–1900 for females in the age group between 60 and 74 years; 1700–1950 for males and 1500–1750 for females in the age group over 75 years [20].

## Recommended Dietary Intake for Proteins

The current RDA for proteins for adults of all ages is 0.8 g/kg body weight [50]. Because older adults are likely to have less lean body tissue per kilogram of body weight than younger people, this protein allowance actually is higher per unit of lean body mass and should allow for any age changes in protein utilisation or metabolism [51]. It is recommended that proteins provide 12–14% of the total energy intake [50].

## Recommended Dietary Intake for Carbohydrates

The current guidelines of the Food and Nutrition Board (1989) [50] suggest that at least half of all kilocalories be supplied by carbohydrates. Normal metabolic function is maintained on a daily intake of 50–100 g of carbohydrate.

## Recommended Dietary Intake for Lipids

A diet that conforms to the recommendations of the Food and Nutrition Board's Committee on Diet and Health (1989) [52] (fat 30% or less of total kilocalories) is appropriate for people of all ages.

## Dietary Fibre Intake

The Food and Nutrition Board's Committee on Diet and Health (1989) [52] suggests that people of all ages eat five or more servings of fruit and vegetables and six or more servings of a combination of legumes, breads and cereals.

## Biochemical Parameters of Nutrition in the Elderly

The epidemiological findings suggest that intakes of particular vitamins are related to the incidence of chronic diseases [53]; so vitamin requirements and metabolism should be studied more closely. Vitamins that act as antioxidants appear to have a role in preventing coronary artery disease and cancer [53]. Current work is focusing on the actions of vitamins as related to immune function, the formation of cataracts, and the development of osteoporosis, all associated with ageing [53]. The Food and Nutrition Board, the Institute of Medicine, and the National Academy of Science and Health of Canada have recently developed a standard set of nutrient recommendations, known as dietary reference intakes (DRIs), which has added, with regard to vitamin intakes, the groups for ages 51–70 years and for 70 years and older [54]. These recommendations are listed in Table 3 [54].

Fat-soluble vitamins are D, E, A and K. Fat-soluble vitamins are harder to deplete than water-soluble vitamins, because humans can store variable amounts in the body. Water-soluble vitamins include vitamin C, the B-complex vitamins and folate.

## Vitamin D

Vitamin D (calciferol) is essential for mineral homeostasis and for normal mineralisation of the skeleton. Vitamin D is a generic name for all steroids that show the biological activity of vitamin D3 (cholecalciferol). It increases the absorption of calcium and phosphates, and influences kidney re-absorption of amino acids [55, 56].

Vitamin D deficiency is particularly important in the elderly population because it is common and has a direct relationship with increased morbidity [54]. The deficiency of vitamin D is linked to osteomalacia, osteoporosis, and increased vertebral and non-vertebral fractures [57].

Vitamin D is obtained from two sources, diet and skin formation: the elderly receive less exposure to sunlight and synthesis in the skin is reduced by about 50% [58]. In fact, an inverse relation exists between the concentrations of provitamin D3 in the epidermis with age [59]. The RDA of vitamin D for older persons is 10 µg (400 IU) per day in males and females (Table 3) [54]. Over two thirds of the elderly have vitamin D intakes that are below two thirds of the RDA [60]. Supplementation has been shown to increase bone mineral density and decrease fracture risk [61]. Excessive intakes cause increased calcium absorption and increased calcium mobilisation from bone, resulting in hypercalcaemia and soft tissue calcification [56].

**Table 3.** Dietary reference intakes

| RDA or AI | A µg | D µg | E mg | K µg | Niacin mg | Thiamin mg | Riboflavin mg | B6 mg | B12 µg | C mg | Folate µg |
|---|---|---|---|---|---|---|---|---|---|---|---|
| Women | | | | | | | | | | | |
| 51-70 years | 700 | 10 | 15 | 90 | 14 | 1.1 | 1.1 | 1.5 | 2.4 | 75 | 400 |
| 70 + years | 700 | 15 | 15 | 90 | 14 | 1.1 | 1.1 | 1.5 | 2.4 | 75 | 400 |
| Men | | | | | | | | | | | |
| 51-70 years | 900 | 10 | 15 | 120 | 16 | 1.2 | 1.3 | 1.7 | 2.4 | 90 | 400 |
| 70 + years | 900 | 15 | 15 | 120 | 16 | 1.2 | 1.3 | 1.7 | 2.4 | 90 | 400 |
| UL | | | | | | | | | | | |
| Men/Women | | | | | | | | | | | |
| 51-70 + years | 3000 | 50 | 1000 | ND* | 35 | ND | ND | 100 | ND | 2000 | 1000 |

Source: National Academy of Science at www.nap.edu
Please note: Vitamin D conversion factor 5 µg = 200 IU Vitamin E conversion factor 15 mg = 22IU of Natural vitamin E 15 mg = 33 IU of synthetic (supplemental) vitamin E
* Not determinable because of lack of data of adverse effects in the age group and concern about inability to handle excess amounts. Source of intake should be food only to prevent high levels of intake
RDA, recommended dietary allowance; AI, adequate intake; UL, tolerable upper intake level; ND, not determinable

## Vitamin E

Alpha-tocopherol is the biologically active form of vitamin E and is probably the major lipid-soluble antioxidant. Vitamin E absorption is not altered with ageing; deficiency of vitamin E has not been reported for healthy elderly people [39]. The RDA of vitamin E is 15 mg (22 IU) (Table 3) [54] and is the same for the elderly and for adults. Low levels of alpha-tocopherol may be associated with an increased risk of cancer mortality [62]. Because of these effects of vitamin E deficiency, the use of supplemental vitamin E has been investigated to prevent cancer. Clear benefit has only been associated with reducing the risk of prostate cancer [63].

## Vitamin A

Vitamin A is the generic name for compounds with the qualitative biological activity of retinol, i.e. retinoids, beta-carotene and provitamin A carotenoids. The RDA of vitamin A is 700 μg for women over age 50 and 900 μg for men over 50 (Table 3) [54]. Low serum retinol levels indicate vitamin A deficiency. The effects of vitamin A deficiency are night blindness (hemeralopy), dry-eye syndrome, keratomalacia, Bitot's spots on the conjunctiva, dry skin and follicular hyperkeratosis. Toxicity has been associated with abuse of vitamin A supplements and with diets extremely high in vitamin A content [39].

## Vitamin K

The forms of vitamin K include phylloquinone, which is found in plants, and the menaquinones, which are synthesised by gut bacteria. Vitamin K is necessary for the synthesis of clotting factors 2, 7, 9 and 10 and for the synthesis of protein C and protein S [64]. Causes of vitamin K deficiency include any source of fat malabsorption and drugs that interfere with vitamin K metabolism, such as anticonvulsants, warfarin and certain antibiotics [64]. The major clinical feature of vitamin K deficiency is bleeding. The RDA of vitamin K is 90 μg per day for women over 50 years and 120 μg per day for men over 50 years (Table 3) [54].

## Vitamin C

Also known as ascorbic acid, vitamin C is obtainable only through dietary sources. It is claimed that five servings of fruit and vegetables per day can supply the RDA [54]. Like vitamin A and E, vitamin C is an antioxidant and reduces harmful free radicals [54]. The conversion of iron from ferric to ferrous form requires vitamin C; without this conversion, methaemoglobin could not be converted to haemoglobin, and iron could not be absorbed in the duodenum [54]. Scurvy is the clinical syndrome of vitamin C deficiency. The RDA of vitamin C is 75 mg per day for women over 50 years and 90 mg per day for men over 50 years (Table 3) [54].

## Vitamin B1 (or Thiamine)

The active form of thiamine, thiamine pyrophosphate, is a coenzyme involved in energy metabolism reactions; the requirement for thiamine is therefore related to energy expenditure [56]. Patients at risk for vitamin B1 deficiency include alcoholics, those on chronic peritoneal dialysis, those re-fed after starvation, and thiamine-depleted persons who are given glucose [64]. The RDA of vitamin B1 is 1.1 mg per day for women over 50 years and 1.2 mg per day for men over 50 years (Table 3) [54]. Patients at high risk, such as alcoholics, may benefit from supplementation [54]. Excessive amounts of ingested thiamine are rapidly cleared by the kidneys. No evidence exists of thiamine toxicity by oral administration [50].

## Vitamin B2

Vitamin B2 is also known as riboflavin. It is an essential component of flavin mononucleotide and flavin adenine dinucleotide, both of which are involved in ATP synthesis [54]. Deficiency may result from insufficient dietary intake or from medical conditions such as chronic diarrhoea, alcoholism, or liver disease [54]. The RDA of vitamin B2 is 1.1 mg per day for women older than 50 years and 1.3 mg per day for men over 50 years (Table 3) [54].

## Vitamin B3

Vitamin B3 is niacin, also known as nicotinic acid. The metabolically active forms of niacin are the pyridine nucleotides, nicotinamide adenine dinucleotide (NAD) and nicotinamide adenine dinucleotide phosphate (NADP) [65]. Free forms of the vitamin are white stable crystalline solids [65]. Only small amounts of the free forms of niacin occur in nature [65]. Most of the niacin in food is present as a component of NAD or NADP [65]. Pellagra is the clinical manifestation of niacin deficiency.

## Vitamin B6

Vitamin B6 occurs in three forms, pyridoxine, pyridoxal and pyridoxamine; all of them are phosphorylated and pyroxal-5'-phospate is the active coenzyme form of many enzymes involved in protein and amino acid metabolism [56]. Deficiency is associated with seborrhoeic dermatitis, epileptiform convulsions and anaemia [56]. The elderly tend to be at greater risk of vitamin B6 deficiency [39], even if it is widely available in most foods. The RDA of vitamin B6 is 1.5 mg per day for women older than 50 years and 1.7 mg per day for men older than 50 years (Table 3) [54].

## Vitamin B12

Vitamin B12 includes the cobalamins, which can be converted to methyl- or 5'-deoxyadenosyl cobalamin, which qualitatively exhibit the biological activity of cyanocobalamin [39]. Deficiencies due to inadequate intake are rare. However, negative vitamin B12 balance is often found in the elderly [66], especially in those with atrophic gastritis, *Helicobacter pylori* infection [67] and use of proton pump inhibitors or other agents that interfere with gastric acidity [54]. A significant increase in malabsorption of vitamin B12 seems to occur with age [54]. The main symptoms of deficiency are anaemia and/or neuropsychological disorders. The RDA of vitamin B12 for the elderly is the same as for adults: 2.0 µg per day in males and females [50].

## Folate

Folate is the generic name for folic acid-related compounds. They are mainly involved in thymidine synthesis. There seem to be no age-related changes in folate metabolism. Folate is ubiquitous in nature and is present in nearly all natural foods. Deficiencies are characterised by anaemia (megaloblastic), depression and dermatological lesions [56]. Alcohol and drug intake increase the risk of deficiency.

Folate deficiency can occur within a few days of insufficient intake [54]. This deficiency is a particular risk in the elderly who have recently been institutionalised [54]. Deficiency in these persons is presumably caused by decreased food choices and possibly by depression [68]. The RDA of folate for adults is 400 µg daily [54].

In conclusion, vitamin supply is essential for all people but especially for the elderly, because they are at higher risk for deficiency than younger adults. Vitamin deficiency is difficult to detect in older people because it can be easily obscured by other morbidities, such as skin, neurological and gait abnormalities.

## Micro(oligo)elements

Micro(oligo)elements play an important role in the maintenance of multiple enzyme reactions and are essential for the maintenance of tissue structure [69]. Table 4 summarises the major functions of some trace elements and the effects of ageing on them.

### Zinc

Zinc is required by enzymes involved in DNA and protein synthesis and is essential for cell growth and repair. Zinc may also have antioxidant and antiatherogenic properties [70, 71]. Zinc plays a key role in several important functions of particular concern in ageing.

The following functional consequences of zinc deficiency are relevant to the elderly: skin lesions, diarrhoea, impaired wound healing and impaired protein metabolism, altered visual function,

**Table 4.** The dietary reference intakes of the four trace mineral discussal

| | |
|---|---|
| *Zinc* | |
| Males | 51-70 years and > 70 years: RDA is 11 mg/day |
| Females | 51-70 years and > 70 years: RDA is 8 mg/day |
| Adults >19 years of age | Tolerable intake level (UL) is 40 mg/day |
| | |
| *Copper* | |
| Males | 51-70 years and > 70 years: RDA is 900 µg/day |
| Females | 51-70 years and > 70 years: RDA is 900 µg/day |
| Adults > 19 years of age | |
| | |
| *Selenium* | |
| Males | 51-70 years and > 70 years: RDA is 55 µg/day |
| Females | 51-70 years and > 70 years: RDA is 55 µg/day |
| Adults > 19 years of age UL is 400 µg/day | |
| | |
| *Chromium* | |
| Males | 51-70 years and > 70 years: adequate intake (AI) Is 30 µg/day |
| Females | 51-70 years and > 70 years: adequate intake (AI) Is 20 µg/day |

A tolerable upper intake level was not determinated for Cr. *AI*, adequate intake; *RDA*, Reccommended dietary allowance; *UL*, upper intake level

anorexia, impaired taste, altered mental function, altered immune function with increased susceptibility to infections, hypogonadism [72]. The mechanisms by which zinc deficiency produces anorexia are currently unclear [73]. The RDA is 11 mg/day for elderly males and 6 mg/day for elderly females (Table 4) [72]. Excess zinc intake (exceeding 10 times the RDA) decreases immunological functions and can induce copper deficiency [39]. However, the elderly per se might still be considered at risk for inadequate zinc intake, due to the decreased food intake and the increased susceptibility to infections related to ageing [39].

## Copper

Copper is a component of several important proteins and enzymes and is essential for erythropoiesis. Most of the copper in blood plasma is bound to ceruloplasmin.

Elevated serum copper levels have been observed in patients with cardiovascular disease and are inversely related to serum high-density lipoprotein cholesterol levels [53].

The elderly have been documented to be at high risk for inadequate copper intake [74].

Moreover, patients on chronic tube feeding such as the institutionalised elderly are at risk for clinical copper deficiency, including haematological complications such as anaemia [75]. The RDA is 900 µg/day for both genders (Table 4) [72]. Excessive copper provokes epigastric pain, nausea, vomiting and diarrhoea, which usually prevents the more serious manifestations of copper toxicity (coma, oliguria, hepatic necrosis, vascular collapse and death) [76].

## Selenium

Selenium is a cofactor for glutathione peroxidase, an enzyme that, in concert with vitamin E, plays an important role in antioxidant function [53]. Selenium deficiency in humans results in a degenerative disease of the myocardium (Keshan disease) identified in young people in areas of China where the soil is lacking in selenium [53, 72]. This cardiomyopathy can be improved or reversed with selenium supplementation [72]. Unfortunately, the role of selenium in cardiovascular diseases and cardiomyopathy in the elderly has received little investigative attention [77], although serum selenium levels decrease with age [78]. The RDA is 55 µg/day for both genders (Table 4) [72]. Selenium is commonly used as a therapeutic agent in certain types of cancer (prostate) [79]. Epidemiological data suggest that men with high selenium and vitamin E intakes have lower risk for prostate cancer [72].

## Chromium

Chromium is essential for maintaining normal glucose metabolism as it influences the interaction of insulin with the receptor site on the cell membrane [53]. The main signs and symptoms of deficiency in mammals include glucose intolerance with peripheral insulin resistance, altered lipid metabolism, neuropathy and encephalopathy [72]. The adequate intake is 30 µg for elderly males and 20 µg for elderly females (Table 4) [72]. Dietary intake of chromium in the USA is frequently inadequate (including in the elderly) [53, 72]. There is considerable controversy in the literature concerning the role of chromium in improving glucose tolerance [72]. In different patient populations including the elderly, some studies have reported an increase in glucose tolerance, while others have reported a decrease in glucose tolerance [72].

## Iron

Iron is one of the most abundant metals in the earth [80]. It is also one of the most useful, both in technology and in biology, for iron compounds are involved in numerous oxidation–reduction reactions [80]. The requirement for iron is sharply reduced in post-menopausal women [81]. Because adult men generally have no problem in meeting their iron requirements, it can be stated that as a general rule, iron status improves as people get older [82]. Despite long and effective intervention activities, iron deficiency is the primary mineral deficiency in the USA and the whole world [83]. Anaemia in older individuals is rarely caused by iron deficiency; when it occurs, chronic blood loss or deficiency of folate or vitamin B12 should be looked for [82]. Whether iron plays a substantial role in the ageing process is not known [82]. After age 50, the RDA for iron is 10 mg for both genders [50]. Recently, it has been suggested that high intakes of iron may be a health concern [83].

With regard to the other trace elements (arsenic, iodine, lithium, molybdenum, silicon, vanadium), no studies on their effect with ageing have been carried out [69].

## Conclusions

The older population differs from younger adults not only in age but also in health status. The elderly group is not a homogeneous population, and their many different health and social problems impact on their nutritional status [84]. Optimal nutrient intake not only meets their needs but prevents some chronic diseases and ameliorates others [84]. Besides the biochemical parameters, attention must be paid to environmental and psychological factors in evaluating nutritional status and interventions.

## References

1. Chen CC, Schilling LS, Lyder CH (2001) A concept analysis of malnutrition in the elderly. J Adv Nurs 36:131–141
2. Anonymous (1995) American Society for Parenteral and Enteral Nutrition: Standards for nutrition support: hospitalized patients. Nutr Clin Pract 10:208–219
3. Coats KG, Morgan SL, Bartolucci AA, Weinsier RL (1993) Hospital-associated malnutrition: a re-evaluation 12 years later. J Am Diet Ass 93:27–33
4. Reilly HM, Martineau JK, Moran A, Kennedy H (1995) Nutritional screening – evaluation and implementation of a simple nutrition risk score. Clin Nutr 14:269–273
5. Tinetti ME, Williams CS, Thomas MG (2000) Dizziness among older adults: a possible geriatric syndrome. Ann Int Med 132:337–344
6. Roncadio Pablo AM, Arroyo Izaga M, Ansotegui Alday L (2003) Assessment of nutritional status on hospital admission: nutritional scores. Eur J Clin Nutr 57:824–831
7. Windsor JA (1993) Under-weight patients and the risks of major surgery. World J Surg 17:165–172
8. Gibbs J, Cull W, Henderson W et al (1999) Preoperative serum albumin level as a predictor of operative mortality and morbidity: results from the National VA Surgical Risk Study. Arch Surg 134:36–42

9.  Berner YN (2003) Assessment tools for nutritional status in the elderly. Isr Med Assoc J 5:365–367

10. Bruun LI, Bosaeus I, Bergstad I, Nygaard K (1999) Prevalence of malnutrition in surgical patients: evaluation of nutritional support and documentation. Clin Nutr 18:141–147

11. Schneider SM, Hebuterne X (2000) Use of nutritional scores to predict clinical outcomes in chronic diseases. Nutr Rev 1:31–38

12. Olde Rikkert MGM, Deurenberg P, Jansen RWWM et al (1997) Validation of multifrequency bioeletrical impedance analysis in detecting changes in fluid balance of geriatric patients. J Am Geriatr Soc 45:1345–1351

13. Steele CM, Greenwood C, Ens I et al (1997) Mealtime difficulties in a home for the aged: not just dysphagia. Dysphagia 12:43–50

14. Khaw KT (1997) Epidemiological aspects of ageing. Philos Trans R Soc Lond B Biol Sci 352:1829–1835

15. Campion EW (1998) Aging better. N Engl J Med 338:1064–1066

16. Fries JF (1980) Aging, natural death, and the compression of morbidity. N Engl J Med 303:130–135

17. Haveman-Nies A, de Groot LCPGM, van Steveren for the Seneca investigators (2001) Relationship of dietary quality, physical activity, and smoking habits to 10-year changes in health status in elderly Europeans of the Seneca study. In: Dietary quality, lifestyle factors and healthy ageing in Europe. Thesis Wageningen University 6: pp 75–88

18. Verbrugge LM, Patrick DL (1995) Seven chronic conditions: their impact on US adults' activity and use of medical services. Am J Public Health 85:173–182

19. Van Staveren WA, De Groot CP, Blauw YH, van der Wielen RP (1994) Assessing diets of elderly people: problems and approaches. Am J Clin Nutr 59:221S–223S

20. Anonymous (2003) Linee Guida per una sana alimentazione italiana. Ministero delle Politiche Agricole e Forestali. INRAN http://www.inran.it/servizi_cittadino/stare_bene/guida_corretta_alimentazione/INRAN%20L.G%20df.pdf

21. Guigoz Y, Lauque S, Vellas B (2002) Identifying the elderly at risk for malnutrition. The Mini Nutritional Assessment. Clin Geriatr Med 18:737–757

22. Rudman D (1989) Nutrition and fitness in elderly people. Am J Clin Nutr 49:1090–1098

23. Doty RL, Shaman P, Applebaum SL et al (1984) Smell identification ability: changes with age. Science 226:1441–1443

24. Schiffman SS (1997) Taste and smell losses in normal aging and disease. JAMA 278:1357–1362

25. Garry PJ (1994) Nutrition and aging. Chapter 5 in Geriatric Clinical Chemistry reference values. Edited by WR Faulkner and S. Meites. American Association for Clinical Chemistry Press, Washington

26. Bollag D, Genton L, Pichard C (2000) Assessment of nutritional status. Ann Med Intern 15:575–583

27. Symreng T, Anderberg B, Kagedal B et al (1983) Nutritional assessment and clinical course in 112 elective surgical patients. Acta Chir Scand 149:657–662

28. Lansey S, Wasilien C, Mulvihill M, Fillit H (1993) The role of anthropometry in the assessment of malnutrition in the hospitalized frail elderly. Gerontology 39:346–353

29. Hegsted DM (1989) Recommended dietary intakes of elderly subjects. Am J Clin Nutr 50:1190–1194

30. Rubenstein LZ (1990) An overview of aging – demographics, epidemiology and health services. In Morley JE, Glick Z, Rubenstein LZ (eds) Geriatric nutrition: a comprehensive review. New York, Raven Press

31. Schlettwein-Gsell D (1992) Nutrition and the quality of life: a measure for the outcome of nutritional intervention? Am J Clin Nutr 55:1263S–1266S

32. De Jong N (2000) Nutrition and senescence: healthy aging for all in the new millennium? Nutrition 16, 7/8:537–533

33. Goldberg GR, Black AE, Jebb SA et al (1991) Critical evaluation of energy intake data using fundamental principles of energy physiology: 1. Derivation of cut-off limits to identify under-recording. Eur J Clin Nutr 45:569–581

34. Labò G, Melchionda N (1986) Le basi della metodologia clinica per la valutazione dello stato nutrizionale nei soggetti anziani. Estratto dalla Rivista 'Gli Ospedali della Vita' XIII 4–5, pp 71–85

35. Inelmen EM, Jimenez GF, Gatto MRA et al (2000) Dietary intake and nutritional status in Italian elderly subjects. J Nutr Health Aging 4:91–101

36. Gatto MRA, Inelmen EM, Ferrari S et al (1995) Nutrients intake in elderly: descriptive results of a cross-sectional study. Age Nutrition 6:16–24

37. Axelson JM, Csernus MM (1983) Reliability and validity of a food frequency checklist. J Am Diet Ass 83:153–154

38. Guigoz Y, Vellas B, Garry PJ (1994) Mini Nutritional Assessment: a practical assessment tool for grading the nutritional status of elderly patients. Facts Res Gerontol (suppl nutrition) 2nd ed, pp 15–59

39. Guigoz Y (1994) Recommended dietary allowances (RDA) for the free-living elderly. Facts Res Gerontol (suppl nutrition) 2nd ed, pp 113–143

40. Gofin J, Kark E, Mainemer N et al (1981) Prevalence of selected health characteristics of women and comparisons with men. A community health survey in Jerusalem. Isr J Med Sci 17:145–159

41. Wahlqvist ML (1990) Vitamins, nutrition and aging. Prog Clin Biol Res 326:175–202

42. Carnovale E, Miuccio FC (1987) Tabelle di composizione degli alimenti. Ministero Agricoltura e Foreste. Istituto Nazionale Nutrizione. Modified in: Sette S, Ferro-Luzzi A, 1987 and LARN (Livelli di Assunzione Raccomandati di Energia e Nutrienti per la popolazione italiana; revisione 1986–87)

43. Munro HN (1982) Nutritional requirements in the elderly. Hosp Pract 17:143–154

44. James WPT, Ralph A, Ferro-Luzzi A (1989) Energy needs of the elderly. A new approach. In: Munro HN,

Danford DE (eds) Nutrition, aging, and the elderly. Plenum Press, New York, pp 129–151

45. Durnin JVGA (1992) Energy metabolism in the elderly. In: Munro HN, Sclierf G (eds) Nutrition of the elderly. Nestlé Nutrition Workshop Series, 29. Nestlé, Vevey / Raven Press, New York, pp 51–63
46. Voorrips LE, van Acker TM, Deurenberg P, van Staveren WA (1993) Energy expenditure at rest and during standardized activities: a comparison between elderly and middle-aged women. Am J Clin Nutr 58:15–20
47. Carnovale E, Miuccio FC (1984) Tabelle di composizione degli alimenti. Ministero Agricoltura e Foreste. Istituto Nazionale Nutrizione. Modified in: Sette S, Ferro-Luzzi A, and LARN (Livelli di Assunzione Raccomandati di Energia e Nutrienti per la popolazione italiana; revisione 1996)
48. Prenctice AM (1992) Energy expenditure in the elderly. Eur J Clin Nutr 46 (Suppl. 3):S21–S28
49. Goran MI, Poehman ET (1992) Total energy expenditure and energy requirements in healthy elderly persons. Metabolism 41:744–753
50. Food and Nutrition Board (1989) Recommended dietary allowances, 10th edn. National Academy of Sciences, Washington DC
51. Munro HN (1989) Protein nutritive and requirements of the elderly. In: Munro HN, Danford DE (eds) Nutrition, aging, and the elderly. New York, Plenum Press, pp 13–23
52. Committee on Diet and Health, Food and Nutrition Board (1989) Diet and Health. Implications for reducing chronic disease risk. National Academy Press, Washington DC
53. Schlenker ED (1993) Vitamins in the aged. In: Smith JM (ed) Nutrition in aging, 2nd edn. Mobsy-Year Book Inc, Saint Louis, pp 123–145
54. Johnson KA, Bernard MA, Funderburg K (2002) Vitamin nutrition in older adults. Clin Geriatr Med 18:773–799
55. Linder MC (1991) Nutrition and metabolism of vitamins. In: Linder MC (ed) Nutritional biochemistry and metabolism with clinical applications, 2nd edn. Elsevier, New York, pp 111–189
56. Combs GF (1992) Vitamin D, chapter 6. In: Combs GF (ed) The vitamins. Fundamental aspects in nutrition and health. Academic Press Inc, San Diego, pp 151–178
57. LeBoff MS, Kohlmeier L, Hurwitz S et al (1999) Occult vitamin D deficiency in postmenopausal US women with acute hip fracture. JAMA 281:1505–1511
58. Holick MF (1987) Photosynthesis of vitamin D in the skin: effect of environmental and life-style variables. Federation Proc 46:1876–1882
59. Mac Laughlin JA, Holick MF (1985) Aging decreases the capacity of human skin to produce vitamin D3. J Clin Invest 76:1536–1538
60. Delvin EE, Imbach A, Copti M (1988) Vitamin D nutritional status and related biochemical indices in an autonomous elderly population. Am J Clin Nutr 48:373–378
61. Gloth FM, Tobin JD (1995) Progress in geriatrics: vitamin D deficiency in older people. J Am Geriatr Soc 43:822–828
62. Knekt P, Aromaa A, Maatela J et al (1988) Serum vitamin E and risk of cancer among Finnish men during a 10-year follow-up. Am J Epidemiol 127:28–41
63. Stephenson J (1998) Vitamin E and prostate cancer. JAMA 279:1153
64. Goljan EF (1998) Disorders of nutrition. In: Pathology. WB Saunders, Philadelphia, pp 115–129
65. Swendseid ME, Jacob RA (1994) Niacin. In: Shils ME, Olson JA, Shike M (eds) Modern nutrition in health and disease. Lippincott Williams, Philadelphia, pp 376–382
66. Herbert V (1994) Staging vitamin B12 (cobalamin) status in vegetarians. Am J Clin Nutr 59:1213S–1222S
67. Kaptan K, Beyan C, Ural AU et al (2000) Helicobacter pylori – is it a novel causative agent in vitamin B12 deficiency? Arch Intern Med 160:1349–1353
68. Essama-Tjani JC, Guilland JC, Potier de Courcy G et al (2000) Folate status worsens in recently institutionalized elderly people without evidence of functional deterioration. J Am Coll Nutr 19:392–404
69. Morley JE (1995) Other trace elements. In: Morley JE, Glick Z, Rubenstein LZ (eds) Geriatric nutrition, 2nd edn. Raven Press, New York, pp 123-131
70. Powell S (2000) The anti-oxidant properties of zinc. J Nutr 130:1447S–1457S
71. Hennig B, Toborek M, McClain CJ, Diana JN (1996) Nutritional implications in vascular endothelial cell metabolism. J Am Coll Nutr 15:345–358
72. McClain CJ, McClain M, Barve S, Boosalis MG (2002) Trace metals and the elderly. Clin Geriatr Med 18:801–818
73. Shay NF, Mangian HF (2000) Neurobiology of zinc-influenced eating behaviour. J Nutr 130:1493S–1499S
74. Ma J, Betts NM (2000) Zinc and copper intakes and their major food sources for older adults in the 1994-96 continuing survey of food intakes by individuals (CSFII). J Nutr 130:2838–2843
75. Masugi J, Amano M, Fukuda T (1994) Copper deficiency anemia and prolonged enteral feeling. Ann Intern Med 12:386
76. Turnlund JR (1994) Future directions for establishing mineral/trace element requirements. J Nutr 124:1765S–1770S
77. Witte KK, Clark AL, Cleland JG (2001) Chronic heart failure and micronutrients. Am Coll Cardiol 37:1765–1774
78. Savarino L, Granchi D, Ciapetti G et al (2001) Serum concentrations of zinc and selenium in elderly people: results in healthy nonagenarians/centenarians. Exp Gerontol 36:327–339
79. Brawley OW, Parnes H (2000) Prostate cancer prevention trials in the USA. Eur J Cancer 36:1312–1315
80. Fairbanks VF (1994) Iron in medicine and nutrition. In: Shils ME, Olson JA, Shike M (eds) Modern nutrition in health and disease. Lippincott Williams, Philadelphia, pp 185–213
81. Morris ER (1987) Iron. In: Mertz W (ed) Trace elements

in human and animal nutrition, 5th edn. Academic Press, San Diego, pp 79–142

82. Mertz W (1992) Trace elements in aging. In: Munro H, Schlierf G (eds) Nutrition of the elderly. Nestlé Nutrition Workshop Series, Vol 29. Nestlé, Vevey - Raven Press, New York, pp 161-167

83. Nielsen FH (2002) Trace mineral deficiencies. In: Berdanier C (ed) Handbook in nutrition and food. CRC Press LLC, Boca Raton, pp 1463–1487

84. Feldman EB (2002) Nutrition in later years. In: Berdanier C (ed) Handbook in nutrition and food. CRC Press LLC, Boca Raton, pp 319–336

# Nitrogen Balance and Protein Requirements: Definition and Measurements

Paolo Tessari

## Introduction

Nitrogen is a main body component and is required for both tissue protein synthesis and the production of several nitrogenous compounds involved in a variety of functions (hormones, immune mediators, neurotransmitters, antioxidant defences, etc.). Thus, the body nitrogen content should be both quantitatively and qualitatively normal, as well as normally maintained, to ensure normal body functions.

Nitrogen homeostasis is a highly regulated function. Nitrogen balance is commonly referred to as the net difference between the intake (and/or the effective absorption) of nitrogen contained in the diet and its excretion. Since nitrogen is contained predominantly in proteins, this term pertains mainly to the balance of proteins and of amino acids [1].

Nitrogen excretion and/or loss can occur through different routes. The principal component is in the urine as urea, ammonia and creatinine (Table 1). Faecal and miscellaneous losses represent an additional route, which may be fairly constant and lower as an absolute amount [1].

Measurements of nitrogen balance usually require an adaptive period of the subject of at least 4–5 days [2], to ensure that equilibration has been achieved and that acute changes do not occur within the time span of measurement.

Apart from intake, the rate of nitrogen excretion is also affected by renal function, the hydration state and the anabolic/catabolic state of the subject [3].

With prolonged fasting, total urinary nitrogen and urea nitrogen excretion diminish, whereas ammonia excretion increases relatively [4]. Such a shift is related to the excretion of acid equivalents, which are produced in excess by ketogenesis during fasting.

Nitrogen excretion cannot be reduced below a certain amount despite reduction to zero intake. This amount is called the 'obligatory nitrogen losses' (ONL), which represent the nitrogen loss that is measurable in subjects fed a protein-free diet for a relatively short period of time (Table 2). These losses have been estimated to be 36 mg/kg/day in the urine, 12 mg/kg/day in faeces and 8 mg/kg/day as miscellaneous nitrogen losses (sweat, sebum, desquamations, nails, hairs and saliva) [5]. Given the equivalence of 6.25 grams of protein per gram of N, ONL thus correspond on the whole to a protein amount of 0.35 g/kg/day [6].

Rand and Young recently pointed out a series of limitations in the estimation of nitrogen bal-

**Table 1.** Urinary nitrogen excretion ('azoturia')

As urea N: urea excretion (in grams) × 0.46
 since: Urea MW = 60; N2 MW = 28; then: urea N = Urea × [28/60] i.e. × [0.46]

Urea usually accounts for 70–90% of urinary nitrogen excretion

As non-urea N: 2 g/day (ammonia, uric acid, creatinine, nitrates, amino acids, etc.)

**Table 2.** Obligatory nitrogen losses

Urine: 36 mg/kg/day N

Faeces: 12 mg/kg/day N

Miscellaneous N losses (sweat, sebum, desquamations, nails, hairs and saliva): 8 mg/kg/day

Total (as protein equivalents): 0.35 g/kg/day

ance [7]. They state that: 'Nitrogen balance estimates are highly dependent on the assumed amount of N miscellaneous losses... further studies on these losses and on the factors that influence them are essential.' They raised the following points: (a) there is a slight difference between large values for N intake and N losses; (b) it is well recognised that the nitrogen balance technique overestimates N intake and underestimates N losses. This is mainly due to the difficulty in the assessment of the N gas losses after denitrification by the colonic microflora, of the N losses through the skin (urea) and in the expired air (ammonia) and of the nitrate content in food and urine, which is not measured using the Kjeldahl method.

The irreversible loss of amino acid nitrogen corresponds to net protein (i.e. amino acid) catabolism. This occurs because nitrogen is firstly and reversibly lost through deamination/transamination of the amino acids. If this step is followed by another step irreversibly catabolising the amino acid carbon skeleton (i.e. oxidation, hydroxylation, etc.), the nitrogen cannot be re-utilised for amino acid re-synthesis (despite the reversibility of transamination reactions), thus it enters the urea cycle and is either excreted as such, or included into ammonia. Therefore, the net nitrogen loss should theoretically correspond to the irreversible catabolism of the amino acids. This assumption has indeed been proven in 24-hour studies using leucine tracer and nitrogen balance measurements [8, 9]. Therefore, nitrogen loss is an integrated measurement of oxidation/catabolism of all amino acids and thus of net protein loss.

## Protein Requirements

Dietary requirements for protein, amino acid and nitrogen depend on the metabolic demand that must be satisfied. They are conditioned by both the amount of proteins needed and their quality. Protein quality in turn depends on the amount of essential amino acids (EAA), but also of the non-essential (NEAA) ones [10, 11]. The link between protein quality and EAA is obvious: since the EAA

cannot, by definition, be synthesised by the body, they must be introduced with the diet in a proportion that will fit with the organism's metabolic needs. On the other hand, in the absence of dietary NEAA, despite the theoretical capability of the body to synthesise them, nitrogen will be needed for their de novo synthesis. This nitrogen in turn must be derived either from EAA catabolism (thus increasing their requirement above theoretical values) or from the diet. In this respect, although NEAA can theoretically be replaced, they are required in nutrition as well.

An evaluation of dietary protein quality must therefore consider not only the quality of the protein itself, but also the various processes involved in amino acid and nitrogen homeostasis, which may vary as regards the individual amino acids and the individual metabolic conditions of a subject.

Nitrogen balance can be used to derive estimates of human nitrogen (i.e. protein) requirements [1, 12]. The usual approach is based upon the regression of nitrogen balance (i.e. the equilibrium between intake and loss) on intake. The subject is adapted for a few days to a diet of a given protein (and energy) content, and nitrogen balance is measured at the end of adaptation. Diets with varying amounts of proteins (and energy) are tested. Requirement is then defined as the intake level that would produce a zero (or a slightly positive) nitrogen balance.

An intake of 0.6 g/kg/day of well-balanced proteins is considered sufficient to achieve a zero (i.e. at equilibrium) nitrogen balance [6] (Table 3). A safety amount is considered to be 0.75 g/kg/day. These values represent the minimum recommended protein intake, derived also from studies investigating the metabolic response to a range of protein intakes between 0.75 and 2 g/kg/day.

Amino acid requirement may increase in many physiological conditions (Table 3). In children [13], the requirement for growth must be integrated in addition to the requirement for maintenance. In the first 6 months of life, a suggested intake is of ≈1.7 g/kg/day, with a further allowance of +25% (+2 SD), leading therefore to a total of ≈2 g/kg/day. Beyond the sixth month of life, suggest-

**Table 3.** Daily protein requirements by age

Adult, weight stable, moderate activity: 0.75 g/kg

Children:          first 6 months: 2 g/kg
                   beyond sixth month: 1.6 g/kg

Between 7 and 14 years: 1 g/kg

Beyond 14 years: 0.75 g/kg

ed intake is 1.6 g/kg/day, resulting from a +50% increase, beyond a suggested intake of 0.8 g/kg/day of the adult, due to individual variability in growth, plus a +30% increase due to variability in utilisation efficiency, +25% (= 2 SD). Between 7 and 14 years, the recommended intake is 1 g/kg/day, and beyond 14 years it is the same as for an adult.

In pregnancy [14], the total nitrogen deposition over the entire period up to delivery is estimated to be ≈925 g. Average rates of nitrogen retention are 0.11 g/kg/day in the first trimester, 0.52 g/kg/day in the second, and 0.92 g/kg/day in the third. In practice, due to a 70% efficiency in nitrogen utilisation, and the still partially unknown effective nitrogen retention in the first trimester, it is suggested to increase the dietary protein intake by 10–12 g/day in each trimester.

During lactation, an extra protein intake of 15–20 g/day in the first 6 months, and of 12 g/day in the subsequent months, is advisable [15].

In the elderly, the maintenance of nitrogen equilibrium by a diet containing 0.8 g/kg/day and a normal energy intake may be difficult, because of a lower efficiency in nitrogen utilisation for anabolic purposes [16].

A surplus of dietary proteins is also recommended for individuals who exercise regularly [17]. Amino acids are oxidised as substrates during prolonged submaximal exercise. In addition, both endurance and resistance training exercise increase skeletal muscle protein synthesis and breakdown in the post-exercise recovery period. In studies using nitrogen balance, it has been confirmed that protein requirements for individuals engaged in regular exercise are increased. Current

recommended intakes of proteins for strength and endurance exercising athletes are 1.6–1.7 g/kg/day and 1.2–1.4 g/kg/day, respectively. It is presently estimated that most athletes consume adequate (if not excessive!) amounts of proteins. Recent research has also pointed out that the timing and nutritional amount of a meal ingested after exercise have synergistic effects on net protein accumulation in body tissues after exercise. It has been suggested that athletes who engage in strenuous activity should consume a meal rich in amino acids and carbohydrates soon after the exercise bout or the training session.

## Protein Requirement and Energy Intake

It has been proposed that protein requirement is, within a certain limit, inversely dependent on energy intake, i.e. the more energy is ingested, the less protein is needed (Table 4). This is because proteins can be used also as energy sources (beyond their structural, regulatory and functional role). Therefore, if their use to produce energy varies, their requirement also varies. Furthermore, alternative energy substrates, such as the carbohydrates, can stimulate insulin secretion, which in turn spares endogenous proteins [18].

A relationship between protein requirement and energy intake is reported in Table 4. The reported amount should be increased by 2 SD for safe allowances.

**Table 4.** Relationship between dietary protein requirement (in grams of protein per kg of body weight), titrated to the achievement of zero nitrogen balance, and energy intake (in kJ per kg of body weight) in a weight-stable healthy adult man [19, 20]

| Protein requirement (g/kg) | Safe allowance (+2 SD) (g/kg) | Energy intake (kJ/kg) |
|---|---|---|
| 0.78 | 1.02 | 9.57 |
| 0.56 | 0.74 | 10.77 |
| 0.51 | 0.62 | 11.48 |
| 0.42 | 0.50 | 13.64 |

## The Fate of Dietary Protein Nitrogen During the Postprandial Phase

The diurnal cycle of feeding and fasting is accompanied by concurrent changes in protein turnover. Protein feeding is necessary to replenish the body protein stores that would be wasted during fasting [21–24]. Because of this, nitrogen retention calculated on a daily basis is lower than that derived just from the postprandial phase [21], and, conversely, dietary protein utilisation calculated as the daily gain is lower than the postprandial gain.

Dietary proteins, once ingested, are digested in the gut and thereafter absorbed as either free amino acids or dipeptides [25]. The absorbed amino acids are subjected to a variable first-pass extraction by splanchnic organs (mainly the liver) [26–28] and then they travel as such through the extracellular spaces before being used by the cells, either for catabolism or for protein synthesis. A minor fraction of amino acids are excreted unmodified into the urine [29].

The acute nitrogen deposition during the postprandial phase is likely to be the most critical in terms of the net deposition of proteins in the tissues, more than the rate of protein synthesis occurring in the postabsorptive periods. Therefore, the assessment of the postprandial utilisation of dietary proteins is a key step to understand net body protein deposition. It also represents an important conditioning factor of the rate of whole-body protein turnover [30].

The key steps of the fate of dietary nitrogen are: (1) the amount of nitrogen that is actually absorbed; (2) the amount that is deaminated and then recovered mainly in the form of urea; and (3) the amount that is retained in the body.

As regards point (1), nitrogen digestibility within the ileum and the short-term retention of dietary protein nitrogen can be measured by the use of $^{15}N$-labelled proteins. By this technique, therefore, it is possible to assess the metabolic utilisation of dietary nitrogen in humans, i.e. the amount that is effectively absorbed [31–35].

As concerns point (2), assuming that whole-body protein turnover is ≈300 g, and that daily protein intake is ≈100–110 g/day, it has been calculated that ≈80 g of the total proteins turned over

(i.e. ≈27% of total) are lost through the oxidative/urea-producing pathways, and ≈14 g within the ileum [21, 22]. The amounts of dietary nitrogen entering the anabolic (i.e. protein synthesis) and oxidative pathways are 70–80 and 13–20 g/day, respectively, i.e. contributing by 30–40% to total anabolism and by 15–25% to total oxidation (Fig. 1).

This indicates that dietary nitrogen (and proteins) is preferentially directed toward anabolic pathways. Such a preferential orientation of dietary nitrogen toward body protein synthesis is strictly linked to the adequacy (i.e. quality) of the dietary protein amino acid composition with respect to that of body protein.

The maintenance of nitrogen homeostasis involves a complex series of changes in whole-body protein turnover, amino acid oxidation, urea production and nitrogen excretion, during the fasting, fed, postprandial and postabsorptive periods of the day. Whole-body processes also represent the additive result of the metabolism of individual organs and tissues, which may be differently affected during physiological and pathological conditions. Therefore, whole-body measurements are crude, although comprehensive, estimates of body protein metabolism, but rarely can they provide information on regional protein turnover.

The usual daily protein consumption is normally greater than the theoretical requirement based on nitrogen balance estimates [36]. Since body proteins cannot be stored in the body, mechanisms exist to dispose of the protein ingested in excess. Thus, the effects of increased protein loads on whole-body nitrogen balance and protein

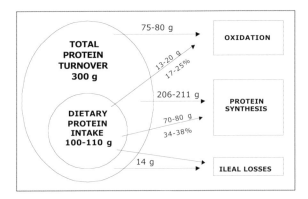

**Fig. 1.** Proportions of nitrogen turnover and utilisation

turnover must be determined. These investigations should involve the study of nitrogen pools likely to be modified by the level of nitrogen intake, the effects linked to the type of protein ingested, as well as the effects of the nitrogen loads on the different nitrogen pathways [37].

An increase in protein intake is followed by adaptive processes: (1) an increase in amino acid oxidation and in the associated nitrogen excretion, mainly as urea, which is especially pronounced in the fed state; (2) a trend toward a disproportionate increase in nitrogen balance when nitrogen intake is increased [38], possibly linked to an enhanced inhibition of protein breakdown by feeding and to an increase in protein synthesis [39]. This likely occurs because whole-body as well as tissue protein synthesis are sensitive to amino acid availability, whereas degradation may be sensitive to an interactive effect by both the amino acid level and insulin [40]. Thus, high protein intakes are associated with a continuous, positive N balance approaching 1–3 g N/day [38, 39, 41, 42]. However, it is not clear whether this apparent retention is a real one or linked to intrinsic errors in calculating N balance.

Interestingly, the amplitude of diurnal body protein cycling increases with an increase in dietary protein intake, with no clear change in the mean daily protein turnover rate [43].

## Nitrogen Metabolism and Dietary Protein Characteristics

Nitrogen balance data measured after adaptation to different protein levels over periods of several days is the usual approach to measure nitrogen retention [2, 44]. Diets containing poor quality proteins are associated with an increase in nitrogen losses, due to the inefficient utilisation of indispensable amino acids in turn linked to unbalanced amino acid composition. The (relative) lack of essential amino acids generates the ineffective utilisation of dietary nitrogen. Furthermore, besides such an insufficient utilisation, it is important to assess the amount of dietary and intestinal nitrogen that is absorbed as free amino acids or dipeptides, or excreted in the faeces, urine or other routes. Finally, the assessment of the anabolic utilisation for protein synthesis is a key step to measure amino acid retention in the body.

As stated above, classic nitrogen balance studies reflect the integrated net result of the diurnal cycling between the fasted and fed states (i.e. phases of nitrogen accretion postprandially and of nitrogen losses postabsorptively).

Other factors may affect nitrogen retention. Differences in the gastric emptying rate of dietary proteins may result in highly variable rates of amino acid absorption in the small intestine [45]. Also, differences in the rate of protein digestion and/or absorption result in relevant differences in amino acid oxidation and postprandial nitrogen accretion [46]. In this regard, the concept of net postprandial protein utilisation (NPPU) has been proposed, which is calculated using true ileal digestibility and true $^{15}$N-labelled protein deamination parameters, adding the dietary nitrogen collected in the urine [22, 47] and that retained in the body in the form of urea.

Using this approach, the NPPU values for milk protein and soy protein, measured over 8 h after the ingestion of a standard meal by healthy human subjects, were reported between 80 and 72%, respectively [47]. These data strongly suggest the existence of differences between the nutritional value of proteins and their utilisation for anabolic purposes. These differences are valuable and should be taken into account when calculating amino acid scores. Finally, differences in interorgan amino acid metabolism may be due to the protein source-dependent difference, as shown in pigs after the administration of either soy or casein [48].

## References

1. Mattews DE (1999) Proteins and amino acids. In: Shills ME, Olson JA, Shine M, Ross AC (eds) Modern nutrition in health and disease, 9th ed. Lippicott Williams & Wilkins, Baltimore, pp 11–48
2. Munro HN, Allinson JB (1964) Mammalian protein metabolism. Academic Press, New York, London
3. Papper S (1971) Renal failure. Med Clin North Am 55:335–357
4. Cahill GF Jr (1976) Starvation in man. Clin Endocrinol Metab 5:397–415
5. Bodwell CE, Schuster EM, Kyle E et al (1979) Obligatory urinary and fecal nitrogen losses in young women, older men, and young men and the factorial estimation of adult human protein requirements. Am J Clin Nutr 32:2450–2459
6. Anonymous (1985) Energy and protein requirements. Report of a joint FAO/WHO/UNU Expert Consultation. World Health Organ Tech Rep Ser 724:1–206
7. Rand WM, Pellett PL, Young VR (2003) Meta-analysis of nitrogen balance studies for estimating protein requirements in healthy adults. Am J Clin Nutr 77:109–127
8. el-Khoury AE, Fukagawa NK, Sanchez M et al (1994) Validation of the tracer-balance concept with reference to leucine: 24-h intravenous tracer studies with L-[1-13C]leucine and [15N-15N]urea. Am J Clin Nutr 59:1000–1011
9. el-Khoury AE, Ajami AM, Fukagawa NK et al (1996) Diurnal pattern of the interrelationships among leucine oxidation, urea production, and hydrolysis in humans. Am J Physiol 271(3 Pt 1):E563–E573
10. Young VR, Borgonha S (2000) Nitrogen and amino acid requirements: the Massachusetts Institute of Technology amino acid requirement pattern. J Nutr 130:1841S–1849S
11. James PJ, Reeds PJ (2003) Protein and amino acid requirements and the composition of complementary foods. J Nutr 133:2953S–2961S
12. Visek WJ (1984) An update of concepts of essential amino acids. Annu Rev Nutr 4:137–155
13. Heird WC (1999) Nutritional requirements during infancy. In: Shills ME, Olson JA, Shike M, Ross AC (eds) Modern nutrition in health and disease, 9th ed. Lippicott Williams & Wilkins, Baltimore, pp 839–855
14. McGanity WJ, Dawson EB, Van Hook JW (1999) Maternal nutrition. In: Shills ME, Olson JA, Shike M, Ross AC (eds) Modern nutrition in health and disease, 9th ed. Lippicott Williams & Wilkins, Baltimore, pp 812–838
15. Sampson DA, Jansen GR (1984) Protein and energy nutrition during lactation. Annu Rev Nutr 4:43–67
16. Kurpad AV, Vaz M (2000) Protein and amino acid requirements in the elderly. Eur J Clin Nutr 54:S131–S142
17. Fielding RA, Parkington J (2002) What are the dietary protein requirements of physically active individuals? New evidence on the effects of exercise on protein utilization during post-exercise recovery. Nutr Clin Care 5:191–196
18. Pellett PL, Young VR (1991) The effects of different levels of energy intake on protein metabolism and of different levels of protein intake on energy metabolism: a statistical evaluation from the published literature. In: Scimshaw NS, Schurch B (eds) Protein Energy Interactions. International dietary energy consultative group, Lausanne, pp 81–136
19. Kishi K, Mitayani S, Inohue G (1978) Requirement and utilization of egg protein by Japanese young men with marginal intakes of energy. J Nutr 108:658–669
20. Food and Nutrition Board (1989) National Research Council: protein and amino acids. In: Recommended dietary allowances, 10th ed. National Academic Press, Washington, pp 52–77
21. Millward DJ (2004) Macronutrient intakes as determinants of dietary protein and amino acid adequacy. J Nutr 134:1588S–1596S
22. Millward DJ, Fereday A, Gibson NR, Pacy PJ (1996) Post-prandial protein metabolism. Baillieres Clin Endocrinol Metab 10:533–549
23. Tessari P, Zanetti M, Barazzoni M et al (1996) Mechanisms of post-prandial protein accretion in human skeletal muscle: insight from leucine and phenylalanine forearm kinetics. J Clin Invest 98:1361–1372
24. Cayol M, Boirie Y, Rambourdin F et al (1997) Influence of protein intake on whole body and splanchnic leucine kinetics in humans. Am J Physiol 272:E584–E591
25. Klein S, Cohn SM, Alpers DH (1999) The alimentary tract in nutrition. In: Shills ME, Olson JA, Shike M, Ross AC (eds) Modern nutrition in health and disease, 9th ed. Lippicott Williams & Wilkins, Baltimore, pp 605–629
26. Biolo G, Tessari P, Inchiostro S et al (1992) Leucine and phenylalanine kinetics during mixed meal ingestion. A multiple tracer approach. Am J Physiol 262:E455–E463
27. Tessari P (2000) Regulation of splanchnic protein synthesis by enteral feeding. In: Furst P, Young V (eds) Proteins, peptides and amino acids in enteral nutrition. Nestlè Nutrition Workshop Series. Clinical & Performance Program, Vol 3. Karger, Basel, pp 47–62
28. Capaldo B, Gastaldelli A, Antoniello S et al (1999) Splanchnic and leg substrate exchange after ingestion of a natural mixed meal in humans. Diabetes 48:958–966
29. Harper HA, Doolan PD (1963) The renal aminoacidurias. Clin Chem 9:19–26
30. Marchini JS, Cortiella J, Hiramatsu T et al (1993) Requirements for indispensable amino acids in adult humans: longer-term amino acid kinetic study with support for the adequacy of the Massachusetts

Institute of Technology amino acid requirement pattern. Am J Clin Nutr 58:670–683

31. Bos C, Mahe S, Gaudichon C et al (1999) Assessment of net postprandial protein utilization of 15N-labelled milk nitrogen in human subjects. Br J Nutr 81:221–226

32. Gaudichon C, Mahe S, Benamouzig R et al (1999) Net postprandial utilization of [15N]-labeled milk protein nitrogen is influenced by diet composition in humans. J Nutr 129:890–895

33. Gausseres N, Mahe S, Benamouzig R et al (1996) The gastro-ileal digestion of 15N-labelled pea nitrogen in adult humans. Br J Nutr 76:75–85

34. Mahe S, Roos N, Benamouzig R et al (1994) True exogenous and endogenous nitrogen fractions in the human jejunum after ingestion of small amounts of 15N-labeled casein. J Nutr 124:548–555

35. Mariotti F, Mahe S, Benamouzig R et al (1999) Nutritional value of [15N]-soy protein isolate assessed from ileal digestibility and postprandial protein utilization in humans. J Nutr 129:1992–1997

36. Beaton GH (1994) Dietary intakes: individual and populations. In: Shills ME, Olson JA, Shike M, Ross AC (eds) Modern nutrition in health and disease, 9th ed. Lippincott Williams & Wilkins, Baltimore, pp 1705–1726

37. Millward DJ (1999) The nutritional value of plant-based diets in relation to human amino acid and protein requirements. Proc Nutr Soc 58:249–260

38. Price GM, Halliday D, Pacy PJ et al (1994) Nitrogen homeostasis in man: influence of protein intake on the amplitude of diurnal cycling of body nitrogen. Clin Sci (Lond) 86:91–102

39. Forslund AH, El-Khoury AE, Olsson RM et al (1999) Effect of protein intake and physical activity on 24-h pattern and rate of macronutrient utilization. Am J Physiol 276:E964–E976

40. Tessari P (1991) Regulation of amino acid and protein metabolism in normal physiology and diabetes mellitus. Diab Nutr Metab 4:57–70

41. Cheng AH, Gomez A, Bergan JG et al (1978) Comparative nitrogen balance study between young and aged adults using three levels of protein intake from a combination wheat-soy-milk mixture. Am J Clin Nutr 31:12–22

42. Oddoye EA, Margen S (1979) Nitrogen balance studies in humans: long-term effect of high nitrogen intake on nitrogen accretion. J Nutr 109:363–377

43. Pacy PJ, Price GM, Halliday D et al (1994) Nitrogen homeostasis in man: the diurnal responses of protein synthesis and degradation and amino acid oxidation to diets with increasing protein intakes. Clin Sci (Lond) 86:103–116

44. Millward DJ, Pavy PJ (1995) Postprandial protein utilization and protein quality assessment in man. Clin Sci (Lond) 88:597–606

45. Gaudichon C, Roos N, Mahe S et al (1994) Gastric emptying regulates the kinetics of nitrogen absorption from 15N-labeled milk and 15N-labeled yogurt in miniature pigs. J Nutr 124:1970–1977

46. Beaufrere B, Dangin M, Boirie Y (2000) The 'fast' and 'slow' protein concept. Nestle Nutr Workshop Ser Clin Perform Programme 3:121–31; discussion 131–133

47. Millward DJ (2001) Protein and amino acid requirements of adults: current controversies. Can J Appl Physiol 26:S130–S140

48. Deutz NE, Bruins MJ, Soeters PB (1998) Infusion of soy and casein protein meals affects interorgan amino acid metabolism and urea kinetics differently in pigs. J Nutr 128:2435–2445

# Plasma Proteins and Protein Catabolism

Paolo Tessari, Renato Millioni

## Introduction

In the adult organism, maintenance of body protein stores is the result of changes linked to a diurnal rhythm of catabolic and anabolic phases [1]. In physiological states a net loss of body proteins occurs in the periods between meals, particularly at night-time, and during exercise [2]. Conversely, a net protein gain occurs during meal absorption, both in the entire body and at muscle level [3]. Recently, the recovery phase after exercise has also been recognised as anabolic [4].

Both protein accretion and loss are the net result of a variety of combinations of changes in protein degradation and synthesis. Thus each process plays a key role in the maintenance of protein homeostasis and balance. As with those occurring at whole-body or muscle level, coordinate changes in protein synthesis and degradation are likely to occur also within the splanchnic bed during the day.

Many protein catabolic conditions are characterised by profound alterations of both visceral and muscular proteins, mostly at advanced stages of the disease, and by alterations of plasma and intracellular amino acid patterns. A list of potential catabolic conditions is reported in Table 1.

In many of these conditions, loss of lean body mass, particularly of skeletal muscle, and decreased concentrations of some plasma proteins that are liver-synthesised, i.e. visceral proteins, such as albumin, are often observed. All these changes reflect both a poor nutritional status and an abnormal regulation of protein turnover.

Proper nutrition is required to maintain a balanced body weight and composition in the adult. It is also necessary to ensure proper physiological growth in the young, developing organism. Nutrition, particularly with proteins and/or amino acids, is necessary to stimulate body tissue protein synthesis. Normal growth requires water, vitamins, oligoelements, electrolytes, carbohydrates, fat and proteins/amino acids. Both the essential and the non-essential amino acids are necessary, although to different degrees. Even though non-essential amino acids can be synthesised de novo, their synthesis requires nitrogen from other sources: therefore, to a certain degree, they are also necessary in nutrition and to maintain an adequate protein accretion. Net protein deposition is the result of two opposite processes: protein synthesis and protein degradation. Whenever protein synthesis exceeds degradation, net protein deposition occurs.

**Table 1.** Catabolic states in human pathology

| |
| --- |
| Liver diseases |
| Cancer |
| Kidney insufficiency |
| Metabolic acidosis |
| Insulin-deficiency or resistance |
| Gastrointestinal diseases |
| Immunodeficiency syndromes |
| Chronic cardiac failure |
| Chronic respiratory insufficiency |
| Inflammation |
| Drug-induced protein catabolism |
| Head trauma |

## Mechanism of Net Protein Gain

Protein synthesis is the result of the incorporation of the amino acids into the newly formed protein, through a series of tightly regulated steps [5–7]. The newly formed protein is then either used inside the cell (such as structural or regulatory protein) or exported as secreted protein. Intracellular amino acids derive from either endogenous protein degradation or external sources. Proteolysis is activated intracellularly by a number of pathways [8–10]. It is usually coupled to a certain degree to intracellular oxidation (and/or catabolism), biotransformation, or reutilisation of the amino acids. Alternatively, the amino acids can be released into the bloodstream.

Theoretically, protein degradation could be set to zero, thus restraining also to zero the need for an external supply of amino acids to maintain body protein turnover and composition. This, however, never occurs for a variety of reasons: (1) there are bioenergetic/entropy reasons to make this possibility not feasible; (2) there is an obligatory loss of amino acids; and/or (3) protein degradation is used to remove aged and perhaps modified proteins that are no longer viable for cell metabolism. Protein synthesis and degradation are regulated differently in different tissues and organs under physiological and pathological conditions. There is an extensive trafficking of amino acids and proteins among and across organs in the living organisms.

## Visceral Proteins as Indexes of Malnutrition

In clinical practice, levels of serum hepatic proteins (albumin, transferrin, prealbumin, etc.) have historically been associated with nutritional status. There are two conventional types of malnutrition: kwashiorkor and marasmus. These conditions were categorised before the role of inflammatory processes of acute and chronic illness on protein turnover was known. Subsequent literature on inflammation and its effects on hepatic protein metabolism has replaced previous knowledge/views suggesting that the nutritional status and protein intake were the relevant factors conditioning serum hepatic protein levels. Recent and compelling evidence suggests that serum hepatic protein levels are excellent correlates of morbidity and mortality. In other words, serum hepatic pro-

tein levels are useful indicators of severity of disease. The concentrations of these proteins help to identify those subjects who are likely to develop malnutrition, even if they were properly nourished prior to trauma or the onset of illness. Furthermore, hepatic protein levels do not accurately measure nutritional repletion. Low serum levels indicate that a patient is very ill and probably requires aggressive and closely monitored medical nutrition therapy.

**Table 2.** Negative and positive acute-phase proteins

**Negative acute-phase proteins**
    Albumin
    Prealbumin (transthyretin)
    Transferrin
    Insulin-like growth factor I
    Thyroxine-binding globulin
    $\alpha_2$-HS glycoprotein
    Alpha-fetoprotein
    Coagulation factor XII

**Positive acute-phase proteins**
    *Proteins of the coagulation cascade and of the fibrinolytic system*
        Fibrinogen, plasminogen
        Tissue plasminogen activator, plasminogen-activator inhibitor
        Urokinase
        Protein S
    *Antiproteases*
        $\alpha_1$-Protease inhibitor
        Inter-$\alpha$-trypsin inhibitors
        $\alpha_1$-Antichymotrypsin
        Pancreatic secretory trypsin inhibitor
    *Proteins of the complement system*
        C1 inhibitor, C3, C4, C4b-binding protein
        Factor B
        Mannose-binding lectin
    *Proteins involved in transport*
        Ceruloplasmin
        Haptoglobulin
        Hemopexin
    *Proteins involved in the inflammatory responses*
        Secreted phospholipase $A_2$
        Lipopolysaccharide-binding protein
        Interleukin-1-receptor antagonist
        Granulocyte colony-stimulating factor
    *Miscellaneous*
        C-reactive protein, serum amyloid A
        $\alpha_1$-Acid glycoprotein
        Fibronectin
        Ferritin

Plasma proteins are usually categorised as negative and positive acute-phase proteins. The former diminish as the result of a stressed condition, the latter behave in the opposite way. A list of these proteins is reported in Table 2.

# Negative Acute-Phase Proteins

## Albumin

Albumin is the most abundant circulating protein, produced only by the liver (see [11] for review). The albumin gene is on chromosome 4. Albumin has a large variety of functions (metabolism, tissue fluid distribution, nutrition, transport of substrates, etc.). Therefore, a decrease of albumin concentrations has a widespread impact.

### Structure of Albumin

The albumin molecule is a single polypeptide chain of 69 KDa arranged predominantly in an α-helix, bound by 17 disulphide bridges. Three α-helices are arranged in parallel and they constitute a *sub-domain*, and two sub-domains facing each other in an antiparallel fashion constitute a *domain*. The outer part of this structure resembling a cylinder is mainly polar, the central part is predominantly apolar. Each sub-domain is allowed to move relative to the other by means of proline molecules. This allows a change in the spatial orientation of the molecule in relation to the substrates bound.

### Functions of Albumin

One of the main functions of albumin is linked to its colloidal properties, regulating fluid distribution through the body [11]. Albumin is responsible for more than three quarters of the normal oncotic pressure. The colloidal property of albumin requires that it is in unbound form. In the skin, which contains a lot of albumin molecules, albumin is largely bound to tissues, therefore it is not effective as regards oncotic pressure. Albumin is responsible for about half of the normal ion gap, and has a key role in substrate binding and transport [11].

### Albumin Pool Size, Secretion, Metabolism, Nutritional and Hormonal Regulation

The concentration of serum albumin is the compounded result of synthesis, catabolism, changes in intra/extravascular distribution, and hydration state. Normal plasma albumin concentration reflects the intravascular portion of the pool, which is about 40% of the total [11]. The total albumin pool (intra- plus extravascular) in a healthy adult human subject is about 200 grams. The extravascular pool is composed of one pool with a faster half life (≈6 h), likely located in organs with discontinuous capillaries (liver, spleen, gut) and another with a slower half life (≈28 h), likely located in organs with continuous capillaries (skeletal muscle, skin). Therefore, three pharmacokinetic compartments of albumin can be identified, one intravascular and two extravascular. Of the total albumin pool, 11–18% (30–40% of the total extravascular pool) is located in the skin, 15% in muscle and 1% in the liver [12, 13].

Little or no albumin is stored within the hepatocytes. Albumin equilibrates rapidly (in 2 min) within the plasma pool. However, complete equilibration between the intra- and the extravascular pools requires 7–10 days. In normal conditions, about 80% of the albumin that has moved into the interstitium comes back into the systemic circulation through the thoracic duct within 48 h.

Between 12 and 25 grams of albumin can be produced daily [11], accounting for a maximum of 50% of total liver protein synthesis at its peak value, but less than 10% of the average daily total protein synthesis by the liver. Approximately 6% of the daily nitrogen intake is required for albumin synthesis. The main regulator of albumin synthesis seems to be the oncotic pressure at the hepatocyte, which in turn is a function of extracellular albumin concentration [11]. The main nutritional factors regulating albumin synthesis are total caloric and protein intake, the route of nutrient administration, and specific amino acids such as tryptophan. Calorie/nutrient deficiencies and, conversely, repletion, have greater effects on the synthesis of albumin than on other proteins. Many hormones (cortisone, thyroid hormones, insulin, growth hormone, sex hormones) have in vitro effects on albumin synthesis, which are additive [13].

The plasma half life of infused albumin is normally 24 h [14]. The total half life of albumin is 17–19 days, and ≈4% of the exchangeable albumin pool is degraded per day. The fractional catabolic rate of albumin is low: however, in absolute terms (grams per day) it is high, because of its large mass [3]. A precise site of albumin catabolism has not been characterised. All organs are likely to be involved in albumin removal, which is a receptor-independent process [11].

### Albumin Kinetics in Vivo in Normal Man

Using tracer methodologies to measure primarily albumin synthesis, the albumin fractional synthesis rate in normal post-absorptive humans has been calculated to be between 6 and 10% per day [11, 15, 16], corresponding to an absolute synthesis rate of 8–10 grams per day (based on the intravascular pool) or 20–25 grams per day (based on the total pool). A balanced, mixed meal of adequate caloric content stimulates albumin synthesis by ≈30–40% above basal [15–18]. Both dietary amino acids and post-prandial insulin are important stimulatory factors [19]. Short-term growth hormone or prednisone administrations did not apparently alter the post-prandial stimulation of albumin synthesis in vivo, contrary to the in vitro findings, in healthy humans [11, 15, 20]. Such an increase in albumin fractional secretion rate post-prandially does not induce appreciable changes in albumin concentrations, because of the low fractional basal albumin synthesis rate, as well as the large total intravascular albumin pool, which would lead to a maximum increase of ≈0.15% of the total pool in 1 h, clearly below common detection limits. It has been proposed that albumin is a carrier of nitrogen from visceral (i.e. the liver) to peripheral (i.e. muscle) organs [15] after a mixed meal ingestion.

Other factors have been shown to regulate albumin synthesis (Table 3).

Inflammation in the rat down-regulated albumin synthesis, consistent with the hypoalbuminaemia found in inflammation [21]. The response of albumin synthesis to this condition is opposite to the observed increase in total liver protein synthesis, likely secondary to the increase of acute-phase proteins [21].

**Table 3.** Factors affecting serum albumin, prealbumin and transferrin

| Factors leading to a decrease | Factors leading to an increase |
|---|---|
| Loss of albumin | Exogenous albumin infusion |
| Excess of intravascular volume | Decrease of intravascular volume |
| Liver diseases, alcohol abuse | Renal failure |
| Nephrotic syndrome, uraemia | (Transferrin) iron deficiency |
| Pregnancy | |
| Hypothyroidism | |
| Tumours | |
| Trauma, inflammation | |

### Transthyretin or Prealbumin

The transthyretin (TTR)/prealbumin molecule is a stable tetramer, composed of four identical subunits, with a total molecular weight (MW) of 55 KDa. Each prealbumin subunit contains 127 amino acid residues [22]. The TTR monomer contains eight antiparallel beta-pleated sheet domains. The molecular structure has been determined by X-ray analysis [23]. TTR was formerly called prealbumin because it migrates anodally to albumin on serum protein electrophoresis, but this name is misleading because TTR is not a precursor of albumin. Its gene has been mapped to chromosome 18q11.2–q12.1 [24], spans 6.9 kb with four exons and three introns.

TTR is mainly synthesised by the liver, the choroid plexuses of the brain, and the retinal pigment epithelia of the eye. It is one of the main proteins synthesised in the choroid plexus, being abundant in cerebrospinal fluid (CSF) [25]. Prealbumin concentration normally ranges between 150 and 400 mg/l.

It has been shown that TTR is a plasma transport protein for the thyroid hormone (TH) thyroxine (T4) and retinol, through the association with retinol-binding protein, and that helps in maintaining their normal levels in the circulating plasma

[26]. It is the main T4 transport protein in CSF, and might contribute to the transport of serum T4 across the blood–brain and blood–choroid plexus–CSF barriers [27]. TTR binds other ligands such as pterins [28] and apolipoprotein ApoA1 [29], but the role of the protein in the metabolism of these ligands has not yet been assessed.

Part of the interest in TTR stems from the occurrence of mutations in the molecule leading to the extracellular deposition in tissues as amyloid. The main sites of deposition are the peripheral nerves and/or the heart, associated with neuropathies and/or cardiomyopathies, respectively [30]. Over 80 different disease-causing mutations in TTR have been reported. The vast majority are inherited in an autosomal-dominant manner and are related to amyloid deposition, affecting predominantly peripheral nerves and/or the heart. A small portion of TTR mutations are apparently non-amyloidogenic. Among these are mutations responsible for hyperthyroxinaemia [31]. Identification and characterisation of TTR mutations in healthy and diseased subjects will help to unravel the unknown pathogenetic mechanisms underlying TTR amyloidosis.

## Thyroxine-Binding Globulin

Thyroxine-binding globulin (TBG), the principal TH transport protein in human serum, is synthesised by the liver and secreted into the bloodstream as a 54 KDa acidic glycoprotein made up of a single polypeptide chain of 395 amino acids and four heterosaccharide units. The carbohydrate chains are important for the correct post-translational folding, secretion and degradation of the molecule, but are not required for hormone binding. TBG, encoded by a single gene copy located on Xq22, consists of five exons spanning 5.5 kb [32, 33].

By virtue of sequence homology, TBG belongs to the superfamily of serine proteinase inhibitors (serpins) [34], which consists of a variety of heterogeneous proteins including $_1$-antitrypsin (also known as proteinase inhibitor, PI), $_1$-antichymotrypsin, antithrombin III and cortisol-binding globulin (CBG) [35]. TBG and CBG are the only serpins that transport small lipophilic molecules having lost the serpin-characteristic function of proteinase inhibition [36].

Cleavage of TBG by a serine protease causes a conformational change that reduces the affinity of TBG for T4. This would allow large concentrations of TH at specific sites. Cleavage also may increase the clearance of TBG.

The normal serum concentration of TBG ranges from 1.1 to 2.1 mg/dl in adults. Although TBG concentrations are far lower than those of the other two TH-binding proteins (i.e., TTR and albumin), it carries approximately 75% of serum T4 and tri-iodothyronine (T3). TBG has a tenfold greater affinity for T4 than T3; its molecule has a single TH-binding site. In normal serum, TBG usually is only 25% saturated with T4 [37].

Several states of deficiency of this protein have been described that are either inherited or acquired [38]. Thyroid function tests (TFTs) in patients with TBG deficiency show normal TSH and free T4, but low total T4, and, occasionally, low total T3 serum concentrations.

Acquired TBG deficiency, which can be caused by protein malnutrition, is encountered frequently in chronic diseases and debilitative states, in liver failure, and in calorie malnutrition. In patients with the nephrotic syndrome, TBG is lost through the glomerular filtrate. The cause of the decrease in TBG concentration associated with glucocorticoid or androgen administration is not clear, but it is believed that the effect is transcriptionally mediated, although cleavage of the protein may also play a role in increasing its clearance.

## Transferrin

Plasma transferrin is a 80 KDa glycoprotein with homologous N-terminal and C-terminal iron-binding domains (called the N- and C-lobes) [39]. The transferrin gene is on chromosome 3. Transferrin is the product of an ancient intragenic duplication that led to homologous carboxyl and amino domains, each of which has one binding site for trivalent iron and two for bicarbonate [40].

The liver synthesises transferrin and secretes it into the plasma. Transferrin is also produced locally in the testes and in the central nervous system [41]. These two sites are relatively inaccessible to proteins in the general circulation (blood:testis barrier, blood:brain barrier). The locally synthesised transferrin could play a role in iron metabolism in these tissues.

Essentially all circulating plasma iron normally is bound to transferrin. In addition, two-thirds of serum transferrin exists as apotransferrin and will quickly capture the free iron which is released from the cell [42]. This chelation serves three purposes: it renders iron soluble under physiologic conditions, it prevents iron-mediated free radical toxicity, and it facilitates transport into cells.

The normal concentration of transferrin in plasma is about 2.2 to 3.5 g/L.

Transferrin carries iron from the intestine, the reticuloendothelial system, and the liver parenchymal cells to all proliferating cells in the body, mostly to erythrocyte precursors in the bone marrow for haemoglobin synthesis [43]. It carries iron into cells through a receptor-mediated endocytosis. After dissociation of iron, transferrin and its receptor return undegraded to the extracellular environment and the cell membrane, respectively.

The blood transferrin level is tested for several reasons: to determine the cause of anaemia, to examine iron metabolism (for example, in iron-deficiency anaemia) and to determine the iron-carrying capacity of blood. Low transferrin can impair haemoglobin production and so lead to anaemia. Low transferrin can be due to poor production of transferrin by the liver (where it is made) or excessive loss of transferrin through the kidneys into the urine. Many conditions including infections and malignancies can depress transferrin levels. The transferrin is abnormally high in iron deficiency anaemia.

## Positive Acute-Phase Proteins

### Fibrinogen

Fibrinogen (factor 1) is a circulating glycoprotein synthesised by the liver. Its MW is 350 kDa. It is present not only in plasma and liver but also in the platelet cytosol. Its plasma half life is 2–4 days [44]. The molecule is constituted by three pairs of polypeptide chains linked by disulphur bridges to form a large molecule with a symmetric structure, with three types of chains defined as Aa, Bb and

gamma. The Aa and Bb chains are subject to thrombin action, which removes the fibrinopeptides A and B, whereas the gamma chains are not cleaved. Removal of fibrinopeptides is associated with clot formation, since the cleaved fibrinogen molecules (the so-called fibrin monomers) spontaneously form a gel phase and aggregate to form insoluble fibrin filaments.

The activation of fibrinogen to fibrin, mediated by thrombin, represents the last step in clot formation. Levels of fibrinogen are increased as an acute-phase response [45] in many pathological states as well as in all acute and chronic inflammation conditions [46]. Horizontal and prospective studies since the 1950s have shown that hypercoagulability and elevated plasma fibrinogen concentrations are associated with the presence of clinical vascular disease [47, 48] and increased vascular events [49–53]. Although most epidemiological studies have strongly documented the independent and powerful role of fibrinogen in cardiovascular risk, in many of them fibrinogen was significantly correlated with other important arteriosclerotic risk factors, such as age, body weight, plasma lipids, hypertension and smoking [54–56]. Thus, hyperfibrinogenaemia and the altered coagulation may mediate the effects of these factors on atherogenesis [56]. Normal fibrinogen concentrations may vary among different laboratories and populations, but usually range between 150 and 500 mg/dl.

Hyperfibrinogenaemia has also been found in diabetes [54–56], and it was correlated with plasma glucose values [57]. In the general population an association with insulin levels has been found [58], thus confirming a relationship between fibrinogen and insulin resistance, a common characteristic in type 2 insulin diabetes [59].

The fibrinogen fractional synthesis rate (FSR) was found to be increased in acute and marked insulin deficiency in type 1 diabetes [59], and it was reduced by insulin infusion in both normal and diabetic individuals [20, 59]. A mixed meal increased fibrinogen FSR, although with a variable statistical significance [17, 19, 60]. We have shown that insulin infusion in type 2 diabetes paradoxically increased fibrinogen FSR, whereas it did not change it in controls [61], thus suggesting a possible link between insulin resistance and hyperfibrinogenaemia at the production level. Glucagon infusion acutely increased fibrinogen production in healthy humans [62]. Since glucagon is a stress hormone [63, 64], these data suggest a link between acute-phase proteins and stress hormones, possibly mediated by proinflammatory interleukins at the liver level.

## C-reactive protein

C-reactive protein (CRP) is an acute-phase protein that is a very sensitive index of inflammation. Its serum level increases as much as 1000-fold during the acute phase of inflammation [65–68]. Structurally, it is a planar pentamer of identical subunits, expressed and synthesised almost exclusively in the liver by the hepatocytes. Its normal concentrations, using a sensitive assay, normally range between 0 and 2.5 mg/l.

Besides being an index of inflammation, CRP concentrations have been associated with morbidity and mortality under a number of conditions. Largely based on the pioneering work of Ridker et al. [65–67], a large bulk of evidence derived from epidemiological studies, from primary and secondary prevention studies and from trials conducted in patients with acute coronary syndromes, has revealed that the plasma concentration of such a relatively simple marker of inflammation, CRP, could predict the risk of a first or of a recurrent coronary event, beyond the contribution of classical risk factors [67].

Evidence has also accumulated that CRP may further play a pivotal role in promoting atherogenesis. It has been shown that CRP increases the release of inflammatory cytokines [69], enhances the binding of monocytes to endothelial cells [70] and favours the formation of macrophage foam cells [71]. In addition, CRP decreases endothelial nitric oxide synthase activation and increases the expression of endothelial cell adhesion molecules, chemokines, endothelin-1, and plasminogen activator inhibitor-1 [72, 73].

Due to these multifaceted actions, the study of factors responsible for the elevated CRP concentrations is important both from public health and clinical perspectives. Therefore, therapeutic options are pursued that can optimally reduce inflammation (along with its most popular marker, CRP).

Many clinical conditions are associated with an inflammatory state and/or profiles. Obesity [74], especially that of the abdominal type [75], is commonly associated with elevated CRP concentrations. The expanded abdominal fat deposits of overweight/obese patients represent a source of inflammatory cytokines (interleukin [IL]-6 and tumour necrosis factor [TNF]-$\alpha$) [76]. The production of CRP by the hepatocytes is stimulated by IL-6 [77], and adipose tissue is a key source of circulating IL-6 in patients with abdominal obesity [78, 79]. Intervention studies have shown that weight loss is associated with a reduction in circulating CRP concentrations, and this reduction is proportional to the extent of weight loss [80, 81].

The degree of physical activity/fitness can also affect CRP concentrations [82]. Individuals with a low cardiorespiratory fitness (who are also often sedentary) exhibit increased CRP levels compared with fit individuals. Such a difference remained significant even after adjustment for the degree of adiposity, assessed by the body mass index (BMI) [83]. Since endurance exercise training affects risk factors for coronary heart disease (glucose tolerance and insulin effectiveness, body composition, plasma lipoprotein levels, fibrinolysis and thrombosis, endothelial function, etc.) [84], it is of interest to evaluate the extent to which exercise training might affect inflammation and, if so, what are the parameters affected by exercise training possibly associated with its beneficial effect on CRP levels.

It has been shown repeatedly that endurance training can reduce CRP concentrations [85, 86]. Part of this effect seems to be mediated by the exercise-associated weight loss. The specific impact of selective loss of visceral adipose tissue [87] associated with endurance exercise training needs to be examined. Interestingly, pharmacotherapy of atherogenic dyslipidaemias with statins and fibrates can also reduce CRP levels [87, 88]. As with abdominal obesity, type 2 diabetes and the metabolic syndrome (which are major correlates of elevated CRP concentrations) have achieved an epidemic status. The importance of targeting the sedentary lifestyle, unfortunately adopted by an increasing number of our population, needs to be further emphasised.

## Fibronectin

Fibronectins (FNs) are high molecular weight gly-coproteins found in plasma, on cell surfaces, and in extracellular matrices [89]. Cell FN (cFN) and plasma FN (pFN) are two different products of a single gene [90]. cFN is synthesised by fibroblasts and other cell types, which secrete it into the extracellular matrix, where it assembles in a fibrillar form. In contrast, pFN is synthesised by hepatocytes and circulates as a soluble molecule in plasma [91]. Both forms are disulphide-linked dimers of 250-Da subunits, taken from a pool of similar but not identical polypeptides. Sequencing studies have revealed that each polypeptide has three different types of internal repeats (homology types I, II and III, which are, on average, 40, 60 and 90 amino acid residues long, respectively) [92, 93]. The primary structural differences between the subunits are the result of a complex pattern of alternative splicing of the precursor mRNA.

By binding macromolecules such as collagen, fibrin, heparin, gelatin [94], as well as cells and bacteria, FNs play an important role in various contact processes such as cell attachment and spreading [95], cell migration, embryonic development, wound healing [96], haemostasis, opsonisation [97] and oncogenic transformation.

Fibronectin is commonly known as cold-insoluble globulin because it precipitates from plasma in the cold with fibrinogen and the factor VIII–von Willebrand factor complex.

## Ferritin

Iron is an essential element for mammalian cell growth. It is a required constituent of numerous enzymes, including iron–sulphur and heme proteins of the respiratory chain, as well as ribonucleotide reductase, which catalyses the rate-limiting step in DNA synthesis. However, 'free' iron has the capacity to participate in oxygen free radical formation via Fenton chemistry [98]. Balancing both the deleterious and beneficial effects of iron thus emerges as an essential aspect of cell survival. Ferritin plays a central role in the maintenance of this delicate intracellular iron balance [99–101]. This protein has the capacity to sequester up to 4500 atoms of iron in a ferrihydrite mineral core, and it functions to store iron not required for immediate metabolic needs.

Its ability to sequester the element gives ferritin the dual functions of iron detoxification and iron reserve.

Ferritin is a 24-subunit protein composed of two subunit types, termed H and L, which perform complementary functions in the protein. The H subunit is thought to play a role in the rapid detoxification of iron (it contains the majority of the ferroxidase activity that oxidises iron to the Fe(III) form for deposition within the core), whereas the L subunit facilitates iron nucleation, mineralisation and long-term iron storage. The ratio of H to L subunits varies depending on tissue type and physiological status, and changes in response to inflammation or infection [102]. Its plasma concentrations usually range between 20 and 300 $\mu$g/l.

Several results support a role of ferritin as a protectant against oxygen free radical-mediated damage. Exposure of endothelial cells to haemin was observed to induce ferritin synthesis and concordantly reduce the cytotoxic response of these cells to toxic doses of $H_2O_2$ [103].

## References

1. Millward DJ, Rivers JPW (1989) The need for indispensable amino acids: the concept of the anabolic drive. Diabetes Metab Rev 5:191–212
2. Wolfe RR, Goodenaugh RD, Wolfe MH et al (1982) Isotopic analysis of leucine and urea metabolism in exercising humans. J Appl Physiol 52:458–466
3. Tessari P, Zanetti M, Barazzoni R et al (1996) Mechanisms of post-prandial protein accretion in human skeletal muscle: insight from leucine and phenylalanine forearm kinetics. J Clin Invest 98:1361–1372
4. Devlin JT, Brodsky I, Scrimgeour A et al (1990) Amino acid metabolism after intense exercise. Am J Physiol 21:E249–E255
5. Kimball SR, Jefferson LS (2004) Regulation of global and specific mRNA translation by oral administration of branched-chain amino acids. Biochem Biophys Res Commun 313:423–427
6. Jefferson LS, Kimball SR (2003) Amino acids as regulators of gene expression at the level of mRNA

translation. J Nutr 133:2046S–2051S

7. Shah OJ, Anthony JC, Kimball SR, Jefferson LS (2000) 4E-BP1 and S6K1: translational integration sites for nutritional and hormonal information in muscle. Am J Physiol Endocrinol Metab 279:E715–E712

8. Munro HN, Crim MC (1988) The proteins and amino acids. In: Shils ME, Young VR (eds) Modern nutrition in health and disease. Lea & Febiger, Philadelphia, pp 1–37

9. Waterlow JC, Garlick PJ, Millward DJ (1978) Protein turnover in mammalian tissues and in the whole body. North Holland, Amsterdam

10. Reeds PJ, Fuller MF, Nicholson BA (1984) Metabolic basis of energy expenditure with particular reference to protein. In: Garrow JS, Halliday D (eds) Substrate and energy metabolism in man. John Libbey, London, pp 46–57

11. Doweiko JP, Nompleggi DJ (1991) Role of albumin in human physiology and pathophysiology. JPEN J Parenter Enteral Nutr 15:207–211

12. Rothschild MA (1972) Albumin synthesis (first of two parts). N Engl J Med 286:748–757

13. Rothschild MA, Oratz M, Schreiber S (1973) Albumin metabolism. Gastroenterology 64:324–337

14. Rothschild MA (1972) Albumin synthesis (second of two parts). N Engl J Med 286:816–820

15. De Feo P, Horber FF, Haymond MW (1992) Meal stimulation of albumin synthesis: a significant contributor to whole-body protein synthesis in humans. Am J Physiol 263:E794–E799

16. Cayol M, Boirie Y, Rambourdin F et al (1997) Influence of protein intake on whole body and splanchnic leucine kinetics in humans. Am J Physiol 272:E584–E591

17. Tessari P, Barazzoni R, Kiwanuka E et al (2002) Impairment of albumin and whole-body postprandial protein synthesis in compensated cirrhosis. Am J Physiol 282:E304–E311

18. Hunter KA, Ballmer PE, Anderson SE et al (1995) Acute stimulation of albumin synthesis rate with oral meal feeding in healthy subjects measured with [ring-2H5]phenylalanine. Clin Sci 88:235–242

19. Volpi E, Lucidi P, Cruciani G et al (1996) Contribution of amino acids and insulin to protein anabolism during meal absorption. Diabetes 45:1245–1252

20. De Feo P, Volpi E, Lucidi P et al (1993) Physiological increments in plasma insulin concentrations have selective and different effects on hepatic protein synthesis in normal humans. Diabetes 42:995–1002

21. Ballmer PE, McNurlan MA, Grant I, Garlick PJ (1995) Down regulation of albumin synthesis in the rat by human recombinant interleukin-1 beta or turpentine and the response to nutrients. JPEN J Parenter Enteral Nutr 19:266–271

22. Kanda Y, Goodman DS, Canfield RE, Morgan FJ (1974) The amino acid sequence of human plasma prealbumin. J Biol Chem 249:6796–6805

23. Blake CCF, Geisow MJ, Swan IDA et al (1974) Structure of human plasma prealbumin at 2.5 A resolution. A preliminary report on the polypeptide chain conformation quaternary structure and thyroxine binding. J Mol Biol 88:1–12

24. Sparkes RS, Sasaki H, Mohandas T ct al (1987) Assignment of the prealbumin (PALB) gene (familial amyloidotic polyneuropathy) to human chromosome region 18q11.2–q12.1. Hum Genet 75:151–154

25. Herbert J, Wilcox JN, Pham KC et al (1986) Transthyretin: a choroid plexus specific transport protein in human brain. Neurology 36:900–911

26. Episkopou V, Maeda S, Nishiguchi S et al (1993) Disruption of the transthyretin gene results in mice with depressed levels of plasma retinol and thyroid hormone. Proc Natl Acad Sci USA 90:2375–2379

27. Schreiber G, Aldred AR, Jaworowski A et al (1990) Thyroxine transport from blood to brain via transthyretin synthesis in choroid plexus. Am J Physiol 258:R338–R345

28. Ernstrom U, Petterson T, Jornvall H (1995) A yellow component associated with human transthyretin has properties like a pterin derivative, 7,8-dihydropterin-6-carboxaldehyde. FEBS Lett 360:177–182

29. Sousa MM, Berglund L, Saraiva MJ (2000) Transthyretin in high density lipoproteins – association via apolipoprotein. A-I. J Lipid Res 41:58–65

30. Shirahama T, Skinner M, Westermark P et al (1982) Senile cerebral amyloid. Prealbumin as a common constituent in the neuritic plaques, in the neurofibrillary tangle and in the microangiopathic lesion. Am J Pathol 107:41–50

31. Saraiva MJM (2001) Transthyretin mutations in hyperthyroxinemia and amyloid diseases. Hum Mutat 17:493–503

32. Refetoff S, Murata Y, Mori Y et al (1996) Thyroxine-binding globulin: organization of the gene and variants. Horm Res 45:128–138

33. Mori Y, Miura Y, Oiso Y et al (1995) Precise localization of the human thyroxine-binding globulin gene to chromosome Xq22.2 by fluorescence in situ hybridization. Hum Genet 96:481–482

34. Schussler GC (2000) The thyroxine-binding proteins. Thyroid 10:141–149

35. Flink IL, Bailey TJ, Gustafson TA et al (1986) Complete amino acid sequence of human thyroxine-binding globulin deduced from cloned DNA: close homology to the serine antiproteases. Proc Natl Acad Sci USA 83:7708–7712

36. Gettins PG (2002) Serpin structure, mechanism, and function. Chem Rev 102:4751–4804

37. Murata Y, Sarne DH, Horwitz AL et al (1985) Characterization of thyroxine-binding globulin secreted by a human hepatoma cell line. J Clin Endocrinol Metab 60:472–478

38. Burr WA, Ramsden DB, Hoffenberg R (1980) Hereditary abnormalities of thyroxine-binding globulin concentration. A study of 19 kindreds with inherited increase or decrease of thyroxine-binding

globulin. Q J Med 49:295–313

39. Huebers HA, Finch CA (1987) The physiology of transferrin and transferrin receptors. Physiol Rev 67:520–582

40. MacGillivray RTA, Moore SA, Chen J et al (1998) Two high-resolution crystal structures of the recombinant N-lobe of human transferrin reveal a structural change implicated in iron release. Biochemistry 37:7919–7928

41. Aldred AR, Dickson PW, Marley PD, Schreiber G (1987) Distribution of transferrin synthesis in brain and other tissue. J Biol Chem 262:5293–5297

42. Ponka P (1999) Cellular iron metabolism. Kidney Int Suppl 69:S2–S11

43. Ponka P (1997) Tissue-specific regulation of iron metabolism and heme synthesis: distinct control mechanisms in erythroid cells. Blood 89:1–25

44. Castaldi G, Liso V (1997) Malattie del sangue e degli organi Ematopoietici. McGraw-Hill, Milan

45. Gordon AH (1976) The acute phase plasma proteins. In: Bianchi R, Mariani G, Mcfarlane AS (eds) Plasma protein turnover. MacMillan Press, London, pp 381–394

46. Morimoto R, Tissieres A, Georgopoulos C (1990) Stress proteins in biology and medicine. Cold Spring Harbor Laboratory Press, Cold Spring Harbor

47. McDonald L, Edgill M (1959) Changes in coagulability of the blood during various phases of ischaemic heart-disease. Lancet 1:1115–1158

48. Dormandy JA, Hoare E, Colley J et al (1973) Clinical, haemodynamic, rhelogical and biochemical findings in 126 patients with intermittent claudication. Br Med J 4:576–581

49. Wilhemsen L, Svardsudd K, Korsan-Bengsten K (1984) Fibrinogen as a risk factor for stroke and myocardial infarction. N Eng J Med 311:501–505

50. Stone MC, Thorp JM (1985) Plasma fibrinogen – a major coronary risk factor. J R Coll Gen Pract 3:565–569

51. Meade TW, Brozovic M, Chakrabarti RR et al (1986) Haemostatic function and ischemic heart disease: principal results of the Northwich Park Heart Study. Lancet 533–537

52. Kannel WB, Wolf PA, Castelli WP, D'Agostino RB (1987) Fibrinogen and risk of cardiovascular disease: the Framingham Study. J Am Med Ass 258:1183–1186

53. Yarnell JW, Baker IA, Sweetnam PM et al (1991) Fibrinogen, viscosity and white cell count are major risk factors for ischemic heart disease. The Caerphilly and Speedwell collaborative heart disease studies. Circulation 83:836–844

54. Kannel WB, D'Agostino RB, Belanger AJ (1987) Fibrinogen, cigarette smoking and risk of cardiovascular disease: insights from the Framingham Study. Am Heart J 113:1006–1010

55. Folsom AR, Wu KK, Davis CE et al (1991) Population correlates of plasma fibrinogen and factor VII, putative cardiovascular risk factors. Atherosclerosis 91:191–205

56. Lee AJ, Lowe GDO, Woodward M, Tunstall-Pedoe H (1993) Fibrinogen in relation to personal history of prevalent hypertension, diabetes, stroke, intermittent claudication, coronary heart disease, and family history. The Scottish Heart Health Study. Br Heart J 69:338–342

57. Kannel WB, McGee DL (1979) Diabetes and cardiovascular disease. The Framingham Study. J Am Med Ass 241:2035–2038

58. DeFronzo R, Ferrannini E (1991) Insulin resistance. A multifaceted syndrome responsible for NIDDM, obesity, hypertension, dyslipidemia, and atherosclerotic cardiovascular disease. Diabetes Care 14:173–194

59. De Feo P, Gan Gaisano M, Haymond MW (1991) Differential effects of insulin deficiency on albumin and fibrinogen synthesis in humans. J Clin Invest 88:833–840

60. Bruttomesso D, Iori E, Kiwanuka E et al (2001) Insulin infusion normalizes fasting and post-prandial albumin and fibrinogen synthesis in Type 1 diabetes mellitus. Diabet Med 18:915–920

61. Barazzoni R, Kiwanuka E, Zanetti M et al (2003) Insulin acutely increases fibrinogen production in type 2 diabetic but not in non diabetic people. Diabetes 52:1851–1856

62. Tessari P, Iori E, Vettore M et al (1997) Evidence for acute stimulation of fibrinogen production by glucagon in humans. Diabetes 46:1368–1371

63. Unger RH (1972) Glucagon and insulin: glucagon ratio in diabetes and the other catabolic illnesses. Diabetes 20:834–838

64. Russell RCG, Walker CJ, Bloom SR (1975) Hyperglucagonemia in the surgical patient. Br Med J 1:10–12

65. Ridker PM, Hennekens CH, Buring JE, Rifai N (2000) C-reactive protein and other markers of inflammation in the prediction of cardiovascular disease in women. N Engl J Med 342:836–843

66. Ridker PM, Buring JE, Shih J et al (1998) Prospective study of C-reactive protein and the risk of future cardiovascular events among apparently healthy women. Circulation 98:731–733

67. Ridker PM (2003) Cardiology Patient Page. C-reactive protein: a simple test to help predict risk of heart attack and stroke. Circulation 108:e81–e85

68. Fuhrman MP, Charney P, Mueller CM (2004) Hepatic proteins and nutrition assessment. Am Diet Assoc 104:1258–1264

69. Ballou SP, Lozanski G (1992) Induction of inflammatory cytokine release from cultured human monocytes by C-reactive protein. Cytokine 4:361–368

70. Woollard KJ, Phillips DC, Griffiths HR (2002) Direct modulatory effect of C-reactive protein on primary human monocyte adhesion to human endothelial cells. Clin Exp Immunol 130:256–262

71. Fu T, Borensztajn J (2002) Macrophage uptake of low-density lipoprotein bound to aggregated C-

reactive protein: possible mechanism of foam-cell formation in atherosclerotic lesions. Biochem J 366:195–201

72. Pasceri V, Willerson JT, Yeh ET (2000) Direct proinflammatory effect of C-reactive protein on human endothelial cells. Circulation 102:2165–2168

73. Devaraj S, Xu DY, Jialal I (2003) C-reactive protein increases plasminogen activator inhibitor-1 expression and activity in human aortic endothelial cells: implications for the metabolic syndrome and athethrombosis. Circulation 107:398–404

74. Hak AE, Stehouwer CD, Bots ML et al (1999) Associations of C-reactive protein with measures of obesity, insulin resistance, and subclinical atherosclerosis in healthy, middle-aged women. Arterioscler Thromb Vasc Biol 19:1986–1991

75. Lemieux I, Pascot A, Prud'homme D et al (2001) Elevated C-reactive protein: another component of the atherothrombotic profile of abdominal obesity. Arterioscler Thromb Vasc Biol 21:961–967

76. Yudkin JS, Stehouwer CD, Emeis JJ, Coppack SW (1999) C-reactive protein in healthy subjects: associations with obesity, insulin resistance, and endothelial dysfunction: a potential role for cytokines originating from adipose tissue? Arterioscler Thromb Vasc Biol 19:972–978

77. Castell JV, Gomez-Lechon MJ, David M et al (1989) IL-6 is the major regulator of acute phase protein synthesis in adult human hepatocytes. FEBS Lett 242:237–239

78. Fried SK, Bunkin DA, Greenberg AS (1998) Omental and subcutaneous adipose tissues of obese subjects release IL-6: depot difference and regulation by glucocorticoid. J Clin Endocrinol Metab 83:847–850

79. Mohamed-Ali V, Goodrick S, Rawesh A et al (1997) Subcutaneous adipose tissue releases IL-6, but not tumor necrosis factor-alpha, in vivo. J Clin Endocrinol Metab 82:4196–4200

80. Heilbronn LK, Noakes M, Clifton PM (2001) Energy restriction and weight loss on very-low-fat diets reduce C-reactive protein concentrations in obese, healthy women. Arterioscler Thromb Vasc Biol 21:968–970

81. Tchernof A, Nolan A, Sites CK et al (2002) Weight loss reduces C-reactive protein levels in obese postmenopausal women. Circulation 105:564–569

82. Church TS, Barlow CE, Earnest CP et al (2002) Associations between cardiorespiratory fitness and C-reactive protein in men. Arterioscler Thromb Vasc Biol 22:1869–1876

83. Després JP, Lamarche B, Bouchard C et al (1995) Exercise and the prevention of dyslipidemia and coronary heart disease. Int J Obes 19:S45–S51

84. Okita K, Nishijima H, Murakami T et al (2004) Can exercise training with weight loss lower serum C-reactive protein levels? Arterioscler Thromb Vasc Biol 24:1868–1873

85. Obisesan TO, Leeuwenburgh C, Phillips T et al (2004) C-reactive protein genotypes affect baseline, but not exercise-training induced changes in C-reactive protein levels. Arterioscler Thromb Vasc Biol 24:1874–1879

86. Ross R, Dagnone D, Jones PJ et al (2000) Reduction in obesity and related comorbid conditions after diet-induced weight loss or exercise-induced weight loss in men. A randomized, controlled trial. Ann Intern Med 133:92–103

87. Staels B, Koenig W, Habib A et al (1998) Activation of human aortic smooth-muscle cells is inhibited by PPAR but not by PPAR activators. Nature 393:790–793

88. Ridker PM, Rifai N, Pfeffer MA et al (1999) Long-term effects of pravastatin on plasma concentration of C-reactive protein. The Cholesterol and Recurrent Events (CARE) Investigators. Circulation 100:230–235

89. Mosher DF (1980) Fibronectin. Prog Hemost Thromb 5:111–151

90. Kornblihtt AR, Vibe-Pedersen K, Baralle FE (1983) Isolation and characterization of cDNA clones for human and bovine fibronectins. Proc Natl Acad Sci USA 11:3218–3222

91. Tamkun JW, Hynes RO (1983) Plasma fibronectin is synthesized and secreted by hepatocytes. J Biol Chem 10258:4641–4647

92. Amrani DL, Homandberg GA, Tooney NM et al (1983) Separation and analysis of the major forms of plasma fibronectin. Biochem Biophys Acta 28748:308–320

93. Petersen TE, Thogersen HC, Skorstengaard K et al (1983) Partial primary structure of bovine plasma fibronectin: three types of internal homology. Proc Natl Acad Sci USA 1:137–141

94. Engvall E, Ruoslahti E (1977) Binding of soluble form of fibroblast surface protein, fibronectin, to collagen. Int J Cancer 1520:1–5

95. Yamada KM (1983) Cell surface interactions with extracellular materials. Annu Rev Biochem 52:761–799

96. Arneson MA, Hammerschmidt DE, Furcht LT, King RA (1980) A new form of Ehlers-Danlos syndrome. Fibronectin corrects defective platelet function. JAMA 244:144–147

97. Blumenstock FA, Saba TM, Weber P, Laffin R (1978) Biochemical and immunological characterization of human opsonic alpha2SB glycoprotein: its identity with cold-insoluble globulin. J Biol Chem 253:4287–4291

98. Linn S (1998) DNA damage by iron and hydrogen peroxide in vitro and in vivo. Drug Metab Rev 30:313–326

99. Harrison PM, Arosio P (1996) The ferritins: molecular properties, iron storage function and cellular regulation. Biochem Biophys Acta 1275:161–203

100. Theil EC (1990) The ferritin family of iron storage proteins. Adv Enzymol Relat Areas Mol Biol 63:421–449

101. Chasteen ND (1998) Ferritin. Uptake, storage, and release of iron. Met Ions Biol Syst 35:479–514

102. Rucker P, Torti FM, Torti SV (1996) Role of H and L subunits in mouse ferritin. J Biol Chem 271:33352–33357

103. Balla G, Jacob HS, Balla J et al (1992) Ferritin: a cytoprotective antioxidant strategem of endothelium. J Biol Chem 267:18148–18153

# Nutritional Status Assessment

Daniele Scevola, Angela Di Matteo, Omar Giglio, Silvia Scevola

## Nutritional Indexes

Malnutrition is not invariably diagnosed by physical findings of nutritional deficits. Malnutrition is a deviation (in excess or defect) from a complex of ideal scores. Paradoxically, a plump, flourishing patient may be affected by malnutrition if he or she exceeds this ideal score.

The nutritional status assessment of the patient enables a physician to correctly manage the patient's energy balance, and it is correlated with the evolution and prognosis of the underlying disease. The assessment includes historical and physical findings, anthropometric measurements, and biochemical and immunological assays, as summarised in Tables 1 and 2 and extensively treated in references [1–3].

## Nitrogenous Balance

The difference between the introduced nitrogen (IN) and urinary (UN), faecal (FN) and sweat (SN) nitrogen represents the nitrogenous balance (NB), as expressed by the equation: NB = IN – (UN + FN + SN). The balance may be positive, negative or null. The urinary daily loss of N is about 70% of IN, while faecal loss ranges between 10 and 20%. A negative balance induces a loss of body free fat mass and reduction of the pool of muscle and visceral proteins. Because 6.25 g of alimentary proteins contain 1 g of N, the nitrogenous balance can be calculated with the equation: NB = introduced proteins (g/6.25) – UN + 4 g*, where * = N loss with urine, sweat and faeces.

**Table 1.** Clinical and anthropometric parameters in nutritional assessment

| Clinical history | Physical examination | Anthropometric parameters |
|---|---|---|
| Involuntary diet restriction (poverty) | General appearance Skin, hair, nails | Height–weight ratio Body surface |
| Anorexia | Tongue, mucous membranes, dentition | Wrist circumference (bone structure) |
| Inadequate diet (alcoholism, vegetarianism) | Muscle masses (temporal, proximal extremity) | Skin folds (fat mass) |
| Gastrointestinal symptoms (dysphagia, vomiting, diarrhoea) | Eyes, loss of vision Neurological system | Mid-arm muscle circumference (lean mass) |
| Chronic illnesses | | |

## Biochemical Parameters

Many biochemical parameters, easy to obtain in clinical practice, are useful for the evaluation of nutritional status (Tables 2, 3).

## Muscle Proteins

Muscle proteins are expressed by two biochemical indexes: 3-methyl-histidine and so-called CHI (24-h urinary creatinine/ideal urinary creatinine with respect to height x 100) (Table 4).

**Table 2.** Biochemical and immunological parameters in nutritional assessment

| Biochemical assays | Immunological assays |
| --- | --- |
| Commonly available lab tests | Lymphocyte count |
| Nitrogenous balance | Skin tests to common recall antigens |
| Muscle proteins | C3 fraction |
| Plasma proteins (albumin, prealbumin, transferrin, retinol-binding protein, fibronectin) | |
| Vitamins and minerals | |

**Table 3.** Biochemical parameters of nutrition

Nitrogenous balance

Muscle proteins

Plasma proteins:

- Albumin

- Prealbumin

- Transferrin

- Retinol-binding-protein

Vitamins and oligoelements

Basic chemical–clinical tests

The amino acid 3-methyl-histidine is produced by degradation of muscle proteins and excreted only in urine. The dosage of this amino acid in urine over 24 h represents the proteic turnover. CHI is the best index of endogenous protein catabolism linked to the muscle mass.

## Plasma Proteins

The plasma values of albumin, prealbumin, transferrin, retinol-binding protein and fibronectin are the usual indexes of visceral (mainly hepatic) synthesis. Examples of different degrees of depletion of albumin, prealbumin and transferrin are reported in Table 5.

## Vitamins and Trace Elements

Physical signs of deficits of vitamins and trace elements are reported in Table 6. The daily

**Table 4.** Ideal urinary creatinine in relation to height in children and adults

| Height (cm) | Creatinine (mg/24 h) | | |
| --- | --- | --- | --- |
| | Children | Adult males | Adult females |
| 50.8 | 38 | | |
| 53.3 | 44 | | |
| 55.9 | 52 | | |
| 58.4 | 60 | | |
| 61.0 | 68 | | |
| 63.5 | 76 | | |
| 66.0 | 84 | | |
| 68.6 | 92 | | |
| 71.1 | 102 | | |
| 73.7 | 113 | | |
| 76.2 | 124 | | |
| 78.7 | 134 | | |
| 81.3 | 145 | | |
| 83,8 | 160 | | |
| 86.4 | 176 | | |
| 88.9 | 193 | | |
| 91.4 | 209 | | |
| 94.0 | 230 | | |
| 96.5 | 253 | | |
| 99.1 | 272 | | |
| 101.6 | 288 | | |
| 104.1 | 300 | | |
| 106.7 | 314 | | |
| 109.2 | 342 | | |
| 111.8 | 373 | | |
| 114.3 | 391 | | |
| 116.8 | 405 | | |
| 119.4 | 446 | | |
| 121.9 | 483 | | |
| 124.5 | 528 | | |
| 127.0 | 577 | | |
| 147.3 | | - | 830 |
| 149.9 | | - | 851 |
| 152.4 | | - | 875 |
| 154.9 | | - | 900 |

*continue* →

**Table 4** *continue*

|  | Children | Adult males | Adult females |
|---|---|---|---|
| 157.5 |  | 1288 | 925 |
| 160.0 |  | 1325 | 949 |
| 162.6 |  | 1359 | 977 |
| 165.1 |  | 1386 | 1006 |
| 167.6 |  | 1426 | 1044 |
| 170.2 |  | 1467 | 1076 |
| 172.7 |  | 1513 | 1109 |
| 175.3 |  | 1555 | 1141 |
| 177.8 |  | 1596 | 1174 |
| 180.3 |  | 1642 | 1206 |
| 182.9 |  | 1691 | 1240 |
| 185.4 |  | 1739 | - |
| 188.0 |  | 1785 | - |
| 190.5 |  | 1831 | - |
| 193.0 |  | 1891 | - |

requirements of vitamins and trace elements are reported in Tables 7 and 8 respectively.

## Basic Nutritional Tests

The main biochemical parameters related to the nutritional status and expression of metabolic functions are reported in Table 9.

Additional functional parameters have been introduced, and several specialised techniques, both invasive and non-invasive ($^3$H-labelled $H_2O$, total potassium measurement, CT scan, PET, MNR, DEXA, sonography, hydrostatic weight, bioelectric impedance analysis), have been developed.

**Table 5.** Concentrations of albumin, prealbumin and transferrin according to level of protein catabolism

| Albumin (g/dl) | Normal >3.5 | Slight depletion 2.8–3.5 | Medium depletion 2.1–2.7 | Severe depletion < 2.1 |
|---|---|---|---|---|
| Prealbumin (mg/dl) | Normal 15–29 | Slight depletion 10–15 | Medium depletion 5–10 | Severe depletion < 5 |
| Transferrin (mg/dl) | Normal 250–300 | Slight depletion 150–250 | Medium depletion 100–150 | Severe depletion < 100 |

**Table 6.** Signs and symptoms of vitamin and/or trace element deficits

| Organs involved | Signs and symptoms | Vitamin and/or trace element deficit |
|---|---|---|
| Hair, nails | Alopecia | Multiple deficits |
|  | Discolouring | Zinc |
|  | Dryness | A, E |
|  | Fragility |  |
| Skin | Pigmentation | Niacin |
|  | Erythema | Niacin |
|  | Acne | A |
|  | Dryness | A |
|  | Petechiae, ecchymoses | K, C |
|  | Scrotal dermatitis | Niacin |
| Eye | Blepharitis | B2 |
|  | Dry conjunctiva | A |
|  | Night blindness | A |
| Mouth | Cheilosis | B2 |
|  | Stomatitis | B12, C |
|  | Glossitis | Niacin, folates, B12 |
|  | Taste bud atrophy | Niacin |
|  | Magenta tongue | B2 |
| Bones, joints | Valgus or varus knee | D |
|  | Rib 'rosary' | D |
|  | Reduction of tendon reflexes | B1, B12 |

**Table 7.** Daily requirements for vitamins

| Vitamin | Requirement | Level in connection with nutritional status | | |
| | | Unit of measure | Severe defect | Marginal | Acceptable |
|---|---|---|---|---|---|
| A | 2,000 IU | µg%ml | < 10 | 10–19 | > 20 |
| Carotene[a] | 4,000 IU | mg%ml | < 20 | 20–39 | > 40 |
| D[b] | 200 IU | ng%ml | < 7 | 10–27 | > 27 |
| E | 10 IU | mg%ml | < 0.2 | 0.2–0.6 | > 0.6 |
| B1 | 3 mg | [c] | < 27 | 7–65 | > 65 |
| B2 | 3.6 mg | [c] | < 27 | 27–79 | > 80 |
| B3 | 15 mg | [c] | < 200 | - | > 200 |
| B5 | 40 mg | mg/g creatinine | < 0.5 | 0.5–1.6 | > 1.6 |
| B6 | 4 mg | [c] | < 20 | - | > 20 |
| B7 | 60 µg | mg/ml | < 0.8 | 0.8–1.4 | > 2.5 |
| B9 | 400 µg | mg/ml | < 2 | 2.1–5.9 | > 6 |
| B12 | 5 µg | pg/ml | < 100 | - | > 100 |
| C | 100 mg | mg%ml | < 0.1 | 0.1–0.2 | > 0.2 |
| K | 5–10 mg | ng/ml | < 1 | 1–3 | > 3 |

[a]1 IU (vit. A = 0.3 µg; beta carotene = 0.6 µg); [b]dosed as 25-OH-vitamin D; [c]urinary levels expressed in µg/g creatinine

**Table 8.** Daily requirements for trace elements

| Trace element | Requirement |
|---|---|
| Sodium (Na) | 50–250 mEq |
| Potassium (K) | 30–200 mEq |
| Chlorine (Cl) | 50–250 mEq |
| Magnesium (Mg) | 10–30 mEq |
| Calcium (Ca) | 10–20 mEq |
| Phosphorus (P) | 10–40 mmol |
| Zinc (Zn) | 2.5–4 mg |
| Copper (Cu) | 0.5–1.5 mg |
| Chromium (Cr) | 10–15 µg |
| Manganese (Mn) | 0.15–0.8 mg |
| Fluorine (F) | 1.5–4 µg |
| Iodine (I) | 150 µg |
| Selenium (Se) | 50 µg |
| Iron (Fe) | 10–18 mg |

## Anthropometric Indexes

The extent of body growth is determined by genetic, environmental and nutritional factors. The anthropometric evaluation of subcutaneous fat, bone structure and muscle mass is the most relevant method in assessing the nutritional status.

## Height and Body Weight

Unclothed measurements must be taken using an anthropometer and weight scales. Body weight is the most obvious index of nutritional status, but, taken alone, it is not an accurate measurement. Actual body weight must be compared with ideal body weight (IBW) and other anthropometric parameters. For example, patients with ascites and/or oedema may have a normal body weight but severe malnutrition. Several approaches are used for estimating the IBW. One simple method consists of measuring body height and wrist circumference as an index of bone structure. The subject is allocated to one of three groups (short-limbed, normal-limbed or long-limbed), and the ideal body weight (Y) is estimated as reported in Table 10a.

Other approaches suggest different methods for the calculation of IBW, for example:
1. IBW = height (cm) – 100 ± 10% for males; IBW = height (cm) – 100/104 ± 10% for females

**Table 9.** Reference values of main biochemical tests used in the study of nutritional status

| Test | Unit of measure | Normal range |
| --- | --- | --- |
| Haemoglobin | g/dl | 14–18 |
| Haematocrit | % | 40–54 |
| Red blood cells | millions/mm$^3$ | 4.5–6 |
| White blood cells | thousands/mm$^3$ | 4.5–8 |
| Lymphocytes | % | 25–35 |
| Iron | µg/dl | 75–175 |
| Sodium | mEq/l | 135–145 |
| Magnesium | mEq/l | 1.5–2.3 |
| Potassium | mEq/l | 3.5–5.0 |
| Phosphates | mg/dl | 2.5–4.5 |
| Chlorine | mEq/l | 98–110 |
| Calcium | mg/dl | 8.5–10 |
| Glucose | mg/dl | 65–110 |
| Total cholesterol | mg/dl | 150–250 |
| Esterified cholesterol | % | 60–80 |
| Free cholesterol | % | 20–40 |
| HDL cholesterol (M) | mg/dl | 45 |
| HDL cholesterol (F) | mg/dl | 55 |
| Total proteins | g/dl | 6–8 |
| Total bilirubin | mg/dl | 0.1–1.1 |
| Aspartate aminotransferase | U/l | 7–40 |
| Alanine aminotransferase | U/l | 10–45 |
| Alkaline phosphatase | U/l | 30–115 |
| Blood urea nitrogen | mg/dl | 7–23 |
| Uric acid | mg/dl | 2.3–7 |
| Total lipids | mg/dl | 400–900 |
| Triglycerides | mg/dl | 36–165 |
| Betalipoproteins | mg/dl | 360–740 |
| Phosphatides | mg/dl | 150–250 |
| Non-esterified fatty acids | mEq%ml | 0.09–0.06 |
| Lipoproteins | % | 6–12 |
| Pre-alpha-lipoproteins (VHDL) | % | 22–32 |
| Alpha-lipoproteins (HDL) | % | 16–24 |
| Pre-beta-lipoproteins (VLDL) | % | 37–51 |
| Chylomicrons | % | 0–2 |
| Alpha/beta ratio | % | 12–25 |

2. IBW = (height – 150) x 0.75 + 50 for males; IBW = (height – 150) x 0.60 + 50 for females
3. IBW = height – 100 – (height – 150)/4 for males; IBW = height – 100 – (height – 150)/2 for females.
An adaptation of the above methods takes into account the subject's age, without gender difference:
1. IBW = 50 + [3 (height – 150)/4] + [(age – 20)/4]
2. IBW = 0.8 x (height – 100) + age/2
3. IBW = 1.012 x height – 107.5.

Table 10b shows IBW values according to height and bone structure.

**Table 10a.** Estimating ideal body weight by anthropometry

|  | Short-limbed | Normal-limbed | Long-limbed |
|---|---|---|---|
| Male | $Y = 75 X – 58.5$ | $Y = 75 X – 63.5$ | $Y = 75 X – 69$ |
| Female | $Y = 68 X – 51.5$ | $Y = 68 X – 58$ | $Y = 68 X – 61$ |
| Short limbed | Male with wrist circumference > 20 cm<br>Female with wrist circumference > 18 cm | | |
| Normal limbed | Male with wrist circumference 16–20 cm<br>Female with wrist circumference 14–18 cm | | |
| Long limbed | Male with wrist circumference < 16 cm<br>Female with wrist circumference < 14 cm | | |

$Y$, ideal weight; $X$, height (metres)

**Table 10b.** Ideal weight (kg) and bone size with respect to skeletal structure

| Male Height (cm) | Skeletal structure | | | Female Height (cm) | Skeletal structure | | |
|---|---|---|---|---|---|---|---|
|  | Light | Middle | Heavy |  | Light | Middle | Heavy |
| 164 | 54.3–57.9 | 57.0–62.5 | 60.2–68.2 | 152 | 43.4–47.0 | 45.6–51.0 | 49.2–56.5 |
| 166 | 55.4–59.2 | 58.1–63.7 | 61.7–69,6 | 154 | 44.4–48.0 | 46.7–52.1 | 50.3–57.6 |
| 168 | 56.5–60.6 | 59.2–65.1 | 62.9–71.1 | 156 | 45.4–49.1 | 47.7–53.2 | 513–58.6 |
| 170 | 57.9–62.0 | 60.7–66.6 | 64.3–72.9 | 158 | 46.5–50.2 | 48.8–54.3 | 52.4–59.7 |
| 172 | 59.4–63.4 | 62.1–68.3 | 66.0–74.7 | 160 | 47.6–51.2 | 49.9–55.3 | 53.5–60.8 |
| 174 | 60.8–64.9 | 63.5–69.9 | 67.6–76.2 | 162 | 48.7–52.3 | 51.0–56.8 | 54.6–612 |
| 176 | 62.2–66.4 | 64.9–71.3 | 69.0–77.6 | 164 | 49.8–53.4 | 52.0–58.2 | 55.9–63.7 |
| 178 | 63.6–68.2 | 66.4–72.8 | 70.4–79.1 | 166 | 50.8–54.6 | 53.3–59.8 | 57.3–65.1 |
| 180 | 65.1–69.6 | 67.8–74.5 | 71.9–80.9 | 168 | 52.0–56.0 | 54.7–61.5 | 58.8–66.5 |
| 182 | 66.5–71.0 | 69.2–76.3 | 73.6–82.7 | 170 | 53.4–57.5 | 56.1–62.9 | 60.2–67.9 |
| 184 | 67.9–72.5 | 70.7–78.1 | 75.2–84.3 | 172 | 54.8–58.9 | 57.5–64.3 | 61.6–69.3 |
| 186 | 69.4–74.0 | 72.1–79.9 | 76.7–86.2 | 174 | 56.3–60.3 | 59.0–65.8 | 63.1–70.8 |
| 188 | 70.8–75.8 | 73.5–81.7 | 78.5–88.0 | 176 | 57.7–61.9 | 60.4–67.2 | 64.5–72.3 |
| 190 | 72.2–77.2 | 75.3–83.5 | 80.3–89.8 | 178 | 59.1–63.6 | 61.8–68.6 | 65.9–74.1 |
| 192 | 73.6–78.6 | 77.1–85.3 | 81.8–91.6 | 180 | 60.5–65.1 | 63.3–70.1 | 67.3–75.9 |
| 194 | 75.1–80.1 | 78.9–87.0 | 83.2–93.4 | 182 | 62.0–66.5 | 64.7–71.5 | 68.8–77.7 |
|  |  |  |  | 184 | 63.4–67.9 | 61.1–72.9 | 70.2–79.5 |

## Body Mass Index

A more recent approach to the evaluation of nutritional status refers to body mass index (BMI). It affords a more accurate measurement, as follows: body weight (kg)/height$^2$ (m$^2$).

The reference table (Table 11) includes only five classes: 0 = < 20 kg/m$^2$, weight deficit; N = 20–24.9 kg/m$^2$, normal; 1 = 25–29.9 kg/m$^2$, mild weight excess; 2 = 30–39.9 kg/m$^2$, obesity; 3 = > 40 kg/m$^2$, severe obesity.

**Table 11.** Body mass index: values of the body classes

| | |
|---|---|
| 0 = < 20.0 kg/m$^2$ | Body mass deficit |
| N = 20.0–24.9 kg/m$^2$ | Normal |
| 1 = 25.0–29.9 kg/m$^2$ | Moderate excess of weight |
| 2 = 30.0–39.9 kg/m$^2$ | Significant excess of weight |
| 3 = > 40.0 kg/m$^2$ | Very significant excess of weight |

Recently it has been proposed that the obesity threshold should be lowered to 25 kg/m$^2$, based on epidemiological studies showing an increase in all-cause, metabolic, cancer and cardiovascular morbidity when BMI is greater than or equal to 25. In normal adults in western countries, the mean is 24, in less developed countries it is 20–21, with a mean of 18 in some cases.

BMI has been used in social and economic studies and a good correlation was observed with lean muscle mass, serum albumin levels, oxygen expenditure, hydrostatic weight measurement, potassium and water content. A statistically significant correlation of BMI and morbidity-mortality from all causes, diabetes, cardiovascular and infectious diseases, and cancer has been shown by unequivocal studies.

## Body Circumferences

Measurement of circumferences of different areas of the body enables the estimation of lean mass and total fatty mass. Mid-arm muscle circumference (MAC) is a good index of lean mass and is estimated by the equation:

MAC (mm) = AC (arm circumference) – (π triceps skin fold) (mm).

The same equation is used for other body sites. Table 12a,b reports percentiles of MAC respectively for males and females.

**Table 12a.** Percentiles of mid-arm circumference (mm) in males aged 1–74 years

| Age (years) | Percentile | | | | | | |
|---|---|---|---|---|---|---|---|
| | 5° | 10° | 25° | 50° | 75° | 90° | 95° |
| 1–1.9 | 110 | 113 | 119 | 127 | 135 | 144 | 147 |
| 2–2.9 | 111 | 114 | 122 | 130 | 140 | 146 | 150 |
| 3–3.9 | 117 | 123 | 131 | 137 | 143 | 148 | 153 |
| 4–4.9 | 123 | 126 | 133 | 141 | 148 | 156 | 159 |
| 5–5.9 | 128 | 133 | 140 | 147 | 154 | 162 | 168 |
| 6–6.9 | 131 | 135 | 142 | 151 | 161 | 170 | 177 |
| 7–7.9 | 137 | 139 | 151 | 160 | 168 | 177 | 190 |
| 8–8.9 | 140 | 145 | 154 | 162 | 170 | 182 | 187 |
| 9–9.9 | 151 | 154 | 161 | 170 | 183 | 196 | 202 |
| 10–10.9 | 156 | 160 | 166 | 180 | 191 | 209 | 221 |
| 11–11.9 | 159 | 165 | 173 | 183 | 195 | 205 | 230 |
| 12–12.9 | 167 | 171 | 182 | 195 | 210 | 223 | 241 |
| 13–13.9 | 172 | 179 | 196 | 211 | 226 | 238 | 245 |
| 14–14.9 | 189 | 199 | 212 | 223 | 240 | 260 | 264 |
| 15–15.9 | 199 | 204 | 218 | 237 | 254 | 266 | 272 |
| 16–16.9 | 213 | 225 | 234 | 249 | 269 | 287 | 296 |
| 17–17.9 | 224 | 231 | 245 | 258 | 273 | 294 | 312 |
| 18–24 | 235 | 244 | 258 | 272 | 289 | 308 | 323 |
| 25–34 | 242 | 253 | 265 | 280 | 300 | 317 | 329 |
| 35–44 | 250 | 256 | 271 | 287 | 303 | 321 | 330 |
| 45–54 | 240 | 249 | 265 | 281 | 298 | 315 | 326 |
| 55–64 | 228 | 244 | 262 | 279 | 296 | 310 | 318 |
| 65–74 | 225 | 237 | 253 | 269 | 285 | 299 | 307 |

**Table 12b.** Percentiles of mid-arm circumference (mm) in females aged 1–74 years

| Age (years) | Percentile | | | | | | |
|---|---|---|---|---|---|---|---|
| | 5° | 10° | 25° | 50° | 75° | 90° | 95° |
| 1–1.9 | 105 | 111 | 117 | 124 | 132 | 139 | 143 |
| 2–2.9 | 111 | 114 | 119 | 126 | 133 | 142 | 147 |
| 3–3.9 | 113 | 119 | 124 | 132 | 140 | 146 | 152 |
| 4–4.9 | 115 | 121 | 128 | 136 | 144 | 152 | 157 |
| 5–5.9 | 125 | 128 | 134 | 142 | 151 | 159 | 165 |
| 6–6.9 | 130 | 133 | 138 | 145 | 154 | 166 | 171 |
| 7–7.9 | 129 | 135 | 142 | 151 | 160 | 171 | 176 |
| 8–8.9 | 138 | 140 | 151 | 160 | 171 | 183 | 194 |
| 9–9.9 | 147 | 150 | 158 | 167 | 180 | 194 | 198 |
| 10–10.9 | 148 | 150 | 159 | 170 | 180 | 190 | 197 |
| 11–11.9 | 150 | 158 | 171 | 181 | 196 | 217 | 223 |
| 12–12.9 | 162 | 166 | 180 | 191 | 201 | 214 | 220 |
| 13–13.9 | 169 | 175 | 183 | 198 | 211 | 226 | 240 |
| 14–14.9 | 174 | 179 | 190 | 201 | 216 | 232 | 247 |
| 15–15.9 | 175 | 178 | 189 | 202 | 215 | 228 | 264 |
| 16–16.9 | 170 | 180 | 190 | 202 | 216 | 234 | 249 |
| 17–24 | 177 | 185 | 194 | 206 | 221 | 236 | 249 |
| 25–34 | 183 | 189 | 200 | 214 | 229 | 249 | 266 |
| 35–44 | 185 | 192 | 206 | 220 | 240 | 261 | 274 |
| 45–54 | 188 | 195 | 207 | 222 | 243 | 266 | 278 |
| 55–64 | 186 | 195 | 208 | 226 | 244 | 263 | 281 |
| 65–74 | 186 | 195 | 208 | 225 | 244 | 265 | 281 |

### Skin Folds

Skin fold measurements in different body sites, where subcutaneous fat is more abundant, estimate fat mass in a non-invasive way, and are obtained by using special calipers. Standard sites and methods of measurement are shown in Table 13.

Percentiles of the most common skin fold thicknesses in healthy people are reported in Tables 14–19.

From multiple measurements of skin folds, the percentage of body fat can be easily calculated by means of the following equation:
% fatty mass = [(4971/body density) – 4519)] x 100
Body density is calculated as follows:
density = c – m x log skin fold thickness (mm);
c and m are constants correlated to the age and the sex, as reported in Tables 20 and 21.

The sum of multiple skin fold measurements affords an accurate estimation of body fat, related to age and sex (Table 22).

### Body Surface

Body surface is an important anthropometric parameter included in the estimation of resting energy expenditure (REE) or basal metabolism (BM) and for drug dosage. Body surface is estimated using body weight and height in the equations:

$$S = W^{0.425} \times H^{0.725} \times 71.84$$
or:
$$S = \log W \times 0.425 + \log H \times 0.725 + 1.8564$$

In this expression, S is surface, W is body weight and H is height. Special nomograms can be derived in this way.

**Table 13.** Skin folds and methods of measurement

| | |
|---|---|
| Triceps skin fold | On dorsal side of left arm relaxed, to medium point of humerus between olecranus and acromion, in vertical direction |
| Biceps skin fold | On median and front line of arm, at the point of measurement of arm circumference, in vertical direction |
| Subscapular skin fold | In left angle subscapular (1–2 cm under), in diagonal direction |
| Iliac skin fold | At the point of contact between axillary median line and iliac crest, in diagonal direction |
| Cheek fold | In the middle of line joining labial commissure to external auditory meatus |
| Meatus fold | Between auditory meatus and hyoid bone |
| Pectoral fold | On big pectoral muscle in correspondence of axillary front pillar, with arm extended laterally |
| Thoracic fold | Corresponding to tenth rib, on medium axillary line |
| Abdominal fold | Corresponding to third medial of line joining umbilicus to iliac spine front upper |
| Thigh skin fold | At the medium point of line joining iliac spine front upper to rotula |
| Knee fold | Onto the rotula |
| Calf fold | Under popliteal cavity with leg semiflexed and fingers on the ground, on median back line, in vertical direction |

**Table 14.** Percentiles of triceps skin fold (mm) in males aged 1–74 years

| Age (years) | Percentile | | | | | | |
|---|---|---|---|---|---|---|---|
| | 5° | 10° | 25° | 50° | 75° | 90° | 95° |
| 1–1.9 | 6 | 7 | 8 | 10 | 12 | 14 | 16 |
| 2–2.9 | 6 | 7 | 8 | 10 | 12 | 14 | 15 |
| 3–3.9 | 6 | 7 | 8 | 10 | 11 | 14 | 15 |
| 4–4.9 | 6 | 6 | 8 | 9 | 11 | 12 | 14 |
| 5–5.9 | 6 | 6 | 8 | 9 | 11 | 14 | 15 |
| 6–6.9 | 5 | 6 | 7 | 8 | 10 | 13 | 16 |
| 7–7.9 | 5 | 6 | 7 | 9 | 12 | 15 | 17 |
| 8–8.9 | 5 | 6 | 7 | 8 | 10 | 13 | 16 |
| 9–9.9 | 6 | 6 | 7 | 10 | 13 | 17 | 18 |
| 10–10.9 | 6 | 6 | 8 | 10 | 14 | 18 | 21 |
| 11–11.9 | 6 | 6 | 8 | 11 | 16 | 20 | 24 |
| 12–12.9 | 6 | 6 | 8 | 11 | 14 | 22 | 28 |
| 13–13.9 | 5 | 5 | 7 | 10 | 14 | 22 | 26 |
| 14–14.9 | 4 | 5 | 7 | 9 | 14 | 21 | 24 |
| 15–15.9 | 4 | 5 | 6 | 8 | 11 | 18 | 24 |
| 16–16.9 | 4 | 5 | 6 | 8 | 12 | 16 | 22 |

*continue* →

**Table 14** *continue*

| Age (years) | | | | Percentile | | | |
|---|---|---|---|---|---|---|---|
| | 5° | 10° | 25° | 50° | 75° | 90° | 95° |
| 17–17.9 | 5 | 5 | 6 | 8 | 12 | 16 | 19 |
| 18–24 | 4 | 5 | 5 | 9.5 | 14 | 20 | 21 |
| 25–34 | 4.5 | 5.5 | 55 | 12 | 16 | 21.5 | 24 |
| 35–44 | 5 | 6 | 6 | 12 | 15.5 | 20 | 23 |
| 45–54 | 5 | 6 | 6 | il | 15 | 20 | 25.5 |
| 55–64 | 5 | 6 | 6 | il | 14 | 18 | 21.5 |
| 65–74 | 4.5 | 5.5 | 5.5 | il | 15 | 19 | 22 |

**Table 15.** Percentiles of triceps skin fold (mm) in females aged 1–74 years

| Age (years) | | | | Percentile | | | |
|---|---|---|---|---|---|---|---|
| | 5° | 10° | 25° | 50° | 75° | 90° | 95° |
| 1–1.9 | 6 | 7 | 8 | 10 | 12 | 14 | 16 |
| 2–2.9 | 6 | 8 | 9 | 10 | 12 | 15 | 16 |
| 3–3.9 | 7 | 8 | 9 | 10 | 12 | 14 | 15 |
| 4–4.9 | 7 | 8 | 8 | 10 | 12 | 14 | 16 |
| 5–5.9 | 6 | 7 | 8 | 10 | 12 | 15 | 18 |
| 6–6.9 | 6 | 6 | 8 | 10 | 12 | 14 | 16 |
| 7–7.9 | 6 | 7 | 9 | il | 13 | 16 | 18 |
| 8–8.9 | 6 | 8 | 9 | 12 | 15 | 18 | 24 |
| 9–9.9 | 8 | 8 | 10 | 13 | 16 | 20 | 22 |
| 10–10.9 | 7 | 8 | 10 | 12 | 17 | 23 | 27 |
| 11–11.9 | 7 | 8 | 10 | 13 | 19 | 24 | 28 |
| 12–12.9 | 8 | 9 | 11 | 14 | 19 | 23 | 27 |
| 13–13.9 | 8 | 8 | 12 | 15 | 21 | 26 | 30 |
| 14–14.9 | 9 | 10 | 13 | 16 | 21 | 26 | 28 |
| 15–15.9 | 8 | 10 | 12 | 17 | 21 | 25 | 32 |
| 16–16.9 | 10 | 12 | 15 | 18 | 22 | 26 | 31 |
| 17–17.9 | 10 | 12 | 13 | 19 | 24 | 30 | 37 |
| 18–24 | 9.4 | 11 | 14 | 18 | 24 | 30 | 34 |
| 25–34 | 10.5 | 12 | 16 | 21 | 26.5 | 31.5 | 37 |
| 35–44 | 12.0 | 14 | 18 | 23 | 29.5 | 39.5 | 39 |
| 45–54 | 13.0 | 15 | 20 | 25 | 30 | 36 | 40 |
| 55–64 | 11.0 | 14 | 19 | 25 | 30.5 | 35 | 39 |
| 65–74 | 11.5 | 14 | 18 | 23 | 28 | 33 | 36 |

**Table 16.** Percentiles of subscapular skin fold (mm) in males aged 18–74 years

| Age (years) | Percentile | | | | | | |
|---|---|---|---|---|---|---|---|
| | 5° | 10° | 25° | 50° | 75° | 90° | 95° |
| 18–24 | 6.0 | 6.5 | 8.0 | 11.0 | 16.0 | 24.0 | 29.0 |
| 25–34 | 6.5 | 7.0 | 10.0 | 14.0 | 20.0 | 26.0 | 30.5 |
| 35–44 | 7.0 | 8.0 | 11.5 | 16.0 | 21.0 | 26.0 | 30.5 |
| 45–54 | 7.0 | 8.0 | 12.0 | 16.5 | 22.0 | 29.0 | 32.0 |
| 55–64 | 6.0 | 7.0 | 11.0 | 15.5 | 21.0 | 27.0 | 30.0 |
| 65–74 | 6.0 | 7.5 | 10.5 | 15.0 | 20.0 | 25.0 | 30.0 |

**Table 17.** Percentiles of subscapular skin fold (mm) in females aged 18–74 years

| Age (years) | Percentile | | | | | | |
|---|---|---|---|---|---|---|---|
| | 5° | 10° | 25° | 50° | 75° | 90° | 95° |
| 18–24 | 6.0 | 7.0 | 9.0 | 13.0 | 19.0 | 27.0 | 31.5 |
| 25–34 | 6.0 | 7.0 | 10.0 | 14.5 | 22.5 | 32.0 | 38.0 |
| 35–44 | 6.5 | 8.0 | 11.0 | 17.0 | 26.5 | 34.0 | 39.0 |
| 45–54 | 7.0 | 8.5 | 12.0 | 20.0 | 28.0 | 35.0 | 40.0 |
| 55–64 | 7.0 | 8.0 | 12.5 | 20.0 | 28.0 | 34.5 | 38.0 |
| 65–74 | 7.0 | 8.0 | 12.0 | 18.0 | 25.0 | 32.5 | 37.0 |

**Table 18.** Percentiles of the sum of triceps skin fold and subscapular skin fold (mm) in males aged 18–74 years

| Age (years) | Percentile | | | | | | |
|---|---|---|---|---|---|---|---|
| | 5° | 10° | 25° | 50° | 75° | 90° | 95° |
| 18–24 | 10.0 | 12.0 | 15.0 | 21.0 | 30.0 | 41.0 | 51.0 |
| 25–34 | 11.5 | 13.5 | 19.0 | 26.0 | 36.5 | 45.0 | 54.0 |
| 35–44 | 12.0 | 15.0 | 21.0 | 28.0 | 36.0 | 44.0 | 48.5 |
| 45–54 | 13.0 | 15.0 | 21.0 | 28.0 | 37.0 | 46.0 | 53.0 |
| 55–64 | 12.0 | 14.0 | 20.0 | 26.0 | 34.0 | 44.0 | 48.0 |
| 65–74 | 11.5 | 14.0 | 19.5 | 26.0 | 34.0 | 42.5 | 49.0 |

**Table 19.** Percentiles of the sum of triceps skin fold and subscapular skin fold (mm) in females aged 18–74 years

| Age (years) | Percentile | | | | | | |
|---|---|---|---|---|---|---|---|
| | 5° | 10° | 25° | 50° | 75° | 90° | 95° |
| 18–24 | 17.0 | 19.0 | 24.0 | 31.0 | 41.5 | 54.5 | 64.0 |
| 25–34 | 18.5 | 20.5 | 26.5 | 35.0 | 48.0 | 64.0 | 73.0 |
| 35–44 | 20.0 | 23.0 | 30.0 | 40.5 | 55.0 | 68.0 | 75.0 |
| 45–54 | 22.0 | 25.0 | 33.5 | 45.0 | 58.0 | 69.5 | 78.5 |
| 55–64 | 19.0 | 25.0 | 33.0 | 46.0 | 58.0 | 68.0 | 73.0 |
| 65–74 | 30.0 | 25.0 | 32.0 | 41.0 | 52.5 | 63.0 | 70.0 |

**Table 20.** Values of c and m of several skin folds in males

| Skin fold | | Age (years) | | | | | |
|---|---|---|---|---|---|---|---|
| | | 17–19 | 20–29 | 30–39 | 40–49 | > 50 | 17–72 |
| Biceps (BSF) | c | 1.1066 | 1.1015 | 1.0781 | 1.0829 | 1.0833 | 1.0997 |
| | m | 0.0686 | 0.0616 | 0.0396 | 0.0508 | 0.0617 | 0.0659 |
| Triceps (TSF) | c | 1.1252 | 1.1131 | 1.0834 | 1.1041 | 1.1027 | 1.1143 |
| | m | 0.0625 | 0.0530 | 0.0361 | 0.0609 | 0.0662 | 0.0618 |
| Subscapular (SSF) | c | 1.1312 | 1.1360 | 1.0978 | 1.1246 | 1.1334 | 1.1369 |
| | m | 0.0670 | 0.0700 | 0.0416 | 0.0686 | 0.0760 | 0.0741 |
| Iliac (ISF) | c | 1.1092 | 1.1117 | 1.1047 | 1.1029 | 1.1193 | 1.1171 |
| | m | 0.0420 | 0.0431 | 0.0432 | 0.0483 | 0.0652 | 0.0530 |
| BSF + TSF | c | 1.1423 | 1.1307 | 1.0995 | 1.1174 | 1.1185 | 1.1356 |
| | m | 0.0687 | 0.0603 | 0.0431 | 0.0614 | 0.0683 | 0.0700 |
| BSF + SSF | c | 1.1457 | 1.1469 | 1.0753 | 1.1341 | 1.1427 | 1.1498 |
| | m | 0.0707 | 0.0709 | 0.0445 | 0.0680 | 0.0762 | 0.0759 |
| BSF + ISF | c | 1.1247 | 1.1259 | 1.1174 | 1.1171 | 1.1307 | 1.1331 |
| | m | 0.0501 | 0.0502 | 0.0486 | 0.0539 | 0.0678 | 0.0601 |
| TSF + SSF | c | 1.1561 | 1.1525 | 1.1165 | 1.1519 | 1.1527 | 1.1625 |
| | m | 0.0711 | 0.0687 | 0.0484 | 0.0771 | 0.0793 | 0.0797 |
| TSF + ISF | c | 1.1370 | 1.1362 | 1.1273 | 1.1383 | 1.1415 | 1.1463 |
| | m | 0.0545 | 0.0538 | 0.0531 | 0.0660 | 0.0718 | 0.0656 |
| SSF + ISF | c | 1.1374 | 1.1429 | 1.1260 | 1.1392 | 1.1592 | 1.1522 |
| | m | 0.0544 | 0.0573 | 0.0497 | 0.0633 | 0.0771 | OD671 |
| BSF + TSF + SSF | c | 1.1643 | 1.1593 | 1.1213 | 1.1530 | 1.1569 | 1.1689 |
| | m | 0.0727 | 0.0694 | 0.0487 | 0.0730 | 0.0780 | 0.0793 |
| BSF + TSF + ISF | c | 1.1466 | 1.1451 | 1.1332 | 1.1422 | 1.1473 | 1.1556 |
| | m | 0.0584 | 0.0572 | 0.0542 | 0.0647 | 0.0718 | 0.0683 |
| BSF + SSF + ISF | c | 1.1469 | 1.1508 | 1.1315 | 1.1452 | 1.1626 | 1.1605 |
| | m | 0.0583 | 0.0599 | 0.0510 | 0.0640 | 0.0768 | 0.0694 |
| TSF + SSF + ISF | c | 1.1555 | 1.1575 | 1.1393 | 1.1604 | 1.1689 | 1.1704 |
| | m | 0.0607 | 0.0617 | 0.0544 | 0.0716 | 0.0787 | 0.0731 |
| BSF + TSF + SSF + ISF | c | 1.1620 | 1.1631 | 1.1422 | 1.1620 | 1.1715 | 1.1765 |
| | m | 0.0630 | 0.0632 | 0.0544 | 0.0700 | 0.0779 | 0.0744 |

**Table 21.** Values of c and m of several skin folds in females

| Skin fold | | Age (years) | | | | | |
|---|---|---|---|---|---|---|---|
| | | 16–19 | 20–29 | 30–39 | 40–49 | > 50 | 16–68 |
| Biceps (BSF) | c | 1.0889 | 1.0903 | 1.0794 | 1.0736 | 1.0682 | 1.0871 |
| | m | 0.0553 | 0.0601 | 0.0511 | 0.0492 | 0.0510 | 0.0593 |
| Triceps (TSF) | c | 1.1159 | 1.1319 | 1.1176 | 1.1121 | 1.1160 | 1.1278 |
| | m | 1.0648 | 1.0776 | 1.0686 | 1.0691 | 1.0762 | 1.0775 |
| Subscapular (SSF) | c | 1.1081 | 1.1184 | 1.0979 | 1.1860 | 1.0899 | 1.1100 |
| | m | 0.0621 | 0.0716 | 0.0567 | 0.0505 | 0.0590 | 0.0669 |
| Iliac (ISF) | c | 1.0931 | 1.0923 | 1.0860 | 1.0691 | 1.0656 | 1.0884 |
| | m | 0.0470 | 0.0509 | 0.0497 | 0.0407 | 0.0419 | 0.0514 |
| BSF + TSF | c | 1.1290 | 1.1398 | 1.1243 | 1.1230 | 1.1226 | 1.1362 |
| | m | 0.0657 | 0.0738 | 0.0646 | 0.0672 | 0.071.0 | 0.0740 |
| BSF + SSF | c | 1.1241 | 1.1314 | 1.1120 | 1.1031 | 1.1029 | 1.1245 |
| | m | 0.0643 | 0.0706 | 0.0581 | 0.0549 | 0.0592 | 0.0674 |
| BSF + ISF | c | 1.1113 | 1.1112 | 1.1020 | 1.0921 | 1.0857 | 1.1090 |
| | m | 0.0537 | 0.0568 | 0.0528 | 0.0494 | 0.0490 | 0.0577 |
| TSF + SSF | c | 1.1468 | 1.1582 | 1.1356 | 1.1230 | 1.1347 | 1.1507 |
| | m | 0.0740 | 0.0813 | 0.0680 | 0.0635 | 0.0742 | 0.0785 |
| TSF + ISF | c | 1.1311 | 1.1377 | 1.1281 | 1.1198 | 1.1158 | 1.1367 |
| | m | 0.0624 | 0.0684 | 0.0644 | 0.0630 | 0.0635 | 0.0704 |
| SSF + ISF | c | 1.1278 | 1.1280 | 1.1132 | 1.0997 | 1.0963 | 1.1234 |
| | m | 0.0616 | 0.0640 | 0.0564 | 0.0509 | 0.0523 | 0.0632 |
| BSF + TSF + SSF | c | 1.1509 | 1.1605 | 1.1385 | 1.1303 | 1.1372 | 1.1543 |
| | m | 0.0715 | 0.0777 | 0.0654 | 0.0635 | 0.0710 | 0.0756 |
| BSF + TSF + ISF | c | 1.1382 | 1.1441 | 1.1319 | 1.1267 | 1.1227 | 1.1432 |
| | m | 0.0628 | 0.0680 | 0.0624 | 0.0626 | 0.0633 | 0.0696 |
| BSF + SSF + ISF | c | 1.1355 | 1.1366 | 1.1212 | 1.1108 | 1.1063 | 1.1530 |
| | m | 0.0622 | 0.0648 | 0.0570 | 0.0536 | 0.0544 | 0.0727 |
| TSF + SSF + ISF | c | 1.1517 | 1.1566 | 1.1397 | 1.1278 | 1.1298 | 1.1327 |
| | m | 0.0689 | 0.0728 | 0.0646 | 0.0609 | 0.0650 | 0.0643 |
| BSF + TSF + SSF + ISF | c | 1.1549 | 1.1599 | 1.1423 | 1.1333 | 1.1339 | 1.1567 |
| | m | 0.0678 | 0.0717 | 0.0632 | 0.0612 | 0.0645 | 0.0717 |

**Table 22.** Percentage body fat estimated by four skin fold measurements (triceps, biceps, subscapular, iliac) in males and females

| Skin folds (mm) | Males | | | | Females | | | |
|---|---|---|---|---|---|---|---|---|
| | | | | Age (years) | | | | |
| | 17–29 | 30–39 | 40–49 | > 50 | 16–29 | 30–39 | 40–49 | > 50 |
| 15 | 4.8 | - | - | - | 10.5 | - | - | - |
| 20 | 8.1 | 12.2 | 12.2 | 12.6 | 14.1 | 17.0 | 19.8 | 21.4 |
| 25 | 10.5 | 14.2 | 15.0 | 15.6 | 16.8 | 19.4 | 22.2 | 24.0 |
| 30 | 12.9 | 16.2 | 17.7 | 18.6 | 19.5 | 21.8 | 24.5 | 26.6 |
| 35 | 14.7 | 17.7 | 19.6 | 20.8 | 21.5 | 23.7 | 26.4 | 28.5 |
| 40 | 16.4 | 19.2 | 21.4 | 22.9 | 23.4 | 25.5 | 28.2 | 30.3 |
| 45 | 17.7 | 20.4 | 23.0 | 24.7 | 25.0 | 26.9 | 29.6 | 31.9 |
| 50 | 19.0 | 21.5 | 24.6 | 26.5 | 26.5 | 28.2 | 31.0 | 33.4 |
| 55 | 20.1 | 22.5 | 25.9 | 27.9 | 27.8 | 29.4 | 32.1 | 34.6 |
| 60 | 21.2 | 23.5 | 27.1 | 29.2 | 29.1 | 30.6 | 33.2 | 35.7 |
| 65 | 22.2 | 24.3 | 28.2 | 30.4 | 30.2 | 31.6 | 34.1 | 36.7 |
| 70 | 23.1 | 25.1 | 29.3 | 31.6 | 31.2 | 32.5 | 35.0 | 37.7 |
| 75 | 24.0 | 25.9 | 30.3 | 32.7 | 32.2 | 33.4 | 35.9 | 38.7 |
| 80 | 24.8 | 26.6 | 31.2 | 33.8 | 33.1 | 34.3 | 36.7 | 38.6 |
| 85 | 25.5 | 27.2 | 32.1 | 34.8 | 34.0 | 35.1 | 37.5 | 40.4 |
| 90 | 26.2 | 27.8 | 33.0 | 35.8 | 34.8 | 35.8 | 38.3 | 41.2 |
| 95 | 26.9 | 28.4 | 33.7 | 36.6 | 35.6 | 36.5 | 39.0 | 41.9 |
| 100 | 27.6 | 29.0 | 34.4 | 37.4 | 36.4 | 37.2 | 39.7 | 42.6 |
| 105 | 28.2 | 29.6 | 35.1 | 38.2 | 37.1 | 37.9 | 40.4 | 43.3 |
| 110 | 28.8 | 30.1 | 35.8 | 39.0 | 37.8 | 38.6 | 41.0 | 43.9 |
| 115 | 29.4 | 30.6 | 36.4 | 39.7 | 38.4 | 39.1 | 41.5 | 44.5 |
| 120 | 30.0 | 31.1 | 37.0 | 40.4 | 39.0 | 39.6 | 42.0 | 45.1 |
| 125 | 30.5 | 31.5 | 37.6 | 41.1 | 39.6 | 40.1 | 42.5 | 45.7 |
| 130 | 31.0 | 31.9 | 38.2 | 41.8 | 40.2 | 40.6 | 43.0 | 46.2 |
| 135 | 31.5 | 32.3 | 38.7 | 42.4 | 40.8 | 41.1 | 43.5 | 46.7 |
| 140 | 32.0 | 32.7 | 39.2 | 43.0 | 41.3 | 41.6 | 44.0 | 47.2 |
| 145 | 32.5 | 33.1 | 39.7 | 43.6 | 41.8 | 42.1 | 44.5 | 47.7 |
| 150 | 32.9 | 33.5 | 40.2 | 44.1 | 42.3 | 42.6 | 45.0 | 48.2 |
| 155 | 33.3 | 33.9 | 40.7 | 44.6 | 42.8 | 43.1 | 45.4 | 48.7 |
| 160 | 33.7 | 34.3 | 41.2 | 45.1 | 43.3 | 43.6 | 45.8 | 49.2 |
| 165 | 34.1 | 34.6 | 41.6 | 45.6 | 43.7 | 44.0 | 46.2 | 49.6 |
| 170 | 34.5 | 34.8 | 42.0 | 46.1 | 44.1 | 44.4 | 46.6 | 50.0 |
| 175 | 34.9 | - | - | - | - | 44.8 | 47.0 | 50.4 |
| 180 | 35.3 | - | - | - | - | 45.2 | 47.4 | 50.8 |
| 185 | 35.6 | - | - | - | - | 45.6 | 47.8 | 51.2 |
| 190 | 35.9 | - | - | - | - | 45.9 | 18.2 | 51.6 |
| 195 | - | - | - | - | - | 46.2 | 48.5 | 52.0 |
| 200 | - | - | - | - | - | 46.5 | 48.8 | 52.4 |
| 205 | - | - | - | - | - | - | 49.1 | 52.7 |
| 210 | - | - | - | - | - | - | 49.4 | 53.0 |

# Functional Parameters

Recently, functional parameters have been introduced to evaluate nutritional status. The most important are listed in Table 23.

Among them, voluntary muscle function (contractile function, tone, stretch reflexes) is easily evaluated by nerve stimulation. For example, in subjects with malnutrition, the thumb adduction after ulnar stimulation is decreased. A non-invasive

**Table 23.** Classification for systems of functional indexes of nutritional assessment

| Systems and evaluable functions | Factors involved |
| --- | --- |
| Structural integrity of cells | |
|    Fragility of erythrocytes | Vitamin E, Se |
|    Fragility of capillary | Vitamin C |
|    Strength of skin tension | Cu |
|    Experimental recovery of wounds | Zn |
|    Collagen accumulation in installed sponge | Zn |
|    Lipoprotein peroxidation | Vitamin E, Se |
| Defence mechanisms | |
|    Leucocyte chemotaxis | P/E, Zn |
|    Leukocyte phagocyte activity | P/E, Fe |
|    Leukocyte bactericide capacity | P/E, Fe, Se |
|    Leucocyte metabolism | P/E |
|    Opsonic activity of serum | P/E |
|    Leucocyte production of interferon | P/E |
|    Blastogenesis of T lymphocytes | P/E |
|    Delayed skin hypersensitivity | P/E |
|    Rebuck's skin window technique | P/E |
| Transport | |
|    *Intestinal absorption:* | |
|    Iron absorption | Fe |
|    Cobalt absorption | Co |
|    *Transport plasma-tissue:* | |
|    Erythrocyte capture of Zn | Zn |
|    Erythrocyte capture of Se | Se |
|    Dosage answer to retinol | Vitamin A |
|    Plasmatic answer of chromium to glucose load | Cr |
|    Urinary answer of chromium to glucose load | Cr |
|    Thyroid capture of radioiodine | I |
| Haemostasis | |
|    Prothrombin time | Vitamin K |

*continue* →

**Table 23** *continue*

| Systems and evaluable functions | Factors involved |
| --- | --- |
| Platelet aggregation | Vitamin E, Zn |
| Reproduction | |
| Count and mobility of spermatozoa | Energy (carnitine), Zn, Vitamin E |
| Neurological functions | |
| Adaptation to obscurity | Vitamin A, Zn |
| Colour recognition | Vitamin A |
| Central scotoma | Vitamin A |
| Olfactory acuity | Vitamin A, B, Zn |
| Taste acuity | Vitamin A, Zn |
| Nervous conductivity | P/E, vitamin B and B12 |
| Skin conductivity | P/E |
| Function of sixth cranial nerve | Vitamin B |
| EEG | P/E |
| Sleeping | P/E |
| Work capacity | |
| Work intensity and duration | P/E, vitamins B12, B2, B6, Fe |
| VO$_2$ max | P/E, Fe |
| Heart rate | P/E, Fe |
| Vasopressory answer | Vitamin C |
| Muscle contraction | P/E |
| Not classified | |
| Suppression test of d-uridine | Folic acid, vitamin B12 |

*P/E*, protein-energy food

approach to muscle function evaluation is dynamometry. The mean hand-grabbing strength is $48 \pm 7$ kg in males and $34 \pm 5$ kg in females; it is greatly decreased in malnourished subjects and in obese subjects on ipocaloric diets. In muscle biopsies, a loss of type II muscle fibres, increased intracellular $Ca^{2+}$ and decreased levels of phosphofructokinase can be demonstrated.

The above-mentioned nutritional parameters have been linked with clinical prognosis by several paradigms. Each paradigm links specific features of malnutrition with some immune functions, since abnormal immune function correlates with increased risk in malnourished subjects. A surgical risk prognostic nutritional index (PNI) predicts postsurgical morbidity on the basis of preoperative levels of serum albumin, transferrin, triceps skin fold thickness, delayed hypersensitivity to skin antigens, as follows:

PNI% = 158 – 16.6 (serum albumin, g/dl) – 0.78 (triceps skin fold, mm) – 0.2 (serum transferrin, mg/dl) (delayed hypersensitivity assay with 0 = anergy, 1 = 5 mm, 2 = > 5 mm).

Other paradigms take into account quality of life, self-evaluated capability of working, performing physical activity, mood, well-being.

In the near future more sophisticated techniques such as total $K^+$ measurement or neutronic activation measurement are expected to be more widely available.

# Special Techniques for Nutritional Assessment

These techniques are used to evaluate energy and protein stores in malnourished patients at baseline assessment or to check the efficacy of nutritional support.

## Bioelectric Impedance Analysis

Bioelectric impedance analysis (BIA) [4] is a method for measurement of body compartments: fat mass, fat free mass (FFM) and total body water (TBW). This method affords a very fast evaluation of body composition, while anthropometric methods (skin fold measurements) are quite time consuming. It also allows the measurement of the TBW content and the intracellular and extracellular water, which are otherwise not evaluable. BIA is reliable enough only to allow total body analysis, while for body district analysis complementary data obtained from skin fold measurements are still needed. BIA is performed by measuring the electric conductivity of a weak current between electrodes placed at both ends of the body. The measurement reflects differences in the impedance to electric current. Bioelectric impedance (Z) is composed of resistance (R) and reactance (Xc). The trigonometric ratio between R and Xc is the phase angle (F). The greatest F is measured by an artificial bioconductor. The human body possesses an individual resistance to the passage of an electric current through it. The current passing through a body is directly proportional to the potential applied and inversely proportional to its resistance. Impedance, resistance and reactance are measured in Ohms. An electric circuit where a tension of 1 Volt sustains a current of 1 Ampere possesses a resistance of 1 Ohm. The intensity of an electric current in a conductor when an electromotive force (potential) is applied to it is measured in Amperes. Reactance is the force that opposes the passage of an alternate current. The phase angle is calculated in relation to the reactance (Xc) and resistance (R). The phase angle may span 0 to 90 degrees, according to whether the body circuit is completely resistive or completely reactive.

The phase angle of a healthy male adult varies between 4 and 15 degrees. The phase angle is a highly prognostic index of cell membrane integrity.

The electric bioimpedance analyser generates a stimulation current of 800 mA, with a frequency of 50 KHz. When current and frequency are maintained constant, and the conductor (namely the body of the subject undergoing the procedure) is unchanged, electric impedance is determined by the volume of the conductor, as follows:

$V = pL/Z$, where Z is impedance ($Z = \sqrt{R^2 + Xc^2}$), p is volume resistivity and L is the length of the conductor. As Xc is much smaller than Z, we can assume $V = pL/R$, where L is the height of the subject undergoing the procedure. Nevertheless, application of such a procedure to living beings with their differences can hardly be so straightforward. When an alternate current is applied to a living body, the fluid portion (including intra- and extracellular fluids) behaves like a resistive conductor, while cell membranes behave like a reactive conductor. In the human body, lean tissues behave like good conductors, because of their high water and electrolyte content, with subsequent low resistance to alternate current.

The cell membrane consists of a double layer of lipids, which is not conductive, between two layers of highly conductive proteins. Cells are highly reactive bodies, behaving as condensers when an alternate current is applied. Bioelectric impedance is measured at the right side of the body, while the subject is lying on his or her back, arms slightly aside, and legs apart enough to avoid thigh contact. The subject may keep his clothes on, but must be requested to remove his shoes and socks, and every metal object.

Widely used models of analyser electrodes are applied, according to the manufacturer's instructions, after thorough cleansing of the skin with ethanol, as follows: *right hand*, the sensor electrode at the midline of the wrist, the stimulating electrode at the third finger, 5 cm from the sensor; *right foot*, the sensor electrode at the midline of the ankle joint, the stimulating electrode at the third finger, 6 cm from the sensor.

A thorough calibration of the analyser is required before each measurement. Software is supplied, which affords 12 successive analyses per patient.

The software requires the following data:
1. Height
2. Actual weight
3. Abdominal circumference
4. Buttock circumferences
5. Proximal thigh circumference
6. The impedance measured.

The elaborated data, on paper and video, afford the following information:
1. Regional determination of fat tissue
2. Lean mass determination (FFM)
3. Fat mass determination (FAT)
4. TBW determination
5. Basal metabolism
6. Ideal body weight
7. Balance weight.

## Regional Determination of Fat Tissue

This is determined by calculating the waist/hip ratio (W/H) and the waist/thigh ratio (W/T), in cm. These measures overlap with the corresponding anthropometric measures.

## Fat-Free Mass Determination

This is measured in kg and as a percentage of the actual weight.

## Fat Mass Determination

Fat mass is measured in kg and as a percentage of the actual weight. The bioimpedance analysis allows measurement of visceral and intra-abdominal fat, which is overlooked by using the skin fold measurement. This is of great importance in assessing the nutritional status and nutritional requirements of individuals. Where available, other methods can be used, such as DEXA, MNR, CT scan or sonography.

## Total Water Determination

Water content is greater in lean tissues, and it changes among individuals according to age, health condition and exercise. Total water is measured in litres, and as a percentage of lean mass. Mean percentage measures are reported between 67.4 and 77.5% of body mass. BIA is a sufficient method to measure TBW.

## Basal Metabolism (Resting Energy Expenditure)

Basal metabolism or REE is inferred by the lean mass of a subject, and is measured as kilocalories (kcal) or Joules. Indirect calorimetry together with anthropometry is a valid method to measure REE.

## Ideal Weight

This is determined by an estimation of equilibrium percentage of fat mass, according to age and sex. The ideal weight for a determined group is the weight associated with the maximal longevity.

## Delta Weight

The balance between ideal weight and the actual weight is the delta weight. This value, along with clinical data and laboratory tests, such as arterial pressure, total and high-density lipoprotein cholesterol, glycaemia, family history, behavioural factors (smoking, lifestyle), allows estimation of the coronary risk rate for the individual patient. This procedure is complemented with a simple cardiac step test such as a treadmill or step-up, and with the spinal flexion test, which allows a good evaluation of the global joint and muscle flexibility.

## References

1. Scevola D, Marinelli M (1991) Dietetica medica. Tipografia Viscontea, Pavia
2. Shils ME (ed) (1999) Modern nutrition in health and disease, 9th edn. Lea and Febiger, Philadelphia
3. Naber TH, Schermer T, de Bree A et al (1997) Prevalence of malnutrition in nonsurgical hospitalized patients and its association with disease complications. Am J Clin Nutr 66:1232–1239
4. Anonymous (1996) Bioelectrical impedance analysis in body composition measurement: National Institutes of Health technology assessment conference statement. Am J Clin Nutr 64:524S–532S

# Immunological Parameters of Nutrition

Clelia Madeddu, Giovanni Mantovani

## Introduction

The interdependency between nutrition and immune function was recognised formally in the 1970s when immunological measures were introduced as part of the assessment of nutritional status [1]. Both the nutritional status and specific nutrients may affect the immune system directly (e.g., by triggering immune cell activation or altering immune cell interactions) or indirectly (e.g., by changing substrates for DNA synthesis, altering energy metabolism, changing the physiological integrity of cells, or altering signals or hormones) [2]. Protein-energy malnutrition is accepted as a major cause of immune deficiency worldwide, and the immune response is considered integral to the pathophysiology of many chronic diseases [3]. Protein-energy malnutrition is associated with a significant impairment of cell-mediated immunity, phagocyte function, complement system, secretory immunoglobulin A antibody concentrations and cytokine production.

Deficiency of single nutrients also results in altered immune response: this is observed even when the deficiency state is relatively mild. Among the micronutrients, zinc, selenium, copper, iron, vitamins A, C, E and B6, and folic acid have important influences on immune responses [4].

Moreover, several immunological mediators (particularly cytokines, such as interleukin [IL]-1, tumour necrosis factor [TNF]-$\alpha$ and IL-6) can drive metabolism and thus body composition in various illnesses, and moreover they also play a homeostatic role in the age-related changes in body composition [5].

Knowledge of the impact of nutritional status on the functioning of the immune system has led to several practical applications, including the use of immunological tests as prognostic indexes in patients undergoing surgery and the use of immunological methods to assess nutritional status and to determine the efficacy and adequacy of nutritional therapy [6].

## Pathophysiology of Immune Response

The immune system (the cells and the molecules responsible for immunity) is defined as part of the host's defence against destructive forces either from outside the body (e.g., bacteria, viruses and parasites) or from within (e.g., malignant and autoreactive cells). Innate (natural) immune defences are those components of the immune system (macrophages, monocytes and neutrophils) that function without relying on prior exposure to a particular antigen. They are the early phases of the host defence that protect the organism during the 4–5 days it takes for lymphocytes to become activated. Adaptive or acquired immune responses develop over the lifetime of a human being in response to environmental challenges (pathogens or antigens). Lymphocytes are the primary cells of the aquired immune system. The T lymphocytes can both modulate the function of other immune cells and directly destroy cells infected with intracellular pathogens. During development, each T cell generates a unique receptor by rearranging its receptor genes, enabling the cell to produce receptors with an almost infinite range of specificities. Once they are mature, T cells migrate from the thymus and perhaps the gut to the periphery, where they encounter antigens presented to them by specialised antigen-presenting cells in the context of a class I or II major histocompatibility complex molecule. An additional signal derived from B cells, macrophages, or dendritic cells is needed to induce lymphocyte proliferation and differentiation [7]. Today, the response by T cells is considered to be not only a factor in acute infections but also an integral component of biological processes such as development and ageing, as well as the pathophysiology of many chronic diseases (e.g., rheumatoid arthritis, type 1 diabetes, coeliac disease, cancer and cardiovascular diseases) [8].

# Metabolic Effects of Immune Response Mediators

When the organism is stressed by an injury, infection or illness, the daily swing of insulin- and glucagon-mediated metabolic shifts between fed and fasted states is disturbed. The organ system charged with recognising and responding to an injury is the immune system, which has the capacity to radically change body protein and energy metabolism and thus body composition [5]. The antigen-presenting cell (APC) of the immune system is typically a macrophage, tissue monocyte or skin dendritic cell. The APC contacts an antigen, phagocytoses it, processes an antigenic determinant, and brings it to its surface in an HLA-restricted manner in order to trigger an immune response. This immune response requires both the presence of a specific epitope from the antigen and the elaboration of one or more non-specific signals, chiefly via secretion of the cytokine IL-1. IL-1 secretion triggers activation of T cells and other portions of the immune response. The subsequent APC-initiated signals include the elaboration of TNF-α and, later, production of IL-6. These three cytokines (IL-1, TNF-α and IL-6) are currently thought to play the most important role in the development of the acute-phase metabolic response, which parallels the acute-phase immune response. Because there are receptors for these cytokines on every cell in the body except red blood cells, these cytokines have profound effects on the hormones that govern metabolism as well as acting directly on the metabolic target organs such as muscle, liver, gut and brain [9]. The result is an increase in resting energy expenditure, a net export of amino acids from muscle to liver, an increase in gluconeogenesis, and a marked shift in liver protein synthesis away from albumin and towards production of acute-phase proteins such as fibrinogen and C-reactive protein [10].

# Proinflammatory Cytokines

Immune response results in a variety of metabolic adjustments that are mediated by cytokines of leukocytic origin. Among cytokines released during an immune response, IL-1, TNF-α and IL-6 are the major mediators of intermediary metabolism. These cytokines act in concert to decrease food intake, increase resting energy expenditure, gluconeogenesis, glucose oxidation, and hepatic synthesis of fatty acids and acute-phase proteins, decrease fatty acid uptake by adipocytes and alter the distribution of zinc, iron and copper. Most of these activities result from direct interactions between the cytokine and the responding cells. IL-1, TNF-α and IL-6 also affect changes in metabolism by changing levels of circulating insulin, glucagon and corticosterone [11].

Proinflammatory cytokine peptides were originally studied for their effect on immunological homeostasis in several areas, but they also exert potent activity towards regulation of metabolic responses [12]. During early post-injury or infectious conditions, the initial cytokine response to such insults likely mediates beneficial protective signalling of the immune system. Nevertheless, prolonged production of cytokines sustains some metabolic effects of the hypercatabolic state. Proinflammatory cytokines may function by autocrine (acting on the same cell), paracrine (acting on cells in the immediate area), or systemic mechanisms of action. They produce local tissue responses by cell-to-cell interaction at very low concentrations but also exert systemic effects at higher concentrations. Among cytokines, the proinflammatory ones (IL-1, IL-6, TNF-α, interferon [IFN]-α and IFN-γ) have been more widely studied from a metabolic perspective [13].

TNF-α is a protein primarily secreted from monocytes and macrophages. However, many other cell types, including adipocytes, synthesise and secrete TNF-α [14]. Although originally isolated as a soluble factor that produced cachexia during infection and in vivo necrosis of some solid tumours [15], this cytokine has been implicated as the initiating signal for a variety of cellular and metabolic events seen in critically ill patients. TNF-α may circulate predominantly as a complex with its soluble receptors, making detection of the bioactive ligand more difficult. Increased levels of these soluble TNF-α receptors are seen in response to diverse inflammatory stimuli including sepsis, cancer and AIDS [16]. Nevertheless, elevated TNF-α levels are detected in many disease states including bacterial infections, cancer, sepsis and AIDS [17]. TNF-α is a metabolic hormone acting both in a paracrine fashion, and, in some istances, as an endocrine hormone [18]. Systemically, TNF-α has been suggested to act in the brain to cause anorexia and subsequent body weight loss [19]. The metabolic effects of TNF-α seem to promote redistribution of body protein and lipid stores. The result is a net loss of peripheral tissue protein with a concomitant increase in hepatic uptake [20]. TNF-α might also act in a paracrine fashion to limit adiposity by causing insulin resistance [14], inhibiting glucose transporter gene expression [21], and decreasing adipose tissue lipoprotein lipase activity [22]. TNF-α alters lipid metabolism in other ways as well, stimulating lipolysis [23], hepatic triglyceride synthesis, and subsequent hypertriglyceridaemia [24]. Because this can lead to futile cycling, these effects are energetically inefficient and direct the organism towards a negative energy balance. The chronic over-production of TNF-α has been suggested to be a factor in cachexia [25]. Several studies have shown that tissue-specific expression of TNF-α is increased in diseases such as AIDS [26] and multiple sclerosis [27]. Furthermore, chronic exposure to TNF-α, by way of a TNF-α-secreting tumour, induced progressive weight loss in mice [19]. The chronic effects of cytokines like TNF-α could cause many of the metabolic symptoms of wasting.

IL-1 is produced by macrophages/monocytes, neutrophils, lymphocytes and keratinocytes [12]. Its production is stimulated by TNF-α and endotoxin, and, like TNF-α, it may represent an early cytokine response to injury. Once released, it exerts multiple immunological and metabolic effects including stimulation of ACTH [28], inducing of fever, hepatic acute-phase protein synthesis, and alteration of energy metabolism [12].

IL-6 is the most frequently detected cytokine in patients with acute infection, injury, cancer and after surgical procedures [13]. The biological actions of this protein include regulation of acute-phase protein synthesis [29, 30] and differentiation of lymphocytes [31]. It also induces fever via prostaglandin production [13]. Administration of IL-6 to humans increases energy expenditure, fatty acid and ketone production, fat oxidation, glucose production, lactate production and glucose oxidation [32]. Such effects account for many of the manifestations of inflammatory stress, implicating IL-6 as the direct cause of them, perhaps the mediator of some of the effects of TNF-α, which secondarily stimulates IL-6 production. IL-6 in turn stimulates production of catecholamines, glucagon and cortisol, which may mediate some or all of the effects of IL-6. Interestingly, IL-6 levels also increase during exercise, another circumstance besides injury in which nutrient mobilisation is essential, and are inhibited by glucocorticoids, underscoring feedback on the cytokine cascade by the adrenal axis, which is potently stimulated by IL-6 [33].

IFN-γ is secreted from lymphocytes and macrophages and exerts antiviral effects as well as protection against bacteria, fungi and parasites. It enhances TNF-α production in response to endotoxin [34] and increases the cytotoxicity of monocytes, possibly by increasing their respiratory burst activity [35]. A direct role for IFN-γ in directing altered metabolic processes has not been defined in humans, although its administration does induce cachexia and loss of protein and lipid stores in animals [36].

Proinflammatory cytokines have been widely studied for their role in the pathogenesis of the cachectic state, particularly cancer-related anorexia cachexia syndrome (CACS) [37]. CACS results from circulating factors produced by the tumour, or by the host immune system in response to the tumour, such as cytokines released by lymphocytes and/or monocytes/macrophages. IL-1, IL-6, TNF-α, IFN-α and IFN-γ have been implicated in the pathogenesis of cachexia associated with human cancer. Direct evidence of a cytokine involvement in CACS is provided by the observation that cachexia can rarely be attributed to any one cytokine, but rather is associated with a set of cytokines that work in concert. These same cytokines seem to play central roles also in cachexia related to inflammation and the acute-phase response [37], congestive heart failure [38], and sarcopenia [39].

## The Acute-Phase Proteins

Nutritional status can be assessed by measuring blood levels of transport proteins, such as albumin, prealbumin, and transferrin. These proteins are known as negative acute-phase proteins and are the main facilitators of protein synthesis under normal circumstances [40]. When a catabolic process occurs, protein synthesis shifts from negative acute-phase reactants to the acute-phase acute reactants such as C-reactive protein and/or fibrinogen [41].

The acute-phase response is a rapid systemic reaction to tissue damage, typically observed during inflammation, infection or trauma, that integrates the elimination of microbes, the control of further tissue damage and the initiation of repair processes [42]. It is characterised by the release of a series of hepatocyte-derived plasma proteins known as acute-phase reactants, including C-reactive protein (CRP), fibrinogen, complement components B, C3 and C4, and by reduced synthesis of albumin and transferrin [37]. IL-1, IL-6 and TNF-$\alpha$ are regarded as the major mediators of acute-phase protein induction in the liver.

In patients with advanced cancer, baseline weight loss and Mini Nutritional Assessment score were strongly correlated to serum CRP. So, testing for the serum concentration of CRP at baseline may identify a subset of patients for whom decline in nutritional status is linked to the presence of an active inflammatory response, a recognised precursor of cachexia [43].

## Leptin and Immune Function

Initially described as an antiobesity hormone, leptin has subsequently been shown also to influence haematopoiesis, thermogenesis, reproduction, angiogenesis and immune response. Circulating levels of this adipocyte-derived hormone are proportional to fat mass, but may be lowered rapidly by fasting. Impaired cell-mediated immunity and reduced levels of leptin are both features of low body weight in humans. There is enough reported evidence to suggest a role for leptin in linking nutritional status to cognate cellular immune function, and to provide a molecular mechanism to account for the immune dysfunction observed in starvation [44]. The decrease in leptin plasma concentrations during food deprivation leads to impaired immune function, whereas the restoration of leptin to normal levels by feeding after starvation is sufficient to ameliorate the immune response and is followed by a significant increase in Th1 activity, supporting further the role of leptin as a nutritional sensor for the immune functions [45]. Therefore, leptin is the signal that connects the energy stores with the immune system, and may play a role in the immunosuppression of starvation. Leptin seems to be a signal for the adaptation of starvation, saving energy for muscle and brain activity [46]. Thus, leptin could be considered a link between nutritional status and the immune system [47].

## Immunological Tests for the Assessment of Nutritional Status

Although a large number of tests are routinely available to assess the immunological status of any individual's immune system, at present there is no one overall measure of immune function, making it difficult to design and assess studies aimed at determining the effect of a nutrient or food component on immunity. Moreover, nutritional changes are not likely to influence only one aspect of the immune system, and even if they do, they may also alter the other components [48].

### In Vivo Measures of Immune Function

The delayed T-cell hypersensitivity (DTH) response is a widely used in vivo assay for assessing an individual's bacterial host defence capability. Suppression of the response signals a failure of one or more components of the host defence system. In this procedure, a series of antigens (ubiquitous antigens derived from bacterial and fungal products as well as 2,4-dinitrochlorobenzene) are injected intradermally in the forearm and the area of induration is measured at 24 and 48 h. The rationale is that Langerhans cells will present the cutaneously encountered antigens to activated or memory T cells. Anergy (loss of cutaneous hypersensitivity) to skin testing is associated with adverse outcome from infections, burns, or surgical trauma and has been used to predict postoperative complications as well as the severity of various types of malnutrition (protein energy, iron, zinc, and vitamins A, C and B6) [49, 50]. Because of large interindividual variation in the response, sequential testing in subjects might be a more valuable use of this technique. The assumption is that improvement in the DTH response represents an increased resistance to infection; a decrease in the response was reported to be strongly associated with sepsis and related mortality in intensive care or trauma patients [51]. Neither the sensitivity nor the value of the DTH response for measuring moderate changes in nutrient intake in healthy persons is clear. However, DTH response appears to have been used successfully in a study that evaluated the efficacy of a nutritional supplement in the elderly [6].

## In Vitro Measures of Immune Function

In humans, studies of nutritional effects on immunity most often concentrate on peripheral blood lymphocytes. Automated peripheral white blood cell counts and differential cell counts are routine clinical measures that have been used as indexes of protein-energy malnutrition [48].

### Identification of Cell Types

Flow cytometry is the most reliable technique to determine the frequencies of different leucocyte types in a sample. Information, in the form of light scatter and fluorescence, is collected to measure a variety of cell characteristics that serve to identify leukocytes as lymphocytes, macrophages, etc. The flexibility of the flow cytometry technique is greatly enhanced by the use of monoclonal antibodies that recognise specific cellular markers. These antibodies, which bind to specific cell-surface epitopes, are conjugated to fluoresceinated materials that, when excited by the laser, serve to identify cell types. Flow cytometry is also used to measure other cellular parameters such as membrane fluidity, DNA content and intracellular $Ca^{2+}$.

### Leukocyte Function

A frequently used in vitro method for assessing the cell-mediated response to nutritional intervention is lymphocyte cellular proliferation (blastogenesis). Isolated immune cells are incubated with and without stimuli (e.g., mitogen, monoclonal antibody, cytokine, hormone, etc.). Briefly, a predetermined number of purified lymphocytes in a cell culture medium are stimulated by mitogens or agents that activate cells in an antigen-non-specific fashion. After a short period of culture (approximately 3 days), the cells are pulsed with $^3$H-thymidine, which is incorporated in the newly synthesised DNA of the proliferating cells and detected by scintillation counting. Alternatively, the expression of activation markers and other proteins on the cell surface in response to stimulation can be used as markers of stimulation. Other possible in vitro measurements of cell-mediated immune function are directed against allogenic histocompatibility antigens such as mixed leukocyte cultures [48].

### Cytokine Assays

During the past 20 years, an astonishing number of soluble factors that influence cells involved in the immune and inflammatory responses have been described. These non-antibody glycoproteins, generated by activated lymphocytes, act as intracellular mediators of the immunological response and are grouped under the term cytokines. Both nutritional status and specific nutrients have been reported to affect the concentration and production of cytokines [52, 53]. Cytokines released by cells in vitro or present in serum/plasma may be measurable by ELISA. However, because cytokines such as the interleukins tend to operate at very short intercellular distances, have very short half-lives, and/or are produced in minute quantities, ELISA detection may be impractical. Alternatively, Northern blot analysis or the polymerase chain reaction may be used to measure the levels of cytokine mRNA in cells, or intracellular cytokines may be detected by fluorescent anticytokine antibodies and quantified by flow cytometry technique.

### Apoptosis and Cell Death

Apoptosis (programmed cell death) is characterised morphologically by increased cytoplasmic granularity, cell shrinkage and nuclear condensation. The most prominent feature of apoptosis is the activation of an endogenous endonuclease that degrades nuclear DNA at linker sections to fragments. It has been suggested that a decrease in the rate of apoptosis plays a role in the pathogenesis and age-related events such as tumorigenesis. Energy restriction increases apoptosis, which may be the mechanism for its effect in suppressing tumours, ameliorating autoimmune diseases, and prolonging life span. Programmed cell death is an endpoint for many cellular events, but it has not been examined in nutrition studies [48].

### Gene Expression

Specific nutrients can affect gene expression and these changes significantly affect cellular function [54]. In immune cells, nutrients can have an impact on the early signals for gene expression and on the message and proteins of genes such as activation markers and cytokine-activation markers [55].

### Cellular Metabolism

The use of energy substrates by immune cells is a new and exciting field of research. Glucose and glutamine are the major energy sources of the immune system. When immune cells are activated, use of these nutrient substrates increases substantially and immune cells are extremely sensitive to changes in substrate availability [56, 57].

Thus, lymphocyte metabolism is a possible biomarker for many nutritional interventions.

### Membrane Composition

In lymphocytes, events associated with the plasma membrane play an important role in signal transduction, the expression of surface-associated molecules, enzymatic activities and cellular activation [58]. In other cell types, modifying the lipid composition of the plasma membrane alters its function [59]. Changing the fatty acid composition of lymphocyte phospholipids may be the mechanism by which fatty acids modulate lymphocyte functions [60]. Changing the n-6 and n-3 content of immune cell lipids affects lymphocyte proliferation, cell-to-cell adhesion, plasma membrane fluidity, the activity of membrane-bound enzymes, cytokine production, and the expression of some activation epitopes [58, 61].

## Influence of Nutritional Status on Immune Response

A survey of the literature shows that most nutritional deficits lead to suppressed immune responses. This is not surprising, since anabolic and catabolic pathways in the immune system require the same sort of building blocks and energy sources as other physiological activities. Caloric restriction is another area of emerging interest, with important implications for human health. In general, moderate caloric restriction appears to have beneficial effects on longevity and disease resistance. However, these trends and generalisations must be approached with some caution [62].

## Protein-Calorie Malnutrition

Protein-calorie malnutrition (PCM) is a major cause of immunodeficiency. Kwashiorkor (protein deficiency) and marasmus (generalised undernutrition or starvation) are the two clinical manifestations of PCM. The immunological manifestations of PCM are broad and include lymphoid tissue atrophy, decreases in lymphocyte count, and abnormally low cellular and humoral immune responses. As a result, PCM is associated with a high incidence of morbidity and mortality from infections [62].

## Proteins and Amino Acids

Inadequacies in general protein intake lead to suboptimal tissue repair and decreased resistance to infections and tumours. Studies on T lymphocytes indicate that protein malnutrition can have selective effects on immune functions [63]. Chronic protein deprivation in mice resulted in diminished IgG and DTH responses after 3 weeks, followed by reinstatement of normal responses by 11 weeks. Additionally, protein deprivation affects oral tolerance to ovoalbumin. Increases in DHT inflammatory responses suggested impaired T-cell suppression of the cell-mediated response [64].

## Arginine

Arginine is a semi-essential amino acid important to the urea cycle, and supports the synthesis of other amino acids and of polyamines, urea and NO [62]. Arginine is important for cell-mediated immunity, and exogenous sources are often required during sepsis. The growth and function of T lymphocytes in culture requires L-arginine. In vivo, arginine has the effect of retarding thymic involution by encouraging production of thymic hormones and thymocyte proliferation. Arginine also promotes leukocyte-mediated cytotoxicity in a number of ways. Growth hormone receptors are widespread in the immune system, and arginine may increase the cytotoxic activities of macrophages, NK cells, cytotoxic T cells, and neutrophils by releasing growth hormone. A product of arginine metabolism, NO, has tumoricidal and microbicidal activities, induces blood vessel dilatation, and influences leukocyte–endothelial cell adhesion.

## Glutamine

Glutamine is the most abundant amino acid in the blood and in the body's free amino acid pool [62].

Lymphocytes and macrophages use glutamine as a source of energy and molecular intermediates for purine and pyrimidine synthesis. As with arginine, glutamine is an essential component of leukocyte cell culture media. Following cellular uptake, a glutaminase in the inner mitochondrial membrane converts glutamine to glutamate and ammonia. Further processing results in production of aspartate and oxidation of about 25% of the glutamine to carbon dioxide. This 'glutaminolysis' pathway works in conjuction with the glycolytic pathway to allow the combined use of glucose and glutamine as energy sources in lymphocytes and macrophages.

The integrity of the intestinal immune system also relies heavily on sufficient glutamine intake. In animals, addition of glutamine to total parenteral nutrition inhibited the mucosal atrophy and leucocyte depletion normally associated with intravenous feeding, reduced bacterial translocation across the gut epithelium, and increased secretory IgA production.

## Nucleic Acids

Preformed purines and pyrimidines in the diet appear necessary to maintain a number of cell-mediated immunological mechanisms [62]. A variety of T-cell-associated processes declined when mice were fed nucleotide-free diets, including DTH responses, graft rejection, IL-2 and IFN-γ production, T-cell proliferation, splenic NK cell cytotoxicity, and impairments of polymorphonuclear leukocyte (PMN) functions. Dietary restriction of nucleotides also slowed the maturation of T lymphocytes. On the other hand, nucleotide supplementation improved human immune responses by increasing NK cell activity in human infants [65]. Among septic or critically ill patients, feeding commercial diets containing nucleotides resulted in shorter hospitalisation than feeding nucleotide-free diets [66].

## Oligoelements
### Copper

In animal and human studies, copper (Cu) deficiency is associated with increased susceptibility to infections. Cu deficiency may impair phagocyte functions, decrease T lymphocyte numbers and activities, lower IL-2 production, and increase B cell numbers [67–69]. A report on human responses to experimental Cu deficiency described a decrease in T-cell proliferation [70]. Explanations of these effects include copper's involvement in complement function, cell membrane integrity, immunoglobulin structure, Cu–Zn superoxide dismutase, and interactions with iron (Fe).

## Iron

A reduction in the plasma iron is considered an important host response to microbial infection. However, a number of T-cell and phagocyte abnormalities follow Fe deficiency [71]. Characteristic changes include reduced inflammatory responses such as the DTH reaction, impairments in neutrophil and macrophage cytotoxic activity, reductions in lymphocyte proliferation, T-cell numbers, cytokine release, antibody production, and lymphoid tissue atrophy. Whitley et al. [72] noted decreased allograft rejection and changes in the migration patterns of T lymphocytes.

The effects of Fe on immune function may be related to its involvement in folate metabolism, mitochondrial energy production, the respiratory burst, and/or its function as a component of many metalloenzymes including NO synthase, cyclooxygenase, lipoxygenase and catalase [73]. In addition, a complex network of interactions link iron metabolism with cellular immune function in the pathogenesis of 'anaemia of chronic disease' [74].

## Magnesium

Animal studies have associated magnesium (Mg) deficiency with increases in thymic cellularity and inflammatory cells (especially eosinophils). Magnesium deficits also elevate plasma concentrations of inflammatory cytokines such as IL-1, IL-6 and TNF-$\alpha$. Conversely, Mg deficiency decreased concentrations of acute-phase molecules [71]. Complement activity depends on an optimum Mg concentration range. In vitro T-cell-mediated lysis of target cells is directly propor-

tional to Mg concentration, an effect possibly mediated via interactions with adhesion molecules [75]. Since T cells may also induce target cell death by release of ATP, low Mg levels enhanced ATP-mediated killing of target cells.

## Manganese

Information on manganese (Mn) and immunity is relatively limited [67, 71]. Manganese is a component of several metalloenzymes that may participate in immune functions, including arginase, peroxidase, catalase and Mn superoxide dismutase [73].

## Selenium

Selenium (Se) deficiency is associated with suppression of a large number of immunological endpoints including resistance to infection, antibody synthesis, cytotoxicity, cytokine secretion and lymphocyte proliferation, and is also associated with a high incidence of cancer. Conversely, experimental Se supplementation increases the most important immune parameters, suggesting that this element has adjuvant properties.

In a recent paper, we demonstrated that $SeO_2$ was effective in inducing a progression of peripheral blood mononuclear cells isolated from advanced cancer patients into the cell cycle, which is an essential prerequisite for the physiological functioning of the immune system and thus positively influence the immune status of advanced cancer patients [76].

Selenium is also an essential component of glutathione peroxidase (GPx), an antioxidant enzyme that, in conjunction with vitamin E, prevents peroxidation of cellular and membrane lipids [71, 77]. As an example of their interaction, lowered antibody production caused by Se deficiency is reversible by vitamin E supplementation. Since phagocytes produce reactive oxygen species, limiting the potential for lipid peroxidation during immune and inflammatory processes is important to prevent autoxidation as well as damage to surrounding tissues. Indeed, excess $H_2O_2$ is neutralised by phagocyte-produced GPx.

In addition, Taylor [78] reported that Se could mediate post-translational modifications of important immune system proteins. A study of human mRNA sequences coding for CD4, CD8 and HLA-DR suggested alternate reading frames that could code for selenoproteins. Taylor hypothesised that redox reactions and selenium availability at these selenocysteine sites may alter the conformation of these proteins.

## Zinc

Insufficient zinc (Zn) intake may be the most common form of mineral deficiency, particularly among people consuming diets high in cereal and low in animal products. The best-documented immunological consequences of Zn deficiency are low thymic weights and T-cell defects [67, 71, 79]. Several T-cell abnormalities are related to Zn deficiency, including reduction in T-cell numbers and responsiveness to mitogenic stimuli; T cells help toward antibody production, DTH reactions, thymic hormone production, T-cell activity and T-cell maturation. Interestingly, Zn deprivation does not affect T-cell response to Con A, while the responses to phytohaemagglutinin and pokeweed mitogen are reduced, suggesting differences in Zn dependency among T-cell subpopulations.

The presence of Zn in many proteins [80] complicates the understanding of Zn-related immune effects. Zn is a widely used structural component: Zn-finger structures are found in transcription factors and nuclear-hormone receptors. Zn is known to influence endocrine function: recently, prolactin was shown to bind Zn [81]. The activity of thymulin is Zn dependent [82], as is the respiratory burst of macrophages [83]. Obviously, a deficiency of Zn may cause numerous irregularities in the immune system.

## Vitamins

Vitamins are important factors in a wide variety of metabolic processes such as gene transcription, enzymatic reactions and redox reactions. Reviews of the literature present a correspondingly broad range of immunological effects related to vitamin deficiencies and excesses [67, 71, 77, 84].

## Vitamin A

A deficiency of vitamin A is associated with increased morbidity and mortality, most likely because of increased severity of infections [85]. Vitamin A and related retinoids maintain the integrity of epithelial boundaries and the production of mucosal secretions. Some of the immunological abnormalities following vitamin A inadequacies include a reduced number of leukocytes, reduced lymphoid organ weights, reduced circulating levels of complement, impaired T-cell functions, and decreased resistance to immunogenic tumours.

Vitamin A supplementation studies showed decreases in respiratory infections and neutrophil counts and increases in reticuloendothelial system function, lymphocyte proliferation, tumour resistance, graft rejection and cytotoxic T-cell activities. Supplementation above that required to maintain normal vitamin A stores results in adjuvant effects. Excess vitamin A increases antibody and cell-mediated immune responses, stimulates Kupffer cells and potentiates some types of liver toxicity and gouty arthritis [86]. The inhibition of T-cell apoptosis by retinoic acid may contribute to its adjuvant effect [87].

The vitamin A precursor β-carotene is generally considered an antioxidant with activities that are independent of its provitamin A function. Some of its reported benefits include protecting host cells and tissues from oxidation by the respiratory burst and promoting lymphocyte proliferation, T-cell functions, cytokine production and cell-mediated cytotoxicity. However, Bates [88] cautioned that carotenoids can exhibit both pro-oxidant and antioxidant activity.

## B Complex Vitamins

Pyridoxine or vitamin B6 deficiency induces lymphocytopenia with decrease in lymphoid tissue weight and reduced proliferative responses to mitogens. There are general deficiencies in cell-mediated immunity, including allograft rejection, IL-2 production, and the DTH response [84]. Humoral immunity is also affected, as seen by lowered antibody responses and depression in antigen-specific secondary responses. The pyridoxine requirement for nucleic acid and protein synthesis during lymphocyte proliferation is probably responsible for the greater effect on lymphocyte than on macrophages or NK cells. Appropriate vitamin B6 supplementation readily restores the immunological deficiencies.

Cianocobalamin (vitamin B12) deficiency and folate deficiency are clinically indistinguishable since both are required for synthesis of thymidylate. Their deficiency depresses a number of immunological parameters including the respiratory burst, phagocytosis by PMNs, DTH reponses and T-cell proliferation by phytohemagglutinin. Biotin deficiency is associated with humoral and cell-mediated immune deficiencies. Depression in thymic weight, antigen-specific antibody responses, and reduced lymphocyte-mediated suppressor activity have been noted. Deficiency in panthotenic acid commonly leads to decreased antibody responses. The biochemical consequence may be an inability to secrete newly synthesised proteins into the extracellular space. Immunological abnormalities associated with vitamin B1 (thiamine) deficiency include increased susceptibility to infectious disease agents, premature thymic atrophy, decreased antibody responses, and reduced PMN mobility [62].

## Vitamin C

Vitamin C functions as a biological reducing agent in regeneration of oxidised vitamin E [89]. Immunological problems associated with vitamin C deficits include impairment in many immunological functions, such as decreased resistance to infections and cancer, reduced phagocyte mobility and phagocytosis, diminished DTH response, reduced skin allograft rejection and wound repair. Studies on people of different age groups demonstrated the ability of vitamin C supplementation to enhance many of the above immunological parameters, including the DTH and antibody responses [90].

## Vitamin D

Vitamin D has both stimulatory and suppressive effects on immune responses because of its influence on mineral metabolism and its hormonal nature. For example, vitamin D stimulates maturation of normal and neoplastic myelomonocytic cells to more differentiated monocytes and macrophages. Receptors of vitamin D present on the surface of activated lymphocytes probably mediate vitamin D's influence on lymphocyte proliferation and function [62].

## Vitamin E

Vitamin E deficiency is relatively rare in human populations and controversy exists about recommended intakes. However, its essential nature derives from its function as a radical scavenger to limit cell membrane peroxidation and its interactions with other antioxidants [91]. Experimentally induced deficiency leads to depressed leukocyte proliferation, lower chemotaxis and phagocytosis by PMNs and macrophages, and decreased tumour resistance. Vitamin E supplementation increased a number of immune parameters including lymphocyte proliferation, antibody levels, the DTH reaction, IL-2 production and phagocytosis. Supplementation also reduced $PGE_2$ synthesis, level of plasma lipid hydroperoxides, and oxidative damage induced by burns in lung tissue. Vitamin E supplementation also restored Th1 activity, and IL-2 and IFN-$\gamma$ production in murine AIDS [92]. Finally, in human populations high vitamin E intake increases resistance to infections among the elderly.

## Lipids

Fatty acids (FA) function as energy sources, as cell membrane components, and as mediators of cell signalling. Since cell membrane composition is partially dependent on the FA species taken through the diet [93], dietary lipids have an important influence on cell function. Among the polyunsaturated fatty acids (PUFAs), the most important dietary sources are the n-3 PUFAs.

The n-3 PUFA eicosapentaenoic acid (EPA) and docosahexaenoic acid (DHA), which are found in fish oils, suppress the production of arachidonic-acid-derived eicosanoids and EPA is a substrate for the synthesis of an alternative family of eicosanoids. Thus, dietary fats that are rich in n-3 PUFAs have the potential to alter cytokine production. Several human studies have shown that supplementation of the diet of healthy volunteers results in reduced ex vivo production of IL-1, IL-6, TNF-α and IL-2 by peripheral blood mononuclear cells. Similar results have been found in patients with rheumatoid arthritis and multiple sclerosis. Animal studies indicate that dietary fish oil reduces the response to endotoxin and to proinflammatory cytokines, resulting in increased survival: such diets have been beneficial in some models of bacterial challenge, chronic inflammation and auto-immunity. These beneficial effects of dietary n-3 PUFAs may be useful as a therapy for acute and chronic inflammation and for disorders that involve an inappropriately activated immune response [94].

In a randomised controlled study, Gogos et al. [95] investigated the effect of dietary omega-3 PUFA plus vitamin E on the immune status and survival of well-nourished and malnourished patients with generalised malignancy. Sixty patients with generalised solid tumours were randomised to receive dietary supplementation with either fish oil (18 g of omega-3 PUFA) or placebo daily until death. Each group included 15 well-nourished and 15 malnourished patients. They found that omega-3 PUFA had a considerable immunomodulating effect by increasing the ratio of T-helper cells to T-suppressor cells in the subgroup of malnourished patients. There were no significant differences in cytokine production among the groups, except for a decrease in TNF-α production in malnourished cancer patients,

which was restored by omega-3 fatty acids. The mean survival was significantly higher for the subgroup of well-nourished patients in both groups, whereas omega-3 fatty acids prolonged the survival of all the patients [95].

## Conclusions

Nutritional status and specific nutrients may impact on the immune system. In addition, altered immune status can impact on nutritional status. For example, immune response to injury (infection, cancer, etc.) can change the efficiency of the body to adsorb and utilise nutrients, alter metabolic rate, modify hormone secretion, alter hepatic synthesis of proteins or lipids, change intracellular enzymes (gluconeogenesis, lipogenesis, etc.). Mediators of immune response such as proinflammatory cytokines and CRP are involved in the pathogenesis of several metabolic disorders (diabetes mellitus, insulin resistance, obesity, cachexia associated with different chronic diseases) and have a well-recognised role as prognostic factors of disease outcome and survival. So, the assessment of immunological parameters has to be included in an exhaustive global assessment of nutritional status, especially with the aim to develop and to monitor the effect of nutritional approaches. Another exciting field of research is the attempt to modulate immunocompetence in health and disease by designing nutritional supplements and diets aimed at modulation of specific immune functions [96].

## References

1. Bistrian BR, Blackburn GL, Sherman M et al (1975) Therapeutic index of nutritional depletion in hospitalized patients. Surg Gynecol Obstet 141:512–516
2. Field CJ (2000) Use of T cell function to determine the effect of physiologically active food components. Am J Clin Nutr 71:1720S–1725S
3. Romagnani S (1994) Lymphokine production by human T cells in disease states. Annu Rev Immunol 12:227–257
4. Chandra RK (2002) Nutrition and the immune system from birth to old age. Eur J Clin Nutr 56:S73–S76
5. Roubenoff R (1997) Inflammatory and hormonal mediators of cachexia. J Nutr 127:1014S–1016S
6. Chandra RK (1997) Graying of the immune system: can nutrient supplements improve immunity in the elderly? JAMA 277:1398–1399
7. Nossal GJV (1993) Life, death and the immune system. Sci Am 269:52–64
8. Field CJ (1996) Using immunological techniques to determine the effect of nutrition on T-cell function. Can J Physiol Pharmacol 74:769–777
9. Pomposelli JJ, Flores EA, Bistrian BR (1988) Role of biochemical mediators in clinical nutrition and surgical metabolism. JPEN J Parenter Enteral Nutr 12:212–218

10. Kushner I (1993) Regulation of the acute phase response by cytokines. Perspect Biol Med 36:611–622

11. Klasing KC (1988) Nutritional aspects of leukocytic cytokines. J Nutr 118:1436–1446

12. Fong Y, Lowry SF (1996) Cytokines and the cellular response to injury and infection. In: Harken AH, Wilmore DW (eds) Care of the surgical patient. Sci Am (Suppl), pp 1–21

13. Smith MK, Lowry SF (1998) The hypercatabolic state. In: Shils ME, Olson JA, Shike M, Ross AC (eds) Modern nutrition in health and disease, 9th ed. Williams and Wilkins, Baltimore, pp 1555–1568

14. Hotamisligil GS, Shargill NS, Spiegelman BM (1993) Adipose expression of tumor necrosis factor-alpha: direct role in obesity-linked insulin resistance. Science 259:87–91

15. Carswell EA, Old LJ, Kassel RL et al (1975) An endotoxin-induced serum factor that causes necrosis of tumors. Proc Natl Acad Sci USA 72:3666–3670

16. Tracey KJ, Cerami A (1993) Tumor necrosis factor, other cytokines and disease. Annu Rev Cell Biol 9:317–343

17. Fong Y, Lowry SF (1993) Metabolic consequences of critical illness. In: Barie PS, Shires GT (eds) Surgical intensive care, vol 1. Little, Brown and Co, Boston, pp 893–905

18. Finck BN, Johnson RW (2000) Tumor necrosis factor-alpha regulates secretion of the adipocyte-derived cytokine, leptin. Microsc Res Tech 50:209–215

19. Oliff A, Defeo-Jones D, Boyer M et al (1987) Tumors secreting human TNF/cachectin induce cachexia in mice. Cell 50:555–563

20. Van der Poll T, Romijn JA, Endert E et al (1991) Tumor necrosis factor mimics the metabolic response to acute infection in healthy humans. Am J Physiol 261:E457–E465

21. Stephens JM, Pekala PH (1991) Transcriptional repression of the GLUT4 and C/EBP genes in 3T3-L1 adipocytes by tumor necrosis factor-alpha. J Biol Chem 266:21839–21845

22. Mackay AG, Oliver JD, Rogers MP (1990) Regulation of lipoprotein lipase activity and mRNA content in rat epididymal adipose tissue in vitro by recombinant tumour necrosis factor. Biochem J 269:123–126

23. Hardardottir I, Doerrler W, Feingold KR, Grunfeld C (1992) Cytokines stimulate lipolysis and decrease lipoprotein lipase activity in cultured fat cells by a prostaglandin independent mechanism. Biochem Biophys Res Commun 186:237–243

24. Adi S, Pollock AS, Shigenaga JK et al (1992) Role for monokines in the metabolic effects of endotoxin. Interferon-gamma restores responsiveness of C3H/HeJ mice in vivo. J Clin Invest 89:1603–1609

25. Beutler B, Cerami A (1986) Cachectin and tumour necrosis factor as two sides of the same biological coin. Nature 320:584–588

26. Jirillo E, Covelli V, Maffione AB et al (1994) Endotoxins, cytokines, and neuroimmune networks with special reference to HIV infection. Ann NY Acad Sci 741:174–184

27. Renno T, Krakowski M, Piccirillo C et al (1995) TNF-alpha expression by resident microglia and infiltrating leukocytes in the central nervous system of mice with experimental allergic encephalomyelitis. Regulation by Th1 cytokines. J Immunol 154:944–953

28. Tracey KJ, Lowry SF (1990) The role of cytokine mediators in septic shock. Adv Surg 23:21–56

29. Helfgott DC, Tatter SB, Santhanam U et al (1989) Multiple forms of IFN-beta 2/IL-6 in serum and body fluids during acute bacterial infection. J Immunol 142:948–953

30. Castell JV, Gomez-Lechon MJ, David M et al (1989) Interleukin-6 is the major regulator of acute phase protein synthesis in adult human hepatocytes. FEBS Lett 242:237–239

31. Garman RD, Jacobs KA, Clark SC, Raulet DH (1987) B-cell-stimulatory factor 2 (beta 2 interferon) functions as a second signal for interleukin 2 production by mature murine T cells. Proc Natl Acad Sci USA 84:7629–33

32. Stouthard JM, Romijn JA, Van der Poll T et al (1995) Endocrinologic and metabolic effects of interleukin-6 in humans. Am J Physiol 268:E813–E819

33. Papanicolaou DA, Petrides JS, Tsigos C et al (1996) Exercise stimulates interleukin-6 secretion: inhibition by glucocorticoids and correlation with catecholamines. Am J Physiol 271:E601–E605

34. Luedke CE, Cerami A (1990) Interferon-gamma overcomes glucocorticoid suppression of cachectin/tumor necrosis factor biosynthesis by murine macrophages. J Clin Invest 86:1234–1240

35. Nathan CF, Murray HW, Wiebe ME, Rubin BY (1983) Identification of interferon-gamma as the lymphokine that activates human macrophage oxidative metabolism and antimicrobial activity. J Exp Med 158:670–689

36. Matthys P, Dijkmans R, Proost P et al (1991) Severe cachexia in mice inoculated with interferon-gamma-producing tumor cells. Int J Cancer 49:77–82

37. Mantovani G, Macciò A, Massa E, Madeddu C (2001) Managing cancer-related anorexia/cachexia. Drugs 61:499–514

38. Freeman LM, Roubenoff R (1994) The nutrition implication of cardiac cachexia. Nutr Rev 52:340–347

39. Morley JE, Baumgartner RN, Roubenoff R et al (2001) Sarcopenia. J Lab Clin Med 137:231–243

40. Heimburger DC, Weinsier RL (1997) Handbook of clinical nutrition. Mosby, St Louis

41. Fearon KC, Barber MD, Falconer JS et al (1999) Pancreatic cancer as a model: inflammatory mediators, acute-phase response, and cancer cachexia. World J Surg 23:584–588

42. Baumann H, Gauldie J (1994) The acute phase response. Immunol Today 15:74–80

43. Slaviero KA, Read JA, Clarke SJ, Rivory LP (2003) Baseline nutritional assessment in advanced cancer patients receiving palliative chemotherapy. Nutr Cancer 46:148–157

44. Lord GM, Matarese G, Howard JK et al (1998) Leptin modulates the T-cell immune response and reverses starvation-induced immunosuppression. Nature 394:897–901

45. Palacio A, Lopez M, Perez-Bravo F et al (2002) Leptin levels are associated with immune response in malnourished infants. J Clin Endocrinol Metab 87:3040–3046

46. Sanchez-Margalet V, Martin-Romero C, Santos-Alvarez J et al (2003) Role of leptin as an immunomodulator of blood mononuclear cells: mechanisms of action. Clin Exp Immunol 133:11–19

47. La Cava A, Alviggi C, Matarese G (2004) Unraveling the multiple roles of leptin in inflammation and autoimmunity. J Mol Med 82:4–11

48. Field CJ (2000) Use of T cell function to determine the effect of physiologically active food components. Am J Clin Nutr 71:1720S–1725S

49. Bistrian BR, Blackburn GL, Sherman M et al (1975) Therapeutic index of nutritional depletion in hospitalized patients. Surg Gynecol Obstet 141:512–516

50. McMurray DN (1984) Cell-mediated immunity in nutritional deficiency. Prog Food Nutr Sci 8:193–228

51. Christou NV, Meakins JL, Gordon J et al (1995) The delayed hypersensitivity response and host resistance in surgical patients. 20 years later. Ann Surg 222:534–538

52. Beisel WR (1995) Herman Award Lecture, 1995: infection-induced malnutrition – from cholera to cytokines. Am J Clin Nutr 62:813–819

53. Jolly CA, Jiang YH, Chapkin RS et al (1997) Dietary (n-3) polyunsaturated fatty acids suppress murine lymphoproliferation, interleukin-2 secretion, and the formation of diacylglycerol and ceramide. J Nutr 127:37–43

54. Docherty K, Clark AR (1994) Nutrient regulation of insulin gene expression. FASEB J 8:20–27

55. Robinson LE, Field CJ (1998) Dietary long chain (n-3) fatty acids facilitate immune cell activation in sedentary, but not exercise-trained rats. J Nutr 128:498–504

56. Wu GY, Field CJ, Marliss EB (1991) Elevated glutamine metabolism in splenocytes from spontaneously diabetic BB rats. Biochem J 274:40–54

57. Yaqoob P, Knapper JA, Webb DH et al (1998) Effect of olive oil on immune function in middle-aged men. Am J Clin Nutr 67:129–135

58. Calder PC, Yaqoob P, Harvey DJ et al (1994) Incorporation of fatty acids by concanavalin A-stimulated lymphocytes and the effect on fatty acid composition and membrane fluidity. Biochem J 300:509–518

59. Clandinin MT, Cheema S, Field CJ et al (1991) Dietary fat: exogenous determination of membrane structure and cell function. FASEB J 5:2761–69

60. Peck MD (1994) Interactions of lipids with immune function II: experimental and clinical studies of lipids and immunity. J Nutr Biochem 5:514–520

61. Meydani M, Meydani SN, Shapiro AC et al (1991) Influence of dietary fat, vitamin E, ethoxyquin and indomethacin on the synthesis of prostaglandin E2 in brain regions of mice. J Nutr 121:438–444

62. Yoshida AH, Keen CL, Ansari AA, Gershwin E (1999) Nutrition and the immune system. In: Schills ME, Olson JA, Shike M, Ross AC (eds) Modern nutrition in health and disease, 9th ed. Williams & Wilkins, Baltimora, pp 725–750

63. Ferguson A (1994) Immunological functions of the gut in relation to nutritional state and mode of delivery of nutrients. Gut 35:S10–S12

64. Weiner HL, Friedman A, Miller A et al (1994) Oral tolerance: immunologic mechanisms and treatment of animal and human organ-specific autoimmune diseases by oral administration of autoantigens. Annu Rev Immunol 12:809–837

65. Carver JD (1994) Dietary nucleotides: cellular immune, intestinal and hepatic system effects. J Nutr 124:144S–148S

66. Van Buren CT, Kulkarni AD, Rudolph FB (1994) The role of nucleotides in adult nutrition. J Nutr 124:160S–164S

67. Newberne PM, Locniskar M (1991) Nutrition and immune status. In: Rowland I (ed) Nutrition, toxicity, and cancer. CRC Press, Boca Raton

68. Kramer TR, Johnson WT (1993) Copper and immunity. In: Cunningham-Rundles S (ed) Nutrient modulation of immune response. Marcel Dekker, New York

69. O'Dell BL (1993) Interleukin-2 production is altered by copper deficiency. Nutr Rev 51:307–309

70. Kelley DS, Daudu PA, Taylor PC et al (1995) Effects of low-copper diets on human immune response. Am J Clin Nutr 62: 412–416

71. Myrvik QN (1994) Immunology and nutrition. In: Shills ME, Olson JA, Shike M (eds) Modern nutrition in health and disease, 8th ed. Lea & Febiger, Philadelphia, pp 623–662

72. Whitley WD, Hancock WW, Kupiec-Weglinski JW et al (1993) Iron chelation suppresses mononuclear cell activation, modifies lymphocyte migration patterns, and prolongs rat cardiac allograft survival in rats. Transplantation 56:1182–1188

73. Karlin KD (1993) Metalloenzymes, structural motifs, and inorganic models. Science 261:701–708

74. Weiss G, Wachter H, Fuchs D (1995) Linkage of cell-mediated immunity to iron metabolism. Immunol Today 16:495–500

75. Redegeld F, Filippini A, Sitkovsky M (1991) Comparative studies of the cytotoxic T lymphocyte-mediated cytotoxicity and of extracellular ATP-

induced cell lysis. Different requirements in extracellular $Mg^{2+}$ and pH. J Immunol 147:3638–3645

76. Mantovani G, Macciò A, Madeddu C et al (2004) Selenium is effective in inducing lymphocyte progression through cell cycle in cancer patients: potential mechanisms for its activity. J Exp Ther Oncol 4: 69–78

77. Kuvibidila S, Yu L, Ode D et al (1993) The immune response in protein-energy malnutrition and single nutrient deficiencies. In: Klurfield DM (ed) Nutrition and immunology. Plenum Press, New York, pp 121–157

78. Taylor EW (1995) Selenium and cellular immunity. Evidence that selenoproteins may be encoded in the +1 reading frame overlapping the human CD4, CD8, and HLA-DR genes. Biol Trace Elem Res 49:85–95

79. Vruwink KG, Keen CL, Gershwin ME et al (1993) The effect of experimental zinc deficiency on development of the immune system. In: Cunningham-Rundles S (ed) Nutrient modulation of the immune response. Marcel Dekker, New York, pp 263–279

80. Berg JM, Shi Y ()1996 The galvanization of biology: a growing appreciation for the roles of zinc. Science 271:1081–1085

81. Lorenson MY, Patel T, Liu JW, Walker AM (1996) Prolactin (PRL) is a zinc-binding protein. I. Zinc interactions with monomeric PRL and divalent cation protection of intragranular PRL cysteine thiols. Endocrinology 137:809–816

82. Hadden JW (1995) The treatment of zinc deficiency is an immunotherapy. Int J Immunopharmacol 17:697–701

83. Cook-Mills JM, Fraker PJ (1993) The role of metals in the production of toxic oxygen metabolites by mononuclear phagocytes. In: Cunningham-Rundles S (ed) Nutrient modulation of the immune response. Marcel Dekker, New York, pp 127–140

84. Blumberg JB (1994) Vitamins. In: Forse RA (ed) Diet, nutrition, and immunity. CRC Press, Boca Raton, p 237

85. Ross AC, Hammerling UG (1994) Retinoids and the immune system. In: Sporn MB, Roberts AB, Goodman DS (eds) The retinoids: biology, chemistry, and medicine, 2nd ed. Raven Press, New York, pp 521a–543a

86. Mawson AR, Onor GI (1991) Gout and vitamin A intoxication: is there a connection? Semin Arthritis Rheum 20:297–304

87. Iwata M, Mukai M, Nakai Y, Iseki R (1992) Retinoic acids inhibit activation-induced apoptosis in T cell hybridomas and thymocytes. J Immunol 149:3302–3308

88. Bates CJ (1995) Vitamin A. Lancet 345:31–35

89. Muggli R (1993) Vitamin C and phagocytes. In: Cunningham-Rundles S (ed) Nutrient modulation of the immune response. Marcel Dekker, New York

90. Cunningham-Rundles WF, Berner Y, Cunningham-Rundles S (1993) Interaction of vitamin C in lymphocyte activation: current status and possible mechanism of action. In: Cunningham-Rundles S (ed) Nutrient modulation of the immune response. Marcel Dekker, New York

91. Meydani SN, Blumberg JB (1993) Vitamin E and the immune response. In: Cunningham-Rundles S (ed) Nutrient modulation of the immune response. Marcel Dekker, New York

92. Wang Y, Huang DS, Eskelson CD, Watson RR (1994) Long-term dietary vitamin E retards development of retrovirus-induced disregulation in cytokine production. Clin Immunol Immunopathol 72:70–75

93. Taraszewski R, Jensen GL (1994) N-6 fatty acids. In: Forse RA (ed) Diet, nutrition, and immunity. CRC Press, Boca Raton, pp 165–177

94. Calder PC (1997) N-3 polyunsaturated fatty acids and cytokine production in health and disease. Ann Nutr Metab 41:203–234

95. Gogos CA, Ginopoulos P, Salsa B et al (1998) Dietary omega-3 polyunsaturated fatty acids plus vitamin E restore immunodeficiency and prolong survival for severely ill patients with generalized malignancy: a randomized control trial. Cancer 82:395–402

96. Gogos CA, Kalfarentzos F (1995) Total parenteral nutrition and immune system activity: a review. Nutrition 11:339–344

# Functional Parameters of Nutrition

Max Dahele, Kenneth C.H. Fearon

## Introduction

Functional assessment is at the heart of understanding how a chronic disease and its therapy impact on patients. It puts into tangible terms what the patient is capable of and brings an understandable 'human context' to the patient burden. Functional status can be a prognostic indicator. It may also have a role in treatment selection for individual patients and be used to enter and stratify patients in clinical trials. It remains to be seen whether it will be possible and practical to use end-points such as function (and other related end-points such as 'quality of life') to direct individual patient management. Using cancer cachexia as a paradigm, this chapter sets out to discuss some of the broader issues in functional patient assessment. New approaches to assessing function and preliminary experience with an emerging technology are also presented.

Traditional end-points such as survival are used because there is certainty over the event and its meaning. However, the translation of other apparently clear-cut outcomes such as tumour response or weight gain in a cachectic patient into tangible patient benefit cannot be taken for granted [1]. There is a requirement for patient-centred end-points in medicine especially when confronted by a chronic disease, when cure may not be a realistic proposition and maximising function and well-being for as long as possible becomes the priority. These end-points should be robust enough to assess objectively individual patients and the therapeutic benefit they are deriving from an intervention and 'user-friendly' enough for both patient and medical staff to complete in a busy environment. For some (physicians and patients alike), acknowledging the shift from 'cure' to 'preservation' represents a significant lowering

of expectation and may be difficult. This may also demand more of 'physician–patient' communication and of their relationship. However such a shift has the potential to assist the patient in making the most of their capabilities. Assessing a disease and its therapy with these end-points may also facilitate an understanding of treatment aims and agreement between the patient and physician on the likelihood of achieving these aims – does greater survival come at the expense of marked morbidity and increased functional dependence? Patients may have different priorities and expectations when assessing treatment options and greater insight into the likely effects of an intervention may assist in their decision-making. An increased understanding of the possible functional effects of a therapy may also raise awareness of the patient, their family and the medical team and allow them to identify problems at an early stage.

In addition to more rigorous and comprehensive individual patient care, a functional approach to assessing illness and intervention offers the possibility of enhancing the profession's understanding of both disease and treatment. There are also wider societal, financial and service costs from the burgeoning number of therapeutic options in medicine. To make health service and policy decisions about the affordability and cost-effectiveness of an intervention requires as clear an understanding as possible of the likely benefits and toxicities to be derived. Functional assessment may hold promise in providing information to assist in making these decisions.

## What is Functional Assessment?

Functional assessment in medicine has been formalised. It involves obtaining information about 'activities of daily living' (ADL) on three levels using tools specific for each of these levels:

1. Basic activities of daily living (BADL), which include bathing, dressing and feeding (e.g. Barthel index [2])
2. Intermediate or instrumental activities of daily living (IADL), which comprise activities such as shopping, housework and finances (e.g. Lawton IADL scale [3])
3. Advanced activities of daily living (AADL), which include more complex personal, family and social roles (e.g. Reuben AADL scale [4]).

In the present chapter, a less restrictive concept of patient function is used. Some of the tools already in widespread clinical use in oncology are less rigorous in their assessment of these different levels of functioning or health domains. However, even abbreviated tools can collect important information with prognostic value.

Although functional assessment is well established in oncology, geriatric medicine exemplifies 'complete' functional assessment. Applying the 'comprehensive geriatric assessment' (CGA) method has been demonstrated to improve patient function [5]. This tool assesses patient function, co-morbidity, nutrition and mental status. There is a growing voice within 'geriatric oncology' to use the CGA or a similar tool to optimise patient management. Some cachectic patients may be biologically older than their chronological age and tools like the CGA therefore deserve further study in cachectic patients.

## Performance Status as a Functional End-Point in Oncology

Assigning a 'performance status' (PS) score to a patient is the most common form of functional assessment in oncology. There are several PS tools in widespread use, providing a formal framework for gathering functional information and influencing treatment decisions. Common examples are the Karnofsky PS score (KPS) [6], an 11-point scale from normal (score = 100) to deceased (0) and the World Health Organisation (WHO) PS score [7], a more succinct five-point scale from normal (0) to completely disabled and confined to

bed/chair (4). These scores assess several variables including patient independence and ability to work and be active. These performance status tools are simple and broadly comparable. They are quick, convenient and readily administered in the clinic and are of prognostic value. They are, however, scored by a third party (e.g. physician) usually from information gleaned in dialogue with the patient (cognitive status permitting) and this has been a point of criticism. In fact the literature on patient–physician agreement is inconclusive. Whilst some find little consistency [8], others [9] find that there is general agreement between oncologist and patient-generated PS scores (in this case using another common tool – the Eastern Co-operative Oncology Group [ECOG] or 'Zubrod' tool [10] – analogous to the WHO tool).

There are other concerns – it has been suggested that PS suffers from being too narrow a tool [11], that inter-observer reliability is only moderate [12] and that conventional PS tools may be less informative in older patients [13]. In addition, it is unclear just how objective and accurate is the information obtained in PS assessment. Undoubtedly there is scope for the further refinement of routine functional assessment – to increase objectivity and information content, to optimise the application and clinical utility of the information that is collected and to develop tools that provide free-living information. However, despite these concerns, it remains the case that by applying these tools widely in oncology, function has rightly assumed an important role in patient assessment and has become established as a means of assessing suitability for therapy and as an entry and stratification criterion for clinical trials.

## Contrasting Performance Status and Quality of Life – Two Patient-Centred, 'Non-survival' End-Points in Common Use in Oncology

In common with PS assessment, quality of life (QoL) tools gather patient-centred information, which may also be of prognostic value. Quality of life questionnaires elicit information on physical functioning and much more. This breadth leads some to consider them more effective and meaningful than simple functional assessment alone, but how do these two non-survival end-points contrast?

Protagonists of QoL methodology point out that it may herald a paradigm shift in medicine away from a disease-oriented and towards a patient-centred perspective [14]. But what is 'quality of life'? This has been a difficult concept to define and although QoL assessment has entered widespread use in oncology, there remains considerable debate about this central issue. What is clear is that it is a multidimensional concept with a broader scope than performance status. The WHO has defined health as a 'state of complete physical, mental and social well-being' [15] and most comprehensive QoL tools will include an assessment of these 'domains'. Health-related QoL (HRQoL) focuses on QoL in the presence of illness and concentrates on gathering information on those parameters most affected by the illness and its treatment. An example of a 'generic' QoL tool is the Medical Outcomes Study Short-Form Health Survey, SF-36 [16] and there are several commonly used oncology-specific tools (e.g. European Organisation for Research and Treatment of Cancer, EORTC [17] and Functional Assessment of Cancer Therapy, FACT [18]).

A recent study by Cohen [19] is informative in discussing what 'quality of life' means to patients. Patients' definitions of QoL were grouped into five domains – the patient's own state, the quality of their palliative care, their physical environment, relationships and outlook – and the authors commented that no single instrument at that time addressed all of these. Relevant to the study of cachexia, Greisinger [20] and Steinhauser [21] have also addressed this issue in patients with a prognosis of 6 months or less. Although attempting to record accurately the patient's experience, most QoL tools use researcher-defined domains (such as physical, functional, social and emotional well-being [22]) and there is a concern that in so doing they may reflect the views of health professionals rather than patients. Waldron [23] studied determinants of QoL and suggested that the emphasis placed on health by many QoL tools might be questionable in patients with advanced cancer.

Whilst the variables assessed by functional or PS tools contribute in some way to QoL, these are not interchangeable or directly comparable methodologies. Performance status correlates with other 'medical variables' in the disease process. However, a greater understanding of what functional information is most appropriate to collect, the relationship of functional assessment to individual QoL domains, whether function alone is a surrogate for overall 'quality of life', how to collect optimally and interpret functional information and whether or not questionnaire-based functional assessment is accurate are all questions that need further study.

Quality of life tools tend to gather subjective data. In contrast, some functional assessment tools (such as the 'Simmonds Functional Assessment', see below) can provide objective information. One of the challenges with tools such as this is how to know that what is measured in a controlled environment reflects the patient's 'free-living' experience in their own environment.

Although there has been increasing interest in and utilisation of QoL tools, both in research and in some aspects of clinical practice, these tools tend to be complex and represent a significant burden for clinician and patient. Shorter tools that give a 'global' QoL score have been shown to give meaningful information [24] but they have not generally been favoured as it has been felt that they provide little understanding of what determines the score. They have also been felt to be less responsive to change over time and they are seen as less helpful in identifying unexpected outcomes. The tendency to favour more comprehensive instruments means that they become more time consuming and are not well suited to routine use in the clinic. They require sophisticated analysis, training in their use and expertise in their application and interpretation. Measuring responses and analysing and interpreting QoL data are also challenging [25]. Although a large amount of information is gathered by QoL tools, it is unclear how this information should best be synthesised – for example, should individual responses or domains be weighted, and if so, how? Selection bias due to drop-out resulting from the complexity of the tools has already been a hurdle in some QoL studies [26]. Common QoL tools are not interchangeable and are unlikely to be directly comparable [27]. It is important to choose the most appropriate QoL tool for the study population as different tools may lead to different results or conclusions. Consideration should also be given as to the timing of data collection [28]. Such complexities have given rise to recent calls for an international consensus on how to assess quality of life in oncology [29]. Finally, it remains unclear how useful QoL tools are in routine practice. In busy clinic settings, logistics may impede the routine collection of QoL data [30] and strategies are needed to overcome this.

Many of these challenges will also be relevant to developing functional assessment as an effective means of gathering sufficient information about cachectic patients to optimise holistic management. Although one method is sometimes presented as superior to the other, PS and QoL tools are different. Given the likely interdependence of function and other aspects of patient well-being, these two methodologies may turn out to be complementary and composite tools may be needed for optimum patient assessment in cachexia.

## Cancer Cachexia: The Importance of Functional Assessment

### What is Cancer Cachexia and how Might It Affect Function?

The workshop 'Clinical Trials for the Treatment of Secondary Wasting and Cachexia: Selection of Appropriate Endpoints' (1997) indicated a lack of consensus as to the definition of cachexia and its evaluation and treatment [31]. Consensus is required to facilitate the rigorous evaluation of patients with cachexia and the assessment of interventions. Non-volitional weight loss has often been used as a surrogate for 'cachexia'. However, this fails to capture the subtleties of the syndrome. Patients may demonstrate metabolic changes in the absence of weight loss [32] and it is unclear how weight change relates to variables like function and quality of life. There remains a need for consensus on a clinical and research defi-

nition of cachexia and recognition of categories of cachexia by prognostic severity. This would facilitate the comparison of studies and assist in the development of targeted therapies. Pragmatic clinical definitions of the syndrome do exist [33] but greater detail and objectivity are needed for research purposes.

The cancer cachexia syndrome is usually diagnosed clinically in patients with advanced cancer who display features of non-volitional weight loss and muscle wasting. Patients may undergo a profound change in body image and often have severe anorexia and chronic nausea. Inanition, depression and fatigue may be compounded by reduced social interaction and loss of independence incurred as the result of muscle wasting (primary and secondary) and loss of physical reserve. Such wasting is not unique to cancer but may also be observed in other chronic illnesses including rheumatoid arthritis, end-stage renal failure, heart failure, HIV/AIDS, chronic obstructive pulmonary disease and chronic liver disease.

Selective loss of skeletal muscle protein mass due to a combination of reduced synthesis and increased degradation is characteristic of cachexia [34]. There is often an increase in whole-body protein turnover [35] and this may reflect increased visceral protein synthesis, particularly in the liver. Proteolysis-inducing factor (PIF) [36] is frequently present in weight-losing cancer patients and may be one mediator of muscle loss, possibly via activation of the ubiquitin–proteasome pathway [34]. Activation of the systemic inflammatory response due to enhanced proinflammatory cytokine release is also common in weight-losing cancer patients and can be inferred from an elevated serum C-reactive protein (CRP). Systemic inflammation is often associated with anorexia, reduced food intake and reduced voluntary activity, which may lead to secondary muscle wasting.

The sequelae of cachexia all tend to impede physical function, making the latter not only an obvious and relevant variable for assessing cachectic patients but also potentially a meaningful study end-point.

### The Functional Impact of Cancer Cachexia

Many of the consequences of cachexia are likely to impact on patient function but as yet this has not been studied in detail. There is, however, a considerable body of knowledge about the importance of weight loss in relation to clinical end-points and treatment variables. Scott [37] studied patients with inoperable non-small-cell lung cancer – about 40% had at least 5% weight loss and almost 80% an elevated CRP. Weight-losing patients had a significantly lower KPS and overall QoL and greater fatigue and pain. An elevated CRP was independently associated with increased fatigue. In patients with advanced gastrointestinal (GI) cancer receiving palliative chemotherapy, Persson [38] showed that those who were losing weight had a reduced global QoL. In addition, on multivariate analysis, poor performance status and weight loss were independently related to decreased survival and a lower probability of responding to treatment.

O'Gorman has published a series of studies in advanced GI cancer [39–41]. Patients with more than 5% weight loss had a higher serum CRP, lower serum albumin, lower anthropometry measures, poorer appetite and lower QoL scores. Both low performance status and elevated CRP were associated with adverse survival independent of weight loss. Over a 6-week period, patients losing more than 3% of their body weight had a higher CRP and lower KPS and anthropometry measures. Patients who gained more than 3% body weight had a higher KPS. The authors suggested that a loss or gain of more than 2.5 kg over 6–8 weeks was required to produce a significant change in performance status in weight-losing patients with GI cancer.

In a one-month study of 24 patients with lung cancer, Sarna [42] used the KPS and two patient self-reported tools to show that in those not receiving chemotherapy physical function worsened. In the sample of 24 patients, one third had difficulty walking one block or more, 79% had serious fatigue and 44% difficulty with household chores. Only 21% were completely satisfied with their level of activity.

A recent study by Yadav [43] has looked at 100 ambulant patients with advanced lung cancer. Functional ability was assessed objectively (Simmonds Functional Assessment and 6-minute walk), KPS recorded and standardised questionnaire data collected (using a fatigue scale and a disease-specific tool). The authors concluded that measurable differences in daily tasks were identifiable when patient data were compared with normative data for middle-aged (30–59 years) and older (over 59 years) controls and that objective functional ability was an independent end-point in this patient population. Simmonds Functional Assessment [44] combines a self-reported questionnaire that collects information on symptoms and function and a panel of nine physical tasks (including tying a belt, putting on a sock and walking tests). In the original analysis, a control group out-performed cancer patients and the questionnaire and physical tasks were complementary. It was suggested that the tool could be useful for patient and outcome assessment.

These and other studies support a relationship between weight loss, decreased performance status, increased symptomatology, reduced tolerance and efficacy of palliative chemotherapy and decreased survival. They illustrate the profound impact that cachexia has on the function, well-being and prognosis of patients with advanced cancer.

### The Importance of Functional Assessment in Advanced Cancer and Cachexia

It goes without saying that the best way to treat cancer cachexia is to treat successfully the patient's cancer. For some patients oncological therapy may be influenced by chronological age [45, 46]. However, it is often recognised that physiological age is perhaps more important. Functional assessment may provide one measure of this robustness and contribute to the shift in medical treatment delivery away from being unduly governed by chronological age and towards a greater use of markers of 'biological age' or risk. Understanding the relationship, therefore, between functional status and overall patient 'fitness' and 'reserve' is important.

Unfortunately, for many of patients with advanced solid malignancy, progression of disease occurs despite active oncological therapy. At this point patients have often been weakened by the catabolic side-effects of anti-cancer therapy and their low performance status requires that any anti-cachexia therapy is non-toxic and will improve function. Understanding the determinants of function (such as cachectic muscle performance or mood) may assist in developing such selective therapies in cachexia.

## Functional End-Points for Regulatory Approval of Anti-cachexia Therapies

The importance of identifying robust, objective functional outcomes is recognised by regulatory bodies [47]. In approving growth hormone for the treatment of AIDS-related wasting, the American Food and Drug Administration (FDA) took account of an improvement in functional status reflected by an increase in treadmill work output compared with placebo [48]. It must be pointed out, however, that the relationship of laboratory-based tools such as the treadmill for assessing the capacity of patients to perform work bears an uncertain relationship to 'free-living' activity. The development of 'intelligent', ambulatory personal activity monitors (see below) may herald a new era in objective functional assessment in the patient's own environment.

## Physical Activity: A Novel, Objective, 'Free-Living' End-Point in Functional Assessment?

### Physical Activity Level

In refining functional patient assessment and deriving objective, 'free-living' end-points in cachexia, 'physical activity level' (PAL) is worthy of further study [49]. Physical activity is influenced not only by several QoL domains, but also by several different specific features of cachexia (e.g. anaemia [50]), giving it validity as an end-point.

A person's total energy expenditure (TEE) is made up of resting energy expenditure (REE) and the energy cost of physical activity (Fig. 1). PAL

represents TEE divided by REE and can be measured accurately using doubly labelled water (to measure TEE) combined with indirect calorimetry (to measure REE). PAL expresses the energy expended on physical activity in relation to an individual's REE without needing to control for age, sex, weight or other parameters and is therefore a convenient way of comparing activity. Technological advances mean that assessing physical activity is now an evolving field and small, lightweight, 'intelligent' personal activity recorders capable of recording activity in considerable detail and possibly of estimating the energy expended on physical activity are now being developed (see below).

In anorectic wasted cancer patients, although REE may be increased, total energy expenditure may actually fall, suggesting a compensatory down-regulation of overall energy demands via a reduction in physical activity [51]. This reduction in physical activity may reach 50% or more [51] and seems likely to affect adversely QoL to a major degree.

Doubly labelled water is the gold-standard for measuring total energy expenditure in free-living people and any new methodology to estimate PAL needs to combine this with indirect calorimetry in order to achieve adequate validation. Doubly labelled water is a relatively simple test to perform

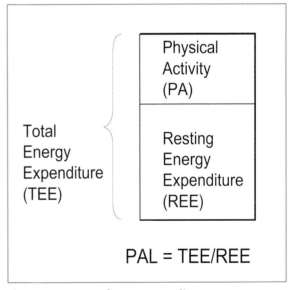

**Fig. 1.** Components of energy expenditure

but the raw materials and analytical equipment are expensive and considerable expertise is required [52]. Stable isotopes $^2H$ and $^{18}O$ are used to enrich the body water pool. These are then lost from this pool as water (in the breath, urine and sweat) and additionally in the case of $^{18}O$, as $CO_2$ in the breath. Samples of urine or blood are collected at the beginning and end of the study period, which is typically of the order of 2 weeks. These are then analysed using mass spectrometry. The washout curve for $^{18}O$ is steeper than for $^2H$ and the difference represents $CO_2$ production – an indirect measure of metabolic rate.

In a recent study of the components of energy expenditure in cachectic cancer patients, resting energy expenditure was shown to be elevated, but total energy expenditure and therefore physical activity level were significantly decreased [53]. In the same study, patients were randomised subsequently to either an n-3 fatty acid enriched or a conventional oral nutritional supplement. The n-3 enriched supplement resulted in the patients achieving normal physical activity levels, whereas there was no significant difference with the control supplement [53]. These results demonstrate the practical application of physical activity level as an objective end-point in prospective randomised trials.

## Ambulatory Monitoring of Physical Activity: A New Way of Assessing Patient Function

Assessing patients' ambulatory function under free-living conditions has long represented a challenge for the bio-medical community. A number of groups have now reported devices capable of discriminating between different postural states, e.g. sitting, lying, standing, stepping [54, 55], although performance is likely to vary between instruments [56]. It has even proved possible to generate a 'behavioural map' of the wearer by incorporating a global positioning system [57].

There are significant challenges in developing these instruments including adequate recording precision, data acquisition and memory, practical energy requirements, fixation methods, device size and weight, and sufficient memory capacity.

Any device that is to be worn for several days will need to be securely attached. It may need to be waterproofed and should be easily removed/replaced by the wearer. To some extent these hurdles are beginning to be overcome.

### *Experience with an Ambulatory 'Physical Activity Meter'*

We are currently undertaking pilot work with an advanced physical activity meter (Fig. 2), the activPAL™ professional 'physical activity logger' (PAL Technologies, Glasgow, Scotland). This records the time that is spent lying/sitting, standing and stepping. In addition it will display the number of up-down/down-up transitions, the stepping cadence and estimated energy expenditure. From this estimated energy expenditure it is possible to derive an estimated PAL (the estimated energy expenditure function has not yet been validated against standard methodologies, e.g. doubly labelled water). The lightweight device is about the size of a matchbox and worn on the front of the thigh. It can record about a week of data, which is downloaded onto a computer, analysed by proprietary software and displayed (Fig. 3).

Table 1 shows preliminary results from nine cachectic patients with upper GI cancer (varying primary sites) who wore the activPAL™ meter for 1 week. Many of the patients were receiving palliative chemotherapy at the time of activity assessment. Their physician-assigned WHO performance status was recorded at the beginning of the week. The total time spent upright (stationary or moving) was combined and used to derive a figure for the average proportion of an idealised 16-hour waking day spent in the vertical position. This was done to allow a provisional comparison to the performance status score. A WHO performance status of 0–2 suggests that the patient is up and about for more than 50% of the waking day; however, from the meter data it appears that patients have a very low level of physical activity, spending on average only about 20% of an idealised day in the vertical position. The estimated PAL is also extremely low. This is only a first-order estimate. Whilst this may reflect a true reduction in physical activity, it might also suggest that this parameter (derived from meter information) may require calibration

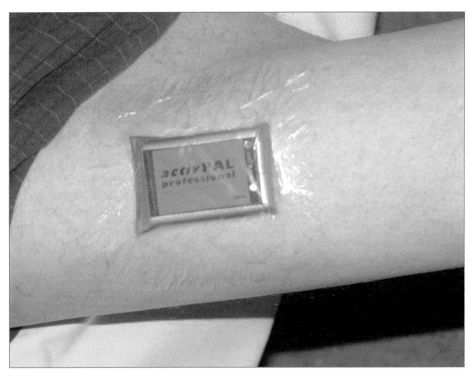

**Fig. 2.** The activPAL™ professional physical activity logger attached to the front of the thigh

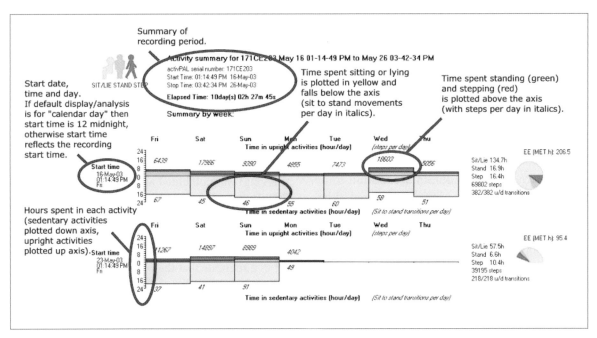

**Fig. 3.** An example of data from the activPAL™ meter. (Reproduced with permission)

from gold-standard measurements using doubly labelled water/indirect calorimetry. Further study is clearly required; however, despite these reserva-tions, the preliminary data raise the suggestion that patients with cancer cachexia may be less active than we realise.

**Table 1.** Performance status and activity assessment in a group of patients with upper gastrointestinal cancer and cachexia

| Age | Sex | %WL | WHO | %UP | ePAL | pPAL |
|-----|-----|-----|-----|-----|------|------|
| 43[a] | M | 10 | 0 | 28 | 1.23 | 1.5 |
| 46[a] | M | 26 | 1 | 32 | 1.15 | 1.5 |
| 47[a] | F | 7 | 0 | 23 | 1.15 | 1.5 |
| 55[a] | M | 39 | 2 | 18 | 1.1 | 1.5 |
| 59[a] | M | 19 | 2 | 36 | 1.23 | 1.5 |
| 62 | M | 19 | 2 | 10 | 1.08 | 1.5 |
| 65[a] | F | 6 | 2 | 2 | 1.01 | 1.5 |
| 69 | F | 44 | 2 | 17 | 1.09 | 1.5 |
| 70[a] | M | 9 | 2 | 12 | 1.09 | 1.5 |

[a]Receiving chemotherapy (not all patients were receiving the same regimen or had their activity recorded at the same point in their treatment schedule)
%WL, per cent of 'usual' weight lost; WHO, physician-assigned World Health Organisation performance status; %UP, Proportion (in per cent) of an 'idealised' 16-h waking day spent upright (either moving about or stationary); ePAL, estimated physical activity level derived from meter information; pPAL, predicted physical activity level; a PAL of 1.5 is typical of a healthy, sedentary adult

There remain appreciable challenges in developing physical activity meter technology. These include determining the acceptability, reliability and practicality of the equipment, deciding which variables should be reported, the appropriate timing, frequency and duration of data collection and how the information should be presented and interpreted. In addition, devices such as the activPAL™ need to be 'tested' in populations with differing levels of activity. As with all assessment tools, it is conceivable that in setting out to measure a variable, its level is inadvertently changed. However, these devices measure activity objectively over a prolonged period of time, which is likely to increase the chances of obtaining an accurate reflection of contemporary activity. The initial experience suggests that the device is acceptable to patients.

## Conclusions

Many cachectic patients lose significant body weight and functionally important tissue (e.g.

skeletal muscle) and they may also experience a number of additional effects of the cachexia syndrome (e.g. fatigue). One consequence of this may be a reduction in activity, which could translate into reduced independence and 'quality of life'. Functional assessment in cachexia has the potential to describe the day-to-day patient burden of the illness and should allow greater understanding of how it affects patients. In turn, this may help in the development of targeted therapies, the robust assessment of interventions and comprehensive patient care. Physical activity level measured by conventional methodology (doubly labelled water/indirect calorimetry) or estimated by an ambulatory physical activity meter offers an objective approach to the free-living assessment of such function in cachectic patients.

### Acknowledgements
We acknowledge our colleague Dr Lucy Wall (Consultant Medical Oncologist, Edinburgh Cancer Centre) and all the patients under her care who have very generously contributed to the work we have described in this chapter.

# References

1. Simons JP, Aaronson NK, Vansteenkiste JF et al (1996) Effects of medroxyprogesterone acetate on appetite, weight, and quality of life in advanced-stage non-hormone-sensitive cancer: a placebo-controlled multicenter study. J Clin Oncol 14:1077–1084

2. Maloney FI, Barthel DW (1965) Functional evaluation: the Barthel Index. MD St Med J 14:61–65

3. Lawton MP, Brody EM (1969) Assessment of older people: self-maintaining and instrumental activities of daily living. Gerontologist 9:179–186

4. Rueben DB, Laliberte L, Hiris J, Mor V (1990) A hierarchical exercise scale to measure function at the advanced activities of daily living (AADL) level. J Am Geriatr Soc 38:855–861

5. Trentini M, Semeraro S, Motta M (2001) Italian Study Group for Geriatric Assessment and Management. Effectiveness of geriatric evaluation and care. One-year results of a multicenter randomized clinical trial. Aging (Milan) 13:395–405

6. Karnofsky DA, Burchenal JH (1949) The clinical evaluation of chemotherapeutic agents in cancer. In: Macleod CM (ed) Evaluation of chemotherapeutic agents. Columbia University Press, New York, pp 199–205

7. Anonymous (1979) WHO Handbook for Reporting Results of Cancer Treatment. World Health Organisation, Geneva

8. Slevin ML, Plant H, Lynch D et al (1988) Who should measure quality of life, the doctor or the patient? Br J Cancer 57:109–112

9. Blagden SP, Charman SC, Sharples LD et al (2003) Performance status score: do patients and their oncologists agree? Br J Cancer 89:1022–1027

10. Zubrod GC, Schneiderman M, Frei E et al (1960) Appraisal of methods for study of chemotherapy of cancer in man: comparative therapeutic trial of nitrogen mustard and triethylene thiophosphamide. J Chron Dis 11:7–33

11. Schaafsma J, Osoba D (1994) The Karnofsky Performance Status Scale re examined: a cross-validation with the EORTC-C30. Qual Life Res 3:413–424

12. Schag CC, Heinrich RL (1984) Karnofsky Performance Status revisited: reliability, validity and guidelines. J Clin Oncol 2:193–197

13. Jatoi A, Hillman S, Stella PJ et al (2003) Daily activities: exploring their spectrum and prognostic impact in older, chemotherapy-treated lung cancer patients. Support Care Cancer 11:460–464

14. Osoba D (1999) What has been learned from measuring health-related quality of life in clinical oncology. Eur J Cancer 35:1565–1570

15. Anonymous (1949) World Health Organisation. Constitution in Basic Documents. World Health Organisation, Geneva

16. McHorney CA, Ware JE, Raczek AE (1993) The MOS 36-Item Short-Form Health Survey (SF-36): II. Psychometric and clinical tests of validity in measuring physical and mental health constructs. Med Care 31:247–263

17. Aaronson NK, Ahmedzai S, Bergman B et al (1993) The European Organisation for Research and Treatment of Cancer QLQ-C30: a quality-of-life instrument for use in international clinical trials in oncology. J Natl Cancer Inst 85:365–376

18. Cella DF, Tulsky DS, Gray G et al (1993) The Functional Assessment of Cancer Therapy scale: development and validation of the general measure. J Clin Onc 11:570–579

19. Cohen SR, Leis A (2002) What determines the quality of life of terminally ill cancer patients from their own perspective? J Palliat Care 18:48–58

20. Greisinger AJ, Lorimor RJ, Aday LA et al (1997) Terminally ill cancer patients. Their most important concerns. Cancer Pract 5:147–154

21. Steinhauser KE, Christakis NA, Clipp EC et al (2000) Factors considered important at the end of life by patients, family, physicians, and other care providers. JAMA 284:2476–2482

22. Cella D, Chang CH, Lai JS, Webster K (2002) Advances in quality of life measurements in oncology patients. Semin Oncol 29(Suppl 8):60–68

23. Waldron D, O'Boyle CA, Kearney M et al (1999) Quality-of-life measurement in advanced cancer: assessing the individual. J Clin Oncol 17:3603–3611

24. Gough IR, Furnival CM, Schilder L, Grove W (1983) Assessment of the quality of life of patients with advanced cancer. Eur J Cancer Clin Oncol 19:1161–1165

25. Nordin K, Steel J, Hoffman K, Glimelius B (2001) Alternative methods of interpreting quality of life data in advanced gastrointestinal cancer patients. Br J Cancer 85:1265–1272

26. Ballatori E (2001) Unsolved problems in evaluating the quality of life of cancer patients. Ann Oncol 12 (Suppl 3):S11–S13

27. Holzner B, Kemmler G, Sperner-Unterweger B et al (2001) Quality of life measurement in oncology – a matter of the assessment instrument? Eur J Cancer 37:2349–2356

28. Hakamies-Blomqvist L, Luoma ML, Sjostrom J et al (2001) Timing of quality of life (QoL) assessments as a source of error in oncological trials. J Adv Nurs 35:709–716

29. Conroy T, Bleiberg H, Glimelius B (2003) Quality of life in patients with advanced colorectal cancer: what has been learnt? Eur J Cancer 39:287–294

30. Wasson J, Keller A, Rubenstein L et al (1992) Benefits and obstacles of health status assessment in ambulatory settings. The clinician's point of view. The Dartmouth Primary Care COOP Project. Med Care 30:MS42–MS49

31. Raiten DJ, Talbot JM (eds) (1999) Proceedings of the workshop 'Clinical Trials for the Treatment of

Secondary Wasting and Cachexia: Selection of Appropriate Endpoints', May 22-23, 1997, Bethesda. J Nutr 129:223S–317S

32. Jatoi A, Daly BD, Hughes VA et al (2001) Do patients with nonmetastatic non-small cell lung cancer demonstrate altered resting energy expenditure? Ann Thorac Surg 72:348–351

33. MacDonald N, Easson AM, Mazurak VC et al (2003) Understanding and managing cancer cachexia. J Am Coll Surg 197:143–161

34. Tisdale MJ (2001) Loss of skeletal muscle in cancer: biochemical mechanisms. Front Biosci 6:D164–D174

35. Fearon KC, Hansell DT, Preston T et al (1988) Influence of whole body protein turnover rate on resting energy expenditure in patients with cancer. Cancer Res 48:2590–2595

36. Todorov P, Cariuk P, McDevitt T et al (1996) Characterization of a cancer cachectic factor. Nature 379:739–742

37. Scott HR, McMillan DC, Brown DJ et al (2003) A prospective study of the impact of weight loss and the systemic inflammatory response on quality of life in patients with inoperable non-small cell lung cancer. Lung Cancer 40:295–299

38. Persson C, Glimelius B (2002) The relevance of weight loss for survival and quality of life in patients with advanced gastrointestinal cancer treated with palliative chemotherapy. Anticancer Res 22:3661–3668

39. O'Gorman P, McMillan DC, McArdle CS (1998) Impact of weight loss, appetite, and the inflammatory response on quality of life in gastrointestinal cancer patients. Nutr Cancer 32:76–80

40. O'Gorman P, McMillan DC, McArdle CS (1999) Longitudinal study of weight, appetite, performance status, and inflammation in advanced gastrointestinal cancer. Nutr Cancer 35:127–129

41. O'Gorman P, McMillan DC, McArdle CS (2000) Prognostic factors in advanced gastrointestinal cancer patients with weight loss. Nutr Cancer 37:36–40

42. Sarna L (1993) Fluctuations in physical function: adults with non-small cell lung cancer. J Adv Nurs 18:714–724

43. Yadav RR, Fossella F, Palmer JL et al (2003) An objective evaluation of functional ability (OEF) in patients with advanced lung cancer. Proc Am Soc Clin Oncol 22:746 (abs)

44. Simmonds MJ (2002) Physical function in patients with cancer: psychometric characteristics and clini-cal usefulness of a physical performance test battery. J Pain Symptom Manage 24:404–414

45. Bennett CL, Greenfield S, Aronow HU et al (1991) Patterns of care related to age of men with prostate cancer. Cancer 67:2633–2641

46. Newschaffer CJ, Penberthy L, Desch CD et al (1996) The effect of age and comorbidity in the treatment of elderly women with nonmetastatic breast cancer. Arch Intern Med 156:85–90

47. Johnson JR, Williams G, Pazdur R (2003) End points and United States Food and Drug Administration approval of oncology drugs. J Clin Oncol 21:1404–1411

48. Schambelan M, Mulligan K, Grunfeld C et al (1996) Recombinant human growth hormone in patients with HIV-associated wasting. A randomized, place-bo-controlled trial. Serostim Study Group. Ann Intern Med 125:873–882

49. Schutz Y, Weinsier RL, Hunter GR (2001) Assessment of free-living physical activity in humans: an overview of currently available and proposed new measures. Obes Res 9:368–379

50. Cella D (1998) Factors influencing quality of life in cancer patients: anemia and fatigue. Semin Oncol 25(3 Suppl 7):43–46

51. Gibney ER (2000) Energy expenditure in disease: time to revisit? Proc Nutr Soc 59:199–207

52. Ritz P, Coward WA (1995) Doubly labelled water measurement of total energy expenditure. Diabete Metab 21:241–251

53. Moses AW, Slater C, Preston T et al (2004) Reduced total energy expenditure and physical activity in cachectic patients with pancreatic cancer can be modulated by an energy and protein dense oral supplement enriched with n-3 fatty acids. Br J Cancer 90:996–1002

54. Ma J, Barbenel JC (1997) A new ambulatory monitoring instrument of posture and mobility related activities. Biomed Sci Instrum 33:88–93

55. Matsuoka S, Yonezawa Y, Maki H et al (2003) A microcomputer-based daily living activity recording system. Biomed Sci Instrum 39:220–223

56. Aminian K, Robert P, Buchser EE et al (1999) Physical activity monitoring based on accelerometry: validation and comparison with video observation. Med Biol Eng Comput 37:304–308

57. Makikawa M, Kurata S, Kawato M et al (1998) Ambulatory physical activity monitoring system. Medinfo 9(Pt 1):277–281

# SECTION 4
# THE DIFFERENT FEATURES OF WASTING IN HUMANS

# Anorexia

Alessandro Laviano, Michael M. Meguid, Filippo Rossi Fanelli

## Introduction

In medicine, specific combinations of symptoms and signs contribute to establishing a diagnosis. However, symptoms or constellations of symptoms (i.e., syndromes) per se may not be specific for a single disease; rather, they are observed during the clinical course of a number of acute and chronic diseases. Among them, anorexia is a highly prevalent syndrome that heavily impacts on the prognosis of patients suffering from acute (i.e. sepsis) and chronic (i.e. cancer, liver cirrhosis, chronic renal failure, chronic obstructive pulmonary [COPD]) diseases.

Anorexia is grossly defined as the loss of the desire to eat and is almost invariably associated with reduced food intake. As a consequence, reduced calorie intake should be considered as the consequence and not part of the clinical definition of anorexia. However, since these two aspects are strictly interconnected, they are often used synonymously.

Anorexia is among the physiological responses prompted in the host by internal/external insults (i.e., immune system activation, increased energy expenditure, etc.). Initially, all these changes are believed to help the host organism to isolate and fight invading cells. As far as anorexia is concerned, the beneficial effect is usually assumed to be related to a number of mechanisms. First, the host saves energy by not moving around in search of food, which also reduces heat loss that would otherwise occur from increased convection. The conserved energy is then available for the body's fight against disease. Second, the suppression of food intake during disease may be important in reducing both the availability of nutrients essential for invading organisms and energy expenditure for digestion. The initial beneficial effect of anorexia during disease is supported by a classic study in which force-feeding of experimentally infected mice increased their mortality [1]. Nevertheless, long-lasting anorexia compromises host defence and ultimately delays recovery.

As a consequence, the clinical relevance of anorexia varies according to the time course of the underlying diseases. In acute clinical states, such as sepsis or influenza infection, anorexia does not represent a therapeutic target, since quick and effective treatment of the underlying disease is the main goal and inevitably leads to an amelioration of eating behaviour. In chronic clinical states, anorexia should be considered and treated because its long-lasting effects on food intake and quality of life impact on patient's prognosis.

## Diagnostic Tools

It is still difficult to clearly define and diagnose anorexia. Sometimes, a visual analogue scale is used, which is a useful tool in epidemiological or prospective studies but may prove quite unreliable if small changes in appetite need to be detected [2]. Very often, the diagnosis of anorexia is based on the presence of reduced energy intake, even if this approach is misleading, since the reduction of ingested calories might be the consequence of dysphagia or depression rather than a sign of true anorexia, as previously mentioned. To reliably assess the presence of anorexia, a number of symptoms reflecting an interference with food intake and likely related to changes in the central nervous system control of energy intake have been identified (Table 1) [3]. Patients reporting at least one of these symptoms are defined as anorectic. However, considering that this diagnostic tool provides only a qualitative assessment of the presence of anorexia, it may be advisable to also quantify the degree of anorexia via the visual analogue scale.

**Table 1.** Symptoms interfering with food intake and related to changes in the central nervous system regulation of energy intake. Patients reporting at least one of these symptoms are defined as anorectic. (Modified from [3])

| Symptoms |
| --- |
| Early satiety |
| Taste alterations |
| Smell alterations |
| Meat aversion |
| Nausea/vomiting |

# Prevalence

As a consequence of the difficulties in clearly defining and diagnosing anorexia, its prevalence in different clinical conditions has yet to be precisely assessed. A clear example is given by the anorexia associated with cancer. In 300 cancer patients, Geels et al. identified the nine most common symptoms using both patients' responses to a quality-of-life questionnaire and graded toxicity data collected on case report forms [4]. Based on the latter, anorexia was detected in approximately 13% of patients, while according to the former 55% of patients were diagnosed as anorectic [4].

## Cancer

An acceptable estimate of the prevalence of cancer anorexia can be derived from a number of papers showing that approximately 50% of cancer patients upon diagnosis report abnormalities of eating behaviour [5, 6]. While this figure may slightly overestimate the actual prevalence of cancer anorexia, it is generally acknowledged that anorexia and reduced food intake are frequently encountered in cancer patients [6]. Moreover, anorexia is usually the symptom urging the patients to refer to their physicians, and its alleviation is perceived as a sign of benign evolution of the disease.

Prevalence data are more reliable in terminally ill cancer patients. In this subset of patients, the prevalence of anorexia ranges between 60% and 65% [7, 8]. Based on these alarming figures and considering that 20% of cancer deaths are due to malnutrition per se [9], it is reasonable to conclude that many cancer patients starve to death.

## Liver Cirrhosis

Similarly to what is observed in the course of neoplastic disease, patients suffering from chronic liver failure frequently experience anorexia. In a recent paper, Marchesini et al. assessed the presence of anorexia in 174 patients with advanced liver cirrhosis (Child-Pugh score ≥ 7; class B or C), using the guiding symptoms previously mentioned. The data showed that more than 50% of patients were anorectic [10].

## Chronic Renal Failure

In this clinical setting, anorexia is among the most important causes of malnutrition. It is pervasive in patients treated conservatively (medical and dietetic) and almost invariably found in patients on haemodialysis [11].

## Chronic Obstructive Pulmonary Disease

In COPD patients, the prevalence of anorexia is particularly high, since most patients suffer from breathlessness, which affects food intake. Recent data indicate that 67% of chronic lung disease patients experience anorexia during the last year of life. This figure is not much different from the prevalence of 76% found among lung cancer patients [12]. More striking, however, are data showing that although COPD patients have physical and psychosocial needs at least as severe as those of lung cancer patients, their symptoms, including anorexia, receive much less attention from health care professionals [12].

## Congestive Heart Failure

In this clinical setting, assessment of the prevalence of anorexia is made difficult by the high proportion of patients suffering from dyspnoea, the incidence of which peaks at 90% in the last stages of the disease [13]. Severe nausea has been reported to affect approximately 10% of congestive heart failure (CHF) patients [14], but the actual prevalence of anorexia may well be higher [15].

## Clinical Impact

The onset of anorexia significantly impacts on the clinical course of the disease. It contributes to the development of malnutrition and cachexia, since it reduces the oral intake of calories, thus further promoting skeletal-muscle wasting. Also, it exacerbates the detrimental effects of disease-related alterations of protein metabolism on nutritional status, eventually leading to increased morbidity and mortality [16]. The metabolic dysregulation associated with cachexia [17] sustains and corroborates the neurochemical alterations responsible for anorexia. Also, the clinical relevance of anorexia is underscored by its role as an independent prognostic factor in terminally ill cancer patients [8], being as reliable in predicting survival as well-defined prognostic factors, including Karnofsky Performance Status and Clinical Prediction of Survival [8, 18]. Finally, anorexia and reduced energy intake impinge on the quality of life, which is now becoming a critical endpoint in the management of patients as well as in designing clinical trials [19].

## Pathogenesis of Anorexia

The pathogenesis of anorexia is multifactorial and related to disturbances of the central physiological mechanisms controlling food intake. The precise neurochemical mechanisms are still matter of debate; however, by understanding how energy intake is physiologically controlled, insights might be obtained.

Under normal conditions energy intake is controlled within the hypothalamus by specific neuronal populations that integrate peripheral signals conveying information on energy and adiposity status [20]. In particular, the arcuate nucleus of the hypothalamus transduces these inputs into neuronal responses and, via second-order neuronal signalling pathways, into behavioural responses. Intuitively, anorexia may be secondary to defective signals arising from the periphery, due to an error in the transduction process, or to a disturbance in the activity of second-order neuronal signalling pathways.

## Role of Peripheral Signals

The hypothesis that peripheral signals are involved in the pathogenesis of anorexia is intriguing. Among the large series of peripheral signals (Table 2), the hormone leptin exerts a strong negative influence on food intake.

**Table 2.** Signals arising from the periphery and influencing food intake

| Signals | |
| --- | --- |
| Adiposity signals | Insulin, Leptin |
| Ghrelin | |
| Cholecystokinin | |
| Polypeptide YY | |
| Energy signals | Intracellular malonyl-CoA |

### Hormones

Leptin is produced primarily by adipocytes in proportion to body fat. It reaches the brain and an increase in circulating levels of the hormone results in inhibition of energy intake. Thus, intuitively, leptin is a likely mediator of anorexia, particularly because its synthesis and secretion appear to be stimulated by cytokines, which are recognised anorexigenic factors [21]. However, results from animal and clinical studies are controversial [22, 23] and do not seem to support this hypothesis. More recently, Bing et al. significantly contributed to the debate by showing in an animal model that anorexia develops despite the normal regulation of leptin synthesis [24]. Consistent with these animal data, Mantovani et al. showed that in anorectic cancer patients circulating leptin levels are lower than those of healthy individuals, while there is no difference between cancer patients and healthy individuals regarding leptin production by peripheral blood mononuclear cells [25]. Recently, Stenvinkel et al. could not demonstrate a role for circulating leptin in the pathogenesis of anorexia in chronic renal failure patients undergoing dialysis [26]; rather, they suggested that leptin in these patients may represent a marker of inflammation [26]. Supporting a common pathophysiologic mechanism for anorexia associated with different diseases, Ben-Ari et al. showed that in chronic liver disease serum leptin appears to be a passive marker and not a cause of anorexia [27]. When considered together, the data suggest that peripheral leptin synthesis is preserved during disease and point to a central dysregulation of the physiological feedback loop.

### Energy Signals

Similar to the changes in fat mass, changes in energy metabolism also influence energy intake in a leptin-independent manner via energy signals. Conceptually, energy signals differ from classic peripheral signals, since they are generated within hypothalamic neurons controlling energy intake. A number of studies have suggested that a metabolic control of food intake also exists, in which biochemical partitioning between fatty-acid oxidation and synthesis represents a key signal indicating catabolic or anabolic energy status [28]. Energy signals are independent from leptin pathway and they inform the brain on the metabolic switch occurring at a subcellular level between fatty-acid oxidation and synthesis [29]. Under physiological conditions, food intake is accompanied by increased intracellular levels of malonyl coenzyme A (malonyl-CoA) [30], a potent signal reducing food intake, via inhibition of the synthesis of the prophagic factor neuropeptide Y (NPY) [29]. It is therefore tempting to speculate that energy signals contribute to anorexia, possibly via a deranged 'sensing' of the energy metabolism during disease. Supporting evidence shows that during tumour growth fat metabolism is altered, leading to decreased fatty-acid oxidation [31] and

possibly increased intracellular malonyl-CoA levels. Also, the supplementation of carnitine, which is involved in fatty acid oxidation, ameliorates anorexia in pathophysiological conditions [32]. Nonetheless, more studies are needed to verify the involvement of energy signals in anorexia.

### Second-Order Neuronal Signalling

The hypothalamic arcuate nucleus, where peripheral signals mainly converge, projects to other hypothalamic areas, thus interacting with a number of neuronal populations [20]. Many pathways serving as second-order neuronal signalling pathways, including those of orexins A and B, have been described but their involvement in the pathogenesis of anorexia has so far received little attention, although it cannot be excluded. In a recent study, Li et al. showed that a loss of renal function in Wistar rats reduced hypothalamic orexin A, a prophagic mediator [33], which in turn may have contributed to the development of anorexia in these animals.

Evidence exists suggesting that disease-associated metabolic changes, and particularly alterations of protein turnover, impact on the neurochemistry in localised brain areas [34]. However, they also appear to have a role in sustaining and corroborating anorexia, while its onset seems to be secondary to the inability of the hypothalamus to recognise and respond appropriately to consistent peripheral signals [35].

### Peptides

Consistent and convincing evidence suggests that disease-associated anorexia is brought about by derangement of the hypothalamic system regarding its ability to transduce peripheral signals into neuronal responses. Under normal conditions, peripheral signals interact with two separate neuronal populations within the arcuate nucleus: the NPY/agouti-related peptide (AgRP) neurons, stimulating food intake, and the pro-opiomelanocortin (POMC)/cocaine- and amphetamine-regulated transcript (CART) neurons, inhibiting food intake (for review see [20]). As a consequence, when energy intake needs to be initiated, peripheral signals activate the NPY/AgRP pathway, simultaneously inhibiting the POMC/CART pathway. When energy intake needs to be inhibited, peripheral signals inhibit the NPY/AgRP pathway while simultaneously activating POMC/CART neurons and thus up-regulating the expression of a number of POMC/CART pathway-related factors, including α-melanocyte stimulating hormone (α-MSH) and corticotropin releasing hormone (CRH).

Because of the central role of these neuronal pathways, they have been postulated as putative mediators of anorexia. A number of studies investigated the role of the prophagic signal NPY in the pathogenesis of anorexia. In cancer, the results obtained in animal models and humans are conflicting [36–39]. However, it seems that a dissociation exists between NPY mRNA levels and actual NPY levels, which are decreased. Indeed, recent data show a decrease of NPY and NPY-immunoreactive neurons in the hypothalamus of anorectic tumour-bearing rats [40, 41]. These data suggest that NPY is involved in cancer anorexia, but it is difficult to assess the extent of the involvement.

In chronic renal failure, animal and human studies consistently show a reduction of NPY [33, 42]. However, as in cancer, it is not clear whether NPY should be considered as a mediator or a marker of anorexia.

Results from studies investigating the role of the hypothalamic anorexigenic pathway POMC/CART in anorexia are more convincing. Unfortunately, this line of investigation has been pursued in cancer anorexia only, but it is likely that the pathophysiological mechanisms hypothesised for cancer anorexia also operates during the clinical course of other diseases. It has been repeatedly demonstrated that by blocking the hypothalamic melanocortin system, using either its physiological inhibitor (AgRP) or the synthetic compound SHU-9119, food intake is restored in tumour-bearing animals, and the development of cachexia is prevented [43, 44]. Similar results have been obtained in melanocortin 4 receptor (MC4-R) knock-out mice. In these mutants, POMC/ CART neurons cannot be completely activated because of the lack of this class of receptors, and tumour growth is not accompanied by the development of

anorexia and cachexia, which occurs in wild-type mice [43].

Thus, it appears that cancer anorexia, and probably anorexia as a whole, is related to the inability of the hypothalamus to respond appropriately to consistent peripheral signals, primarily due to hyperactivation of the melanocortin system. This derangement could be triggered by cytokines.

## Role of Cytokines

A number of studies have indicated that cytokines are involved in anorexia [45, 46]. In the Fischer rat/MCA sarcoma model, brain interleukin-1 (IL-1) levels inversely correlate with food intake [47] while intra-hypothalamic IL-1 receptor antagonist microinjection increases energy intake [48]. In Lobund-Wistar rats bearing prostate adenocarcinoma tumour cells, early anorexia is associated with an up-regulation of brain IL-1β mRNA [38]. In chronic renal failure patients, several groups have found increased levels of cytokines [42, 49]. In cancer patients, cytokines and anorexia are intuitively connected, but compelling evidence is lacking since the biological effects of cytokines are largely mediated by paracrine and autocrine influences. Thus, the level of circulating cytokines may not reliably reflect their role in determining specific biological responses [50] but may instead suggest their involvement. However, it must be acknowledged that there are also studies that failed to demonstrate a direct role of cytokines in experimental models of cancer anorexia, while suggesting the involvement of the nitric oxide system and systemic or local production of eicosanoids [51, 52].

## Role of Hypothalamic Neuro-immune Interactions

The mechanisms by which cytokines negatively influence energy intake are currently under investigation. As proposed by Inui, cytokines may play a pivotal role in long-term inhibition of feeding by mimicking the hypothalamic effect of excessive negative-feedback signalling [53]. This could be done by inhibition of the NPY/AgRP orexigenic network as well as by persistent stimulation of the

POMC/CART anorexigenic pathway.

Recent data suggested that hypothalamic serotonergic neurotransmission may be critical in linking cytokines and the melanocortin system. Fenfluramine is a serotonin agonist once widely prescribed in the treatment of obesity. It has been recently shown that fenfluramine raises hypothalamic serotonin levels, which in turn activate POMC/CART neurons in the arcuate nucleus, therefore inducing anorexia and reduced food intake [54]. It is also well-documented that cytokines, and particularly IL-1, stimulate the release of hypothalamic serotonin [55]. Thus, it could be speculated that during disease cytokines increase hypothalamic serotonergic activity, which in turn contributes to persistent activation of POMC/CART neurons, leading to the onset of anorexia and reduced food intake. Supporting the role of serotonin in the pathogenesis of anorexia, we demonstrated that in anorectic tumour-bearing animals hypothalamic serotonin levels are increased when compared with the levels in control rats [56]. After tumour removal, hypothalamic serotonin levels normalised and food intake improved [56]. In the same experimental model, intrahypothalamic microinjections of mianserin, a serotonin antagonist, improved food intake [48]. In cancer patients, the activity of hypothalamic serotonergic system is inferred by cerebrospinal fluid (CSF) levels of tryptophan, a precursor of serotonin, the synthesis of which is strictly dependent on the availability of tryptophan [57]. In anorectic cancer patients, plasma and especially CSF concentrations of tryptophan are increased when compared to concentrations in controls and in non-anorectic cancer patients [3, 58]. After tumour removal, plasma tryptophan normalises and food intake improves [50].

Similar data suggesting increased serotonergic activity in the presence of anorexia have been obtained in patients suffering from either chronic renal failure [11, 34, 46] or liver cirrhosis [59], thus supporting the view that anorexia associated with different diseases shares a similar pathophysiologic mechanism. It must be acknowledged that partial brain serotonin depletion and antagonism did not result in improved food intake of tumour-bearing animals [52, 60]. However, it is not clear whether the failure to influence food intake in these models was secondary to incomplete depletion of brain serotonin or to the lack of any involvement of serotonin in cancer anorexia [61]. When considered together, we believe that these data suggest that brain serotonin could represent a key factor in the pathogenesis of disease-associated anorexia and thus provide an interesting therapeutic target.

## Therapy

The detrimental effects of anorexia on nutritional status and quality of life can be counteracted by a well-designed therapeutic strategy that includes both nutritional counselling and a pharmacological approach (Table 3).

**Table 3.** Therapeutic strategies in cancer anorexia

| Dietary counselling | Drugs |
| --- | --- |
| Small but frequent meals | Cannabinoids (dronabinol) |
| Energy-dense food | Corticosteroids (dexamethasone) |
| Limit fat intake | Progestagens (MA, MPA) |
| Avoid extremes in taste | |
| Avoid extremes in smell | |
| Pleasant environment | |
| Presentation of food | |

*MA*, megestrol acetate; *MPA*, medroxylprogesterone acetate

### Dietary Habits

In anorectic patients, nutritional counselling may significantly improve food intake. For example, food intake can be improved by providing small and frequent meals that are energy-dense and easy to eat. Patients should eat in pleasant surroundings and attention should be given to the presentation of food. It is advisable to avoid high-fat food, since fat delays gastric emptying and thus may worsen anorexia symptoms. Since changes in taste/smell may occur in anorectic patients, extremes in temperature and flavour should be avoided [6].

## Drug Therapy

The optimal therapeutic approach to anorexia should be aimed at counteracting its pathophysiologic mechanisms. Therefore, considering their involvement in anorexia, cytokines represent the ideal therapeutic target. A series of animal studies support this approach by showing that intrahypothalamic IL-1 blockade results in amelioration of anorexia and improves food intake [48, 62]. In humans, cytokine therapeutic targeting is achieved by the use of agents that interfere with their synthesis and release. They include progestagens [63–65], cannabinoids [66], and corticosteroids [67].

## Perspectives

The n-3 polyunsaturated fatty acids eicosapentaenoic acid (EPA) and docosahexaenoic acid (DHA) suppress the production of proinflammatory cytokines [68]. Thus, the effects of EPA supplementation on anorexia have been investigated specifically in patients with advanced cancer and have yielded contrasting results [69].

Anorexia might be therapeutically approached by interfering with the neurochemical events downstream of cytokine activation, particularly with serotonergic hypothalamic neurotransmission (see Chapter 10.8).

As previously mentioned, the nitric oxide system and the production of eicosanoids might be of importance for the pathogenesis of anorexia, and particularly cancer anorexia. Supporting this view, animal and clinical studies have shown that nitric oxide synthase and cyclooxygenase inhibitors, including indomethacin, decrease tumour growth and improve anorexia [70, 71]. However, evidence that nitric oxide and eicosanoids act directly on cells in the central nervous system is lacking. Also, the nitric oxide mechanism may involve tumour growth and thereby secondarily influence appetite. Finally, nitric oxide and eicosanoid influences on appetite appear to be related to serotonin metabolism [72, 73], and the prostaglandin $E_2$ receptor EP3 has been identified on serotonergic neuronal cell bodies in the raphe nucleus [74]. Thus, nitric oxide and eicosanoid pathways could not be completely alien from the cytokine–monoamine system.

## Conclusions

Anorexia is a syndrome that is pervasive among patients suffering from acute and chronic diseases. The pathogenesis is multifactorial, but it appears to be related to the hyperactivation of hypothalamic inhibitory pathways, which in turn may be triggered by cytokine-driven stimulation of the hypothalamic serotonergic system. Anorexia can be effectively treated, although it is not known whether amelioration of anorexia results in a long-term benefit for patients, leading to reduced morbidity and mortality. However, it should be always remembered that improving anorexia and energy intake has a positive impact on the quality of life: this could be enough for many patients.

## References

1. Murray MJ, Murray AB (1979) Anorexia of infection as a mechanism of host defense. Am J Clin Nutr 32:593–596
2. Stubbs RJ, Hughes DA, Johnstone AM et al (2000) The use of visual analogue scales to assess motivation to eat in human subjects: a review of their reliability and validity with an evaluation of new handheld computerized systems for temporal tracking of appetite ratings. Br J Nutr 84:405–415
3. Rossi Fanelli F, Cangiano C, Ceci F et al (1986) Plasma tryptophan and anorexia in human cancer. Eur J Cancer Clin Oncol 22:89–95
4. Geels P, Eisenhauer E, Bezjak A et al (2000) Palliative effect of chemotherapy: objective tumor response is associated with symptom improvement in patients with metastatic breast cancer. J Clin Oncol 18:2395–2405
5. DeWys WD, Begg C, Lavin PT et al (1980) Prognostic effect of weight loss prior to chemotherapy in cancer patients. Eastern Cooperative Oncology Group. Am J Med 69:491–497
6. Sutton LM, Demark-Wahnefried W, Clipp EC (2003) Management of terminal cancer in elderly patients. Lancet Oncol 4:149–157

7. Pirovano M, Maltoni M, Nanni O et al (1999) A new palliative score: a first step for the staging of terminally ill cancer patients. Italian Multicenter and Study Group on Palliative Care. J Pain Symptom Manage 17:231–239

8. Maltoni M, Nanni O, Pirovano M et al (1999) Successful validation of the palliative prognostic score in terminally ill cancer patients. Italian Multicenter Study Group on Palliative Care. J Pain Symptom Manage 17:240–247

9. Daly JM, Redmond HP, Gallagher H (1992) Perioperative nutrition in cancer patients. JPEN 16(Suppl 6):100S–105S

10. Marchesini G, Bianchi G, Merli M et al for the Italian BCAA Study Group (2003) Nutritional supplementation with branched-chain amino acids in advanced cirrhosis: a double-blind, randomized trial. Gastroenterology 124:1792–1801

11. Hiroshige K, Sonta T, Suda T et al (2001) Oral supplementation of branched-chain amino acid improves nutritional status in elderly patients on chronic haemodialysis. Nephrol Dial Transplant 16:1856–1862

12. Edmonds P, Karlsen S, Khan S, Addington-Hall J (2001) A comparison of the palliative care needs of patients dying from chronic respiratory diseases and lung cancer. Palliat Med 15:287–295

13. Nordgren L, Sorensen S (2003) Symptoms experienced in the last six months of life in patients with end-stage heart failure. Eur J Cardiovasc Nurs 2:213–217

14. Lynn J, Teno JM, Phillips RS et al (1997) Perceptions by family members of the dying experience of older and seriously ill patients. SUPPORT investigators. Study to Understand Prognoses and Preferences for Outcomes and Risks of Treatments. Ann Int Med 126:97–106

15. Gibbs JS, McCoy AS, Gibbs LM et al (2002) Living with and dying from heart failure: the role of palliative care. Heart 88(Suppl 2):ii36–ii39

16. Rossi Fanelli F, Muscaritoli M, Cangiano C et al (1999) The basis for a rational nutritional approach to patients with cancer. In: Abraham NG, Tabilio A, Martelli M et al (eds) Molecular biology of hematopoiesis. Kluwer Academic/Plenum Publishers, New York, pp 229–234

17. Tisdale MJ (2002) Cachexia in cancer patients. Nat Rev Cancer 2:862–871

18. Maltoni M, Pirovano M, Scarpi E et al (1995) Prediction of survival of patients terminally ill with cancer. Results of an Italian prospective multicentric study. Cancer 75:2613–2622

19. Apolone G, De Carli G, Brunetti M, Garattini S (2001) Health-related quality of life (HR-QOL) and regulatory issues. An assessment of the European Agency for the Evaluation of Medicinal Products (EMEA) recommendations on the use of HR-QOL measures in drug approval. Pharmacoeconomics 19:1727–1729

20. Schwartz MW, Woods SC, Porte D Jr et al (2000) Central nervous system control of food intake. Nature 404:661–671

21. Janik JE, Curti BD, Considine RV et al (1997) Interleukin-1 alpha increases serum leptin concentrations in humans. J Clin Endocrinol Metab 82:3084–3086

22. Chance WT, Sheriff S, Moore J et al (1998) Reciprocal changes in hypothalamic receptor binding and circulating leptin in anorectic tumor-bearing rats. Brain Res 803:27–33

23. Simons JP, Schols AM, Campfield LA et al (1997) Plasma concentration of total leptin and human lung-cancer-associated cachexia. Clin Sci 93:273–277

24. Bing C, Taylor S, Tisdale MJ, Williams G (2001) Cachexia in MAC 16 adenocarcinoma: suppression of hunger despite normal regulation of leptin, insulin and hypothalamic neuropeptide Y. J Neurochem 79:1004–1012

25. Mantovani G, Macciò A, Mura L et al (2000) Serum levels of leptin and proinflammatory cytokines in patients with advanced-stage cancer at different sites. J Mol Med 78:554–561

26. Stenvinkel P, Lindholm B, Lonnqvist F et al (2000) Increases in serum leptin levels during peritoneal dialysis are associated with inflammation and a decrease in lean body mass. J Am Soc Nephrol 11:1303–1309

27. Ben-Ari Z, Schafer Z, Sulkes J et al (2002) Alterations in serum leptin in chronic liver disease. Dig Dis Sci 47:183–189

28. Kahler A, Zimmermann M, Langhans W (1999) Suppression of hepatic fatty acid oxidation and food intake in men. Nutrition 15:819–828

29. Loftus TM, Jaworsky DE, Frehywot GL et al (2000) Reduced food intake and body weight in mice treated with fatty acid synthase inhibitors. Science 288:2379–2381

30. Rasmussen BB, Holmback UC, Volpi E et al (2002) Malonyl coenzyme A and the regulation of functional carnitine palmitoyltransferase-1 activity and fat oxidation in human skeletal muscle. J Clin Invest 110:1687–1693

31. Peluso G, Nicolai R, Reda E et al (2000) Cancer and anticancer therapy-induced modification on metabolism mediated by carnitine system. J Cell Physiol 182:339–350

32. Laviano A, Meguid MM, Renvyle T et al (1996) Carnitine supplementation accelerates normalization of food intake depressed during TPN. Physiol Behav 60:317–320

33. Li JL, Zheng FL, Tan HB et al (2003) Orexin A and neuropeptide Y in plasma and hypothalamus of rats with chronic renal failure. Zhonghua Yi Xue Za Zhi 83:992–995

34. Rossi Fanelli F, Cangiano C (1991) Increased availability of tryptophan in brain as common pathogenic mechanism for anorexia associated with different diseases. Nutrition 7:364–367

35. Laviano A, Meguid MM, Yang Z-J et al (1996) Cracking the riddle of cancer anorexia. Nutrition 12:706–710

36. Chance WT, Balasubramaniam A, Fischer JE (1995) Neuropeptide Y and the development of cancer anorexia. Ann Surg 221:579–587

37. Chance WT, Sheriff S, Kasckow JW et al (1998) NPY messenger RNA is increased in medial hypothalamus of anorectic tumor-bearing rats. Regul Pept 75–76:347–353

38. Plata-Salaman CR, Ilyin SE, Gayle D (1998) Brain cytokine mRNAs in anorectic rats bearing prostate adenocarcinoma tumor cells. Am J Physiol 275:R566–R573

39. Jatoi A, Loprinzi CL, Sloan JA et al (2001) Neuropeptide Y, leptin, and cholecystokinin 8 in patients with advanced cancer and anorexia: a North Central Treatment Group exploratory investigation. Cancer 92:629–633

40. Meguid MM, Ramos EJ, Laviano A et al (2004) Tumor anorexia: effects on neuropeptide Y and monoamines in paraventricular nucleus. Peptides 25:261–266

41. Makarenko IG, Meguid MM, Gatto L et al (2003) Decreased NPY innervation of the hypothalamic nuclei in rats with cancer anorexia. Brain Res 961:100–108

42. Aguilera A, Codoceo R, Selgas R et al (1998) Anorexigen (TNF-alpha, cholecystokinin) and orexigen (neuropeptide Y) plasma levels in peritoneal dialysis (PD) patients: their relationship with nutritional parameters. Nephrol Dial Transplant 13:1476–1483

43. Marks DL, Ling N, Cone RD (2001) Role of central melanocortin system in cachexia. Cancer Res 61:1432–1438

44. Wisse BE, Frayo RS, Schwartz MW, Cummings DE (2001) Reversal of cancer anorexia by blockade of central melanocortin receptors in rats. Endocrinology 142:3292–3301

45. Plata-Salaman CR (1996) Anorexia during acute and chronic disease. Nutrition 12:69–78

46. Aguilera A, Selgas R, Codoceo R, Bajo A (2000) Uremic anorexia: a consequence of persistently high brain serotonin levels? The tryptophan/serotonin disorder hypothesis. Perit Dial Int 20:810–816

47. Opara EI, Laviano A, Meguid MM, Yang Z-J (1995) Correlation between food intake and CSF IL-1a in anorectic tumor bearing rats. Neuroreport 6:750–752

48. Laviano A, Gleason JR, Meguid MM et al (2000) Effects of intra-VMN mianserin and IL-1ra on meal number in anorectic tumor-bearing rats. J Investig Med 48:40–48

49. Pereira BJ, Shapiro L, King AJ et al (1994) Plasma levels of IL-1 beta, TNF-alpha and their specific inhibitors in undialyzed chronic renal failure, CAPD and hemodialysis patients. Kidney Int 45:890–896

50. Cangiano C, Testa U, Muscaritoli M et al (1994) Cytokines, tryptophan and anorexia in cancer patients before and after surgical tumor ablation. Anticancer Res 14:1451–1456

51. Wang W, Lonnroth C, Svanberg E, Lundholm K (2001) Cytokine and cyclooxigenase-2 protein in brain areas of tumor-bearing mice with prostanoid-related anorexia. Cancer Res 61:4707–4715

52. Wang W, Danielsson A, Svanberg E, Lundholm K (2003) Lack of effects by tricyclic antidepressant and serotonin inhibitors on anorexia in MCG 101 tumor bearing mice with eicosanoid-related anorexia. Nutrition 19:47–53

53. Inui A (1999) Cancer anorexia-cachexia syndrome: are neuropeptides the key? Cancer Res 59:4493–4501

54. Heisler LK, Cowley MA, Tecott LH et al (2002) Activation of central melanocortin pathways by fenfluramine. Science 297:609–611

55. Shintani F, Kanba S, Nakaki T et al (1993) Interleukin-1beta augments release of norepinephrine, dopamine and serotonin in the rat anterior hypothalamus. J Neurosci 13:3574–3581

56. Blaha V, Yang ZJ, Meguid MM et al (1998) Ventromedial nucleus of hypothalamus is related to the development of cancer-induced anorexia: in vivo microdialysis study. Acta Medica (Hradec Kralove) 41:3–11

57. Diksic M, Young SN (2001) Study of the brain serotonergic system with labelled a-methyl-L-tryptophan. J Neurochem 78:1185–1200

58. Cangiano C, Cascino A, Ceci F et al (1990) Plasma and CSF tryptophan in cancer anorexia. J Neural Transm (Gen Sect) 81:225–233

59. Laviano A, Cangiano C, Preziosa I et al (1997) Plasma tryptophan and anorexia in liver cirrhosis. Int J Eating Disord 21:181–186

60. Chance WT, von Meyenfeldt M, Fischer JE (1983) Serotonin depletion by 5,7-dihydroxytryptamine or para-chloroamphetamine does not affect cancer anorexia. Pharmacol Biochem Behav 18:115–121

61. Laviano A, Rossi Fanelli F (2003) Pathogenesis of cancer anorexia. Still doubts after all these years? Nutrition 19:67–68

62. Torelli GF, Meguid MM, Moldawer LL et al (1999) Use of recombinant human soluble TNF receptor in anorectic tumor-bearing rats. Am J Physiol 277:R850–R855

63. Inui A (2002) Cancer anorexia-cachexia syndrome: current issues in research and management. CA Cancer J Clin 52:72–91

64. Mantovani G, Macciò A, Bianchi A et al (1995) Megestrol acetate in neoplastic anorexia/cachexia: clinical evaluation and comparison with cytokine levels in patients with head and neck carcinoma treated with neoadjuvant chemotherapy. Int J Clin Lab Res 25:135–141

65. Mantovani G, Macciò A, Esu S et al (1997) Medroxyprogesterone acetate reduces the in vitro production of cytokines and serotonin involved in anorexia/cachexia and emesis by peripheral blood mono-

nuclear cells of cancer patients. Eur J Cancer 33:602–607

66. Jatoi A, Windschitl HE, Loprinzi CL et al (2002) Dronabinol versus megestrol acetate versus combination therapy for cancer-associated anorexia: a North Central Cancer treatment Group study. J Clin Oncol 20:567–573

67. Loprinzi CL, Kugler JW, Sloan JA et al (1999) Randomized comparison of megestrol acetate versus dexamethasone versus fluoxymesterone for the treatment of cancer anorexia/cachexia. J Clin Oncol 17:3299–3306

68. Calder PC (2002) Dietary modifications of inflammation with lipids. Proc Nutr Soc 61:345–358

69. Bruera E, Strasser F, Palmer JL et al (2003) Effect of fish oil on appetite and other symptoms in patients with advanced cancer and anorexia/cachexia: a double-blind, placebo-controlled study. J Clin Oncol 21:129–134

70. Cahlin C, Gelin J, Delbro D et al (2000) Effect of cyclooxigenase and nitric oxide synthase inhibitors on tumor growth in mouse tumor models with and without cachexia related to prostanoids. Cancer Res 60:1742–1749

71. Lundholm K, Gelin J, Hyltander A et al (1994) Anti-inflammatory treatment may prolong survival in undernourished patients with metastatic solid tumors. Cancer Res 54:5602–5606

72. Squadrito F, Calapai G, Altavilla D et al (1994) Central serotoninergic system involvement in the anorexia induced by NG-nitro-L-arginine, an inhibitor of nitric oxide synthase. Eur J Pharmacol 255:51–55

73. Lugarini F, Hrupka BJ, Schwartz GJ et al (2002) A role for cyclooxygenase-2 in lipopolysaccharide-induced anorexia in rats. Am J Physiol Regul Integr Comp Physiol 283:R862–R868

74. Nakamura K, Li YQ, Kaneko T et al (2001) Prostaglandin E3 receptor protein in serotonin and catecholamine cell groups: a double immunofluorescence study in the rat brain. Neuroscience 103:763–775

# Starvation: Social, Voluntary, and Involuntary Causes of Weight Loss

Daniele Scevola, Angela Di Matteo, Omar Giglio, Filippo Uberti

## Introduction

Under physiological conditions, body weight remains remarkably stable because of the importance of maintaining energy stores. A complex network of neural and hormonal factors regulates appetite and metabolism. A fundamental role is played by hypothalamic centres of feeding and satiety. Neuropeptides induce anorexia by acting on the satiety centre; gastrointestinal peptides, such as glucagon, somatostatin, and cholecystokinin, induce anorexia by vagal signalling; hypoglycaemia inhibits satiety centre. Leptin, produced by adipose tissue, acts on the hypothalamus to decrease food intake and increase energy expenditure, thus achieving long-term weight homoeostasis [1].

## Voluntary and Involuntary Weight Loss

An intake of protein calories and/or any of the 39 essential nutrients that is less than the minimal required threshold leads to disruption of the balance between energy expenditure and nutrient requirements, resulting in various undernutrition syndromes and weight loss. Still, weight loss may be an ambiguous finding, as the presence of oedema may mask depletions in fat or lean body mass, or, conversely, a gain in fat and lean body mass may not be apparent in the presence of massive diuresis. Undernutrition may be *primary,* due to an inadequate dietary supply of essential nutrients, or *secondary*, in which nutrient intake is adequate but disease or excessive utilisation prevents adequate absorption or metabolism. Although primary and secondary mechanisms often reinforce each other, the respective pathways to weight loss are different. The secondary form takes place as a consequence of a hypercatabolic state, leading to progressive 'self-cannibalism' [2, 3]. When examining a patient with weight loss, a physician should ascertain whether it is voluntary or unintentional.

In the majority of individuals, approximately 50% of the energy introduced by the consumption of food is utilised for maintenance of basal metabolism, such as body temperature; 40% is utilised for physical activity (50% in the extremely vigorous activity performed by athletes); and 10% is used for dietary thermogenesis, i.e. the energy required for digestion, absorption, and metabolism of food.

Weight loss may be a result of decreased food intake, malabsorption, loss of calories, or increasing energy expenditure. A deficit of 3500 Kcal correlates with a loss of 0.45 kg of body fat, but water gained or lost must also be taken into account. During the first few days of restricted food intake, most weight loss is attributable to water loss. In a historical experiment, Brozek [4] studied the kinetics of weight loss in young healthy volunteers on a hypocaloric diet (1010 Kcal daily) over a 24-day period (Table 1). On days 1–3 , 70% of the weight lost by the volunteers consisted of water, and 1 kg lost correlated with a deficit of 2596 Kcal. On days 11–13, weight losses were due to a reduction of fat tissue, and 1 kg lost correlated with a deficit of 7043 Kcal. On days 22–24, weight losses were due almost exclusively to reductions of fat and muscle tissue, and 1 kg lost correlated with a deficit of 8700 Kcal.

Involuntary weight loss (IWL) is defined as a clinically significant and progressive loss of at least 4.5 kg or > 5% of the usual body weight over a period of 24–48 weeks [5]. A weight loss > 10-20% represents the condition known as protein-energy malnutrition (PEM). A more correct reference than usual body weight to measure

**Table 1.** Weight loss of young volunteers consuming a diet of 1010 Kcal/day during a period of 24 days

| Period | Days 1–3 | Days 11–13 | Days 22–24 |
|---|---|---|---|
| Losses kg/day | 0.80 | 0.23 | 0.17 |
| $H_2O$ (%) | 70 | 19 | 0 |
| Fat body mass (%) | 25 | 69 | 85 |
| Lean body mass (%) | 5 | 12 | 15 |
| Caloric deficit (Kcal/kg loss) | 2596 | 7043 | 8700 |

normality or a gain or loss of weight is ideal body weight (IBW). IBW is defined as the weight that corresponds to the maximal expectancy of life. IWL results acutely from impaired absorption and utilisation of energy and protein, or gradually from a prolonged deprivation of nutrients (starvation). A rapid and frequently dramatic weight loss, including loss of total body water, fat, lean body and skeletal mass is associated with traumatic injury, infections, burns, major surgery, pulmonary diseases, and cancer [6, 7]. IWL and PEM may develop together, increasing morbidity and the mortality rates of underlying diseases.

## The Magnitude of the Problem and Associated Conditions

The occurrence of IWL/PEM is increased among several high-risk patient groups: 15–40% of patients admitted to the hospital are at risk of PEM, reaching 46, 45, 39 and 43–60% in medical,

respiratory, orthopaedic, and elderly patients, respectively [8, 9]. A catabolic state induced by severe wounds, major surgery, burn, sepsis, defective immunity, elderly, cancer, HIV, and other chronic infections leads to PEM and IWL, as especially documented in nursing-home residents and in patients newly admitted to long-term care facilities; among such patients, the prevalence of malnutrition has been reported to be 23–85% [10, 11].

## Social Causes of Weight Loss

In developing countries, malnutrition takes on different forms of multiple or partial deficiencies, ranging from simple undernourishment to denutrition and cachexia. High rates of malnutrition persist, in spite of progress in the production, preservation, and distribution of food, and in sanitary measures and education.

UNO, FAO, WHO and UNICEF data collected in the 1990s (Table 2) show that 20% of the popu-

**Table 2.** Prevalence of undernourishment in developing countries (source: FAO)

| Countries | Total population | Number of undernourished people | Proportion of total | Proportion of total | Proportion of total |
|---|---|---|---|---|---|
| | 1997 (millions) | 1996–1998 (millions) | 1979–1981 (%) | 1990–1992 (%) | 1996–1998 (%) |
| Developing world | 4 501.2 | 791.9 | 29 | 21 | 18 |
| Asia and Pacific | 3 091.2 | 515.2 | 32 | 21 | 17 |
| East Asia | 1 321.9 | 155.0 | 29 | 16 | 12 |
| China | 1 244.1 | 140.1 | 30 | 17 | 11 |
| China, Hong Kong | 6.5 | 0.1 | … | … | … |
| North Korea | 23.0 | 13.2 | 19 | 19 | 57 |
| South Korea | 45.7 | 0.5 | … | … | … |
| Mongolia | 2.5 | 1.1 | 16 | 34 | |

lations of developing countries, particularly in the group of least-developed countries (LDCs), comprising more than 800 million people, eats an amount of food that is only enough to guarantee energy for a sedentary life (1.2–1.4 times the basal metabolism). More than 192 million children suffer from PEM and 2000 million people lack various micronutrients (vitamins, minerals, essential amino acids)!

In Western countries, where an enormous surplus of food exists, many people belonging to various groups (the poor, the elderly, drug-addicts, pregnant women, as well as hepatopathic, nephropathic, gastroenteropathic, neoplastic, and AIDS patients) have nutritional deficits that are either unknown or evident.

An insufficient intake of food is the first cause of malnutrition, but a lack of nourishment is often associated with other aggravating factors. These can be the main cause of undernourishment, such as is the case in patients with infectious or parasitic diseases [12, 13], poor alimentary habits, traumas, burns, neoplasms, or who have undergone surgery [14, 7].

Infectious diseases produce a series of metabolic alterations [15] that either separately or jointly give rise to malnutrition (Table 3).

'Hospital malnutrition,' due to incongruous alimentary habits before hospitalisation or to the irrational diets of some health-care organisations, deserves special attention [16, 17]. It is calculated that 20–40% of patients admitted to medical wards and 20–25% of surgical patients show signs of protein-caloric malnutrition, which usually increases after 7–10 days of hospitalisation or after surgery. Malnutrition is a common feature in hospitalised AIDS patients, who take in only 70% of resting energy expenditure (REE) needs and 65% of protein needs, excluding the extra needs resulting from the hypermetabolism associated with fever, acute infections, and physical activity. Dietetic deficits in protein and calorie consumption interfere with the natural course of the main disease, emphasising subjective symptoms such as sickness, asthenia, anorexia, emesis, and constipation, which in turn interfere with feeding. A close relationship exists between susceptibility to infectious diseases and nutritional status: regular nutrition and general good health make individuals more resistant to infections. Similarly, anergy to cutaneous tests (PPD, candidin, DNCB, etc.) is closely related to body-weight insufficiency and hypoalbuminaemia. The pre-surgical correction of denutrition reduces the incidence of post-surgical infectious complications, favouring the healing of the wounds and a quicker return to health [18–20].

Diseases that are usually benign in Western countries (measles, pertussis, TBC) are particularly serious in developing countries [21]. The individual effects of undernourishment/denutrition consist of a progressive loss of weight, lack of body development, anaemia, loss of muscular strength and working capacity, blindness, and a greater susceptibility to diseases. The general effects are economic and social, as well as health-related, as, in a vicious circle, entire populations in some regions are not able to work and produce food because of undernourishment.

## Dimension of the Nutritional Problem in the World

International organisations (UNO, FAO, WHO, UNICEF, World Bank) have established methods of evaluating available foods, the consumption of food, and nutritional status by taking into consideration parameters of agricultural production, anthropometrical measurements, birth-rate, mortality and morbidity rates, and clinical, immunological, haematological, and biochemical parameters.

One of the most frequently used comprehensive indexes of alimentary and nutritional condi-

**Table 3.** Metabolic disturbances induced by infectious diseases

Hypercatabolism

High consumption of $O_2$

Loss of potassium, phosphorous and magnesium

Hydric-saline retention

Hypertriglyceridaemia

Hypoglycaemia

Negative nitrogen balance

tion is the DES (dietary energy supply). The DES expresses the daily average of available energy per person, taking into account all the alimentary sources of a country during a certain period. However, because of the unequal distribution of available food among social classes, age groups, and those with special physiological needs (pregnancy, childhood, old age, and illness), the DES underestimates the real alimentary needs.

DES tables are produced by the FAO based on food balance sheets (FBS), which track the supply and use of food worldwide but do not indicate actual consumption or equity in the distribution of available supplies. Nevertheless, trends in food and energy supplies at the national and regional levels are well-expressed by the FBS. Accordingly, the diets of 800 million people lack 100–400 kcal per day, but most of these people are not dying of starvation; they become thin but are not emaciated (Fig. 1).

Evidence of chronic hunger is not always apparent because the body compensates by slowing down metabolism and physical activity. In children, growth and school activity are compromised, susceptibility to disease is increased.

Mothers may give birth to underweight babies. The situation is particularly serious in sub-Saharan Africa, where acute malnutrition occurs more often, while the majority of chronically hungry people is in Asia and the Pacific area.

In 46% of countries, the undernourished have an average deficit of more than 300 kcal/person/day, including deficits in every nutrient, particularly the starchy staple foods (carbohydrate-rich maize, potatoes, rice, wheat, and cassava) that usually provide the greatest part of energy. About 11 countries have a DES that is less than 2000 kcal per person. While some people generally get enough of the staple foods, they lack other foods, including legumes, meat, fish, oils, dairy products, vegetables, and fruit, which provide protein, fat, micronutrients, and energy.

The global availability of food in the world has increased in the last few years, except in the poorest developing countries, including the sub-Sahara, which is afflicted by frequent famine for climatic and social reasons. About 18 million inhabitants of these regions seriously risk starving to death.

Moreover, 60% of the world population con-

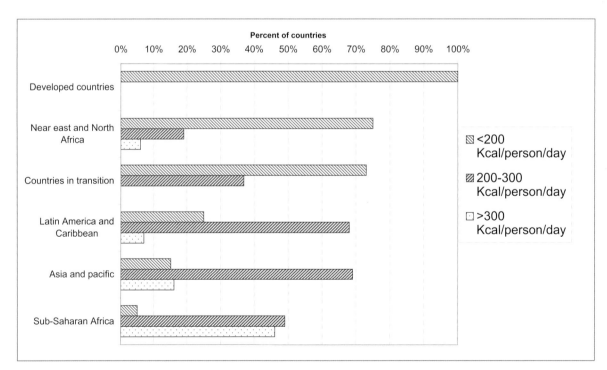

**Fig. 1.** Average food deficit in the world

sumes about 2600 Kcal per person per day, which is considered barely sufficient for limited activity. In 41 developing countries, food intake is more than 2600 Kcal per day per person, while in 15 countries it is more than 3000 Kcal/inhabitant per day. In 11 countries, the DES is less than 2000 Kcal/person/per day, resulting in the inevitable development of severe malnutrition (Table 4).

ity between more and less affluent countries is growing. At the same time, the income gap is growing within most countries, both developed and developing. Concurrently, epidemiological, demographic, and nutritional transitions are taking place in many countries. Current information on malnutrition and the consequences of socioeconomic disparities on global nutrition and

**Table 4.** Dietary energy supply (Kcal/person/day) in the world from the 1970s to the 1990s (source: FAO)

| Countries | 1970s | 1980s | 1990s |
|---|---|---|---|
| *World* | 2430 | 2580 | 2700 |
| *Developed countries* | 3190 | 3290 | 3400 |
| North America | 3230 | 3330 | 3600 |
| Europe | 3240 | 3370 | 3450 |
| Oceania | 3290 | 3160 | 3330 |
| Former USSR | 3320 | 3370 | 3380 |
| *Developing countries* | 2120 | 2330 | 2470 |
| Asia and the Pacific | 2040 | 2250 | 2450 |
| South America and the Caribbean | 2500 | 2690 | 2690 |
| Near East | 2420 | 2810 | 2920 |
| *Least-developed countries* | 2030 | 2060 | 2070 |

To identify the groups and individuals who are most affected by denutrition within a population, methods have been established that estimate chronic alimentary defects and long-term needs, with reference to basal metabolism and during working activity. The FAO World Food Survey has fixed the new limit of the minimum alimentary need at 1.54 times the basal metabolic rate (BMR), previously 1.2–1.4 times the BMR. The earlier value expressed a person's energy expenditure before meals and at complete rest, whereas the more recent index corresponds, in a more realistic manner, to the energy level required to maintain body weight and carry out light physical activity. Raising the value of the minimum amount of energy needed automatically increases the number of undernourished people in the world. Malnutrition, both under and over, can no longer be addressed without considering global food insecurity; socioeconomic disparity, both globally and nationally; and global cultural, social, and epidemiological transitions. The economic dispar-

health reveal dramatic trends. One-third of young children residing in the world's lowest-income countries suffer from growth deficits and rickets because of malnutrition. One-half of all deaths among young children are, at least in part, a consequence of malnutrition. In the developing world, 40% of women suffer from iron deficiency anaemia, a major cause of maternal mortality and low birth weight infants. Despite such worrying trends, there have been significant increases in life expectancy in almost all countries of the world. The proportion of malnourished children has generally decreased, although the actual numbers have not changed in sub-Saharan Africa and southern Asia. However, inequalities are increasing between the richest developed countries and the poorest developing countries. Social inequality is an important factor in differential mortality in both developed and developing countries. Pockets of malnutrition and a high morbidity and mortality of children are emerging in many countries, while the prevalence of obesity and noncommunicable diseases (NCDs) is increasing. Not infrequently, it is the poor and relatively disadvantaged people who suffer both. In developed countries, the overall cardiovascular disease incidence has declined, but less so in the poorer socioeconomic classes.

Hunger and malnutrition are devastating problems afflicting poor people worldwide, in spite of increasing progress in food production and distribution during the 1980s and 1990s [22] (Fig. 2). At one end of the energy malnutrition spectrum is the problem of undernourishment and undernutrition, often described in terms of *macronutrients*. Low dietary energy supply, wasting, stunting, underweight, and low BMI are all used to identify the problem.

However, at the other end of the spectrum is the problem of overnourishment, leading to overweight and obesity. A high BMI is one indicator of the problem. Already a well-known phenomenon in developed countries, obesity is increasing among new urban dwellers in the developing world. Concomitantly, various weight control practices are becoming increasingly common [23]. It should be emphasised that obesity is a multifactorial, chronic disorder that warrants a

continuous, complex model of intervention. Evidence linking voluntary weight loss to decreased mortality is still insufficient to recommend weight loss as a priority in the treatment of obesity. Moreover, current recommendations could be biased by social pressure [24]. The consequences of obesity, i.e. decreased productivity and increased risk of heart disease, hypertension, diabetes and certain cancers, can be as serious as those of underweight.

A diet unbalanced in macronutrients, which are the energy-providing food components, is also a cause for concern, even when total energy intake is adequate. The healthy range of macronutrient intake, expressed as a percent of total energy, can be broad: 55–75% from carbohydrates, 15–35% from fats, and 10–15% from proteins. A more modern balance of energy intake should be suggested, for example 40% from carbohydrates, 30% from proteins, and 30% from fats.

Superimposed upon the energy intake spectrum is the global problem of *micronutrient malnutrition*. Iron deficiency anaemia affects approximately 1.5 billion people, mostly women and children. Iodine deficiency disorders affect about 740 million people worldwide. Vitamin A deficiency-

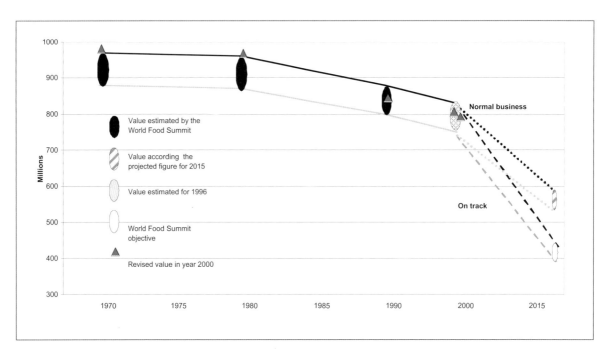

**Fig. 2.** Number of undernourished people in the developing world: observed and projected values (source: FAO)

induced blindness affects around 2.8 million children under 5 years of age. More than 200 million people are considered vitamin A deficient. Calcium deficiency in pregnant and lactating women can affect the development of their children, and appears as osteoporosis later in life. Severe vitamin C deficiency (scurvy) is mostly a problem in the extremely deprived, such as refugees populations. Micronutrients – minerals and vitamins – are needed for proper growth, development, and body function. Deficiencies are particularly common among women of reproductive age, children, and the immunocomprised, such as people with AIDS. Some micronutrient deficiencies affect people whose energy intake is low, but those consuming too much energy can also suffer from it.

Specific requirements have been established for most micronutrients. In most cases, deficiencies can be corrected by consuming a well-balanced diet. Variety is the key to prevention. Women are at greater risk of malnutrition and need appropriate nutritional support. They are more vulnerable than men to food unbalance because of their specific physiological requirements. Women usually have lower metabolic rates and less muscle mass than men and thus require about 25% less dietary energy per day, but they have to eat a much higher proportion of nutrient-rich foods. Women require more vitamins and minerals than men in proportion to total dietary energy intake (Table 5).

Pregnant or lactating women, need foods that are richer in energy and nutrients. During pregnancy, a woman needs an additional 300 kcal per day after the first trimester, and 500 kcal more while lactating. Compared to a non-pregnant woman, she requires almost as much protein as a man (60 g vs. 63 g per day) and more when lactating (65 g/day), up to four times more iron, 1.5 times more folate, and 20% more calcium. A lactating mother needs 40% more vitamin A and C, at least 15% more vitamin B12, and extra levels of micronutrients. Lack of access to adequate amounts and variety of food places pregnant women at greater risk of complications during pregnancy and delivery. The deaths of many infant and young children in developing countries are attributable to the poor nutritional status of their mothers.

Because they are growing rapidly, infants and young children, especially under 2 years old, need foods rich in energy and nutrients. Poor diets prevent children from achieving their full genetic potential. Severe malnutrition can cause early death, permanent disabilities, and increased susceptibility to life-threatening illnesses. A child's growth is a good indicator of his or her overall health status. Figure 3 shows the prevalence of undernutrition among young children in developing countries.

**Table 5.** Nutrient requirements per day for women[a] and men. (Data from [25])

| Nutrient | Adult female | Adult male | Adult male per 1000 kcal[b] | Adult female per 1000 kcal[c] |
|---|---|---|---|---|
| Calcium (mg) | 1000 | 1000 | 500 | 350 |
| Iron (mg)[d] | 24 | 11 | 12 | 4 |
| Vitamin A (μg RE) | 500 | 600 | 250 | 210 |
| Vitamin C (mg) | 45 | 45 | 23 | 16 |
| Vitamin E (mg) | 7.5 | 10 | 3.6 | 3.6 |
| Niacin (mg) | 14 | 16 | 7 | 6 |
| Protein (g) | 50 | 63 | 25 | 22.5 |

[a]The needs of pregnant and lactating women are not included
[b]Based on total dietary energy intake of 2000 kcal/day
[c]Based on total dietary energy intake of 2800 kcal/day
[d]Based on 12% bioavailability

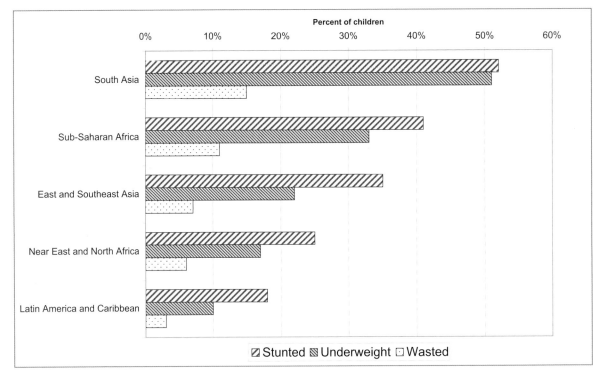

**Fig. 3.** Undernutrition in children in developing countries

Teenage mothers and their babies are particularly vulnerable to malnutrition. Girls generally grow in height and weight until the age of 18 and do not achieve peak bone mass until about 25. The diet of a chronically hungry adolescent girl cannot support adequately both her own growth and that of her foetus. Malnourished young women often give birth to underweight babies.

## Body Mass Index

Body mass index (BMI) is an anthropometric standard measure defining the body composition of men and women. Initially it was used to measure obesity in developed countries, but it is now applied to underweight and overweight adults throughout the world. BMI provides a simple, convenient and relatively inexpensive indicator for assessing whether a person is taking in too little or too much energy. However, BMI is a crude measure of nutritional status, and additional information is needed to determine a person's health status. In addition, the values may have to be adapted for specific groups of adults, such as adolescents, pregnant women, and the elderly.

BMI is calculated by as: BMI = body weight (kg) / height$^2$ (m$^2$). The healthy range of BMI for adults, as recommended by FAO, the WHO, and the International Dietary Energy Consultative Group, is considered 18.5–25. Figures 4 and 5 show a range of BMI scores from severely underweight (< 16) to severely obese (> 40) adult men and women. The risk of health problems is greater for people with BMI at either end of the spectrum than for those in the middle range (18.5–25). Nonetheless, the cut-off points of 18.5, defining underweight, and 25, defining overweight, are not universally accepted. Some researchers believe that cut-off points based on country-specific reference groups should be established to reflect differences in height and muscle mass. Concerns about the universal applicability of the BMI should be kept in mind when interpreting the prevalence of underweight and overweight people in selected countries and groups.

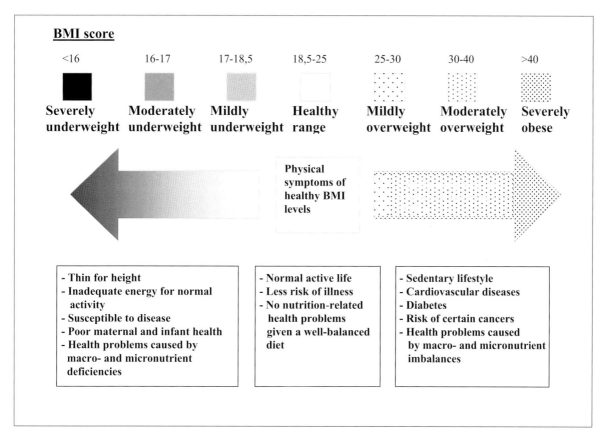

**Fig. 4.** The body mass index (BMI) in adults under normal and clinical conditions

## Expected Changes

The people and the productivity of the land and water are the two greatest resources in most poor, food-insecure countries. Without investments in both people and productivity, chronic hunger and poverty cannot be reversed. People need investments in education, clean water supplies, and health and social services and, in some cases, direct food and nutrition support. In rural areas, such expenditures are essential if the corresponding investments in agriculture and its productive subcompartments are to pay off.

Reducing hunger not only has a humanitarian justification but also a strong economic rationale. The economic cost of hunger and malnutrition, resulting in lost productivity, illness, and death, is extremely high. Undernourishment significantly lowers physical ability, cognitive development, and learning achievement. It not only blights the lives of individuals and families but also reduces the return on investment in social and economic progress.

A recent study sponsored by the FAO examined 110 countries from 1960 to 1990 using statistical techniques to investigate the links between economic growth and nutritional well-being. The results showed that if all countries with average DES below the minimum requirement in 1960 had eliminated hunger by raising average per capita DES to 2770 Kcal per day, their gross domestic product (GDP) growth rates would have been significantly higher. This growth can be quite large. Per capita GDP in sub-Saharan Africa could have reached levels of US $1000 to US $3500 by 1990 if undernourishment had been eliminated. Instead, the region's average GDP per capita in 1990 was just US $800 per year (Fig. 6). The FAO's projections for the next 15 years indicate that, if agricultural innovation continues at a reasonable rate,

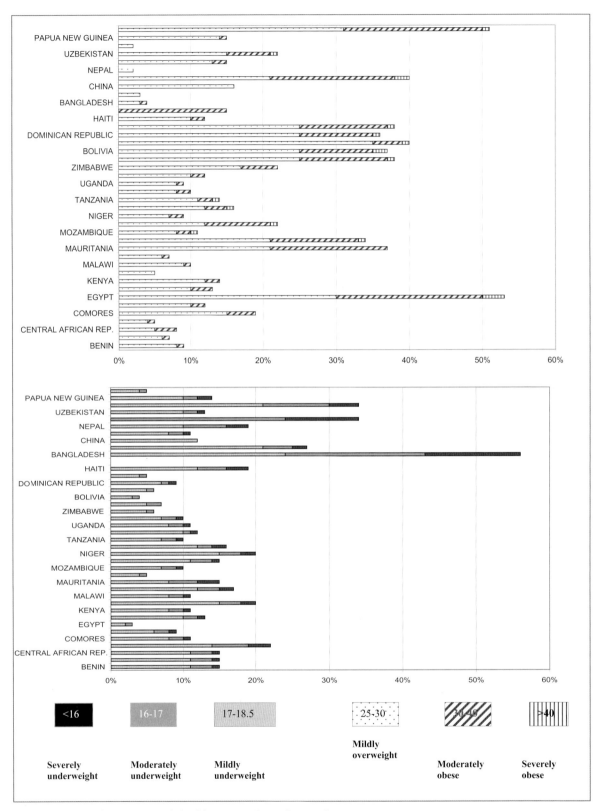

**Fig. 5.** Percentage of women outside healthy range of BMI (18.5–25)

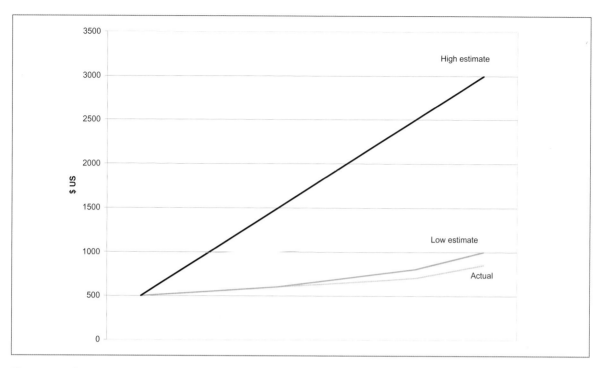

**Fig. 6.** Gross domestic product (GDP) (mean $ US per capita) in sub-Saharan Africa and estimates assuming no undernourishment. (Data from [26])

food production can increase by 2% per year in the developing world. Without this growth, the goals set out by the World Food Summit cannot be met. But overall growth is not enough – it must be directed to the hungriest.

For countries that are still largely rural, investment in small-scale agriculture is one way to target growth that benefits the poor. The importance of putting resources into the agricultural research in production and post-production processes is now well recognised. Funding for agricultural research is particularly vital for commodities and farming systems that can provide growth opportunities for the poor.

Even if the anticipated growth in food production is achieved, nearly 600 million people will remain undernourished in 2015, unless the growth takes place in areas where food insecurity is worst and public policies are implemented that make elimination of food insecurity their primary objective.

## Reducing Hunger Through Basic Crop Research

A study by the Impact Assessment and Evaluation Group of the Consultative Group on International Agricultural Research (CGIAR) [27] emphasised the benefits of international agricultural research in reducing undernourishment among children by improving crop variety and productivity.

Between 1970 and 1995, international agricultural research centres released a large number of new crop varieties resulting from their breeding programmes on staple food crops, including wheat, rice, maize, sorghum, pearl millet, cassava, potatoes, barley, and lentils. According to the study, this represented 70–100 new varieties per year and led to additional productivity gains of 0.5% per year. The resulting additional food production brought a reduction in grain prices of 27–41%. As a direct consequence, 1–3% fewer children were undernourished than would have been without this research.

# References

1. Ramos EJ, Suzuky S,Marks D et al (2004) Cancer anorexiacachexia syndrome: cytokines and neuropeptides. Curr Opin Clin Nutr Metab Care 7:427–434
2. Douglas RG, Shaw JHF (1989) Metabolic response to sepsis and trauma. Br J Surg 76:115–122
3. Tisdale MJ. Cancer cachexia (1991) Br J Cancer 63:337–342
4. Brozek J, Grande F, Taylor HL et al (1957) Changes in body weight and body dimensions in men performing work on a low calorie carbohydrate diet. J Appl Physiol 10:412
5. Bouras EP, Lange SM, Scolapio JS (2001) Rational approach to patients with unintentional weight loss. Mayo Clin Proc 76:923–929
6. Collins N (2003) Protein-energy malnutrition and involuntary weight loss: nutritional and pharmacological strategies to enhance wound healing. Expert Opin Pharmacother 4:1121–1140
7. Laviano A, Russo M, Freda F et al (2002) Neurochemical mechanism for cancer anorexia. Nutrition 18:100–105
8. Mcwhirter JP, Pennington CR (1994) Incidence and recognition of malnutrition in hospital. Br Med J 308:945–948
9. Sullivan DH, Sun S,Walls RC (1999) Protein-energy undernutrition among elderly hospitalized patients: a prospective study. JAMA 281:2013–2019
10. Silver AJ, Morley JE, Strome LS et al (1988) Nutritional status in an academic nursing home. J Am Geriatr Soc 36:487–491
11. Thomas DR, Zdrowski CD, Wilson MM et al (2002) Malnutrition in subacute care. Am J Clin Nutr 75:308–313
12. Tomkins A (1981) Nutritional status and severity of diarrhoea among preschool children in rural Nigeria. Lancet 1:860–862
13. Lifshitz F (1982) Infections and undernutrition. Nutr Rev 40: 119–126
14. Scevola D (1994) Patologia d'organo. Apparato gastrointestinale. In: Dianzani F, Ippolito G, Moroni M (eds) Il libro italiano dell'AIDS. McGraw-Hill, Milano, pp 305–312
15. Beisel WR, Powanda MC (2003) Metabolic effects of infection on protein and energy status. J Nutr 133:3225–3275
16. Nixon DW, Heymsfield SB, Cohen AE et al (1980) Proteincalorie undernutrition in hospitalized cancer patients. Am J Med 68: 683–690
17. Mc Laren DS (1988) A fresh look at protein-energy malnutrition in the hospitalized patient. Nutrition 4:1–6
18. Macfie J,Yule AG, Hill GL (1981) Effect of added insulin on body composition of gastroenterologic patients receiving intravenous nutrition: a controlled clinical trial. Gastroenterology 81:285–289
19. Bozzetti F (1989) Effects of artificial nutrition on the nutritional status of cancer patients. J Parenter Enter Nutr 13:406–420
20. Wilmore DW (1991) Catabolic illness:strategies for enhancing recovery. N Engl J Med 325:695–702
21. Ambrus JL Sr, Ambrus JL Jr (2004) Nutrition and infectious diseases in Developing Countries and problems of acquired immunodeficiency syndrome. Exp Biol Med (Maywood) 229:464–472
22. Lopez A (2004) Malnutrition and the burden of diseases. Asia Pac J Clin Nutr 13:57
23. Goodrick GK, Poston WS 2nd, Foreyt JP (1996) Methods for voluntary weight loss and control: update 1996. Nutrition 12:672–676
24. Heini A (2000) Contraindications to weight reduction. Ther Umsch 57:537–541
25. Anonymous (2002) Human vitamin and mineral requirements. Report of a joint FAO/WHO expert consultation. Bangkok, Thailand. Available at: http://www.fao.org/documents/show_cdr.asp?url_file=/DOCREP/004/Y2809E/y2809e00.htm
26. Arcand JL (2000) Malnutrition and growth: the efficiency cost of hunger. FAO. Epub available at www.fao.org/documents
27. Evenson RE (2000) Crop genetic improvement and agricultural development. Prepared for the Technical Advisory Group of the CGIAR for the May 21-26, 2000 meeting of the CGIAR, Dresden, Germany. Document No SDR/TAC:IAR/00/17

# Cachexia Related to Multiple Causes

Giovanni Mantovani, Clelia Madeddu

Despite the long and widespread interest in this topic, there is not an univocal definition for cachexia [1]. The term derives from the Greek *kakòs,* which means 'bad,' and from *hexis,* meaning 'condition.' The clinical syndrome of cachexia is characterised by anorexia, tissue wasting, loss of body weight accompanied by a decrease in muscle mass and adipose tissue, and poor performance status that often precedes death [2–5]. Cachexia can occur as part of many chronic or end-stage diseases, such as infections, cancer, AIDS, congestive heart failure, rheumatoid arthritis, tuberculosis, chronic obstructive pulmonary disease, cystic fibrosis, and Crohn's disease. It may develop also in a proportion of elderly persons without obvious diseases. A literature search using the term 'cachexia' yielded more than 1000 articles published over the past 5 years [1].

Multiple mechanisms appear to be involved in the development of cachexia, including anorexia, decreased physical activity, decreased secretion of host anabolic hormones, and altered host metabolic response with abnormalities in protein, lipid, and carbohydrate metabolism [6]. Anorexia, one of the main features of the cachectic syndrome, may be so significant that spontaneous nutrition is totally inhibited. The pathogenesis of anorexia is most certainly multifactorial but is not yet well-understood. It seems to be attributable, in part, to intermediary metabolites (e.g. lactate, ketones, oligonucleotides) that accumulate along an abnormal metabolic pathway, or to other substances released, such as acute phase response proteins [3], by normal body cells. Indeed, nutritional supplementation alone is not able to effectively reverse the process of cachexia. An increased resting energy expenditure may contribute to the loss of body weight in cachectic patients and may explain the increased oxidation of fat tissue. Futile energy-consuming cycles, such as the Cori cycle, may also play a role in the increased energy demand. Unlike starvation, body-weight loss in cachectic patients arises equally from loss of muscle and fat, characterised by increased catabolism of skeletal muscle and decreased protein synthesis [7]. Catabolic factors capable of direct breakdown of muscle and adipose tissue appear to be secreted in cachexia and may play an active part in tissue degeneration [7].

The degree of wasting is an important prognostic factor, with a loss to 66% of ideal body weight being predictive of death regardless of the specific cause of the weight loss [8]. Therefore, a more thorough understanding of the pathogenesis of cachexia may lead to further therapeutic options that theoretically could improve survival. Neither the infective burden nor the tumour size correlate with the degree of wasting; rather, the host response, via endogenous mediators, appears to affect the cachectic response in diseased patients. Much research has focused on possible mediators of cachexia induced by disease [6].

The causes of cachexia are multiple and differ, at least in part, in different diseases, but some of them are common and they constitute the main background on which the symptoms of cachexia are based. Among the common causes of cachexia, the most well-recognised are: (1) proinflammatory cytokines with related metabolic symptoms and hypermetabolism; (2) neurotransmitters, (3) hormone changes, and (4) anorexia. Proinflammatory cytokines certainly play a central role in non-cancer-related cachexia, but more particularly in cancer cachexia. Neurotransmitters are represented mainly by neuropeptide Y and an endogenous antagonist of α-MSH, the agouti-related protein (AgRP). The hormones that play the most significant role in weight maintenance and homeostasis are leptin, also referred to as a satiety signal hormone, which is released from white adipose tissue, and ghrelin, a hunger signal hormone that is released from the stomach [9]. Both neurotransmitters and hormones, and their abnormalities, may be involved in cachexia.

## References

1. Kotler DP (2000) Cachexia. Ann Intern Med 133:622–634
2. Heber D, Byerley LO, Chi J (1986) Pathophysiology of malnutrition in the adult cancer patient. Cancer Res 58:1867–1873
3. Bruera E (1992) Clinical management of anorexia and cachexia in patients with advanced cancer. Oncology 49(Suppl 2): 35–42
4. Brennan MR (1997) Uncomplicated starvation vs cancer cachexia. Cancer Res 37:2359–2364
5. Nelson K, Walsh D (1991) Management of the anorexia/cachexia syndrome. Cancer Bull 43:403–406
6. Smith MK, Lowry SF (1999) The hypercatabolic state. In: Shils ME, Olson JA, Shike M, Ross AC (eds) Modern nutrition in health and disease, 9th ed. Lippincott Williams & Wilkins, Philadelphia, pp 1555–1568
7. Tisdale MJ (1997) Cancer cachexia: metabolic alterations and clinical manifestations. Nutrition 13:1–7
8. Kotler DP (1992) Nutritional effects and support in the patient with acquired immunodeficiency syndrome. J Nutr 122:723–727
9. Horvath TL, Diano S, Sotonyi P et al (2001) Minireview: ghrelin and the regulation of energy balance – a hypothalamic perspective. Endocrinology 142:4163–4169

# Non-AIDS Lipodystrophy Syndrome

Giuliano Enzi, Luca Busetto, Giuseppe Sergi, Sabrina Pigozzo

## Lipodystrophies

Lipodystrophies (LDs) are clinically heterogeneous acquired or inherited disorders characterised by a generalised or regional loss of adipose tissue. Generalised LDs, both inherited and acquired, are associated with peripheral insulin resistance, glucose intolerance or overt diabetes, acanthosis nigricans, dyslipidaemia. Bone demineralisation and polycystic ovary syndrome are also part of these diseases. LDs can be classified as acquired or congenital, and generalised or partial (Table 1).

**Table 1.** Classification of lipodystrophies (LDs)

A. Acquired LDs
 1. Acquired generalised LD or Lawrence syndrome

 2. Acquired partial LD or Barraquer-Simons syndrome

 3. Acquired localised LD
   c. Hemifacial LD
   b. Cranial LD or Romberg syndrome
   c. Other localised LDs

B. Congenital LDs
 1. Congenital generalised LD or Berardinelli-Seip syndrome
   a. Type 1
   b. Type 2

 2. Congenital partial LDs
   a. Type 1 or Dunningam syndrome
   b. Type 2

 3. Mandibuloacral dystrophy

 4. Other inherited partial LDs

 5. LD associated with multiple symmetric lipomatosis

## Acquired Lipodystrophies

### Acquired Generalised Lipodystrophy (Lipoatrophic Diabetes or Lawrence Syndrome)

Acquired generalised lipodystrophy (AGLD) is a rare, juvenile-onset lipodystrophy, first fully described by Lawrence in 1946 [1], who reported on a young female subject with 'lipodystrophy, and hepatomegaly with diabetes, lipaemia and other metabolic disturbances.' To date, approximately 80 patients with AGLD have been reported [2]. Like others LDs, AGLD is prevalent in females. Lipoatrophy develops over a number of years, in childhood or in adolescence, so that the onset of the condition is later than that of congenital generalised lipodystrophy (CGLD). Extended areas of subcutaneous fat are involved, including the face, arms, and legs. Less frequently mesenteric, retroperitoneal, perirenal and mediastinal fat depots are involved, while retroorbital fat seems to be spared. Muscle mass, evaluated by dual energy X-ray analysis (DEXA), is preserved or even increased compared to age-, sex- and body mass index (BMI)-matched subjects. Therefore, in spite of the generalised atrophy of fat tissue the BMI in the majority of lipodystrophic patients falls into the low-normal range. Resting energy expenditure, independent of hyperthyroidism, is increased. This syndrome is associated with hyperinsulinaemia, insulin resistance, and acanthosis nigricans, soon resulting in overt, non-ketotic diabetes mellitus. Hyperlipidaemia, namely hypertriglyceridaemia, is a further metabolic abnormality associated with AGLD. Liver steatosis, autoimmune hepatitis, splenomegaly, and, ultimately, liver cirrhosis occur in some 20% of patients, often beginning in childhood [3, 4]. Other autoimmune diseases, such as Sjögren's syndrome and dermatomyositis, have been reported in association with AGLD, suggesting an immunomediated fat loss as a possible pathogenetic basis [3]. Panniculitis, characterised by a granulomatous infiltration of adipose tissue, may be an early manifestation of the disease [5]. Acute viral infections often precede AGLD onset. A higher frequency than casually expected of astrocytomas of the third ventricle have been reported. Low levels of leptin and adiponectin have also been described in these patients [6].

## Acquired Partial Lipodystrophy (Barraquer-Simons Syndrome)

Acquired partial lipodystrophy (APLD) was first described by Mitchell in 1885 [7] as a 'singular case of absence of adipose tissue in the upper part of the body,' and then as segmental atrophy of the subcutaneous fat layer by Barraquer [8] in 1907, and as 'lipodystrofia progressiva' by Simons in 1911 [9]. APLD is phenotypically characterised by a loss of fat in the upper body segment, namely, in the face, trunk, and arms. In the lower body segment, the subcutaneous fat depots are spared or even increased. Bichat's fat pad is also involved, giving the face an extremely lean appearance (Fig. 1). Women are affected three times more frequently than men. A mesangiocapillary glomerulonephritis [10] develops in some 30% of affected subjects within 8–15 years after the onset of the disease, leading to renal failure [10], associated with low levels of serum C3 complement fraction [11–13]. A slight increase of a circulating polyclonal IgG, a C3 nephritic factor, causes activation of the alternative complement pathway and increased consumption of the C3 fraction. C3 nephritic factor could induce fat cell lysis, and then a loss of subcutaneous fat [14]. Other autoimmune disorders, such as rheumatoid arthritis, temporal arteritis, dermatomyositis, thyroiditis, coeliac disease, and systemic lupus erythematosus, have been reported to be associated with APLD [15–18]. No information has been offered so far to explain the segmental involvement of subcutaneous fat and the female prevalence, and no effective therapy is currently available. Cosmetic surgical procedures

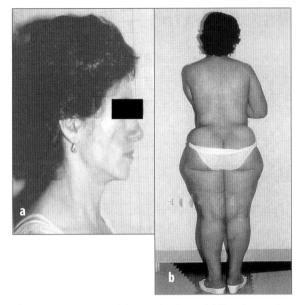

**Fig. 1a, b.** A patient with acquired partial lipodystrophy. Lipoatrophy exclusively involves the upper body segment and face (**a**), while a marked increase in subcutaneous fat depots is evident in the lower body segment (**b**)

may be suggested when psychological discomfort impairs the patient's quality of life.

## Acquired Localised Lipodystrophies

### Hemifacial Lipoatrophy

Hemifacial lipoatrophy (HFLD) asymmetrically involves the left or right half of the face. No peculiar symptoms are associated with HFLD, and aesthetic discomfort is the main consequence. HFLD affects mainly females of any age, from childhood to adulthood.

Atrophy of the subcutaneous fat makes the face asymmetrical due to depression of the cheek and the supramandibular region. Cutis, muscles, and bones are unaffected. No renal, neurological, or autoimmune diseases have been reported in association with HFLD. Skull X-ray rules out involvement of the facial bones. Electromyography reveals no sensory or motor abnormalities of the facial muscles. Lipofilling procedures can improve the aesthetic appearance.

### Progressive Cranial Lipodystrophy (Romberg Disease)

Progressive cranial lipodystrophy (PCLD) represents the most important differential diagnosis from HFLD. PCLD is characterised by abnormality of the cranial basal angle, with monolateral atrophy of all the structures of the face, including muscles, bones, cartilaginous tissues, and subcutaneous fat. Damage of the nerves manifests as trigeminal neuropathy and facial palsy. Cranial X-ray and electromyography easily discriminate between PCLD and HFLD.

### Other Acquired Localised Lipoatrophies

Other atrophies of small, circumscribed areas of subcutaneous fat layers can appear after a local trauma or prolonged pressure, or at the site of drug (mainly of protein structure) injection. Extractive hormones, e.g. bovine insulin, growth hormone, ACTH, calcitonin, and vasopressin, have been reported to be responsible for this form of fat atrophy at injection sites. Local formation of immunocomplexes, or protein precipitate or activation of complement fractions could induce a local lipolytic response mediated by inflammatory agents, and may explain the zonal loss of subcutaneous fat. Tumour necrosis factor (TNF)-$\alpha$ release induced by insulin may mediate adipocyte atrophy [19]. An asymptomatic, discoid or funnel-shaped depression appears. Microscopic examination of biopsy samples of tissue from atrophic area shows the disappearance of fat cells. A dedifferentiation of fat cells to fibroblast-like cells can be postulated, rather than adipocyte necrosis. In fact, the subcutaneous fat may reappear spontaneously or after topical steroid treatment. Recently, the recombinant technology used for hormonal drug production has made local fat atrophy unusual.

Localised lipoatrophies of unknown origin, not belonging to any of other previously reported LD, have been defined as localised involutional LDs. For example, in 1984, Imamura et al.

described several cases of a progressive centrifugal loss of subcutaneous fat at the abdominal wall [20]. The age of onset is infancy. Histological studies show an accumulation of lymphocytes and histiocytes at the edge of the lipoatrophic area, with a satellite lymphadenopathy. The disease usually regresses spontaneously in a few months or years. The aetiology is unknown, but an inflammatory reaction to unknown agents seems to be the most credible hypothesis.

## Congenital Lipodystrophies

### Congenital Generalised Lipodystrophy (Berardinelli–Seip Syndrome or Lipoatrophic Diabetes)

Congenital generalised lipodystrophy (CGLD) is an autosomal recessive, transmitted disease characterised by a pronounced loss of subcutaneous and visceral fat tissue manifested since birth. The condition is associated with acromegalic traits (Fig. 2), accelerated growth with normal hGH

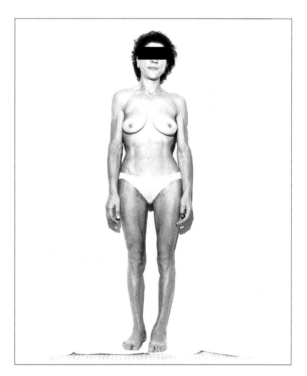

**Fig. 2.** A patient with congenital lipodystrophy or lipoatrophic diabetes. There is evidence of a pronounced loss of subcutaneous fat, acromegaloid aspect, and phlebomegaly (for details, see Table 3, patient GF)

plasma levels, hypertrichosis, mild virilisation, liver enlargement, reduced glucose tolerance or overt diabetes, heat intolerance, and increased perspiration (Table 2) [21–23].

The loss of fat involves the mesenteric, perirenal, and paracardiac adipose tissue depots [24]. Orbital and perirenal fat depots are spared. Acanthosis nigricans and hyperinsulinaemia are the rule. Accelerated growth in early childhood and advanced bone development compared with age-matched controls have been reported, but adult body height is normal or only slightly increased. In one patient (e.g., DMM, Table 3) a defect in adipose tissue lipoprotein lipase in a small residual lobule of omental tissue obtained during surgery was observed [25]. In all four patients in our series, post-heparin plasma lipoprotein lipase activity was blunted or near absent. Elevated triglyceride and reduced HDL cholesterol plasma levels are part of the syndrome. Total cholesterol levels are not constantly increased, but occasionally can be remarkably high [25] (Table 3). Muscle mass, evaluated by DEXA, is preserved on even increased compared with age-, sex- and BMI-matched subjects. The increase in resting energy expenditure is related to the higher fat-free mass/body mass ratio. Two subtypes of CGLD have been identified and are distinguished according to the mode of inheritance [26–29]. Type 1 CGLD is related to an autosomal recessive genetic defect in AGPAT2 isoform. This enzyme, involved in the biosynthesis of triglycerides and phospholipids, is expressed at high levels in adipose tissue. Thus, a defect in AGAPT function may reduce triglyceride synthesis in fat cells. Type 2 CGLD is related to an autosomal recessive involvement of seipin, a protein of unknown function [30]. Mutation of the seipin gene has been reported to cluster in a large consanguineous pedi-

**Table 2.** Clinical aspects of the most important lipodystrophies (LDs)

|  | Generalised congenital LD | Partial congenital LD | Generalised acquired LD | Partial acquired LD |
|---|---|---|---|---|
| Eponym | Berardinelli Seip syndrome | Dunningam syndrome | Lawrence syndrome | Barraquer Simons syndrome |
| Inheritance | Autosomal recessive | Autosomal dominant | - | - |
| Gene involved |  |  |  |  |
| Type 1 | AGPAT2 | LMNA |  |  |
| Type 2 | Seipin | PPARγ |  |  |
| Age at onset | Birth | Puberty | Any age | Youth |
| Sex prevalence | = | Women | Women | Women |
| Insulin resistance | Usual | Usual | Frequent | Unusual |
| Glucose tolerance | Reduced | Reduced | Reduced | Normal |
| Acanthosis nigricans | Frequent | Frequent | Unusual | Absent |
| Hypertrichosis | Frequent | Frequent | Unusual | Absent |
| Genital hypertrophy | Frequent | Frequent | Unusual | Absent |
| Somatic growth (if early manifestation) | Precocious | Normal | Precocious | Normal |
| Liver enlargement | Frequent | Frequent | Frequent | Absent |
| Hypertriglyceridaemia | Usual | Usual | Usual | Absent |
| Basal metabolic rate | Increased | Increased | Increased | Normal |
| Polycystic ovary syndrome | Frequent | Frequent | Frequent | Absent |
| C3 deficiency | Absent | Absent | Absent | Frequent |

gree [31]. A high level of seipin RNA expression in the brain of affected subjects suggests an involvement of the cerebral nervous system. This hypothesis seems to be supported by the association of type 2 CGLD with mild mental retardation.

CGLD can manifest with different expression of signs and symptoms and with different degrees of severity of the metabolic abnormalities (Table 3). Insulin resistance usually evolves into overt diabetes. Micro- and macroangiopathies and ketosis are unusual in lipoatrophic diabetes. An increased resting energy expenditure without abnormalities of thyroid function has been reported. Liver steatosis, liver fibrosis, portal hypertension, and oesophageal varices are late-onset complications, possibly leading to death.

## Congenital Partial Lipodystrophy: Type 1 (Dunningam Syndrome)

This LD variety was first described by Dunningam in 1974 [32] in females belonging to two families

in Scotland. An autosomal dominant transmission of the disease was reported in five families. To date, some 200 cases of the disease have been reported, with a higher prevalence in females.

Atrophy of the subcutaneous fat layer usually manifests at puberty, involving the arms, legs, and buttocks. The subcutaneous adipose tissue of the face, neck, and intra-abdominal area may be preserved, giving patients a silhouette of visceral obesity. An increase in intramuscular fat has been reported. Insulin resistance, reduced glucose tolerance, overt diabetes, hypertriglyceridaemia, and low levels of HDL cholesterol are associated with Dunningam syndrome and lead to early onset of atherosclerotic vascular diseases. Acute pancreatitis and liver steatosis may complicate the clinical picture. The identification of missense mutations on chromosome 1q 21–22, involving genes encoding lamins A and C, in affected members of a family suggests the molecular basis of the disease [33]. Lamins provide structural integrity to the nuclear membrane, such that mutations in the

**Table 3.** Main clinical aspects of four patients with congenital lipoatrophic generalised lipodystrophy

|  | DMM | GF | GI | TV |
|---|---|---|---|---|
| Sex | F | F | F | F |
| Age (years) | 18 | 35 | 31 | 24 |
| BMI | 22.0 | 21.6 | 22.2 | 15.5 |
| Glucose tolerance | Diabetes | Diabetes | Reduced glucose tolerance | Diabetes |
| Blood glucose | 335 | 168 | 106 | 165 |
| Plasma insulin | 28 | 20 | 16 | 37 |
| Total cholesterol | 415 | 154 | 158 | 250 |
| HDL cholesterol | 18 | 30 | 35 | 24 |
| Triglycerides | 471 | 201 | 270 | 310 |
| Uric acid | 9.3 | 5.4 | 5.8 | 6.8 |
| Lipoatrophy | +++ | ++ - | ++ - | +++ |
| Resting energy expenditure | +28% | +14% | +18% | +16% |
| Muscle hypertrophy | +++ | +-- | +++ | --- |
| Liver steatosis | +++ | +-- | ++ - | +-- |
| Bone cysts | +++ | ++- | +-- | --- |

GF and GI: sisters. DMM: cousin of GF and GI. The father of GF and GI and the mother of DMM are cousins

gene could result in disruption of the nuclear lamina in adipocytes and subsequently cell death. The Dunningam's variety of familial partial LD seems to be a heterogeneous disorder with a slightly different clinical expression. The site of missense mutations could explain these differences. A variety of this congenital LD was described by Köbberling in 1975 [34].

## Familial Partial Lipodystrophy Associated with a PPARγ Gene Mutation

Garg et al. recently reported on a missense heterozygous mutation, Arg397Cys, in peroxisome-proliferator-activated receptor-gamma (PPARγ) gene in a 64-year-old woman with diabetes, hypertriglyceridaemia, hypertension, hirsutism, and marked subcutaneous fat loss, more prominent in her forearms and calves than in her upper arms and thighs [35].

Other heterozygous mutations in the PPARγ gene were subsequently recognised in subjects with familial partial LD [36, 37]. PPARγ is highly expressed in adipose tissue and plays a role in adipogenesis and adipocyte differentiation. However, the localised atrophy of adipose tissue has yet to be explained.

## Familial Partial Lipodystrophy Associated with Mandibuloacral Dysplasia

This type of dystrophy was first identified by Young et al. in 1971 [38] as 'a new syndrome manifested by mandibular hypoplasia, acroosteolysis (at the extremities), stiff joints and cutaneous atrophy, a bird-like face associated to lipoatrophy at the arms and legs, in two unrelated boys.' Metabolic abnormalities, namely insulin-resistant diabetes mellitus, hypermetabolism, and the molecular basis of the disease were subsequently demonstrated [39, 40]. Two different patterns of mandibuloacral dysplasia (MAD) have been reported. Type A is characterised by a homozygous Arg527His mutation in the LMNA gene [40]. Type B heterozygous mutations in the zinc metalloproteinase ZMPSTE24 gene [41] were observed in a patient whose generalised LD and MAD were associated with progeria and renal failure.

## Other Inherited Partial Lipodystrophies

Other varieties of LD have been described in small series of patients. A syndrome characterised by a low birth weight, short stature, defective ocular development, mental retardation, delayed teething, hyperextensible joints, and atrophy of the subcutaneous fat layer at the arms and trunk, sparing any other site, called the SHORT syndrome, was reported by Sensenbrenner et al. in 1975 [42].

A LD characterised by a near absence of subcutaneous fat from birth, sparing the adipose tissue of the sacral and gluteal fat deposits, has been reported in newborns affected by a neonatal progeroid syndrome [43].

Recently, a new clinical condition was reported, characterised by generalised lipoatrophy, insulin-resistant diabetes, disseminated leukomelanodermal papules, liver steatosis, and cardiomyopathy. The condition was linked to lamin A and C mutations [44].

## Lipoatrophy Associated with Multiple Symmetric Lipomatosis (Launois-Bensaude Syndrome or Madelung Collar)

Multiple symmetric lipomatosis (MSL) is characterised by the growth of fat masses symmetrically located at the neck, shoulders, deltoid and suprascapular regions, proximal segments of the arms and legs, and at the thoracic inlet, a distribution reminiscent of the location of brown adipose tissue in the foetus. The remaining subcutaneous fat layer is markedly atrophic, allowing MSL to be included in the group of LDs (Fig. 3). MSL is reported to be highly prevalent in men, but several cases of MSL in women have recently been reported [45].

In a series of 69 patients, the male to female ratio was 7:1. MSL appears in adulthood (range: 29–65 years), has a slowly progressive course, and is an autosomal dominant inherited disorder that primarily affects adipose tissue. Previous observations suggested lipomatous cells as brown-adipose-tissue-derived cells [46, 47]. Almost all patients have a high alcohol intake, usually red wine, suggesting a specific role for ethanol or

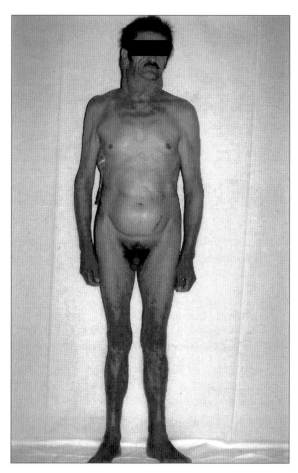

**Fig. 3.** A patient with multiple symmetric lipomatosis. The presence of lipomatous masses localised at the neck, occipital region, and lower part of the abdomen is associated with a marked loss of the subcutaneous fat layer at the limbs

pharyngeal accumulation of fat tissue. In some 20% of MSL patients, fat infiltration of the pharyngeal and tracheal wall was found to be responsible for an obstructive apnoea syndrome during sleep. Metabolic abnormalities include hypertriglyceridaemia and high levels of circulating HDL cholesterol. Hyperuricaemia and reduced glucose tolerance or overt diabetes occur at a frequency slightly higher than casually expected. A defect in adrenergic-stimulated lipolysis [50] and an increase in lipoprotein lipase activity of adipose tissue [51] have been demonstrated in samples of lipomatous tissue. No information is available on the metabolic activity in uninvolved subcutaneous adipose tissue, due to the fat atrophy which makes fat sampling extremely difficult.

There is evidence for a mitochondrial dysfunction in muscle fibres. Levels of respiratory-chain enzyme show a significant decrease of cytochrome-c oxidase, succinic dehydrogenase, and citrate synthase activity [52]. Reduced mitochondrial enzyme activity could provide the pathogenetic basis of the multisystemic clinical manifestations of MSL. Cultured MSL adipocytes synthesise UCP-1, the selective marker of brown adipocyte, but unlike in normally functioning brown fat cells, UCP-1 gene expression was not significantly induced by noradrenaline. Thus, MSL may be the consequence of a defective noradrenergic modulation of proliferation and differentiation of brown fat cells [53].

other wine components in revealing a genetic defect. MSL was considered slowly progressive and benign, but a recent longitudinal study demonstrated a significant disease-specific mortality [48]. The main complications include mediastinal occupation by lipomatous tissue, with compression and infiltration of the muscles of the neck and mediastinal structures, and a somatic and autonomic neuropathy. Symptoms of sensory and autonomic neuropathies are frequently associated with the disease [49]. In a 15-year follow-up of 70 patients, sudden death, in the absence of coronary heart disease, was recorded in three out of 11 patients, related to severe autonomic neuropathy [48]. A further clinical sign of MSL is the

## Therapeutic Approaches to Lipodystrophies

No specific treatment is currently available for LD. In some patients, therapy has to be addressed to coexisting comorbidities or to correcting cosmetic appearance.

Hyperglycaemia is treated with conventional medication. Insulin is used for overt diabetes. High doses of regular or long-acting insulin may be required when a pronounced resistance is present. Metformin has been suggested to improve insulin sensitivity and the control of hyperphagia. Liver steatosis and polycystic ovary syndrome may be additional indications for metformin treatment.

Dyslipidaemia requires close adherence to a low-fat diet (no more than 15% of calories). Adequate control of diabetes will improve or even normalise plasma lipid levels. Hypertriglyceridaemia occurs in the majority of congenital LD patients. Fibrates and high doses of ω-3 polyunsaturated fatty acids are mandatory to minimise the risk of vascular disease and liver steatosis. Alcoholic beverages should be avoided. Cosmetic appearance can only be improved in localised LD, as in Barraquer-Simons syndrome and HFLD. Cosmetic surgery including silicon or collagen implants or isolated fat-cell transplantation from the gluteal region can be used to correct sunken cheeks and asymmetry.

## References

1. Lawrence RD (1946) Lipodystrophy and hepatomegaly with diabetes, lipemia and other metabolic disturbances. Lancet 1:724–731
2. Misra A, Garg A (2003) Clinical features and metabolic derangements in acquired generalized lipodistrophy: case reports and review of the literature. Medicine 82:129–146
3. Garg A (2000) Lipodistrophies. Am J Med 108:143–152
4. Huemer C, Kitson H, Realleson PN et al (2001) Lipodystrophy in patients with juvenile dermatomyositis. Evaluation of clinical and metabolic abnormalities. J Rheumatol 28:610–615
5. Billings JK, Milgraum SS, Gupta AK et al (1987) Lipoatrophic panniculitis: a possible autoimmune inflammatory disease of fat: report of three cases. Arch Dermatol 123:1662–1666
6. Hacque WA, Shimomura I, Matsuzawa Y, Garg A (2002) Serum adiponectin and leptin levels in patients with lipodystrophies. J Clin Endocrinol Metab 87:2395–8
7. Mitchell SW (1885) Singular case of absence of adipose matter in the upper half of the body. Am J Med Sci 90:105–106
8. Barraquer L (1907) Histoire clinique d'un cas d'atrophie du tissue celluloadipeux. Neurolog Centralblatt 26:1072
9. Simons A (1911) Eine seltnen throphoneurose ('Lipodystrophia progressiva'). Z Gesamte Neurol Psychiatr 5:29–38
10. Eisinger AJ, Shortland JR, Moorhead PJ (1972) Renal disease in partial lipodostrophy. QJ Med 41:343–354
11. Peters DK, Charlesworth JA, Sissons JG et al (1973) Mesangiocapillary nephritis, partial lipodystrophy and hypocomplementaemia. Lancet 2:538–539
12. Williams DG, Bartlett A, Duffus P (1978) Identification of nephritic factor as an immunoglobulin. Clin Exp Immunol 33:425–429
13. Wrst CD, McAdams AJ (1999) The alternative pathway C3 convertase and glomerular deposits. Pediatr Nephrol 13:448–453
14. Mathieson PW, Wurzner R, Oliveria DB et al (1993) Complement-mediated adipocyte lysis by nephritic factor sera. J Exp Med 177:1827–1831
15. Walport MJ, Davies KA, Botto M et al (1994) C3 nephritic factor, and SLE: report of four cases and review of the literature. QJ Med 87:609–615
16. Font J, Herrero C, Bosch X et al (1990) Systematic lupus erythematosus in a patient with partial lipodystrophy. J Am Acad Dermatol 22:337–340
17. Cronin CC, Higgins T, Mollory M (1995) Lupus, C3 nephritic factor and partial lipodystrophy. QJ Med 88:298–299
18. Torrelo A, Espana A, Boixeda P, Ledo A (1991) Partial lipodistrophy and dermatomyositis. Arch Dermatol 127:1846–47
19. Atlan Gepner C, Bongrand P, Fornasier C et al (1996) Insulin induced lipoatrophy in type I diabetes. A possible tumor necrosis factor alpha-mediated differentiation of adipocytes. Diabetes Care 19:1283–1285
20. Imamura S, Yamada M, Yamamoto K (1984) Lipodystrophya centrifugalis abdominalis infantilis. A follow-up study. J Am Acad Dermatol 11:203–209
21. Berardinelli W (1954) An undiagnosed endocrino-metabolic syndrome report of 2 cases. J Clin Endocrinol Metab 14:193–204
22. Seip M (1959) Lipodystrophy and gigantism with associated endocrine manifestation: a new diencephalic syndrome? Acta Paediatr 48:555–574
23. Seip M, Trygstad O (1996) Generalized lipodystrophy, congenital and acquired (lipoatrophy). Acta Paediatr 413:2–28
24. Garg A, Flecknstein JL, Peshork RM, Grundy SM (1992) Peculiar distribution of adipose tissue in patients with congenital generalized lipodystrophy. J Clin Endocrinol Metab 75:358–361
25. Enzi G, Cominacini L, Dodi G et al (1988) Lipid metabolism in lipoatrophic diabetes. Horm Metab Res 20:587–591
26. Agarwal AK, Arioglu A, de Almeida S et al (2002) AGPA2 is mutated in congenital generalized lipodystrophy linked to chromosome 9q34. Nat Genet 31:21–23
27. Agarwal AK, Simha V, Oral EA et al (2003) Phenotypic and genetic heterogeneity in congenital generalized lipodystrophy. J Clin Endocrinol Metab 88:4840–4847
28. Simha V, Garg A (2003) Phenotypic heterogeneity in body fat distribution in patient with congenital generalized lipodystrophy caused by mutation in the AGPAT2 or Seipin genes. J Clin Endocrinol Metab 88:5433–5437

29. Van Maldergem L, Magre J, Khallonf E et al (2003) Genotype-phenotype relationships in Berardinelli-Seip congenital lipodystrophy. J Med Genet 40:150

30. Magre J, Delpine M, Khallonf E et al (2001) Identification of the gene altered in Berardinelli-Seip congenital lipodystrophy on chromosome 11q13. Nat Genet 28:365–370

31. Garg A, Wilson R, Barnes R et al (1994) A gene for congenital generalized lipodystrophy maps to human chromosome 9q34. J Clin Endocrinol Metab 84:3390–3394

32. Dunningam MG, Cochrane MA, Kelly A, Scott JW (1974) Familial lipoatrophic diabetes with dominant transmission: a new syndrome. QJ Med 49:33–48

33. Peters JM, Bannes R, Bennet L et al (1998) Localization of the gene for familial partial lipodystrophy (Dunningan variety) to chromosome 1q21–22. Nature Genet 18:292–295

34. Kobberling J, Willms B, Katterman R, Creutzfeld W (1975) Lipodystrophy of the extremities. A dominant inherited syndrome associated with lipoatrophyc diabetes. Humangenetik 29:111–120

35. Agarwal AK, Garg A (2002) A novel heterozygous mutation in perixosome proliferators activated receptor-gamma gene in a patient with familial partial lipodystrophy. J Clin Endocrinol Metab 87:418–411

36. Barroso I, Gurnell M, Crowley VE et al (1999) Dominant negative mutation in human PPAR-gamma associated with severe insulin resistance, diabetes mellitus and hypertension. Nature 402:880–883

37. Garg A, Vinaitherthan M, Weatherale PT, Boncork AM (2001) Phenotypic heterogeneity in patients with familial partial lipodystrophy (Dunningan variety) related to the site of missense mutation in lamin A/C gene. J Clin Endocrinol Metab 86:59–65

38. Young LW, Radebaugh JF, Rubin P et al (1971) New syndrome manifested by mandibular hypoplasia, acroosteolysis, still joints and cutaneous atrophy (mandibuloacral dysplasia) in two unrelated boys. Birth defects 7:291–297

39. Simba V, Garg A (2002) Bodyfat distribution and metabolic derangements in patients with familial partial lipodystrophy associated with mandibuloacral dysplasia. J Clin Endocrinol Metab 87:776–785

40. Novelli G, Munchir A, Sangiuolo F et al (2002) Mandibuloacral dysplasia is caused by a mutation in LMNA-encoding lamin A/C. Am J Hum Genet 71:426–431

41. Agarwal AK, Fryns JP, Auchus RJ, Garg A (2003) Zinc metalloproteinase ZMPSTE 24 is mutated in mandibuloacral dysplasia. Hum Mol Genet 12:1995–2001

42. Sensenbrenner JA, Hussels IE, Levin LS (1975) A low birth weight syndrome, Riegen syndrome? Birth Defects Orig Artic Ser 11:423–426

43. Pivnick EK, Angle B, Kaufman RA et al (2000) Neonatal progeroid (Wiedemann-Rautenstrauch) syndrome: report of five new cases and review. Am J Med Genet 90:131–140

44. Caux F, Dubosclard E, Lascols O et al (2003) A new clinical condition linked to a novel mutation in lamin A and C with generalized lipodystrophy, insulin resistant diabetes, disseminated leukomelanodermic papules, liver steatosis and cardiomyopathy. J Clin Endocrinol Metab 88:1006–1013

45. Busetto L, Sträter D, Enzi G et al (2003) Differential clinical expression of multiple symmetric lipomatosis in men and women. Int J Obesity 27:1419–1422

46. Zancanaro C, Sbarbati A, Morrini M et al (1990) Multiple symmetric lipomatosis. Ultrastructural investigation of the tissue and preadipocytes in primary culture. Lab Invest 63:253–258

47. Cinti S, Enzi G, Cigolini M, Bosello O (1983) Ultrastructural features of cultured mature adipocyte precursors from adipose tissue in multiple symmetric lipomatosis. Ultrastruct Pathol 5:145–152

48. Enzi G, Busetto L, Ceschin E et al (2002) Multiple symmetric lipomatosis: clinical aspects and outcome in a long-term longitudinal study. Int J Obesity 26:253–261

49. Enzi G, Angelini C, Negrin P et al (1986) Sensory, motor and autonomic neuropathy in patients with multiple symmetric lipomatosis. Medicine 64:388–393

50. Enzi G, Dorigo P, Prosdocimi M et al (1977) Multiple symmetric lipomatosis: a defect in adrenergic stimulated lipolysis. J Clin Invest 60:1221–1229

51. Enzi G, Martini S, Baggio G et al (1985) Lipoprotein metabolism in patients with elevated lipoprotein-lipase activity in adipose tissue. Int J Obesity 9:173–176

52. Coin A, Enzi G, Bussolotto M et al (2000) Multiple symmetric lipomatosis: evidence for mitochondrial dysfunction. J Clin Neuromusc Dis 1:124–130

53. Nisoli E, Regianini L, Briscini L et al (2002) Multiple symmetric lipomatosis may be the consequence of detective noradrenergic modulation of proliferation of brown fat cells. J Pathol 198:378–387

# SECTION 5
# PATHOPHYSIOLOGY OF WASTING/CACHEXIA

# Body Composition: Physiology, Pathophysiology and Methods of Evaluation

Giuseppe Sergi, Pietro Bonometto, Alessandra Coin, Giuliano Enzi

## Introduction

Estimating body compartments is fundamental in performing nutritional assessments. In recent years, highly reliable and minimally invasive methods have become available for quantifying body fluids, fat-free mass and fat mass. These measurements integrate the clinical evaluation, overcoming the drawbacks of anthropometric measurements used as indirect parameters of nutritional status and body composition.

Fat-free mass (FFM) is composed of all non-fat tissues. It represents the main active component, from a metabolic point of view, and it is responsible for the majority of resting energy expenditure [1]. The main function of fat mass is as an energy reserve, because it is composed of triglycerides, which have a high caloric power.

A correct nutritional balance maintains an adequate FFM in relation to the subject's height and a good ratio of fat to fat-free mass. This proportion varies according to gender, age and genetics. In a normal adult, fat-free soft mass, fat mass and bone minerals represent 75, 18 and 7% of the body weight, respectively. Muscle mass and non-muscle lean tissue represent 25 and 14% of the fat-free soft tissue, respectively [2].

Evaluating body fluids is very important in clinical practice because many nutritional and pathological conditions are associated with water disorders. Nowadays, total body water (TBW) and extracellular water (ECW) can be determined by non-invasive methods such as bioelectrical impedance analysis (BIA). This enables the monitoring of several clinical conditions characterised by an altered water homeostasis, e.g. dehydration or water retention states.

In an adult subject with a normal nutritional status, TBW accounts for up to 60% of the total body weight, while ECW is around 25% [3].

## Body Composition and Cachexia

In a condition of negative energy balance, i.e. when the nutrient intake does not match the energy expenditure, the body primarily uses fat mass as an energy source. If the caloric deficit persists, fat-free tissues are also used, with a consequent further weight loss. While a loss of fat mass has no negative consequences because it only cuts into the energy reserves, the loss of fat-free mass has a negative prognostic value.

The loss of body mass may follow three basic models depending on the body compartment most affected: starvation, cachexia and sarcopenia.

Starvation is caused by a reduction in calorie intake. The body goes through a metabolic adaptation in order to preserve FFM and increase lipid metabolism, with secondary fat loss. Fat reserves are preferentially used and the brain adapts to using ketones instead of glucose from gluconeogenesis. These changes are reversible with an appropriate refeeding programme.

Cachexia is associated with inflammatory and neoplastic conditions, which induce an acute-phase response. It is caused by chronic or terminal diseases, such as infections, neoplasms, heart failure, chronic inflammatory diseases and chronic obstructive pulmonary disease. In the elderly it can also develop in the absence of any overt disease. The changes in body composition, characterised by a reduction in both fat mass and fat-free mass, are not reversible with refeeding.

Sarcopenia is characterised by a reduction in skeletal muscle mass. Apart from body composition changes in the elderly, this term is also used in the case of weight loss from repeated dieting, in patients with growth hormone deficiencies, and in subjects with a severe motility impairment.

Cachexia is a model of body composition changes because it enables a better basic characterisation of both tissue and biomolecular processes.

Cachectic patients equally lose fat and fat-free mass. The loss of fat-free mass mainly involves the skeletal muscle and it reflects a decrease in body cell mass and intracellular potassium, thus indicating a bioenergetic defect. These evidences are confirmed in pathological conditions such as neoplasms [4], chronic heart failure [5], terminal renal failure [6] and rheumatoid arthritis [7]. Cachexia is a pathophysiological condition that produces a so-called 'acute-phase response', usually based on a process of tissue damage. This process is self-maintaining with a positive feedback and includes a marked protein synthesis by the liver. The proteins secreted are mainly opsonines, protease inhibitors, complement factors, apoproteins, fibrinogen and others. The acute-phase response demands a great deal of energy and essential amino acids, obtained directly from skeletal muscle.

At muscle level, white fibres are less involved than red fibres, and myofibrillar proteins are mainly affected [8]. In cachexia, however, unlike the situation in starvation, there is an increase in liver mass and the synthesis of visceral proteins [9]. A 15% reduction in FFM interferes with organic and physiological functions, while a decrease beyond 30% is usually fatal.

The loss of fat mass is due more to an increased lipolysis than to a decreased lipogenesis [10]. For example, in neoplastic cachexia there is a remarkable mobilisation of the fatty acids even before weight loss becomes established [11]. These effects can partly be explained by an increased beta-adrenergic activity, which has been demonstrated experimentally [12]. From a finalistic point of view, the aim is to convert the organic priorities from offensive to defensive, using the most extensive protein reserve. But this adaptive effect, effective over the short term, becomes damaging in the long term, because a depletion in muscle mass contributes increasingly to morbidity and mortality.

## Body Composition: Measurement Methods

The whole body can be distinguished into separate homogeneous fractions based on different chemical and physical characteristics, depending on the method used for body composition study. The whole body can be considered on four different levels, i.e. the atomic, the molecular, the cellular and the tissue-system (Fig. 1).

Most methods for measurement of body composition are based on a bicompartmental model, according to which the body is divided into two distinct chemical compartments, fat mass and fat-free mass. Fat mass is composed entirely of lipids and fat-free mass is composed of water, proteins, minerals and glycogen. Having measured one compartment, the other is usually taken to be the difference [13, 14]. The bicompartmental model is defined by the following relationship:

Body mass = fat mass + fat-free mass (alipidic mass)

Fat-free mass or alipidic mass has a density of 1.1 g/cm$^3$, a water content of 73.2%, and a potassium content of 60–70 mmol/kg in the male and 50–60 mmol/kg in the female. It is composed of skeletal and extraskeletal muscles, other lean tissues and the skeleton [15]. Fat mass has a density of 0.9 g/cm$^3$ and, in normal subjects, it represents around 15–18% and 25–28% of the male and female body weight, respectively. It is water- and potassium-free.

The ideal method for estimating the body compartments should offer maximal accuracy together with minimal invasiveness. Some methods are precise, but they are invasive and they are only used to validate easier methods. Only a few methods offer an acceptable compromise between accuracy and invasiveness, making them suitable for use in epidemiological studies and clinical practice.

Some methods, e.g. the dilution method and BIA, are used to measure body fluids. Other methods evaluate fat-free mass, bone mass and fat mass. Among the latter, dual-energy X-ray absorptiometry (DEXA) enables the body composition

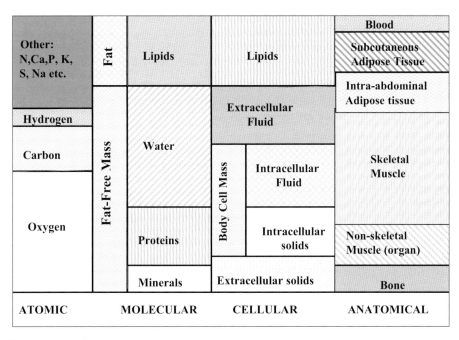

**Fig. 1.** Model of body composition

## Body Fluids

### Isotope Dilution Methods

All classic methods for measuring TBW and ECW are based on the dilution principle, which demands a tracer that is not noxious, that becomes uniformly distributed throughout the unknown compartment and that does not interfere with the distribution of water or other substances. The volume of each compartment is calculated from the ratio between the quantity of the tracer administered and its concentration in the distribution volume at the equilibrium time.

To measure TBW, deuterium is used as a tracer because it is a stable isotope of hydrogen and can be given to children and women in pregnancy. The subject receives a known oral dose of deuterium oxide ($D_2O$, approx. 50 g of a 20% solution)

and venous blood samples are drawn 3 hours later (equilibrium time) [16].

The TBW is obtained in litres by the following formula:

$$TBW = A/B \times 0.928$$

where A is the quantity of $D_2O$ administered in milligrams, B is the plasma $D_2O$ concentration in ppm at the equilibrium time; 0.928 is the correction factor for non-aqueous exchangeable hydrogen in the body [17].

Fat-free mass can be determined from TBW by the following formula, assuming it contains a constant fraction (73.2%) of TBW [18]:

$$FFM\ (kg) = TBW/0.732$$

Fat mass is calculated from the difference between body weight and FFM.

The value of 73.2% assumed for FFM hydration derives from chemical analyses on a few cadavers [19] and it represents the mean of values ranging from 69 to 82%. Later in vivo studies confirmed a wide individual variability in FFM hydration in healthy subjects that increases with age [20] and in fluid imbalance conditions [21].

To estimate extracellular water, the subject is given about 35 mg/kg body weight of sodium bromide. The bromide concentration in the blood reaches an equilibrium about 3 hours after its administration [22]. ECW can be estimated as the corrected bromide space (CBS), which is calculated according to the following formula [3]:

CBS = Br dose (mmol)/Br in plasma (mmol/l) × 0.90 × 0.95 × 0.94

where 0.90 is the correction factor for the bromide distribution in the non-extracellular sites (mainly red blood cells); 0.95 is the correction factor for the Donnan equilibrium; 0.94 is the correction factor for the concentration of water in the plasma, which is about 94%.

## Bioelectrical Impedance Analysis

Bioelectrical impedance analysis is a simple, non-invasive and portable method for estimating fluid compartments and fat-free mass. This method is based on the bioelectrical principle that lean tissues containing the majority of the body's water and electrolytes are good electrical conductors, whereas fat mass (which is almost dry) acts as an insulator and is a poor electrical conductor (Fig. 2).

The human body is considered as a conductor, which opposes an obstruction of defined impedance (Z) to an alternating current. Impedance is the vectorial sum of the resistance (R) and reactance (Xc). Resistance is defined as the pure opposition of the body to the alternating current and reactance (Xc) is the resistive effect related to capacities produced by tissue interfaces and cell membranes [23].

The volume (V) of a cylindrical conductor through which an electric current flows can be calculated according to Ohm's second law as a function of the length of the conductor (L), the bioelectrical resistance (R), and the specific resistivity ($\rho$, i.e. indicating the tissue intrinsic property to behave as resistors) of the lean mass:

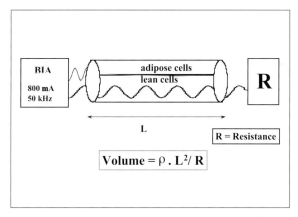

**Fig. 2.** Bioelectrical impedance analysis: theoretical bases

$V = \rho \times L^2/R$

Applying this model to the human body, a strong correlation was found between bioelectrical volume (height²/resistance) and the fluid compartments determined by dilution methods.

Intracellular and extracellular fluids are electrical conductors, while cell membranes act as capacitors [24]. At low frequencies (5 kHz) the current flows almost exclusively through the extracellular compartments. At higher frequencies ($\geq$ 50 kHz) it exceeds the cell membranes and flows through both the extracellular and the intracellular fluids. On the basis of this principle, low and high frequencies are applied respectively to estimate ECW and TBW.

Instruments for BIA generally use a single frequency (50 kHz, 800 mA) with a tetrapolar placement of electrodes on the dorsal surface of the right hand (two electrodes) and foot (two electrodes) [25].

The strong correlation between bioelectrical parameters and water volumes has enabled the development of reliable BIA equations for predicting TBW. Moreover, multiple regression equations for estimating fat-free mass from resistance, weight, height, gender and age have been developed by comparison with a reference method such as DEXA, hydrodensitometry, etc. Table 1 shows some common BIA formulae used for estimating TBW and FFM [25–32].

The main limits of the BIA method have to do

**Table 1.** Bioelectrical impedance analysis formulae used for the estimation of total body water (*TBW*) and fat-free mass (*FFM*)

| Author | Formulae for TBW |
|---|---|
| Kushner [25] | M: $0.396 \times$ (stature$^2$/resistance) $+ 0.143 \times$ weight $+ 8.399$ |
| | F: $0.382 \times$ (stature$^2$/resistance) $+ 0.105 \times$ weight $+ 8.315$ |
| Kushner [26] | $0.593 \times$ (stature$^2$/resistance) $+ 0.065 \times$ weight $+ 0.04$ |
| Visser [27] | M: $8.3 + 0.323 \times$ (stature$^2$/resistance) $+ 0.165 \times$ weight |
| | F: $11.9 + 0.272 \times$ (stature$^2$/resistance) $+ 0.109 \times$ weight |
| Sun [28] | M: $1.20 + 0.45$ stature$^2$/resistance $+ 0.18$ weight |
| | F: $3.75 + 0.45$ stature2/resistance $+ 0.11$ weight |
| | **Formulae for FFM** |
| Segal [29] | M: $0.0006636 \times$ stature$^2$ $- 0.2117 \times$ resistance $+ 0.62854 \times$ weight $- 0.1238 \times$ age $+ 9.33285$ |
| | F: $0.00064602 \times$ stature$^2$ $- 0.01397 \times$ resistance $+ 0.42087 \times$ weight $+ 10.43485$ |
| Rising [30] | $13.74 + 0.34 \times$ (stature$^2$/resistance) $+ 0.33 \times$ weight $- 0.14 \times$ age $+ 6.18$ if M |
| Roubenoff [31] | M: $9.15 + 0.43 \times$ (stature$^2$/resistance) $+ 0.2 \times$ weight $+ 0.07 \times$ reactance |
| | F: $7.74 + 0.45 \times$ (stature$^2$/resistance) $+ 0.12 \times$ weight $+ 0.05 \times$ reactance |
| Kyle [32] | $-4.104 + 0.518 \times$ (stature$^2$/resistance) $+ 0.231 \times$ weight $+ 0.130 \times$ reactance $+ 4.229$ if M |
| Sun [28] | M: $-10.68 + 0.65 \times$ (stature$^2$/resistance) $+ 0.26$ weight $+ 0.02$ resistance |
| | F: $-9.53 + 0.69 \times$ (stature$^2$/resistance) $+ 0.17$ weight $+ 0.02$ resistance |

*M*, males; *F*, females; stature in m, weight in kg

with the influence of hydration status on its reliability in estimating fat-free mass. FFM hydration is already highly variable in healthy subjects, becoming more so with age [26]. When water imbalance occurs, BIA can underestimate and overestimate the FFM in dehydration and fluid retention states, respectively.

A recent study of ours demonstrated that BIA is reliable in evaluating body composition in underweight elderly men, but it seems to have intrinsic weaknesses in assessing underweight women [33].

A further application of BIA is to evaluate ECW and the distribution of intracellular and extracellular fluids, using low-frequency analysers (< 5 kHz) [34] or multifrequency systems [35].

## Fat-Free Mass and Fat Mass

### Total Body Potassium

Quantifying total body potassium (TBK) enables an indirect estimate of fat-free mass because potassium is an intracellular cation (99%) that is not present in stored triglycerides.

The method used most often for measuring TBK is whole-body $^{40}K$ determination. $^{40}K$ exists in the body in a known concentration (0.012%), it emits a characteristic gamma-ray at 1.46 MeV and it can be measured in vivo by external whole-body counters, consisting in a large, shielded room containing a gamma-ray detection system.

The error in TBK estimation using the $^{40}K$ method ranges from 3 to 5% [36]. FFM is calculated from TBK, assuming that the potassium content per kilogram of FFM is 2.66 g for men and 2.50 g for women [37].

This method cannot be used routinely, however, because of the high cost of the instrumentation and technical support required.

## Dual-Energy X-ray Absorptiometry

Dual-energy X-ray absorptiometry (DEXA) is a method originally used to determine bone mineral density. For a few years now, it has also been used to study body composition, and to quantify fat and fat-free mass in particular.

DEXA explores the body regions of interest by X-ray emissions at two different energy levels [38]. The different photon attenuation at the two levels depends on the different tissue composition, enabling the bone mineral content and soft tissues to be extrapolated. The different relationship between low- and high-energy photon attenuation enables fat and fat-free mass in the soft tissues to be distinguished.

DEXA yields a high resolution and accuracy with a short acquisition time and consequently with minimal exposure (1.5 mR). The method had a good reproducibility (coefficient of variation) for total body fat mass (2–3%), total body fat-free mass, total body lean soft tissue (1–2%), arm lean soft tissue (3–4%), and leg lean soft tissue (1–2%) [39–41]. Moreover, it is sensitive in assessing minimal changes in body composition [42]. The method has been validated against multislice computed tomography scans, magnetic resonance imaging and a four-compartment model in young and older people [40, 43, 44].

Measurement of body compartments using DEXA is theoretically independent of FFM hydration status, but variations in the relationship between TBW and FFM may interfere with the accuracy of the method. Recent studies have reported, however, on the validity of DEXA in detecting variations in FFM due to hydration disorders.

The method requires little effort on the part of the subject, thus allowing for frail subjects to be also evaluated.

Unlike many other body composition methods, moreover, DEXA has the potential for assessing the composition of the whole body as well as body regions [45]. At the present time, for example, appendicular skeletal muscle mass (ASMM) evaluation, measured as the sum of the fat-free soft tissue masses of arms and legs, as detected by DEXA, is considered the gold standard for the diagnosis of sarcopenia [46, 47]. Subjects are considered sarcopenic when they have ASMMI (ASMM divided by height squared) values 2 standard deviations below the mean ASMMI values (7.26 for males and 5.45 for females) for a young adult referral population from the Rosetta study [47].

## Neutron Activation Analysis

Neutron activation analysis (NAA) measures the multi-elemental composition of the human body in vivo. It can determine the content of certain chemical elements, e.g. calcium, sodium, chlorine, phosphorus and nitrogen.

In the NAA techniques used for body composition studies, a beam of fast neutrons is passed through the human body and the capture of these neutrons by atoms of the target elements creates unstable isotopes, such as $^{49}Ca$, $^{15}Na$, etc. The isotopes revert to a stable condition by emitting gamma rays with an energy characteristic to each element and the radio spectrum of this emission is recorded. The energy levels identify the elements and the levels of activity enable their quantification [48].

The importance of this method lies in its ability to determine total body nitrogen (TBN) in vivo. TBN can be used to derive the body protein mass, assuming it contains 16% of nitrogen. The accuracy of nitrogen determination in phantoms and the precision of repeated measures in humans is about 3% [49].

Some authors have suggested associating TBN determined by NAA and TBK derived from measuring $^{40}K$ to estimate muscle and non-muscle components of lean mass [50]. However, given its high cost, methodological complexity and use of ionising radiations, NAA cannot be used routinely for nutritional assessment or in clinical practice.

## Computerised Axial Tomography

Computerised axial tomography (CAT) is an imaging method enabling a regional analysis of body composition. This technique relies on the relationship between small differences in X-ray attenuation and differences in the physical density of tissues. A two-dimensional image is created of the anatomical structures in the area being scanned. CAT can be applied mainly to evaluating fat distribution in the subcutaneous and visceral tissues [51, 52].

An evolution of this technique, called peripheral quantitative computerised tomography (pQCT), enables the single site density and bone strength to be analysed [53]. pQCT can also be used to assess body composition of the limbs, particularly the volume and morphology of skeletal muscle mass, and subcutaneous and intermuscular adipose tissue [54]. pQCT is fast and reproducible, and the radiating dose per limb is extremely low, so it is an important technique for studying sarcopenia and cachexia in both the adult and the elderly.

## Magnetic Nuclear Resonance

Magnetic nuclear resonance (MNR) is a non-invasive method that can offer an important contribution to district body composition studies. It is non-invasive, so it can be used instead of CAT, which exposes the subjects to ionising radiations. It is already used to investigate the quantity and distribution of adipose tissue. Total adipose tissue can be estimated within a 5–7% error using multiple-body scans at chest and abdomen levels [55].

MNR has also been proposed as a method for quantifying muscle mass [56], but it is too expensive and time-consuming (about an hour for a whole body scan) for routine use [57]. In addition, its accuracy in estimating body composition is still debatable in malnourished and cachectic subjects.

# References

1.  Nelson KM, Weinsier RL, Long CL, Schutz Y (1992) Prediction of resting energy expenditure from fat-free mass and fat mass. Am J Clin Nutr 56:848–856
2.  Ellis KJ, Jasumura S, Morgan WD (eds) (1987) In vivo body composition studies. Institute of Physical Science in Medicine, London
3.  Vaisman N, Pencharz PB, Koren G, Johnson JK (1987) Comparison of oral and intravenous Heitmann administration of sodium bromide for extracellular water measurements. Am J Clin Nutr 46:1–4
4.  Shike M, Russel DM, Detsky AS et al (1984) Changes in body composition in patients with small-cell cancer. The effect of total parenteral nutrition as an adjunct to chemotherapy. Ann Intern Med 101:303–309
5.  Toth MJ, Gottlieb SS, Goran MI et al (1997) Daily energy expenditure in free-living heart failure patients. Am J Physiol 272:E469–E475
6.  Mitch WE (1998) Mechanisms causing loss of lean body mass in kidney disease. Robert H Herman Memorial Award in Clinical Nutrition Lecture 1997. Am J Clin Nutr 67:359–366
7.  Roubenoff R, Roubenoff RA, Cannon JG et al (1994) Rheumatoid cachexia: cytokine-driven hypermetabolism accompanying reduced body cell mass in chronic inflammation. J Clin Invest 93:2379–2386
8.  Mitch WE, Goldberg AL (1996) Mechanisms of muscle wasting. The role of the ubiquitin-proteasome pathway. NEJM 335:1897–1905
9.  Fong Y, Moldawer LL, Marano M et al (1989) Cachectin/TNF or IL-1 alpha induces cachexia with redistribution of body proteins. Am J Physiol 256:R659–R665
10. Tisdale MJ (2002) Cachexia in cancer patients. Nat Rev Cancer 2:862–871
11. Kaibara A, Moshyedi A, Auffenberg T et al (1998) Leptin produces anorexia and weight loss without inducing an acute phase response or protein wasting. Am J Physiol 274:R1518–R1525
12. Hyltander A, Daneryd P, Sandstrom R et al (2000) Beta-adrenoceptor activity and resting energy metabolism in weight losing cancer patients. Eur J Cancer 36:330–334
13. Keys A, Brozek J (1953) Body fat in adult men. Physiol Rev 33:245–325
14. Brozek J, Grande F, Anderson JT, Keys A (1963) Densitometric analysis of body composition: revision of some quantitative assumptions. Ann NY Acad Sci 110:113–140
15. Burkinshaw L, Cotes JE (1973) Body potassium and fat-free mass. Clin Sci 44:621–625
16. Sergi G, Bertani R, Calliari I et al (2003) Total body water and extracellular water measurements through in vivo dilution of D2O and bromide as tracers. Spectroscopy 17:603–611
17. Bartoli WP, Davis JM, Pate RR et al (1993) Weekly variability in total body water using 2H2O dilution in college-age males. Med Sci Sports Exerc 25:1422–1428
18. Pace N, Rathburn EN (1945) Studies on body composition. III The body water and chemically combined nitrogen content in relation to fat content. J Biol Chem 158:685–691

19. Sheng HP, Huggins RA (1979) A review of body composition studies with emphasis on total body water and fat. Am J Clin Nutr 32:630–647

20. Sergi G, Perini P, Bussolotto M et al (1993) Body composition study in the elderly: comparison between tritium dilution method and dual photon absorptiometry. J Gerontol 48:M244–M248

21. Sergi G, Lupoli L, Volpato S et al (2004) Body fluid distribution in elderly subjects affected with congestive heart failure. Ann Clin Lab Sci 34:416–422

22. Shao HR, Liu QX, Enzi G et al (1990) Evaluation of the extracellular water in human body by determination of Br concentration in blood plasma. Nucl Instrum Meth Phys Res B49:238–240

23. Heitmann BL (1994) Impedance: a valid method in assessment of body composition? Eur J Clin Nutr 48:228–240

24. Thomasset A (1963) Bio-electric properties of tissues. Estimation by measurement of impedance of extracellular ionic strength and intracellular ionic strength in the clinic. Lyon Med 209:1325–1350

25. Kushner RF, Schoeller MD (1986) Estimation of total body water by bioelectrical impedance analysis. Am J Clin Nutr 44:417–424

26. Kushner RF, Schoeller DA, Fjeld CR, Danford L (1992) Is the impedance index (Ht/R) significant in predicting total body water? Am J Clin Nutr 56:835–839

27. Visser M, Deurenberg P, van Staveren WA (1995) Multi-frequency bioelectrical impedance for assessing total body water and extracellular water in elderly subjects. Eur J Clin Nutr 49:256–266

28. Sun SS, Chumlea WC, Heymsfield SB et al (2003) Development of bioelectrical impedance analysis prediction equations for body composition with the use of a multicomponent model for use in epidemiologic surveys. Am J Clin Nutr 77:331–340

29. Segal KR, van Loan M, Fitzgerald PI et al (1988) Lean body mass estimation by bioelectrical impedance analysis: a four-site cross-validation study. Am J Clin Nutr 47:7–14

30. Rising R, Swinburn B, Larson K, Ravussin E (1991) Body composition in Pima Indians: validation of bioelectrical resistance. Am J Clin Nutr 53:594–598

31. Roubenoff R, Baumgartner RN, Harris TB et al (1997) Application of bioelectrical impedance analysis to elderly populations. J Gerontol A Biol Sci Med Sci 52:M129–M136

32. Kyle UG, Genton L, Karsegard L et al (2001) Single prediction equation for bioelectrical impedance analysis in adults 20–94 years. Nutrition 17:248–253

33. Lupoli L, Sergi G, Coin A et al (2004) Body composition in underweight elderly subjects: reliability of bioelectrical impedance analysis. Clin Nutr 23:1371–1380

34. Sergi G, Bussolotto M, Perini P et al (1994) Accuracy of bioelectrical impedance analysis in estimation of extracellular space in healthy subjects and in fluid retention states. Ann Nutr Metab 38:158–165

35. Gudivaka R, Schoeller DA, Kushner RF et al (1999) Single- and multifrequency models for bioelectrical impedance analysis of body water compartments. J Appl Physiol 87:1087–1096

36. Cohn SH, Palmer HE (1974) Recent advances in whole body counting: a review. J Nucl Biol Med 1:155–165

37. Forbes GB, Gallup J, Hursh JB (1961) Estimation of total body fat from potassium-40 content. Sciences 133:101–102

38. Van Loan MD, Mayclin PL (1992) Body composition assessment: dual energy X ray absorptiometry (DEXA) compared to reference methods. Eur J Clin Nutr 46:125–130

39. Economos CD, Nelson ME, Fiatarone MA et al (1997) A multi-center comparison of dual energy X-ray absorptiometers: in vivo and in vitro soft tissue measurement. Eur J Clin Nutr 51:312–317

40. Figueroa-Colon R, Mayo MS, Treuth MS et al (1998) Reproducibility of dual-energy X-ray absorptiometry measurements in prepubertal girls. Obes Res 6:262–267

41. Fuller NJ, Hardingham CR, Graves M et al (1999) Assessment of limb muscle and adipose tissue by dual-energy X-ray absorptiometry using magnetic resonance imaging for comparison. Int J Obes Relat Metab Disord 23:1295–1302

42. Houtkooper LB, Going SB, Sproul J et al (2000) Comparison of methods for assessing body-composition changes over 1 y in postmenopausal women. Am J Clin Nutr 72:401–406

43. Salamone LM, Fuerst T, Visser M et al (2000) Measurement of fat mass using DEXA: a validation study in elderly adults. J Appl Physiol 89:345–352

44. Visser M, Fuerst T, Lang T et al (1999) Validity of fan-beam dual-energy X-ray absorptiometry for measuring fat-free mass and leg muscle mass. J Appl Physiol 87:1513–1520

45. Visser M, Pahor M, Tylavsky F et al (2003) One- and two-year change in body composition as measured by DXA in a population-based cohort of older men and women. J Appl Physiol 94:2368–2374

46. Heymsfield SB, Smith R, Aulet M et al (1990) Appendicular skeletal muscle mass: measurement by dual-photon absorptiometry. Am J Clin Nutr 52:214–218

47. Baumgartner RN, Koehler KM, Gallagher D et al (1998) Epidemiology of sarcopenia among the elderly in New Mexico. Am J Epidemiol 147:755–763

48. Lukaski HC (1987) Methods for the assessment of human body composition: traditional and new. Am J Clin Nutr 46:537–556

49. Vartsky D, Ellis KJ, Vaswani AN et al (1984) An improved calibration for the in vivo determination of body nitrogen, hydrogen, and fat. Phys Med Biol 29:209–218

50. Cohn SH, Vartsky D, Yasumura S et al (1983) Indexes of body cell mass: nitrogen versus potassium. Am J Physiol 244:E305–E310

51. Borkan GA, Gerzof SG, Robbins AH et al (1982) Assessment of abdominal fat content by computed tomography. Am J Clin Nutr 36:172–177
52. Borkan GA, Hults DE, Gerzof SG, Robbins AH (1985) Comparison of body composition in middle-aged and elderly males using computed tomography. Am J Phys Anthropol 66:289–295
53. Ebbesen EN, Thomsen JS, Beck-Nielsen H et al (1999) Lumbar vertebral body compressive strength evaluated by dual-energy X-ray absorptiometry, quantitative computed tomography, and ashing. Bone 25:713–724
54. Penninx BW, Pahor M, Cesari M et al (2004) Anemia is associated with disability and decreased physical performance and muscle strength in the elderly. J Am Geriatr Soc 52:719–724
55. Fowler PA, Fuller MF, Glasbey CA et al (1991) Total and subcutaneous adipose tissue in women: the measurement of distribution and accurate prediction of quantity by using magnetic resonance imaging. Am J Clin Nutr 54:18–25
56. Murphy WA, Totty WG, Caroll JE (1986) MRI of normal and pathologic skeletal muscle. Am J Roentoenol 146:565–574
57. Ross R, Shaw KD, Martel Y et al (1993) Adipose tissue distribution measured by magnetic resonance imaging in obese women. Am J Med Nutr 57:470–475

# Protein Metabolism in Cachexia

Michael J. Tisdale

## Introduction

Cachexia is characterised by a specific loss of skeletal muscle, while the non-muscle protein compartment is relatively preserved [1]. This loss can be very large. Thus in lung cancer patients who had lost 30% of their pre-illness stable weight there was a 75% fall in skeletal muscle protein mass. This leads to a general muscle weakness (asthenia) and death from immobility and hypostatic pneumonia [1]. For a 70-kg adult, the lean body mass is about 5.8 kg, of which the majority (4.2 kg) is found in muscle and the remainder in cells of the splancnic organs and gut. During total starvation protein is initially broken down at a rate of about 75 g per day, falling to about 20 g per day after 5–6 weeks, which is related to a reduction in the requirement for glucose by the brain. During cachexia of cancer, injury or sepsis there is interference with the normal process of starvation adaption and the rate of protein degradation continues at the high rate. That loss of lean body mass in cachexia differs from that in starvation is reflected by the inability to reverse the process by simple nutritional supplementation. Thus when individuals with HIV were given parenteral nutrition, an increase in weight was observed, but this represented fat tissue rather than accrual of lean body mass [2]. A similar situation is seen in sepsis [3] and in cancer cachexia [4], and is also seen with appetite stimulants such as megestrol acetate [5]. This suggests that the normal metabolic controls operating to regulate skeletal muscle mass in starvation are by-passed during the process of cachexia.

## Regulation of Muscle Mass

Muscle mass is a balance between the rate of protein synthesis and the rate of protein degradation. In young mammals protein synthesis exceeds degradation and muscle mass increases, while in mature mammals protein synthesis and degradation are roughly equal so that muscle mass remains constant. In cancer cachexia there is both a reduction in protein synthesis [6] and an increase in protein degradation in skeletal muscle [7]. Although reduced protein synthesis and inhibited uptake of amino acids contribute to the atrophy, increased protein degradation and in particular breakdown of the myofibrillar proteins actin and myosin is probably the most important factor. A change in muscle myosin isoform expression has also been reported in cancer cachexia [8] with a decrease in type I and an increase in fast (type II) isoform expression.

There are three main pathways for protein degradation in skeletal muscle: lysosomal (cathepsins), calcium-activated proteases (calpains) and the ubiquitin-proteasome proteolytic pathway. A large number of studies have shown the ubiquitin-proteasome pathway to be of major importance in the development of cachexia in sepsis, metabolic acidosis, weightlessness, severe injury including burn injury, denervation atrophy, cancer [9] and diabetes [10]. Disuse atrophy as occurs in space travel also arises through activation of the ubiquitin-proteasome pathway [11]. The proteasome does not degrade intact myofibrils and the calcium-dependent enzyme calpain is responsible for breakdown of the Z-bands in muscle, with the subsequent loss of actin and myosin from the sarcomeres [12]. Thus muscle catabolism in septic rats is blocked by dantrolene, which inhibits the release of calcium from intracellular stores [13]. These results suggest that calcium-dependent proteolysis is the first step in breakdown of skeletal muscle, followed by degradation of actin and myosin to peptides by the proteasome. These peptides are further broken down into tripeptides by the giant protease tripeptidyl peptidase II, the activity of which has been reported to be elevated in muscle from septic rats [14]. Although this enzyme is not rate-limiting for overall proteolysis, it is important because the accumulation of abnormal peptides may be injurious to the muscle cell.

Although the expression of the ubiquitin-proteasome pathway is increased in a range of different cachexias, expression of the ATPase subunits of the 19S complex seems to vary according to the type of wasting condition. Thus MSS1 and P45 are ATPase subunits of the 19S complex thought to provide energy to inject the substrate into the proteolytic chamber of the 20S proteasome. In wasting muscle of rats bearing the Yoshida sarcoma, mRNA for MSS1, but not P45, was found to be increased, but both MSS1 and P45 increased in atrophying muscle from unweighted rats [15]. An increased expression of the non-ATPase subunit, P112-L, was only seen in unweighted rats, but not in cancer cachexia. These results suggest that expression of the various proteasome subunits is regulated independently. Proteasome catalytic activity rather than substrate ubiquitination has been suggested [16] to be the rate-limiting step in protein degradation by the ubiquitin-proteasome pathway. Nevertheless the ubiquitin protein ligases (E3) are very important in the recognition of specific cellular proteins and the targeting of these for degradation. Two E3s, Muscle Ring Finger 1 (MURF1) and Muscle Atrophy F box (MAFbx), are elevated in skeletal muscle under immobilisation, denervation and hindlimb suspension [17]. In addition muscle from MAFbx- and MURF1-deficient mice have a decreased loss of muscle mass after denervation, showing the importance of these E3 proteins in targeting actin and myosin for degradation within the proteasome. The factors responsible for the increased expression of the ubiquitin-proteasome pathway have recently been identified.

## Factors Regulating Proteasome Expression in Cachexia

A number of diverse factors appear to regulate proteasome expression.

### Oxidative Stress

Experiments on hindlimb unloading in rats indicate that disuse results in a disruption of antioxidant status, elevation of hydroperoxides and an increase in oxidative stress [18]. In mice transplanted with CHO cells transfected with cDNA for the cytokine tumour necrosis factor (TNF)-$\alpha$, muscle wasting was also associated with oxidative stress and increased nitric oxide synthase in skeletal muscle [19]. The decreased body weight, muscle wasting and skeletal muscle molecular abnormalities were prevented by treatment with antioxidants, or the nitric oxide synthase inhibitor nitro-L-arginine, suggesting that the oxidative stress was directly responsible for the increased muscle protein breakdown.

Induction of mild oxidative stress in skeletal muscle myotubes led to an increase in proteasome chymotrypsin-like enzyme activity, and increased expression of 20S proteasome $\alpha$ subunits, p42, an ATPase subunit of the 19S regulator and the ubiquitin-conjugating enzyme E2$_{14k}$ [20]. The mechanism by which mild oxidative stress induces expression of genes for the ubiquitin-proteasome proteolytic pathway is not known, but exogenous hydrogen peroxide has been shown to stimulate binding of the transcription factor nuclear factor-$\kappa$B (NF-$\kappa$B) to its targeted DNA sequence and to stimulate degradation of the inhibitor protein I-$\kappa$B$\alpha$ [21]. There is evidence to suggest that other factors inducing proteasome gene expression also activate NF-$\kappa$B.

### Cytokines

Certain cytokines such as TNF-$\alpha$, interleukins-1 and -6 (IL-1 and IL-6), interferon-$\gamma$ (IFN-$\gamma$) and leukaemia inhibitory factor (LIF) have been identified from experimental studies as possible cofactors in the onset of cachexia. Treatment of rats with TNF-$\alpha$ enhances protein degradation in skeletal muscle, associated with an increased proteasome gene expression and higher levels of free and conjugated ubiquitin [22]. Acute TNF-$\alpha$ treatment caused an enhanced proteolytic rate and decreased protein synthesis in red-type muscle such as soleus, while little effects were seen in white-type muscle such as extensor digitorum longus [23]. In vitro studies show that protein degradation induced by TNF-$\alpha$ is mediated through activation of NF-$\kappa$B [24].

Atrophy of skeletal muscles is also observed in IL-6 transgenic mice, which is completely blocked by anti-mouse IL-6 receptor antibody [25]. The muscle atrophy is associated with increased mRNA levels for cathepsins (B and L) and mRNA levels of ubiquitins (mono and poly). However, this may be an indirect effect, since intravenous administration of IL-6 to rats had no effect on ubiquitin gene expression [26] and repeated administration of IL-6 to healthy mice over a 7-day period had no effect on body weight [27].

Severe cachexia has been shown to develop rapidly in nude mice inoculated with CHO cells constitutively producing murine IFN-$\gamma$ [28]. As with TNF-$\alpha$ [26], intravenous administration of IFN-$\gamma$ to rats caused an increased expression of both the 1.2- and 2.4-kb transcripts of ubiquitin, although there were no measurements on the expression of proteasome subunits. These results suggest that some, but not all, cytokines increase protein degradation through an increase in expression of the ubiquitin-proteasome proteolytic pathway.

## Proteolysis-Inducing Factor

Proteolysis-inducing factor (PIF) is a 24-kDa sulphated glycoprotein secreted by cachexia-inducing murine and human tumours [29]. Administration of PIF to normal mice causes atrophy of skeletal muscle by an inhibition of protein synthesis and an increase of protein degradation [30]. The increased protein degradation arises from an increased expression of the ubiquitin-proteasome proteolytic pathway [31]. As with

TNF-$\alpha$ [24], upregulation of the pathway involves the transcription factor NF-$\kappa$B [32].

## Glucocorticoids

Glucocorticoids have been suggested to be important mediators of muscle catabolism in metabolic acidosis, acute diabetes, sepsis and starvation [33]. As with other inducers of protein degradation in skeletal muscle, glucocorticoids increase the expression of the ubiquitin-proteasome system [34]. However, unlike the other mediators, it has been suggested that NF-$\kappa$B acts as a suppressor of genes in the proteasome pathway, and that glucocorticoids increase proteolysis by downregulating NF-$\kappa$B activity [35].

## Apoptosis as a Factor in Muscle Loss in Cachexia

Apoptosis has been found to be associated with atrophy of skeletal muscle in hindlimb unweighting in rats [36] and in motor neuron disorders [37]. Increased DNA fragmentation has also been found in the skeletal muscle of rats bearing the cachexia-inducing Yoshida AH-130 ascites hepatoma [38] and in the early stage of tumour development in rabbits bearing the VX2 carcinoma cells, together with increased expression of the apoptosis-promoting protein bax [39]. In the latter model there was an early increase in apoptotic index when the loss of lean body mass amounted to 18%, but a decrease at higher weight loss (up to 30%) [40]. The authors suggest two mechanisms of muscle depletion during tumour growth, apoptosis in the early stage and metabolic abnormalities in the late stage. Using an in vitro model of skeletal muscle, PIF was shown to stimulate the activity of the apoptotic initiator caspases-8 and -9, and the apoptotic effector caspases-2, -3 and -6, at the same concentrations as those inducing muscle protein degradation [41]. In addition PIF increased the cytosolic content of both cytochrome C and bax and increased DNA fragmentation. The relative importance of apoptosis compared with other mechanisms of muscle atrophy is not known.

## Fate of Amino Acids Released from Skeletal Muscle

Proteolysis of muscle results in the release of amino acids, particularly alanine and glutamine, which represent more than 50% of the amino acids exported by skeletal muscle [42]. Alanine is channelled to the liver for gluconeogenesis and acute-phase protein (APP) synthesis (see later), while glutamine is taken up by the tumour to sustain the energy and nitrogen demands. The amide nitrogen of glutamine is utilised in the synthesis of purine and pyrimidine bases and for aminosugars. Glutamine is the prime source of nitrogen for tumours and a marked decrease has been observed in rats bearing a rapidly growing hepatoma, which was attributed to an increased activity of glutamine-utilising enzymes [43]. Patients with progressive cancer have increased glucose synthesis from alanine [44]. Both glutamine and alanine are produced in muscle from the metabolism of other amino acids, mainly branched-chain amino acids (BCAA) and aspartate. The BCAA (leucine, isoleucine and valine) are often increased in cancer cachexia and their turnover rates altered. The carbon skeletons of BCAA arising from transamination provide a major source of metabolic fuel for skeletal muscle. In addition the BCAA, and leucine in particular, stimulate protein synthesis and inhibit protein degradation in skeletal muscle. In cancer cachexia, but not in starvation, leucine inhibits the expression of genes of the proteasome pathway [45], while BCAA directly inhibit proteasome chy-

motrypsin-like enzyme activity in muscle, but not in liver [46].

Although protein synthesis in skeletal muscle is depressed in patients with cachexia, liver protein synthesis is enhanced due to APP synthesis. Thus liver protein synthesis shifts from the synthesis of albumin to APP such as C-reactive protein (CRP), fibrinogen, serum amyloid A, 2-macroglobulin and $\alpha$-1 antitrypsin [47]. There is an association between a chronic inflammatory response and the rate of loss of body mass in lung and gastrointestinal cancers [48], while elevated levels of fibrinogen were correlated with a reduced survival in patients with pancreatic cancer [49]. It is possible that enhanced APP synthesis in the liver inhibits synthesis of myofibrillar proteins in muscle by reducing the pool size of critical amino acids.

## Conclusions

Atrophy of skeletal muscle in cachexia results from an increased protein degradation coupled with a reduced protein synthesis. Increased protein degradation appears to result from an increased expression and activity of the ubiquitin-proteasome proteolytic pathway due to a range of factors in the different cachexias. The situation differs from starvation in that liver protein synthesis is elevated due to APP production. Release of amino acids from muscle may be important in the synthesis of APP, while certain amino acids may be essential for tumour growth.

## References

1. Fearon KCH (1992) The mechanisms and treatment of weight loss in cancer. Proc Nutr Soc 51:251–265
2. Kotler DP, Tiemey AR, Culpepper-Morgan JA et al (1990) Effect of home total parenteral nutrition on body composition in patients with acquired immunodeficiency syndrome. J Parent Enteral Nutr 14:454–458
3. Strent SJ, Beddoe AH, Hill GL (1987) Aggressive nutritional support does not prevent protein loss despite fat gain in septic intensive care patients. J Trauma 27:262–266
4. Evans WK, Makuch R, Clamon GH et al (1985) Limited impact of total parenteral nutrition on nutritional status during treatment for small cell lung cancer. Cancer Res 45:3347–3353
5. Loprinzi CL, Schaid DJ, Dose AM et al (1993) Body composition changes in patients who gain weight while receiving megestrol acetate. J Clin Oncol 11:152–154
6. Lundholm K, Bylund AC, Holm J, Schersten T (1976) Skeletal muscle metabolism in patients with malignant tumour. Eur J Cancer 12:465–473
7. Lundholm K, Bennegard K, Eden E, Rennie MJ (1982) Efflux of 3-methylhistidine from the leg of cancer patients who experience weight loss. Cancer Res 42:4809–4818

8. Diffee GM, Kalfos K, Al-Majid S, McCarthy DO (2002) Altered expression of skeletal muscle myosin isoforms in cancer cachexia. Am J Physiol 283:C1376–C1382

9. Lecker SH, Solomon V, Mitch WE, Goldberg AL (1999) Muscle protein breakdown and the critical role of the ubiquitin-proteasome pathway in normal and disease states. J Nutr 129:227S–237S

10. Calban VD, Evangelista EA, Migliorini RH, Kettlehut IC (2001) Role of ubiquitin-proteasome-dependent proteolytic process in degradation of muscle protein from diabetic rats. Mol Cell Biochem 225:35–41

11. Ikemoto M, Nikawa T, Takeda S et al (2001) Space shuttle flight (STS 90) enhances degradation of rat myosin heavy chain in association with activation of ubiquitin-proteasome pathway. FASEB J 10:1096

12. Hasselgren P-O, Fischer JE (2001) Muscle cachexia: current concepts of intracellular mechanisms and molecular regulation. Ann Surg 233:9–17

13. Fischer DR, Sun XY, Williams AB (2001) Dantrolene reduces serum TNF alpha and corticosterone levels and muscle calcium, calpain gene expression and protein breakdown in septic rats. Shock 15:200–207

14. Hasselgren P-O, Wray C, Mammen J (2002) Molecular regulation of muscle cachexia: it may be more than the proteasome. Biochem Biophys Res Commun 290:1–10

15. Attaix D, Taillandier D, Combaret L et al (1997) Expression of subunits of the 19S complex and of the P28 activator in rat skeletal muscle. Mol Biol Rep 24:95–98

16. Temparis S, Asensi M, Taillandier D et al (1994) Increased ATP-ubiquitin-dependent proteolysis in skeletal muscles of tumor-bearing rats. Cancer Res 54:5568–5573

17. Bodine SC, Latres E, Baumhueter Si et al (2001) Identification of ubiquitin ligases required for skeletal muscle atrophy. Science 294:1704–1708

18. Lawler JM, Song W, Demaree SR (2003) Hindlimb unloading increases oxidative stress and disrupts antioxidant capacity in skeletal muscle. Free Radical Biol Med 35:9–16

19. Buck M, Chojkier M (1996) Muscle wasting and dedifferentiation induced by oxidative stress in a murine model of cachexia is prevented by inhibitors of nitric oxide synthesis and antioxidants. EMBO J 15:1753–1765

20. Gomes-Marcondes MCC, Tisdale MJ (2002) Induction of protein catabolism and the ubiquitin-proteasome pathway by mild oxidative stress. Cancer Lett 180:69–74

21. Li YP, Schwartz RJ, Waddell ID et al (1998) Skeletal muscle myocytes undergo protein loss and reactive oxygen-mediated NF-kappaB activation in response to tumor necrosis factor alpha. FASEB J 12:871–880

22. Llovera M, Lopez-Soriano FJ, Argilés JM (1993) Effects of tumor necrosis factor-a on muscle protein turnover in female Wistar rats. J Natl Cancer Inst 85:1334–1339

23. Garcia-Martinez C, Lopez-Soriano FJ, Argiles JM (1993) Acute treatment with tumour necrosis factor-α induces changes in protein metabolism in rat skeletal muscle. Mol Cell Biochem 125:11–18

24. Li Y-P, Reid MB (2000) NF-κB mediates the protein loss induced by TNF-α in differentiated skeletal muscle myotubes. Am J Physiol 279:R1165–R1170

25. Tsujinaka T, Fujita J, Ebisui C et al (1996) Interleukin 6 receptor antibody inhibits muscle atrophy and modulates proteolytic systems in interleukin-6 transgenic mice. J Clin Invest 97:244–249

26. Llovera M, Carbo N, Lopez-Soriano J et al (1998) Different cytokines modulate ubiquitin gene expression in rat skeletal muscle. Cancer Lett 133:83–87

27. Espat NJ, Auffenberg T, Rosenberg JJ et al (1996) Ciliary neurotrophic factor is catabolic and shares with IL-6 the capacity to induce an acute phase response. Am J Physiol 271:R185–R190

28. Matthys P, Dijkmans R, Proost P et al (1991) Severe cachexia in mice inoculated with interferon-γ-producing tumour cells. Int J Cancer 49:77–82

29. Todorov P, Cariuk P, McDevitt T et al (1996) Characterization of a cancer cachectic factor. Nature 379:739–742

30. Lorite MJ, Cariuk P, Tisdale MJ (1997) Induction of muscle protein degradation by a tumour factor. Br J Cancer 76:1035–1040

31. Lorite MJ, Smith HJ, Arnold JA et al (2001) Activation of ATP-ubiquitin-dependent proteolysis in skeletal muscle in vivo and murine myoblasts in vitro by a proteolysis-inducing factor (PIF). Br J Cancer 85:297–302

32. Whitehouse AS, Tisdale MJ (2003) Increased expression of the ubiquitin-proteasome pathway in murine myotubes by proteolysis-inducing factor (PIF) is associated with activation of the transcription factor NF-κB. Br J Cancer 89:1116–1122

33. Kettlehut IC, Wing SS, Goldberg AL (1988) Endocrine regulation of protein breakdown in skeletal muscle. Diabetes Metab Rev 8:751–772

34. Auclair D, Garrel RD, Zerouala AC, Ferland LH (1997) Activation of the ubiquitin pathway in rat skeletal muscle by catabolic doses of glucocorticoids. Am J Physiol 272:C1007–C1016

35. Du J, Mitch WE, Wang X, Price SR (2000) Glucocorticoids induce proteasome C3 subunit expression in L6 muscle cells by opposing the suppression of its transcription by NF-κB. J Biol Chem 275:19661–19666

36. Allen DL, Linderman JK, Roy RR et al (1997) Apoptosis: a mechanism contributing to the remodeling of skeletal muscle in response to hindlimb unweighting. Am J Physiol 273:C579–C587

37. Tews DS, Gobel HH, Meinck HM (1997) DNA fragmentation and apoptosis-related proteins of muscle cells in motor neuron disorders. Acta Neurol Scand 96:380–386

38. van Rogen M, Carbo N, Busquets S et al (2000) DNA fragmentation occurs in skeletal muscle during

tumour growth: a link with cancer cachexia? Biochem Biophys Res Commun 270:533–537

39.  Yoshida H, Ishiko O, Sumi T et al (2001) Expression of apoptosis regulatory proteins in the skeletal muscle of tumor-bearing rabbits. Jpn J Cancer Res 92:631–637

40.  Ishiko O, Sumi T, Hirai K et al (2001) Apoptosis of muscle cells causes weight loss prior to impairment of DNA synthesis in tumor-bearing rabbits. Jpn J Cancer Res 92:30–35

41.  Smith HJ, Tisdale MJ (2003) Induction of apoptosis by a cachectic-factor in murine myotubes and inhibition by eicosapentaenoic acid. Apoptosis 8:161–169

42.  Felig P (1975) Amino acid metabolism in man. Ann Rev Biochem 44:933–955

43.  Weber G, Prajda N, Lui MS et al (1982) Multi-enzyme-targeted chemotherapy by acivicin and actinomycin. Adv Enzyme Regul 20:75–96

44.  Lundholm K, Holm G, Schersten T (1979) Gluconeogenesis from alanine in patients with progressive ma-

lignant disease. Cancer Res 39:1968–1972

45.  Busquets S, Alvarez B, Lopez-Soriano FJ, Argiles JM (2002) Branched-chain amino acids: a role in skeletal muscle proteolysis in catabolic states? J Cell Physiol 19:283–289

46.  Hamel FG, Upward JL, Siford GL, Duckworth WC (2003) Inhibition of proteasome activity by selected amino acids. Metabolism 52:810–814

47.  Fearon KCH, Falconer JS, Slater C et al (1998) Albumin synthesis rates are not decreased in hypoalbuminemic cachectic cancer patients with an ongoing acute-phase protein response. Ann Surg 227:249–254

48.  McMillan DC, Scott HR, Watson WS et al (1998) Longitudinal study of body cell mass depletion and the inflammatory response in cancer patients. Nutr Cancer 31:101–105

49.  Falconer JS, Fearon KC, Ross JA et al (1995) Acute phase protein response and survival duration of patients with pancreatic cancer. Cancer 74:2077–2082

# Lipid Metabolism in Cachexia

Enzo Manzato, Giovanna Romanato

In this chapter we will review the alterations of lipoprotein metabolism observed in cachexia. Other aspects of lipid metabolism in cachexia, in particular those regarding adipose tissue, are covered in other chapters. Lipoproteins are macromolecules circulating in blood and they are quite easily measured in the clinical chemistry laboratory. For this reason lipoproteins can be used to monitor the alterations of lipid metabolism in several clinical conditions, including cachexia.

All lipids, except free (non-esterified) fatty acids (FFA), are transported in blood in the form of lipoproteins in association with specific proteins (apolipoproteins). The major lipids found in human plasma lipoproteins are triglycerides, phospholipids and cholesterol (free and esterified) [1].

FFA are transported from their storage site (i.e. adipose tissue) to the sites of utilisation (liver and muscles). The release of FFA from adipose tissue is regulated by a hormone–sensitive lipase (which is activated by noradrenaline and glucocorticoid hormones) and is promoted by prolonged fasting, acute stress, and lack of insulin. The adipose tissue hormone–sensitive lipase is thus involved in removing FFA from the triglycerides present within the adipocytes.

Triglycerides are esters of glycerol with fatty acids and they are produced in the small intestine during fat absorption or in the liver and in the adipose tissue. Triglycerides have a relatively short half–life in the plasma and they are hydrolysed by lipolytic enzymes (lipoprotein lipase) in various organs (adipose tissue, muscles, liver). The lipoprotein lipases are involved in extraction of fatty acids from plasma triglycerides and these FFA are used for storage in adipose tissue, for energy production in several organs, or for lipid synthesis in the liver.

Several phospholipids are found in plasma but the two most abundant are phosphatidylcholine (also called lecithin) and sphingomyelin. Most of the plasma phosholipids are synthesised in the liver. Phospholipids are essential components of all cellular membranes and they have a key role in maintaining non-polar lipids (like triglycerides and cholesterol esters) in a soluble state within lipoproteins.

Cholesterol is a sterol containing a hydroxyl group that can be non-esterified (free cholesterol) or esterified with one of several long–chain fatty acids (mostly linoleic and oleic acid). Free cholesterol is an essential component of all cell membranes, while two thirds of the cholesterol present in plasma is esterified. Plasma cholesterol is produced by the liver and in part it is derived from intestinal absorption. The major metabolites of cholesterol are the bile acids, which are synthesised exclusively by the liver.

To form lipoproteins, lipids are associated with apolipoproteins. The role of apolipoproteins is both structural and functional. In fact, apolipoproteins have amphipatic properties, i.e. they can solubilise apolar lipids (triglycerides and cholesterol esters) in an aqueous environment. The most important apolipoproteins found in human plasma are apo AI, AII, B100, B48, CI, CII, CIII and E. Some apolipoproteins are cofactors of important enzymes involved in lipoprotein metabolism (e.g. apo CII for lipoprotein lipase, apo AI for lecithin–cholesterol acyl transferase) or are involved in the receptor-mediated lipoprotein uptake (e.g. apo B100 and apo E for the low-density lipoprotein [LDL] receptor).

Four major classes of lipoproteins can be isolated from plasma: chylomicrons, very-low-density lipoproteins (VLDL), LDL and high-density lipoproteins (HDL). Chylomicrons are produced by the small intestine during fat absorption: they consist mainly of triglycerides that are catabolised by lipoprotein lipase. VLDL are triglyceride-rich lipoproteins produced by the liver, which are transformed into LDL by lipoprotein lipase. LDL are cholesterol-rich lipoproteins that can be used by peripheral tissues for cholesterol supply or by the liver for cholesterol catabolism through biliary acids. LDL are the major cholesterol-carrying lipoproteins of human plasma, containing about two thirds of plasma cholesterol. HDL contain mainly phospholipids and small amounts of cholesterol that is acquired from peripheral tissue to be released to the liver ('inverse' cholesterol transport).

Plasma lipid and lipoprotein concentrations are regulated by genetic, metabolic and dietary factors. Several genetic (primary) forms of both hyperlipidaemia and hypolipidaemia have been described, as well as secondary (or acquired) forms due to systemic disease such as diabetes, endocrine diseases (thyroid, hypophysis) or organ failure (liver, kidney)(Table 1) [2]. Secondary hyperlipidaemias are also produced by some drugs. In association with genetic background, dietary habits have an important role in modulating plasma lipid concentrations: therefore, the alterations of lipid metabolism in cachexia must be considered taking into account all these factors.

Since cachexia is a common feature of several different illnesses (including cancer, sepsis, chronic heart failure, thyroid diseases, severe liver diseases, rheumatoid arthritis and AIDS), the alterations of lipid metabolism observed in these patients may have different causes, related to specific organ involvement, dietary modifications, fat absorption or drugs.

The main lipid abnormalities found in cachexia are related to reduced food intake, enhanced lipid mobilisation from the adipose tissue, reduced lipogenesis in the liver, and reduced lipoprotein lipase activities (Table 2). The mechanisms responsible for the lipid alterations are malabsorption, dietary deficiency and metabolic dysfunctions. Anorexia can be related to the primary disease or to side-effects of drugs. These abnormalities are usually associated with low HDL cholesterol and variable triglyceride concentrations [3].

In patients with a variety of tumours, VLDL triglycerides accumulate in plasma as a result of decreased lipoprotein lipase activity. In fact, both the extrahepatic and hepatic lipoprotein lipase activities are decreased in cancer patients with varying degrees of weight loss, the levels of these activities being correlated with the per cent body weight lost [4]. On the other hand, fasting in healthy humans is associated with increased lipase activities and reduced triglyceride levels [5].

In patients with cachexia, the production of cytokines is frequently altered. Several cytokines inhibit the lipoprotein lipase activities, thus reducing plasma triglyceride catabolism and preventing fatty acid deposition in the adipose tissue [6].

Interleukin-6 (IL-6) reduces lipase activities and may play a role in inducing cancer cachexia, but in cancer patients IL-6 does not correlate with lipase activities and therefore IL-6 does not seem to be involved in the lipid alterations of these patients [7].

**Table 1.** Secondary causes of lipoprotein abnormalities that may be present in patients with cachexia

1. Reduced LDL cholesterol: chronic infections (AIDS, tuberculosis), chronic liver diseases, hyperthyroidism, malabsorption (short bowel, blind-loop syndrome, coeliac disease, pancreatic exocrine insufficiency, giardiasis), malnutrition, monoclonal gammopathy, myeloproliferative diseases
2. Increased LDL cholesterol: anorexia nervosa, drugs (cyclosporine, progestogens, thiazides), obstructive liver disease
3. Increased VLDL (hypertriglyceridaemia): alcohol, chronic renal failure, drugs (beta blockers, oestrogen, glucocorticoids, isotretinoin, protease inhibitors, thiazides), monoclonal gammopathy (lymphoma, multiple myeloma), ileal bypass surgery, lipodystrophy, poorly controlled diabetes mellitus, sepsis, stress, systemic lupus erythematosus
4. Reduced HDL cholesterol: anabolic steroids, beta blockers, cigarette smoking, malnutrition

**Table 2.** Pathophysiological alterations involved in the lipid abnormalities of patients with cachexia

Impaired lipoprotein lipase activities

Increased lipolysis from adipose tissue

Reduced total body lipids

Reduced fat synthesis

Interleukin-2 (IL-2), when used to treat refractory cancers, causes severe hypocholesterolaemia, associated with reduction of both lipoprotein lipase and lecithin:cholesteryl acyltransferase (LCAT) activities. The LCAT reduction has been associated with the presence of abnormal lipoproteins in plasma [8].

Tumour necrosis factor (TNF)-α inhibits lipoprotein lipase by down-regulation of the protein expression of this lipase [9], thus reducing the tryglyceride catabolism in VLDL [10] and the fatty acid deposition in the adipocytes. These observations may explain why hypertriglyceridaemia is sometimes present in patients with cachexia. On the other hand, TNF-α can increase the activity of the adipose tissue hormone-sensitive lipase, thus leading to an increased lipolysis from the adipocytes [11].

Hypocholesterolaemia is commonly found in patients with acute leukaemia, lung cancer and solid tumours, due to the high LDL-receptor activity of cancer cells. In some of these patients, the LDL-receptor activity is inversely correlated with plasma-cholesterol concentration. It has been hypothesised that this hypocholesterolaemia might be due to three different mechanisms: (1) enhanced uptake of plasma LDL by cancer cells; (2) increased transport of cholesterol from cancer cells to the liver; (3) reduced conversion of cholesterol to bile acids, which may result in a decreased intestinal absorption of cholesterol and subsequent hypocholesterolaemia. During chemotherapy, cholesterol levels may increase [12].

Hypocholesterolaemia has been shown to be associated with a poor prognosis in several clinical conditions associated with cachexia, such as chronic heart failure, cancer, dialysis and AIDS [13]. However, the increased LDL uptake by cancer cells could be useful for introducing drugs incorporated in LDL particles into malignant cells.

Advanced HIV disease and immune deficiency are accompanied by changes in lipoprotein metabolism characterised by decreased levels of total, LDL-cholesterol and HDL-cholesterol as well as decreased apolipoprotein B. Progression to AIDS is associated with elevated triglyceride levels. Patients taking HIV protease inhibitors frequently have hypercholesterolaemia and hypertriglyceridaemia, with increased VLDL concentrations and increased concentrations of apolipoprotein B [14].

In conclusion, lipoprotein alterations in cachexia are easily monitored in the clinical chemistry lab and are useful to evaluate the clinical evolution of the diseases responsible for this syndrome. These alterations might also be used to improve our current therapy in these patients.

# References

1. Durrington P (2003) Dyslipidemia. Lancet 362:717–731
2. Ginsberg HN, Goldberg IJ (2001) Disorders of lipoprotein metabolism. In: Braunwald E, Hauser SL, Fauci AS et al (eds) Principles of internal medicine. McGraw Hill, New York, pp 2245–2257
3. Tisdale MJ (2002) Cachexia in cancer patients. Nat Rev Cancer 2:862–871
4. Vlassara H, Spiegel RJ, San Doval D, Cerami A (1986) Reduced plasma lipoprotein lipase activity in patients with malignancy-associated weight loss. Horm Metabol Res 18:698–703
5. Ruge T, Svensson A, Eriksson JW et al (2001) Food deprivation increases post-heparin lipoprotein lipase activity in humans. Eur J Clin Invest 31:1040–1047
6. Inui A (2002) Cancer anorexia-cachexia syndrome: current issues in research and management. CA Cancer J Clin 52:72–91
7. Nomura K, Noguchi Y, Yoshikawa T, Kondo J (1997) Plasma interleukin-6 is not a mediator of changes in lipoprotein lipase activity in cancer patients. Hepatogastroenterology 44:1519–1526
8. Kwong LK, Ridinger DN, Bandhauer M et al (1997) Acute dyslipoproteinemia induced by interleukin-2 lecithin:cholesteryl acyltransferase, lipoprotein lipase, hepatic lipase deficiencies. J Clin Endocrinol Metab 82:1572–1581
9. Hauner H, Petruschke T, Russ M et al (1995) Effects of tumour necrosis factor alpha (TNF alpha) on glucose transport and lipid metabolism of newly-differentiated human fat cells in cell culture. Diabetologia 38:764–771
10. Kern PA, Saghizadeh M, Ong JM et al (1995) The expression of tumor necrosis factor in human adipose tissue. Regulation by obesity, weight loss, and relationship to lipoprotein lipase. J Clin Invest 95:2111–2119
11. Sethi JK, Hotamisligil GS (1999) The role of TNF-α in adipocyte metabolism. Semin Cell Dev Biol 10:19–29
12. Tatidis L, Vitols S, Gruber A et al (2001) Cholesterol catabolism in patients with acute myelogenous leu-

kemia and hypocholesterolemia: suppressed levels of a circulating marker for bile acid synthesis. Cancer Letters 170:169–175

13. Kalantar-Zadek K, Block G, Horwich T, Fonarow GC (2004) Reverse epidemiology of conventional cardiovascular risk factors in patients with chronic heart failure. J Am Coll Cardiol 43:1439–1444

14. Grunfeld C, Pang M, Doerrler W et al (1992) Lipids, lipoproteins, triglyceride clearance, and cytokines in human immunodeficiency virus infection and the acquired immunodeficiency syndrome. J Clin Endocrinol Metab 74:1045–1052

# Glucose Metabolism

Antonio Macciò, Clelia Madeddu, Giovanni Mantovani

In 1919, glucose intolerance became the earliest recognised metabolic abnormality in cancer patients. Prior to the development of severe malnutrition, patients with colon, gastric, sarcoma, endometrial, prostate, localised head, neck and lung cancer had many of the metabolic abnormalities of type II (non-insulin-dependent) diabetes mellitus. These metabolic abnormalities included glucose intolerance, an increase in both hepatic glucose production (HGP) and glucose recycling, and insulin resistance. In a study of over 600 cancer patients, a diabetic pattern of glucose tolerance test was noted in over one-third of the patients [1].

Changes in energy metabolism consisting of increased resting energy expenditure associated with alterations of glucose, lipid and protein metabolism are typical of cancer-related anorexia/cachexia syndrome (CACS).

The tumour growth and the chronic activation of the immune system (to counteract the tumour growth) are responsible for an increased energy expenditure and thus for a continuous consumption of energetic substrates, especially glucose [2]. In fact, the oxidation of glucose into $CO_2$ and $H_2O$ through the Krebs' cycle is a well-known major source of energy and plays a key role in the biosynthesis of ATP, DNA, RNA and phospholipids. Glucose is also necessary for the pentose-phosphate pathway and the synthesis of reducing compounds such as NADPH.

In advanced cancer patients, energy metabolism is severely compromised by the occurrence during the disease progression of symptoms such as anorexia, nausea and vomiting, which do not allow for a normal nutrition and so a regular supply of carbohydrates, proteins, amino acids and vitamins. In addition to the reduced food intake, important changes of energy metabolism and bio-chemical/metabolic abnormalities in carbohydrate, protein and lipid biochemistry and metabolism have been observed, which may account for CACS [3].

## Glucose Metabolism Changes in CACS

Glucose is the most important energetic substrate of the human body. Neoplastic cells preferentially metabolise glucose through anaerobic glycolysis.

In cancer patients, glucose intake is severely compromised by the presence of symptoms such as nausea, vomiting and anorexia. The reduced glucose intake induces the activation of gluconeogenesis from lactate, muscle amino acids and free fatty acids, finally leading to depletion of fat and protein stores. The cycle converting lactate to pyruvate and glucose is named the Cory cycle. The Cory cycle activity is increased from 20% (value observed in healthy subjects) to 50% in cancer patients with CACS.

The utilisation of lactate and glycogenetic amino acids for the synthesis of glucose in the liver is a process associated with high energy consumption. Increased gluconeogenesis has been proposed as the main cause of increased energy expenditure of cancer patients. The increase of glucose turnover is strictly related to histotype, stage of disease and grade of cachexia. Several studies have analysed the relationship between glucose metabolism and changes of body weight. Patients without weight loss have a normal Cory cycle activity, whilst those with progressive weight loss have an increased Cory cycle activity associated with an increased lactate production. However, the compensatory increased gluconeogenesis is associated with reduced synthesis of insulin and insulin resistance. In fact, the most important carbohydrate abnormalities observed in cachectic cancer patients are increased glucose synthesis, gluconeogenesis and Cory cycle activity, insulin resistance, and decreased glucose tolerance [3].

This adaptation redirects glucose to the liver and other viscera and away from skeletal muscle because hepatic glucokinase is not affected by insulin, unlike hexokinase in myocytes and elsewhere. The energy needs of muscle are met by oxidation of non-essential amino acids, which contributes to negative nitrogen balance [4].

In addition to having increased glucose production and glucose intolerance, cancer patients show a clear insulin resistance that involves adipose tissue, skeletal muscle and liver. The increased hepatic glucose production is partially the result of a lack of inhibition of gluconeogenesis by insulin due to a certain degree of liver insulin resistance. Similarly, glucose utilisation by skeletal muscle is reduced both in experimental animals and cancer patients, this being the result of clear insulin resistance [5]. In addition, increases in counter-regulatory hormones, such as glucocorticoids or glucagons, also seem to be involved [6]. The decreased stimulation of glucose uptake does not seem to be the consequence of a defect in insulin binding but rather a post-receptor defect. The insulin resistance observed in skeletal muscle also affects glycogen synthesis, which is clearly reduced in cancer patients [7].

Peripheral insulin resistance is mediated by proinflammatory cytokines. Insulin resistance is associated with increases in circulating tumour necrosis factor (TNF)-α in several pathological situations, such as endotoxaemia, trauma and cancer [8]. Clinical administration of TNF-α in healthy humans has been reported to reduce insulin sensitivity, by inducing hyperglycaemia without lowering insulin levels [9].

## Mediators Involved in Glucose Abnormalities

### Proinflammatory Cytokines

It has been suggested that the chronic action of mediators released by tumour cells and immune cells counteracting tumour is the main cause of the metabolic abnormalities characterising the cachectic neoplastic patient. Indeed, several experimental and clinical researches confirm the central role exerted by proinflammatory cytokines, especially interleukin (IL)-1, IL-6 and TNF-α, in the pathogenesis of CACS. Chronically elevated levels for these factors, either alone or in combination, are capable of reproducing the different features of CACS [10, 11]. More direct evidence of a cytokine involvement in CACS is provided by the observation that cachexia in animal experimental models can be relieved by administration of specific cytokine antagonists [11–13]. These studies revealed that CACS can rarely be attributed to any one cytokine but rather is associated with a set of cytokines that work in concert [3].

The role of IL-1 in the pathogenesis of CACS has been clearly elucidated. IL-1 exerts a specific effect on reducing food intake and influences meal size, meal duration and meal frequency [14, 15]. Hypothalamic IL-1 is increased either through access from the median eminence (a circumventricular nucleus without a blood–brain barrier proximal to the arcuate nucleus) or is generated within the hypothalamus [16]. IL-1 has an anorectic action by directly decreasing neuropeptide Y (NPY) neurotransmission and secondarily by increasing corticotropin-releasing factor (CRF), which in turn acts on the satiety circuitry inhibiting food intake. In rat models, IL-1 has been demonstrated to inhibit serum levels of growth hormone (GH) by increasing CRF and somatostatin levels [17]. The reduced synthesis of GH leads to reduced synthesis of the insulin-like growth factors (IGFs), which in turn influence the muscle protein turnover and the autocrine and paracrine regulation of muscle mass proliferation [18]. In vitro studies have demonstrated that IGF-1 induces muscle glucose synthesis and amino acid uptake and inhibits protein catabolism [19–21]. Studies on experimental models of rats bearing cachectic tumour showed that the administration of IGF-1 was able to prevent weight loss, muscle wasting and loss of muscle protein. IL-1 also acts peripherally on pancreatic beta cells, which have specific receptors for IL-1 [22]. IL-1 on beta cells first induces the release and synthesis of insulin and, secondarily, inhibits the synthesis and release of insulin [23].

TNF-α has been shown to promote lipolysis and inhibit lipogenesis and plays a key role in the depletion of adipose tissue mass seen in cachexia. It has been proposed that an elevation in plasma levels of TNF-α is responsible for the metabolic alterations in adipose tissue seen in cachexia [24]. Lipid metabolism is a complex sequence of events that determine whether the triglyceride pool within the adipocyte increases, due to the processes of free fatty acid (FFA) uptake and lipogenesis, or decreases, due to the process of lipolysis. Circulating lipoproteins and triglycerides are first converted into FFA by the action of lipoprotein lipase (LPL), which is secreted by the adipocyte. FFA can then enter the adipocyte via a fatty acid transporter. Once inside the adipocyte, the FFA is converted into the triglyceride by a multi-step-regulated enzymatic reaction, one of the enzymes involved being acyl-CoA synthetase. In addition, triglyceride can be formed from the uptake of glucose, via glucose transporters (GLUT)1 and 4, into the adipocyte. The glucose can then be converted into triglyceride by the actions of a series of enzymes, which include acetyl-CoA carboxylase and fatty acid synthase. A large body of evidence now supports a role for TNF-α in modulating these processes [25]. Studies utilising mammary adipose tissue from human subjects have now shown that TNF-α inhibits LPL activity by down-regulating its protein expression [26]. Indeed, increasing TNF-α mRNA levels are correlated with decreasing LPL activity in human subcutaneous adipose tissue [27]. In addition, TNF-α has been shown to reduce the expression of FFA transporters in adipose tissue of the Syrian hamster [28]. TNF-α could thus hinder the synthesis and entry of FFA into the adipocyte, curtailing an increase in the intracellular triglyceride pool size. Studies have also suggested that TNF-α may decrease the expression of enzymes involved in lipogenesis. Specifically, it has been suggested that acetyl-CoA carboxylase and fatty acid synthase are down-regulated. However, it is unclear if this occurs in mature adipocytes [25]. Acyl-CoA synthase expression and activity have also been suggested

to be down-regulated by TNF-α [29]. TNF-α has been found to promote lipolysis. However, the mechanisms by which this is achieved are unclear. TNF-α administration also induces increase of cortisol, glucagon and insulin levels and these effects seem to be mediated by IL-1; the concomitant administration of recombinant IGF-1 reduces the percentage of protein loss by 15% with an associated improvement of glucose metabolism. TNF-α has been implicated as a factor associated with the development of insulin resistance. Studies in women have found a positive association between plasma insulin levels and TNF-α mRNA from subcutaneous adipose tissue [30], which is supported by a study showing increased adipose TNF-α secretion in obese patients with insulin resistance [27]. Extensive research has highlighted several potential mechanisms by which TNF-α induces insulin resistance. These include: accelerated lipolysis and a concomitant increase in circulating FFA concentrations, down-regulation of GLUT4 synthesis, down-regulation of insulin receptor, insulin receptor substrate-1 (IRS-1) synthesis and increased Ser/Thr phosphorylation of IRS-1 [31].

Interleukin-6 is another proinflammatory cytokine with cachectic effects. In an experimental animal model, Strassmann et al. [32] demonstrated that the presence of tumour in mouse models was associated with early CACS and production of IL-6, dosable in the serum. Serum IL-6 levels correlated with the severity of CACS. Moreover, the administration of anti-IL-6 antibody inhibits the appearance of CACS symptoms. In vitro studies have demonstrated that IL-6 induces, similarly to IL-1, the hypothalamic release of CRF. Moreover, IL-6 acts on beta pancreatic cells similarly to IL-1 [33].

Thus, proinflammatory cytokines IL-1, TNF-α and IL-6 play a central role in the pathogenesis of metabolic derangements associated with CACS. It may be hypothesised that, during the initial phases of neoplastic disease, the synthesis of proinflammatory cytokines leads to an efficient antineoplastic effect. However, their chronic activity leads to severe alterations of cell metabolism, with deleterious effects on body composition, nutritional status and immune system efficiency.

## Leptin

A fundamental advance in our understanding of control of energy balance came with the discovery of the adipocyte-derived hormone leptin. Leptin is a 164-kDa protein that is transcribed in adipocytes of a variety of species, including humans, and after cleavage of a signal peptide, it is secreted into the bloodstream where it circulates at concentrations proportional to body fat stores [34]. Leptin production is regulated by the peripheral signal pathway from the adipose tissue to the hypothalamus, which is involved in the regulation of feeding and energy balance [35]. Thus, leptin is the major peripheral regulator of long-term body composition and is responsible for self-correcting changes in energy intake and expenditure [36].

Several in vitro and in vivo studies showed high serum levels of leptin during acute inflammatory diseases. So, this hormone has been hypothesised to be responsible for anorexia and weight loss occurring in chronic inflammatory disease [37, 38]. By contrast, several studies, including our own [39–42], carried out in a population of cancer patients, demonstrated that leptin levels in cancer patients are lower than those in healthy individuals. Specifically, we demonstrated that circulating leptin concentrations in advanced cancer patients are inversely related to the intensity of the inflammatory response (C-reactive protein [CRP], fibrinogen, IL-6, TNF-α). In addition, the lowest leptin levels were found in patients at advanced stages and with the most compromised performance status, and were associated with impairment of the immune system and low levels of IL-2 [39, 40].

We hypothesise that low serum leptin levels have a primary physiological role as a signal of depletion of energy stores rather than as a suppressor of body fat involved in the onset of cancer cachexia [43, 44] and they may be evidence of the alterations of energy metabolism occurring in CACS. The low serum leptin levels observed in advanced cancer patients are related to the increased energy expenditure induced by tumour during the progression of disease and to the appearance of anorexia with consequent reduced intake of energy substrates.

In advanced cancer patients, and especially in cachectic patients, characterised by severe alterations of energy metabolism, impairment of energy utilisation and increased energy expenditure, the activation of leptin feedback may be a biological defence of the body that limits the use of energy when energy is scarce. Decrease of leptin synthesis and release should induce lowering of metabolic rate and a powerful drive to eat more, in an effort to prevent weight loss induced by several mediators, proinflammatory cytokines first of all.

In fact, several recent studies showed that leptin production is strictly related to glucose utilisation [45]. Data from experiments in isolated adipocytes and from clinical studies in human subjects support the hypothesis that insulin increases leptin production indirectly via its effects to increase glucose utilisation and oxidative glucose metabolism in adipocytes [46, 47].

Havel et al. demonstrated that changes of leptin concentrations during periods of energy restriction were related to an index of what was happening in the adipocyte metabolically [48, 49]. These metabolic manifestations include decreased available glucose, decreased insulin-induced glucose utilisation and increased lipolysis. Glucose in the cells can go through glycolysis and be converted anaerobically to lactate, or it can enter the tricarboxylic acid cycle and, through the activity of pyruvate dehydrogenase, be converted to acetyl-CoA. From there it can go onto lipogenesis or be oxidised to generate adenosine triphosphate (ATP). Insulin causes a concentration-dependent decrease in the amount of glucose that is anaerobically metabolised to lactate without affecting the proportion of glucose that enters lipogenesis. Thus, in response to insulin activity, when less glucose is metabolised to lactate, more leptin is produced; on the other hand, the greater the proportion of glucose converted to lactate, the less leptin is produced [50]. From these findings the authors hypothesised that aerobic glucose metabolism is likely to be involved in the stimulation of leptin production through either the production of ATP via insulin-mediated glucose oxidation or the effect of glucose oxidation on cellular redox status and pyruvate cycling [51].

This evidence obtained by in vitro experiments (on cultured adipocytes) provides a strong support to our hypothesis that in advanced cancer patients, and especially those with CACS, low leptin levels function as a signal of negative energy balance and low energy reserves [47] consequent to the reduced intake and the impaired utilisation of energy substrates, particularly glucose.

Leptin as the major signal of energy substrates is strictly related to oxidative stress. In one of our papers we demonstrated that in advanced cancer patients with tumours at different sites, low leptin levels were associated with high levels of reactive oxygen species (ROS) and reduced antioxidant enzyme activity (e.g. glutathione [GSH] peroxidase and superoxide dismutase [SOD]) [50]. Therefore, we can consider oxidative stress to be the consequent manifestation of the impairment of metabolism of cancer patients *signalled* by leptin levels.

## Consequences of Altered Glucose Metabolism

### Oxidative Stress

Oxidative stress is defined as an imbalance between oxidants and antioxidants in favour of the oxidants. The oxidants, also termed ROS, are present as a normal product of aerobic metabolism but can be produced at elevated rates under pathophysiological conditions. They are intermediate compounds derived from the univalent reduction of molecular oxygen (by electrons and protons), characterised by a spared electron in the external orbital, which confers them a particular instability (anion superoxide $O_2^-$; hydroxyl radical $OH^-$); or compounds such as hydrogen peroxide ($H_2O_2$), which react with oxidable functional groups. Anion superoxide and hydrogen peroxide are poorly reactive but in the presence of the transitional form of some metals, such as $Fe^{3+}$, they generate the more reactive hydroxyl radical. These compounds are partially useful but potentially toxic, so the body is provided with several systems to counteract their activity. These systems include antioxidants produced in the body, both endogenous and exogenous, supplied from the diet. Endogenous antioxidants include both enzymatic defences, such as Se-GSH peroxidase, catalase and

SOD, as well as non-enzymatic defences, such as GSH, histidine peptides, the iron-binding proteins transferrin and ferritin, dihydrolipoic acid and reduced CoQ10 [50].

Glucose, through the pentose phosphate pathway, plays a key role in the synthesis of reducing compounds such as the reduced GSH, which is required to maintain the normal reduced state of the cells and to counteract all the deleterious effects of oxidative stress. GSH is synthesised inside the cells through a complex biochemical pathway composed of several well-known enzymes. During the reaction of $H_2O_2$ scavenging, GSH is oxidised to GSH disulphide (GSSG) by the enzyme GSH peroxidase. The reduction of GSSG to GSH is catalysed by GSSG reductase, which uses NADPH as reducing potential. NADPH is also required for the formation of active catalase tetramers. This latter enzyme catalyses the reduction of $H_2O_2$ to $H_2O$ and $O_2$. The NADPH required for the production of both GSH and catalase is produced by the pentose phosphate pathway. Glucose-6-phosphate dehydrogenase (G6PD) is the first and rate-limiting enzyme of the pentose phosphate pathway and recent results have demonstrated that this enzyme plays a protective role against ROS [52].

Reactive oxygen species, if not detoxified by the antioxidant systems, exert a toxic action on polyunsaturated fatty acids, circulating proteins, proteins of cell surface, enzymes and nucleic acid (DNA), leading to irreversible damage of cell structure and functions. Thus, an adequate presence and functioning of antioxidant systems is paramount for cell activity. In advanced cancer patients the high levels of ROS are caused by:

1. An increased production due to hypermetabolism, increased activation of the immune system and chronic inflammation with the associated release of proinflammatory cytokines, CRP and fibrinogen
2. An inadequate detoxification due to altered glucose metabolism in addition to symptoms such as anorexia/cachexia, nausea, and vomiting, that prevent a normal nutrition and thereby a normal supply of nutrients such as glucose, proteins and vitamins, leading to accumulation of ROS [53].
   In a series of our recently published studies

[50, 53, 54] we have demonstrated that patients with cancer at advanced stage showed a condition of oxidative stress characterised by high blood levels of ROS and reduced erythrocyte GSH peroxidase and SOD activity. Antioxidant activity was significantly reduced in patients with the most advanced stage (IV) and compromised performance status (EGOG PS 2-3). Moreover, oxidative stress was associated with high levels of proinflammatory cytokines IL-6 and TNF-α, and CRP, and low levels of leptin [51]. The inverse correlation between leptin levels and the parameters of oxidative stress (ROS) strongly suggests that leptin is a signal of negative energy balance and low energy reserves and that oxidative stress is a consequence of the metabolic derangements, particularly of glucose metabolism.

## Impairment of the Immune System

Immunodepression is a key feature of patients with CACS. The severity of immunodepression is related to stage of disease and severity of cachexia. Several of our studies demonstrated that the immune system of cancer patients shows an impaired blastic response to mitogens. The reduced proliferative response to mitogens (such as PHA, anti-CD3 antibody and recombinant IL-2) of peripheral blood mononuclear cells (PBMCs) isolated from cancer patients has to be considered as an index of more complex functional alterations. In normal circumstances (PBMCs isolated from healthy individuals) the above-cited mitogens induce cell cascade events similar to those occurring after antigen activation: production and release of cytokines, synthesis and release of IL-2 from CD4+ cells and surface expression of IL-2 receptor by lymphocytes. Thus, the blastic response depends on the amount of cytokines, IL-2 receptor expression and interaction between IL-2 and its receptor [55]. Patients with advanced cancer often exhibit a poorly functioning immune system manifested by anergy to skin-test antigens, decreased T-cell proliferation, alterations in signal transducing molecules, and reduced production of IL-2.

These defective functions correlate with the severity of disease and poor survival [56] and are actually considered a consequence of the oxidative

stress, which in turn is an effect of the cell's impaired glucose metabolism. In advanced cancer patients, the altered energy metabolism and particularly the defective glucose utilisation are responsible for the reduced synthesis of reducing compounds by the pentose-phosphate pathway. However, the correct immune cell functioning requires adequate concentrations of intracellular reducing compounds and particularly GSH. In fact, several studies have widely demonstrated that GSH is essential for the progression of activated lymphocytes into the cell cycle from G1 to S phase; the supplementation of GSH to the medium of cultured T cells increases the IL-2 receptor expression as well as its internalisation and degradation and ameliorates the blastic response of lymphocytes to PHA, anti-CD3 and recombinant IL-2.

Moreover, in addition to reduced antioxidant defences, increased levels of ROS sustained by the cancer-related chronic inflammation directly induce T-cell hyporesponsiveness and alter the expression levels of key T-cell-signalling molecules such as TCR-ζ and the TCR-dependent activation [57].

These hypotheses have been confirmed by several of our in vitro experiments, which demonstrated that, by adding the antioxidants N-acetyl cysteine, alpha lipoic acid and amifostine to the medium of cultured PBMCs isolated from advanced cancer patients, we were able to reverse in vitro the most significant functional defects of immune cells, such as response to mitogen (PHA) and antigens (anti CD3), the expression of surface activation markers (CD25 and CD95) and cell cycle progression (from G1 to S phase) [55, 58].

These findings confirm that impairment of energy metabolism, by inducing oxidative stress, is responsible for defective immune functions shown in advanced cancer patients and that correction of oxidative stress by appropriate antioxidants may reverse immunological deficits.

Leptin is a marker consistent with energy reserves and may be the signal that connects energy stores with the immune system. Moreover, several studies showed that leptin plays a role in immunosuppression: the decrease in leptin plasma concentrations during food deprivation leads to impaired immune function, whereas the restoration of leptin to normal levels by feeding after starvation is sufficient to ameliorate the immune response and is followed by a significant increase in Th1 activity, further supporting the role of leptin as a nutritional sensor for the immune functions [59, 60].

This evidence demonstrates that immunodepression in advanced cancer patients is a consequence of increased energy expenditure, altered energy metabolism pathways and reduced availability of energy substrates that are reflected by leptin levels and of which oxidative stress is the main manifestation.

## References

1. Tayek JA (1992) A review of cancer cachexia and abnormal glucose metabolism in humans with cancer. J Am Coll Nutr 11:445–456
2. Mantovani G, Macciò A, Lai P et al (1998) Cytokine activity in cancer-related anorexia/cachexia: role of megestrol acetate and medroxyprogesterone acetate. Semin Oncol 25(Suppl 6):45–52
3. Mantovani G, Macciò A, Massa E, Madeddu C (2001) Managing cancer-related anorexia/cachexia. Drugs 61:499–514
4. Kotler DP (2000) Cachexia. Ann Intern Med 133:622–634
5. Glicksman AS, Rawson RW (1956) Diabetes and altered carbohydrate metabolism in patients with cancer. Cancer 9:1127–1134
6. Werk EE Jr, Macgee J, Sholiton IJ (1964) Altered cortisol metabolism in advanced cancer and other terminal illnesses: excretion of 6-hydroxycortisol. Metabolism 13:1425–1438
7. Lundholm K, Holm G, Schersten T (1978) Insulin resistance in patients with cancer. Cancer Res 38:4665–4670
8. Argiles JM, Lopez-Soriano FJ (1999) The role of cytokines in cancer cachexia. Med Res Rev 19:223–248
9. Van der Poll T, Romijn JA, Endert E et al (1991) Tumor necrosis factor mimics the metabolic response to acute infection in healthy humans. Am J Physiol 261:E457–E465
10. Strassmann G, Fong M, Kenney JS, Jacob CO (1992) Evidence for the involvement of interleukin 6 in experimental cancer cachexia. J Clin Invest 89:1681–1684
11. Gelin J, Moldawer LL, Lonnroth C et al (1991) Role of endogenous tumor necrosis factor alpha and interleukin 1 for experimental tumor growth and the development of cancer cachexia. Cancer Res 51:415–421
12. Noguchi Y, Yoshikawa T, Matsumoto A et al (1996) Are cytokines possible mediators of cancer cachexia? Surg Today 26:467–475
13. Matthys P, Billiau A (1997) Cytokines and cachexia. Nutrition 13:763–770
14. Laviano A, Russo M, Freda F, Rossi Fanelli F (2002) Neurochemical mechanisms for cancer anorexia. Nutrition 18:100–105
15. Plata-Salaman CR (1998) Cytokine-induced anorexia. Behavioral, cellular, and molecular mechanisms. Ann NY Acad Sci 856:160–170
16. Sonti G, Ilyin SE, Plata-Salaman CR (1996) Anorexia induced by cytokine interactions at pathophysiological concentrations. Am J Physiol 270:R1394–R1402
17. Morley JE, Silver AJ, Miller DK, Rubenstein LZ (1989) The anorexia of the elderly. Ann NY Acad Sci 575:50–58
18. Jennische E, Skottner A, Hansson HA (1987) Satellite cells express the trophic factor IGF-1 in regenerating skeletal muscle. Acta Physiol Scand 129:9–15
19. Poggi C, Le Marchand-Brustel Y, Zapf J et al (1979) Effects and binding of insulin-like growth factor I in the isolated soleus muscle of lean and obese mice: comparison with insulin. Endocrinology 105:723–730
20. Yu KT, Czech MP (1984) The type I insulin-like growth factor receptor mediates the rapid effects of multiplication-stimulating activity on membrane transport systems in rat soleus muscle. J Biol Chem 259:3090–3095
21. Beguinot F, Kahn CR, Moses AC, Smith RJ (1985) Distinct biologically active receptors for insulin, insulin-like growth factor I, and insulin-like growth factor II in cultured skeletal muscle cells. J Biol Chem 260:15892–15898
22. Ng EH, Rock CS, Lazarus DD et al (1992) Insulin-like growth factor I preserves host lean tissue mass in cancer cachexia. Am J Physiol 262:R426–R431
23. Barbosa J, Bach FH (1987) Cell-mediated autoimmunity in type I diabetes. Diabetes Metab Rev 3:981–1004
24. Argiles JM, Lopez-Soriano J, Busquets S, Lopez-Soriano FJ (1997) Journey from cachexia to obesity by TNF. FASEB J 11:743–751
25. Sethi JK, Hotamisligil GS (1999) The role of TNF alpha in adipocyte metabolism. Semin Cell Dev Biol 10:19–29
26. Hauner H, Petruschke T, Russ M et al (1995) Effects of tumour necrosis factor alpha (TNF alpha) on glucose transport and lipid metabolism of newly-differentiated human fat cells in cell culture. Diabetologia 38:764–771
27. Kern PA, Ranganathan S, Li C et al (2002) Adipose tissue tumor necrosis factor and interleukin-6 expression in human obesity and insulin resistance. Am J Physiol Endocrinol Metab 280:E745–E751

28. Memon RA, Feingold KR, Moser AH et al (1998) Regulation of fatty acid transport protein and fatty acid translocase mRNA levels by endotoxin and cytokines. Am J Physiol 274:E210–E217

29. Memon RA, Fuller J, Moser AH et al (1998) In vivo regulation of acyl-CoA synthetase mRNA and activity by endotoxin and cytokines. Am J Physiol 275:E64–E72

30. Hotamisligil GS, Arner P, Caro JF et al (1995) Increased adipose tissue expression of tumor necrosis factor-alpha in human obesity and insulin resistance. J Clin Invest 95:2409–2415

31. Moller DE (2000) Potential role of TNF-alpha in the pathogenesis of insulin resistance and type 2 diabetes. Trends Endocrinol Metab 11:212–217

32. Strassmann G, Fong M, Kenney JS, Jacob CO (1992) Evidence for the involvement of interleukin 6 in experimental cancer cachexia. J Clin Invest 89:1681–1684

33. Navarra P, Pozzoli G, Brunetti L et al (1992) Interleukin-1 beta and interleukin-6 specifically increase the release of prostaglandin E2 from rat hypothalamic explants in vitro. Neuroendocrinology 56:61–68

34. Schwartz MW, Baskin DG, Kaiyala KJ, Woods SC (1999) Model for the regulation of energy balance and adiposity by the central nervous system. Am J Clin Nutr 69:584–596

35. Hukshorn CJ, Saris WH (2004) Leptin and energy expenditure. Curr Opin Clin Nutr Metab Care 7:629–633

36. Leibel RL, Rosenbaum M, Hirsch J (1995) Changes in energy expenditure resulting from altered body weight. N Engl J Med 332:621–628

37. Bornstein SR, Licinio J, Tauchnitz R et al (1998) Plasma leptin levels are increased in survivors of acute sepsis: associated loss of diurnal rhythm, in cortisol and leptin secretion. J Clin Endocrinol Metab 83:280–283

38. Zumbach MS, Boehme MW, Wahl P et al (1997) Tumor necrosis factor increases serum leptin levels in humans. J Clin Endocrinol Metab 82:4080–4082

39. Mantovani G, Macciò A, Mura L et al (2000) Serum levels of leptin and proinflammatory cytokines in patients with advanced-stage cancer at different sites. J Mol Med 78:554–561

40. Mantovani G, Macciò A, Madeddu C et al (2001) Serum values of proinflammatory cytokines are inversely correlated with serum leptin levels in patients with advanced stage cancer at different sites. J Mol Med 79:406–414

41. Aleman MR, Santolaria F, Batista N et al (2002) Leptin role in advanced lung cancer. A mediator of the acute phase response or a marker of the status of nutrition? Cytokine 19:21–26

42. Simons JP, Schols AM, Campfield LA et al (1997) Plasma concentration of total leptin and human lung-cancer-associated cachexia. Clin Sci (Lond) 93:273–277

43. Rosenbaum M, Nicolson M, Hirsch J et al (1997) Effects of weight change on plasma leptin concentrations and energy expenditure. J Clin Endocrinol Metab 82:3647–3654

44. Considine RV, Sinha MK, Heiman ML et al (1996) Serum immunoreactive-leptin concentrations in normal-weight and obese humans. N Engl J Med 334:292–295

45. Pi-Sunyer FX (2000) Overnutrition and undernutrition as modifiers of metabolic processes in disease states. Am J Clin Nutr 72:533S–537S

46. Havel PJ (2001) Peripheral signals conveying metabolic information to the brain: short-term and long-term regulation of food intake and energy homeostasis. Exp Biol Med (Maywood) 226:963–977

47. Havel PJ (2004) Update on adipocyte hormones: regulation of energy balance and carbohydrate/lipid metabolism. Diabetes 53:S1443–S1451

48. Keim NL, Stern JS, Havel PJ (1998) Relation between circulating leptin concentrations and appetite during a prolonged, moderate energy deficit in women. Am J Clin Nutr 68:794–801

49. Dubuc GR, Phinney SD, Stern JS, Havel PJ (1998) Changes of serum leptin and endocrine and metabolic parameters after 7 days of energy restriction in men and women. Metabolism 47:429–434

50. Mantovani G, Macciò A, Madeddu C et al (2002) Quantitative evaluation of oxidative stress, chronic inflammatory indices and leptin in cancer patients: correlation with stage and performance status. Int J Cancer 98:84–91

51. Mueller WM, Stanhope KL, Gregoire F et al (2000) Effects of metformin and vanadium on leptin secretion from cultured rat adipocytes. Obes Res 8:530–539

52. Salvemini F, Franze A, Iervolino A et al (1999) Enhanced glutathione levels and oxidoresistance mediated by increased glucose-6-phosphate dehydrogenase expression. J Biol Chem 274:2750–2757

53. Mantovani G, Madeddu C, Macciò A et al (2004) Cancer-related anorexia/cachexia syndrome and oxidative stress: an innovative approach beyond current treatment. Cancer Epidemiol Biomarkers Prev 13:1651–1659

54. Mantovani G, Macciò A, Madeddu C et al (2003) The impact of different antioxidant agents alone or in combination on reactive oxygen species, antioxidant enzymes and cytokines in a series of advanced cancer patients at different sites: correlation with disease progression. Free Radic Res 37:213–223

55. Mantovani G, Macciò A, Melis G et al (2000) Restoration of functional defects in peripheral blood mononuclear cells isolated from cancer patients by thiol antioxidants alpha-lipoic acid and N-acetyl cysteine. Int J Cancer 86:842–847

56. Malmberg KJ, Lenkei R, Petersson M et al (2002) A short-term dietary supplementation of high doses of vitamin E increases T helper 1 cytokine production in patients with advanced colorectal cancer. Clin

Cancer Res 8:1772–1778

57. Cemerski S, Cantagrel A, Van Meerwijk JP, Romagnoli P (2002) Reactive oxygen species differentially affect T cell receptor-signaling pathways. J Biol Chem 277:19585–19593

58. Mantovani G, Macciò A, Madeddu C et al (2003) Antioxidant agents are effective in inducing lymphocyte progression through cell cycle in advanced cancer patients: assessment of the most important laboratory indexes of cachexia and oxidative stress. J Mol Med 81:664–673

59. Palacio A, Lopez M, Perez-Bravo F et al (2002) Leptin levels are associated with immune response in malnourished infants. J Clin Endocrinol Metab 87:3040–3046

60. Faggioni R, Feingold KR, Grunfeld C (2001) Leptin regulation of the immune response and the immunodeficiency of malnutrition. FASEB J 15:2565–2571

# Cytokines in Cachexia

Giovanni Mantovani

## The Role of Acute-Phase Response in Cachexia

Tissue damage is a threat to well-being because it is self-promoting; that is, hydrolases released from inflammatory or injured cells cause further injury and provide substrate for formation and propagation of free radicals. For this reason, the body must localise and limit the injury and clear tissue debris. To perform these functions, the organism has developed an acute-phase response that includes stereotyped, coordinated adaptations ranging from behavioural to physiological [1]. The acute-phase response includes the hepatic synthesis of large quantities of proteins. The functions of the acute-phase proteins vary widely and include binding proteins (opsonins), protease inhibitors, complement factors, apoproteins, fibrinogen, and others.

For example, a cycle involving C-reactive protein, complement and interleukin-6 has been described [2]. C-reactive protein, which was named for its ability to bind to a specific bacterial lipopolysaccharide, circulates in low quantities in healthy persons; however, its levels increase in response to inflammatory or neoplastic processes. C-reactive protein is an opsonin that binds to denatured proteins, lipopolysaccharides and nucleic acids. Binding leads to local complement activation and phagocytosis by macrophages through their complement receptors. The complement-split products stimulate release of interleukin-6 by macrophages, which in turn stimulates the synthesis and secretion of more C-reactive protein in the liver. This completes a positive feedback loop. The intensity of this response is quantitatively related to the amount of tissue debris; the response extinguishes itself after tissue debris is cleared.

The acute-phase response has nutritional implications. It is energy-intensive with high rates of hepatic protein synthesis and requires large quantities of essential amino acids. The need for essential amino acids drives the loss of skeletal muscle. The survival value is obvious: an injured animal has an impaired ability to obtain exogenous protein, and skeletal muscle, which represents approximately 40% of body weight in men and approximately 33% in women, is the largest available pool of protein. The tradeoff may be viewed as a shift in the body's priorities from offensive to defensive. The adaptation is effective over the short term because skeletal muscle is replaced rapidly as recovery is completed. Problems ensue when the process is chronic because skeletal muscle depletion contributes increasingly to morbidity and mortality.

## Changes in Intermediary Metabolism During the Acute-Phase Response

The acute-phase response includes coordinated adaptations in intermediary metabolism, which differ from those of starvation. A major difference is an increase in protein degradation in skeletal muscle. Recent studies have partially defined the mechanisms by which cellular protein turnover is regulated. Turnover rates vary for individual proteins. Regulatory proteins, such as those that control the cell cycle, have extremely rapid turnover; for others, such as myofibrillar proteins in skeletal muscle, turnover is slower. Of the various cellular proteolytic pathways, the adenosine triphosphate-dependent ubiquitin–proteasome pathway has the predominant role in the regulation of protein turnover [3]. Cachexia is also characterised by changes in fat metabolism, including hypertriglyceridaemia, increased hepatic secretion of very-low-density lipoproteins, decreased lipoprotein lipase activity, increased de novo triglyceride synthesis and esterification, increased release of free fatty acid from the periphery, and a futile cycle of fatty acids between the liver and adipose tissue beds. These changes, which are promoted by a variety of cytokines, maintain serum lipid concentrations despite the presence of anorexia [4].

Alterations in carbohydrate metabolism include peripheral insulin resistance, which is also mediated by proinflammatory cytokines.

## Cytokine Regulation of the Acute-Phase Response

The realisation that the response to illness and injury is an endogenous, not exogenous, process was a milestone in the understanding of cachexia. Our understanding that cytokines regulate the acute-phase response and cachexia resulted from several observations. For example, studies of hypertriglyceridaemia in experimental infections suggested indirect, or endogenous, control; the degree of hypertriglyceridaemia was not necessarily correlated with infectious or tumour burden, and metabolic effects of infection could be reproduced with dead organisms or even with supernatants of macrophage cultures stimulated in vitro. The responsible protein was sought, isolated, and named cachectin, and its sequence was found to be identical to that reported for tumour necrosis factor (TNF) [5]. These studies concluded that this molecule was the mediator of cachexia. At approximately the same time, other investigators demonstrated that proteolysis in animals occurred after infusion of a leukocyte-derived factor [6], in keeping with the notion of an endogenous mediator of the acute-phase response [7]. This mediator was found after diverse stresses, ranging from vaccination to sepsis. The circulatory nature of a cachectic factor was shown by using parabiotic rats – that is, animals grown with a surgically produced shared vascular supply. Cancer implanted in one rat led to anorexia and cachexia in both rats [8]. Analysis of the components of leukocyte endogenous mediator yielded interleukin-1 and other proinflammatory cytokines. Further studies have shown that many cytokines are capable of inducing metabolic changes [4], although some specificity among cytokines can be demonstrated by using experimentally altered animal models.

Proinflammatory cytokines are protein mediators that are secreted from immunocompetent cells and other cells and that mediate the acute-phase response, among other functions. As noted, metabolic effects of cytokines can be distinguished from those of starvation by pair-feeding. One implication of combining immunological and nutritional signal functions within a single molecule is that the intensity of the nutritional adaptation parallels the other cytokine effects. Most experimental work has concentrated on TNF, interleukin-1 and interleukin-6, although other cytokines and chemokines also mediate the acute-phase response. The mode of action is predominantly paracrine and autocrine. A series of animal studies demonstrated that the predominant cytokine effect is local. Central infusion of TNF led to predominant anorexia, and peripheral production of TNF produced predominant metabolic losses of protein [9].

Cytokines do mediate systemic effects, however. Among the proinflammatory cytokines, interleukin-6 has the longest serum half-life and may have important endocrine effects. Circulation of mononuclear cells that secrete cytokines in a target organ is an alternate way to achieve a classic endocrine effect. Such a mechanism might be especially important in transmission of cytokine signals through the blood–brain barrier.

Proinflammatory cytokines exert a variety of behavioural and physiological effects in addition to their immunological and nutritional functions. Anorexia results from proinflammatory cytokine activity and has both central and peripheral elements. The central effect is at the level of the hypothalamic nuclei, which control feeding behaviour.

Several cytokines affect food intake directly or through other mediators, such as corticotropin-releasing hormone, serotonin or leptin. Leptin, a cytokine secreted from adipocytes, which has prominent effects on feeding behaviour and energy balance, is believed to be a major peripheral regulator of long-term body composition. It is also thought to be responsible for self-correcting changes in energy intake and expenditure that can be demonstrated after voluntary overfeeding and underfeeding [10]. However, animal studies demonstrated that endotoxin leads to a dose-dependent increase in plasma leptin and white fat leptin mRNA, which implies that leptin might be a mediator of anorexia in cachexia. There is a normal relationship between plasma leptin concentration and body fat content in healthy persons as well as in patients with AIDS, cancer and chronic obstructive pulmonary disease [11–15]. Leptin does not mediate the metabolic changes of the acute-phase response [16].

Several alterations in gastrointestinal function that indirectly affect nutritional status have been ascribed to proinflammatory cytokines, including altered gastric emptying. Decreases in intestinal blood flow, changes in small bowel motility, changes in cellular proliferation, and altered ion fluxes have also been described.

## References

1. Kushner I (1993) Regulation of the acute phase response by cytokines. Perspect Biol Med 36:611–622
2. Gotschlich EC (1989) C-reactive protein. A historical overview. Ann NY Acad Sci 557:9-18
3. Mitch WE, Goldberg AL (1996) Mechanisms of muscle wasting. The role of the ubiquitin-proteasome pathway. N Engl J Med 335:1897–1905
4. Feingold KR, Soued M, Serio MK et al (1989) Multiple cytokines stimulate hepatic lipid synthesis in vivo. Endocrinology 125:267–274
5. Beutler B, Greenwald D, Hulmes JD et al (1985) Identity of tumour necrosis factor and the macrophage-secreted factor cachectin. Nature 316:552–554
6. Baracos V, Rodemann HP, Dinarello CA et al (1983) Stimulation of muscle protein degradation and prostaglandin E2 release by leukocytic pyrogen (interleukin-1). N Engl J Med 308:553–558
7. Powanda MC, Beisel WR (1982) Hypothesis: leukocyte endogenous mediator/endogenous pyrogen/lymphocyte-activating factor modulates the development of nonspecific and specific immunity and affects nutritional status. Am J Clin Nutr 35:762–768
8. Norton JA, Moley JF, Green MV et al (1985) Parabiotic transfer of cancer anorexia/cachexia in male rats. Cancer Res 45:5547–5552
9. Tracey KJ, Morgello S, Koplin B et al (1990) Metabolic effects of cachectin/tumor necrosis factor are modified by site of production. Cachectin/tumor necrosis factor-secreting tumor in skeletal muscle induces chronic cachexia, while implantation in brain induces predominantly acute anorexia. J Clin Invest 86:2014–2024
10. Leibel RL, Rosenbaum M, Hirsch J (1995) Changes in energy expenditure resulting from altered body weight. N Engl J Med 332:621–628
11. Grunfeld C, Pang M, Shigenaga JK et al (1996) Serum leptin levels in the acquired immunodeficiency syndrome. J Clin Endocrinol Metab 81:4342–4346
12. Simons JP, Schols AM, Campfield LA et al (1997) Plasma concentration of total leptin and human lung-cancer-associated cachexia. Clin Sci (Colch) 93:273–277
13. Wallace AM, Sattar N, McMillan DC (1998) Effect of weight loss and the inflammatory response on leptin concentrations in gastrointestinal cancer patients. Clin Cancer Res 4:2977–2979
14. Takabatake N, Nakamura H, Abe S et al (1999) Circulating leptin in patients with chronic obstructive pulmonary disease. Am J Respir Crit Care Med 159:1215–1219
15. Schols AM, Creutzberg EC, Buurman WA et al (1999) Plasma leptin is related to proinflammatory status and dietary intake in patients with chronic obstructive pulmonary disease. Am J Respir Crit Care Med 160:1220–1226
16. Kaibara A, Moshyedi A, Auffenberg T et al (1998) Leptin produces anorexia and weight loss without inducing an acute phase response or protein wasting. Am J Physiol 274:R1518–R1525

# Cytokines in Chronic Inflammation

Wolfgang Langhans

With the tremendous increase in scientific knowledge about cytokines and their immune functions, it has also become clear that cytokines have systemic and local effects that are only partly related to their coordinating functions in the immune system. Thus, proinflammatory cytokines are the major endogenous mediators of anorexia and cachexia during chronic diseases. They have substantial hypermetabolic effects, which are at the core of the organism's fever reaction, and, last but not least, they are implicated in the metabolic disturbances and several other comorbidities of obesity, in particular by contributing to insulin resistance. This chapter summarises current knowledge of these effects: it describes studies including different levels of scientific analysis, from the molecular through cellular to the systemic and behavioural levels, which reveal interesting features of the role of cytokines in these phenomena.

## Introduction

The term inflammation describes a complex series of events, many of which are coordinated by cytokines. More than 100 structurally identified cytokines with unique and redundant actions have been identified (see [1] for review). Several cytokines share receptors or intracellular signalling mechanisms, and this presumably accounts for part of their redundant actions. Cytokine production is not constitutive, but triggered by many different stimuli. Virtually all cells can produce cytokines, with production cycles usually lasting from a few hours to a few days, but cytokine production may be prolonged if the stimulus persists in a chronic disease. The high potency of cytokines is related to the high affinity

of their receptors and to the fact that signalling requires only low (often < 10%) receptor occupancy [1]. Cytokines are broadly categorised as being proinflammatory or anti-inflammatory: i.e., cytokines are involved in both pathogenesis of and protection against the disease [2]. In addition to their immune-related effects, cytokines affect other physiological functions and cause central nervous system (CNS)-mediated effects such as fever, sleep, and an activation of the hypothalamic–pituitary–adrenal axis. This chapter provides a brief overview of the role of proinflammatory cytokines in three main phenomena associated with chronic inflammation and/or infection, i.e., anorexia, hypermetabolism and changes in insulin action.

## Cytokines and Anorexia

### General

Several proinflammatory cytokines, including interleukin-1 (IL-1), IL-2, IL-6, IL-8, tumour necrosis factor-$\alpha$ (TNF-$\alpha$) and interferon-$\gamma$ (IFN-$\gamma$), reduce food intake after peripheral or central administration in laboratory animals [3, 4]. Some cytokines suppress feeding synergistically [3, 4]. The anorectic effects of cytokines are pathophysiologically relevant because acute antagonism of particular cytokines and/or their receptors often attenuates anorexia in various diseases or models of disease [5]. Furthermore, several immune challenges reduce food intake less in mice that are genetically deficient in a particular cytokine or cytokine receptor than in control animals (see below). Failure to establish a role for a particular cytokine in disease-related anorexia with genetic knock-out (KO) mice [5] is presumably due to the redundant and overlapping actions of cytokines, which allow for developmental compensation. Interestingly, the feeding-suppressive effect of proinflammatory cytokines appears to be enhanced by oestradiol [6], which fits the well-known modulatory effect of ovarian hormones on immune system activity and the responsiveness to cytokines in female mammals [7]. Anhedonic effects of cytokines may contribute to or enhance anorexia under certain circumstances [5, 8], but do not appear to be the major cause of their anorectic effects [5].

## Central Cytokines

Glia cells and neurons in various brain areas express proinflammatory cytokines and cytokine receptors [9, 10]. Acute and chronic CNS diseases (e.g., meningitis, encephalitis, multiple sclerosis, Alzheimer's disease, stroke and brain tumours) stimulate CNS cytokine production [11, 12]. Cytokines produced within the blood–brain barrier (BBB) can act directly on neural circuitries controlling energy balance, and intracerebroventricular (ICV) administration of proinflammatory cytokines presumably models the clinical features of such diseases, e.g. anorexia. Peripheral immune stimulation may increase de novo proinflammatory cytokine synthesis in the brain, and this may contribute to anorexia in some of these conditions [3, 13–15]. Often, however, centrally produced cytokines may not be essential in the anorexia of systemic immune challenges because a crucial cytokine is not expressed in the brain [16], the cytokine expression pattern does not fit a role in the anorexia [17], and only unnaturally strong peripheral stimuli induce CNS cytokine synthesis [17]. Finally, peripheral immune stimulation may increase cytokines but reduces cytokine receptor expression in the brain [18], and the latter effect may attenuate any net effect of centrally produced cytokines on food intake.

## Peripheral Cytokines

Cytokines produced outside the BBB have local catabolic effects (proteolysis, lipolysis) (see [19] for review) and can influence CNS-mediated functions by activating afferent nerves, by releasing other peripheral mediators, by acting at the BBB, or by being transported into the brain. Figure 1 shows a rough scheme of how peripheral cytokines are able to affect CNS-mediated functions. We have shown that afferent autonomic nerves from below the diaphragm are not necessary for the anorectic effect of intraperitoneally (IP) injected IL-1β (see [20] for review). Also, leptin does not appear to be a necessary mediator of peripheral IL-1β anorectic effect because IP-injected IL-1β reduced food intake similarly in obese and lean Zucker rats [21]. Yet, IL-1β increases leptin expression [22], and the multiple interactions between IL-1β and leptin may also result in modulation of the effects of both peptides on energy balance. In addition to activating afferent nerves or triggering the release of other humoral mediators in the periphery, circulating cytokines may get direct access to the brain through circumventricular organs and active transport mechanisms [23]. Finally, IL-1β and other cytokines may trigger the release of downstream mediators by acting through receptors on BBB capillary endothelial cells. In these cells, proinflammatory cytokines cause activation of the transcription factor NF-κB [24, 25], increase cyclo-oxygenase-2 (COX-2) mRNA expression [26–28], and trigger the release of neuromodulators such as nitric oxide or prostanoids [26, 29]. Together with cytokines, which are also produced by BBB endothelial cells, these mediators can affect neurons involved in control of energy balance. Activation of COX-2 and the subsequent release of prostanoids appears to be particularly important in this context [30–32] and is involved in the anorectic effect of IL-1β [32, 33] as well as in cancer cachexia and anorexia [30]. PGE 2 and/or other prostanoids act on prostanoid receptors on neurons that project to brain sites involved in food intake control, in particular to the paraventricular (PVN) and arcuate (ARC) nuclei of the hypothalamus [5].

## Central Neural Mediation of Cytokine-Induced Anorexia

Peripherally administered IL-1β induces c-fos immunoreactivity in the PVN and ARC of the hypothalamus [34]. The ARC is considered to be the major hypothalamic detection site for blood-derived signals. Yet, severing the ARC from PVN or its connections with the PVN only slightly attenuated peripheral IL-1β-induced anorexia [35], indicating that the ARC is involved but not necessary for peripheral IL-1β-induced anorexia. Several lines of evidence [20] implicate activation of hindbrain to forebrain aminergic neurons in the feeding suppression and hypermetabolic effects of circulating IL-1β. IL-1β-induced anorexia may in part be mediated through prostaglandin E2-dependent activation of serotoninergic neurons originating in the raphe nuclei and projecting to the hypothalamus [36]. In line with this idea, systemic administration of a serotonin (5-HT$_{2C}$) receptor antagonist and microinjection of the 5-HT$_{1A}$ autoreceptor agonist 8-hydroxy-2-(di-n-propylamino)tetraline (8-OH-DPAT) directly into the raphe nucleus both markedly attenuated the feeding-suppressive effect of peripherally injected IL-1-β [3]. Interestingly, anorexia induced by experimental colitis in rats is mediated, in part, by the stimulatory effect of IL-1 on medial hypothalamic 5-HT [37]. It is still largely unknown whether TNF-α inhibits feeding through the same mechanisms as IL-1β. It has been shown, however, that both cytokines can replace each other in mediating infection-induced anorexia [38]. These and other results suggest that cytokines act in concert to inhibit eating [5]. In addition to 5-HT, melanocortins are involved in the anorexia and weight loss associated with inflammatory and neoplastic disease processes. Studies using melanocortin antagonists (SHU9119 or agouti-related peptide) or genetic approaches (melanocortin-4 receptor KO mice) suggest that melanocortin action is required for anorexia and weight loss induced by injected lipopolysaccharide (LPS, an inflammatory gram-negative bacterial cell wall product) or by implantation of prostate or lung cancer cells. Although the precise mechanisms for the effects of peripheral inflammation or neoplasia on the melanocortin system remain unknown, it is reasonable to assume that proinflammatory cytokines (IL-1β, IL-6, TNF-α) play a role [39, 40].

Interestingly, 5-HT and the melanocortin system appear to jointly contribute to the anorexia in chronic inflammation and infection. Most recent data indicate that activation of 5-HTergic neurons ultimately influences the hypothalamic melanocortin pathways of energy balance regulation and that activation of the melanocortin system is necessary to produce the complete anorectic effect of 5-HTergic activation [41]. In line with this hypothesis, anorectic 5-HTergic drugs activated pro-opiomelanocortin (POMC) neurons in the ARC, and this effect appeared to be mediated by the 5-HT$_{2C}$ receptor expressed on POMC neurons [41]. The exact mechanisms of this interaction between 5-HT and the melanocortin pathway still need to be determined.

Also, IL-1β appears to be essential for the production of ciliary neurotrophic factor (CNTF) in response to brain injury or trauma [42]. CNTF was first characterised as a trophic factor for motor neurons in the ciliary ganglion and spinal cord and subsequently found to markedly reduce food intake and body weight [43]. This makes CNTF a possible mediator of IL-1β effects on food intake and energy expenditure. Some data suggest that CNTF ultimately affects energy balance by markedly reducing the expression and action of NPY [44]. A reduction of hypothalamic NPY has also been implicated in the feeding-suppressive effect of IL-1β [45]. Summarising, several lines of evidence suggest that the pathways of cytokine-induced suppression of feeding and stimulation of energy expenditure ultimately converge on the well-characterised hypothalamic neuropeptide systems that control energy balance.

## Cytokines and Hypermetabolism

Hypermetabolism, i.e. an increase in resting energy expenditure, occurs in many cachectic diseases [46]. Several cytokines, including TNF-α, IL-1β and IL-6 [47–49], have been shown to stimulate energy expenditure and to induce fever as part of their effects on CNS mechanisms of defence and/or energy balance control.

Similar to the cytokine anorectic effects (see above), cytokine-induced hypermetabolism appears to result from synergistic and sequential interactions [50] and to involve the same principles of action of circulating cytokines on the CNS [51–53] (see Fig. 1 and above). Some discrepancy exists as to whether the vagus is involved in the hypermetabolic effect of cytokines. Whereas some studies provide evidence for a vagal mediation [54–56], others do not [57, 58]. Different routes of administration (i.e., intraperitoneal vs. intravenous) [59] and/or different doses [60] of the involved cytokine may contribute to some of the observed discrepancies. In addition, the time and duration of measurement may be crucial because some evidence suggests that vagal afferents are involved in the immediate fever effect of peripheral cytokines, but not in their longer-term actions [55].

An alternative pathway of metabolic stimulation has recently been demonstrated for IFNγ. A study in experimentally induced murine toxoplasmosis showed that the hypermetabolism in this animal model depends on IFN-γ and is due to a stimulation of extramitochondrial lipid oxidation in macrophage-rich tissues [61]. This suggests that IFN-γ-dependent stimulation of the oxidative burst in macrophages can be a major contributor to the hypermetabolic response in some pathological situations.

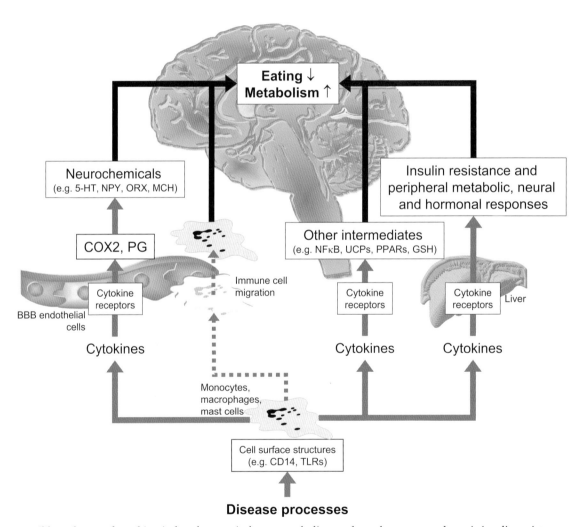

**Fig. 1.** Possible pathways of cytokine-induced anorexia, hypermetabolism and, to a lesser extent, hepatic insulin resistance. See text for further details. *5-HT*, serotonin; *ARC*, arcuate nucleus; *BBB*, blood–brain barrier; *COX-2*, cyclo-oxygenase-2; *GSH*, glutathione; *MCH*, melanin-concentrating hormone; *NF-κB*, transcription factor nuclear factor-κB; *NPY*, neuropeptide Y; *ORX*, orexin; *PG*, prostaglandins; *PPARs*, peroxisome proliferator-activated receptors; *TLRs*, toll-like receptors; *UCPs*, uncoupling proteins

Moreover, IP administration of LPS or tumour burden increased UCP2 gene expression in the brain, and this was also observed after LPS treatment in TNF-1 receptor and TNF-2 receptor KO mice. Thus, the brain may contribute significantly to the increase in energy expenditure associated with fever and tumour burden, and TNF-α does not appear to be a necessary mediator of this response [62]. Yet, another study in genetically modified mice implicated natural killer cells and IFN-γ as well as TNF-α in the metabolic alterations induced by LPS [16]. Exogenous TNF-α has also been shown to induce thermogenesis and UCP2 mRNA expression in broadly distributed tissues in rats, including brown and white adipose tissue as well as skeletal muscle [63]. Overall, it appears safe to say that the common proinflammatory cytokines TNF-α, IL-1β and IFN-γ all contribute to hypermetabolism in chronic disease/inflammation through different, presumably overlapping mechanisms.

An interesting new discovery related to the hypermetabolism in chronic inflammation is that proinflammatory cytokines activate the transcriptional peroxisome proliferator-activated receptor gamma (PPARγ) coactivator-1 (PGC-1): this activation is mediated through phosphorylation by p38 kinase. The PGC-1 is considered to be a master regulator of oxidative metabolism.

Activation of PGC-1 in cultured muscle cells or muscle in vivo causes increased respiration and expression of genes linked to mitochondrial uncoupling and energy expenditure. Thus, PGC-1, which is expressed in normal skeletal muscle, may provide a new link between proinflammatory cytokines and increased energy expenditure [64].

## Cytokines and Insulin Resistance

In addition to their well-known anorectic and hypermetabolic effects, cytokines appear to be involved in obesity-related disorders such as insulin resistance and vascular diseases [65]. Epidemiological findings support the hypothesis that the metabolic syndrome, type II diabetes and cardiovascular diseases have an inflammatory component mediated by cytokines [66, 67]. Thus, overweight and obese children as well as adults

have elevated serum levels of C-reactive protein, IL-6 and TNF-α, which are known markers of inflammation, closely associated with cardiovascular risk factors as well as cardiovascular and non-cardiovascular causes of death [66]. The inflammatory mediators and/or cytokines involved may originate from adipose tissue.

TNF-α was among the first substances to be implicated in fat cell insulin resistance [68]. Adipose tissue TNF-α expression is increased in obese subjects, and TNF-α may limit an increase in adipocyte size by inhibiting lipoprotein lipase (LPL) and increasing insulin resistance [68]. A p55 TNF-α receptor-mediated phosphorylation of serine residues on the insulin receptor substrate-1 (IRS-1) appears to be an important mechanism for the induction of insulin resistance by TNF-α [69, 70]. The genetic deficiency of TNF-α or TNF-α signalling resulted in improved insulin sensitivity, lower levels of circulating free fatty acids, and protection from the obesity-related reduction in the insulin receptor signalling in muscle and fat tissues. All these results indicate that TNF-α is an important mediator of insulin resistance in obesity through its effects on several important sites of insulin action [71, 72].

The expression of the proinflammatory cytokine IL-6, like that of TNF-α and IL-8, is increased in human fat cells from insulin-resistant individuals, and IL-6 is also associated with the insulin resistance of obesity and type II diabetes [73]. Interestingly, TNF-α markedly increases IL-6 mRNA and protein secretion. Chronic IL-6 treatment selectively impaired hepatic insulin signalling in vivo, further supporting a role for IL-6 in hepatic insulin resistance. IL-6, like TNF-α, exerts long-term inhibitory effects on the gene transcription of IRS-1, glucose transporter-4 (GLUT-4) and PPARγ. Moreover, IL-6 reduced GLUT-4 mRNA and insulin-stimulated glucose transport in vivo [74]. IL-6 also decreased refeeding-dependent glucokinase mRNA induction and reduced insulin sensitivity. This decrease was characterised by a reduction in tyrosine phosphorylation of IRS-1 and a decreased association of the p85 subunit of phosphatidylinositol 3-kinase with IRS-1 in response to physiological insulin levels. In addition, insulin-dependent activation of

Akt, important in mediating insulin downstream metabolic actions, was markedly inhibited by IL-6. These and other data suggest that IL-6 plays a direct role in insulin resistance at the cellular level in the liver (see Fig. 1) and may contribute to insulin resistance and type II diabetes [75].

Another possible mechanism for the effect of proinflammatory cytokines, and in particular of IL-6, on insulin resistance is by induction of suppressors of cytokine signalling (SOCS) [76]. Members of the SOCS family associate with the insulin receptor (IR), and their ectopic expression inhibits IR signalling. Several SOCS proteins are induced by IL-6, and SOCS-3 induction in the liver by IL-6 may be an important mechanism of IL-6-mediated insulin resistance. Cell culture studies in 3T3-L1 adipocytes revealed that insulin resistance-inducing cytokines also increase the expression of SOCS-1 and SOCS-3 in adipocytes, which may be important intracellular mediators of insulin resistance in fat cells and a potential pharmacological target for the treatment of impaired insulin sensitivity [77]. These results suggest that SOCS proteins may be inhibitors of IR signalling and could mediate cytokine-induced insulin resistance, thus contributing to the pathogenesis of type II diabetes [78].

Finally, proinflammatory cytokines may induce insulin resistance in part by increasing the expression of resistin, a polypeptide that induces insulin resistance in rodents. In rodents, resistin is predominantly expressed in adipocytes, whereas in humans, peripheral blood mononuclear cells (PBMC) seem to be a major source of resistin. Proinflammatory cytokines (IL-1, IL-6, TNF-$\alpha$) strongly increase PBMC resistin mRNA expression. Thus, in humans, resistin may be among the factors that link chronic inflammation and insulin resistance [79]. A reduced secretion of adiponectin may also contribute to the increased cardiovascular risk factors and manifestation of metabolic syndrome in obese individuals. TNF-$\alpha$ and adiponectin appear to be antagonistic in stimulating NF-$\kappa$B activation. Thus, TNF-$\alpha$ induces oxidative stress, which exacerbates pathological processes leading to oxidised low-density lipoproteins and dyslipidaemia, glucose intolerance, insulin resistance, hypertension, endothelial dysfunction and atherogenesis. NF-$\kappa$B activation further stimulates the production of additional inflammatory cytokines, along with adhesion molecules, which promote endothelial dysfunction. Elevated free fatty acids, glucose and insulin levels enhance this NF-$\kappa$B activation and further downstream modulate specific clinical manifestations of metabolic syndrome [80].

# References

1. Oppenheim JJ, Feldmann M (2001) Introduction to the role of cytokines in innate host defense and adaptive immunity. In: Oppenheim JJ, Feldmann M (eds) Cytokine Reference, Volume 1: Ligands. Academic Press, San Diego, pp 3–20
2. Feldmann M, Saklatvala J (2001) Proinflammatory cytokines. In: Oppenheim JJ, Feldmann M (eds) Cytokine Reference, Volume 1: Ligands. Academic Press, San Diego, pp 291–305
3. Langhans W, Hrupka BJ (2003) Cytokines and appetite. In: Kronfol Z (ed) Cytokines and mental health. Kluwer/Academic Publishers, Boston, pp 167–224
4. Plata-Salamàn CR (1995) Cytokines and feeding suppression: an integrative view from neurologic to molecular levels. Nutrition 11:674–677
5. Langhans W (2004) Anorexia during disease. Neurobiology of food and fluid intake. In: Stricker E, Woods SC (eds) Handbook of Behavioral Neurobiology, 2nd ed. Kluwer Academic/Plenum Publishers, London, pp 347–379
6. Butera PC, Doerflinger AL, Roberto F (2002) Cyclic estradiol treatment enhances the effects of interleukin-1 beta on food intake in female rats. Brain Behav Immun 16:275–281
7. Geary N (2001) Sex differences in disease anorexia. Nutrition 17:499–507
8. Merali Z, Brennan K, Brau P, Anisman H (2003) Dissociating anorexia and anhedonia elicited by interleukin-1 beta: antidepressant and gender effects on responding for 'free chow' and 'earned' sucrose intake. Psychopharmacology (Berl) 165:413–418
9. Gayle D, Ilyin SE, Plata-Salamàn CR (1997) Interleukin-1 receptor type mRNA levels in brain regions from male and female rats. Brain Res Bull 42:463–467
10. Vitkovic L, Bockaert J, Jacque C (2000) 'Inflammatory' cytokines: neuromodulators in nor-

mal brain? J Neurochem 74:457–471

11. Plata-Salamàn CR, Turrin NP (1999) Cytokine interactions and cytokine balance in the brain: relevance to neurology and psychiatry. Mol Psychiatry 4:303–306

12. Rothwell NJ (1999) Cytokines - killers in the brain? J Physiol 514:3–17

13. Laviano A, Renvyle T, Meguid MM et al (1995) Relationship between interleukin-1 and cancer anorexia. Nutrition 11:680–683

14. Mchugh KJ, Collins SM, Weingarten HP (1994) Central interleukin-1 receptors contribute to suppression of feeding after acute colitis in the rat. Am J Physiol 266:R1659–R1663

15. Plata-Salamàn CR, Ilyin SE, Gayle D (1998) Brain cytokine mRNAs in anorectic rats bearing prostate adenocarcinoma tumor cells. Am J Physiol 44:R566–R573

16. Arsenijevic D, Garcia I, Vesin C et al (2000) Differential roles of tumor necrosis factor-alpha and interferon-gamma in mouse hypermetabolic and anorectic responses induced by LPS. Eur Cytokine Netw 11:662–668

17. Eriksson C, Nobel S, Winblad B, Schultzberg M (2000) Expression of interleukin-1 alpha and beta, and interleukin-1 receptor antagonist mRNA in the rat central nervous system after peripheral administration of lipopolysaccharides. Cytokine 12:423–431

18. Haour F, Marquette C, Ban E et al (1995) Receptors for interleukin-1 in the central nervous and neuroendocrine systems - role in infection and stress. Ann Endocrinol (Paris) 56:173–179

19. Langhans W (2002) Peripheral mechanisms involved with catabolism. Curr Opin Clin Nutr Metab Care 5:419–426

20. Langhans W (2000) Anorexia of infection: current prospects. Nutrition 16:996–1005

21. Lugarini F, Hrupka BJ, Schwartz GJ et al (2005) Acute and chronic administrtion of immunomodultors induces anorexia in obese (fa/fa) and lean (fa/?) Zucker rats. Physiol Behav 84:165–173

22. Grunfeld C, Zhao C, Fuller J et al (1996) Endotoxin and cytokines induce expression of leptin, the ob gene product, in hamsters - A role for leptin in the anorexia of infection. J Clin Invest 97:2152–2157

23. Banks WA, Kastin AJ (1996) Passage of peptides across the blood-brain barrier: pathophysiological perspectives. Life Sci 59:1923–1943

24. Bierhaus A, Chen J, Liliensiek B, Nawroth PP (2000) LPS and cytokine-activated endothelium. Semin Thromb Hemost 26:571–587

25. Laflamme N, Lacroix S, Rivest S (1999) An essential role of interleukin-1 beta in mediating NF-kappa B activity and COX-2 transcription in cells of the blood-brain barrier in response to a systemic and localized inflammation but not during endotoxemia. J Neurosci 19:10923–10930

26. Cao CY, Matsumura K, Yamagata K, Watanabe Y (1996) Endothelial cells of the rat brain vasculature express cyclooxygenase-2 mRNA in response to systemic interleukin-1 beta: a possible site of prostaglandin synthesis responsible for fever. Brain Res 733:263–272

27. Kalaria RN (1999) Cerebral endothelial activation and signal transduction mechanisms during inflammation and infectious disease. Am J Pathol 154:1311–1314

28. Lacroix S, Rivest S (1998) Effect of acute systemic inflammatory response and cytokines on the transcription of the genes encoding cyclooxygenase enzymes (COX-1 and COX-2) in the rat brain. J Neurochem 70:452–466

29. Nadeau S, Rivest S (1999) Effects of circulating tumor necrosis factor on the neuronal activity and expression of the genes encoding the tumor necrosis factor receptors (p55 and p75) in the rat brain: a view from the blood-brain barrier. Neuroscience 93:1449–1464

30. Cahlin C, Korner A, Axelsson H et al (2000) Experimental cancer cachexia: the role of host-derived cytokines interleukin (IL)-6, IL-12, interferon-gamma, and tumor necrosis factor alpha evaluated in gene knockout, tumor-bearing mice on C57 Bl background and eicosanoid-dependent cachexia. Cancer Res 60:5488–5493

31. Lugarini F, Hrupka BJ, Schwartz GJ et al (2002) A role for cyclooxygenase-2 in lipopolysaccharide-induced anorexia in rats. Am J Physiol 283:R862–R868

32. Swiergiel AH, Dunn AJ (2002) Distinct roles for cyclooxygenases 1 and 2 in interleukin-1-induced behavioral changes. J Pharmacol Exp Ther 302:1031–1036

33. Langhans W, Savoldelli D, Weingarten S (1993) Comparison of the feeding responses to bacterial lipopolysaccharide and interleukin-1beta. Physiol Behav 53:643–649

34. Herkenham M, Lee HY, Baker RA (1998) Temporal and spatial patterns of c-fos mRNA induced by intravenous interleukin-1: a cascade of non-neuronal cellular activation at the blood-brain barrier. J Comp Neurol 400:175-196

35. Reyes TM, Sawchenko PE (2002) Involvement of the arcuate nucleus of the hypothalamus in interleukin-1-induced anorexia. J Neurosci 22:5091-5099

36. Ericsson A, Arias C, Sawchenko PE (1997) Evidence for an intramedullary prostaglandin-dependent mechanism in the activation of stress-related neuroendocrine circuitry by intravenous interleukin-1. J Neurosci 17:7166-7179

37. El Haj T, Poole S, Farthing MJG, Ballinger AB (2002) Anorexia in a rat model of colitis: interaction of interleukin- 1 and hypothalamic serotonin. Brain Res 927:1-7

38. Bluthe RM, Laye S, Michaud B et al (2000) Role of interleukin-1 beta and tumour necrosis factor-alpha in lipopolysaccharide-induced sickness behaviour: a study with interleukin-1 type I receptor-deficient

mice. Eur J Neurosci 12:4447–4456

39. Marks DL, Butler AA, Turner R et al (2003) Differential role of melanocortin receptor subtypes in cachexia. Endocrinology 144:1513–1523

40. Wisse BE, Schwartz MW, Cummings DE (2003) Melanocortin signaling and anorexia in chronic disease states. Ann NY Acad Sci 994:275–281

41. Heisler LK, Cowley MA, Kishi T et al (2003) Central serotonin and melanocortin pathways regulating energy homeostasis. Ann NY Acad Sci 994:169–174

42. Herx LM, Rivest S, Yong VW (2000) Central nervous system-initiated inflammation and neurotrophism in trauma: IL-1 beta is required for the production of ciliary neurotrophic factor. J Immunol 165:2232–2239

43. Lambert PD, Anderson KD, Sleeman MW et al (2001) Ciliary neurotrophic factor activates leptin-like pathways and reduces body fat, without cachexia or rebound weight gain, even in leptin-resistant obesity. Proc Natl Acad Sci USA 98:4652–4657

44. Xu B, Dube MG, Kalra PS et al (1998) Anorectic effects of the cytokine, ciliary neurotropic factor, are mediated by hypothalamic neuropeptide Y: Comparison with leptin. Endocrinology 139:466–473

45. Gayle D, Ilyin SE, Plata SC (1997) Central nervous system IL-1 beta system and neuropeptide Y mRNAs during IL-1 beta-induced anorexia in rats. Brain Res Bull 44:311–317

46. Pi-Sunyer FX (2000) Overnutrition and undernutrition as modifiers of metabolic processes in disease states. Am J Clin Nutr 72:533S–537S

47. Caldwell FT, Graves DB, Wallace BH (1998) Studies on the mechanism of fever after intravenous administration of endotoxin. J Trauma 44:304–312

48. Jansky L, Vybiral S, Pospisilova D et al (1995) Production of systemic and hypothalamic cytokines during the early phase of endotoxin fever. Neuroendocrinology 62:55–61

49. Kluger MJ, Kozak W, Leon LR, Conn CA (1998) The use of knockout mice to understand the role of cytokines in fever. Clin Exp Pharmacol Physiol 25:141–144

50. Cartmell T, Poole S, Turnbull AV et al (2000) Circulating interleukin-6 mediates the febrile response to localised inflammation in rats. J Physiol 526:653–661

51. Blatteis CM, Sehic E, Li SX (2000) Pyrogen sensing and signaling: old views and new concepts. Clin Infect Dis 31(Suppl 5):S168–S177

52. Miller AJ, Hopkins SJ, Luheshi GN (1997) Sites of action of IL-1 in the development of fever and cytokine responses to tissue inflammation in the rat. Br J Clin Pharmacol 120:1274–1279

53. Netea MG, Kullberg BJ, Van Der Meer JW (1999) Do only circulating pyrogenic cytokines act as mediators in the febrile response? A hypothesis. Eur J Clin Invest 29:351–356

54. Gaykema RPA, Goehler LE, Hansen MK et al (2000) Subdiaphragmatic vagotomy blocks interleukin-1 beta-induced fever but does not reduce IL-1 beta levels in the circulation. Auton Neurosci 85:72–77

55. Szekely M, Balasko M, Kulchitsky VA et al (2000) Multiple neural mechanisms of fever. Auton Neurosci 85:78–82

56. Watkins LR, Goehler LE, Relton JK et al (1995) Blockade of interleukin-1 induced hyperthermia by subdiaphragmatic vagotomy: evidence for vagal mediation of immune brain communication. Neurosci Lett 183:27–31

57. Caldwell FT, Graves DB, Wallace BH (1999) Humoral versus neural pathways for fever production in rats after administration of lipopolysaccharide. J Trauma 47:120–129

58. Luheshi GN, Bluthe RM, Rushforth D et al (2000) Vagotomy attenuates the behavioural but not the pyrogenic effects of interleukin-1 in rats. Auton Neurosci 85:127–132

59. Goldbach JM, Roth J, Zeisberger E (1997) Fever suppression by subdiaphragmatic vagotomy in guinea pigs depends on the route of pyrogen administration. Am J Physiol 41:R675–R681

60. Romanovsky AA, Simons CT, Szekely M, Kulchitsky VA (1997) The vagus nerve in the thermoregulatory response to systemic inflammation. Am J Physiol 42:R407–R413

61. Arsenijevic D, de Bilbao F, Giannkopoulos P et al (2002) Role for interferon-gamma in the hypermetabolic response to murine toxoplasmosis. Eur Cytokine Netw 12:518–527

62. Busquets S, Alvarez B, Van Royen M et al (2001) Increased uncoupling protein-2 gene expression in brain of lipopolysaccharide-injected mice: role of tumour necrosis factor-alpha? Biochim Biophys Acta 1499:249–256

63. Masaki T, Yoshimatsu H, Kakuma T et al (1999) Induction of rat uncoupling protein-2 gene treated with tumour necrosis factor alpha in vivo. Eur J Clin Invest 29:76–82

64. Puigserver P, Rhee J, Lin JD et al (2001) Cytokine stimulation of energy expenditure through p38 MAP kinase activation of PPAR gamma coactivator-1. Mol Cell 8:971–982

65. Yudkin JS (2003) Adipose tissue, insulin action and vascular disease: inflammatory signals. Int J Obes 27:S25–S28

66. Das UN (2001) Is obesity an inflammatory condition? Nutrition 17:953–966

67. Schmidt MI, Duncan BB (2003) Diabesity: an inflammatory metabolic condition. Clin Chem Lab Med 41:1120–1130

68. Kern PA (1997) Potential role of TNF alpha and lipoprotein lipase as candidate genes for obesity. J Nutr 127:S1917–S1922

69. Hostamisligil GS (1999) Mechanisms of TNF-alpha-induced insulin resistance. Exp Clin Endocrinol Diabetes 107:119–125

70. Uysal KT, Wiesbrock SM, Hotamisligil GS (1998) Functional analysis of tumor necrosis factor (TNF)

receptors in TNF-alpha-mediated insulin resistance in genetic obesity. Endocrinology 139:4832–4838

71. Hotamisligil GS (2000) Molecular mechanisms of insulin resistance and the role of the adipocyte. Int J Obes 24:S23–S27

72. Uysal KT, Wiesbrock SM, Marino MW, Hotamisligil GS (1997) Protection from obesity-induced insulin resistance in mice lacking TNF-alpha function. Nature 389:610–614

73. Klover PJ, Zimmers TA, Koniaris LG, Mooney RA (2003) Chronic exposure to interleukin-6 causes hepatic insulin resistance in mice. Diabetes 52:2784–2789

74. Rotter V, Nagaev I, Smith U (2003) Interleukin-6 (IL-6) induces insulin resistance in 3T3-L1 adipocytes and is, like IL-8 and tumor necrosis factor-alpha, overexpressed in human fat cells from insulin-resistant subjects. J Biol Chem 278:45777–45784

75. Senn JJ, Klover PJ, Nowak IA, Mooney RA (2002) Interleukin-6 induces cellular insulin resistance in hepatocytes. Diabetes 51:3391–3399

76. Senn JJ, Klover PJ, Nowak IA et al (2003) Suppressor of cytokine signaling-3 (SOCS-3), a potential mediator of interleukin-6-dependent insulin resistance in hepatocytes. J Biol Chem 278:13740–13746

77. Fasshauer M, Kralisch S, Klier M et al (2004) Insulin resistance-inducing cytokines differentially regulate SOCS mRNA expression via growth factor- and Jak/Stat-signaling pathways in 3T3-L1 adipocytes. J Endocrinol 181:129–138

78. Mooney RA, Senn J, Cameron S et al (2001) Suppressors of cytokine signaling-1 and-6 associate with and inhibit the insulin receptor - A potential mechanism for cytokine-mediated insulin resistance. J Biol Chem 276:25889–25893

79. Kaser S, Kaser A, Sandhofer A et al (2003) Resistin messenger-RNA expression is increased by proinflammatory cytokines in vitro. Biochem Biophys Res Commun 309:286–290

80. Sonnenberg GE, Krakower GR, Kissebah AH (2004) A novel pathway to the manifestations of metabolic syndrome. Obes Res 12:180–186

# Biochemistry of the Growth Hormone-Releasing Peptides, Secretagogues and Ghrelin

Cyril Y. Bowers, Jaw-Kang Chang, Shaoxing Wu, Klaus D. Linse, David L. Hurley, Johannes D. Veldhuis

## Overview

A general chronology of growth hormone-releasing peptide (GHRP) and ghrelin and their shared receptor is shown in Table 1 [1–3]. The discovery of the natural hormone ghrelin appears to be the exciting beginning of a new unusual hormone system. Initially, in 1980, GH-releasing activity of the unnatural GHRPs was thought to represent the activity of the as-yet unidentified natural hypophysiotrophic hormone GH-releasing hormone (GHRH). However, in 1982, GHRH was isolated from a pancreatic tumour and the hypothalamus and chemically identified as 44 and 40 amino acid linear peptides. Although the GH-releasing activity of GHRPs and GHRH are similar, it is also apparent that they are definitely chemically and functionally different because of the uniqueness of the action of GHRP on GH secretion in vitro as well as in vivo in a variety of animal species. In 1984, it was postulated that GHRP reflected the activity of another new hypothalamic hormone involved in the increased secretion of GH and thus was in need of isolation. Further support of this conclusion was presented between 1989 and 1993 with the demonstration of differential specific in vitro GHRP and GHRH binding results utilising peripheral membrane fragments from rat hypothalami and pituitaries. It was also shown that the primary GHRP/ghrelin pituitary intracellular signalling pathway is via phospholipase C, inositoltriphosphate and protein kinase C, while that of GHRH is via adenyl cyclase, cAMP and protein kinase A. This was followed by the cloning of the GHRP/GHS (growth hormone secretagogue) receptor by the Merck group in 1996 [4]. Ultimately, Kojima et al. achieved the isolation and identification of the natural GHRP in 1999. They designated the peptide with the euphonic name

ghrelin, derived from the word ghre (Proto-Indo-European root), meaning grow [5]. With the identification of ghrelin and its receptor, the unnatural GHRPs were no longer orphans after a 23-year adolescence [6].

**Table 1a.** Historical milestones of unnatural growth hormone-releasing peptide (GHRP)

| | |
|---|---|
| 1976 | First GHRP |
| 1984 | New hypothalamic hormone |
| 1989–91 | GH release (H) |
| 1993 | Pulsatile GH secretion (H) |
| 1995–96 | Food intake |
| 2003 | Food intake (H) |

*H*, human; *GH*, growth hormone

**Table 1b.** Historical milestones of natural growth hormone-releasing peptide (GHRP)

| | |
|---|---|
| 1996 | GHRP/GHS receptor (H) |
| 1999 | Ghrelin |
| 2000–04 | Ghrelin and GHRP actions same |
| 2001 | Food intake (H) |
| 2004 | Pulsatile GH secretion (H) |

*H*, human, *GH*, growth hormone

In a first among peptide hormones, the 28 amino acid ghrelin linear peptide was post-translationally modified with an ester bond to an eight carbon atom saturated chain carboxylic acid, *n*-octanoyl. Octanoylation has had a major impact on the chemistry and particularly the biology of ghrelin. Although the characterisation and/or identification of the mechanism involved in the octanoylation of the ghrelin peptide has not been achieved, it has significantly guided our conceptualisation of the ghrelin system. Octanoylation not only is a critical determinant of the bioactive chemical conformation of the ghrelin molecule but, in addition, it is envisioned as a critical determinant of the biological regulation of the ghrelin hormone, presumably via the presence and activity of a putative specific octanoylating enzyme complex. This particular octanoylating enzyme complex is presumed to be responsible for esterification of the 28 amino acid ghrelin peptide by the octanoyl group, which is the major regulatory determinant of where, when, how and to what degree the ghrelin peptide is activated.

In terms of therapeutic potential, one of the most valuable GH-releasing actions of GHRP in humans is considered to be the increased normal physiological pattern of pulsatile GH secretion, which occurs during the prolonged continuous subcutaneous (sc) infusion of GHRP. As recorded in Fig. 1, 24-h continuous sc ghrelin infusion in humans produces the same effect as GHRP-2 (Fig. 2) and when GHRP-2 or ghrelin is infused together with GHRH, the pulsatile GH secretion pattern is unchanged but the amplitude of the GH pulse is further increased.

During a 30-day continuous infusion of GHRP-2 to older men and women with low serum insulin-like growth factor-1 (IGF-1) levels, the sustained augmentation of GH secretion in turn increased plasma levels of IGF-1 and its binding proteins BP3 and 5 but not BP4 or the plasma level of IGF-II (Table 2) [7]. In addition, cortisol, prolactin, leptin and adiponectin levels were

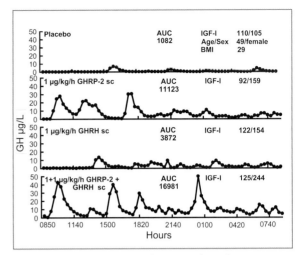

**Fig. 2.** Continuous infusion of GHRP-2 for 24 hours

unchanged. This overall physiological action on the function of the GH–IGF-1 axis is in contrast to the pharmacological effects on this axis when recombinant GH is administered once daily, intermittently or continuously sc.

## Reverse Pharmacology

Reverse pharmacology is the terminology proposed by Conn and Bowers in 1996 to describe the chemical biological approach utilised in accomplishing the development from unnatural GHRP to natural ghrelin. The first GHRP we developed was the DTrp[2] pentapeptide listed in Table 3.

DTrp[2] was only active in vitro and was low in potency, but released only GH and not prolactin, adrenocorticotropin (ACTH), luteinising hormone (LH), follicle-stimulating hormone (FSH) or thyroid-stimulating hormone (TSH). The four chemical classes of GHRPs that became chemical templates for us as well as other investigators were developed in the subsequent 3 years. Highly potent GHRPs have been developed from each of these four classes of GHRP chemical templates that are active in releasing GH in vivo. The chemistry of three of our highly potent GHRPs derived from the DTrp[2]LTrp[4] chemical class is recorded in Table 4.

The comparative GH-releasing activity in humans of the three GHRPs (Table 3) relative to

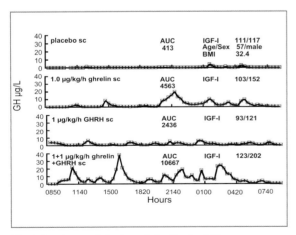

**Fig. 1.** Continuous infusion of ghrelin for 24 hours

**Table 2a.** 30-Day continuous subcutaneous infusion of 1 µg/kg/h growth hormone-releasing peptide (GHRP)-2

| | Day | AUC·24 h (µg/l±SEM) | | |
| | | GH | IGF-1 | IGF-II |
|---|---|---|---|---|
| Placebo | -3 | 824 ± 153 | 105 ± 9 | 356 ± 14 |
| GHRP-2 | 0 | 4544 ± 764[a] | 173 ± 15[a] | 357 ± 16 |
| GHRP-2 | 14 | 1764 ± 198[a] | 175 ± 16[b] | 393 ± 36 |
| GHRP-2 | 30 | 1699 ± 201[b] | 177 ± 16[a] | 369 ± 30 |
| – | 60 | – | 99 ± 14 | 333 ± 26 |

Age 64 ± 2.8, BMI 26 ± 1.1, $n = 17$, values are mean of single determinations at end of infusion, $p$ value = [a] < 0.001, [b] < 0.01. *IGF*, insuline-like growth factor; *GH*, growth hormone

**Table 2b.** 30-Day continuous subcutaneous infusion of 1µg/kg/h growth hormone-releasing peptide (GHRP)-2

| | Day | AUC·24 h (µg/l±SEM) | | |
| | | IGF BP3 | IGF BP4 | IGF BP5 |
|---|---|---|---|---|
| Placebo | -3 | 2483 ± 207 | 545 ± 35 | 313 ± 16 |
| GHRP-2 | 0 | 2937 ± 253 | 554 ± 23 | 393 ± 27[c] |
| GHRP-2 | 14 | 3677 ± 253[b] | 542 ± 34 | 377 ± 30 |
| GHRP-2 | 30 | 3462 ± 311[c] | 516 ± 38 | 385 ± 21[c] |
| – | 60 | 2623 ± 327 | 452 ± 44 | 324 ±10 |

Age 64 ± 2.8, BMI 26 ± 1.1, $n = 17$, values are mean of single determinations at end of infusion, $p$ value = [b] < 0.01, [c] < 0.02. *IGF*, insuline-like growth factor

**Table 3.** In vitro active growth hormone-releasing peptides (1976–1985)

| Amino acid sequence | Abbreviation |
|---|---|
| TyrDTrp[2]GlyPheMetNH$_2$ | DTrp[2] |
| TyrAlaDTrp[3]PheMetNH$_2$ | DTrp[3] |
| TyrDTrp[2]DTrp[3]PheNH$_2$ | DTrp[2,3] |
| TyrDTrp[2]AlaTrp[4]DPheNH$_2$ | DTrp[2]LTrp[4] |

activity of ghrelin and GHRP, which further underscores the independency and interdependency of their in vivo actions.

The high potency, effectiveness and chemical stability of the GHRPs can be deduced by the results in Fig. 4, which reveal that GHRP-2 very effectively releases GH in normal men by various routes of administration. It is particularly of clinical interest that this release is increased by oral administration, even at the low dose of 10 mg. In

each other and to GHRH is shown in Fig. 3. The results were notable in that while GHRH was at its maximal dosage, each of the unnatural GHRPs stimulated more GH release than GHRH alone. Therefore, these GHRPs were acting differently from GHRH to release GH. Parenthetically, it must be noted that intact endogenous GHRH is an absolute determinant of the in vivo GH-releasing

**Table 4.** In vivo active growth hormone-releasing peptides (*GHRPs*)

| GHRP | Amino acid sequence |
|---|---|
| GHRP-6 | His[1]DTrp[2]Ala[3]Trp[4]DPhe[5]Lys[6]NH$_2$ |
| GHRP-1 | Ala[1]His[2]DβNal[3]Ala[4]Trp[5]DPhe[6]Lys[7]NH$_2$ |
| GHRP-2 | DAla[1]DβNal[2]Ala[3]Trp[4]DPhe[5]Lys[6]NH$_2$ |

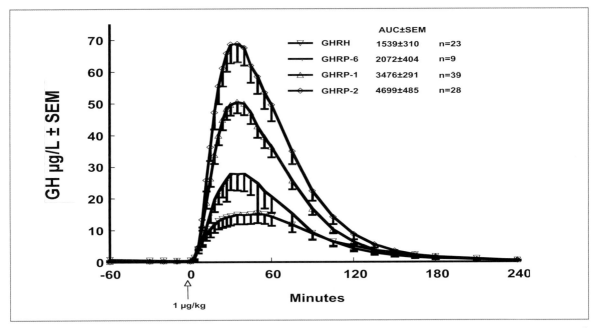

**Fig. 3.** Comparative GH responses to 1 μg/kg intravenous bolus administration of GHRH 1–44NH$_2$, GHRP-6, GHRP-1 and GHRP-2 in normal young men. Values are means ± SEM. (Modified from [1])

contrast, when GHRPs are administered in high pharmacological dosages, as recorded in Fig. 4, ACTH/cortisol and prolactin release is increased via a hypothalamic action.

Thus, GHRP showed clinical potential in several ways: defining a pathway complementary to that of GHRH (vide infra); displaying oral activi-

ty; and having high potency. This potential was furthered when the ghrelin molecule was isolated and then validated as the natural GHRP hormone. The interesting 28 amino acid structure of ghrelin is shown below (Fig. 5).

As has been discussed (vide infra), the covalent linked octanoyl group addition to the Ser[3]

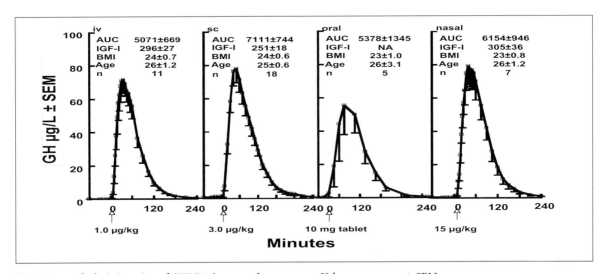

**Fig. 4.** Route of administration of GHRP-2 in normal young men. Values are means ± SEM

amino acid side chain via an ester bond is a first in peptide hormone chemistry. The ghrelin molecule with the octanoic carboxylic acid is just as exciting biologically as it is chemically because the desoctanoyl ghrelin (without the octanoyl group attached) no longer binds to the ghrelin type 1a receptor. Thus, the octanoyl group is a critical determinant for attaining a complementary receptor conformation by the ghrelin molecule.

In spite of the very different chemistry of the unnatural GHRPs and natural ghrelin, each of these two very different classes of peptides binds with high affinity to the same natural GHS/GHRP/ghrelin receptor. This is further demonstrated by the results in Fig. 6, where both GHRP-2 and ghrelin have the same acute GH-releasing actions in normal young men alone and synergistically with GHRH [8]. Therefore, the bio-

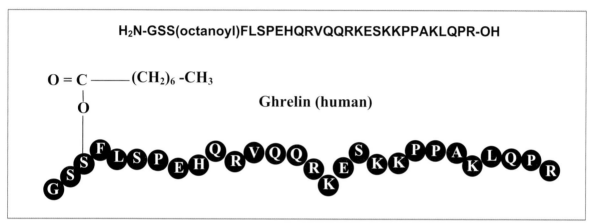

**Fig. 5.** Amino acid sequence of human ghrelin

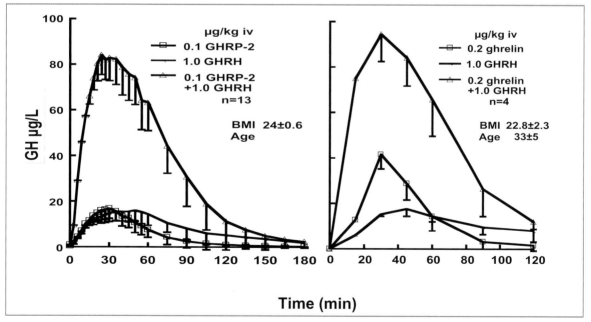

**Fig. 6.** Ghrelin and GHRP each synergise similarly with GHRH to stimulate GH release. Low-dose sensitisation of GHRP-2 (*left panel*) and ghrelin (*right panel*) in normal young men. Values are means ± SEM. (Data from [8])

logical isolation of the natural hormone ghrelin did not alter the interesting attributes of the GHRP and GHS compounds; rather, it stimulated further new biochemical analysis to understand the novel functionality of this uniquely octanoylated peptide.

Because the chemistry of the ghrelin molecule and its bioactivity on the ghrelin GHS receptor type 1a are only achievable after the post-translational octanoyl addition, it is apparent that a mixture of special strategies, approaches and techniques was required for the isolation and identification of ghrelin. This included the unnatural GHRPs, the cloned GHRP/GHS receptor, the classical purification of ghrelin from stomach extracts and finally mass spectrometry. Even a seemingly simple decision based on conceptualisation and strategy guiding the approaches may profoundly influence the success of the isolation of a natural hormone. For example, because of the bioactive dependency of the ghrelin octanoylation step and because octanoylation is a post-translational step, a singular recombinant molecular cDNA approach would have been unsuccessful. Additionally, our studies of unnatural GHRPs encouraged us to believe that the putative natural GHRP hormone would be another hypothalamic hypophysiotropic hormone and for that reason the ideal tissue from which to isolate the natural hormone would be the hypothalamus. Thus for several years we pursued the same classical isolation procedure and approaches from thousands of porcine hypothalami as utilised for TRH and LHRH, but this was unsuccessful. Several years later, Kojima et al. showed that the primary anatomical origin of ghrelin is the stomach and not the hypothalamus, which again emphasised the role and importance of conceptualisation and strategy in the isolation process of a new hormone. Furthermore, before the isolation of ghrelin was accomplished, the focus of the GHRPs was on increasing GH secretion, although limited studies in rats and mice had already demonstrated that GHRPs also increased food intake. However, once ghrelin was isolated and its origin was found to be primarily from the stomach, the focus on the biological role of ghrelin and GHRP increasingly has been on food intake.

## Ghrelin System

At last the GHRP/ghrelin circle, together with their biological actions, has been completed with a high degree of definitiveness as a result of the cloning of the natural ghrelin receptor and the isolation of the natural hormone ghrelin. The unique and biologically meaningful actions of GHRP on the regulation of GH secretion and food intake gradually have been revealed to be the same for ghrelin in animals and humans. The complexity of evaluating the central nervous system (CNS) ghrelin system emanates from the regulation of GH secretion and food intake by ghrelin within a hypothalamic network involving a number of other hormones, several different hypothalamic nuclei and also brain stem nuclei.

Although many of the central CNS actions of GHRP and ghrelin are well established, their possible peripheral actions and roles are much less established. Nevertheless, the existence of a functional peripheral ghrelin system seems most likely. Some findings in support of this conclusion are: bioactive ghrelin is delivered directly to peripheral tissues as it is secreted into the circulation from the stomach; although in low amounts, evidence supports synthesis of ghrelin and its receptors in peripheral tissues and organs and the actions of GHRP and ghrelin at peripheral anatomical sites have been demonstrated. A number of complexities and unknown factors prevent the direct analysis of a putative but seemingly likely peripheral ghrelin system. Some issues requiring further understanding are: (1) what might be the consequences when bioactive ghrelin originates from two anatomical sites of synthesis, i.e., the stomach as well as peripheral tissues; (2) what might be the mechanism of octanoylation of the ghrelin peptide and its regulation at two anatomical sites of synthesis; (3) what might be the action, regulation and physiological and/or pharmacological role(s) of ghrelin in peripheral tissues.

Recent findings that add to the complexity of ghrelin activity are the results indicating that the hypothalamic and pituitary intracellular signalling pathways are different from each other, at least in regard to the neuropeptide Y (NPY) arcuate neurons involved in increased food intake compared to the somatotrophs involved in GH secretion. Substantial evidence obtained by Kohno et al. indicates ghrelin activation of NPY neurons is elicited by $Ca^{2+}$ signalling via protein kinase A and N-type $Ca^{2+}$ channel-dependent mechanisms [9]. The fact that ghrelin stimulated NPY arcuate neurons at a low $10^{-10}$ mol/l concentration supports the physiological relevance of this effect and also indicates that the ghrelin receptor on the arcuate neuron is not a type 1a receptor, which is in agreement with genomic results. A different intracellular signalling pathway is certainly of fundamental interest in regard to the regulation of food intake by ghrelin. Parenthetically, it will be important to determine the type of intracellular signalling pathway in the hypothalamic arcuate neurons that mediates increase of GH secretion by ghrelin.

As Kohno et al. envisioned, stimulation of the cAMP pathway in the arcuate neurons may be specifically relevant to the increase of food intake by ghrelin for the following reasons: induction of the cAMP response element-mediated gene(s) in NPY arcuate neurons that results from fasting and is decreased by leptin; fasting increases ghrelin secretion; leptin inhibits ghrelin stimulation of NPY arcuate neurons; and the possibility that ghrelin-induced $Ca^{2+}$ signalling in NPY neurons may depend on basal protein kinase A activity or the activation of protein kinase A. As discussed (vide infra), the GHRP/ghrelin GHS type 1a receptor constitutively functions at a high signalling rate in the absence of stimulation by ghrelin and, in addition, fasting increases the number of GHS type 1a receptors in the hypothalamus. Collectively, this would result in the high activity of these receptors since the receptor number, the constitutive signalling rate, and the basal protein kinase A activity of NPY neurons may be increased independent of the ghrelin concentration. The ghrelin increase of intracellular $Ca^{2+}$ concentration may depend on the basal activity of protein kinase C and/or cAMP protein kinase A may be involved in the $Ca^{2+}$ influx.

Still unexplained is that in vitro GHRP, unlike GHRH, does not increase pituitary cAMP, although in vivo the two peptides together synergistically raise pituitary cAMP levels. In vivo GHRP alone slightly increases and GHRH alone markedly increases pituitary cAMP; together the effect on cAMP is synergistic. Other disparate findings include a number of incompletely understood actions of GHRP and ghrelin, especially on the sensitisation and desensitisation of secretion and synthesis of GH both in vitro and in vivo in animals and humans.

## Structure Activity of Ghrelin

Recorded in Table 5 are the results of Matsumoto et al. on the in vitro structure–activity relationships (SAR) of mainly carboxylic acids of different carbon atom chain lengths that have been substituted for the octanoic carboxylic acid at $Ser^3$ and covalently linked by an ester bond formed between the carboxyl group of the straight chain saturated carboxylic acid or fatty acid and the hydroxyl group on the side chain of the $Ser^3$ amino acid residue of natural rat and human ghrelin [10].

These studies were performed in vitro in a cell line in which the ghrelin GHS receptor type 1a had been transfected and calcium mobilisation was utilised as the index of response. We have considered these results to be potentially most provocative and instructive in terms of conceptualisation. In comparison to ghrelin with an eight carbon atom chain carboxylic acid (octanoic acid) covalently linked to the $Ser^3$ amino acid, substitutions of shorter carbon atom chain length carboxylic acids, i.e., acetyl, butyryl, hexanoyl, were much less active, while the longer carbon chain substitutions were much nearer the activity of natural octanoylated ghrelin. What seems potentially so meaningful is that carboxylic acids of different chain lengths substituted at $Ser^3$ have a variable effect on the bioactivity of the ghrelin in vitro via the GHRP/ghrelin GHS receptor, type 1a, which very possibly is the result of altering the conformation of the ghrelin peptide as a function of the carbon chain length of the carboxylic acid. We have conceptualised that the 'ubiquitous' octanoylation of the ghrelin peptide has occurred in evolution by natural selection not just for chemical reasons but also for yet to be established

**Table 5.** Property of Ser$^3$ side chain of ghrelin and activity

| No. | Peptide | Structure | EC$_{50}$ (nM)[a] |
|---|---|---|---|
| 2 | Rat ghrelin | GSS(O-CO-C$_7$H$_{15}$)FLSPEHQKAQQRKESKKPPAKLQPR | 1.5 |
| 4 | [des-acyl]-Rat ghrelin | GSSFLSPEHQKAQQRKESKKPPAKLQPR | 3500 |
| 13 | [Ser$^3$(acetyl)]-Rat ghrelin | GSS(O-CO-CH$_3$)FLSPEHQKAQQRKESKKPPAKLQPR | 780 |
| 14 | [Ser$^3$(butyryl)]-Rat ghrelin | GSS(O-CO-C$_3$H$_7$)FLSPEHQKAQQRKESKKPPAKLQPR | 280 |
| 15 | [Ser$^3$(hexanoyl)]-Rat ghrelin | GSS(O-CO-C$_5$H$_{11}$)FLSPEHQKAQQRKESKKPPAKLQPR | 16 |
| 16 | [Ser$^3$(decanoyl)]-Rat ghrelin | GSS(O-CO-C$_9$H$_{19}$)FLSPEHQKAQQRKESKKPPAKLQPR | 1.7 |
| 17 | [Ser$^3$(lauroyl)]-Rat ghrelin | GSS(O-CO-C$_{11}$H$_{23}$)FLSPEHQKAQQRKESKKPPAKLQPR | 2.4 |
| 18 | [Ser$^3$(palmitoyl)]-Rat ghrelin | GSS(O-CO-C$_{15}$H$_{31}$)FLSPEHQKAQRKESKKPPAKLQPR | 6.5 |
| 19 | [Ser$^3$(3-octenoyl)]-(H)[b] ghrelin | GSS(O-COCH$_2$CH==CH(CH$_2$)$_3$CH$_3$)FLSPEHQRVQQRKESKKPPAKLQPR | 1.7 |
| 20 | [Ser$^3$(4-methylpentanoyl)]-(H) ghrelin | GSS(O-CO-CH$_2$CH$_2$CH(CH$_3$)$_2$)FLSPEHQRVQQRKESKKPPAKLQPR | 4.4 |
| 21 | [Ser$^3$(3-phenylpropionyl)]-(H) ghrelin | GSS(O-CO-CH$_2$ CH$_2$Ph)FLSPEHQKAQQRKESKKPPAKLQPR | 1.4 |
| 22 | [Ser$^3$(octyl)]-(H) ghrelin | GSS(O-C$_8$H$_{17}$)FLSPEHQRVQQRKESKKPPAKLQPR | 1.2 |
| 23 | [Cys$^3$(octyl)]-Rat ghrelin | GSS(S-C$_8$H$_{17}$)FLSPEHQKAQQRKESKKPPAKLQPR | 5.4 |

[a] EC$_{50}$ is the concentration of peptides or peptide derivatives at [Ca$^{2+}$]$_i$ increase on GHS-R-expressing cells; [b] $H$, human. (Data from [9])

specific biological reasons. Octanoylation of the ghrelin peptide is a premier step that concomitantly subserves the chemistry and also the biology of the intact full-length ghrelin molecule in unique and novel independent ways.

Other notable SAR ghrelin results of Matsumoto et al. revealed that thioether and ether bonds for linking octanoic acid to $Ser^3$ result in high activity of the ghrelin molecule [10, 11]. Also our results (Chang, Bowers) reveal that when an amide bond is substituted for the ester bond of ghrelin, the in vivo GH-releasing potency of this peptide and ghrelin is the same in rats.

To what degree substitutions of various carboxylic acids of different carbon atom chain lengths and/or amino acid alternatives at or for the $Ser^3$ residue may influence the in vivo activity at the physiological and/or pharmacological levels has not been reported, but this could change the chemical conformation of the ghrelin molecule, which may activate putative subtypes of ghrelin receptors as well as alter the ghrelin pharmacokinetics or pharmacodynamics. Substitutions of $Trp^3$ and $Nal^3$ but not $DNal^3$, $Val^3$, $Leu^3$, $Ile^3$ or $Nle^3$ have relatively high in vitro activity. The relatively high receptor binding of $Trp^3$ ghrelin compared to octanoylated ghrelin (33-fold less active) emphasises the uniqueness of the octanoyl addition for biological regulation as well as for the receptor conformation of the ghrelin molecule.

Evaluation of the bioactivity of truncated octanoylated ghrelin peptides with a free acid at the C terminus revealed the in vitro activity of the 1–15, 1–11, 1–10 and 1–9 fragments to be about 6-, 11-, 17- and 30-fold less active than human ghrelin 1–28, while fragments 1–8 and 1–4 were 97- and 460-fold less active, respectively [10]. The N terminus tetrapeptide with octanoylation of $Ser^3$ and amidation at the C terminus was the smallest fragment with in vitro activity [11, 12]. The most active in vitro small ghrelin analogue synthesised by this group was 5-aminopentanoyl-Ser (octyl)-Phe-Leu aminoethylamide [11].

The C-terminal amide versus the C-terminal free acid of truncated octanoylated ghrelin 1–8 was nine-fold more active in vitro [11]. Results of these various truncated octanoylated ghrelin fragments with free acids in contrast to C-terminal amides are relevant because only the C-terminal free acid and not C-terminal amide truncated ghrelin is produced in vivo from partial proteolytic degradation of the bioactive full-length ghrelin 1–28 molecule. Although the fragments may not be secreted into the peripheral circulation, they may be formed in the circulation and act peripherally or may be formed at peripheral tissue sites and act in a paracrine/autocrine manner. Another additional issue of clinical relevance could be the possible cross-reactions that these proteolytic-derived ghrelin fragments may have on the ghrelin radioimmunoassays (RIAs) that have been developed already and probably those that will be developed in the future.

## Octanoylation of Ghrelin

Collectively, the chemistry-driven conceptualisation of the ghrelin system compellingly fuses the chemistry and biology of bioactive ghrelin into a very special interdependence. The control of regulation of the octanoylating enzyme complex by a potential array of specific metabolic, nutritional and hormonal factors will require elucidating.

Octanoylation of the 28 amino acid ghrelin peptide requires the extraordinary specificity of performing three major precise chemical steps presumably by a specialised enzyme complex that has yet to be characterised or identified. The three steps include addition of only the octanoic carboxylic or fatty acid and presumably not any other carboxylic or fatty acid to the ghrelin peptide, specific addition of the octanoic carboxylic acid to only the ghrelin peptide and not any other peptide hormone, and specifically covalently linking the octanoic carboxylic acid to the hydroxyl group of the side chain of only the $Ser^3$ but not $Ser^2$ of ghrelin via an ester bond. Furthermore, the octanoylating enzyme complex must be distributed at key anatomical sites where the ghrelin peptide is synthesised, likely at intracellular locations and perhaps as a functional complex within vesicles. Because of the envisioned multiple components and requirements of the enzyme complex, octanoylation of the desoctanoyl ghrelin peptide seems unlikely to occur in plasma.

Whether the relatively high concentration of des-octanoylated ghrelin in peripheral plasma originating from the stomach and delivered to the peripheral tissues provides a substrate for the presumed octanoyl enzyme complex in tissues is an important unknown. If this seemingly special enzyme complex function occurs only intracellularly, desoctanoyl ghrelin from plasma would be unlikely to be the substrate for the enzyme complex because of the difficulty of delivering it to a specific enzyme octanoylation site within the cell and in an appropriate amount.

In principle, it is necessary to consider a possible biological role for the desoctanoyl ghrelin, the full-length ghrelin peptide without an octanoyl modification. It is secreted from the stomach directly into the peripheral circulation where it is present in higher concentrations than octanoylated ghrelin. Molecular evidence further supports that the desoctanoylated ghrelin peptide is synthesised in many tissues of the body, but whether this ghrelin peptide becomes octanoylated is unknown. Although gene expression data indicated that only low concentrations of desoctanoylated ghrelin are synthesised in peripheral tissue, this may dramatically change in select tissues or organs as a function of metabolism, nutrition and/or hormonal secretion.

The first possible biological in vivo action of desoctanoylated ghrelin was recently reported by Thompson et al. [13]. In this novel study, bone marrow fat was increased after the direct continuous infusion of desoctanoyl ghrelin into the tibial marrow cavity of rats for 7 days. However, since infusion of octanoylated ghrelin produced this same effect, the provocative possibility is raised of whether the infused desoctanoylated ghrelin became octanoylated. The studies of Choi et al. demonstrate that ghrelin increases the genesis of rat adipocytes in vitro via the type 1a GHS receptor [14]. More important is that these studies may result in many new conceptual thoughts, strategies and experimental approaches. Because it is known that desoctanoylated ghrelin is not active on the GHS type 1a receptor, while several studies indicate the action of desoctanoyl ghrelin occurs in vitro [15, 16], it will be necessary to re-evaluate

approaches to disentangle des- from octanoylated ghrelin actions.

At present, the role and action of ghrelin are frequently indirectly surmised from peripheral plasma immunoactivity levels of 'ghrelin' obtained by various RIAs, each of which have inherent limitations or are incompletely validated for specifically measuring the concentration of the intact bioactive ghrelin molecule. It has been reported by Nagaya et al. that the half-life of ghrelin after intravenous administration is about 10 minutes. Plasma desoctanoylated ghrelin levels are variable, about five-fold or more greater than plasma octanoylated ghrelin levels. These levels likely vary under pathophysiological conditions or even during normal metabolic, nutritional and hormonal states. In addition to the limitation of this methodology, it is necessary to consider the list of factors in Table 6, which may directly and/or indirectly modulate the level of desoctanoyl ghrelin in peripheral plasma and/or the sensitivity of the ghrelin/GHRP action on GH secretion and food intake. The analysis of the effects of these factors will be focal to the interpretation of the physiological and pathophysiological roles of ghrelin.

To date, only octanoylated ghrelin 1–27 has been identified in peripheral human plasma and the stomach by Hosoda et al. [17]. It originates from octanoylated ghrelin 1–28 by cleavage of the $Pro^{27}-Arg^{28}$ C-terminal bond and has the same

**Table 6.** Relevant mechanisms of the actions of ghrelin

| | |
|----|----------------------------------|
| 1 | Ghrelin gene |
| 2 | Octanoylation enzyme complex |
| 3 | Secretion rate of bioactive ghrelin |
| 4 | Desoctanoylation plasma enzyme |
| 5 | Plasma ghrelin binding proteins |
| 6 | Clearance by kidney or liver |
| 7 | Blood–brain barrier |
| 8 | Expression of ghrelin receptor |
| 9 | Intracellular signalling |
| 10 | Interacting hormones |

high in vitro and in vivo activity as ghrelin 1–28. Other relevant findings in humans consist of n-decanoylated ghrelin in the stomach and plasma and preliminary evidence that immunoreactive ghrelin in peripheral plasma rapidly decreases to 35% of normal control levels following total gastrectomy. Because ghrelin levels in plasma are not lower after total gastrectomy, the anatomical origin may be the intestinal tract, where immunoreactive ghrelin has been identified. However, the chemical point arises in regard to what degree the full-length ghrelin peptide is present, as well as the octanoylation status in the intestine, plasma and peripheral tissues.

## Putative New Natural Ghrelin Hormones and Companion Receptor Subtypes

The seminal chemical-biological role of octanoylation as the initial immediate critical chemical step in determining the bioactive receptor conformation of the ghrelin peptide for the GHS type 1a receptor is notable and intriguing. We are currently working with Shaoxing Wu to study the effect of octanoylation on the ghrelin conformation determined from NMR analysis in conjunction with ghrelin conformation as determined from theoretical molecular modelling. The long-term objective is to evaluate changes in ghrelin conformation following substitution of shorter and longer carboxylic acids of the octanoyl group. It is hypothesised that at certain anatomical peripheral tissue sites, carboxylic acids other than octanoic acid are covalently linked to Ser$^3$ of ghrelin, which produce ghrelin molecules with different conformations that act on the putative ghrelin receptor subtypes. Novel in this hypothesis is that ghrelin molecular subtypes are generated without changing the open reading frame of the gene for the ghrelin peptide. If this occurs, the effects on the physiology of the ghrelin system would be major. If this hypothesis is incorrect, it could be because the special octanoylation enzyme complex is so specific in action that it only links octanoic carboxylic acid to Ser$^3$ of the full-length ghrelin peptide. So far this key important specific enzyme complex has

neither been directly demonstrated to exist nor its regulation characterised. Unknown is whether the specificity of this enzyme may be only for the ghrelin peptide and only selective for the Ser$^3$ amino acid residue, while the esterification reaction may be more permissive. Envisioned is the possibility that carboxylic acids of different chain lengths may be substituted at Ser$^3$, which are tissue, metabolic and nutrition dependent.

Several findings have led to this possible broader, less restrictive 'carboxylic acid hypothesis'. These include the following points. (1) Octanoylation as the critical immediate determinant of the bioactive chemical conformation of the ghrelin peptide raises the possibility that different carboxylic acids added at Ser$^3$ may occur and may induce different conformations of the ghrelin molecule that bind to select ghrelin subtype receptors. (2) Octanoylation of the ghrelin peptide has been directly established and validated chemically only for ghrelin synthesised in the stomach but not at other anatomical tissue and organ sites, where only mRNA or in situ hybridisation evidence of the ghrelin peptide exists and/or that immunohistochemistry evidence specifically detects full-length bioactive octanoylated ghrelin. Thus, at peripheral anatomical sites other than the stomach, the ghrelin peptide may be desoctanoyl ghrelin or may have a different carboxylic acid covalently linked to the Ser$^3$ residue. (3) Putative ghrelin receptor subtypes have been proposed as a result of different biological profiles of select GHRPs. (4) Binding affinities for the ghrelin GHS receptor vary from high to low as a function of the carbon atom chain length of the carboxylic acid substituted for the octanoyl group of the ghrelin molecule. This may suggest the spectrum and number of ghrelin receptor types could be considerable since the receptor binding affinities were so variable for the type 1a ghrelin receptor when different carboxylic acids were substituted for the octanoyl group on the Ser$^3$ residue of the full-length ghrelin peptide. It is possible to envision that these variable binding affinities may indicate different subtypes of ghrelin. The ghrelin molecule subtypes and ghrelin receptor subtypes may both exist in the putative peripheral ghrelin system as well as the CNS system, but they may be regulated by the metabolic, nutritional and hormonal status. Additionally, another molecular form of ghrelin itself has been identified in the stomach, i.e., des[Gln[14]]-ghrelin in a 27 amino acid Ser[3] octanoylated peptide, which is the result of alternative splicing of the ghrelin gene. It has the same bioactivity of the primary 28 amino acid octanoylated ghrelin.

Besides the GHRP/ghrelin GHS type 1a receptor, the Merck group cloned another related GHS receptor designated type 1b in 1997. The type 1b receptor is a truncated version of the type 1a GHS receptor because only TM-1 through TM-5 domains are encoded. Its function is still unknown. Neither the GHRPs nor ghrelin bind to this receptor and the type 1a and 1b receptors are localised to separate chromosomes. When selective, sensitive hybridisation probes for the type 1a and 1b receptors were utilised, the mRNA distribution in normal human tissues demonstrates the truncated type 1b receptor is widely distributed while the type 1a GHRP/ghrelin active receptor is much more restricted, i.e., predominantly in the pituitary gland but also in the thyroid gland, pancreas, spleen, myocardium and adrenal gland. In contrast to the distribution of the active type 1a receptor, the expression of the mRNA distribution of the ghrelin peptide is widespread in human tissues, which suggests that ghrelin may be acting on selected receptor subtypes in peripheral tissues [18]. These results indicate the necessity of utilising subtype-specific probes in order to distinguish the widespread but inactive truncated receptor from the active GHS receptor, as well as the need to attempt to identify additional ghrelin receptor subtypes.

Tomassetto et al. identified the motilin-related peptide from the stomach in a separate study via a recombinant cDNA approach, in contrast to the GHS-type 1a receptor approach utilised by Kojima et al., which identified octanoylated ghrelin [19]. Significantly, the motilin-related peptide is chemically but not biologically identical to desoctanoyl ghrelin, particularly since octanoylation of the 28 amino acid ghrelin peptide is essential for binding to the type 1a ghrelin receptor and its enhancement of GH release and food intake. Additionally,

on the basis of chemical similarities between octanoylated ghrelin, motilin-related peptide and the duodenal hormone motilin, an important regulator of gastrointestinal motility, it is reasonable to project that octanoylated ghrelin also may have a motilin-like effect on gastrointestinal motility. Most informative and meaningful are the recent studies and detailed discussion of Inui et al. in support of the unique and potent physiological gastro-prokinetic effect of ghrelin and its relationship to the increase of food intake by ghrelin [20]. A special aspect is the functional interdependency of the stomach and hypothalamus for the integration of feeding and associated autonomic, neuroendocrine and gastrointestinal functions emphasised by Inui. It becomes apparent that the route of administration or the anatomical origin of endogenous secretion of ghrelin is a basic issue that must be considered. Peripheral versus central intracerebroventricular (ICV) administration may produce differing effects on gastric acid secretion, motility or food intake. Inui et al. and others (vide infra) bring out the potential physiological functional significance of only a very small amount of 'ghrelin' synthesised in the hypothalamus, particularly the arcuate nucleus [20, 21]. A basic point still in need of chemical validation is whether bioactive octanoylated ghrelin is produced in the hypothalamus because desoctanoyl ghrelin is non-functional in regard to these effects. Obviously, these are convoluted biological regulatory issues, suggesting that a coordinated approach will be required to resolve these complex issues, i.e., whether the bioactive ghrelin molecule is synthesised in the hypothalamus.

NMR studies of ghrelin and five of its truncated analogues in solution detail that all of them behave as random coils [22]. NMR comparison of the N-terminal octanoylated C-terminal amidated pentapeptide ghrelin fragment, active in vitro, with the N-terminal portion of the full-length ghrelin further indicates that they are similar. An exception is the presence of two additional nuclear Overhauser effects (NOE) between the Phe[4] NH proton and the protons of the beta-methylene of the Ser[3] residue of this pentapeptide fragment. Circular dichroism spectroscopy of ghrelin pentapeptides in water also indicates a conformation as random coils. However, molecular modelling of GHRP-6 and ghrelin with the incorporation of these NMR results did not account for nor agree with the binding of these peptides to the ghrelin GHS type 1a receptor.

In 1998, Scott Feighner and his Merck collaborators published mutation studies on the human GHS 7 transmembrane (TM) domain G-protein coupled receptor. They found that mutation of amino acids on TM 2, 3 and 5, 6 both affect and activate the GHS receptor [23]. This group developed a three-dimensional docking model of the Merck benzolactam and spiropiperidine non-peptide GHSs as well as GHRP-6. Mutating glutamic acid to glutamine at position 124 in TM 3 resulted in a non-functional receptor for each of the three different dissimilar chemical types of GHRP/GHSs. Since each GHRP has an essential positive-charged atom at the N-terminus, the non-functional receptor with the glutamic acid to glutamine mutation was explained by eliminating the counter ion interaction between these three GHSs and the receptor. Furthermore, the TM 2, 5 and 6 mutations induced different effects on the binding and activation of these three chemically different GHRP/GHSs. This led to the speculation by this group that these three GHSs probably bind to the same receptor site in different molecular orientations.

## High Constitutive Signalling of the Ghrelin Receptor

Although obtained only in vitro, the recent results of Holst et al. convincingly demonstrated that the transfected ghrelin GHS receptor Type 1a in HEK or COS cells has a constitutively high signalling rate [24]. This property of the receptor was shown to be due to an inherent high on-rate of the receptor alone, even when devoid of any ligand. The authors theorised that the molecular mechanism of this constitutive activation was due to the tilting or the direct approximation of the receptor TM 3 and TM 6 domains to each other through a counter ion interaction at the side chains of a specific pair of amino acids in TM 3 and TM 6. In studies performed in parallel with the transfected homologous motilin receptor, which functioned

only at a low constitutive signalling rate, it was concluded that the motilin receptor was functionally distinctively different from the transfected ghrelin receptor in spite of the strong structural homology between these receptors. Furthermore, this group showed that the $[DArg^1,DPhe^5,DTrp^{7,9},Leu^{11}]$-substance P peptide, which we had characterised as an in vitro and in vivo GHRP and ghrelin weak receptor antagonist, acted as a potent inverse agonist. At 5 nM, there was complete inhibition of the high constitutive signalling activity of the transfected ghrelin receptor. Also, this GHRP/ghrelin receptor antagonist only weakly inhibited the activity of this transfected receptor when stimulated by ghrelin; the $IC_{50}$ of the substance-P antagonist was 650 nM in inhibiting in vitro ghrelin activation. In competitive binding receptor studies using $^{125}I$-ghrelin as tracer, the Kd of $[DArg^1,DPhe^5,DTrp^{7,9},Leu^{11}]$-substance P was 45 nM while that of ghrelin was 0.36 nM. These latter results again underscore that this substance-P analogue acts in different roles as an inverse agonist and as a ghrelin competitive receptor antagonist.

A number of potentially important conceptual ideas have evolved from these studies suggesting the meaningful influences on how the ghrelin system functions physiologically, particularly the biochemical and molecular mechanisms imparting high constitutive signalling to the ghrelin receptor that can also be hormonally regulated. Regulation of GH secretion and food intake may be modulated not only by the secretion of ghrelin but possibly by the presence, location and number of ghrelin receptors, even at subthreshold levels of ghrelin. The high constitutive signalling of the ghrelin receptor may even explain in part why mice with knock-out of the ghrelin receptor grow less and weigh less than mice with knock-out of the ghrelin hormone. For instance, tonically activated ghrelin receptor unstimulated by ghrelin may maintain or heighten hunger between meals and may raise basal GH secretion between GH pulses. If this occurs, these results will encourage development of specifically acting inverse agonists to the ghrelin receptor, as such compounds would appear to very effectively decrease the high constitutive signalling. Pertinent is the report of

Kim et al. that rats fasted for 48 h had increased ghrelin mRNA levels in the stomach, which were reduced by refeeding [25]. In addition, ghrelin receptor mRNA levels increased eight-fold in the hypothalamus and three-fold in the pituitary after 48 h of fasting in comparison to fed rats; the constitutive activity of the receptor may heighten and/or maintain the hunger for food by tonically activating arcuate NPY/AgRP neurons responsible for mediating food intake, even without an increase in ghrelin itself. Also, basal GH secretion may be maintained or increased by the high constitutive signalling of this receptor, and pituitary responsiveness to the GH-releasing actions of ghrelin may be enhanced. Taken together, regulation of the ghrelin system by the high constitutive signalling of the receptor, with or without ghrelin, appears to require reconsideration of how the ghrelin system functions. If the major function of the ghrelin system is to enhance and maintain food intake and GH secretion during fasting and starvation, a high constitutive activity of the receptor would seem to be teleologically a unique and novel mechanism for both animals and humans.

The degree that the Holst in vitro data (vide infra) translate to in vivo results and the circumstances under which this occurs may significantly depend on whether leptin and/or SRIF inhibit the high constitutive signalling activity of the ghrelin receptor in vivo. If these two hormones are inhibitory this would be an additional mechanism for explaining how the ghrelin system is activated during starvation and GH secretion and food intake are increased.

Neuroendocrine and neuroanatomical mechanistic studies evolving from the decreased action of ghrelin on the NPY/AgRP hypothalamic arcuate neurons caused by leptin are considered of special relevance. When leptin was administered to leptin-deficient mice during critical periods of early development, Bouret et al. observed that the hypothalamic arcuate nucleus architecture was altered [26]. This again appears to be an example of hormonal hypothalamic imprinting on the developing brain that possibly results from the neonate surge of leptin secretion. This action has been reported previously and also may forecast that a

similar but opposite action of ghrelin may occur at this critical period when ghrelin is increased in amount. Pinto et al. further observed not only that leptin and ghrelin administration to mice acutely (6 h) altered the neural connections within the hypothalamic arcuate nucleus without a change in the neuron number, but also that these synaptic neural connections were increased by ghrelin and decreased by leptin [27]. Although the ghrelin receptor has been reported to be co-localised on most of the arcuate NPY neurons in the Pinto et al. study, ghrelin acted only on the pro-opiomelanocortin (POMC) and not the NPY neurons, which again emphasises the dynamic structural and functional plasticity of the CNS neurons. Since secretion of leptin decreases and ghrelin increases during restricted energy balance, these fundamental results are considered to be substantive support for one of the roles, or possibly the major regulatory physiological role, of the ghrelin system.

## Conclusions

The chemistry of unnatural GHRPs and natural ghrelin and its receptor is predicted to have unique as well as novel complementary effects on the physiological and pathophysiological dimensions of the new ghrelin system. In spite of the different chemistries of the peptide and non-peptidyl GHRPs that have been developed, as well as between natural ghrelin and the non-natural GHRPs, it is amazing that they target the same receptor and produce the same biological actions of increasing GH secretion and food intake in animals and humans. The conceptualisation of the GHRP action during the first 20 years of this story focused on GH secretion. Since the identification of ghrelin 6 years ago, the emphasis has evolved to the enhancement of food intake and the possible role of the ghrelin system in overnutrition, as in obesity, and malnutrition, as in anorexia nervosa and cancer. Understanding the physiological role and dimensions of ghrelin actions from the stomach to CNS to pituitary and to peripheral adipose tissue, the ghrelin system has an exciting future. This future includes the determination of complementary biological actions of GHRP/ghrelin on GH secretion and food intake, a better chemical orientation on the variability of these compounds, a more in-depth appreciation of the possible selective actions of the unnatural ghrelin peptides, partial peptides, non-peptides and whether different receptors may be involved, and further understanding of the seminal chemistry of ghrelin with the indispensable octanoyl carboxylic acid addition for the bioactive chemical conformation of the ghrelin molecule and the characterisation and identification of the special enzyme complex responsible for the octanoylation of ghrelin. New branches are sprouting from the trunk of the ghrelin/GHRP/GHS path in several unexpected directions complementing existing evidence of the potential value of GHRP for clinical diagnostic and therapeutic purposes.

### Acknowledgements

This work was supported in part by the National Center for Research Resources and National Institutes of Health (Bethesda, MD) via the General Clinical Research grant MO1 RR05096 (C.Y.B.) and the National Science Foundation CAREER Award IBN9600805 (D.L.H.). The authors are grateful to G.A. Reynolds, K. Friedman and C. Maier for technical assistance and to Kaken Pharmaceutical Co for supplying GHRP-2.

## References

1. Bowers CY (1999) GH releasing peptides (GHRPs). In: Kostyo J, Goodman H (eds) Handbook of Physiology. Oxford University Press, New York, vol 7, pp 267–297
2. Bowers CY (1998) Growth hormone releasing peptide (GHRP). Cell Mol Life Sci 54:1316–1329
3. Veldhuis JD, Bowers CY (2003) Sex-steroid modulation of growth hormone (GH) secretory control. Endocrine 22:25–39
4. Howard AD, Feighner SD, Cully DF et al (1966) A receptor in pituitary and hypothalamus and functions in growth hormone release. Science 273:974–977
5. Kojima M, Hosada H, Date Y et al (1999) Ghrelin is a growth-hormone releasing acylated peptide from stomach. Nature 402:656–660
6. Bowers CY (2001) Unnatural growth hormone-releasing peptide begets natural ghrelin. J Clin Endocrinol Metab 86:1464–1469
7. Bowers CY, Granda-Ayala R, Mohan S et al (2004) Sustained elevation of pulsatile growth hormone (GH) secretion and insulin-like growth factor I (IGF-1), IGF-binding protein-3 (IGFBP-3), and IGFBP-5 concentrations during 30-day continuous subcutaneous infusion of GH-releasing peptide-2 in older men and women. J Clin Endocrinol Metab 89:2290–2300
8. Hataya Y, Akamizu T, Kazuhiko T et al (2001) A low dose of ghrelin stimulates growth hormone (GH) release synergistically with GH-releasing hormone in humans. J Clin Endocrinol Metab 86:4552–4555
9. Kohno D, Gao H-Z, Muroya S et al (2004) Ghrelin directly interacts with neuropeptide Y-containing neurons in the rat arcuate nucleus. Diabetes 52:948–956
10. Matsumoto M, Hosoda H, Kitajima Y et al (2001) Structure-activity relationship of ghrelin: Pharmacological study of ghrelin peptides. Biochem Biophys Res Commun 287:142–146
11. Matsumoto M, Kitajima Y, Iwanami T et al (2001) Structural similarity of ghrelin derivatives to peptidyl growth hormone secretagogues. Biochem Biophys Res Commun 284:655–659
12. Bednarek MA, Feighner SD, Pong SS et al (2000) Structure-function studies on the new growth hormone-releasing peptide, ghrelin: minimal sequence of ghrelin necessary for activation of growth hormone secretagogue receptor 1a. J Med Chem 43:4370–4376
13. Thompson N, Gill DAS, Davies R et al (2004) Ghrelin and des-octanoyl ghrelin promote adipogenesis directly in vivo by a mechanism independent of the type 1a growth hormone secretagogue receptor. Endocrinology 145:234–242
14. Choi K, Roh SG, Hong YH et al (2003) The role of ghrelin and growth hormone secretagogues receptor on rat adipogenesis. Endocrinology 144:754–759
15. Cassoni P, Papotti M, Ghe C et al (2001) Identification, characterization, and biological activity of specific receptors for natural (ghrelin) and synthetic growth hormone secretagogues and analogs in human breast carcinomas and cell lines. J Clin Endocrinol Metab 86:1738–1745
16. Baldanzi G, Filigheddu N, Cutrupi S et al (2002) Ghrelin and des-acyl ghrelin inhibit cell death in cardiomyocytes and endothelial cells through ERK1/2 and PI 3-Kinase/AKT. J Cell Biol 159:1029–1037
17. Hosoda H, Kojima M, Mizushima T et al (2003) Structural divergence of human ghrelin. Identification of multiple ghrelin-derived molecules produced by post-translational processing. J Biol Chem 278:64–70
18. Gnanapavan S, Kola B, Bustin SA et al (2002) The tissue distribution of the mRNA of ghrelin and subtypes of its receptor, GHS-R, in humans. J Clin Endocrinol Metab 87:2988–2991

19. Tomassetto C, Karam SM, Ribieras S et al (2000) Identification and characterization of a novel gastric peptide hormone: the motilin-related peptide. Gastroenterology 119:395–405
20. Inui A, Asakawa A, Bowers CY et al (2004) Appetite and growth - the emerging role of the stomach as an endocrine gland. FASEB J 18:439–456
21. Lu S, Guan JL, Wang, QP et al (2002) Immunocytochemical observation of ghrelin-containing neurons in the rat arcuate nucleus. Neurosci Lett 321:157–160
22. Silva Elipe MV, Bednarek MA, Gao YD (2001) 1H NMR structural analysis of human ghrelin and its six truncated analogs. Biopolymers 59:489–501
23. Feighner SD, Howard AD, Prendergast K et al (1998) Structural requirements for the activation of the human growth hormone secretagogue receptor by peptide and non-peptide secretagogues. Mol Endocrinol 12:137–145
24. Holst B, Cygankiewicz A, Jensen TH et al (2003) High constitutive signalling of the ghrelin receptor - identification of a potent inverse agonist. Mol Endocrinol 17:2201–2210
25. Kim M-S, Yoon C-Y, Park K-H et al (2003) Changes in ghrelin and ghrelin receptor expression according to feeding status. Neuroreport 14:1317–1320
26. Bouret SG, Draper SJ, Simerly RB (2004) Trophic action of leptin on hypothalamic neurons that regulate feeding. Science 304:108–110
27. Pinto S, Roseberry AG, Hongyan L et al (2004) Rapid rewiring of arcuate nucleus feeding circuits by leptin. Science 304:110–115

# Ghrelin as a New Factor in the Central Network Controlling Appetite and Food Intake

Fabio Broglio, Cristina Gottero, Flavia Prodam, Elisa Me, Silvia Destefanis, Fabrizio Riganti, Federico Ragazzoni, Maria Angela Seardo, Aart J. van der Lely, Ezio Ghigo

## Introduction

Ghrelin is a 28 amino acid peptide predominantly produced by the stomach, although it is also expressed in many other central and peripheral endocrine and non-endocrine tissues [1–3]. Ghrelin displays strong growth hormone (GH)-releasing activity mediated by the activation of the GH secretagogue receptor type 1a (GHS-R 1a) [1, 3]. Prior to the discovery of ghrelin, this orphan receptor had been shown to be specific for a family of synthetic peptidyl and non-peptidyl molecules known as GH secretagogues (GHS) [1, 3, 4]. GHS-R are concentrated in the hypothalamic-pituitary unit but are also distributed in other central and peripheral tissues [1–4]. Apart from the potent GH-releasing effect, ghrelin exhibits additional actions including stimulation of prolactin and ACTH secretion, negative influence on gonadal axis, stimulation of appetite and positive influence on energy balance, endocrine and non-endocrine gastro-entero-pancreatic functions, cardiovascular actions and modulation of cell viability [3, 5, 6]. Given this wide spectrum of biological activities, it is clear that the discovery of ghrelin opened new perspectives of research in endocrinology but also in other areas of internal medicine.

## From GH-Releasing Peptides to Ghrelin

Growth hormone-releasing peptide-6 (GHRP-6) was the first peptidyl GHS able to release GH in vivo even after oral administration in humans [3, 4]. Further research led to the synthesis of other peptidyl and non-peptidyl GHS; the spiroindoline MK-0677 was one of the most powerful, being able to enhance 24-h GH secretion and insulin-like growth factor-1 (IGF-1) levels even after single oral administration [3, 4].

In 1996, in agreement with data from binding studies, a specific GHS receptor expressed by a single gene found at chromosomal location 3q26.2 was cloned [3, 4]. Two types of GHS receptor complementary DNA (cDNA), as the result of alternate processing of a pre-mRNA, encode for two different receptors, the GHS receptor type 1a, which consists of 366 amino acids with seven transmembrane regions, and the GHS receptor type 1b, of 289 amino acids with only five transmembrane regions. Whereas the GHS-R 1b does not bind GHS and therefore its functional role remains unknown, ghrelin as well as synthetic peptidyl and non-peptidyl GHS exhibit high binding affinity to the GHS-R 1a [1–4].

Studies focusing on GHS-R distribution revealed particular concentration not only in the hypothalamic–pituitary area but also in other central and peripheral tissues [2–4], thus explaining the GH-releasing effect and the other endocrine and non-endocrine actions of GHS [3].

Ghrelin, discovered in 1999 as a natural ligand of the GHS-R 1a [7], is a 28 amino acid peptide predominantly produced by the stomach, but also expressed in bowel, pancreas, kidney, lung, placenta, thyroid, testis, ovary, pituitary and hypothalamus. Within the stomach, ghrelin is produced by enteroendocrine cells, probably the X/A-like cells, a major endocrine population in the oxyntic mucosa, the hormonal product of which had not previously been clarified [3, 8].

Ghrelin is the first peptide isolated from natural sources in which the hydroxyl group of one of its serine residues is acylated by a n-octanoic acid [3, 7]. The acylation of the peptide is essential for its binding to the GHS-R type 1a and for its endocrine actions [3, 7, 9]: however, non-acylated ghrelin, which circulates in amounts far higher than the acylated form, is not biologically inactive. Non-acylated ghrelin is able to exert some non-endocrine actions including cardiovascular, anti-proliferative and adipogenetic effects probably binding different GHS-R subtypes [3, 10].

Besides 28 amino acid acylated ghrelin, other endogenous ligands of the GHS-R 1a have been described, among which are several acylated ghrelin variants: adenosine, which acts as a weak agonist [11] and cortistatin, a neuropeptide homologous to somatostatin, which, in turn, is unable to recognise this receptor [12]. It has been suggested that different molecules are able to bind different pockets of the GHS-R 1a but not necessarily to activate it; however, further studies are required to clarify whether ghrelin is the sole ligand or one of a number of ligands activating GHS-R and whether the GHS-R used for ghrelin isolation is the sole receptor or one of a group of receptors for one or more than one ligand.

## Physiological Control of Ghrelin Secretion

Circulating ghrelin levels, mostly represented by its acylated form, are rapidly reduced by 80% after total gastrectomy but gradually recover thereafter, indicating that the stomach is the major source of circulating ghrelin but that other tissues can compensate for the loss of ghrelin production after gastrectomy [13].

Ghrelin is secreted in a pulsatile manner [14]. Notably, there is no strict correlation between ghrelin and GH levels, while ghrelin pulses are correlated with food intake episodes and sleep cycles [14].

Specifically, ghrelin secretion in humans has been shown to follow a circadian rhythm with superimposed increases before meals and decreases after food intake [15]. Such a secretory profile suggested that food intake may be triggered by ghrelin increases [15] and, on the other hand, revealed that ghrelin secretion mainly undergoes a metabolic control [16]. In fact, ghrelin secretion is markedly inhibited by food intake but not by simple gastric distension [17, 18].

Among nutrients, glucose, after either oral or intravenous administration, has been shown to exert the most potent inhibitory effect on ghrelin secretion, while the role of free fatty acids and arginine load has not yet been fully established [18–20].

Evidence of a clear negative association between ghrelin and insulin secretion [15] suggested an inhibitory influence of insulin on ghrelin secretion in agreement with data showing a direct modulation of gastric ghrelin expression by insulin itself [21]. Indeed, during both euglycaemic and hypoglycaemic clamp, the steady-state increase in insulin levels is associated with a clear reduction in circulating ghrelin levels [22, 23]. Recently, it has been shown that post-prandial hyperinsulinaemia is a decisive signal for meal-related ghrelin suppression [16]. In insulin-resistant states there is a lower decrement in post-prandial circulating ghrelin concentrations suggesting a negative cycle that augments nutrient intake in obese and type 2 diabetic subjects [16].

Moreover, further confirming the major role of metabolic and nutritional factors in the regulation of ghrelin secretion, several other factors involved in the regulation of food intake and metabolic balance have also been reported as being able to inhibit ghrelin secretion, such as glucagon-like peptide 1 [24], gastrin [24], urocortin-1 [25], PYY [26] and oxyntomodulin [27], or to increase it, such as gastrin [24].

Notably, although playing a functional complementary role in the regulation of appetite at the hypothalamic level, leptin has been shown to be devoid of any modulatory effect on ghrelin secretion [28].

However, the most remarkable inhibitory input on ghrelin secretion reported so far is represented by the activation of somatostatin receptors by somatostatin as well as by its natural analogue cortistatin [29].

Overall, evidence that insulin and somatostatin exert a critical inhibitory action on ghrelin secretion indicates that the latter is under major control from the endocrine pancreas, which, in turn, is under the influence of ghrelin. In fact, in humans, acute intravenous ghrelin administration has been reported to increase circulating somatostatin levels [30] and to induce a transient inhibition of insulin secretion that is coupled, although mediated by independent mechanisms, with an increase of circulating glucose levels [30, 31].

In agreement with the major influence of nutrition on ghrelin secretion, circulating ghrelin levels are inversely related to body mass index (BMI), i.e. increased in anorexia and cachexia while reduced in obesity and overfeeding, a notable exception being patients with Prader-Willi syndrome (PWS) [3, 32, 33]. In particular, ghrelin hypersecretion has been suggested to be responsible for the hyperphagia and weight excess commonly present in this syndrome [32, 33].

In both anorexia and obesity, ghrelin secretion is normalised by recovery of ideal body weight [18, 34, 35]. These changes are opposite to those of leptin, suggesting that both ghrelin and leptin are hormones signalling the metabolic balance and managing the neuroendocrine and metabolic response to starvation [3, 35, 36].

In humans, ghrelin secretion has been reported to occur throughout the lifespan, with some age-related variations. In particular, ghrelin secretion significantly increases after birth, peaking during the first two years of life, then decreases until the end of puberty [37]. Moreover, a further decrease of ghrelin levels in elderly subjects has also been reported recently [38].

Gender-dependent differences have been found by some authors [39] but not by others [40].

This general picture of the control of ghrelin secretion generally comes from evaluating total circulating ghrelin levels. As endocrine actions are displayed by acylated ghrelin only, more appropriate information about the control of ghrelin secretion and its functional significance could come from distinguishing plasma variations in acylated and unacylated ghrelin.

## Ghrelin as a New Factor in the Control of Energy Balance, Appetite and Food Intake

Among all the biological actions of ghrelin, particular attention has been focused on its role in the regulation of appetite and energy balance.

Long before ghrelin was discovered, different reports in rodents indicated that some GHS pos-

sess orexigenic activity [41]. Moreover, in the last decade, a substantial amount of data showed that GHS were able to activate neurons in hypothalamic areas strictly involved in the control of energy balance [41, 42]. Accordingly, ghrelin emerged as one of the most powerful orexigenic and adipogenic agents known so far [3, 6, 15, 43]. At first, it was puzzling to link adipogenic effects to a hormone that was originally discovered as a potent secretagogue of GH, a lipolytic hormone, but progressively, ghrelin resulted as a previously unidentified interface between energy balance regulation, glucose homeostasis, and hypothalamic neuropeptides [3, 6, 43].

Ghrelin dose-dependently stimulates food intake in rodents, particularly after central administration [17, 44]. Unlike other potent orexigenic agents (e.g. neuropeptide Y [NPY], agouti-related protein [AgRP], melanin-concentrating hormone [MCH]) that are active only when injected intracerebroventricularly, ghrelin has orexigenic and adipogenic effects even after systemic administration [45]. The efficacy of ghrelin as an orexigenic agent after peripheral administration would be explained by its transport across the blood–brain barrier in a blood-to-brain direction. The hypothalamic areas playing a crucial role in the regulation of energy homeostasis, such as the ventromedial part of the arcuate nucleus, are not completely protected by the blood–brain barrier, contain neurons expressing GHS-R [3], and might therefore mediate ghrelin effects [45, 46].

It has also been demonstrated that ghrelin's influence on appetite and energy balance is, at least partially, mediated by hypothalamic leptin-responsive neurons [46–51].

Among the major hypothalamic pathways mediating ghrelin's influence on energy balance [48, 49, 51], one involves NPY neurons [52, 53] and the other involves melanocortin receptors [54]. Ghrelin increases AgRP and NPY expression after both acute and chronic administration in rats [47, 48, 51, 53]. Thus, NPY and AgRP likely co-mediate ghrelin's effects on energy balance; NPY might be more important for acute effects while AgRP might be involved in both chronic and acute ghrelin action in the hypothalamus [46].

Accordingly, whereas deletion of either NPY or

AgRP causes only a modest effect on the orexigenic effect of ghrelin, simultaneous genetic ablation completely abolishes ghrelin's modulatory action on food intake [55]. However, other agents are likely to be involved in mediating the impact of ghrelin on appetite, food intake and energy balance; these include orexins, pro-opiomelanocortin (POMC), cocaine- and amphetamine-related transcript (CART), MCH, ciliary neurotropic factor (CNTF), gamma amino butyric acid (GABA), galanin, corticotropin-releasing hormone (CRH) and somatostatin [46, 50, 56]. Besides the increase of appetite and food intake, reduced cellular fat oxidation and promotion of adipogenesis reportedly contributes to increased fat mass induced by ghrelin [10, 50].

It is noteworthy that ghrelin regulation of energy homeostasis seems to be mediated by efferent and afferent fibres of the vagal nerve [57]. Intravenously administered ghrelin decreases the afferent activity of the gastric vagal nerve at low doses [57]. Moreover, the blockade of the gastric vagal afferent fibres abolishes ghrelin-induced feeding, GH secretion, and activation of NPY-producing and growht hormone-releasing hormone (GHRH)-producing neurons in rats. Cholinergic influence on systemic ghrelin secretion has already been reported both in animals and humans [20, 58–60]. Nevertheless, cholinergic agonists and antagonists do not influence the endocrine response to ghrelin administration in humans [61].

Overall, as a result of central and peripheral actions, ghrelin administration in rodents causes weight gain [3, 6, 17, 43]. This effect is not due to longitudinal growth or an increase in lean mass as one would expect to occur after stimulation of GH secretion [62]. Data in rodents clearly showed that ghrelin-induced weight gain is based on accretion of fat mass without changes in longitudinal skeletal growth and with a decrease of lean mass [17].

Despite all these data, it has to be taken into account that ghrelin-null mice do not differ from controls in terms of food intake, size, growth rate and body composition [63] and even GHS-R-null mice show normal appetite and body composition, with only a mild reduction in body weight compared with controls [64].

## Ghrelin and Cachexia

Cachexia is a clinical condition frequently associated with neoplastic disease and chronic heart failure characterised by loss of body weight, negative nitrogen balance and fatigue that significantly affects patients' quality of life, morbidity and survival.

Taking into account the important role of ghrelin in the regulation of food intake and energy metabolism, several studies investigated the possible role of ghrelin as a factor involved in the development of cachexia or as a potential tool in its treatment.

In cachectic nude mice bearing human G361 melanoma cells, plasma ghrelin concentration as well as both ghrelin peptide and mRNA in the stomach have been reported to increase with the progression of cachexia [65].

Interestingly, in a different mouse model of cancer cachexia induced by the inoculation of human SEKI melanoma cells, one-week intraperitoneal ghrelin administration suppressed weight loss and increased food intake [66]. Moreover, ghrelin administration increased the weight of white adipose tissue and plasma leptin concentration, thus suggesting a potential therapeutic ability to ameliorate cancer cachexia [66].

In humans, plasma ghrelin levels have been reported to be significantly higher in patients affected by lung cancer with cachexia than in those without cachexia in whom, on the other hand, ghrelin levels were similar to those in healthy subjects [67].

Furthermore, an increase of circulating ghrelin levels was also observed in those patients developing anorexia after chemotherapy treatment [67].

Taken together, these data suggest that measurement of plasma ghrelin may be a simple and non-invasive method to assess the development of cachexia and, potentially, chemotherapy-induced toxicity.

Besides neoplastic cachexia, increased ghrelin levels have also been reported in cachectic syndromes of other aetiologies.

Independently from the aetiology of the liver disease, ghrelin levels have been reported to be significantly increased in Child C cirrhosis, showing high correlation with clinical complications of liver disease, but not with indexes of liver function [68].

Similarly, patients with cardiac cachexia suffering from chronic heart failure show increased ghrelin levels; in rats with chronic heart failure, chronic subcutaneous ghrelin administration, besides exerting its well-known positive cardiotropic effect, also prevented cardiac cachexia, as shown by increased body weight and preserved muscle-to-bone ratio [5, 69].

Overall, these data suggest that, considering ghrelin-induced positive effects on energy balance, the increase of ghrelin levels may represent a compensatory mechanism under catabolic–anabolic imbalance in cachectic patients of different aetiologies.

## Ghrelin and Anorexia Nervosa

Anorexia nervosa is a psychiatric disorder characterised by patient-induced and maintained weight loss that leads to progressive malnutrition and specific pathophysiological signs (disturbance of body image and fear of obesity). Based on the presence or not of bulimic symptoms, anorexia nervosa appears in two specific subtypes, restricting and binge-eating/purging [70]. Complications in many organ systems can occur, including cardiovascular, gastrointestinal, haematological, renal, skeletal, endocrine and metabolic systems. These alterations are not only related to the state of malnutrition, but also to the behaviour of these patients to control their weight. The endocrine disturbances include hypothalamic amenorrhoea, hyperactivity of the hypothalamus–pituitary–adrenal (HPA) axis, low T3 syndrome and alterations in the activity of the GH/IGF-1 axis [71–73]. Exaggerated GH secretion coupled with reduced IGF-1 levels are common findings in anorexia nervosa as well as in other catabolic states, reflecting malnutrition-induced peripheral GH resistance and implying reduced IGF-1 feedback action on somatotropic secretion [73, 74]. Primary or secondary alterations in the neuroendocrine control of GH secretion have also been hypothesised and are likely to include GHRH hyperactivity coupled with reduced somatostatin-

ergic tone [71–73]. Accordingly, an exaggerated GH response to GHRH has been reported by many studies [58, 71–73, 75].

As anticipated, ghrelin levels in anorexia nervosa have been reported to be clearly high, in agreement with evidence showing that ghrelin levels are inversely related to BMI [18, 34, 76–78]. A difference in ghrelin levels between restricting or purging-type anorectic patients has been reported by some studies [79], but not others [80].

Interestingly, however, despite the elevated plasma ghrelin levels, in anorexia nervosa, the sensitivity of ghrelin secretion to the inhibitory effect of glucose seems to be preserved, although some differences among the different subtypes of anorexia have been reported [80–82].

In fact, oral glucose load has been reported to reduce circulating total and acylated ghrelin levels in women with anorexia nervosa to a similar extent as in normal subjects, despite absolute ghrelin levels in anorexia nervosa persisting higher than in controls [81, 82].

Another study showed that while the inhibitory effect of oral glucose load is preserved in patients with anorexia of purging type, although with delayed nadir, such effect seems to be markedly blunted in women with anorexia of restricting type, thus suggesting that differences in eating behaviour may influence the metabolic control of ghrelin secretion [80].

Interestingly, previous reports showed that, differently from normal subjects, in patients with anorexia nervosa, ghrelin secretion is not inhibited by food intake [83]. The reasons for these discrepant data are at present unexplained and may reflect a different sensitivity to different types of nutrient intake [84]. One hypothesis is that, due to the chronic food restriction and the consequent adaptation, a single physiological meal could be insufficient to suppress the drive to eat, in order to regain a normal weight and replenish energy stores [83]. However, weight gain in anorectic patients is associated with decreased plasma ghrelin levels [78]. It is therefore possible that in these patients the correction of the abnormal feeding behaviour over a prolonged period of time may restore the normal acute response of plasma ghrelin to single meals [78].

Notably, though the reduced food intake in anorexia nervosa might seem discordant with a ghrelin hypersecretory state, it has to be emphasised that this condition is not characterised by lack of appetite; on the contrary, appetite is often increased, leading to a stressful condition [85].

The possibility that ghrelin hypersecretion could play a major role in GH hypersecretion in anorexia nervosa has been hypothesised. To support this hypothesis, there is evidence that fasting-induced GH hypersecretion is anticipated by an increase in ghrelin levels, at least in humans [86]. Interestingly, however, anorexia nervosa shows a selective reduction of the GH response to ghrelin administration and, differently from normal women, in anorectic patients ghrelin does not significantly increase glucose levels [87].

Evidence of a blunted GH response to ghrelin is remarkable considering that anorexia nervosa is associated with elevated circulating ghrelin levels coupled with both basal and GHRH-induced GH hypersecretion.

Notably, the GH hyporesponsiveness to ghrelin administration in anorexia nervosa represented an unexpected finding. In fact, several common hormonal alterations in anorexia nervosa, such as enhanced endogenous GHRH activity, reduced IGF-1 feedback action and reduced somatostatinergic tone, could have induced an enhanced GH responsiveness to ghrelin [71, 73, 88, 89].

However, the possibility that in anorexia nervosa chronic exposure to elevated circulating ghrelin levels may induce desensitisation to the GH-releasing effect of ghrelin itself has also to be taken into account [90, 91].

On the other hand, the absence of a hyperglycaemic effect of ghrelin in anorexia nervosa, which in normal subjects has been suggested to reflect a direct or indirect glycogenolytic effect, might simply reflect exhaustion of glycogen stores in the liver due to chronic starvation [92].

## Ghrelin and Weight Loss in Obesity

Obesity is a chronic disease that is causally related to serious medical illnesses such as type 2 diabetes mellitus, hypertension, hyperlipidaemia, sleep apnoea and orthopaedic complications.

Based on evidence of the potent orexigenic action of ghrelin, its levels were at first expected to be increased in obesity. On the contrary, ghrelin levels turned out to be inversely related to body mass index.

At present, the exact peripheral signals leading to a reduced ghrelin secretion in obesity have not yet been identified. The most likely hypothesis is that low ghrelin levels in obesity might represent a signal to the hypothalamic centres regulating food intake that energy stores are filled [34].

Ghrelin gene polymorphisms have been described by several groups; linkage analysis studies, however, failed to prove a solid association between ghrelin and obesity [76, 93, 94].

While diet-induced human obesity, as well as polygenic (e.g. Pima Indians) or monogenic (e.g. MC4-R defect) causes of human obesity all present with low plasma ghrelin levels [34, 77], severely obese patients with PWS show markedly increased plasma ghrelin levels [32, 33, 95]. PWS is the most frequent known cause of genetically induced obesity and is associated with a defect on the short arm of chromosome 15, while the exact pathophysiological mechanisms leading to the obesity syndrome in PWS remain unclear [96]. Apart from their adiposity, patients with PWS suffer from a severe hunger syndrome, decreased locomotory activity, impaired GH secretion, increased sleepiness and relative hypoinsulinaemia [97, 98]. Although it appears intriguing that hyperghrelinaemia in PWS might be responsible, at least in part, for the majority of symptoms characterising this disease, the biological significance of the link between ghrelin and PWS remains at present unexplained [32, 33, 95].

However, independently from whatever the pathophysiological mechanisms underlying ghrelin hypersecretion in PWS may be [99], several data indicate that ghrelin hyposecretion in essential obesity is only a functional impairment.

In fact, a significant increase of ghrelin levels has been reported after weight loss induced by either diet or lifestyle modifications [77].

Given the potent orexigenic effect of ghrelin, the implication of these findings is that an increase in ghrelin levels caused by weight loss may help to promote regaining weight. In this context, it has been hypothesised that methods of weight loss that fail to trigger a compensatory rise in ghrelin levels might help sustain weight loss on a long-term basis.

Among the different surgical treatments of obesity, Roux-en-Y gastric bypass (RYGB) surgery is the most effective approved treatment for morbid obesity [100, 101]. This procedure restricts the gastric volume that is capable of storing food, bypassing most of the stomach and all of the duodenum (i.e. the majority of ghrelin-producing tissue) with a gastrojejunal anastomosis.

Importantly, the ultimate mechanisms by which this technique induces weight loss have not yet been defined but, notably, restrictive vertical-banded gastroplasty, which induces similar reduction of gastric volume, is less effective at maintaining long-term weight loss [100].

Interestingly, patients who undergo RYGB typically experience a generalised loss of appetite, suggesting that different mechanisms influencing appetite beyond simple gastric restriction may occur after this surgical treatment [100]. For these reasons, the existence of peculiar alterations of ghrelin secretion after RYGB has been hypothesised.

In fact, most authors reported that, despite inducing a marked weight loss, RYBG surgery is not followed by normalisation of ghrelin secretion and, according to some authors, even induces a further reduction of its circulating levels [104]. On the other hand, weight loss induced by biliopancreatic diversion [102] or adjustable gastric binding [103] is associated with an increase of circulating ghrelin levels, in agreement with the reported inverse relationship between BMI and ghrelin levels [104].

The pathophysiological mechanisms leading to the apparently inappropriate ghrelin hyposecretion after RYBG have not been described so far. The most convincing hypothesis is that the majority of ghrelin-producing cells, when chronically isolated from contact with enteral nutrients, undergo overriden inhibition [104]. According to this model, the condition of an empty stomach and duodenum, which acutely stimulates ghrelin production, paradoxically inhibits it when present continuously after RYGB [101].

If this model is valid, the location of the staple line that partitions the stomach into upper and lower compartments in RYGB may be a critical determinant of ghrelin suppression [101]. In fact, the persistence of some ghrelin-producing cells in intermittent contact with food would fail to be silenced through overriden inhibition.

This hypothesis would explain why bariatric surgery that does not exclude major ghrelin-producing tissues, such as the fundus, from contact with food would be ineffective at suppressing ghrelin.

Normal concentrations of ghrelin might also be sustained in RYGB variants with a short biliopancreatic intestinal limb because intermittent retrograde flow of ingested nutrients from the anastomosis could reach the duodenum and stomach, where ghrelin is mainly produced [102, 104].

An alternative hypothesis to reconcile discordant reports regarding the effect of different techniques of bariatric surgery on ghrelin levels pertains to variable surgical treatment of the autonomic nervous input to ghrelin-producing tissue in the foregut, since an important modulatory role of gastric vagal (parasympathetic) innervation on ghrelin secretion has been clearly demonstrated [105].

## Conclusions

Ghrelin, a 28 amino acid acylated peptide predominantly produced by the stomach, displays strong GH-releasing activity mediated by the hypothalamic–pituitary GHS receptors, which have been shown to be specific for a family of synthetic, orally active molecules known as GHS. However, ghrelin and GHS, acting on central and peripheral receptors, also exert different actions including orexigenic effects, an influence on exocrine and endocrine gastro-entero-pancreatic functions, cardiovascular and antiproliferative effects and manage the neuroendocrine and metabolic response to starvation. In particular, the effect of ghrelin in promoting food intake and modulating energy metabolism strongly suggests the possibility that ghrelin could be involved in the pathophysiological or metabolic and neuro-hormonal alterations commonly reported in cachexia, eating disorders and obesity and that ghrelin analogues acting as GHS-R agonists or antagonists could have a potential role in clinical practice. However, at present, although specific alterations in ghrelin secretion and/or action in

cachexia, anorexia nervosa and obesity have already been reported, there is no definitive evidence that ghrelin analogues may, in the near future, represent a useful therapeutic tool for these pathological conditions.

## References

1. Kojima M, Hosoda H, Kangawa K (2001) Purification and distribution of ghrelin: the natural endogenous ligand for the growth hormone secretagogue receptor. Horm Res 56(Suppl 1):93–97
2. Gnanapavan S, Kola B, Bustin SA et al (2002) The tissue distribution of the mRNA of ghrelin and subtypes of its receptor, GHS-R, in humans. J Clin Endocrinol Metab 87:2988
3. Muccioli G, Tschop M, Papotti M et al (2002) Neuroendocrine and peripheral activities of ghrelin: implications in metabolism and obesity. Eur J Pharmacol 440:235–254
4. Smith RG, Van der Ploeg LH, Howard AD et al (1997) Peptidomimetic regulation of growth hormone secretion. Endocr Rev 18:621–645
5. Nagaya N, Kangawa K (2003) Ghrelin improves left ventricular dysfunction and cardiac cachexia in heart failure. Curr Opin Pharmacol 3:146–151
6. Zigman JM, Elmquist JK (2003) Minireview: From anorexia to obesity—the yin and yang of body weight control. Endocrinology 144:3749–3756
7. Kojima M, Hosoda H, Matsuo H, Kangawa K (2001) Ghrelin: discovery of the natural endogenous ligand for the growth hormone secretagogue receptor. Trends Endocrinol Metab 12:118–122
8. Date Y, Kojima M, Hosoda H et al (2000) Ghrelin, a novel growth hormone-releasing acylated peptide, is synthesized in a distinct endocrine cell type in the gastrointestinal tracts of rats and humans. Endocrinology 141:4255–4261
9. Broglio F, Benso A, Gottero C et al (2003) Non-acylated ghrelin does not possess the pituitaric and pancreatic endocrine activity of acylated ghrelin in humans. J Endocrinol Invest 26:192–196
10. Thompson NM, Gill DA, Davies R et al (2003) Ghrelin and des-octanoyl ghrelin promote adipogenesis directly in vivo by a mechanism independent of the type 1a growth hormone secretagogue receptor. Endocrinology 145:234–242
11. Smith RG, Leonard R, Bailey AR et al (2001) Growth hormone secretagogue receptor family members and ligands. Endocrine 14:9–14
12. Deghenghi R, Papotti M, Ghigo E, Muccioli G (2001) Cortistatin, but not somatostatin, binds to growth hormone secretagogue (GHS) receptors of human pituitary gland. J Endocrinol Invest 24:RC1-RC3
13. Hosoda H, Kojima M, Mizushima T et al (2002) Structural divergence of human ghrelin.
14. Tolle V, Bassant MH, Zizzari P et al (2002) Ultradian rhythmicity of ghrelin secretion in relation with GH, feeding behavior, and sleep-wake patterns in rats. Endocrinology 143:1353–1361
15. Cummings DE, Purnell JQ, Frayo RS et al (2001) A preprandial rise in plasma ghrelin levels suggests a role in meal initiation in humans. Diabetes 50:1714–1719
16. Murdolo G, Lucidi P, Di Loreto C et al (2003) Insulin is required for prandial ghrelin suppression in humans. Diabetes 52:2923–2927
17. Tschop M, Smiley DL, Heiman ML (2000) Ghrelin induces adiposity in rodents. Nature 407:908–913
18. Shiiya T, Nakazato M, Mizuta M et al (2002) Plasma ghrelin levels in lean and obese humans and the effect of glucose on ghrelin secretion. J Clin Endocrinol Metab 87:240–244
19. Greenman Y, Golani N, Gilad S et al (2004) Ghrelin secretion is modulated in a nutrient- and gender-specific manner. Clin Endocrinol 60:382–388
20. Lee HM, Wang G, Englander EW et al (2002) Ghrelin, a new gastrointestinal endocrine peptide that stimulates insulin secretion: enteric distribution, ontogeny, influence of endocrine, and dietary manipulations. Endocrinology 143:185–190
21. Toshinai K, Mondal MS, Nakazato M et al (2001) Upregulation of ghrelin expression in the stomach upon fasting, insulin-induced hypoglycemia, and leptin administration. Biochem Biophys Res Commun 281:1220–1225
22. Flanagan DE, Evans ML, Monsod TP et al (2003) The influence of insulin on circulating ghrelin. Am J Physiol Endocrinol Metab 284:E313–E316
23. Lucidi P, Murdolo G, Di Loreto C et al (2002) Ghrelin is not necessary for adequate hormonal counterregulation of insulin-induced hypoglycemia. Diabetes 51:2911–2914
24. Lippl F, Kircher F, Erdmann J et al (2004) Effect of GIP, GLP-1, insulin and gastrin on ghrelin release in the isolated rat stomach. Regul Pept 119:93–98
25. Davis ME, Pemberton CJ, Yandle TG (2004) Urocortin-1 infusion in normal humans. J Clin Endocrinol Metab 89:1402–1409
26. Batterham RL, Cohen MA, Ellis SM et al (2003) Inhibition of food intake in obese subjects by pep-

Identification of multiple ghrelin-derived molecules produced by post-translational processing. J Biol Chem 278:64–70

tide YY3-36. N Engl J Med 349:941–948

27. Cohen MA, Ellis SM, Le Roux CW et al (2003) Oxyntomodulin suppresses appetite and reduces food intake in humans. J Clin Endocrinol Metab 88:4696–4701

28. Chan JL, Bullen J, Lee JH et al (2004) Ghrelin levels are not regulated by recombinant leptin administration and/or three days of fasting in healthy subjects. J Clin Endocrinol Metab 89:335–343

29. Broglio F, van Koetsveld P, Benso A et al (2002) Ghrelin secretion is inhibited by either somatostatin or cortistatin in humans. J Clin Endocrinol Metab 87:4829–4832

30. Arosio M, Ronchi CL, Gebbia C et al (2003) Stimulatory effects of ghrelin on circulating somatostatin and pancreatic polypeptide levels. J Clin Endocrinol Metab 88:701–704

31. Broglio F, Arvat E, Benso A et al (2001) Ghrelin, a natural GH secretagogue produced by the stomach, induces hyperglycemia and reduces insulin secretion in humans. J Clin Endocrinol Metab 86:5083–5086

32. Cummings DE, Clement K, Purnell JQ et al (2002) Elevated plasma ghrelin levels in Prader Willi syndrome. Nat Med 8:643–644

33. Haqq AM, Farooqi IS, O'Rahilly S et al (2003) Serum ghrelin levels are inversely correlated with body mass index, age, and insulin concentrations in normal children and are markedly increased in Prader-Willi syndrome. J Clin Endocrinol Metab 88:174–178

34. Tschop M, Weyer C, Tataranni PA et al (2001) Circulating ghrelin levels are decreased in human obesity. Diabetes 50:707–709

35. Cummings DE, Schwartz MW (2003) Genetics and pathophysiology of human obesity. Annu Rev Med 54:453–471

36. Yoshihara F, Kojima M, Hosoda H et al (2002) Ghrelin: a novel peptide for growth hormone release and feeding regulation. Curr Opin Clin Nutr Metab Care 5:391–395

37. Soriano-Guillen L, Barrios V, Chowen JA et al (2004) Ghrelin levels from fetal life through early adulthood: relationship with endocrine and metabolic and anthropometric measures. J Pediatr 144:30–35

38. Rigamonti AE, Pincelli AI, Corra B et al (2002) Plasma ghrelin concentrations in elderly subjects: comparison with anorexic and obese patients. J Endocrinol 175:R1–R5

39. Barkan AL, Dimaraki EV, Jessup SK et al (2003) Ghrelin secretion in humans is sexually dimorphic, suppressed by somatostatin, and not affected by the ambient growth hormone levels. J Clin Endocrinol Metab 88:2180–2184

40. Bellone S, Rapa A, Vivenza D et al (2003) Circulating ghrelin levels in newborns are not associated to gender, body weight and hormonal parameters but depend on the type of delivery. J Endocrinol Invest 26:RC9–RC11

41. Ghigo E, Aimaretti G, Arvat E, Camanni F (2001) Growth hormone-releasing hormone combined with arginine or growth hormone secretagogues for the diagnosis of growth hormone deficiency in adults. Endocrine 15:29–38

42. Bowers CY (1998) Growth hormone-releasing peptide (GHRP). Cell Mol Life Sci 54:1316–1329

43. Cummings DE, Schwartz MW (2001) Genetics and pathophysiology of human obesity. Ann Rev Med 54:453–471

44. Wren AM, Small CJ, Abbott CR et al (2001) Ghrelin causes hyperphagia and obesity in rats. Diabetes 50:2540–2547

45. Bowers CY (2001) Unnatural growth hormone-releasing peptide begets natural ghrelin. J Clin Endocrinol Metab 86:1464–1469

46. Horvath TL, Diano S, Sotonyi P et al (2001) Minireview: ghrelin and the regulation of energy balance - a hypothalamic perspective. Endocrinology 142:4163–4169

47. Kamegai J, Tamura H, Shimizu T et al (2000) Central effect of ghrelin, an endogenous growth hormone secretagogue, on hypothalamic peptide gene expression. Endocrinology 141:4797–4800

48. Nakazato M, Murakami N, Date Y et al (2001) A role for ghrelin in the central regulation of feeding. Nature 409: 194–198

49. Shintani M, Ogawa Y, Ebihara K et al (2001) Ghrelin, an endogenous growth hormone secretagogue, is a novel orexigenic peptide that antagonizes leptin action through the activation of hypothalamic neuropeptide Y/Y1 receptor pathway. Diabetes 50:227–232

50. Spiegelman BM, Flier JS (2001) Obesity and the regulation of energy balance. Cell 104:531–543

51. Tschop M, Castaneda T, Pagotto U, Tataranni PA (2004) Ghrelin food intake and energy balance. In: Ghigo E (ed) Ghrelin (more than simply a natural GH secretagogue and/or an orexigenic factor). Kluver Academic Publishers, Boston-Dordrecht-London, pp 31-141

52. Gehlert DR (1999) Role of hypothalamic neuropeptide Y in feeding and obesity. Neuropeptides 33:329–338

53. Kamegai J, Tamura H, Shimizu T et al (2001) Chronic central infusion of ghrelin increases hypothalamic neuropeptide Y and agouti-related protein mRNA levels and body weight in rats. Diabetes 50:2438–2443

54. Marks DL, Cone RD (2001) Central melanocortins and the regulation of weight during acute and chronic disease. Recent Prog Horm Res 56:359–375

55. Chen HY, Trumbauer ME, Chen AS et al (2004) Orexigenic action of peripheral ghrelin is mediated by neuropeptide Y (NPY) and agouti-related protein (AgRP). Endocrinology 145:2607–2612

56. Ahima RS, Osei SY (2001) Molecular regulation of eating behavior: new insights and prospects for therapeutic strategies. Trends Mol Med 7:205–213

57. Asakawa A, Inui A, Kaga T et al (2001) Ghrelin is an appetite-stimulatory signal from stomach with structural resemblance to motilin. Gastroenterology 120:337–345

58. Masuda A, Shibasaki T, Hotta M et al (1988) Study on the mechanism of abnormal growth hormone (GH) secretion in anorexia nervosa:no evidence of involvement of a low somatomedin-C level in the abnormal GH secretion. J Endocrinol Invest 11:297–302

59. Sugino T, Yamaura J, Yamagishi M et al (2003) Involvement of cholinergic neurons in the regulation of the ghrelin secretory response to feeding in sheep. Biochem Biophys Res Commun 304:308–312

60. Broglio F, Gottero C, Van Koetsveld P et al (2004) Acetylcholine regulates ghrelin secretion in humans. J Clin Endocrinol Metab 89:2429–2433

61. Broglio F, Gottero C, Benso A et al (2003) Acetylcholine does not play a major role in mediating the endocrine responses to ghrelin, a natural ligand of the GH secretagogue receptor, in humans. Clin Endocrinol (Oxf) 58:92–98

62. Lissett CA, Shalet SM (2000) Effects of growth hormone on bone and muscle. Growth Horm IGF Res 10(Suppl B):S95–S101

63. Sun Y, Ahmed S, Smith RG (2003) Deletion of ghrelin impairs neither growth nor appetite. Mol Cell Biol 23:7973–7981

64. Sun Y, Wang P, Zheng H, Smith RG (2004) Ghrelin stimulation of growth hormone release and appetite is mediated through the growth hormone secretagogue receptor. Proc Natl Acad Sci USA 101:4679–4684

65. Hanada T, Toshinai K, Date Y et al (2004) Upregulation of ghrelin expression in cachectic nude mice bearing human melanoma cells. Metabolism 53:84–88

66. Hanada T, Toshinai K, Kajimura N et al (2003) Anticachectic effect of ghrelin in nude mice bearing human melanoma cells. Biochem Biophys Res Commun 301:275–279

67. Shimizu Y, Nagaya N, Isobe T et al (2003) Increased plasma ghrelin level in lung cancer cachexia. Clin Cancer Res 9:774–778

68. Tacke F, Brabant G, Kruck E et al (2003) Ghrelin in chronic liver disease. J Hepatol 38:447–454

69. Nagaya N, Uematsu M, Kojima M et al (2001) Elevated circulating level of ghrelin in cachexia associated with chronic heart failure: relationships between ghrelin and anabolic/catabolic factors. Circulation 104:2034–2038

70. Foster DW (1998) Anorexia nervosa and bulimia. In: Fauci AS, Braunwald E, Iesselbacher KJ et al (eds) Harrison's principles of internal medicine, 14th ed. McGraw-Hill, New York, pp 534-538

71. Stoving RK, Veldhuis JD, Flyvbjerg A et al (1999) Jointly amplified basal and pulsatile growth hormone (GH) secretion and increased process irregu-

larity in women with anorexia nervosa: indirect evidence for disruption of feedback regulation within the GH-insulin-like growth factor I axis. J Clin Endocrinol Metab 81:2056–2063

72. Stoving RK, Hangaard J, Habsen-Nord M, Hagen C (1999) A review of endocrine change in anorexia nervosa. J Psychiatr Res 33:139–152

73. Gianotti L, Lanfranco F, Ramunni J et al (2002) GH/IGF-1 axis in anorexia nervosa. Eating and Weight Disorders 7:94–105

74. Argente J, Caballo N, Barrios V et al (1997) Multiple endocrine abnormalities of the growth hormone and insulin-like growth factor axis in patients with anorexia nervosa:effect of short- and long-term weight recuperation. J Clin Endocrinol Metab 82:2084–2092

75. Rolla M, Andreoni A, Belliti D et al (1991) Blockade of cholinergic muscarinic receptors by pirenzepine and GHRH-induced GH secretion in the acute and recovery phase of anorexia nervosa and atypical eating disorders. Biol Psychiatry 29:1079–1091

76. Ukkola O, Poykko S (2002) Ghrelin, growth and obesity. Ann Med 34:102–108

77. Cummings DE, Weigle DS, Frayo RS et al (2002) Plasma ghrelin levels after diet-induced weight loss or gastric bypass surgery. N Engl J Med 346:1623–1630

78. Otto B, Cuntz U, Fruehauf E et al (2001) Weight gain decreases elevated plasma ghrelin concentrations of patients with anorexia nervosa. Eur J Endocrinol 145:669–673

79. Tanaka M, Naruo T, Yasuhara D et al (2003) Fasting plasma ghrelin levels in subtypes of anorexia nervosa. Psychoneuroendocrinology 28:829–835

80. Tanaka M, Naruo T, Nagai N et al (2003) Habitual binge/purge behavior influences circulating ghrelin levels in eating disorders. J Psychiatr Res 37:17–22

81. Nakai Y, Hosoda H, Nin K et al (2003) Plasma levels of active form of ghrelin during oral glucose tolerance test in patients with anorexia nervosa. Eur J Endocrinol 149:R1–R3

82. Misra M, Miller KK, Herzog DB et al (2004) Growth hormone and ghrelin responses to an oral glucose load in adolescent girls with anorexia nervosa and controls. J Clin Endocrinol Metab 89:1605–1612

83. Nedvidkova J, Krykorkova I, Bartak V et al (2003) Loss of meal-induced decrease in plasma ghrelin levels in patients with anorexia nervosa. J Clin Endocrinol Metab 88:1678–1682

84. Gottero C, Bellone S, Rapa A et al (2003) Standard light breakfast inhibits circulating ghrelin levels to the same extent of oral glucose load in humans, despite different impact on glucose and insulin levels. J Endocrinol Invest 26:1203–1207

85. Anonymous (2000) Practice guideline for the treatment of patients with eating disorders (revision). American Psychiatric Association Work Group on Eating Disorders. Am J Psychiatry 157:1–39

86. Muller AF, Lamberts SW, Janssen JA et al (2002) Ghrelin drives GH secretion during fasting in man. Eur J Endocrinol 146:203–207

87. Broglio F, Gianotti L, Destefanis S et al (2004) The endocrine response to acute ghrelin administration is blunted in patients with anorexia nervosa, a ghrelin hypersecretory state. Clin Endocrinol (Oxf) 60:592–599

88. Arvat E, Maccario M, Di Vito L et al (2001) Endocrine activities of ghrelin, a natural growth hormone secretagogue (GHS), in humans:comparison and interaction with hexarelin, a nonnatural peptide GHS, and GH-releasing hormone. J Clin Endocrinol Metab 85:4908–4911

89. Hataya Y, Akamizu T, Takaya K et al (2001) A low dose of ghrelin stimulates growth hormone (GH) release synergistically with GH-releasing hormone in humans. J Clin Endocrinol Metab 86:4552

90. Yamazaki M, Nakamura K, Kobayashi H et al (2002) Regulational effect of ghrelin on growth hormone secretion from perifused rat anterior pituitary cells. J Neuroendocrinol 14:156–162

91. Camina JP, Carreira MC, El Messari S et al (2004) Desensitization and endocytosis mechanisms of ghrelin-activated growth hormone secretagogue receptor 1a. Endocrinology 145:930–940

92. Sasano H (1998) Glycogen and liver dysfunction in anorexia nervosa. Internal Med 37:652–657

93. Hinney A, Hoch A, Geller F et al (2002) Ghrelin gene: identification of missense variants and a frameshift mutation in extremely obese children and adolescents and healthy normal weight students. J Clin Endocrinol Metab 87:2716

94. Korbonits M, Gueorguiev M, O'Grady E et al (2002) A variation in the ghrelin gene increases weight and decreases insulin secretion in tall, obese children. J Clin Endocrinol Metab 87:4005–4008

95. Del Parigi A, Tschop M, Heiman ML et al (2002) High circulating ghrelin: a potential cause for hyperphagia and obesity in Prader-Willi syndrome. J Clin Endocrinol Metab 87:5461–5464

96. Nativio DG (2002) The genetics, diagnosis, and management of Prader-Willi syndrome. J Pediatr Health Care 16:298–303

97. Burman P, Ritzen EM, Lindgren AC (2001) Endocrine dysfunction in Prader-Willi syndrome: a review with special reference to GH. Endocr Rev 22:787–799

98. Eiholzer U, Nordmann Y, L'Allemand D et al (2003) Improving body composition and physical activity in Prader-Willi syndrome. J Pediatr 142:73–78

99. Goldstone AP, Thomas EL, Brynes AE et al (2004) Elevated fasting plasma ghrelin in Prader-Willi syndrome adults is not solely explained by their reduced visceral adiposity and insulin resistance. J Clin Endocrinol Metab 89:1718–1726

100. Msika S (2002) Surgical treatment of morbid obesity by gastrojejunal bypass using laparoscopic roux-en-Y (gastric short circuit). J Chir (Paris) 139:214–217

101. Cummings DE, Shannon MH (2003) Ghrelin and gastric bypass: is there a hormonal contribution to surgical weight loss? J Clin Endocrinol Metab 88:2999–3002

102. Adami GF, Cordera R, Marinari G et al (2003) Plasma ghrelin concentration in the short-term following biliopancreatic diversion. Obes Surg 13:889–892

103. Fruhbeck G, Diez Caballero A, Gil MJ (2004) Fundus functionality and ghrelin concentrations after bariatric surgery. N Engl J Med 350:308–309

104. Adami GF, Cordera R, Andraghetti G et al (2004) Changes in serum ghrelin concentration following biliopancreatic diversion for obesity. Obes Res 12:684–687

105. Date Y, Murakami N, Toshinai K et al (2003) The role of the gastric afferent vagal nerve in ghrelin-induced feeding and growth hormone secretion in rats. Gastroenterology 123:1120-1128, 2002 diversion. Obes Surg 13:889–892

# Leptin and Des-acyl Ghrelin: Their Role in Physiological Body Weight Regulation and in the Pathological State

Simona Perboni, Giovanni Mantovani, Akio Inui

## Introduction

Obesity, eating disorders and cachexia endanger the lives of millions of people worldwide. Fortunately, during the past decade, there has been a rapid and substantial progress toward uncovering the molecular and neural mechanisms by which energy imbalance develops. Central to this research has been the identification and characterisation of certain peripheral metabolic signals, such as leptin and ghrelin, which serve as fundamental indices of energy sufficiency [1].

## Des-acyl Ghrelin: A 'New' Peptide

In 1999, acyl ghrelin was discovered in the stomach as an appetite stimulatory signal from the periphery with structural resemblance to motilin [2]. Ghrelin molecules exist in two major molecular forms: acylated ghrelin, which has *n*-octanoylated serine in position 3, and des-acyl ghrelin, which is the major circulating isoform [3]. A recent study has shown that both the molecular forms are localised to the hypothalamic arcuate nucleus of rodents [4], as seen in the stomach [5]. The glucoprivic state of the hypothalamus, induced by fasting and 2-deoxy-D-glucose, a selective blocker of carbohydrate metabolism, stimulates des-acyl ghrelin secretion from ghrelin-producing neurons [6].

Deacylation of ghrelin to des-acyl ghrelin, which rapidly occurs in the plasma, is responsible for the reduced half-life of ghrelin. Two enzymes involved in the deacylation of ghrelin have been identified: high-density lipoprotein (HDL)-associated paraoxonase functions in the plasma while lysophospholipase I, a thioesterase active against palmitoyl-Gsα and palmitoyl-CoA, functions in the stomach [7]. In contrast, the enzyme that catalyses the acyl modification of ghrelin has not been identified. It has been seen that ingested medium-chain fatty acids are directly utilised for the acyl modification of ghrelin [8]. The ratio of des-acyl ghrelin to acylated ghrelin decreased in food-restricted mice compared with ad libitum fed mice [9].

The increased hydrophobicity of the acyl side-chain may explain why acyl ghrelin circulates bound to larger plasma proteins, particularly HDL species, whereas des-acylated ghrelin circulates as free peptide. This could be important in the transport of ghrelin to centres of appetite control [10].

### Physiological Role of Des-acyl Ghrelin

To date, very little is known about the physiological role of des-acyl ghrelin. Some authors have suggested that des-acyl ghrelin may have an anorexigenic activity that is contrary to the orexigenic activity of acylated ghrelin [2, 11]. Conversely, a recent study showed that both ghrelin and des-acyl ghrelin function as orexigenic peptides in the hypothalamus [12].

Since the acylation of ghrelin is required for the activation of the type 1a growth hormone secretagogue-receptor (GHS-R), it was assumed that des-acyl ghrelin was void of endocrine properties [13]. The des-acyl ghrelin showed no effect on the elevation of intracellular $Ca^{2+}$ concentrations in cells that express the GHS-R and for increasing plasma GH concentrations in rats [14, 15]. Later, a paper reported that des-acyl ghrelin is able to antagonise the metabolic but not the neuroendocrine response elicited by acylated ghrelin in humans [16]. Serum GH levels correlated closely with plasma acylated, rather than des-acylated ghrelin [17]. However, transgenic mice overexpressing des-acyl ghrelin showed small pheno-type, which is not attributed to poor nutritional condition. It has been found that overexpressed des-acyl ghrelin acts in the pituitary and in the hypothalamus in transgenic mice, suggesting a role of des-acyl ghrelin in the regulation of GH secretion [18]. Moreover, recent studies indicated that ghrelin and des-acyl ghrelin exhibit similar GHS-R-independent biological activities, including a cytoprotective effect on cultured cardiomyocytes and endothelial cells [19], the inhibition of cell proliferation in human breast and prostate cancer lines [20, 21], the reduction of glycerol released from rat epididymal adipocytes [22], and the promotion of adipogenesis directly in vivo in bone marrow fat [23]. Overall, these findings suggest that the action of des-acyl ghrelin is mediated by an as-yet unknown receptor that is different from GHS-R1a.

## Des-acyl Ghrelin as an Orexigenic Peptide

Des-acyl ghrelin is thought to stimulate feeding via a mechanism independent of GHS-R. In rats, the intracerebroventricular administration of des-acyl ghrelin increased feeding and locomotor activity, suggesting that des-acyl ghrelin may increase wakefulness and locomotor activity for food seeking by stimulating orexin neurons in the lateral area of the hypothalamus. Orexin-A and -B are involved in the hypothalamic regulation of feeding, energy homeostasis and arousal. It has been found that des-acyl ghrelin does not compete with ghrelin for binding to the GHS-R in orexin neurons. Thus, there are three possible subtypes of orexin neurons: those expressing the GHS-R as a receptor for ghrelin, those expressing an as-yet unknown receptor or target protein of des-acyl ghrelin and those possessing both proteins [24].

## Des-acyl Ghrelin as an Anorexigenic Peptide

Several studies have shown that des-acyl ghrelin induces a state of negative energy balance and reduced body weight by decreasing food intake and delaying gastric emptying in mice. The effect is mediated in the hypothalamus, since the peripheral administration of des-acyl ghrelin showed an increase in c-Fos expression in the hypothalamic arcuate nucleus and in the paraventricular nucleus. The anorexigenic cocaine- and amphetamine-regulated transcript (CART) and urocortin [25], as well as corticotropin-releasing factor type 2 receptor, but not type 1, are involved in this action [26]. Peripheral des-acyl ghrelin may directly activate the brain receptor by crossing the blood–brain barrier [27] but not by the activation of vagal afferent pathways [2, 25]. According to these results, the intracisternal administration of des-acyl ghrelin decreased food intake in food-deprived rats and inhibited gastric emptying without altering small intestine transit [11].

Des-acyl ghrelin-overexpressing mice exhibited a decrease in body weight, food intake and fat pad mass weight accompanied by moderately decreased linear growth. Gastric emptying was also decreased in these mice [25].

## Des-acyl Ghrelin and Glucose and Lipid Metabolism

The ghrelin system, using both the acylated and des-acylated molecules, is actively involved in the acute and long-term control of glucose metabolism and insulin concentrations [16]. It has been demonstrated that glucose output by primary hepatocytes is time- and dose-dependently stimulated by acyl ghrelin and inhibited by des-acyl ghrelin. Furthermore, it has been reported that des-acyl ghrelin is able to antagonise acyl ghrelin-induced glucose output. These actions might be mediated by a different receptor from GHS-R1a, which is not expressed in the hepatocytes, and apparently the two forms of peptides must be considered as separate hormones able to modify each other's actions on glucose handling, at least in the liver [28].

In humans, the acute administration of acyl ghrelin induced a rapid rise of glucose and insulin levels. The acute administration of des-acyl ghrelin has no effect on insulin secretion in humans, but it prevented the acyl ghrelin-induced rise of insulin and glucose when co-administered. The combination of acylated and des-acylated ghrelin significantly improved insulin sensitivity, which might lead to a new treatment for the many disorders in which insulin sensitivity is disturbed [29].

Ghrelin as well as des-acyl ghrelin promotes bone marrow adipogenesis in vivo by a direct peripheral action, via a receptor other than GHS-R1a. The ratio of ghrelin and des-acyl ghrelin production could help to regulate the balance between adipogenesis and lipolysis in response to nutritional status [22, 23].

## Leptin

Leptin, from the Greek *leptos*, meaning thin, is a product of the obese gene that was originally identified because its absence resulted in a syndrome of severe obesity in mice [30]. It is a hormone that provides information to the brain about the status of energy reserves of the organism, regulating feeding, substrate utilisation, energy balance, and the endocrine and immune systems [31]. Moreover, independent of its role in body weight regulation, it exerts effects on metabolism, cardiovascular and renal functions [32].

Leptin is a 16-kDa protein predominantly produced and secreted by adipocytes in white adipose tissue. Gastrointestinal tract, brain, placenta and skeletal muscle are additional sources [33]. Leptin acts throughout the leptin receptor [34], which is a type 1 cytokine receptor. It exerts its effects by activating the janus-kinase/signal transducer and activator of transcription-3 (STAT-3) pathways [1]. Among the six known leptin receptor spliced variants, the long form or signalling form contains a single trans-membrane domain, which is essential for normal energy homeostasis [35]. The long form of the receptor is expressed at high levels in hypothalamic neurons of the arcuate, paraventricular, dorsomedial, ventromedial nuclei and lateral area, each of which is important in regulating energy homeostasis [36]. The short form functions in the transport of leptin across the blood–brain barrier via a saturable process across the capillary endothelial cells [37]. The functional implications are that, in circumstances of chronic hyperleptinaemia such as obesity, relatively few adiposity signals would be available to the central nervous system [38], resulting in a chronic stimulation of excessive food intake [39].

These findings seem to favour the view that ancestral levels of leptin are much lower than those currently considered normal and that the biological impact of leptin is more pronounced when leptin levels are decreasing than when circulating leptin concentrations are elevated [40]. Supporting this view is the observation that when endogenous leptin levels were chronically decreased in women during prolonged consumption of a moderately energy-restricted diet, their increased sensations of hunger correlated with reduction of plasma leptin levels [41].

### Plasma Leptin Concentration

Plasma leptin concentrations correlate with adiposity, being high in obesity and decreasing after weight loss. Elevation of serum leptin in obesity appears to result from both increased fat mass and increased leptin release from larger adipocytes [42]. However, leptin levels are not constant in blood. They are considered to be pulsatile, with a frequency of about one pulse every 45 min [32]. In healthy subjects, circulating leptin concentrations exhibit a diurnal pattern, with a nadir in the mid-morning and a late-night nocturnal peak [5, 43]. The diurnal leptin pattern is dependent on insulin responses to meals and is therefore influenced by meal timing [44] and dietary macronutrient composition [45].

Gender-dependent differences have been found. The distribution of fat in the body differs between the male and female sexes. Females have more body fat and higher plasma leptin levels per gram of fat. Moreover, the brains of male and female rats are differentially sensitive to the catabolic action of small doses of leptin (and insulin) [46].

### Leptin Interacts with Ghrelin and Insulin

It is commonly assumed that the effects of leptin and ghrelin on metabolism, including food intake, are exactly opposite. Ghrelin is considered to be a hunger hormone, whereas leptin is a satiety signal [47]. Rising ghrelin levels in concert with falling leptin levels may serve as a critical signal to induce hunger during fasting [48]. It has been observed that leptin exerts a restraint on the orexigenic effects of ghrelin in two ways, centrally by counteracting its appetite-promoting effects at the level of neuropeptide Y (NPY) signalling in the hypothalamus and peripherally by attenuating gastric ghrelin secretion [49]. Moreover, there is evidence suggesting that leptin and ghrelin may also work via the hindbrain [42].

Leptin and insulin interact with each other. Insulin plays a major role in the regulation of leptin production, stimulating the transcriptional activity of the leptin promoter, increasing leptin gene expression and elevating leptin circulating concentrations. These effects are all mediated by actions of insulin to promote glucose uptake and oxidative metabolism in adipocytes [50].

On the other hand, leptin can down-modulate insulin signalling in adipocytes in two different ways. Leptin may modulate the pancreatic insulin and glucose homeostasis acting in the hypothalamus throughout the activation of neuronal circuits and the autonomic nervous system [49], but it also exerts a direct effect on the adipocytes. In animals with elevated serum leptin concentrations, leptin inhibits insulin signalling, impairing insulin receptor autophosphorylation. This modulation of adipocyte insulin signalling could be relevant in physiological situations of hyperleptinaemia and central leptin resistance, such as ageing and obesity [51]. In addition, leptin exerts a tonic restraint to the adipocytes for the secretion of adiponectin, a hormone implicated in insulin resistance [49].

## Leptin and Energy Homeostasis

Leptin is an anorexigenic hormone. It acts through or in concert with several neuropeptides, monoamines and other transmitter substances that affect food intake in the brain–gut axis [52]. Leptin has multiple actions to influence food intake and body weight: a rapid and acute response perhaps mediated by gastric leptin acting on vagal afferent endings, and more sustained effects mediated by adipose release of leptin acting on the hypothalamus and/or the hindbrain sites [53].

## Leptin and Central Regulation of Appetite

The hypothalamus is the major site of leptin action in energy homeostasis [54]. Fasting causes a rapid decrease in endogenous leptin level. It is this acute decrease in leptin that signals to the hypothalamus that energy stores may be compromised, resulting in an increase in NPY and agouti-related protein (AgRP) gene expression, which stimulates food intake. At the same time, leptin inhibits the firing of neurons co-expressing the catabolic neuropeptides α-melanocyte-stimulating hormone (α-MSH) (derived from pro-opiomelanocortin, POMC) and CART [37, 55]. The AgRP-NPY and POMC-CART neurons synapse on each other; both project rostrally to second-order neurons in the hypothalamic paraventricular nucleus and caudally to other second-order hypothalamic and extra-hypothalamic sites that are involved in the autonomic and behavioural processes that regulate energy balance [56].

Leptin decreases melanin-concentrating hormone (MCH), galanin and orexin gene expression and increases galanin-like peptide (GALP), neurotensin, and corticotropin-releasing factor gene expression in the hypothalamus. Anorectic prolactin-releasing peptide (PrRP) neurons express leptin receptors and interact with leptin to reduce food intake [57].

In the arcuate nucleus of the hypothalamus, leptin may modulate the hypothalamic neuronal populations, not only by direct action at leptin receptors, but also as a consequence of differential effects of the hormone on synaptic input to NPY and POMC neurons [58]. Leptin can modulate both synapse number and activity of NPY and POMC neurons in the hypothalamus of *ob/ob* mice, resulting in alteration in NPY and POMC hypothalamic tone. It has been suggested that leptin, acting as a long-term programmer of hypothalamic neurons, may underlie the theoretical body weight 'set-point' about which it is proposed that weight is rigorously maintained [59]. Moreover, a mass of evidence shows that leptin plays a neurotrophic role for the development of the hypothalamic pathways for feeding. Some findings have demonstrated that leptin receptors are present and functional in the arcuate nucleus of the hypothalamus during the postnatal period. During the neonatal period, plasma leptin levels are relatively high, although food intake must be maximised to support growth. The general thinking has been that the neonatal brain is relatively insensitive to leptin and may present leptin resistance. In *ob/ob* mice the neuronal projection pathways from the arcuate nucleus of the hypothalamus are permanently disrupted. Treatment with exogenous leptin rescues the development of the arcuate nucleus of the hypothalamus neuronal projections in neonates but not in adult mice [60, 61].

## Leptin and Reward Behaviour

Collective findings are consistent and compelling for the possible role of adiposity signals in modulating reward behaviour. Leptin may act directly at the midbrain ventral tegmental area (VTA) and also indirectly via signalling at the medial hypothalamus, with subsequent activation of pathways that project to the limbic circuitry. It is possible that the efficacy of leptin at low concentrations, such as levels that reflect the switch from fasting to fed status, is predominantly in the VTA, altering the reward threshold. With post-prandial elevations of leptin, the recruitment of inputs via the medial hypothalamus and via the limbic system may be inhibited in a synergic manner, resulting in decreased appetite or ingestive behaviour. It is possible that palatability and hedonic attributes of food may lead to enhanced activation of motivation circuitry, temporarily overriding the effectiveness of the adiposity signals in the hypothalamus [38].

Some studies provide evidence that a specific brain system, involving connections between the basolateral amygdala (BLA) and the lateral hypothalamus, is crucial for allowing learned cues to override satiety and promote eating in sated rats [62]. Leptin and the signalling form of leptin receptor mRNA increased in BLA following conditioned taste aversion formation, indicating that leptin and its receptors may take part in conditioned taste aversion learning and it may act as a mediating factor between feeding and taste in rats. The neuronal projections from the amygdala to the arcuate nucleus of the hypothalamus are possible neuroanatomic substrates [63].

## Leptin and Satiety

Satiety is a condition defined by a feeling of fullness and disappearance of appetite after a meal. In humans, leptin is not considered a primary satiety factor because changes in food intake do not induce short-term changes in blood leptin concentration [64]. On the other hand, leptin may play a permissive effect on satiety, by sufficiently inhibiting the central nervous system orexigenic neurons and allowing satiety signals from gut hormones and baroreceptors to affect eating behaviour [65]. Acting in the forebrain (for example in the arcuate nucleus of the hypothalamus), leptin controls meal size by modulating the hindbrain (for example the nucleus of solitary tract) response to satiety signals such as cholecystokinin (CCK) [66]. This mechanism explains how long-term signals operate to affect short-term signals [67]. A recent study has demonstrated that acute increases in central leptin levels may potently augment post-prandial satiety and influence body fluid homeostasis in rats [68]. Moreover, it has been found that leptin acts on vagal afferent fibres that transport the satiety signal to the hindbrain in rats [53] and that the intraperitoneal administration of an antagonist of CCK-A receptor blocks the effects of leptin on short-term food intake [69].

Humans with congenital deficiency of leptin are constantly hungry and demand food continuously. The administration of leptin and the consequent normalisation of serum leptin concentrations decreased fasting ghrelin concentrations, decreased caloric intake, increased satiety time, and influenced subjective perceptions of hunger, fullness, and desire to eat in these patients [39, 65].

## Leptin and Energy Expenditure

In an attempt to maintain adequate energy stores, mammals increase energy expenditure during periods of abundance. In rodents, it is known that leptin increases energy expenditure through the induction of the mitochondrial uncoupling protein-1 (UCP-1) and the newly identified mitochondrial uncoupling protein-2 (UCP-2) and mitochondrial uncoupling protein-3 (UCP-3) through the sympathetic nervous system [70] in both white and brown adipose tissue [71].

Increasing evidence from human studies suggests that leptin predominantly influences the human energy balance through appetite changes, but it appears not to be involved in regulating energy expenditure [72]. None of the expected factors, such as resting metabolic rate, total diurnal energy expenditure or dietary-induced thermogenesis, was related to blood leptin concentrations [73].

## Leptin and Congenital Leptin Deficiency

Congenital leptin deficiency due to mutations in the leptin gene or receptor is a rare, but treatable, cause of severe early-onset obesity and various endocrine disturbances in both rodents and humans [74, 75]. According to the lypostatic theory, a state of 'perceived starvation' might exist in these subjects and results in a chronic stimulation of excessive food intake [39]. Leptin therapy has shown to have dramatically beneficial effects on weight, fat mass and appetite, hyperinsulinaemia and lipid levels, as well as on neuroendocrine phenotypes and immune functions in these subjects [76, 77]. Leptin treatment blunts the changes in circulating thyroid hormone and corticosterone levels that are normally associated with food deprivation. It has been suggested that the inhibition of thyroid hormone secretion may have evolved to limit energy expenditure and prevent protein catabolism during starvation [78]. The effect of leptin on circulating thyroid hormone can be explained at least in part by the high expression of leptin receptor in the arcuate nucleus of the hypothalamus and by the known projection of the arcuate nucleus to the paraventricular nucleus, where the thyroid-releasing hormone neurons are localised [79].

Total leptin deficiency or insensitivity is associated with hypothalamic hypogonadism in humans and rodents. Leptin treatment restored luteinising hormone secretion and pubertal development in leptin-deficient patients, confirming its critical role in reproduction. It was proposed that high levels of leptin observed in children might reflect leptin resistance, as seen in obesity, serving to maintain sufficient food intake and growth and prevent the onset of premature puberty. Central leptin administration decreases the expression of

NPY in the hypothalamus and consequently removes the inhibitory action of NPY on growth hormone-releasing hormone (GHRH) release. Leptin stimulates the synthesis and release of luteinising hormone and follicle-stimulating hormone in animals. Ovarian follicular cells are regulated directly by leptin, indicating that it is able to control the hypothalamic–pituitary–gonadal axis at multiple levels [79, 80]. These results show that leptin is not only an adipostat signal, but it acts as a metabolic switch, informing the brain when fat reserves are adequate to direct energy expenditure towards activities other than seeking calories [37].

## Leptin and Diet-Induced Obesity

After the discovery of leptin, the initial hypothesis that human obesity results from a deficiency in leptin has failed. Obese humans have high plasma leptin concentrations related to the size of adipose tissue, but this elevated leptin signal does not induce the expected response. This fact suggests that obese humans are resistant to the effects of endogenous leptin. The resistance is also shown by the lack of effect of exogenous administration to induce weight loss in obese patients [64]. Leptin resistance may be defined as reduced sensitivity or complete insensitivity to leptin action, as occurs for insulin in type 2 diabetes [57].

Human and rodent studies indicate that the major cause of this resistance arises from an inability of leptin to cross the blood–brain barrier [81]. The leptin transporter is a saturable system: beyond a certain plasma leptin level, increased production by the growing fat mass would be futile. Furthermore, severe hyperleptinaemia might down-regulate the leptin transporters and make the situation worse [82]. This mechanism may explain why the exogenous administration of leptin to treat obesity might be ineffective if endogenous leptin has already saturated its transporters. However, the blood–brain barrier resistance is acquired and to some extent it is reversible with weight loss [37]. In rodents, it is well known that the down-regulation of leptin signalling receptor is one of the mechanisms by which the effects of leptin are lost [83]. The hypothalamic leptin receptor signalling is not down-regulated in obese patients. Probably, for the presence of the blood–brain barrier saturable system, the hypothalamic interstitial leptin concentration may only be mildly elevated, at least compared with the leptin serum concentration [82].

It is also possible that resistance is determined by chronic elevation of hypothalamic leptin tone, as studied in rats, or by suppressing intracellular signalling [42, 57]. The presence of negative regulators of leptin signalling such as SH2-containing protein tyrosine phosphatase-2 (SHP-2) and protein tyrosine phosphatase-1B (PTP-1B) has been observed in diet-induced obese animals. It has been found that deficiency of the suppressor of cytokine signalling-3 (SOCS-3) is associated with increased leptin sensitivity in the brain and has conferred resistance to diet-induced obesity in animals [84]. This widespread occurrence of leptin resistance could reflect the fact that the inability to store energy efficiently at times of abundance is evolutionarily disadvantageous [73]. Leptin may therefore play an important role during periods of starvation, but may be less significant when food is freely available [85].

### Leptin and Anorexia in Ageing

Ageing appears to be associated with leptin resistance. It has been found that the relatively hyperleptinaemic state of ageing animals blunts the sensitivity of the hypothalamic energy regulatory system, thus decreasing appetite even during episodes of negative energy balance. It has been found that age-associated decreased levels of orexigenic signalling through AgRP and NPY neurons in the arcuate nucleus of the hypothalamus are accompanied by increased levels of anorexigenic signalling through POMC/CART neurons. This pattern of neuropeptide gene expression may contribute to the loss of appetite and anorexia associated with ageing [56].

### Leptin and Cancer Anorexia/Cachexia

Progressive wasting is common in many types of cancer and is one of the most important factors leading to death in cancer patients. Weight loss is a potent stimulus to food intake in normal humans and animals. The persistence of anorexia and the onset of cachexia in cancer patients, therefore, implies a failure of this adaptive feeding response [86]. Leptin, a member of the gp 130 family of cytokines, induces a strong T helper-1 lymphocyte response and is regarded as a proinflammatory inducer [87]. Several data suggested a role of leptin in inflammatory diseases. Proinflammatory cytokines up-regulate leptin expression in white adipose tissue and increase plasma leptin levels in hamsters and mice [88]. However, in many common diseases associated with cachexia, such as chronic obstructive pulmonary disease and chronic inflammatory bowel disease, there is an inflammatory status caused by high proinflammatory cytokine levels, whereby leptin concentrations are decreased related to body fat mass. In patients with advanced non-small-cell lung cancer, serum leptin levels were lower than in controls and lower still in those who were cachectic who also showed an increase of proinflammatory cytokines and acute-phase reactants [32, 88]. In 29 advanced-stage patients with cancer at different sites, an inverse correlation was found between serum levels of leptin (low) and proinflammatory cytokines (high). Additionally there was an inverse correlation between the Eastern Cooperative Oncology Group performance status scale and serum levels of leptin. Regarding survival, patients with very high serum levels of proinflammatory cytokines and very low levels of leptin had very short survival [89–94].

In tumour-bearing rats, leptin concentrations decreased in plasma and adipose depots 4 days after the tumour cell injections. It has been suggested that leptin synthesis in visceral white adipose tissue of tumour-bearing rats might be modulated by tumour necrosis factor-alpha (TNF-$\alpha$) or prostaglandin E2 produced by infiltrating macrophages present in the early stage of cachexia [31]. In tumour-bearing mice, leptin production is decreased while the hypothalamic leptin receptor and NPY expression are increased in response to fat depletion [95]. Overall, these findings suggest that peripheral adipocyte leptin synthesis is preserved in cancer patients and tumour animal models, and point to a central dysregulation of the physiological feedback loop.

## Conclusions

Comprehensively, all the data show the diverse roles of leptin in the interaction of multiple hormone signals involved in the development of obesity and metabolic disorders [49]. Further studies examining the physiological and neuroanatomical interactions between des-acyl ghrelin and its target will establish the role of ghrelin peptides in the regulation of feeding and energy homeostasis [10]. Eating abnormalities are associated with various diseases including obesity, diabetes, anorexia nervosa and cachexia. Better understanding of the physiology and pathophysiology of ghrelin peptides may provide an entirely new therapeutic approach for the treatment of various diseases, which have become increasingly prevalent throughout the world.

## References

1. Zigman JM, Elmquist JK (2003) Minireview: from anorexia to obesity – the yin and yang of body weight control. Endocrinology 144:3749–3756
2. Asakawa A, Inui A, Kaga T et al (2003) Antagonism of ghrelin receptor reduces food intake and body weight gain in mice. Gut 52:947–952
3. Kojima M, Hosoda H, Date Y et al (1999) Ghrelin is a growth-hormone-releasing acylated peptide from stomach. Nature 402:656–660
4. Mondal MS, Date Y, Yamaguchi H et al (2005) Identification of ghrelin and its receptor in neurons of the rat arcuate nucleus. Regul Pept 126:55–59
5. Date Y, Kojima M, Hosoda H et al (2000) Ghrelin, a novel growth hormone-releasing acylated peptide, is synthesized in a distinct endocrine cell type in the gastrointestinal tracts of rats and humans. Endocrinology 141:4255–4266
6. Sato T, Fukue Y, Teranishi H et al (2005) Molecular forms of hypothalamic ghrelin and its regulation by fasting and 2-deoxy-D-glucose administration. Endocrinology 146:2510–2516
7. Beaumont NJ, Skinner VO, Tan TM et al (2003) Ghrelin can bind to a species of high density lipoprotein associated with paraoxonase. J Biol Chem 278:8877–8880
8. Nishi Y, Hiejima H, Hosoda H et al (2005) Ingested medium-chain fatty acids are directly utilized for the acyl modification of ghrelin. Endocrinology 146:2255–2264
9. Ariyasu H, Takaya K, Hosoda H et al (2002) Delayed short-term secretory regulation of ghrelin in obese animals: evidenced by a specific RIA for the active form of ghrelin. Endocrinology 143:3341–3350
10. Patterson M, Murphy KG, le Roux CW et al (2005) Characterization of ghrelin-like immunoreactivity in human plasma. J Clin Endocrinol Metab 90:2205–2211
11. Chen CY, Chao Y, Chang FY et al (2005) Intracisternal des-acyl ghrelin inhibits food intake and non-nutrient gastric emptying in conscious rats. Int J Mol Med 16:695–699
12. Toshinai K, Yamaguchi H, Sun Y et al (2006) Des-acyl ghrelin induced food intake by a mechanism independent of the growth hormone secretagogue receptor. Endocrinology (in press)
13. Hosoda H, Kojima M, Matsuo H et al (2000) Ghrelin and des-acyl ghrelin: two major forms of rat ghrelin peptide in gastrointestinal tissue. Biochem Biophys Res Commun 281:1220–1225
14. Inui A (2001) Ghrelin: an orexigenic and somatotrophic signal from the stomach. Nat Rev Neurosci 2:1–11
15. Matsumoto M, Hosoda H, Kitajima Y et al (2001) Structure-activity relationship of ghrelin: pharmacological study of ghrelin peptides. Biochem Biophys Res Comun 287:142–146
16. Broglio F, Gottero C, Prodam F et al (2004) Non-acylated ghrelin counteracts the metabolic but not neuroendocrine response to acylated ghrelin in humans. J Endocrinol Invest 89:3062–3065
17. Akamizu T, Shimomiya T, Irako T et al (2005) Separate measurement of plasma levels of acylated and desacylated ghrelin in healthy subjects using a new direct ELISA assay. J Clin Endocrinol Metab 90:6–9
18. Ariyasu H, Takaya K, Iwakura H et al (2005) Transgenic mice overexpressing des-acyl ghrelin show small phenotype. Endocrinology 146:355–364
19. Balzani G, Filigheddu N, Cutrupi S et al (2004) Ghrelin and de-acyl ghrelin inhibit cell death in cardiomyocytes and endothelial cells through ERK1/2 and PI 3-kinase/AKT. J Cell Biol 159:1029–1037
20. Cassoni P, Papotti M, Ghe C et al (2001) Identification, characterization, and biological activity of specific receptors for natural (ghrelin) and synthetic growth hormone secretagogues and analogs in human breast carcinomas and cell lines. Eur J Endocrinol 150:173–184
21. Cassoni P, Ghe C, Marrocco T et al (2004) Expression of ghrelin and biological activity of specific receptors for ghrelin and des-acyl ghrelin in human prostate neoplasms and related cell line. Eur J Endocrinol 150:173–184
22. Muccioli G, Pons N, Ghe C et al (2004) Ghrelin and des-acyl ghrelin both inhibit isoproterenol-induced lipolysis in rat adipocytes via a non-type 1 growth hormone secretagogue receptor. Eur J Pharmacol 498:27–35

23. Thompson NM, Gill DAS, Davies R et al (2004) Ghrelin and des-octanoyl ghrelin promote adipogenesis directly in vivo by a mechanism independent of the type 1 growth hormone secretagogue receptor. Endocrinology 145:234–242

24. Toshinai K, Date Y, Muratami N et al (2003) Ghrelin induced food intake is mediated via the orexin pathway. Endocrinology 144:1506–1512

25. Asakawa A, Inui A, Fujimiya M et al (2005) Stomach regulates energy balance via acylated ghrelin and desacyl ghrelin. Gut 54:18–24

26. Chen CY, Inui A, Asakawa A et al (2005) Des-acyl ghrelin acts by CRF type 2 receptors to disrupt fasted stomach motility in conscious rats. Gastroenterology 129:8–25

27. Banks WA, Tschop M, Robinson SM et al (2002) Extent and direction of ghrelin transport across the blood-brain barrier is determined by its unique primary structure. J Pharmacol Exp Ther 302:822–827

28. Gauna G, Delhanty PJ, Hofland LJ et al (2005) Ghrelin stimulates, whereas des-octanoyl ghrelin inhibits, glucose output by primary hepatocytes. J Clin Endocrinol Metab 90:1055–1060

29. Gauna C, Meyler FM, Janssen MJ et al (2004) Administration of acylated ghrelin reduces insulin sensitivity, whereas the combination of acylated plus unacylated ghrelin strongly improves insulin sensitivity. J Clin Endocrinol Metab 89:5035–5042

30. Zhang Y, Proenca R, Maffei M et al (1994) Positional cloning of the mouse obese gene and its human homologue. Nature 372:425–432

31. Machado AP, Costa Rosa LF, Seelaender MC (2004) Adipose tissue in Walker 256 tumour-induced cachexia: possible association between decreased leptin concentration and mononuclear cell infiltration. Cell Tissue Res 318:503–514

32. Somasundar P, McFadden DW, Hileman SM et al (2004) Leptin is a growth factor in cancer. J Surg Res 116:337–349

33. Bates SH, Stearns WH, Dundon TA et al (2003) STAT3 signaling is required for leptin regulation of energy balance but not reproduction. Nature 421:856–859

34. Tartaglia LA, Dembski M, Weng X et al (1995) Identification and expression cloning of a leptin receptor, OB-R. Cell 83:1263–1271

35. Friedman JM, Halaas JL (1998) Leptin and the regulation of body weight in mammals. Nature 395:763–770

36. Inui A (1999) Cancer anorexia-cachexia syndrome: are neuropeptides the key? Cancer Res 59:4493–4501

37. Banks WA (2004) The many lives of leptin. Peptides 25:331–338

38. Figlewicz DP (2003) Adiposity signals and food reward: expanding the CNS roles of insulin and leptin. Am J Physiol Regul Comp Physiol 284:R882 R892

39. Montague CT, Farooqi IS, Whitehead JP et al (1997) Congenital leptin deficiency is associated with severe early-onset obesity in humans. Nature 387:903–908

40. Neary NM, Small CJ, Bloom SR (2003) Gut and mind. Gut 52:918–921

41. Schwartz MW, Woods SC, Seeley RJ et al (2003) Is the energy homeostasis system inherently biased toward weight gain? Diabetes 52:232–238

42. Popovic V, Duntas LH (2005) Brain somatic crosstalk: ghrelin, leptin and ultimate challengers of obesity. Nutr Neurosci 8:1–5

43. Havel PJ (2000) Role of adipose tissue in body-weight regulation: mechanisms regulating leptin production and energy balance. Proc Nutr Soc 59:359–371

44. Havel PJ, Townsend R, Chaump L et al (1999) High-fat meals reduce 24-h circulating leptin concentrations in women. Diabetes 48:334–341

45. Havel PJ (2001) Peripheral signals conveying metabolic information to the brain: short-term and long-term regulation of food intake and energy homeostasis. Exp Biol Med 226:963–977

46. Clegg DJ, Riedy CA, Blake Smith KA et al (2003) Differential sensitivity to central leptin and insulin in male and female rats. Diabetes 52:682–687

47. Ukkola O (2004) Peripheral regulation of food intake: new insights. J Endocrinol Invest 27:96–98

48. Saper CB, Chou TC, Elmquist JK (2002) The need to feed: homeostatic and hedonic control of eating. Neuron 36:199–211

49. Ueno N, Dube MG, Inui A et al (2004) Leptin modulates orexigenic effects of ghrelin and attenuates adiponectin and insulin levels and selectively the dark-phase feeling as revealed by central leptin gene therapy. Endocrinology 145:4176–4184

50. Griffen SC, Oostema K, Stanhope KL et al (2006) Administration of Lispro insulin with meals improves glycemic control, increases circulating leptin, and suppresses ghrelin, compared with regular/NPH insulin in female patients with type 1 diabetes. J Clin Endocrinol Metab 91:485–491

51. Perez C, Fernandez-Galaz C, Fernandez-Agullo T et al (2004) Leptin impairs insulin signaling in rat adipocytes. Diabetes 53:347–353

52. Banks WA, Kastin AJ, Huang W et al (1996) Leptin enters brain by a saturable system independent of insulin. Peptides 17:305–311

53. Peters JH, McKay BM, Simasko SM et al (2005) Leptin-induced satiation mediated by abdominal vagal afferents. Am J Physiol Regul Integr Comp Physiol 288:R879–R884

54. Halaas JL, Friedman JM (1997) Leptin and its receptor. J Endocrinol 155:215–216

55. Cowley MA, Smart JL, Rubinstein M et al (2001) Leptin activates anorexigenic POMC neurons through a neuronal network in the arcuate nucleus. Nature 411:480–484

56. Wolden-Hanson T, Marck BT, Matsumoto AM (2004) Blunted hypothalamic neuropeptide gene expression in response to fasting, but preservation of fee-

ding response to AgRP in aging male Brown Norway rats. Am J Physiol Regul Integr Comp Physiol 287:R138–R146

57. Sahu A (2004) Minireview: a hypothalamic role in energy balance with special emphasis on leptin. Endocrinology 145:2613–2620

58. Pinto S, Roseberry AG, Liu H et al (2004) Rapid rewiring of arcuate nucleus feeding circuits by leptin. Science 304:110–115

59. Harrold JA (2004) Leptin leads hypothalamic feeding circuits in a new direction. BioEssays 26:1043–1045

60. Bouret SG, Draper SJ, Simerly RB (2004) Trophic action of leptin on hypothalamic neurons that regulate feeding. Nature 304:108–110

61. Bouret SG, Simerly RB (2004) Minirevew: leptin and development of hypothalamic feeding circuits. Endocrinology 145:2621–2626

62. Petrovich GD, Setlow B, Holland PC et al (2002) Amygdalo-hypothalamic circuit allows learned cues to override satiety and promote eating. J Neurosci 22:8748–8753

63. Han Z, Yan JQ, Luo GG et al (2003) Leptin receptor expression in the basolateral nucleus of amygdala of conditioned taste aversion rats. World J Gastroenterol 9:1034–1037

64. Jequier E (2002) Leptin signaling, adiposity and energy balance. Ann NY Acad Sci 967:378–388

65. McDuffie JR, Riggs PA, Calis KA et al (2004) Effects of exogenous leptin on satiety and satiation in patients with lipodystrophy and leptin insufficiency. J Clin Endocrinol 89:4258–4263

66. Morton GJ, Blevins JE, Williams DL et al (2005) Leptin action in the forebrain regulates the hindbrain response to satiety signals. J Clin Invest 115:703–710

67. de Graaf C, Bloom WAM, Smeets PAM et al (2004) Biomarkers of satiation and satiety. Am J Clin Nutr 79:946–961

68. Zorrilla EP, Inoue K, Valdez GR et al (2005) Leptin and post-prandial satiety: acute central leptin more potently reduces meal frequency than meal size in the rat. Psychopharmacology 177:324–335

69. Blevins JE, Schwartz MW, Baskin DG (2002) Peptide signals regulating food intake and energy homeostasis. Can J Physiol Pharmacol 80:396–406

70. Inui A (2000) Transgenic approach to the study of body weight regulation. Pharmacol Rev 52:35–62

71. Scarpace PJ, Nicolson M, Matheny M (1998) UCP2, UCP3 and leptin gene expression: modulation by food restriction and leptin. J Endocrinol 15:349–357

72. Nagy TM, Gower BA, Shewchuk RM et al (1997) Serum leptin and energy expenditure in children. J Clin Endocrinol Metab 82:4149–4153

73. Hukshorn CJ, Saris WH (2004) Leptin and energy expenditure.Curr Opin Clin Nutr Metab Care 7:629–633

74. Lahlou N, Issad T, Lebouc Y et al (2002) Mutations in the human leptin and leptin receptor genes as models of serum leptin receptor regulation. Diabetes 51:980–985

75. Farooqi IS, Keogh JM, Kamath S et al (2001) Partial leptin deficiency and human adiposity. Nature 414:34–35

76. Gibson WT, Farooqi IS, Moreau M et al (2004) Congenital leptin deficiency due to homozygosity for the D133G mutation: report of another case and evaluation of response to four years of leptin therapy. J Clin Endocrinol Metab 89:4821–4826

77. Licinio J, Caglayan S, Ozata M et al (2004) Phenotypic effects of leptin replacement on morbid obesity, diabetes mellitus, hypogonadism, and behaviour in leptin-deficient adults. Proc Natl Acad Sci USA 101:4531–4536

78. Ahima RS, Osei SY (2004) Leptin signaling. Physiol Behav 81:223–241

79. Sarkar S, Legradi G, Lechan RM (2002) Intracerebroventricular administration of a-melanocyte stimulating hormone increases phosphorylation of CREB in TRH- and CRH-producing neurons of the hypothalamic paraventricular nucleus. Brain Res 945:50–59

80. Moran O, Phillip M (2003) Leptin: obesity, diabetes and other peripheral effects – a review. Pediatr Diabetes 4:101–109

81. Banks WA (2003) Is obesity a disease of the blood-brain barrier? Physiological, pathological and evolutionary considerations. Curr Pharmac Design 9:801–809

82. Caro JF, Kolaczynski JW, Nyce MR et al (1996) Decreased cerebrospinal-fluid/serum leptin ratio in obesity: a possible mechanism for leptin resistance. Lancet 348:159–161

83. Martin RL, Perez E, He YJ et al (2000) Leptin resistance is associated with hypothalamic leptin receptor mRNA and protein downregulation. Metabolism 49:1479–1484

84. Mori H, Hanada R, Hanada T et al (2004) Socs3 deficiency in the brain elevates leptin sensitivity and confers resistance to diet-induced obesity. Nat Med 10:739–743

85. Murphy KG, Bloom SR (2004) Gut hormones in the control of appetite. Exp Physiol 89:507–516

86. Inui A (2002) Cancer anorexia-cachexia syndrome: current issues in research and management. CA Cancer J Clin 52:72–91

87. Dixit VD, Schaffer EM, Pyle RS et al (2004) Ghrelin inhibits leptin- and activation-induced proinflammatory cytokine expression by human monocytes and T cells. J Clin Invest 114:57–66

88. Lugarini F, Hrupka BJ, Schwartz GJ et al (2005) Acute and chronic administration of immunomodulators induces anorexia in Zucker rats. Physiol Behav 84:165–173

89. Aleman MR, Santolaria F, Batista N et al (2002) Leptin role in advanced lung cancer. A mediator of the acute phase response or a marker of the status of nutrition? Cytokine 19:21–26

90. Simons JP, Schols AM, Campfield LA et al (1997)

Plasma concentration of total leptin and human lung-cancer-associated cachexia. Clin Sci (Lond) 93:273–277

91. Brown DR, Berkowitz DE, Breslow MJ (2001) Weight loss is not associated with hyperleptinemia in humans with pancreatic cancer. J Clin Endocrinol Metab 86:162–166

92. Wallace AM, Sattar N, McMillan DC (1998) Effect of weight loss and the inflammatory response on leptin concentrations in gastrointestinal cancer patients. Clin Cancer Res 4:2977–2979

93. Mantovani G, Macciò A, Mura L et al (2000) Serum

levels of leptin and proinflammatory cytokines in patients with advanced-stage cancer at different sites. J Mol Med 78:554–561

94. Mantovani G, Macciò A, Madeddu C et al (2001) Serum values of proinflammatory cytokines are inversely correlated with serum leptin levels in patients with advanced stage cancer at different sites. J Mol Med 79:406–414

95. Bing C, Taylor S, Tisdale MJ et al (2001) Cachexia in MAC16 adenocarcinoma: suppression of hunger despite normal regulation of leptin, insulin and hypothalamic neuropeptide Y. J Neurochem 79:1004–1012

# Brain Mechanisms in Wasting and Cachexia

Carlos R. Plata-Salaman

## Introduction

As summarised in previous chapters, chronic (neoplastic, necrotic, infectious) pathophysiological processes of various systems are frequently accompanied by wasting and cachexia. The pathophysiology of wasting and cachexia is complex [1–10] and multiple brain mechanisms [11–13] can be involved including neurological, psychiatric, psychological, physiological, biochemical/metabolic, immunological, and chemical per se (e.g. neurotransmitter-, neuropeptide- and cytokine-related). These mechanisms can interact/synergise with peripheral/systemic processes or dysfunctions (e.g. gastrointestinal malabsorption and body losses such as via ulcers, effusions, haemorrhage).

Wasting and cachexia may also interact/synergise with neuropsychiatric manifestations that frequently accompany chronic disorders [14]. For instance, anorexia, early satiety, chronic pain, depression or anxiety, drowsiness and cognitive impairment and delirium, agitation, hypogeusia and hyposmia (and other taste and olfaction abnormalities), chronic nausea, fatigue and asthenia may in fact exacerbate – or in some cases induce – wasting and cachexia. The symptomatology (e.g. anorexia) may be involved as partly the cause and partly the consequence of wasting and cachexia such as in the cachexia–anorexia syndrome. During treatment (e.g. chemotherapy, radiotherapy, immunotherapy) various neuropsychiatric manifestations can be exacerbated.

Conceptually, the profile of brain mechanisms in wasting and cachexia varies depending on the underlying disease condition, but importantly, overlap or interaction of various mechanisms in the pathophysiological dysregulation may be piv-otal in dissimilar diseases such as human immunodeficiency virus infection, cancer, chronic inflammatory bowel disease, chronic liver disease, rheumatoid arthritis, chronic bacterial and parasitic diseases, chronic cardiovascular disease, chronic obstructive pulmonary disease and end-stage renal disease, all representing conditions associated with wasting and cachexia.

Although multiple peripheral and brain mechanisms may be involved in wasting and cachexia, peripheral mechanisms that affect behavioural responses (e.g. induction of anorexia) could be the result of signalling to a pathway that depends on brain mechanisms (i.e. conscious and decision-making processes). Thus, in specific cases, peripheral mechanisms final operational endpoint would be via brain outputs. Fatigue and asthenia during wasting and cachexia could have underlying peripheral (catabolic) and brain components.

Interaction of autonomic nervous system outflows with peripheral metabolic shifts and catabolism is another example of linkage with brain mechanisms.

The output of brain mechanisms would also reflect on many aspects of the quality of life of a patient with wasting and cachexia, including the interactions of these patients with their environment, relatives and caregivers.

## Main Proposed Brain Mechanisms in Wasting and Cachexia

Multiple models have been proposed mediated either by the pathophysiological process itself (e.g. a tumour, chronic infections) or by host-derived chemical factors. The following brief description focuses on 'mediator mechanisms' in wasting and cachexia that can affect brain function directly or indirectly. It is accepted that, in many cases, the magnitude of anorexia does not have a relationship with the severity of wasting and cachexia and degree of malnutrition. Here, metabolic abnormalities and prevalence of catabolic pathway activation play a pivotal role. In addition, although the brain monitors the status of peripheral energy stores and fuel availability, it is unknown how the fine modulation of anabolic and catabolic processes and energy homeostasis/balance interact on a moment-to-moment basis with the profile mentioned below.

## Metabolic Factors

Relevant comments in other chapters of this book relate to the biochemical and metabolic derangements and tumour-derived products including lipid-mobilising factors and proteolysis-inducing factors that have been implicated in the development and/or progression of wasting and cachexia in animal models and humans [4, 15]. Through a variety of mechanisms, cytokines can also contribute to the metabolic dysregulation and insulin resistance in wasting and cachexia [3, 4, 16].

Factors that induce catabolism and shift metabolism may indirectly affect brain mechanisms by changing the availability of nutrient substrates to the brain or the transport of substrates for neurotransmitter synthesis across the blood–brain barrier. For instance, fatty acids and amino acids released during breakdown of adipose tissue and protein, respectively, can affect central nervous system (CNS) function including feeding responses. Neuropsychiatric symptoms and signs could also involve, at least in part, activities resulting directly from the catabolic process.

The involvement of other mechanisms of energy metabolism in brain responses such as uncoupling proteins needs to be characterised based on observations of up-regulation of uncoupling protein subtypes in various tumour-bearing animal models [4, 17]. The same applies to accumulating evidence on ubiquitin-proteasome-dependent proteolysis [5, 6].

## Humoral Factors

Endogenous chemical factors produced in response to the disease condition are involved in wasting and cachexia [1, 3, 8, 18–21]. Two key aspects relate to: (1) factors that can be produced by the pathological process per se, e.g. chemicals released by tumours such as cytokines, bombesin (e.g. produced by small cell lung carcinoma) and serotonin (e.g. produced by bronchial and gastrointestinal carcinoid tumours), or by normal cells responding to an insult (e.g. cytokines produced by the immune system); and (2) the fact that various of these factors can act on the brain or peripheral target organs that signal to the brain to induce a behavioural, endocrine, autonomic, or other relevant CNS response.

Thus, based on the pleiotropic pathophysiology that occurs during wasting and cachexia, brain mechanisms may involve those: (a) activated within the brain, (b) generated in peripheral tissues/organs that can signal to and act on the brain, and (c) resulting from the combination of (a) and (b). Examples may encompass different classes of neurotransmitters, neuropeptides and cytokines.

## Neurotransmitters

This field has been studied extensively. For instance, serotonin is proposed to have a relevant role in cancer anorexia by direct action in the CNS [8, 22]. In cases where wasting and cachexia are associated with anorexia (e.g. the cachexia–anorexia syndrome), activities of anorexigenic neurotransmitters could be involved in the underlying pathophysiology.

## Neuropeptides

Changes of neuropeptides that act in the hypothalamus have been involved in wasting and cachexia including neuropeptide Y [23] (see below) and the melanocortin system. Various classes of inflammatory and neoplastic insults/challenges can activate the melanocortin system. Proinflammatory cytokines generated within the brain play a role in this activation and stimulation of pro-opiomelanocortin synthesis and ACTH secretion by the pituitary [24]. Brain administration of melanocortin 3/4 receptor antagonists ameliorates the anorexia and body weight loss of experimental models of oncological wasting and cachexia including rats bearing prostate gland carcinoma cells or sarcoma tumours [24–26].

## Cytokines

### General Comments

Cytokine activities in brain have a profound impact on neuroregulation, neurochemistry, behavioural manifestations, modulation of the neuroendocrine and autonomic systems, and neurophysiological responses [27]. Cytokines also modulate peripheral gastrointestinal, metabolic (catabolic) and endocrine systems that can impact CNS responses. In diseases associated with wasting and cachexia such as cancer, cytokine deregulation has been extensively studied.

Endogenous cytokines are aberrantly produced in many cancers and by endogenous organs/tissues. In cancer, cytokines can serve as paracrine/autocrine factors (within the neoplastic process and within organs including the brain) or as endocrine signals (from the periphery to brain).

Data suggest that peripherally and centrally (brain) derived cytokines (e.g. IL-1) play a key role in the induction of behavioural and neurological manifestations. Brain cytokine action on neural networks processing can be direct, via modulation of neurons (through glial–neuronal interactions or via modulation of neuronal ion channels, e.g. calcium, sodium, potassium), or indirect, via neurochemical modifications [11, 27].

Multiple classes of cytokines have been proposed to participate in the induction and development of wasting and cachexia including via brain mechanisms. These comprise: IL-1, IL-6 subfamily members including CNTF and leukaemia inhibitory factor, IFN-γ, TNF-α and BDNF, which in many cases also induce anorexia [9, 11, 14, 28]. Studies have shown that intratumoral administration of IL-1 receptor antagonist significantly

reduces the cachexia associated with a colon tumour [29], and that treatment of rodents bearing methylcholanthrene-induced sarcoma with monoclonal antibodies against the IL-1 receptor inhibits tumour growth and improves their food intake [30]. In addition to these examples of inoculation with cytokine-producing tumour cells and passive immunisation against cytokines, other relevant data are available from transgenic animals overexpressing cytokines and from transplants of malignant tumours.

Cytokine production triggered within brain – including that activated in brain in response to a peripheral insult – can result in a multi-cytokine interaction network. This brain network can be sustained through positive feedback systems and paracrine/autocrine interactions among brain cells [21, 31].

Proinflammatory cytokines modulate gastrointestinal activities (e.g. gastric motility and emptying) including via brain mechanisms by signalling through autonomic nervous system outflow. Cytokines also induce the release of other mediators such as hormones including corticotropin-releasing factor, cholecystokinin, glucagon and insulin. As mentioned, cytokines also induce metabolic changes and alterations in lipid, carbohydrate and amino acid metabolism. These cytokine-mediated endocrine and metabolic alterations could be involved in modulating brain responses during wasting and cachexia. Since increased resting energy expenditure can occur during wasting and cachexia, even with a reduced dietary intake, a systemic dysregulation of host metabolism could certainly be influenced by autonomic nervous system outflows.

### Behavioral Responses

Early satiety can be observed during wasting and cachexia. Certain cytokines (e.g. IL-1β), at appropriate concentrations estimated to be within the pathophysiological range, induce an eating pattern consistent with early satiety in animal models. This has been assessed with computerised analyses of the microstructure of eating [11, 27]. Action within the CNS has also been demonstrated due to the fact that brain administration of a cytokine requires 500- to 1000-fold lower doses to induce behavioural responses relative to the doses needed when using peripheral routes of administration.

### Neurophysiological Responses

The behavioural mode of action of cytokines has been found to be consistent with the neurophysiological pattern induced by a cytokine [11, 27]. For instance, IL-1β activates specifically and reversibly the glucosensitive neurons in the ventromedial hypothalamic nucleus or VMN (a site involved in the integrative control of meal termination). This would predict changes of meal size and meal duration as those induced by IL-1β. Based on the data of IL-1β-induced inhibition of the inward calcium channel current (and hence calcium permeability), a model has been proposed that would be consistent with an IL-1β long-lasting VMN neuronal activity modulation that may be associated with the long-term anorexia induced by the cytokine. A decrease of calcium influx in VMN glucose-sensitive neurons may inhibit the defined calcium-dependent potassium conductance in these neurons, leading to maintenance of intracellular potassium, depolarisation and increase in neuronal activity.

### Specificity of Action

Cytokine-induced behavioural (including anorexia), neurophysiological and cellular responses can be blocked with the appropriate receptor antagonists, monoclonal antibodies, and other cytokine inhibitors [e.g. 14, 27]. These data suggest specificity of cytokine action in the CNS.

### Cytokines in Body Fluids and Organ/Tissues

Various clinical studies have associated pathological processes with increased levels of circulating cytokines. These include various types of cancer, the human immunodeficiency virus infection syndrome, chronic inflammatory bowel disease, chronic liver disease, chronic obstructive pul-

monary disease, cardiac cachexia (during congestive heart failure), the flaring phase of rheumatoid cachexia and juvenile rheumatoid arthritis. A specific example is that patients with advanced prostate carcinoma – which is frequently accompanied by wasting and cachexia – have increased serum levels of TNF-α, IL-6 and IL-8 [18]. However, there have been inconsistent findings on the measurement of circulating cytokines. Other than methodological issues, one critical aspect is that cytokine levels in body fluids may not reflect cytokine production, action (paracrine/autocrine/intracrine) and dynamics within an organ or tissue, including the brain. Cytokine production within an organ can occur independently of cytokine concentrations in the circulation if the organ has the capacity to activate its own positive feedback.

### Cytokine Model in Brain Responses

In various clinical conditions, 'blood/circulating' and 'organ/tissue' cytokines could cooperate and this has implications for an integrative cytokine involvement in disease. Thus, proinflammatory cytokines produced and released within brain can interact with cytokines from systemic origin to modulate metabolic outputs and neuropsychiatric manifestations associated with wasting and cachexia.

The simultaneous up-regulation of cytokines in peripheral organs and brain regions in response to a peripheral pathophysiological process has been reported during peripheral tumour development, peripheral cytokine administration, peripheral inflammation, and peripheral bacterial products challenge. For instance, rats bearing prostate gland adenocarcinoma cells exhibit cytokine mRNA (as an index of local production) up-regulation in the peripheral tumour, in peripheral organs such as the spleen and in discrete brain regions [31]. This cytokine up-regulation in the periphery and brain has also been observed in a non-hormone-dependent (non-adenocarcinoma) methylcholanthrene tumour model in rats [32]. In this model, intrahypothalamic administration of IL-1 receptor antagonist improved feeding [33]. There are also model-dependent differences, e.g. in tumour-bearing mice with prostanoid-related anorexia, cytokine alterations seemed secondary to anorexia and not the driver of the process [34].

Data also support that cytokines are relevant to cancer anorexia and cachexia in mice bearing experimentally induced brain tumours. Negri et al. [19] used athymic mice bearing human tumour cells that enable direct identification of the origin of the cytokines from the host or tumour. Anorexia quickly developed in mice bearing human A431 epidermoid carcinoma or human OVCAR 3 ovarian carcinoma in the brain [19]. Anorexia was independent from tumour mass in the lateral cerebral ventricle. Brains exhibited significant up-regulation of IL-1α, IL-1β and leukaemia inhibitory factor (A431), and IL-6, TNF-α, and leukaemia inhibitory factor (OVCAR 3). This indicates that different cytokines were up-regulated depending on the tumour cell type [19].

Conceptually, the data suggest that a peripheral tumour induces a series of events that result in local organ (peripheral and brain) production of cytokines including IL-1β that eventually activate brain responses. This important concept of local production of cytokines in the brain, and cytokines as mediators of neurological and neuropsychiatric manifestations of disease has broad implications. Data obtained from rodents bearing peripheral tumours show that paracrine interactions within the brain represent a predominant mode of cytokine action. Once the network is activated within the brain through positive feedback systems, paracrine interactions can sustain cytokine production. In fact, data suggest that cancer-induced up-regulation of brain cytokines–due to local production–may occur earlier than in other organs [35], and that constitutive expression of cytokines in brain induces changes in gene expression that could be characteristic of chronic inflammation, which may lead to wasting and cachexia [20]. The model is also consistent with the cascade pattern associated with cytokine production. Thus, CNS-related cancer clinical manifestations – without involving metastasis – due to local synthesis of cytokines in brain regions may recapitulate previous inconsistent findings.

## How Do Peripheral Cytokines Signal to the Brain?

This is proposed to occur in different ways including via: (1) transport of cytokines from the peripheral circulation to the brain across the blood–brain barrier and circumventricular organs (which lack blood–brain barrier); (2) release of cytokines from immune system cells that cross a compromised blood–brain barrier during pathophysiological conditions; (3) retrograde axonal cytokine transport; (4) cytokine-induced generation of chemical mediators (e.g. prostaglandins and nitric oxide from the cerebrovascular endothelium, meningeal macrophages and perivascular microglia; and mediators generated from circumventricular organs); and (5) peripheral-to-brain communication through afferent neural fibre signalling. Various of these models, however, have not been established conclusively. On the other hand, the brain production of cytokines (e.g. from microglia, astrocytes, endothelial cells from the cerebrovasculature) as well as direct cytokine CNS action are clearly recognised mechanisms.

## Brain Functional Proinflammatory (Stimulatory) and Anti-inflammatory (Inhibitory) Cytokine Balance

Data continue to accumulate that cytokine positive and negative feedback systems and a balance between stimulatory and inhibitory cytokines may be pivotal for an appropriate modulation of cellular responses in the brain. An unopposed proinflammatory cytokine response cascade could aggravate the magnitude of neurological and neuropsychiatric manifestations and may influence wasting and cachexia [36]. This relevant concept that focuses on the temporal profile of proinflammatory and anti-inflammatory cytokines and their relationship/balance during a pathophysiological process or disease condition is applicable to all systems. The notion of proinflammatory/anti-inflammatory cytokine balance (e.g. IL-1β/IL-1 receptor antagonist) could be extended to a model of pro-catabolic/pro-anabolic cytokine balance based on new accumulating evidence. For instance, IL-1β and TNF-α act as pro-catabolic and IL-15 as pro-anabolic cytokines. IL-15 in fact inhibits skeletal muscle wasting in tumour-bearing rodents [37].

## Integrative Model of Humoral Interactions

The modulation of brain chemistry by cytokines involves relevant cytokine–cytokine, cytokine–neurotransmitter, and cytokine–neuropeptide/hormone interactions. These influences can be reciprocal.

### Cytokine–Neurotransmitter Interactions

Cytokines affect neurotransmitter release, metabolism and/or action (e.g. monoamines including histamine, serotonin, norepinephrine and dopamine; and excitatory amino acids) [8, 9]. Neurotransmitters, in turn, can modulate cytokine production and action. Cytokines and neurotransmitters can also act in coordination.

### Cytokine–Peptide Interactions

Modulation of the neuroendocrine system by cytokines is robust and has been discussed previously in multiple elegant papers. Cytokine-neuropeptide interactions can also be antagonistic. IL-1β blocks neuropeptide Y-induced feeding and neuropeptide Y blocks IL-1β-induced anorexia; IL-1β stimulates vasopressin release and vasopressin inhibits IL-1β-induced fever. In cancer models, a CNS dysregulation of neuropeptide Y mechanisms associated with an enhanced IL-1 activity and serotonin concentrations has been proposed [8, 9, 22].

Other endogenous cytokine–peptide interactions relevant to wasting, cachexia and the cachexia–anorexia syndrome include reciprocal cytokine–leptin (a member of the long-chain helical cytokine family)–neuropeptide Y–corticotropin-releasing hormone–glucocorticoid interactions, and perhaps also among cytokines and other CNS neuropeptide regulators involved in the control of energy balance including cocaine- and amphetamine-regulated transcript, melanin-concentrating hormone, agouti-related protein, α-melanocyte-stimulating hormone, and hypocretins/orexins [8, 10, 12, 22, 27]. Various of these can affect metabolic processes directly (e.g. gluconeogenesis, glycogenolysis).

The hypothalamus plays a critical role with multiple neuronal groups involved, including the arcuate nucleus, the paraventricular nucleus, the ventromedial nucleus, and the lateral hypothalamus. The arcuate nucleus has leptin-responsive neurons with different functions, e.g. the pro-opiomelanocortin-producing neurons that co-express the cocaine and amphetamine-regulated transcript, and the agouti-related peptide neurons that co-express neuropeptide Y.

There has also been significant interest in the proinflammatory cytokine up-regulation of gp 130 molecules and the suppressors-of-cytokine-signalling (SOCS) protein family members in brain. Other hypothalamic systems such as the endogenous cannabinoids, which modulate energy balance, could also be involved in wasting and cachexia [38]. As mentioned, the brain melanocortin signalling system also may have an important contributory role [24–26].

## Mode of Communication

In relation to gut–brain peptides/neuropeptides that affect brain mechanisms involved in wasting and cachexia, an alternate route of action may involve afferent neural signalling through the vagus that would generate outputs of communication to other brain regions involved in energy balance regulation and behaviour. This afferent signalling has been demonstrated and validated for various hormones and peptides and is proposed for different classes of cytokines.

## Compensatory Mechanisms

The analysis of interactions among endogenous chemical factors also needs to consider compensatory mechanisms that are activated during pro-catabolic activities or overriding anabolic processes. For instance, circulating ghrelin – a positive modulator of energy balance via orexigenic, adipogenic and growth hormone releaser activities [39, 40] – levels are elevated in patients with wasting and cachexia and this elevation can be associated with increases in TNF-α [41]. The potential anti-cachectic activity of melatonin [42] is described by Lissoni et al. in Chapter 9.10.

## Transducing Mechanisms and Functional Synergy

Various key interactions (e.g. among IL-1β, TNF-α, IL-6, IL-8, that is, molecules that use different transducing systems) display functional synergistic activity. One mechanism for this synergism is convergence of different signalling pathways onto common downstream mediators, e.g. IL-1β and TNF-α modulation of NF-κB-inducing kinase, a MAP3K-related kinase. This convergence results in the synergistic activation of transcriptional mechanisms. NF-κB is also activated by IL-6, and a synergistic response to IL-1β, IL-6 plus TNF-α can involve a similar convergence of intracellular mechanisms via JAK-STAT (IL-6) and MAPK-NF-κB (IL-1β, TNF-α) pathways. Brain cytokines also induce the production of other cytokine components including ligands, receptors, and transducing molecules in discrete brain regions, further amplifying the cellular responses [21, 27]. Interestingly, a proteolysis-inducing factor has been reported to activate NF-κB and STAT3, which results in up-regulation of IL-6 and IL-8 production [4].

Prostaglandin-dependent mechanisms that can be modulated by proinflammatory cytokines including the brain is another example of interactions involved in wasting and cachexia. Cyclooxygenase-2 has been proposed to be involved in cancer-associated wasting and up-regulation of proinflammatory cytokine expression [43]. This is also consistent with the role proposed for cyclooxygenase-2 as a mediator of anorectic responses to peripheral insults that require the involvement of prostaglandin E2 in the brain [44].

## Transducing Mechanisms and Functional Antagonism

Signalling mechanisms provide multiple levels of interaction in brain responses to cytokines. These could be region specific. For example, the G-protein α-subunit O (GαO) subclass represents an important transductional requirement for the regulation of energy balance, and IL-1β-induced brain action is associated with a significant decrease of the GαO protein content in the ventromedial hypothalamic nucleus [11]. This effect of IL-1β is blocked by the IL-1 receptor antagonist

and is indirect since IL-1 receptors are not G-protein coupled. Receptors coupled to GαO that respond to feeding-stimulatory signals include receptors for galanin, endogenous opioids, and neuropeptide Y. Thus, IL-1β-induced modulation of GαO protein may be involved in IL-1β-induced brain activities and anorexia including antagonism of neuropeptide Y action.

The consequence of this cytokine mode of action is broad. G-protein-coupled receptors that have been associated with energy balance regulation by the brain include receptors for catecholamines, serotonin, histamine, neuropeptide Y, hypocretins/orexins, melanin-concentrating hormone, agouti-related protein, α-melanocyte stimulating hormone, IL-8 and other chemokines/intercrines, cholecystokinin, opioids, glucagon and others. Cytokines have the ability to modulate mechanisms associated with all of these endogenous substances, and therefore, the potential of cytokine-induced modulation of G-proteins – the interface between convergence of multiple chemical signals and divergence to intracellular messengers – in CNS-associated sites may be involved in cachexia–anorexia.

Changes in brain signalling during wasting and cachexia may also involve dysregulation of ion channel subtypes. For instance, brains of tumour-bearing animals (Yoshida AH-130 ascites hepatoma) exhibit a significant down-regulation of the expression of the delayed rectifier as well as the A-type potassium channels, and in the same animals, TNF-α levels are elevated [45].

## Conclusions

Overall, it is important to consider the interrelationships among cytokines, cytokine/growth factors, growth factors, neurotransmitters, neuropeptides/peptides and hormones as well as modifications of signal transducing and intracellular mediator events in the induction and progression of brain modulatory responses that could be involved in wasting and cachexia. Brain interactive functional and chemical models are consistent with the multifaceted and redundant pathophysiology that occurs in wasting and cachexia.

## Ten Aspects To Consider for Future Research into Brain Mechanisms Involved in Wasting and Cachexia

1. The important concept of local brain production of cytokines and their functions as mediators of CNS neurological and neuropsychiatric manifestations of disease that can interact with other mechanisms involved in the induction, progression, maintenance, and/or exacerbation of wasting and cachexia. In practical terms, a tri-dimensional dynamics needs to be considered for cytokines acting in the brain: cytokines originated from the periphery, cytokines produced in cells of the blood–brain barrier, and cytokines produced by brain cells. The first two also impact interface mechanisms at the blood–brain barrier by cytokine-induced generation of neuromediators from endothelial and adjacent cells of the cerebrovasculature. Cytokine production/action in circumventricular organs linked to neuroendocrine and behavioural responses and energy balance regulation such as the median eminence and the area postrema can also be involved in brain responses during wasting and cachexia.

2. Characterisation of brain region cytokines and their system components (ligands, receptors, soluble receptors, signalling proteins) profiles in disease conditions associated with wasting and cachexia of different aetiologies. This includes cerebrospinal fluid profile in clinical subpopulations and clinical stages, and during treatment.

3. Peripheral and brain cytokines can robustly modulate autonomic nervous system outflow and this modulation and associated feedback systems need to be better studied to characterise their relevancy to wasting and cachexia.

4. A pivotal area of research will continue to be on the cytokine balance characterisation and on how cytokines interact sequentially and in parallel during wasting and cachexia. The concepts of proinflammatory/anti-inflammatory and pro-catabolic/pro-anabolic cytokine balance remain a key area to define contributory mechanisms in wasting and cachexia.

5. Cytokine systems interact in a chemical milieu of factors that modulate brain responses and present a multilayered network of cytokines, neurotransmitters, peptides/neuropeptides and hormones. Further analysis of these interactions is critical to understand feedback mechanisms and cause–effect in wasting and cachexia. Analyses need to consider potential additive or synergistic (and antagonistic) activities when: (a) molecules work in parallel on their respective signalling systems or when their signalling cascades converge on downstream mediators, and (b) generating a sequential response. The same concept would apply to functional interactions when neurotransmitters or neuropeptides are primary factors.

6. There is a need to enhance our understanding of the impact of chemical mediation on neurophysiological responses associated with neuronal activity and neural network dynamics that result in supracellular and behavioural responses, and how these relate to the neuropsychiatric manifestations of wasting and cachexia.

7. Even with all data currently available, a case can still be made for the following questions: are cytokines involved in the induction of wasting and cachexia in addition to their contribution potentiating or facilitating pathophysiological cascades? What is the level of recapitulation of brain mechanisms from observations of wasting and cachexia in animal models to those obtained from clinical populations?

8. Links and feedbacks exist among neurological, psychological and psychiatric manifestations of diseases accompanied by wasting and cachexia. Symptoms or signs such as anxiety, depression, cognitive impairment, fatigue and asthenia, and anorexia can exacerbate wasting and cachexia due to deleterious positive feedback cycles. This increases the frequency of complications, decreases the quality of life and activities of daily living and performance, and has an impact on overall morbidity and mortality. What are the main mechanistic interactions and magnitude of the individual contributions responsible for symptomatology interface?

9. Because of the complexity of the pathophysiology involved in wasting and cachexia, caution is essential when interpreting one or various mechanisms in isolation. Mechanisms with apparent limited effects individually could induce a relevant response when interacting and generating additive or synergistic outputs.

10. Various drugs or agents used for wasting and cachexia (e.g. appetite and body weight enhancers such as the progestogens) have been shown to modulate proinflammatory cytokine and neuropeptide expression and responses. Also preliminary studies have been obtained with amino acid manipulations that may reduce brain serotonin synthesis and release. These data sets suggest that interventional strategies that modulate cytokine-, neurotransmitter-, and/or relevant neuropeptide-associated mechanisms could generate novel therapeutics for wasting and cachexia.

### Acknowledgements

The author expresses great appreciation and gratitude to all his co-workers over the years. The author thanks the many laboratories that have contributed with elegant research to the study of mechanisms involved in the pathophysiology of wasting and cachexia. The author apologises that many important contributions could not be included in this brief commentary.

# References

1. Mantovani G, Macciò A, Madeddu C, Massa E (2003) Cancer-related cachexia and oxidative stress: beyond current therapeutic options. Expert Rev Anticancer Ther 3:381–392

2. Argiles JM, Moore-Carrasco R, Busquets S, Lopez-Soriano FJ (2003) Catabolic mediators as targets for cancer cachexia. Drug Discov Today 15:838–844

3. Langhans W (2002) Peripheral mechanisms involved with catabolism. Curr Opin Clin Nutr Metab Care 5:419–426

4. Tisdale MJ (2002) Cachexia in cancer patients. Nat Rev Cancer 2:862–871

5. Hasselgren PO, Wray C, Mammen J (2002) Molecular regulation of muscle cachexia: it may be more than the proteasome. Biochem Biophys Res Commun 290:1–10

6. Costelli P, Baccino FM (2003) Mechanisms of skeletal muscle depletion in wasting syndromes: role of ATP-ubiquitin-dependent proteolysis. Curr Opin Clin Nutr Metab Care 6:407–412

7. Inui A, Meguid MM (2003) Cachexia and obesity: two sides of one coin? Curr Opin Clin Nutr Metab Care 6:395–399

8. Laviano A, Russo M, Freda F, Rossi Fanelli F (2002) Neurochemical mechanisms for cancer anorexia. Nutrition 18:100–105

9. Laviano A, Meguid MM, Rossi Fanelli F (2003) Cancer anorexia: clinical implications, pathogenesis, and therapeutic strategies. Lancet Oncol 4:686–694

10. Nandi J, Meguid MM, Inui A et al (2002) Central mechanisms involved with catabolism. Curr Opin Clin Nutr Metab Care 5:407–418

11. Plata-Salaman CR (2000) Central nervous system mechanisms contributing to the cachexia-anorexia syndrome. Nutrition 16:1009–1012

12. Plata-Salaman CR (1997) Anorexia during acute and chronic disease: relevance of neurotransmitter-peptide-cytokine interactions. Nutrition 13:159–160

13. Plata-Salaman CR (2001) Brain cytokine production and action in anorexia and cachexia. Cytokine 15:1–3

14. Plata-Salaman CR (1996) Anorexia during acute and chronic disease. Nutrition 12:69–78

15. Sanders PM, Tisdale MJ (2004) Role of lipid-mobilising factor (LMF) in protecting tumour cells from oxidative damage. Br J Cancer 90:1274–1278

16. Ryden M, Arvidsson E, Blomqvist L et al (2004) Targets for TNF-$\alpha$-induced lipolysis in human adipocytes. Biochem Biophys Res Commun 318:168–175

17. Argiles JM, Busquets S, Lopez-Soriano FJ (2002) The role of uncoupling proteins in pathophysiological states. Biochem Biophys Res Commun 293:1145–1152

18. Pfitzenmaier J, Vessella R, Higano CS et al (2003) Elevation of cytokine levels in cachectic patients with prostate carcinoma. Cancer 97:1211–1216

19. Negri DR, Mezzanzanica D, Sacco S et al (2001) Role of cytokines in cancer cachexia in a murine model of intracerebral injection of human tumours. Cytokine 15:27–38

20. Prima V, Tennant M, Gorbatyuk OS et al (2004) Differential modulation of energy balance by leptin, ciliary neurotrophic factor, and leukemia inhibitory factor gene delivery: microarray deoxyribonucleic acid-chip analysis of gene expression. Endocrinology 145:2035–2045

21. Plata-Salaman CR (2002) Brain cytokines and disease. Acta Neuropsychiatrica 14:262–278

22. Meguid MM, Ramos EJ, Laviano A et al (2004) Tumor anorexia: effects on neuropeptide Y and monoamines in paraventricular nucleus. Peptides 25:261–266

23. Inui A (1999) Neuropeptide Y: a key molecule in anorexia and cachexia in wasting disorders? Mol Med Today 5:79–85

24. Wisse BE, Schwartz MW, Cummings DE (2003) Melanocortin signaling and anorexia in chronic disease states. Ann NY Acad Sci 994:275–281

25. Marks DL, Cone RD (2003) The role of the melanocortin-3 receptor in cachexia. Ann NY Acad Sci 994:258–266

26. Marks DL, Ling N, Cone RD (2001) Role of the central melanocortin system in cachexia. Cancer Res 61:1432–1438

27. Plata-Salaman CR (1998) Cytokine-induced anorexia: behavioral, cellular and molecular mechanisms. Ann NY Acad Sci 856:160–170

28. Kelley KW, Bluthe RM, Dantzer R et al (2003) Cytokine-induced sickness behavior. Brain Behav Immun 17 (Suppl 1):S112-118

29. Strassmann G, Jacob CO, Evans R et al (1992) Mechanisms of experimental cancer cachexia. Interaction between mononuclear phagocytes and colon-26 carcinoma and its relevance to IL-6-mediated cancer cachexia. J Immunol 148:3674–3678

30. Gelin J, Moldawer LL, Lonnroth C et al (1991) Role of endogenous tumor necrosis factor a and interleukin 1 for experimental tumor growth and the development of cancer cachexia. Cancer Res 51:415–421

31. Plata-Salaman CR, Ilyin SE, Gayle D (1998) Brain cytokine mRNAs in anorectic rats bearing prostate adenocarcinoma tumor cells. Am J Physiol 275:R566–R573

32. Turrin NP, Ilyin SE, Gayle DA et al (2004) Interleukin-1b system in anorectic catabolic tumor-bearing rats. Curr Opin Clin Nutr Metab Care 7:419–426

33. Laviano A, Renvyle T, Meguid MM et al (1995) Relationship between interleukin-1 and cancer anorexia. Nutrition 11:S680–S683

34. Wang W, Lonnroth C, Svanberg E, Lundholm K (2001) Cytokine and cyclooxygenase-2 protein in brain areas of tumor-bearing mice with prostanoid-related anorexia. Cancer Res 61:4707–4715

35. Ozaki K, Yoshida S, Ishibashi N et al (2001) Effect of tumor weight and tube feeding on TNF-α and IL-1b mRNA expression in the brain of mice. J Parenter Enteral Nutr 25:317–322

36. Plata-Salaman CR, Turrin NP (1999) Cytokine interactions and cytokine balance in the brain: relevance to neurology and psychiatry. Mol Psychiatry 4:303–306

37. Quinn LS, Anderson BG, Drivdahl RH et al (2002) Overexpression of interleukin-15 induces skeletal muscle hypertrophy in vitro: implications for treatment of muscle wasting disorders. Exp Cell Res 280:55–63

38. Harrold JA, Williams G (2003) The cannabinoid system: a role in both the homeostatic and hedonic control of eating? Br J Nutr 90:729–734

39. Wu JT, Kral JG (2004) Ghrelin: integrative neuroendocrine peptide in health and disease. Ann Surg 239:464–474

40. Broglio F, Gottero C, Arvat E, Ghigo E (2003) Endocrine and non-endocrine actions of ghrelin. Horm Res 59:109–117

41. Nagaya N, Uematsu M, Kojima M et al (2001) Elevated circulating level of ghrelin in cachexia associated with chronic heart failure: relationships between ghrelin and anabolic/catabolic factors. Circulation 104:2034–2038

42. Lissoni P (2002) Is there a role for melatonin in supportive care? Support Care Cancer 10:110–116

43. Davis TW, Zweifel BS, O'Neal JM et al (2004) Inhibition of cyclooxygenase-2 by celecoxib reverses tumor-induced wasting. J Pharmacol Exp Ther 308:929–934

44. Lugarini F, Hrupka BJ, Schwartz GJ et al (2002) A role for cyclooxygenase-2 in lipopolysaccharide-induced anorexia in rats. Am J Physiol 283:R862–R868

45. Coma M, Vicente R, Busquets S et al (2003) Impaired voltage-gated K+ channel expression in brain during experimental cancer cachexia. FEBS Lett 536:45–50

# Body Weight Regulation and Hypothalamic Neuropeptides

Flavia Prodam, Elisa Me, Fabrizio Riganti, Maria Angela Seardo, Barbara Lucatello, Mario Maccario, Ezio Ghigo, Fabio Broglio

## Introduction

The epidemic increasing incidence and prevalence of obesity and diabetes mellitus have underlined the necessity of understanding the regulation and control of appetite and energy metabolism.

The regulation of body weight can be considered a homeostatic system characterised by a strict balance between caloric intake and energy expenditure.

It is well known in the literature that body weight is stable over long periods in humans, in spite of daily variations in food intake and energy expenditure, thus revealing the existence of short- and long-term control pathways [1].

Within the central nervous system (CNS), the hypothalamus has been shown to have an emerging and central role in the control of appetite and energy metabolism. Notably the activity of the hypothalamus eventually derives from a complex integration of different central and peripheral modulator inputs such as nutrients, but is also affected by sight, smell, experience, lifestyle and environmental conditions [2].

In particular, numerous recent papers have focused on the role of several gastrointestinal hormones and neurotransmitters involved in the control of these vital functions.

## The Hypothalamus: The Regulatory Key

The hypothalamus is divided into nuclei with several functions and connected with other central areas of the brain stem and peripheral tissues.

Both the arcuate nucleus (ARC) and the tractus solitarius nucleus (TNS) have been described as emerging areas in the central modulation of energetic storage and utilisation. Moreover, the paraventricular (PVN) and lateral nuclei are well known to play an important metabolic role, being constituted by glucose-sensitive neurons and free fatty acid (FFA) and amino acid-responsive pathways.

In fact, many hypothalamic neuropeptides play a key role in the regulation of body weight, acting either as orexigenic or anorectic factors in a complex multisystemic redundant network of central and peripheral signals.

### Neuropeptide Y and Agouti-Related Protein

Neuropeptide Y (NPY) is a 36 amino acid neuropeptide expressed in the CNS and, in particular, in the ARC, representing one of the most potent orexigenic factors studied so far [3].

The intracerebroventricular administration of NPY stimulates food intake in rodents after acute injection [2], while chronic treatment induces hyperphagia and weight gain, coupled with decrease in energy expenditure [2, 4]. Interestingly, NPY administration also inhibits luteinising hormone (LH) secretion [5], underlining the tight relationship between energy balance, fat mass and the activity of the reproductive system. Among the physiological regulators, fasting has been shown to be an important stimulator of NPY expression in animals. In fact, maximal NPY concentration in PVN is observed before and during feeding, suggesting a possible role in meal initiation [2].

Notably, despite the clear orexigenic effects of NPY administration, NPY knockout mice have normal body weight and show weight variation similar to control animals in both overfeeding and fasting conditions [2, 6, 7], likely as a consequence of the activation of other orexigenic pathways aimed to preserve the feeling of hunger.

NPY exerts its actions via five specific receptor subtypes, of which the Y5 receptor has been described as the most important for the activity of the peptide [2, 8].

Neurons secreting NPY also co-express agouti-related protein (AgRP) [9], a 132 amino acid protein endowed with remarkable NPY-independent orexigenic actions [2, 10]. Specifically, AgRP increases food intake, acting as an endogenous antagonist of melanocortin (MC) 3 and MC4 receptors, thus inhibiting the anorectic action of α-melanocyte-stimulating hormone (MSH) [2, 7].

The acute intracerebroventricular administration of AgRP in rodents increases food intake for up to 6 days [2] and chronic treatment determines an important weight gain [11].

NPY/AgRP neurons represent the most important target of central and peripheral orexigenic and anorectic signals. In particular, they are inhibited by leptin and insulin and activated by the orexigenic peptide ghrelin [12–14]. Interestingly, an intestinal peptide, named PYY, the chemical structure of which closely resembles that of NPY [2, 10, 15], has been reported to exert its anorectic effect acting as an antagonist of the NPY Y2 receptor. In fact, its administration is devoid of any effect in Y2 knockout mice [15].

## The Melanocortins

The transcript of the pro-opiomelanocortin (POMC) molecule is the precursor of several biologically active molecules: α-, β-, and γ-MSH, adrenocorticotropin (ACTH), β-endorphin and lipotropins. The POMC gene is expressed in different tissues such as hypothalamus, pituitary, immune system and skin [16]. In the hypothalamus, POMC is expressed in particular in the ARC and TNS [16].

Within the CNS, α-MSH is a potent inhibitor of food intake [2, 7, 16], acting via MC3 and MC4 receptors [16], antagonising the effect of AgRP [2, 16, 17].

In animals, the central administration of α-MSH inhibits feeding and reduces body weight [3].

POMC knockout mice show obese and hyperphagic phenotype and suffer from adrenal hypoplasia and altered skin pigmentation [18]. In this experimental model, chronic daily administration of α-MSH reverses these effects and determines a prompt weight decrease [19]. Similarly, the intranasal chronic administration of a synthetic α-MSH fragment (MSH/ACTH4-10) causes a mild but persistent decrease in body fat in humans [20].

Urocortin is a member of the corticotropin-releasing hormone (CRH) family, expressed at both peripheral and central levels, in particular in PVN and lateral septum [21]. Its administration has been shown to induce a dose-dependent inhibition of food intake in animals and humans, even after acute administration [22]. A similar anorectic effect has been observed in animals, even after the intracerebroventricular administration of CRH [23].

Neuromedin-U (NMU) is a 23 amino acid peptide expressed in central and peripheral tissues, such as hypothalamus, in particular in noradrenergic neurons in the nucleus of the solitary tract (NTS), and gastrointestinal tract [24]. It shows several activities: it increases blood pressure, decreases gastric secretion and emptying, and seems to play a role in the modulation of the hypothalamus–pituitary–adrenal (HPA) axis [24].

The central administration of NMU is followed by inhibition of food intake in fasted rats [24–26] and increase in plasmatic ACTH and corticosterone levels [25]. Both these effects are likely mediated by CRH neurons in hypothalamic PVN [24, 25]. In addition, NMU plays a role in the control of circadian rhythms: in fact, it inhibits much more overnight food consumption [24, 26], and time spent in feeding. NMU expression in the brain and particularly at the pituitary levels is lower than in controls in *ob/ob* mice and in *fa/fa* Zucker rats [24], in agreement with the known stimulator effect of leptin on NMU secretion in hypothalamic cells in vitro [26]. MNU knockout mice show increased body weight and adipose tissue, hyperphagia and decreased energy expenditure [27]. These mice develop hyperleptinaemia, hyperinsulinaemia, late-onset hyperglycaemia and hyperlipidaemia [27].

Mahogany is a single trans-membrane protein that is expressed in many tissues, including the hypothalamus [26], in particular in those areas identified as critical for the control of feeding and energy expenditure [28].

Several data suggest an important role of this protein in the regulation of action of the melanocortin system [16]. Moreover, mahogany seems also to play a modulatory action on agouti protein and AgRP functions, as shown in experimental transgenic model [16, 29].

Syndecan is a new family of four transmembrane proteoglycans, acting in cell-adhesion regulation and modulation of binding of growth factors [16, 30]. Recently these peptides have been reported also to have a role in the regulation of feeding. In fact, syndecan-3 is expressed in those hypothalamic areas involved in feeding regulation, and transgenic syndecan-1 overexpression determines hyperphagia and obese phenotype in mutant mice [16, 31]. Moreover, food deprivation causes an increase in the hypothalamic expression of syndecan-3 [16, 31], coupled with an increase in AgRP levels [16]. Animal models characterised by syndecan-3 deficiency lack the hyperphagia reflex after a prolonged fasting period [16, 31]. This evidence suggests that syndecan molecules might participate in the antagonistic function exerted by AgRP on $\alpha$-MSH.

## Orexin A and B

Orexin A (OXA) and B (OXB) are two peptides mainly expressed in the lateral hypothalamus [22], although recent data show the presence of OXA and orexin receptor (OX-1) immunoreactivity also in gastrointestinal submucosa, myenteric plexus and pancreatic islets [32].

Orexins, in particular OXA, possess an important central orexigenic effect, coupled with modulation of peripheral signals [22]. In humans, OXA plasma levels increase during fasting and hypoglycaemia [7]. In fasting conditions, OXA inhibits gastrointestinal motility and the vagal responses to cholecystokinin [32], and is involved in the modulation of insulin and glucagon secretion [34]. Interestingly, however, OXA plasma levels have been shown to be decreased in obesity [33].

OXA and OXB also inhibit CRH-induced ACTH release [35], while central urocortin administration suppresses food intake in food deprivation state as well as after OXA injection [36].

It is interesting to underline that orexins knockout mice are narcoleptic, indicating that these peptides seem to participate not only in the control of feeding and weight homeostasis, but also in the control of sleep [7, 10].

## Opioid Peptides, Cannabinoids and Cocaine- and Amphetamine-Regulated Transcript

Opioid peptides, in particular the endogenous agonists of κ opioid receptor, increase food intake [37]. It has also been hypothesised that these molecules are involved in reward and pleasure feelings related with food [7].

The appetite-stimulating effect of marijuana in humans has been well known for centuries [38]. Endogenous cannabinoids, in particular anandamide, increase appetite and food intake via the activation of specific receptors known as CB1 [39], which are expressed in hypothalamic and central areas involved in the control of feeding behaviour [40, 41]. In fact, CB1 receptor mRNA is co-expressed with CRH, cocaine- and amphetamine-regulated transcript (CART), melanin-concentrating hormone (MCH) and prepro-orexin [42].

Central leptin administration is followed by a decrease in hypothalamic endocannabinoid levels [41–43]. Moreover, the blockade of CB1 receptor inhibits starvation-induced hyperphagia in rodents [43].

CB1 deletion in mice determines a decrease in body weight and fat mass, coupled with hypophagia [41, 42]. Interestingly, since both NPY and AgRP knockout models do not induce a lean phenotype, likely due to the existence of redundant anabolic signals [6], the experimental demonstration of lower body mass in CB1 receptor knockout mice strongly suggests a crucial role of endocannabinoids in the regulation of food intake and energy balance [41, 42].

Notably, cannabinoids regulate energy metabolism even at the peripheral level. In fact, CB1 receptors are also expressed in mouse adipocytes

[42] and their activation seems to increase lipogenesis in primary adipocyte cultures [42].

Cocaine- and amphetamine-regulated transcript is co-expressed in ARC in POMC neurons [3, 44], and is directly modulated by leptin [44]. It is also expressed in PVN, NTS, lateral and dorsomedial hypothalamus and nucleus accumbens [45]. At the peripheral level, CART is expressed in the myenteric gut plexus, vagus nerve, pancreatic somatostatin cells, and antral gastrin cells [45]. Until now, no specific receptors for CART have been identified [45], thus a full description of the activities of this peptide is still lacking.

The intracerebroventricular injection of CART is followed by reduction in food intake [45, 46], even in co-administration with NPY [46], coupled with a decrease in plasma insulin and leptin and an increase in lipid oxidation [47]. However, other experimental models showed that chronic CART over-expression in ARC neurons determines significant weight gain and reduction in thyrotropin levels in rats [48], and the *anx/anx* mice, characterised by anorexia, low body weight, abnormal movement, hyperactivity and early death, present lower hypothalamic CART levels [49]. These disparate data suggest the existence of some central and peripheral resistance mechanisms to CART that need further elucidation.

CART is also able to reduce gastric emptying and motility [45].

Recent studies demonstrate that glucocorticoids regulate CART expression at the hypothalamus and pituitary levels [45]. On the other hand, CART seems to modulate the HPA axis, probably via corticotropin-releasing factor [50].

Thus, CART seems to be another putative peptide involved in the regulation of body mass. However, despite gene polymorphisms having been identified in some obese families, CART-deficient mice do not show a spontaneous obese phenotype in experimental conditions [45].

## Galanin and Galanin-Like Peptide

Galanin is a 30 amino acid peptide with widespread distribution in the CNS [51]. Three distinct galanin receptor subtypes, GalR1, GalR2 and GalR3, have been described at the hypothalamic level [52], in neurons also expressing leptin receptor [51]. Both galanin and galanin receptor have also been demonstrated in adipose tissue in rats [53].

The intracerebroventricular administration of galanin induces food intake [54]. This effect has been suggested to be mediated by modulation of leptin expression and levels [51, 54]. Some studies affirm that galanin increases, in particular, fat ingestion [55]. Galanin administration inhibits leptin levels and its expression in adipose tissue increases during fasting [53]. However, the chronic administration of galanin does not induce hyperphagic behaviour or weight gain [56], in agreement with the observation that galanin knockout mice or galanin over-expressing mice maintain normal weight [51]. In all, this peptide seems to be much more involved in the short-term regulation of feeding rather than in long-term metabolic balance [51, 54].

Galanin-like peptide (GALP) is a 60 amino acid molecule recently isolated and structurally related to galanin [57]. It binds GalR2 and, with lower affinity, GalR1 [51, 57].

Similarly to POMC and unlike galanin, the central expression of GALP is negatively regulated by fasting and is reduced in transgenic models of leptin deficiency [51, 58]. Intracerebroventricular GALP administration reduces energy intake and increases energy expenditure in mice [59].

Moreover, GALP stimulates LH secretion in rodents, suggesting an involvement together with leptin in the functional relationship between energy metabolism and the reproductive system [51, 59].

## Serotonin and Nitric Oxide

Serotonin (5-HT) is a neurotransmitter acting on several receptor subtypes expressed in particular in the limbic system and in the hypothalamus [60]. 5-HT stimulates adrenaline secretion and plays an important role in controlling behaviour [2].

Synthetic agonists of the 5-HT receptors inhibit 5-HT re-uptake and decrease food intake [2, 7]. Accordingly, $5\text{-HT}_{2c}$ receptor knockout mice have been shown to be hyperphagic and obese [61]. Notably, however, chronic treatment with $5\text{-HT}_{2c}$ receptor antagonist does not determine an obese phenotype, probably as a result of other counter-acting signals [2, 7, 10].

Nitric oxide (NO) has also been recently proposed as a neuromodulator of the central pathways of appetite control. Central blockade of NO production inhibits food intake [62]. This condition is reversed by administration of NO donors (L-arginine) [7]. NO seems also to be involved in many central feedback systems, such as those of leptin and 5-HT [63].

## Gastroenteropancreatic Signalling: The Peripheral Balance

As anticipated, energy balance is a complex system in which the hypothalamic network receives many excitatory and inhibitory signals even from peripheral tissues. All these peripheral signals allow the existence of a fine-timing system regulating short-term as well as long-term control of energy metabolism.

### The Positive Peripheral Feedback: Hunger Signals

#### Ghrelin

Ghrelin is a 28 amino acid peptide, recently isolated in the stomach, but also expressed in other tissues, such as pancreas, kidney, testes, placenta, pituitary and hypothalamic ARC and PVN [14, 64, 65].

Ghrelin has been identified as an endogenous ligand of the orphan GH secretagogue (GHS) receptor type 1a [64].

In animals and humans, ghrelin has been reported to exert several biological activities such as: (a) stimulation of growth hormone, prolactin and ACTH release; (b) influence on the pituitary–gonadal axis; (c) influence on sleep and behaviour; (d) control of gastric motility and acid secretion; (e) modulation of exocrine and endocrine pancreatic functions [14, 66].

Moreover, since its discovery, ghrelin has emerged as a player in the regulation of food intake and energy expenditure, being the most potent peripheral orexigenic hormone known so far [65].

In animals and humans, ghrelin, after both central and peripheral administration, has been shown to induce appetite and food intake [14, 65, 67]. This effect has been shown to be mainly mediated by NPY and AgRP [65, 68], but, more recently, POMC, CART, MCH, orexin system, gamma amino butyric acid (GABA) and galanin have also been reported to play a role [14].

Despite these clear orexigenic effects under experimental pharmacological conditions, the actual physiological role of ghrelin in the regulation of appetite is still a matter for debate [14, 69, 70].

Notably, however, it has been clearly shown that, besides the central actions, ghrelin also influences energy metabolism at the peripheral level, likely influencing fat oxidation [13, 71].

### The Negative Peripheral Feedback: Satiety Signals

#### Signals from the Adipocytes

##### Leptin, Adiponectin and Resistin

Leptin is a peptide expressed and secreted by white adipose tissue, proportionally to fat body mass [2, 7]. Both leptin and its receptor have also been isolated in human gastric mucosa [32], suggesting a possible paracrine regulation of the other gastric peptides [10, 32].

Leptin plays a central role in the regulation of energy intake and expenditure. Leptin increases some hours before meals in rodents and after several days of overeating in humans [72], while it decreases during fasting [2].

The main activity of leptin is exerted at the central level, in particular in ARC and PVN [7], via the activation of specific receptors named OB-Rb [73]. Specifically, leptin inhibits NPY and AgRP neurons, achieving a decrease in food intake [2, 7, 32].

Leptin (*ob/ob*)- or leptin receptor (*db/db*)-knockout mice are obese, hyperphagic and hyperinsulinaemic [73, 74]. As in mice, genic mutations leading to leptin deficiency have also been described in humans as a rare cause of obesity that fully normalises during leptin replacement therapy [2]. However, not all obese phenotypes derive from leptin deficiency. In fact, in humans obesity is strongly associated with high plasma leptin levels, suggesting a condition of leptin resistance [75].

Leptin secretion is regulated by several hormonal and metabolic signals [2, 14, 15, 76].

Noteworthy, the gastric release of leptin is also stimulated by the activation of vagal afferents, thus suggesting this hormone to be involved not only in the long-term maintenance of weight balance but also in the cephalic phase of gastric function [32, 77].

Adiponectin is a peptide produced exclusively by adipocytes [78]; it shows structural homology with the tumour necrosis factor family [32], cytokines characterised by negative effects on energy balance [7].

Unlike leptin, adiponectin levels do not follow circadian rhythms and seem not to be affected by feeding behaviour [79]. However, it is negatively correlated with body mass index [80] and is decreased in *ob/ob* mice [32]. The evidence, showing lower adiponectin levels in obese diabetic subjects than in obese non-diabetic subjects, suggests its major role in the development of insulin resistance [32].

Resistin is secreted by adipose tissue and exerts its own activity on several peripheral tissues, such as liver and muscle [32]. It seems to possess inversely related effects to adiponectin: higher levels can increase insulin resistance [81].

### Signals from the Gut

#### Glucagon-Like Peptide-1 and -2, Oxyntomodulin and Amylin

Glucagon-like peptide-1 (GLP-1) is a peptide of 30 amino acids expressed and secreted from endocrine L-cells of intestinal mucosa at ileum and colon level [82]. GLP-1 derives from the same precursor of glucagon [2]. GLP-1 shows several activities, among others a role in enhancing insulin secretion and suppressing glucagon secretion in the postprandial phase [2, 32, 83]. In animals and in humans GLP-1 slows gastric emptying [86, 84] and therefore blunts the meal-induced insulin response [85].

GLP-1 also plays a role in mediating appetite and feeding behaviour [84]. A reduction in hunger feeling, coupled with a sensation of fullness, has been reported after its administration [84]. Moreover, intracerebroventricular GLP-1 injection in rodents is followed by inhibition of food and water intake [32, 82, 84], coupled with

an increase in *c-fos* expression in hypothalamic PVN [86]. These data are confirmed by the finding that the administration of exendin(9-39)amide, a GLP-1 receptor antagonist, determines an increase in food intake in fed rats, but not in fasted rats [86]. Indeed, a significant weight gain has been recorded during chronic exendin(9-39)amide treatment [32].

Consistently with data in animals, in humans GLP-1 induces a mild but significant dose-dependent inhibition of food intake in both lean and obese subjects [87].

GLP-2 is also produced by the endocrine L-cells by post-translational processing of proglucagon and is secreted in response to food intake together with GLP-1 [88]. In contrast to GLP-1, the role of GLP-2 in the regulation of feeding and fasting balance is unclear.

GLP-2 is a trophic peptide of intestinal mucosa and seems to act on gastric motility in pigs [32]. GLP-2 mRNA-expressing neurons have been observed in hypothalamic TNS [89] and its central administration decreases food ingestion in rodents [32, 89]. However, in humans no variation in feeding behaviour or in gastric emptying has been observed after its administration [32, 90].

Oxyntomodulin (OXM) is a 37 amino acid peptide deriving from the post-translational processing of the proglucagon molecule in intestinal cells, in particular in the distal portion of the small bowel [15]. OXM co-localises with GLP-1 expression and secretion [91].

OXM acts as an anorectic peptide in the short-term regulation of food intake [15]. It is released into the circulation after food ingestion proportionally to the caloric amount [92]. The mechanisms of action of OXM are unknown at present. In particular, it is unknown if this peptide is able to cross the blood–brain barrier to exert a putative effect at the hypothalamic level [15]. In rats its intracerebroventricular administration determines an anorectic effect, which is blocked by co-administration of the GLP-1 antagonist exendin(9-39)amide [93], in agreement with data in vitro showing that OXM is able to bind GLP-1 receptor [94]. Noteworthy, the existence of still unknown specific receptors for OXM cannot be ruled out [91].

In humans, OXM administration induces a

prompt decrease of hunger feeling, food intake and gastric emptying [15, 91, 95]. These effects are associated with a suppression of plasma ghrelin levels [15, 93], without variations in leptin [15] and insulin levels [91]. However, after the intravenous injection of OXM, no variations in daily cumulative energy expenditure are observed [91].

Amylin is another peripherally generated peptide, which is co-secreted with insulin [22]. Amylin modulates the regulation of food intake, acting via specific receptors and also via $D_2$ dopamine receptors in the CNS, expressed in particular in the nucleus accumbens [22, 96]. After amylin administration, even in fasting conditions, a strong inhibition of food intake and gastric emptying has been observed [97].

### Cholecystokinin

Cholecystokinin (CCK) was the first gut hormone described as an inhibitor of food intake in rodents [98]. CCK is widely expressed at both central and peripheral levels, in particular in I-cells in the duodenum and jejunum mucosa [99]. CCK is also detectable in the bloodstream in different forms, in particular CCK-8, CCK-33 and CCK-39 [15].

Two CCK receptor subtypes have been isolated: $CCK_A$ receptor expressed in the vagus nerve, enteric neurons, pancreas and at central level [99] and $CCK_B$ expressed in the afferent vagus nerves, CNS and stomach [99].

CCK possesses several activities on different tissues, including the well-known stimulatory effect on pancreatic enzyme excretion and the induction of gallbladder contraction [2].

CCK has been demonstrated to be a satiety signal, in particular in the short-term regulation of feeding behaviour [15, 76, 99]. It acts, synergistically with leptin [15, 100], on hypothalamic PVN and NTS [99, 100] and it can stimulate amylin secretion [32, 99]. Its effect is reduced by vagotomy and vagal afferent disruption [15, 76, 99].

Peripheral CCK administration is followed by a rapid, but short-term effect on inhibition of food intake, with an activity peak at 30 minutes [99]. High doses of CCK determine nausea, vomiting and taste aversion [101]. The inhibition of meal ingestion is specific for the $CCK_A$ receptor [99, 102]. $CCK_A$ receptor synthetic antagonists,

administered before a meal, cause increased solid and liquid intake both in animals and humans [76, 99, 103]. It is important to underline that CCK inhibits food intake, in particular fat ingestion [104]. Interestingly, the inhibitory effect of CCK on food intake undergoes a functional desensitisation after high-dose administration as well as during continuous infusion [99, 105]. When administered intermittently before eating, CCK maintains its anorectic effect, but a compensatory effect is observed by increasing the daily number of meals, with only a mild result on total food intake and body weight [106].

Otsuka Long Evans Tokushima Fatty (OLEFT) rats, which have a deletion in the $CCK_A$ receptor gene resulting in the absence of $CCK_A$ receptors, are hyperphagic, hyperglycaemic, hyperinsulinaemic and obese [99, 107]. The OLEFT hyperphagia is characterised by greater meal sizes [99, 108]. The absence of $CCK_A$ receptors in the OLEFT rats results in several phenotypes [99]. In fact, some mice, with a different genetic mutation for the $CCK_A$ receptor, are insensitive to the feeding inhibitory action of CCK, but show normal daily food intake and body weight [109].

Overall, this evidence suggests a role of CCK in the short-term regulation of feeding, much more than in long-term control of energy balance.

### Peptide YY 3-36

Peptide YY (PYY) is a 36 amino acid peptide, a member of the NPY family and secreted from the L-cells of small and large bowel, including rectum [3] and released in the circulation as PYY1-36 or PYY3-36 [110].

PYY itself has been defined an orexigenic peptide [111], but PYY3-36, the most abundant form circulating in the bloodstream, shows anorectic effects [15, 32]. PYY3-36 exerts its modulator effect on food intake acting on the $Y_2$ receptor at the hypothalamic level, and, consequently, suppressing the orexigenic effect of NPY [15, 32]. Accordingly, PYY3-36 does not reduce food intake in $Y_2$ knockout mice [15].

Plasma PYY3-36 levels increase after meal ingestion [15, 112]. In humans the administration of PYY3-36 is followed by a reduction of 30% of the amount of ingested nutrients compared to placebo [112] and is coupled with fullness sensation [15, 76].

Fasting plasma PYY3-36 levels are lower in obese than in lean subjects [113] and show a slower and delayed increase after meals in obese subjects [15]. These data suggest an involvement of the peptide in the control of food and energy intake and in the long-term control of weight.

PYY3-36 seems to counteract ghrelin activity [14, 15], probably both at vagal afferent and hypothalamic levels, in particular at ARC [14, 15, 114]. It is interesting to note that obese subjects show lower ghrelin as well as PYY3-36 levels [113, 115].

PYY3-36 shows a synergic action with CCK in inhibiting food intake, although their effects on the pancreas are opposite [15].

GLP-1, which is co-secreted with PYY at least in a subpopulation of L-cells [2], shows a feeding decrease similar to that of PYY3-36 [32] and an additive inhibitory effect on food intake [82, 84]. GLP-1 administration determines a negative feedback on PYY secretion [82, 84], suggesting a complex interplay between these two hormones that is still largely unclear [32, 82, 84].

OXM is co-secreted with GLP-1 and PYY3-36 [91]. OXM administration, differently from GLP-1, does not inhibit PYY levels [15, 91]. Few data are available about a possible feedback system among these peptides.

## Conclusions

The intriguing complexity of the biology and physiology of the system makes it difficult to synthesise effective drugs to treat obesity and metabolic syndrome and strongly suggests the need for a multi-target approach [2, 7, 10].

Feeding behaviour, energy expenditure and body weight are regulated by the tight interplay of several signals coming from the brain and the periphery. Given the vital importance of these functions, this regulatory system is characterised by an impressive redundancy of both stimulatory and inhibitory inputs able to functionally replace each other.

This chapter has focused on those substances on which enough information has been collected to hypothesise future clinical implications. Nevertheless, a much longer list of other compounds involved in the regulation of feeding behaviour is known to basic scientists working in this field, including bombesin/gastrin-releasing peptide$_{1-27}$ [116], neurotensin [117] and oleylethanolamide [118]; this list is likely to increase further.

## References

1. Edholm OG (1977) Energy balance in man: studies carried out by the Division of Human Physiology, National Institute for Medical Research. J Hum Nutr 31:413–431
2. Neary NM, Goldstone AP, Bloom SR (2004) Appetite regulation: from the gut to the hypothalamus. Clin Endocrinol 60:153–160
3. Allen YS, Adrian TE, Allen JM et al (1983) Neuropeptide Y distribution in the rat brain. Science 221:877–879
4. Schwartz MW, Seeley RJ, Campfield LA et al (1996) Identification of targets of leptin action in rat hypothalamus. J Clin Invest 98:1101–1106
5. McDonald JK, Lumpkin MD, Samson WK et al (1985) Neuropeptide Y affects secretion of luteinising hormone and growth hormone in ovariectomised rats. Proc Natl Acad Sci USA 82:561–564
6. Qian S, Chen H, Weingarth D et al (2002) Neither agouti-related protein nor neuropeptide Y is critically required for the regulation of energy homeostasis in mice. Mol Cell Biol 22:5027–5035
7. Wilding JP (2002) Neuropeptides and appetite control. Diabet Med 19:619–627
8. Schaffhauser AO, Stricker-Krongrad A, Brunner L et al (1997) Inhibition of food intake by neuropeptide Y Y5 receptor antisense oligodeoxynucleotides. Diabetes 46:1792–1798
9. Sawchenko PE, Pfeiffer SW (1988) Ultrastructural localisation of neuropeptide Y and galanin immunoreactivity in the paraventricular nucleus of the hypothalamus in the rat. Brain Res 474:231–245
10. Wynne K, Stanley S, McGowan B et al (2005) Appetite control. J Endocrinol 184:291–318
11. Small CJ, Kim MS, Stanley SA et al (2001) Effects of chronic central nervous system administration of agouti-related protein in pair-fed animals. Diabetes 50:248–254
12. Kalra SP, Dube MG, Pu S et al (1999) Interacting appetite-regulating pathways in the hypothalamic regulation of body weight. Endocr Rev 20:68–100
13. Nakazato M, Murakami N, Date Y et al (2001) A role for ghrelin in the central regulation of feeding.

Nature 409:194–198

14. van der Lely AJ, Tschop M, Heiman ML et al (2004) Biological, physiological, pathophysiological, and pharmacological aspects of ghrelin. Endocr Rev 25:426–457

15. Konturek SJ, Konturek JW, Pawlik T et al (2004) Brain-gut axis and its role in the control of food intake. J Physiol Pharmacol 55:137–154

16. Yang YK, Harmon CM (2003) Recent developments in our understanding of melanocortin system in the regulation of food intake. Obes Rev 4:239–248

17. Ollmann MM, Wilson BD, Yang YK et al (1997) Antagonism of central melanocortin receptors in vitro and in vivo by agouti-related protein. Science 278:135–138

18. Yaswen L, Diehl N, Brennan MB et al (1999) Obesity in the mouse model of pro-opiomelanocortin deficiency responds to peripheral melanocortin. Nat Med 5:1066–1070

19. Marsh DJ, Hollopeter G, Huszar D et al (1999) Response of melanocortin-4 receptor-deficient mice to anorectic and orexigenic peptides. Nat Genet 21:119–122

20. Fehm HL, Smolnik R, Kern W et al (2001) The melanocortin melanocyte-stimulating hormone/adrenocorticotropin(4-10) decreases body fat in humans. J Clin Endocrinol Metab 86:1144–1148

21. Wank SA, Pisegna JR, de Weerth A (1992) Brain and gastrointestinal cholecystokinin receptor family: structure and functional expression. Proc Natl Acad Sci USA 15(89):8691–8695

22. Cupples WA (2003) Regulating food intake. Am J Physiol Regul Integr Comp Physiol 284:R652–R654

23. Richardson RD, Omachi K, Kermani R et al (2002) Intraventricular insulin potentiates the anorexic effect of corticotropin releasing hormone in rats. Am J Physiol Regul Integr Comp Physiol 283:R1321–R1326

24. Ivanov TR, Le Rouzic P, Stanley PJ et al (2004) Neuromedin U neurones in the rat nucleus of the tractus solitarius are catecholaminergic and respond to peripheral cholecystokinin. J Neuroendocrinol 16:612–619

25. Thompson EL, Murphy KG, Todd JF et al (2004) Chronic administration of NMU into the paraventricular nucleus stimulates the HPA axis but does not influence food intake or body weight. Biochem Biophys Res Commun 323:65–71

26. Wren AM, Small CJ, Abbott CR et al (2002) Hypothalamic actions of neuromedin U. Endocrinology 143:4227–4234

27. Hanada R, Teranishi H, Pearson JT et al (2004) Neuromedin U has a novel anorexigenic effect independent of the leptin signaling pathway. Nat Med 10:1067–1073

28. Nagle DL, McGrail SH, Vitale J et al (1999) The mahogany protein is a receptor involved in suppression of obesity. Nature 398:148–152

29. Gunn TM, Miller KA, He L et al (1999) The mouse mahogany locus encodes a transmembrane form of human attractin. Nature 398:152–156

30. Rapraeger AC, Ott VL (1998) Molecular interactions of the syndecan core proteins. Curr Opin Cell Biol 10:620–628

31. Reizes O, Lincecum J, Wang Z et al (2001) Transgenic expression of syndecan-1 uncovers a physiological control of feeding behavior by syndecan-3. Cell 106:105–116

32. Hellstrom PM, Geliebter A, Naslund E et al (2004) Peripheral and central signals in the control of eating in normal, obese and binge-eating human subjects. Br J Nutr 92:S47–S57

33. Ouedraogo R, Naslund E, Kirchgessner AL (2003) Glucose regulates the release of orexin-a from the endocrine pancreas. Diabetes 52:111–117

34. Adam JA, Menheere PP, van Dielen FM et al (2002) Decreased plasma orexin-A levels in obese individuals. Int J Obes Relat Metab Disord 26:274–276

35. Samson WK, Taylor MM (2001) Hypocretin/orexin suppresses corticotroph responsiveness in vitro. Am J Physiol Regul Integr Comp Physiol 281:R1140–R1145

36. Wang C, Kotz CM (2002) Urocortin in the lateral septal area modulates feeding induced by orexin A in the lateral hypothalamus. Am J Physiol Regul Integr Comp Physiol 283:R358–R367

37. Lambert PD, Wilding JP, al-Dokhayel AA et al (1993) The effect of central blockade of kappa-opioid receptors on neuropeptide Y-induced feeding in the rat. Brain Res 629:146–148

38. Abel EL (1975) Cannabis: effects on hunger and thirst. Behav Biol 15:255–281

39. Williams CM, Kirkham TC (1999) Anandamide induces overeating: mediation by central cannabinoid (CB1) receptors. Psychopharmacology 143:315–317

40. Gomez R, Navarro M, Ferrer B et al (2002) A peripheral mechanism for CB1 cannabinoid receptor-dependent modulation of feeding. J Neurosc 22:9612–9617

41. Cota D, Marsicano G, Lutz B et al (2003) Endogenous cannabinoid system as a modulator of food intake. Int J Obes Relat Metab Disord 27:289–301

42. Cota D, Marsicano G, Tschop M et al (2003) The endogenous cannabinoid system affects energy balance via central orexigenic drive and peripheral lipogenesis. J Clin Invest 112:423–431

43. Di Marzo V, Goparaju SK, Wang L et al (2001) Leptin-regulated endocannabinoids are involved in maintaining food intake. Nature 410:822–825

44. Cowley MA, Smart JL, Rubinstein M et al (2001) Leptin activates anorexigenic POMC neurons through a neural network in the arcuate nucleus. Nature 411:480–484

45. Hunter RG, Philpot K, Vicentic A et al (2004) CART in feeding and obesity. Trends Endocrinol Metab 15:454–459

46. Kristensen P, Judge ME, Thim L et al (1998) Hypothalamic CART is a new anorectic peptide regulated by leptin. Nature 393:72–76

47. Rohner-Jeanrenaud F, Craft LS, Bridwell J et al (2002) Chronic central infusion of cocaine- and amphetamine-regulated transcript (CART 55-102): effects on body weight homeostasis in lean and high-fat-fed obese rats. Int J Obes Relat Metab Disord 26:143–149

48. Kong WM, Stanley S, Gardiner J et al (2003) A role for arcuate cocaine and amphetamine-regulated transcript in hyperphagia, thermogenesis, and cold adaptation. FASEB J 17:1688–1690

49. Johansen JE, Broberger C, Lavebratt C et al (2000) Hypothalamic CART and serum leptin levels are reduced in the anorectic (anx/anx) mouse. Brain Res Mol Brain Res 84:97–105

50. Smith BK, York DA, Bray GA (1994) Chronic cerebroventricular galanin does not induce sustained hyperphagia or obesity. Peptides 15:1267–1272

51. Heiman ML, Statnick MA (2003) Galanin-like peptide functions more like leptin than like galanin. Endocrinology 144:4707–4708

52. Gundlach AL (2002) Galanin/GALP and galanin receptors: role in central control of feeding, body weight/obesity and reproduction? Eur J Pharmacol 440:255–268

53. Li RY, Song HD, Shi WJ et al (2004) Galanin inhibits leptin expression and secretion in rat adipose tissue and 3T3-L1 adipocytes. J Mol Endocrinol 33:11–19

54. Kyrkouli SE, Stanley BG, Seirafi RD et al (1990) Stimulation of feeding by galanin: anatomical localization and behavioral specificity of this peptide's effects in the brain. Peptides 11:995–1001

55. Tempel DL, Leibowitz KJ, Leibowitz SF (1988) Effects of PVN galanin on macronutrient selection. Peptides 9:309–314

56. Smith BK, York DA, Bray GA (1994) Chronic cerebroventricular galanin does not induce sustained hyperphagia or obesity. Peptides 15:1267–1272

57. Cunningham MJ (2004) Galanin-like peptide as a link between metabolism and reproduction. J Neuroendocrinol 16:717–723

58. Jureus A, Cunningham MJ, Li D et al (2001) Distribution and regulation of galanin-like peptide (GALP) in the hypothalamus of the mouse. Endocrinology 142:5140–5144

59. Krasnow SM, Fraley GS, Schuh SM et al (2003) A role for galanin-like peptide in the integration of feeding, body weight regulation, and reproduction in the mouse. Endocrinology 144:813–822

60. Blundell JE (1984) Serotonin and appetite. Neuropharmacology 23:1537–1551

61. Tecott LH, Sun LM, Akana SF et al (1995) Eating disorder and epilepsy in mice lacking 5-HT2c serotonin receptors. Nature 374:542–546

62. Morley JE, Flood JF (1992) Competitive antagonism of nitric oxide synthetase causes weight loss in mice. Life Sci 51:1285–1289

63. Calapai G, Corica F, Allegra A et al (1998) Effects of intracerebroventricular leptin administration on food intake, body weight gain and diencephalic nitric oxide synthase activity in the mouse. Br J Pharmacol 125:798–802

64. Kojima M, Hosoda H, Date Y et al (1999) Ghrelin is a growth-hormone-releasing acylated peptide from stomach. Nature 402:656–660

65. Muccioli G, Tschop M, Papotti M et al (2002) Neuroendocrine and peripheral activities of ghrelin: implications in metabolism and obesity. Eur J Pharmacol 440:235–254

66. Arvat E, Maccario M, Di Vito L et al (2001) Endocrine activities of ghrelin, a natural growth hormone secretagogue (GHS), in humans: comparison and interactions with hexarelin, a nonnatural peptidyl GHS, and GH-releasing hormone. J Clin Endocrinol Metab 86:1169–1174

67. Horvath TL, Diano S, Sotonyi P et al (2001) Minireview: ghrelin and the regulation of energy balance – a hypothalamic perspective. Endocrinology 142:4163–4169

68. Hewson AK, Dickson SL (2000) Systemic administration of ghrelin induces Fos and Egr-1 proteins in the hypothalamic arcuate nucleus of fasted and fed rats. J Neuroendocrinol 12:1047–1049

69. Cummings DE, Purnell JQ, Frayo RS et al (2001) A preprandial rise in plasma ghrelin levels suggests a role in meal initiation in humans. Diabetes 50:1714–1719

70. Broglio F, Gottero C, Benso A et al (2003) Ghrelin and the endocrine pancreas. Endocrine 22:19–24

71. Choi K, Roh SG, Hong YH et al (2003) The role of ghrelin and growth hormone secretagogues receptor on rat adipogenesis. Endocrinology 144:754–759

72. Kolaczynski JW, Ohannesian JP, Considine RV et al (1996) Response of leptin to short-term and prolonged overfeeding in humans. J Clin Endocrinol Metab 81:4162–4165

73. Zhang Y, Proenca R, Maffei M et al (1994) Positional cloning of the mouse obese gene and its human homologue. Nature 372:425–432

74. Chua SC Jr, Chung WK, Wu-Peng XS et al (1996) Phenotypes of mouse diabetes and rat fatty due to mutations in the OB (leptin) receptor. Science 271:994–996

75. Considine RV, Sinha MK, Heiman ML et al (1996) Serum immunoreactive-leptin concentrations in normal-weight and obese humans. N Engl J Med 334:292–295

76. Woods SC (2004) Gastrointestinal satiety signals I. An overview of gastrointestinal signals that influence food intake. Am J Physiol Gastrointest Liver Physiol 286:G7–G13

77. Sobhani I, Buyse M, Goiot H et al (2002) Vagal stimulation rapidly increases leptin secretion in human stomach. Gastroenterology 122:259–263

78. Scherer PE, Williams S, Fogliano M et al (1995) A novel serum protein similar to C1q, produced exclu-

sively in adipocytes. J Biol Chem 270:26746–26749
79. Hotta K, Funahashi T, Arita Y et al (2000) Plasma concentrations of a novel, adipose-specific protein, adiponectin, in type 2 diabetic patients. Arterioscler Thromb Vasc Biol 20:1595–1599
80. Matsubara M, Maruoka S, Katayose S (2002) Inverse relationship between plasma adiponectin and leptin concentrations in normal-weight and obese women. Eur J Endocrinol 147:173–180
81. Steppan CM, Bailey ST, Bhat S et al (2001) The hormone resistin links obesity to diabetes. Nature 409:307–312
82. Naslund E, Bogefors J, Skogar S et al (1999) GLP-1 slows solid gastric emptying and inhibits insulin, glucagon, and PYY release in humans. Am J Physiol 277:R910–R916
83. Orskov C (1992) Glucagon-like peptide-1, a new hormone of the entero-insular axis. Diabetologia 35:701–711
84. Naslund E, Barkeling B, King N et al (1999) Energy intake and appetite are suppressed by glucagon-like peptide-1 (GLP-1) in obese men. Int J Obes Relat Metab Disord 23:304–311
85. Nauck MA, Niedereichholz U, Ettler R et al (1997) Glucagon-like peptide 1 inhibition of gastric emptying outweighs its insulinotropic effects in healthy humans. Am J Physiol 273:E981–E988
86. Turton MD, O'Shea D, Gunn I et al (1996) A role for glucagon-like peptide-1 in the central regulation of feeding. Nature 379:69–72
87. Verdich C, Flint A, Gutzwiller JP et al (2001) A meta-analysis of the effect of glucagon-like peptide-1 (7-36) amide on ad libitum energy intake in humans. J Clin Endocrinol Metab 86:4382–4389
88. Hartmann B, Johnsen AH, Orskov C et al (2000) Structure, measurement, and secretion of human glucagon-like peptide-2. Peptides 21:73–80
89. Tang-Christensen M, Larsen PJ, Thulesen J et al (2000) The proglucagon-derived peptide, glucagon-like peptide-2, is a neurotransmitter involved in the regulation of food intake. Nat Med 6:802–807
90. Schmidt PT, Naslund E, Gryback P et al (2005) Peripheral administration of GLP-2 to humans has no effect on gastric emptying or satiety. Regul Pept 116:21–25
91. Cohen MA, Ellis SM, Le Roux CW et al (2003) Oxyntomodulin suppresses appetite and reduces food intake in humans. J Clin Endocrinol Metab 88:4696–4701
92. Le Quellec A, Kervran A, Blache P et al (1992) Oxyntomodulin-like immunoreactivity: diurnal profile of a new potential enterogastrone. J Clin Endocrinol Metab 74:1405–1409
93. Dakin CL, Gunn I, Small CJ et al (2001) Oxyntomodulin inhibits food intake in the rat. Endocrinology 142:4244–4250
94. Gros L, Thorens B, Bataille D et al (1993) Glucagon-like peptide-1-(7-36) amide, oxyntomodulin, and glucagon interact with a common receptor in a somatostatin-secreting cell line. Endocrinology 133:631–638
95. Schjoldager B, Mortensen PE, Myhre J et al (1989) Oxyntomodulin from distal gut. Role in regulation of gastric and pancreatic functions. Dig Dis Sci 34:1411–1419
96. Lutz TA, Tschudy S, Mollet A et al (2001) Dopamine D(2) receptors mediate amylin's acute satiety effect. Am J Physiol Regul Integr Comp Physiol 280:R1697–R1703
97. Reidelberger RD, Arnelo U, Granqvist L et al (2001) Comparative effects of amylin and cholecystokinin on food intake and gastric emptying in rats. Am J Physiol Regul Integr Comp Physiol 280:R605–R611
98. Gibbs J, Young RC, Smith GP (1973) Cholecystokinin decreases food intake in rats. J Comp Physiol Psychol 84:488–495
99. Moran TH (2000) Cholecystokinin and satiety: current perspectives. Nutrition 16:858–865
100. Emond M, Schwartz GJ, Ladenheim EE et al (1999) Central leptin modulates behavioral and neural responsivity to CCK. Am J Physiol 276:R1545–R1549
101. West DB, Greenwood MR, Marshall KA et al (1987) Lithium chloride, cholecystokinin and meal patterns: evidence that cholecystokinin suppresses meal size in rats without causing malaise. Appetite 8:221–227
102. Funakoshi A, Miyasaka K, Shinozaki H et al (1995) An animal model of congenital defect of gene expression of cholecystokinin (CCK)-A receptor. Biochem Biophys Res Commun 210:787–796
103. Reidelberger RD, Varga G, Solomon TE (1991) Effects of selective cholecystokinin antagonists L364,718 and L365,260 on food intake in rats. Peptides 12:1215–1221
104. Covasa M, Marcuson JK, Ritter RC (2001) Diminished satiation in rats exposed to elevated levels of endogenous or exogenous cholecystokinin. Am J Physiol Regul Integr Comp Physiol 280:R331–R337
105. Crawley JN, Beinfeld MC (1983) Rapid development of tolerance to the behavioural actions of cholecystokinin. Nature 302:703–706
106. West DB, Fey D, Woods SC (1984) Cholecystokinin persistently suppresses meal size but not food intake in free-feeding rats. Am J Physiol 246:R776–R787
107. Kawano K, Hirashima T, Mori S et al (1992) Spontaneous long-term hyperglycemic rat with diabetic complications. Otsuka Long-Evans Tokushima Fatty (OLETF) strain. Diabetes 41:1422–1428
108. Moran TH, Katz LF, Plata-Salaman CR et al (1998) Disordered food intake and obesity in rats lacking cholecystokinin A receptors. Am J Physiol 274:R618–R625
109. Kopin AS, Mathes WF, McBride EW et al (1999) The cholecystokinin-A receptor mediates inhibition of food intake yet is not essential for the maintenance of body weight. J Clin Invest 103:383–391
110. Grandt D, Schimiczek M, Beglinger C et al (1994) Two molecular forms of peptide YY (PYY) are abun-

dant in human blood: characterization of a radioim-munoassay recognizing PYY 1-36 and PYY 3-36. Regul Pept 51:151–159

111. Hagan MM (2002) Peptide YY: a key mediator of orexigenic behavior. Peptides 23:377–382

112. Batterham RL, Cowley MA, Small CJ et al (2002) Gut hormone PYY(3-36) physiologically inhibits food intake. Nature 418:650–654

113. Batterham RL, Cohen MA, Ellis SM et al (2003) Inhibition of food intake in obese subjects by pepti-de YY3-36. N Engl J Med 349:941–948

114. Cone RD, Cowley MA, Butler AA et al (2001) The arcuate nucleus as a conduit for diverse signals relevant to energy homeostasis. Int J Obes Relat Metab Disord 25:S63–S67

115. Tschop M, Weyer C, Tataranni PA et al (2001) Circulating ghrelin levels are decreased in human obesity. Diabetes 50:707–709

116. Rushing PA, Henderson RP, Gibbs J (1998) Prolongation of the postprandial intermeal interval by gastrin-releasing peptide1-27 in spontaneously feeding rats. Peptides 19:175–177

117. Ohinata K, Shimano T, Yamauchi R et al (2004) The anorectic effect of neurotensin is mediated via a histamine H1 receptor in mice. Peptides 25:2135–2138

118. Rosen ED (2003) Energy balance: a new role for PPARalpha. Curr Biol 13:R961–R963

# SECTION 6
# MEDICAL CAUSES OF WASTING/CACHEXIA

# Diabetes

Takeshi Ohara

## Insulin and Diabetes Mellitus

Energy is constantly required in human life, whereas it is supplied only by intermittent food intake. Therefore, food is usually ingested in excess of the immediate caloric needs, and the extra calories are stored in the form of hepatic and muscle glycogen, adipose tissue triglycerides, and to a certain extent as muscle protein. In turn, these fuel reservoirs are broken down during starvation to provide energy for the body. The amount of glycogen stored in skeletal muscle is about 400 g (1600 Kcal), the amount of glycogen in liver is about 75 g (300 Kcal), and the amount of triglycerides stored in adipose tissue is about 15 000 g (141 000 Kcal), at overnight fasting state in healthy men.

Glucose and free fatty acids, which are stored as glycogen and triglycerides, respectively, are the two principal circulating fuels in humans. Endogenous glucose is produced by gluconeogenesis in the liver and glycogenolysis not in skeletal muscle but in the liver [1].

Energy reservoirs in humans are built up and broken down in response to hormonal messages. Insulin is the principal hormonal messenger and has an anabolic effect. It is a major regulator of glycogen storage and its most important action is to enhance glycogen synthesis [2, 3]. In the metabolism of fat, insulin inhibits lipolysis and induces the storage of triglycerides in adipose tissue [4].

Diabetes mellitus is a syndrome characterised by chronic hyperglycaemia and disturbances of carbohydrate, fat, and protein metabolism associated with absolute or relative deficiencies in insulin secretion and/or insulin action. Diabetes mellitus has been classified into four groups: type 1, type 2, other specific types, and gestational diabetes. Type 1 diabetes results from destruction of the beta-cells of the pancreas, usually leading to absolute insulin deficiency. There are two forms of type 1 diabetes, immune-mediated diabetes and idiopathic diabetes. Type 2 diabetes refers to individuals who have insulin resistance and, usually, relative insulin deficiency. There are probably many different causes of type 2 diabetes. Other specific types of diabetes include those induced by genetic defects of beta-cell function, genetic defects in insulin action, diseases of the exocrine pancreas, endocrinopathies, drug- or chemical-induced diabetes, infections, uncommon forms of immune-mediated diabetes, and other genetic syndromes [5].

Whereas the metabolic disorders in type 1 diabetes may be explained by a lack of insulin, the basis for the metabolic abnormalities in type 2 diabetes is unclear but may be the end result of several defects in insulin action. Type 2 diabetes appears to develop in patients with acquired (diet- or obesity-related) and genetically programmed insulin resistance, when the pancreatic beta-cells are no longer able to produce extra insulin to counteract the effects of resistance [6].

Weight loss is one of the major symptoms of diabetes with marked hyperglycaemia, in addition to polyuria, polydipsia, sometimes polyphagia, and blurred vision.

As beta-cell dysfunction progresses, plasma glucose levels increase even in the fasted state because of increased hepatic glucose production. With more severe insulin deficiency, plasma free fatty acid levels increase as a consequence of enhanced lipolysis. The most extreme form of poorly controlled diabetes mellitus is diabetic ketoacidosis. The combined effects of the insulin deficiency and the increase in the levels of counter-insulin hormones result in an increase in the break down of glycogen, triglycerides, and protein beyond the fuel needs of the patient. Furthermore, the ability of peripheral tissues to utilise glucose and ketone bodies is impaired. Therefore, large quantities of these fuels are lost in the urine, resulting in weight loss in diabetic patients.

## Energy Expenditure in Diabetes Mellitus

Urinary glucose loss may be a more important cause of negative energy balance and weight loss in diabetic patients. However, the basal metabolic rate (BMR) of diabetic patients without glycosuria is higher than that of normal subjects. Increased resting energy expenditure may be another mechanism contributing to weight loss in diabetic subjects, in addition to caloric losses due to glycosuria.

The basal energy expenditure of type 1 diabetic patients (2042 Kcal/24 h) was found to be significantly higher than that of control subjects (1774 Kcal/24 h), and intravenous insulin treatment significantly reduced energy expenditure to 1728 Kcal/24 h, which matched predicted values [7].

The basal energy expenditure of obese subjects with type 2 diabetes was also found to be higher than that of obese subjects with normal glucose tolerance. The mean resting metabolic rate (RMR) of diabetic subjects (32.9 Kcal/day/kg fat-free mass) was 5% higher than that of nondiabetic subjects (31.4 Kcal/day/kg fat-free mass). A 5% higher resting energy expenditure can result in a net daily caloric deficit of about 100 Kcal/day, or 3000 Kcal/month [8]. However, resting energy expenditure accounts for only about 70% of the 24-h energy expenditure, which includes other factors, such as the thermic effect of food and exercise. Fontvieille et al. [9] reported that 24-h energy expenditure, BMR, and sleeping metabolic rate were significantly higher in diabetic patients than in control subjects. Spontaneous physical activity was similar in both group whereas the thermic effect of food was significantly lower in type 2 diabetic patients. Adjusted values of 24-h energy expenditure, BMR, and sleeping metabolic rate were correlated with endogenous glucose production in the liver.

Fasting blood glucose levels are increased as a consequence of increased hepatic glucose production [10], which is primarily due to an increased rate of gluconeogenesis [11]. The production of glucose by gluconeogenesis is an energy-expensive process, since the production of 1 mol glucose from pyruvate requires 6 mol ATP. Therefore, increased gluconeogenesis could easily contribute to the increase in energy expenditure observed in diabetic patients [12, 13].

Lipid oxidation was also increased in type 2 diabetic patients compared with control subjects and decreased significantly after insulin therapy. The rate of lipid oxidation correlated positively with BMR both in type 2 diabetic patients and in control subjects. These data demonstrate that BMR, rate of hepatic glucose production, and lipid oxidation are interrelated in type 2 diabetic patients [14]. Increased basal and sleeping metabolic rates resulting in an increased 24-h sedentary energy expenditure may thus play a role in the weight loss so often observed in type 2 diabetic subjects in addition to the energy loss from glycosuria.

## Protein Metabolism in Diabetes Mellitus

Proteins are one of the major body fuels; however, despite the large size of the protein pool, only about 15–20% of daily calorie consumption is accounted for by protein oxidation, while fat accounts for about 30% and carbohydrates for 50% or more. There is no 'storage' form for amino acids – in contrast to glycogen and triglycerides, which are the storage forms for glucose and free fatty acids, respectively. Body proteins are not a fuel reservoir in themselves; instead, protein molecules have specific roles in maintaining organ structure and function. Both the synthesis and the degradation of proteins are metabolically expensive relative to other fuels, i.e. glycogen and triglycerides. Glycogen synthesis requires 3 ATP per glucose added, and one of these ATP is recovered during glycogenolysis. Triglycerides synthesis requires only 2 ATP per fatty acid molecule added. Formation of just one peptide bound requires at least four high-energy phosphates that are not recovered when a protein is subsequently degraded to its constituent amino acids. Furthermore, the degradation process itself requires energy. Thus, on the basis of energy cost to move one unit of monomer into and out of a protein, glycogen, or triglyceride, the flux of amino acids into a protein requires the most energy [15].

Animal and in vitro studies have shown that insulin inhibits muscle protein breakdown and enhances protein synthesis [16, 17].

The results of studies performed in humans do not always agree with those conducted in vitro and in vivo in animals. In human studies, whole-body protein synthesis is estimated by measuring the nonoxidative disposal of branched-chain, essential amino acids during the primed constant infusion of $[1-^{13}C]$Leu or $[1-^{14}C]$Leu. Protein breakdown is usually estimated from the release into plasma of essential amino acids, such as leucine or phenylalanine, while net protein loss is determined from the irreversible loss of any essential amino acid that occurred by oxidation or hydroxylation. Increased rates of leucine flux were found in type 1 diabetic patients, indicating increased protein breakdown. Leucine oxidation also increased, suggesting increased net protein loss. In contrast, the rate of non-oxidised leucine disposal, i.e. the fraction of leucine entering protein, was either normal or increased, but not decreased [18–22]. The anabolic effect of insulin in type 1 diabetic patient is mediated via the reduction of proteolysis rather than by an increase in protein synthesis [23, 24].

Protein metabolism differs in peripheral tissue and in splanchnic tissue in diabetics. Insulin deficiency resulted in a net negative leucine and protein balance as measured in the human leg. Leg protein breakdown was increased, whereas protein synthesis was not decreased. In contrast, net protein balance was positive across the splanchnic area, because proteins synthesis was increased, whereas protein breakdown was unchanged [25]. Protein metabolism within the splanchnic area is further complicated by the different response of two liver-secreted proteins, albumin and fibrinogen, to insulin deficiency and reinfusion. In type 1 diabetic subjects, insulin deficiency reduced the albumin fractional synthetic rate, whereas that of

fibrinogen was increased [26, 27].

The role of insulin in protein metabolism in type 2 diabetes remains uncertain. The flux of essential amino acids (leucine and phenylalanine) in normal-weight or moderately obese type 2 diabetic patients has been found to be normal, indicating no alteration in endogenous protein breakdown. In addition, no resistance to insulin with respect to amino acid kinetics has been shown in type 2 diabetic patients, although under basal conditions these patients were found to be relatively unresponsive to insulin [28, 29]. In contrast, Gougeon et al. recently reported that protein metabolism was accelerated in moderately hyperglycaemic obese diabetic subjects when compared with an obese control group during a weight-maintaining diet. The administration of oral hypoglycaemic agents during an isoenergetic diet corrected protein turnover in relation to glycaemia [30, 31].

As part of its function as an anabolic hormone, insulin has a profound effect on protein turnover through its dual role as a stimulator of protein synthesis and an inhibitor of protein degradation. Protein turnover is dramatically turned to catabolism following either total or marked insulin withdrawal in type 1 diabetes mellitus, when total body protein is lost, which is particularly evident as muscle wasting.

## Diabetes Mellitus Linked to Malnutrition, Fat Loss, and Cachexia

### Malnutrition-Related Pancreatic Diabetes Mellitus

In tropical countries, there is another type of diabetes with many atypical clinical features. Hugh-Jones, in Jamaica, described the features of this type of diabetes and named it type J diabetes [32]. The features of this type include early-age onset of diabetes, a lack of ketosis, a relatively large insulin requirement, and lean body. Although many variants have been reported, the common features of this type of diabetes are malnutrition and protein deficiency.

In 1985, a World Health Organisation study group identified two main subgroups of pancreatic diabetes: protein-deficient diabetes mellitus

(PDDM), and fibrocalculous pancreatic diabetes (FCPD). In patients with the latter, there was no history of alcohol, biliary disease, or other known cause of pancreatitis. Clinically, malnutrition-related diabetes differs from chronic alcoholic pancreatitis in several respects. The disease occurs at an earlier age (usually before age 30) and is related to malnutrition, particularly in childhood. The pancreatitis is progressive and may eventually involve the entire pancreas.

A cross-sectional study showed that the beta-cell loss in FCPD was related to the exocrine loss, which suggested that FCPD is secondary to pancreatitis or that a common factor acts simultaneously on both components [33]. This type of diabetes is now classified as fibrocalculous pancreatopathy in diseases of the exocrine pancreas [5].

Although many theories relating malnutrition to diabetes have been proposed, none of them has been proven yet. Protein deficiency might make beta-cells susceptible to damage by toxic, viral, or autoimmune factors.

## Lipodystrophic Syndrome

Diabetes with lipodystrophy comprises a heterogeneous group of rare syndromes characterised by insulin-resistant diabetes mellitus associated with an absence of subcutaneous adipose tissue.

Several types of lipodystrophy have been reported and are distinguished according to mode of inheritance, and extent and regional distribution of fat loss. Patients with congenital lipoatrophic diabetes demonstrate insulin resistance, elevated BMR, and hepatomegaly. The absence of subcutaneous fat is noted in early infancy, although the diabetes typically appears later, with a mean onset at 12 years. In acquired generalised lipodystrophy, clinical diabetes typically follows the onset of lipoatrophy by an average of 4 years. Although acquired lipodystrophy in human immunodeficiency virus (HIV)-infected patients is the most prevalent type of lipodystrophy, the development of hyperglycaemia appears to be uncommon [34].

The mechanisms of insulin resistance and metabolic complications in patients with lipodystrophies are unclear. These features are observed in patients with various types of lipodystrophy and in several animal models. Since the extent of fat loss determines the severity of the complications, a common mechanism seems likely. Only limited quantities of triglycerides can be stored in unaffected fat depots in patients with marked fat loss. Excess triglycerides may then accumulate in the liver and skeletal muscles, contributing to insulin resistance. Although hyperinsulinaemia may initially compensate for insulin resistance and maintain euglycaemia, gradual progression of beta-cell dysfunction can lead to overt hyperglycaemia [35].

Recently, Oral et al. [36] reported that treatment with recombinant leptin was safe and effective in the treatment of lipodystrophy. Fasting blood glucose and glycosylated haemoglobin values decreased markedly after 4 months of therapy in the eight patients with diabetes, and serum triglyceride levels declined in all nine with lipodystrophies. Leptin therapy appeared to reduce hepatic steatosis, decrease intramyocellular lipid contents, and improve insulin sensitivity [37, 38].

## Diabetic Neuropathy and Digestive System Dysfunction

Dysfunction of the digestive system in diabetic subjects usually results from complications associated with the disease. Neuropathies are also a common complication of diabetes, with the prevalence after diagnosis approaching 50% at 25 years. Diabetic enteric neuropathy plays an important role in many gastrointestinal abnormalities. The symptoms of nausea and vomiting in diabetic patients may be due to diabetic gastroparesis, which is associated with delayed gastric emptying of foods. Metoclopramide, domperidone, cisapride, and motilin agonists such as erythromycin derivatives are thought to be useful for treatment of diabetic gastroparesis [39–43]. Diabetic diarrhoea is a clinical syndrome of unexplained diarrhoea in patients with insulin-dependent diabetes mellitus [44]. As almost patients with this disorder have both peripheral and autonomic neuropathy, autonomic neuropathy is thought to be a plausible cause.

Diabetic neuropathic cachexia is a much rarer form of peripheral neuropathy and is characterised by profound weight loss, painful dysaesthesias over the limbs and trunk with spontaneous resolution usually occurring within a year. In 1974, Ellenberg reported on six patients with diabetic neuropathy who complained of profound weight loss and severe neuropathic pain. These patients were all males, chiefly in the sixth decade of life, had bilateral symmetrical peripheral neuropathy, severe emotional disturbance, anorexia, impotence, mild diabetes, simultaneous onset of neuropathy and diabetes, the absence of other specific diabetic complications, and a uniformly spontaneous recovery in about 1 year. Neurologic examination revealed severe muscle wasting and atrophy in all patients. Motor nerve conduction velocity studies and electromyographic studies corroborated the presence of neuropathy in all cases. Biopsies of muscle and nerve showed neurogenic atrophy in muscle and marked involvement of the nerves, with decrease of axon fibres. Ellenberg coined the term 'diabetic neuropathic cachexia' to describe this syndrome [45]. Several cases including female patients, type 1 diabetic patients, and a patient with recurrent episodes have since been reported [46–51].

Notable weight loss of as much as 60% of total body weight is a constant feature in this syndrome. Weight loss occurs rapidly, usually over a period of 3–6 months, and is generally not related to the control of the diabetes mellitus. The cause of diabetic neuropathic cachexia remains unknown, and treatment is primarily supportive and symptomatic. Gade et al. [52] reported that combination therapy with amitriptyline and fluphenazine was effective for neuropathic pain. Some cases of diabetic neuropathic cachexia appeared to be associated with malabsorption, which may be due to pancreatic dysfunction. Intensive enteral nutritional support and pancreatic supplement may be useful for the management of these patients [53, 54].

## References

1. Chipkin SR, Kelly KL, Ruderman NB (1994) Hormone-fuel interrelationships: fed state, starvation, and diabetes mellitus. In: Kahn CR, Weir GC (ed) Joslin's Diabetes Mellitus 13th ed. Lea & Febiger, Malvern, Pennsylvania, pp 97–115
2. Petersen KF, Laurent D, Rothman DL et al (1998) Mechanism by which glucose and insulin inhibit net hepatic glycogenolysis in humans. J Clin Invest 101:1203–1209
3. Liu Z, Gardner LB, Barrett EJ (1993) Insulin and glucose suppress hepatic glycogenolysis by distinct enzymatic mechanisms. Metabolism 42:1546–1551
4. Bonadonna RC, Groop LC, Zych K et al (1990) Dose-dependent effect of insulin on plasma free fatty acid turnover and oxidation in humans. Am J Physiol 259:E736–E750
5. Alberti KGMM, Zimmet PZ for the WHO Consultation (1998) Definition, diagnosis and classification of diabetes mellitus and its complications. Part 1: diagnosis and classification of diabetes mellitus. Provisional report of a WHO consultation. Diabet Med 15:539–553
6. Defronzo RA, Ferrannini E (1991) Insulin resistance: a multifaceted syndrome responsible for NIDDM, obesity, hypertension, dyslipidemia and atherosclerotic cardiovascular disease. Diabetes Care 14:173–194
7. Nair KS, Halliday D, Garrow JS (1984) Increased energy expenditure in poorly controlled type 1 (insulin-dependent) diabetic patients. Diabetologia 27:13–16
8. Bogardus C, Taskinen MR, Zawadzki J et al (1986) Increased resting metabolic rates in obese subjects with non-insulin-dependent diabetes mellitus and the effect of sulfonylurea therapy. Diabetes 35:1–5
9. Fontvieille AM, Lillioja S, Ferraro RT et al (1992) Twenty-four-hour energy expenditure in Pima Indians with type 2 (non-insulin-dependent) diabetes mellitus. Diabetologia 35:753–759
10. De Fronzo RA (1988) The triumvirate: α-cell, muscle, liver: a collusion responsible for NIDDM. Diabetes 37:667–683
11. Consoli A, Nurjhan N, Capani F, Gerich J (1989) Predominant role of gluconeogenesis in increased hepatic glucose production in NIDDM. Diabetes 38:550–557
12. Ruderman NC, Toews JD, Shafrir E (1969) Role of free fatty acids in glucose homeostasis. Arch Intern Med 123:299–313
13. Ravussin E, Bogardus C, Schwartz RS et al (1983) Thermic effect of glucose and insulin infusion in man. J Clin Invest 72:893–902
14. Franssila-Kallunki A, Groop L (1992) Factors associated with basal metabolic rate in patients with type 2 (non-insulin-dependent) diabetes mellitus. Diabetologia 35:962–966
15. Liu Z, Long W, Hillier T et al (1999) Insulin regulation of protein metabolism in vivo. Diab Nutr Metab 12:420–428
16. Jefferson LS (1980) Role of insulin in the regulation of protein synthesis. Diabetes 29:487–496
17. Rodriguez T, Alvarez B, Busquets S et al (1997) The

increased skeletal muscle protein turnover of the streptozotocin diabetic rat is associated with high concentrations of branched-chain amino acids. Biochem Mol Med 61:87–94

18. Robert JJ, Beaufrere B, Koziet J (1985) Whole-body de novo amino acid synthesis in type 1 (insulin-dependent) diabetes studied with stable isotope labelled leucine, alanine, and glycine. Diabetes 34:67–73

19. Nair KS, Garrow JS, Ford C et al (1983) Effect of poor diabetic control and obesity on whole body protein metabolism in man. Diabetologia 25:400–403

20. Umpleby AM, Boroujerdi MA, Brown PM et al (1986) The effect of metabolic control on leucine metabolism in type 1 (insulin-dependent) diabetic patients. Diabetologia 29:131–141

21. Luzi L, Castellino P, Simonson DC et al (1990) Leucine metabolism in IDDM. Role of insulin and substrate availability. Diabetes 39:38–48

22. Tessari P, Pehling G, Nissen SL et al (1988) Regulation of whole-body leucine metabolism with insulin during mixed meal absorption in normal and diabetic humans. Diabetes 37:512–519

23. Pacy PJ, Nair KS, Ford C, Halliday D (1989) Failure of insulin infusion to stimulate fractional muscle protein synthesis in type 1 diabetic patients. Diabetes 38:618–624

24. Bennet WM, Connacher AA, Smith K et al (1990) Inability to stimulate skeletal muscle or whole body protein synthesis in type 1 (insulin-dependent) diabetic patients by insulin-plus-glucose during amino acid infusion: studies of incorporation and turnover of tracer L-[1–13C] leucine. Diabetologia 33:43–51

25. Nair KS, Ford C, Ekberg K et al (1995) Protein dynamics in whole body and in splanchnic and leg tissues in type 1 diabetic patients. J Clin Invest 95:2926–2937

26. De Feo P, Gan Gaisano M, Haymond MW (1991) Differential effects of insulin deficiency on albumin and fibrinogen synthesis in humans. J Clin Invest 88:833–840

27. De Feo P, Volpi E, Lucidi P et al (1993) Physiological increments in plasma insulin concentration have selective and different effects on synthesis of hepatic proteins in normal humans. Diabetes 42:995–1002

28. Luzi L, Petrides AS, DeFronzo RA (1993) Different sensitivity of glucose and amino acid metabolism to insulin in NIDDM. Diabetes 42:1868–1877

29. Staten MA, Matthews DE, Bier DM (1986) Leucine metabolism in type II diabetes mellitus. Diabetes 35:1249–1253

30. Gougeon R, Pencharz PB, Marliss EB (1994) Effect of NIDDM on the kinetics of whole-body protein metabolism. Diabetes 43:318–328

31. Gougeon R, Styhler K, Morais JA et al (2000) Effect of oral hypoglycemic agents and diet on protein metabolism in type 2 diabetes. Diabetes Care 23:1–8

32. Hugh-Jones P (1955) Diabetes in Jamaica. Lancet 269:891–897

33. Yajnik CS, Shelgikar KM, Sahasrabudhe RA et al (1990) The spectrum of pancreatic exocrine and endocrine (beta-cell) function in tropical calcific pancreatitis. Diabetologia 33:417–421

34. Dube MP, Johnson DL, Currier JS, Leedom JM (1997) Protease inhibitor-associated hyperglycemia. Lancet 350:713–714

35. Garg A (2004) Acquired and inherited lipodystrophies. N Engl J Med 350:1220–1234

36. Oral EA, Simha V, Ruiz E, et al (2002) Leptin-replacement therapy for lipodystrophy. N Engl J Med 346:570–578

37. Petersen KF, Oral EA, Dufour S et al (2002) Leptin reverses insulin resistance and hepatic steatosis in patients with severe lipodystrophy. J Clin Invest 109:1345–1350

38. Simha V, Szczepaniak LS, Wagner AJ et al (2003) Effect of leptin replacement on intrahepatic and intramyocellular lipid content in patients with generalized lipodystrophy. Diabetes Care 26:30–35

39. Snape WJ Jr, Battle WM, Schwartz SS et al (1982) Metoclopramide to treat gastroparesis due to diabetes mellitus: a double-blind controlled trial. Ann Intern Med 96:444–446

40. Heer M, Muller-Duysing W, Benes I et al (1983) Diabetic gastroparesis: treatment with domperidone – a double-blind placebo-controlled trial. Digestion. 27:214–217

41. Horowitz M, Roberts AP (1990) Long-term efficacy of cisapride in diabetic gastroparesis. Am J Med 88:195–196

42. Itoh Z, Nakaya M, Suzuki T et al (1984) Erythromycin mimics exogenous motilin in gastrointestinal contractile activity in the dog. Am J Physiol 247:G688–G694

43. Okano H, Inui A, Ueno N et al (1996) EM523L, a nonpeptide motilin agonist, stimulates gastric emptying and pancreatic polypeptide secretion. Peptide 17:895–900

44. Ogbonnaya KI, Arem R (1990) Diabetic diarrhea. Arch Intern Med 150:262–267

45. Ellenberg M (1974) Diabetic neuropathic cachexia. Diabetes 23:418–423

46. Archer AG, Watkins PJ, ThomasPK et al (1983) The natural history of acute painful neuropathy in diabetes mellitus. J Neurol Neurosurg Psychiatry 46:491–499

47. Blau RH (1983) Diabetic neuropathic cachexia. Report of a women with this syndrome and review of the literature. Arch Intern Med 143:2011–2012

48. Godil A, Berriman D, Knapik S et al (1996) Diabetic neuropathic cachexia. West J Med 165:382–385

49. Weintrob N, Josefsberg Z, Galazer A et al (1997) Acute painful neuropathic cachexia in a young type 1 diabetic woman. Diabetes Care 20:290–291

50. Yuen KCJ, Day JL, Flannagan DW, Rayman G (2001) Diabetic neuropathic cachexia and acute bilateral cataract formation following rapid glycaemic con-

trol in a newly diagnosed type 1 diabetic patient. Diabet Med 18:854–857

51.  Jackson CE, Barohn RJ (1998) Diabetic neuropathic cachexia: report of a recurrent case. J Neurol Neurosurg Psych 64:785–787

52.  Gade GN, Hofeldt FD, Treece GL (1980) Diabetic neuropathic cachexia. Benefical response to combination therapy with amitriptyline and fluphenazine.

JAMA 243:1160–1161

53.  D'Costa DF, Price DE, Burden AC (1992) Diabetic neuropathic cachexia associated with malabsorption. Diabet Med 9:203–205

54.  Van Heel DA, Levitt NS, Winter TA (1998) Diabetic neuropathic cachexia: the importance of positive recognition and early nutritional support. Int J Clin Pract 52:591–592

# Endocrine Disorders

Laura Gianotti, Andrea Picu, Fabio Lanfranco, Francesco Tassone, Matteo Baldi, Roberta Giordano, Ezio Ghigo, Mauro Maccario

## Introduction

Body weight is determined by the complex inter-action of caloric intake, absorption and utilisation of nutrients. Multiple factors (age, health status, neural, hormonal and metabolic influences, and medications) influence this interaction. The major site of this integration is represented by the hypo-thalamic area, where complex and specific neural circuits receive feedback from peripheral signals and coordinate the response in terms of stimula-tion or inhibition of food intake and energy bal-ance [1–3]. Among these peripheral signals, the adipocyte-derived hormone leptin informs the brain regarding the need to inhibit food intake and limit fat accumulation [4, 5]. In contrast, the gastric hormone ghrelin (see chapter by Broglio et al.) induces a sensation of hunger and is involved in energy homeostasis by inducing the storage of fat in adipose tissue [6].

Body weight is regulated within a narrow, indi-vidualised range, the level of which is determined by a combination of genetic, hormonal, and envi-ronmental factors. Among the most compelling data demonstrating this regulation is the observa-tion that people in western countries show little weight gain per year during most of their lives [3], despite the day-to-day energy imbalances charac-teristic of most humans. Thus, cumulative energy intake and expenditure are precisely matched over long periods of time. Generally, among healthy people, total body weight tends to peak in the fifth to sixth decade of life. Once peak weight has been reached, there is relative stability, with longitudi-nal studies demonstrating a decrease of only 1–2 kg per decade thereafter [7, 8].

Clinically important weight loss can be defined as the loss of 4.5 kg, or more than 5% of the usual body weight over a period of 6–12 months. Weight loss greater than 10% is considered to represent protein-energy malnutrition, which is associated with impaired cell-mediated and humoral immu-nity. Weight loss greater than 20% implies severe protein-energy malnutrition and is associated with severe organ dysfunctions [8].

Weight loss may be characterised by the decrease in lean body mass relative to body fat. Excessive loss of lean body mass results in skeletal- and cardiac-muscle wasting and loss of visceral proteins [9]. As a cumulative effect, low body weight and weight loss are powerful predictors of morbidi-ty and mortality [10–12].

Unintentional weight loss is a non-specific finding that can be associated with a great num-ber of pathological conditions [8]. The aetiology can be multifactorial or sometimes idiopathic. It is encountered frequently in clinical practice and is found in up to 12% of elderly outpatients and 50–60% of nursing-home residents [8]. Some patients may be undisturbed by their weight loss, some may welcome it or attribute it to their own change of eating style. Particularly, elderly patients often do not pay attention to a change in weight until it becomes serious. Therefore, regu-lar control and monitoring of body weight is an important strategy in any primary-care practice.

Among the organic aetiologies most common-ly identified in patients with unintentional weight loss, endocrine disorders follow, in order of fre-quency, cancer and gastroenterological disorders [8]. Diabetes mellitus and thyroid disorders are the most common endocrinopathies that cause weight loss. Less common disorders inducing weight loss are adrenal hypofunction, pheocromo-cytoma, pituitary disorders, and hormonal secre-tion of neoplastic origin such as neuroendocrine tumours. In this chapter, we will not discuss dia-betes mellitus as a cause of weight loss as it is covered in Chapter 6.1.

When dealing with endocrine disorders and weight loss, it must be considered that weight loss per se is associated with important endocrine consequences, including hypothyroidism, hypogonadism (with amenorrhoea in women), hypercortisolism, and exaggerated spontaneous growth hormone (GH) secretion with reduced insulin-like growth factor (IGF)-1 levels [13–15]. Weight loss and wasting syndrome associated with critical illness have also been extensively investigated in recent years, and several studies indicate that a reduced function of hypothalamus-pituitary-adrenal axis activity following critical illness, such as sepsis or trauma, may impair survival in critically ill patients [16, 17]. Thus, there is a close and reciprocal link between endocrinological disorders and weight loss that must always be considered in the presence of acute or chronic weight-loss-associated conditions.

## Thyroid Disorders

### Thyrotoxicosis

The term thyrotoxicosis (TS) refers to the biochemical and physiological manifestations of excessive quantities of thyroid hormones. TS may be due to sustained hormone overproduction (hyperthyroidism) or to excessive circulating hormone levels not associated with hyperthyroidism (Table 1). The effects of TS on the major organ systems are the same regardless of the underlying origin, and weight loss is a common feature in the presence of intermediate and severe TS.

**Table 1.** Classification of thyrotoxicosis

**Associated with hyperthyroidism**
Graves' disease
Toxic multinodular goitre
Toxic adenoma
Iodine-induced increased TSH secretion
Trophoblastic tumour

**Not associated with hyperthyroidism**
Thyrotoxicosis factitia
Chronic thyroiditis
Subacute thyroiditis
Ectopic thyroid tissue (struma ovarii, metastatic thyroid cancer)

Weight loss is a common manifestation of hyperthyroidism and is present in about 90% of such patients (Table 2). TS-induced weight loss is the result of the effects of thyroid hormones on different organs and on metabolism, particularly on the cardiovascular system, the sympathetic nervous system, the alimentary system, muscle, and energy metabolism [18]. Interestingly, a direct effect of thyroid hormones on adipocytes is unknown, while an indirect effect mediated by catecholamines has been identified. In fact, by affecting local norepinephrine (NE) levels and adrenergic postreceptor signalling, thyroid hormones may influence the lipolysis rate in abdominal subcutaneous (sc) adipose tissue [19].

In patients with TS, weight loss is commonly associated with increased appetite [20, 21]. The increased food intake is, however, usually inadequate to balance the increased caloric requirements and weight is lost at a variable rate. In the

**Table 2.** Symptoms of thyrotoxicosis

| Symptom | % | Symptom | % |
|---|---|---|---|
| Nervousness | 99 | Increased appetite | 65 |
| Sweating | 91 | Visual disturbances | 50 |
| Hypersensitivity to heat | 89 | Diarrhoea | 25–30 |
| Tachycardia | 85 | Anorexia | 10 |
| Fatigue | 88 | Constipation | < 5 |
| Weight loss | 85 | Weight gain | 1–2 |
| Dyspnoea | 75 | | |
| Weakness | 70 | | |

occasional, usually younger patient with mild disease, weight gain may occur when caloric intake exceeds metabolic demand [18]. Anorexia, rather than hyperphagia, occurs in about one-third of elderly TS patients and contributes to the picture of apathetic TS [22].

Although appetite and food intake are generally increased in patients with TS, ghrelin levels, unexpectedly, are reduced and can be normalised by medical antithyroid treatment. This indicates that circulating ghrelin is not the mediator of the hyperphagia associated with hyperthyroidism [23].

The increased appetite is associated with increased intestinal motility. Diarrhoea is, however, uncommon, while increased gastric emptying and intestinal motility can be responsible for slight fat malabsorption, which is reversed after recovery and thyroid hormones normalisation.

Celiac disease may occur more frequently in patients with autoimmune thyroid disease and represents an associated cause of malabsorption and weight loss [24]. Recent evidence suggests that the association between autoimmune thyroid diseases and celiac disease is quite similar to that between diabetes mellitus type 1 and celiac disease [24]. In an earlier series, about 5% of patients with celiac disease were found to suffer from hyper- or hypothyroidism even though the percentages are highly variable, with clinical hyperthyroidism in celiac disease ranging from 0% up to 7% in different studies [24]. Moreover, gastric achlorydria and autoantibodies against gastric parietal cells are detectable in about one-third of patients with Graves' disease [18, 24]. Hepatic dysfunction also occurs, particularly when TS is severe; hypoproteinaemia and increase of AST and ALP may be present [18].

Generally, TS-induced weight loss is promptly reversed after therapy is started and euthyroidism is reached.

### Effects on Metabolism and Energy Expenditure

As already mentioned, most of the effects of thyroid hormones (TH) are exerted on energy metabolism, including protein, carbohydrate, and lipid metabolism [18]. The stimulation of energy metabolism and heat production is reflected by the increased basal metabolic rate (BMR), increased appetite, heat intolerance and slightly elevated basal body temperature that occur during TS. Despite the increased food intake, a state of chronic caloric and nutritional inadequacy often ensues, depending on the degree of the TS–induced increase of metabolism.

Both the synthesis and the degradation of proteins are increased, the latter to a greater extent than the former, with the result that there is a net decrease in tissue proteins, as indicated by negative nitrogen balance, weight loss, muscle wasting, weakness, and mild hypoalbuminaemia [18].

As regards glucose metabolism, increased insulin resistance is common in TS and pre-existing diabetes is commonly aggravated by TS.

Both the synthesis and the degradation of triglycerides and cholesterol are increased in TS, but the net effect is one of lipid degradation, as reflected by an increase in the plasma concentrations of free fatty acids and glycerol, and the decrease of serum cholesterol level. Serum triglyceride levels are usually slightly decreased [18].

### Effects on Adipose Tissue

Thyroid hormones play a major role in lipid metabolism; however, whether they directly affect lipolysis locally in the adipose tissue remains unknown. It has been shown that TH may influence the lipolysis rate in the abdominal sc adipose tissue in humans, by affecting local NE levels and adrenergic postreceptor signalling [19].

### Effects on Muscle

The effect of TS on muscle is sometimes deleterious, with proximal muscle wasting (thyrotoxic myopathy). Myopathy affects men with TS more commonly than women and may overshadow the other manifestations of TS syndrome. Fortunately, thyrotoxic myopathy is uncommon, with weakness and fatigability more common and related to the generalised wasting associated with loss of weight than to a true myopathy [18].

## Hypothyroidism and Weight Loss

Weight loss is uncommon in hypothyroidism, although appetite is usually reduced. Most patients manifest a gain in weight due to retention of fluid by hydrophilic glycoprotein deposits in the tissues.

The effect of hypothyroidism on energy metabolism is opposite to that of hyperthyroidism and is characterised by a general decrease of energy metabolism and heat production. This is reflected in a reduced BMR, decreased appetite, cold intolerance, and slightly lower basal body temperature [18].

Some cases of weight loss associated with hypothyroidism have been reported, most frequently in elderly patients. In these cases, weight loss can also be induced by malabsorption [18, 24] or hypothalamic or pituitary insufficiency in the case of central hypothyroidism. In these cases, the hyposecretion of TSH is accompanied by a decrease in the secretion of other pituitary hormones, with combined gonadal and corticoid insufficiency.

## Diseases of the Adrenal Gland

Diseases of the adrenal gland can affect the cortex and/or the medulla, with different clinical pictures.

The main products of the adrenal cortex, glucocorticoids (GC) and mineralcorticoids (MC) exert important actions on fluid balance and metabolism. MC regulate electrolyte transport and fluid homeostasis, with the main target tissues being kidney, colon, and salivary glands. The main effects of GC are exerted on metabolism, immunologic functions, and musculoskeletal and connective tissues. GC also affects behaviour as well as the gastrointestinal system and development [25].

The adrenal medulla is composed almost entirely of chromaffin cells, where the synthesis, storage, and secretion of catecholamines take place. In humans, 85% of the adrenomedullary catecholamine store is epinephrine [26]. Catecholamines influence virtually all tissues and many functions, depending on the interaction between catecholamines and the surface receptors of effector cells, $\alpha$ and $\beta$ receptors ($\alpha$1 and $\alpha$2, $\beta$1, $\beta$2, and $\beta$3). In particular, $\alpha$1 receptors mediate vasoconstriction, intestinal relaxation, uterine contraction, and papillary dilatation; $\beta$1 mediate increases of heart rate and lipolysis, $\beta$2 induce smooth muscle relaxation and increase glycogenolysis in skeletal muscle, while $\beta$3 increases brown-fat thermogenesis and lipolysis [26].

Diseases of the adrenal cortex have important and sometimes dramatic consequences on general metabolism and different organs and systems. Weight loss is commonly associated with adrenal insufficiency, although also adrenal hyperfunction (particularly when induced by paraneoplastic andrenocorticotropic hormone [ACTH] secretion) may be associated with catabolic effects on muscle, connective, and bone tissue with loss of body weight mainly due to the loss of lean mass.

Among adrenal diseases inducing weight loss, pheochromocytoma (PCC) – a tumour originating from the adrenal medulla – must also be considered, despite the fact that the clinical presentation of patients with PH mainly consists of hypertension and paroxysmal attacks consequent to an abnormal catecholamine release from the tumour.

## Adrenal Insufficiency and Weight Loss

Adrenal insufficiency with subsequent weight loss may be caused by destruction of the adrenal cortex (Addison's disease), deficient pituitary ACTH secretion (secondary adrenal insufficiency), or deficient hypothalamic secretion of corticotropin releasing hormone (CRH) (tertiary adrenal insufficiency).

Primary adrenal insufficiency is infrequent (the prevalence is 40–110 cases per 1 million adults, and the incidence is 6 cases per 1 million adults per year), but it causes considerable morbidity and frequent mortality. In this form, adrenal insufficiency is characterised by symptoms of weakness, fatigue, weight loss, and gastrointestinal complaints that are, however, common to many other disorders. For this reason, adrenal insufficiency must be considered in their differential diagnosis [25]. The clinical presentation of adrenal insufficiency depends on the rate and degree of loss of adrenal function, on whether mineralocorticoid production is preserved (as in the case of secondary adrenal insufficiency), and on the degree of physiological stress. Adrenal insufficiency is often insidious at the onset and may go undetected until concurrent illness or stress precipitates a crisis.

Primary adrenal insufficiency can develop as acute adrenal insufficiency or adrenal crisis, in which shock and gastrointestinal symptoms are prominent, or as a slow process characterised by weight loss (commonly associated with nausea, vomiting, and anorexia), hyperpigmentation of the skin and mucosae, and electrolyte disturbances. Thus, nausea, vomiting, and a history of weight loss and anorexia, coupled with dehydration and hypotension represent some of the clinical features suggesting adrenal insufficiency [25, 27].

Major clinical manifestations in patients with primary adrenal insufficiency are listed in Table 3.

Weight loss is present in nearly all adult patients. In children, the clinical presentation is similar to that in adults, but the weight loss is not as prominent.

**Table 3.** Manifestations of primary adrenal insufficiency

|  | Frequency (%) |
|---|---|
| **Symptoms** | |
| Weakness, tiredness, fatigue | 100 |
| Anorexia | 100 |
| Gastrointestinal symptoms | 92 |
| Nausea | 86 |
| Vomiting | 75 |
| Constipation | 33 |
| Abdominal pain | 31 |
| Diarrhoea | 16 |
| Salt craving | 16 |
| Postural dizziness | 12 |
| Muscle or joint pains | 6–13 |
| **Signs** | |
| Weight loss | 100 |
| Hyperpigmentation | 94 |
| Hypotension | 88–94 |
| Vitiligo | 10–20 |
| Auricular calcification | 5 |
| **Laboratory findings** | |
| Hyponatraemia | 88 |
| Hyperkalaiemia | 64 |
| Anaemia | 40 |
| Eosinophilia | 17 |

Autoimmune pathogenesis accounts for 70–90% of primary adrenal insufficiency and about 50% of patients affected have one or more other autoimmune endocrine disorders, situation referred to as polyglandular autoimmune syndrome (PGA I and II). In the more common PGA II, primary adrenal insufficiency is the principal manifestation. Other autoimmune manifestations are diabetes mellitus type 1, hypoparathyroidism, pernicious anaemia, and celiac disease. While each of these manifestations can induce weight loss [28, 29], the weight is rapidly recovered once substitutive treatment is started [25].

### Ectopic ACTH Syndrome and Weight Loss

Most patients affected by ectopic ACTH syndrome have malignant tumours, half of them being small-cell lung carcinoma. The metabolic manifestations appear suddenly and progress rapidly while the typical Cushing's habitus is absent. Anorexia, weight loss, and anaemia are frequent and comprise the picture of neoplastic cachexia [30, 31].

About 20% of patients have more benign tumours, such as bronchial, thymic, and pancreatic carcinoid tumours or medullary carcinoma of the thyroid. In these cases, the clinical manifestations may be indistinguishable from those of patients with Cushing's disease [30, 31].

### Pheochromocytoma and Weight Loss

Pheochromocytoma is a tumour that produces catecholamines and is usually derived from adrenomedullary chromaffin cells. When it arises from extra-adrenal chromaffin cells, the tumours are called extra-adrenal PCC or paragangliomas. Similar clinical manifestations may occur in other related tumours that secrete catecholamines, such as chemodectomas and ganglioneuromas [26, 31]. The rarity of PCCs (fewer than 1% of hypertensive patients) should not reduce the importance of these tumours. In fact, when diagnosed and treated, PCC is curable, while when misdiagnosed it can be fatal. Most PCC (90%) are benign. Occasionally PH is inherited as an autosomal dominant trait and may be part of a multiple endocrine neoplasia (MEN) syndrome. PCCs occur at any age, but the incidence increases throughout life, in women more than in men [31, 32].

The clinical manifestations of PCC are due to the effects of the catecholamines that are stored and released in an uncontrolled way and in large amounts by the tumours [32, 33]. They include: (1) sustained hypertension resistant to conventional treatment, (2) hypertensive crisis with malignant hypertension, (3) paroxysmal attacks suggestive of seizure disorders, anxiety attacks, or hyperventilation. Less common manifestations are orthostatic hypotension and shock, cardiac manifestations (ischaemic manifestations or cardiomyopathy), and metabolic manifestations, including weight loss.

Weight loss in PCC patients is usual, although obesity cannot exclude the diagnosis. The weight reduction is partly due to increased metabolic rate, excessive sweating, and heat intolerance. Fever may also be present [31–33]. Weight loss is sustained by an activation of lipolysis in white adipose tissue. An activation of brown fat is also evident in patients with PCC [34]. It is noteworthy that, while adipose tissue constitutes the bulk of body fat stores and primarily has as an energy storage function, brown adipose tissue functions principally to generate heat in humans and many other species [34].

Gastrointestinal symptoms can also contribute to weight loss. They include nausea, vomiting, abdominal pain, and, occasionally, constipation or diarrhoea. Constipation may reflect direct inhibitory effects of catecholamines on gut smooth-muscle contraction. The so-called watery diarrhoea, hypokalaemia, achlorydria syndrome ([WDHA], also known as Verner-Morrison syndrome) in patients with PCC is secondary to the ectopic production of vasoactive intestinal polypeptide (VIP) [35]. These symptoms, including weight loss, resolve after the tumour is removed [26, 35].

## Hypothalamus and Pituitary Disorders

Hypothalamic and/or pituitary disorders can result from different kinds of lesions, most commonly tumours, trauma, congenital brain defects, infections or inflammation, radiation therapy, vascular damage or malformation, familiar disorders, granulomatoses.

In addition, they can originate from the hypothalamus or from suprahypothalamic structures and secondarily cause pituitary dysfunction, or take origin directly in the pituitary gland, most commonly when pituitary tumours develop [36] .

## Hypothalamic Diseases and Weight Loss

Besides pituitary dysfunction, diseases of the hypothalamus can cause abnormal mental function and behavioural disorders, including hyperphagia which leads to marked obesity or anorexia with weight loss [36].

Indeed, the hypothalamus is involved in the regulation of diverse functions and behaviours – in particular, social behaviours, sleep, sexuality, body temperature, and eating patterns. The abnormal eating pattern in subjects affected by hypothalamic lesions include exaggerated and uncontrolled food intake (binge eating, or bulimia) or profound anorexia with cachexia, as in Simmond's disease [37]. These are analogous to syndromes of hyperphagia produced in rats by destruction of the ventromedial nucleus or of connections to the paraventricular nucleus, while lateral hypothalamic damage causes profound anorexia [36].

## Pituitary Disorders and Weight Loss

### Hypopituitarism

Total or partial hypopituitarism may occur in patients with pituitary adenomas, following pituitary surgery or radiation, or after head injury. Deficiency of any or all of the six major hormones (lutheinising hormone [LH], follicle stimulating hormone [FSH], thyroid, GH, thyroid stimulating hormone [TSH], ACTN, and prolactin) can occur. The most common symptom in both men and women is secondary hypogonadism, because of LH and FSH deficiencies or secondary to hyperprolactinaemia. In children, cessation of growth and delayed puberty are common.

Among the uncommon manifestations of anterior pituitary hormone deficiency, weight loss is associated with corticotropin deficiency. In this case, the loss of weight is less severe and rapid than that in primary adrenal insufficiency. Typical symptoms and signs of hypopituitarism include malaise, loss of energy and libido, reduced muscle mass, and increased fat mass with weight gain, anorexia, postural hypotension, orthostatic dizziness, and sometimes headache [36, 38].

### Acromegaly

Though GH exerts a lipolytic effect, patients affected by acromegaly generally do not show significant weight loss. However, a decreased fat mass has been reported [39]. The most common somatic findings include acral growth (gigantism if acromegaly has a prepubertal onset), facial changes, voice reduction, arthralgias, excessive sweating, weakness, and malocclusion. Hypertension, reduced glucose tolerance or diabetes mellitus, and dyslipidaemia (hypertrygliceridaemia) commonly occur. Although GH exerts an anabolic effect on muscle, patients with acromegaly often suffer from myopathy, with muscular weakness [36].

## Neuroendocrine Tumors

Neuroendocrine tumours (NET) constitute a heterogeneous group of neoplasms that originate from endocrine glands, such as the pituitary, parathyroids, and adrenals, as well as endocrine islets within glandular tissue (thyroid or pancreatic) and cells dispersed between exocrine cells, such as the endocrine cells of the digestive and respiratory tracts [31]. NET can be divided into four groups: (a) carcinoid tumours, (b) islet cell tumours, (c) chromaffin cell tumours (PHs and paragangliomas), and (d) medullary thyroid carcinoma (MTC).

NETs can occur sporadically or in a familial context of autosomal dominant inherited syndromes, such as MEN. Most NET-predisposing genes have been related to inactivation of tumour growth suppressor genes, except in MEN II and in the inherited form of MTC, which is due to dominant activation of the RET proto-oncogene.

Weight loss can be one of the symptoms in the clinical presentation of NETs [31]. It can be associated with carcinoid tumours (particularly in gastric carcinoids associated with the Zollinger-Ellison syndrome, in pancreatic and pulmonary carcinoids), in islet cell tumours (particularly in gastrinoma, glucagonoma, VIPoma, and somatostatinoma), and in other rare forms of islet cell tumours, such as ACTHomas, GRFomas, and tumours secreting calcitonin, cholecistokinin (CCK), LH, or ghrelin [31, 40, 41].

Also in PHs and paragangliomas, as reported (see above), weight loss is one of the common but less characteristic symptoms of these conditions [31–33].

The classical carcinoid syndrome that can connote NET is usually the consequence of a synergistic interaction of tumour factors, including 5HT, kinins, kallikrein, prostaglandins, and endocrine factors, including growth hormone-releasing hormone (GHRH) and ACTH.

Patients with the more common classic carcinoid syndrome usually present with flushing (90%), diarrhoea (70%), abdominal pain (40%), and weight loss (40%). The latter is more commonly a consequence of diarrhoea associated with carcinoid syndrome or a consequence of neoplastic cachexia in case of malignant or metastatic NET [31].

Among islet cell tumours, nearly all gastrinomas, glucagonomas, VIPomas, and somatostatinomas are characterised by weight loss, which is more dramatic in gastrinomas and glucagonomas [42].

## Primary Hyperparathyroidism

Among endocrine disorders inducing weight change, and theoretically weight loss, primary hyperparathyroidism (PHPT) must be mentioned. PHPT is a common endocrine disorder that predominantly affects post-menopausal women [43]. It is mostly caused by solitary adenomas of the parathyroid gland and is characterised by hypersecretion of parathyroid hormone (PTH) and consequently by hypercalcaemia. In addition to regulating calcium concentrations, PTH exerts metabolic effects, including a stimulatory effect on lipolysis. This effect has been demonstrated both in animal and in human adipose tissue [44, 45]. However, PHPT is not commonly characterised by significant weight loss and there is contrasting evidence in the literature concerning this effect. For instance, it has been reported that PTH excess may promote weight gain by impeding catecholamine-induced lipolysis [46]. In a study by Grey et al., it was reported that post-menopausal women with mild untreated PHPT are markedly heavier than age-matched controls [47]. Thus, PHPT cannot be definitively considered as an endocrine cause of weight loss, although a lipolytic effect of PTH has been described.

## Conclusions

Body weight is controlled by several key factors. Since the endocrine system has a fundamental role in controlling body weight, food intake, and energy expenditure, when deranged, it may be responsible for abnormal weight loss.

Thyroid, adrenal, and hypothalamic-pituitary disorders, besides diabetes mellitus, are the most common endocrine causes of weight loss. Among them, hyperthyroidism is one of the most common causes of unintentional weight loss.

A rationale stepwise approach to patients presenting with unintentional weight loss should always include a thyroid function study. A basal evaluation of adrenal and pituitary function should be considered on the basis of the patient history and physical examination.

## References

1. Woods SC, Seeley RJ (2000) Adiposity signals and the control of energy homeostasis. Nutrition 16:894–902
2. Altman J (2002) Weight in the balance. Neuroendocrinol 76:131–136
3. Cummings DE, Scwartz MW (2003) Genetics and pathophysiology of human obesity. Ann Rev Med 54:453–471
4. Friedman JM (2002) The function of leptin in nutrition, weight, and physiology. Nutr Rev 60:S11–S14; S68–S84, S85–S87
5. Ukkola O (2004) Peripheral regulation of food intake: new insights. J Endocrinol Invest 27:96–98
6. Van der Lely AJ, Tschop M, Heiman ML, Ghigo E (2004) Biological, physiological, pathophysiological and pharmacological aspects of ghrelin. Endocr Rev 25:426–457
7. Williamson DF (1993) Descriptive epidemiology of body weight and weight change in US adults. Ann Intern Med 119:646–649
8. Bouras EP, Lange SM, Scolapio JS (2001) Rational approach to patients with unintentional weight loss. Mayo Clin Proc 76:923–929
9. Keys A, Brozek J, Henschel A et al (1950) The biology of human starvation. University of Minnesota Press, Minneapolis
10. Tayback M, Kumanyika S, Chee E (1990) Body weight as a risk factor in the elderly. Arch Intern Med 150:1065–1072
11. Stevens J, Cai J, Pamuk ER et al (1998) The effect of age on the association between body mass index and mortality. N Engl J Med 338:1–7
12. Payette H, Coulombe C, Boiutier V, Gray-Donald K (1999) Weight loss and mortality among free-living frail elders: a prospective study. J Gerontol A Biol Sci Med Sci 54:M440–M445
13. Stoving RK, Hanggard J, Hansen-Nord M, Haagen C (1999) A review of endocrine changes in anorexia nervosa. J Psych Res 33:139–152
14. Gianotti L, Lanfranco F, Ramunni J et al (2002) GH/IGF-1 axis in anorexia nervosa. Eat Weight Dis 7:94–105
15. Lanfranco F, Gianotti L, Destefanis S et al (2003) Endocrine abnormalities in anorexia nervosa. Minerva Endocrinol 28:169–180
16. Nylen ES, Muller B (2004) Endocrine changes in critical illness. J Intensive Care Med 19:67–82
17. Prigent H, Maxime V, Annane D (2004) Clinical review: corticotherapy in sepsis. Crit Care 8:122–129
18. Reed Larsen P, Davies TF, Hay ID (1998) The thyroid gland. In: Wilson JD, Foster DW, Kronenberg HM, Larsen PR (eds) Williams textbook of endocrinology, 9th ed. WB Saunders, Philadelphia, pp 389–515
19. Haluzik M, Nedvidkova J, Bartak V et al (2003) Effects of hypo- and hyperthyroidism on noradrenergic activity and glycerol concentrations in human subcutaneous abdominal adipose tissue assessed with microdialysis. J Clin Endocrinol Metab 88:5605–5608
20. Cugini P, Paggi A, Cristina G et al (1999) Hunger sensation in Graves' disease before and after pharmacological therapy. Clin Ther 150:115–119
21. Pijl H, de Meijer PH, Langius J et al (2001) Food choice in hyperthyroidism: potential influence of the autonomic nervous system and brain serotonin precursor availability. J Clin Endocrinol Metab 86:5848–5853
22. Trivalle C, Doucet J, Chassagne P et al (1996) Differences in the signs and symptoms of hyperthyroidism in older and younger patients. J Am Geriatr Soc 44:50–53
23. Dalkjaer AL, Hansen TK, Moller N et al (2003) Hyperthyroidism is associated with suppressed circu-

lating ghrelin levels. J Clin Endocrinol Metab 88:853–857

24. Collin P, Kaukinen K, Valimaki M, Salmi J (2002) Endocrinological disorders and celiac disease. End Rev 23:464–483

25. Orth DN, Kovacs WJ (1998) The adrenal cortex. In: Wilson JD, Foster DW, Kronenberg HM, Larsen PR (eds) Williams textbook of endocrinology, 9th ed. WB Saunders, Philadelphia, pp 517–562

26. Young JB, Landsberg L (1998) Catecholamines and the adrenal medulla. In: Wilson JD, Foster DW, Kronenberg HM, Larsen PR (eds) Williams textbook of endocrinology, 9th ed. WB Saunders, Philadelphia, pp 665–728

27. Nieman LK (2003) Dynamic evaluation of adrenal hypofunction. J Endocrinol Invest 26:74–82

28. Saenger P, Levine LS, Irvine WJ et al (1982) Progressive adrenal failure in polyglandular autoimmune disease. J Clin Endocrinol Metab 54:863–868

29. Betterle C, Scalici C, Presotto F et al (1988) The natural history of adrenal function in autoimmune patients with adrenal autoantibodies. J Endocrinol 117:467–475

30. Terzolo M, Reimondo G, Alì A et al (2001) Ectopic ACTH syndrome: molecular bases and clinical heterogeneity. Ann Oncol 12:S83–S87

31. Kaltsas GA, Besser GM, Grossman AB (2004) The diagnosis and medical management of advanced neuroendocrine tumors. End Rev 25:458–511

32. Veglio F, Morello F, Morra Di Cella S et al (2003) Recent advances in diagnosis and treatment of pheochromocytoma. Minerva Med 94:267–271

33. Ross EJ, Griffith DNW (1989) The clinical presentation of pheochromocytoma. Q J Med 71:485–496

34. Garruti G, Ricquier D (1992) Analysis of uncoupling protein and its mRNA in adipose tissue deposits of adult humans. Int J Obes 16:383–390

35. Smith SL, Slappy AL, Fox TP, Scolapio JS (2002) Pheochromocytoma producing vasoactive intestinal peptide. Mayo Clin Proc 77:97–100

36. Thorner MO, Lee Vance M, Laws RE Jr et al (1998) The anterior pituitary. In: Wilson JD, Foster DW, Kronenberg HM, Larsen PR (eds) Williams textbook of endocrinology, 9th ed. WB Saunders, Philadelphia, pp 249–340

37. Tasca C, Filip Z, Dimitriu R, Popescu P (1983) Simmond's disease following chronic sclerosing hypophysitis. Morphol Embryol 29:267–270

38. Mersebach H, Svendsen OL, Holst JJ et al (2003) Comparisons of leptin, incretins and body composition in obese and lean patients with hypopituitarism and healthy individuals. J Clin Endocrinol Metab 58:65–71

39. O'Sullivan AJ, Kelly JJ, Hoffman DM et al (1994) Body composition and energy expenditure in acromegaly. J Clin Endocrinol Metab 78: 81–386

40. Papotti M, Cassoni P, Volante M et al (2001) Ghrelin-producing tumors of the stomach and intestine. J Clin Endocrinol Metab 86:5052–5059

41. Volante M, Allia E, Gugliotta P et al (2002) Expression of ghrelin and of the GH secretagogue receptor by pancreatic islet cells and related endocrine tumors. J Clin Endocrinol Metab 87:1300–1308

42. Chastain MA (2001) The glucagonoma syndrome: a review of its features and discussion of new perspectives. Am J Med Sci 321:306–320

43. Miedlich S, Krohn K, Paschke R (2003) Update on genetic and clinical aspects of primary hyperparathyroidism. Clin Endocrinol 59:539–554

44. Lanicour B, Basile C, Drueke T, Funck-Brentano JL (1982) Parathyroid function and lipid metabolism in the rat. Miner Electrolyte Metab 7:157–165

45. Taniguchi A, Kataoka K, Kono T et al (1987) Parathyroid hormone-induced lipolysis in human adipose tissue. J Lipid Res 28:490–494

46. McCarty MF, Thomas CA (2003) PTH excess may promote weight gain by impeding catecholamine-induced lipolysis-implications for the impact of calcium, vitamin D, and alcohol on body weight. Med Hypotheses 61:535–542

47. Grey AB, Evans MC, Stapleton JP, Reid IR (1994) Body weight and bone mineral density in postmenopausal women with primary hyperparathyroidism. Ann Intern Med 121:745–749

# Psychiatric Diseases and Depression

Adelio Lucca, Enrico Smeraldi

## Introduction

Changes in appetite and weight loss are commonly occurring symptoms in various psychiatric diseases; however, it is clear that a disturbance of appetite is a cardinal feature of depressive disorders. There is a large amount of data available about the epidemiology, phenomenology, associated neurobiological findings, and pharmacological interventions that bear on the links between mood disorders and appetite. The findings may ultimately contribute to our understanding of appetite regulation per se.

Many investigators have considered the possibility that a disturbance in mood is secondary to eating disorders, such as anorexia nervosa, both at presentation and after variable periods of follow-up [1]. This may involve the somatic effects of low weight and it has been claimed that the depressive symptoms are largely secondary to the severe weight loss [2].

Weight loss, a condition of wasting, and even starvation may be found in some forms of psychotic depression or delusional disorders, such as Cotard's syndrome.

Nutritional status is one of the biological risk factors for late life depression [3]. Moreover, an association of depression with malnutrition is common in chronic haemodialysis patients [4] and in those with Alzheimer's disease [5].

It is noteworthy that in all these psychiatric conditions weight loss is not always associated with a reduction in appetite; body weight may be related to a level of neuroticism without showing any relationship to one or several symptoms or to the overall intensity of the disease.

## Depression

Disturbances in appetite are reported by 77–90% of all depressed patients. Among depressed patients with symptoms of appetite disturbance, about four out of five will have a decrease in appetite and one out of five an increase, a relationship that appears to be constant across cultures. In particular, patients with melancholic features are characterised by significant anorexia or weight loss and those with atypical features by significant weight gain or increase in appetite [6]. Several scales that are used to rate depression (e.g. Hamilton depression rating scale, Newcastle scale, Beck depression inventory) contain items related to appetite and weight changes.

The neurochemical and neurophysiological mechanisms that regulate appetite may be closely linked to some forms of depression. Increased serotoninergic activity is generally associated with decreased food intake, whereas norepinephrine reduces satiety. Part of the discrepancy between the role of 5-HT in appetite regulation and the hyposerotonin hypothesis of depression may be due to incomplete knowledge of the complex ways in which 5-HT modulates food intake. One possible explanation is that increased stimulation of the 5-HT1A autoreceptor causes appetite loss during depression by ultimately decreasing serotoninergic neurotransmission.

Item 12 of the Hamilton depression rating scale records appetite disturbances and considers different gastrointestinal symptoms, such as constipation, diarrhoea, or a heavy feeling in the abdomen, as a whole. Nonetheless, simple selection according to this item leads to a subgroup of untreated depressed patients with or without gastrointestinal symptoms. In a recent study [7], the authors compared platelet 5-HT concentration and apparent kinetic parameters of 5-HT uptake in these two subgroups in order to test the hypothesis that platelet serotonergic parameters are affected by certain somatic symptoms of major depression. The results could provide important information, because 5-HT in the gut seems to be a mucosal transmitter that stimulates sensory nerves and initiates peristaltic and secretory reflexes [8]. Based on findings that 5HT knock-out mice (lack of serotonin transporter) show an increase in intestinal motility (diarrhoea) along with episodes of decreased motility (constipation) [9], the same authors suggested that the low apparent $V_{max}$ of platelet 5-HT uptake reflects low expression of the 5-HT transporter not only in platelets, but also in the gut mucosa and enteric serotoninergic neurons, which probably increase the risk of typical gastrointestinal symptoms, such as appetite loss and nausea, occurring in some depressed patients.

The evidence that depression is frequently associated with poor oral intake involves both central and peripheral mechanisms. The increased feelings of satiety appears to arise from signals in the stomach, but is also related to changes in the central feeding drive, in particular a decrease in the opioid rewarding properties for fatty food [10]. Clinical and experimental studies on animals indicate that depression is associated with increased plasma cytokine acute-phase protein concentration and hypothalamic-pituitary-adrenal axis (HPA) activation [11]. Increased cytokines may further exacerbate the anorexia seen in late-life depression, especially in patients on long-term haemodialysis, in whom depression, strictly related to nutritional status, is the most common psychological complication and could be an independent mortality risk factor [4].

It is often difficult to determine whether certain symptoms (e.g. weight loss, insomnia, fatigue) represent a mood disturbance or are a direct manifestation of a general medical condition (e.g. cancer, stroke, myocardial infarction, diabetes). A variety of general medical conditions may cause mood symptoms. These conditions include degenerative neurological illnesses (e.g. Parkinson and Huntington diseases), stroke, metabolic conditions (e.g. vitamin B12 deficiency), endocrine conditions (e.g. hyper- and hypothyroidism, hyper- and hypoadrenocorticism), autoimmune conditions (e.g. systemic lupus erythematosus), viral or other infections (e.g. hepatitis, mononucleosis, human immunodeficiency virus), and certain cancers (e.g. carcinoma of the pancreas). The associated physical examination findings, laboratory findings, and pattern of prevalence or onset reflect the aetiological general medical condition, the management of which is more complex and the prognosis less favourable if major depressive disorder is present.

## Alzheimer's Disease

Weight loss is common in elderly people with dementia, particularly those with Alzheimer's disease (AD), and feeding difficulties are major issues in their care in the later stages of the disease. The aetiology is still uncertain and appears multifactorial. Hypotheses to explain the weight loss have been suggested (e.g. atrophy of the mesial temporal cortex, biological disturbances, and higher energy expenditure), but none has been proven. More than half of the AD patients of one recent study [5] developed body-weight loss; overall, the AD patients were significantly thinner than non-demented subjects. Anthropometric and laboratory measures suggested a poorer nutritional status and fewer daily physical activities in AD patients. While most of them had poor appetite, their daily calorie intake was not significantly different from that of the control group. In fact, patients with body weight loss consumed more calories per body weight kilogram per day. In the food composition analysis, AD patients consumed more carbohydrates than controls. The authors concluded that the pathophysiological process in AD gives rise to changes of appetite and metabolic state in AD patients, and that these changes contribute to weight loss.

In another longitudinal study [12], the authors studied the changes in nutritional variables in a cohort of patients with a probable diagnosis of

AD. All subjects were submitted to nutritional, neuropsychological, and functional evaluation. The results showed that only the interview and the checklist that explored caregiver burden predicted weight loss in AD patients, suggesting the possibility that caregivers who consider themselves overburdened by the disease process are not willing to invest adequate resources to allow AD patients to properly nourish themselves.

Clinical observation, among AD patients, of periods of weight gain, periods of acute weight loss, and greater fluctuations in weight suggest that the natural history of weight change in AD may be characterised by dysfunction in body weight regulation. However, it remains a fundamental concept that a nutritional education program for caregivers of AD patients is the best way to prevent weight loss and improve the nutritional status of these patients.

## Cotard's Syndrome

This clinical condition was first described by Jules Cotard, in 1880, as a type of severe and agitated melancholia, in which the prevailing symptom is *delire de negation* (nihilistic delusion). In its complete form, this symptom leads the patient to deny his own existence and that of the external world. Cotard described various degrees of severity from mild states characterised by feelings of despair and self-loathing, to severe forms of the disorder in which the sufferer experiences a feeling of change both inside and outside himself, to the most severe type of all in which denial of the very existence of oneself occurs. Simultaneously, ideas of subjective negation may lead the patient to deny the existence of parts of his body or their functions.

Cotard's syndrome may be seen as a separate clinical entity but it may occur in a variety of mental illnesses, especially depressive disorders. In an analysis of 100 patients with Cotard's syndrome, depression was present in 89% of subjects [13]; the most common nihilistic delusions concerned the body (86%) and existence (69%). Anxiety (65%) and guilt (63%) were also common, followed by hypochondriacal delusion (58%)

and delusion of immortality (55%). Other psychiatric symptoms associated with nihilistic delusion are: paranoia, guilt, fear of demonic possession, auditory hallucinations, delusion of omnipotence, and suicidal complex. Somatisation includes: hyperkinesias, muscular rigidity, and alternating retention of urine and faeces and incontinence. Some patients with Cotard's syndrome reportedly refused to eat or drink, claiming that their muscles and nerves were not cooperating. These patients improved dramatically after electroshock therapy, which may be one of the best treatments for the depressive type of Cotard's syndrome.

## Anorexia Nervosa

Anorexia nervosa (AN) is characterised by a deliberate reduction of food intake in order to achieve an 'ideal' body weight and due to constant fear of getting fat. People affected by this disorder are constantly concerned with their body weight; they try to reduce their body size and do not consider their weight loss as abnormal. AN patients have an altered way of experiencing their own body; they 'feel they are fat,' even though they are underweight, and believe that some parts of their body are 'too fat,' even if they are objectively underweight. Table 1 lists the main criteria for the diagnosis of AN.

**Table 1.** Diagnostic criteria for anorexia nervosa (DSM-IV)

A. Refusal to maintain body weight at or above a minimally normal weight for age and height (e.g. weight loss leading to maintenance of body weight less than 85% of that expected, or failure to make expected weight gain during a period of growth, leading to body weight less than 85% of that expected)

B. Intense fear of gaining weight or becoming fat, even though underweight

C. Disturbance in the way in which one's body weight or shape is experienced, undue influence of body weight or shape on self-evaluation, or denial of the seriousness of the current low body weight

D. In postmenarcheal females, amenorrhoea, i.e., the absence of at least three consecutive menstrual cycles. (A woman is considered to have amenorrhoea if her periods occur only following hormone, e.g. oestrogen, administration)

In the restricting type of AN, the affected person has not regularly engaged in binge eating or purging behaviour during his or her active episode of the disease (i.e. self-induced vomiting or the misuse of laxatives, diuretics, or enemas). By contrast, in the binge-eating/purging type of AN, the affected person has regularly engaged in binge eating or purging behaviour (i.e. self-induced vomiting or the misuse of laxatives, diuretics, or enemas).

Prevalence studies among females in late adolescence and early adulthood (between age 13 and 18) have found rates of 0.5–1%; more than 95% of cases occur in females.

The course and outcome are highly variable. Some individuals recover fully after a single episode, some exhibit a fluctuating pattern of weight gain followed by relapse, others experience a chronically deteriorating course of illness over many years.

The most obvious finding on physical examination is emaciation, hypotension, hypothermia, and dryness of skin.

Hospitalisation may be required to restore weight and to address fluid and electrolyte imbalances. The most serious and frequently documented is potassium loss, due to self-induced vomiting and diuretic or laxative abuse. Hypokalaemia can result in cardiac symptoms, specifically, arrhythmias and EKG abnormalities. Low serum magnesium levels are also common and correlate with muscular weakness, diminished concentration, muscular cramping, paraesthesias, arrhythmias, and recent memory loss.

Amenorrhoea is a classic feature of AN and is considered to be not only a result of caloric restriction and weight loss, but also a dysfunction of the hypothalamic-pituitary-gonadal (HPG) system. Sustained elevations of cortisol levels and subnormal triiodothyronine (T3) have been documented in AN patients in multiple studies. For a more extensive discussion, see the review by Lyn [15].

AN has the highest mortality of any psychiatric diagnosis, estimated at 10% and occurring within 10 years of diagnosis. It is the leading cause of death in young females 15–24 years of age. Death is most often due to suicide, infection, or the effects of chronic starvation or electrolyte imbalance.

## References

1. Ivarsson T, Rastam M, Wentz E et al (2000) Depressive disorders in teenage-onset anorexia nervosa: a controlled longitudinal, partly-community-based study. Compr Psychiatry 41:398–403
2. Cooper Z (1995) The development and maintenance of eating disorders. In: Brownell KD, Fairburn CG (ed) Eating disorders and obesity. The Guilford Press, New York, pp 199–206
3. Tiemeier H (2003) Biological risk factors for late life depression. Eur J Epidemiol 18:745–750
4. Koo JR, Yoon JW, Kim SG et al (2003) Association of depression with malnutrition in chronic hemodialysis patient. Am J Kidney Dis 41:1037–1042
5. Wang PN, Yang CL, Lin KN et al (2004) Weight loss, nutritional status and physical activity in patients with Alzheimer's Disease: a controlled study. J Neurol 251:314–320
6. Anonymous (1994) American Psychiatric Association. Diagnostic and statistical manual of mental disorders, DSM-IV. American Psychiatric Association, Washington DC
7. Franke L, Schewe HJ, Uebelhack R et al (2003) Platelet-5HT uptake and gastrointestinal symptoms in patients suffering from major depression. Life Sci 74:521–531
8. Gershon MD (1999) Review article: roles played by 5-hydroxytryptamine in the physiology of the bowel. Aliment Pharmacol Ther 13(Suppl 2):15–30
9. Chen JJ, Li Z, Pan H et al (2001) Maintenance of serotonin in the intestinal mucosa and ganglia of mice that lack the high-affinity serotonin transporter: abnormal intestinal motility and the expression of cation transporters. J Neurosci 15:6348–6361
10. Morley JE, Miller DK, Perry HM 3rd et al (1999) Anorexia of aging, leptin, and the Mini Nutritional Assessment. Nestle Nutr Workshop Ser Clin Perform Programme 1:67–76
11. Dubas-Slemp H, Marmurowska-Michalowska H, Szuster-Ciesielska A et al (2003) The role of cytokines in depression. Psychiatr Pol 37:787–798
12. Gillette-Guyonnet S, Nourhashemi F, Andrieu S et al (2000) Weight loss in Alzheimer disease. Am J Clin Nutr 71:637S–642S
13. Berrios GE, Luque R (1995) Cotard's syndrome: analysis of 100 cases. Acta Psychiatr Scand 91:185–188
14. Anonymous (1993) World Health Organization. ICD-10 classification of mental and behavioural disorders: diagnostic criteria for research. Geneva, Switzerland
15. Lyn P (2002) Eating disorders: a review of the literature with emphasis on medical complications and clinical nutrition. Altern Med Rev 7:184–202

# Cachexia in Chronic Kidney Disease: Malnutrition-Inflammation Complex and Reverse Epidemiology

Kamyar Kalantar-Zadeh, Joel D. Kopple

## Introduction

Chronic kidney disease (CKD) is an irreversible and progressive disease state leading to renal dysfunction and related morbidity [1]. According to the National Kidney Foundation (NKF) Kidney Disease Outcome Quality Initiative (K/DOQI) guidelines, CKD is defined as a chronic disease state in that irreversible, structural, or functional abnormalities of the kidney, with or without a decreased glomerular filtration rate (GFR), are present for at least three consecutive months [1]. The degree of renal insufficiency, based on the magnitude of the estimated GFR for 1.73 m² body surface, is used to classify the CKD into five stages: (1) GFR > 90 ml/min, (2) GFR 60–89 ml/min, (3) GFR 30–59 ml/min, (4) GFR 15–29 ml/min, and (5) GFR < 15 ml/min [1]. If they survive long enough, CKD patients eventually reach stage 5 CKD, also known as end-stage renal disease (ESRD), in which life prolongation is exclusively dependent upon renal replacement therapy, i.e. maintenance haemodialysis or peritoneal dialysis treatment and/or kidney transplantation. However, the majority of CKD patients die before reaching ESRD [2].

Epidemiological data indicate that there are currently at least 20 million individuals with CKD in the US [3], including over 300 000 ESRD patients who undergo maintenance dialysis. Diabetes mellitus accounts for half of all cases of ESRD in industrialised nations [4]. According to the estimates of the US Renal Data System (USRDS), the number of ESRD patients will surpass one-half million by 2010 and will be between 1.5 and 3.1 million by 2030, whereas the US population will grow only from 280 to 350 million over the same 30-year period [4]. This exponential growth has major public health implications, especially since ESRD patients consume a disproportionately large component of the US Medicare budget, due to their requirement for continuous renal replacement therapy and their frequent morbidity [5, 6]. Despite many years of efforts and improvement in dialysis technique and patient care, the mortality rate in maintenance dialysis patients in the US and most industrialized countries continues to be unacceptably high, currently still approximately 20% per year in the US and 10–15% in Europe and Japan [7–9]. CKD and ESRD patients also commonly have a high hospitalisation rate and a low self-reported quality of life [10–13]. Cardiovascular, cerebral-vascular, and peripheral vascular diseases comprise the bulk of the severe morbidity and mortality in CKD patients [14, 15]. Indeed even a slight increase in serum creatinine (an often clinically used marker of renal insufficiency) has been shown to be an independent risk factor for cardiovascular disease and atherosclerosis in the general population [16–18].

Among potential candidates to explain the high rate of morbidity and mortality and cardiovascular disease in CKD patients, wasting syndrome and cachexia continue to top the list. Epidemiological studies have repeatedly and consistently shown a strong association between clinical outcome and measures of both protein-energy malnutrition [19–22] and inflammation in CKD patients [23, 24]. Hypoalbuminaemia, rather than such conventional risk factors as hypertension and hypercholesterolaemia, is one of the strongest risk factors for mortality among dialysis patients (Fig. 1). Almost half of all dialysis patients have a serum albumin < 3.8 g/dl, which has been shown to be associated with at least a two-fold increase in mortality [25]. However, it is not known whether hypoalbuminaemia is a reflection of malnutrition, inflammation, or both. Many

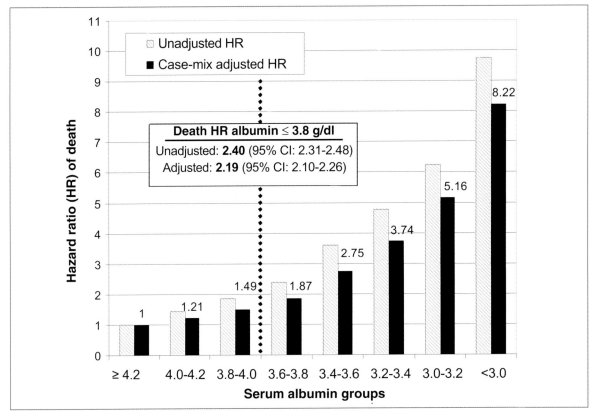

**Fig. 1.** Association between serum albumin concentration and all-cause mortality in a 2-year cohort of 56 920 mainte-nance haemodialysis patients [25]. After dichotomising albumin values based on the cutoff level of 3.8 g/dl, the unadjust-ed and case-mix adjusted HR for serum albumin ≤ 3.8 g/dl was 2.40 (95% CI: 2.31–2.48) and 2.19 (95% CI: 2.10–2.26), respectively [25]

investigators have observed that these two condi-tions tend to occur concurrently and coexist in individuals with CKD, and many factors that engender one of these conditions also lead to the other [22, 23, 26, 27]. Therefore the term 'malnu-trition-inflammation complex (or cachexia) syn-drome' (MICS) [22, 28] or 'malnutrition-inflam-mation-atherosclerosis' (MIA) syndrome [29] has been proposed to indicate the combination of these two conditions in such patients and their associations with atherosclerotic cardiovascular disease and poor outcome (see below).

## Chronic Inflammation as a Cause of Cachexia in CKD Patients

Inflammation is defined as a localised adaptive response elicited by injury or destruction of tis-sues that serves to destroy, dilute, or sequester

both the injurious agent and the injured tissue [30, 31]. The acute-phase response (or reaction) is a major pathophysiological phenomenon that accompanies inflammation and is associated with increased activity of pro-inflammatory cytokines [32]. With this reaction, normal homeostatic mechanisms are replaced by new set points that presumably contribute to defensive or adaptive capabilities [33]. Hence, inflammation is a physio-logical response, and as an acute response to infections, trauma, or toxic injury, it helps the body to defend against pathophysiological insults [34, 35]. Inflammation can become more subtle and less organ-specific and may involve many body organs or the entire organism. If inflamma-tion becomes prolonged in the form of the chron-ic acute-phase reaction, it may lead to adverse consequences, such as a chronic decline in appetite, increased rate of protein depletion in skeletal muscle and other tissues, muscle and fat wasting, hypercatabolism, endothelial dysfunction, and atherosclerosis [35]. Inflammatory processes are common in CKD patients. Approximately 30–60% of North American [36, 37] and European [24, 38] maintenance dialysis patients have increased inflammatory markers, whereas long-term dialysis patients in Asian countries have a lower prevalence of inflammation [39, 40].

A recent study of 331 maintenance haemodialysis patients showed a strong association between anorexia and high levels of pro-inflammatory cytokines [41]. In this study, an appetite questionnaire was used, and the subjectively reported appetite was scored from 1 to 4, corresponding to normal to poor appetite. Inflammatory markers including serum concentrations of high-sensitivity C-reactive protein (hs-CRP), tumour necrosis factor (TNF)-$\alpha$ and interleukin-(IL)-6 were measured. Markers of inflammation were progressively higher in association with declining grades of appetite. There were statistically significant negative correlations between appetite score and serum CRP and TNF-$\alpha$, and these correlations remained

significant after case-mix multivariate adjustment for age, sex, race, and diabetes. After dichotomising the appetite score, the odds ratio (OR) of anorexia, controlled for case mix and other pertinent covariates, for each 10 pg increase in serum TNF-$\alpha$/ml was 1.75 (confidence interval [CI] 1.12–2.74, $p = 0.01$) and for each 10 mg increase in hs-CRP/l the OR was 2.31 (CI: 1.47–3.62, $p < 0.001$) [41]. Hence, inflammation is strongly associated with anorexia in dialysis patients.

In recent years, more attention has been focused on inflammatory processes as the possible cause of accelerated atherosclerosis as well as protein-energy malnutrition and concurrent wasting syndrome, all of which lead to a poor outcome in those with underlying kidney disease. As mentioned above, chronic renal insufficiency per se is now considered as an independent risk factor for cardiovascular diseases [16, 18, 42]. It is believed that inflammation may play an important role in the increased prevalence of cardiovascular disease and mortality associated with renal insufficiency [23, 24, 27, 28, 43]. Renal failure may lead to increased inflammatory responses through a

**Table 1.** Possible causes of chronic inflammation and wasting syndrome in chronic kidney disease (*CKD*) patients

---

A. Causes of inflammation due to CKD or decreased GFR
  1. Decreased clearance of pro-inflammatory cytokines
  2. Volume overload[a]
  3. Oxidative stress (e.g. oxygen radicals)[a]
  4. Carbonyl stress (e.g. pentosidine and advanced glycation end-products)
  5. Decreased levels of antioxidants (e.g. vitamin E, vitamin C, carotenoids, selenium, glutathione)[a]
  6. Deteriorating protein-energy nutritional state and food intake[a]
B. Coexistence of comorbid conditions
  1. Inflammatory diseases with kidney involvement (SLE, HIV, etc.)
  2. Increased prevalence of comorbid conditions[a]
C. Additional inflammatory factors related to dialysis treatment
  1. Haemodialysis
    a. Exposure to dialysis tubing
    b. Dialysis membranes with decreased biocompatiblility (e.g. cuprophane)
    c. Impurities in dialysis water and/or dialysate
    d. Back-filtration or back-diffusion of contaminants
    e. Foreign bodies (such as PTFE) in dialysis access grafts
    f. Intravenous catheter
  D. Peritoneal dialysis
    1. Episodes of overt or latent peritonitis[a]
    2. PD-catheter as a foreign body and its related infections
    3. Constant exposure to PD solution

---

[a]These factors may also be associated with protein-energy malnutrition. *GFR*, glomerular filtration rate; *SLE*, systemic lupus erythematosus; *HIV*, human immune deficiency virus; *PTFE*, polytetrafluoroethylene; *PD*, peritoneal dialysis

number of mechanisms that are listed in Table 1 and reviewed comprehensively elsewhere [44–47]. As indicated in Table 1, some of these factors may also result in protein-energy malnutrition and cachexia and consequently cause an overlap between malnutrition and inflammation. Comorbid conditions may contribute considerably to the development and maintenance of inflammation in dialysis patients. Due to the very high prevalence of comorbid conditions in these individuals, it is difficult at present to ascertain the role of inflammation in the absence of pre-existing comorbidity.

There is no uniform approach for assessing the degree of severity of inflammation in individuals with kidney disease [48]. Positive acute-phase reactants, such as serum CRP or ferritin, are markers whose levels are elevated during an acute episode of inflammation. The serum levels of negative acute-phase reactants, such as albumin or transferrin, decrease during an inflammatory process [34, 35, 44, 47]. Many negative acute-phase reactants are also traditionally known as nutritional markers, since their serum levels also decrease when there is a decline in nutritional status. Hence, it is not clear whether these markers have any specificity in the detection of either of these two conditions. Among pro-inflammatory cytokines, IL-6 is reported to have a central role in the pathophysiology of the adverse effects of inflammation in patients with renal disease [49–51]. These pro-inflammatory cytokines also may be engendered during oxidative stress, which per se can happen in the setting of protein-energy malnutrition [52].

## Protein-Energy Malnutrition and Cachexia in CKD

Protein-energy malnutrition in CKD patients is a state of decreased body pools of protein with or without fat depletion, or a state of diminished functional capacity. It is caused at least partly by inadequate nutrient intake relative to nutrient demand and is improved by nutritional repletion [31]. Hence, protein-energy malnutrition is engendered when the body's need for protein or

energy fuels or both cannot be satisfied by the individual's nutrient intake diet [53]. Protein-energy malnutrition is a common phenomenon in CKD patients and intensifies progressively as CKD stages advance over time (Fig. 2) [54, 55]. Protein-energy malnutrition is a risk factor for poor quality of life and increased morbidity and mortality, including cardiovascular death, in these individuals [56, 57]. Various studies with different criteria have been used to establish the presence of protein-energy malnutrition in the CKD population, which has been studied more thoroughly in maintenance dialysis patients than among other CKD groups. Its reported prevalence varies between 18 and 75% among these individuals according to the type of dialysis modality, nutritional assessment tools, and origin of patient population [22, 58, 59]. Although protein-energy malnutrition per se neither requires nor precludes micronutrient malnutrition, many malnourished dialysis patients may also have a deficiency of various vitamins or trace elements [60, 61].

The aetiology of protein-energy malnutrition in CKD patients is probably multifaceted. Some probable causes are listed in Table 2 and have been reviewed in detail elsewhere [62–66]. As it is evident from Table 2, some of these factors can also lead to inflammation. Hence, the known overlap between malnutrition and inflammation in CKD patients may have its root at the aetiological level. The origin of protein-energy malnutrition generally precedes the need for dialysis treatment, and it is engendered progressively as the GFR falls below 60 ml/min, i.e. CKD stage 3 and above [55, 67]. Hypoalbuminaemia and hypocholesterolaemia have been shown to develop along with the progression of CKD stages, as shown in the Modification of Diet in Renal Disease (MDRD) Study [55] (Fig. 2) and other studies [67].

## Assessment of MICS

Classically, three major lines of inquiry, i.e. dietary intake, biochemical measures, and body composition, are used to assess the protein-energy nutritional status; a fourth category of nutritional assessment, composite indices that include a com-

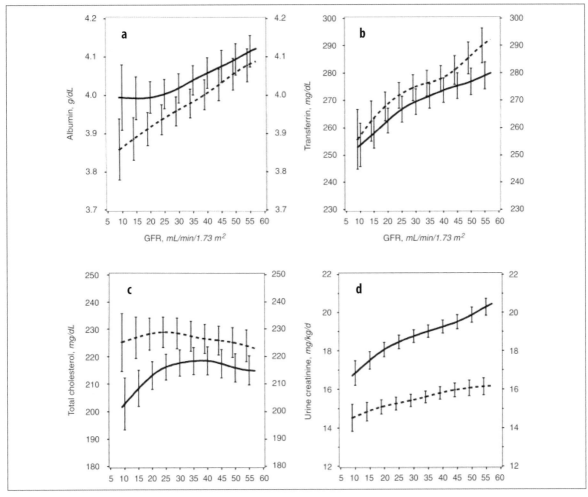

**Fig. 2.** Mean levels of biochemical measures of nutritional status as a function of glomerular filtration rate (GFR) in MDRD Study. The estimated mean levels with 95% confidence limits of biochemical nutritional markers are shown as a function of GFR (males *solid line*, females *dashed line*) controlling for age, race, and use of protein and energy restricted diets. In men, the slope of the relationship was greater at GFR = 12 than GFR = 55 ml/min/1.73 m$^2$ for serum total cholesterol ($p = 0.014$). **a** Males, $N = 1065$ ($p = 0.004$); females, $N = 698$ ($p < 0.001$). **b** Males, $N = 1065$ ($p < 0.001$); females, $N = 698$ ($p < 0.001$). **c** Males, $N = 1063$ ($p = 0.052$); females, $N = 694$ ($p = 0.63$). **d** Males, $N = 1017$ ($p < 0.001$); females, $N = 664$ ($p < 0.001$). (Modified from [54, 55])

bination of assessment measures within these categories, are also utilised, especially the Subjective Global Assessment of Nutrition (SGA) [68, 69] and Malnutrition-Inflammation Score (MIS) [28, 70]. The four categories of nutritional assessment tools are described in Table 3 and have been reviewed in detail elsewhere [22, 71]. As indicated in Table 3, many of these nutritional assessment tools are also designed to detect a combination of protein-energy malnutrition and inflammation and to grade their severity. Hence, the overlap between malnutrition and inflammation also

exists at the diagnostic level, in addition to their overlapping aetiologies.

No uniform approach has been agreed upon for rating the overall severity of protein-energy malnutrition. Among all four categories, dietary assessment is probably the most nutrition-specific entity. Another, rather nutrition-focused measure is the normalised protein equivalent of total nitrogen appearance (nPNA), also known as protein catabolic rate (nPCR); a low nPNA is associated with increased hospitalisation and mortality in haemodialysis patients even when the dose of

**Table 2.** Conditions related to protein-energy malnutrition as a cause of wasting syndrome in CKD patients

A. Inadequate nutrient intake
   1. Anorexia[a]
     a. Due to uraemic toxicity
     b. Due to impaired gastric emptying
     c. Due to inflammation with or without comorbid conditions[a]
     d. Due to emotional and/or psychological disorders
   2. Dietary restrictions
     a. Prescribed restrictions: low-potassium, low-phosphate regimens
     b. Social constraints: poverty, inadequate dietary support
     c. Physical incapacity: inability to acquire or prepare food or to eat
B. Nutrient losses during dialysis
   1. Loss through haemodialysis membrane into haemodialysate
   2. Adherence to haemodialysis membrane or tubing
   3. Loss into peritoneal dialysate
C. Hypercatabolism due to comorbid illnesses
   1. Cardiovascular diseases[a]
   2. Diabetic complications
   3. Infection and/or sepsis[a]
   4. Other comorbid conditions[a]
D. Hypercatabolism associated with dialysis treatment
   1. Negative protein balance
   2. Negative energy balance
E. Endocrine disorders of uraemia
   1. Resistance to insulin
   2. Resistance to growth hormone and/or IGF-1
   3. Increased serum level of or sensitivity to glucagons
   4. Hyperparathyroidism
   5. Other endocrine disorders
F. Acidaemia with metabolic acidosis
G. Concurrent nutrient loss with frequent blood losses

[a]These factors may also be associated with inflammation; *IGF-1,* insulin-like growth factor 1

dialysis is standard or high ($K_t/V_{sp} > 1.20$) [20]. Although, as discussed above, it has been argued that appetite can be suppressed by inflammation and particularly by two pro-inflammatory cytokines, IL-6 and TNF-$\alpha$ [41, 72], the reduced nutritional state is still expected to induce malnutrition and its consequences regardless of the cause of anorexia.

Some more frequently studied indicators of malnutrition in dialysis patients that are associated with clinical outcome include decreased dietary protein and energy intake [20, 60]; reduced weight-for-height [57], body mass index (BMI) [73–75] and total body fat percentage [76, 77]; decreased total body nitrogen [78, 79] and total body potassium [80]; reduced mid-arm muscle mass and skinfold thicknesses [81]; low serum concentrations of albumin [82], prealbumin (transthyretin) [83, 84], transferrin (TIBC) [68, 85], cholesterol [86, 87], and creatinine [88]; and a more abnormal score by such nutritional assessment tools as the SGA [89, 90] and MIS [28]. Although the foregoing measures of nutritional status have practical value, it should be recognised that each of these methods has its limitations. For example, serum albumin, transferrin, and prealbumin are negative acute-phase reactants and may reflect inflammation [46, 68, 91]. The SGA may also be a marker of the degree of sickness and comorbidity in maintenance dialysis patients [68]. During acute catabolic states and hypercatabolism, the urea nitrogen appearance may transiently increase independently of food intake [92]. More elaborate nutritional measures that have

**Table 3.** Assessment tools for the evaluation of protein-energy malnutrition in CKD patients. (Data from [22, 71])

A. Nutritional intake
      1. Direct: diet recalls and diaries, food frequency questionnaires
      2. Indirect: based on urea nitrogen appearance: nPNA (nPCR)
B. Body composition
      1. Weight based measures: BMI, weight-for-height, oedema-free/fat-free weight
      2. Skin and muscle anthropometry via caliper: skinfolds, extremity muscle mass
      3. Total body elements: total body potassium
      4. Energy-beam based methods: DEXA, BIA, NIR
      5. Other energy-beam related methods: total body nitrogen
      6. Other methods: underwater weighing
C. Laboratory values
      1. Visceral proteins (negative acute-phase reactants): albumin, prealbumin, transferrin[a]
      2. Lipids: cholesterol, triglycerides, other lipids, and lipoproteins[a]
      3. Somatic proteins and nitrogen surrogates: creatinine, SUN
      4. Growth factors: IGF-1, leptin
      5. Peripheral blood cell count: lymphocyte count
D. Scoring systems
      1. Conventional SGA and its modifications (e.g. DMS, MIS, and CANUSA)[a]
      2. Other scores: HD-PNI, others (e.g. Wolfson, Merkus, Merckman)[a]

[a]These tools may also detect inflammation

*nPNA*, Normalised protein nitrogen appearance; *nPCR*, normalised protein catabolic rate; *BMI*, body mass index; *DEXA*, dual energy X-ray absorptiometry; *BIA*, bioelectrical impedance analysis; *NIR*, near infra-red interactance; *SGA*, subjective global assessment of nutritional status; *DMS*, dialysis malnutrition score; *MIS*, malnutrition inflammation score; *CANUSA*, Canada-USA study based modification of the SGA; *HD-PNI*, haemodialysis prognostic nutritional index; *SUN*, serum urea nitrogen; *IGF-1*, insuline-like growth factor 1

been used in dialysis and CKD patients include dual energy X-ray absorptiometry (DEXA) [93, 94], total body nitrogen or potassium measurements [79, 80, 95], underwater weighing [96], bioelectrical impedance analysis (BIA) [94], and near infra-red interactance (NIR) [76, 97].

# Malnutrition-Inflammation Complex Syndrome

The foregoing discussion, which is summarised in Tables 1–3, indicates that there is a major overlap among both possible aetiologic factors and the assessment tools for protein-energy malnutrition and inflammation in CKD patients. The link between protein-energy malnutrition and inflammation in CKD population may be an explanation for malnutrition-associated mortality [22, 23, 91]. Indeed, several investigators suggest that protein-energy malnutrition and subsequent wasting syndrome and cachexia are a consequence of chronic inflammatory processes in patients with renal insufficiency [26, 98–100]. Thus, chronic inflammation may be the missing link that causally ties protein-energy malnutrition to morbidity and mortality in these individuals. The following arguments have been proposed to indicate that the development of protein-energy malnutrition is secondary to inflammation: (1) Pro-inflammatory cytokines such as TNF-$\alpha$ not only promote catabolic processes, engendering both protein degradation and suppression of protein synthesis, but also induce anorexia [101–103]. Low appetite has been shown to be associated with increased inflammatory markers in haemodialysis patients [41, 72]. (2) Dialysis patients with signs of inflammation are reported to develop weight loss and a negative protein balance even with an intact appetite, since there may be a shift in protein synthesis from muscle to acute-phase proteins as renal function declines [100]. (3) In both CKD and ESRD patients, albumin synthesis is suppressed when serum CRP is elevated [91, 104]. (4) Inflammation may also lead to hypocholesterolaemia, a strong mortality risk factor in ESRD patients and also a marker of poor nutritional status [49].

The following counter-arguments have questioned the role of inflammation as a primary cause of protein-energy malnutrition: (1) In several studies, serum albumin and other indicators of protein-energy nutritional status correlate with indicators of protein intake independently of inflammatory status [104–106]. (2) In dialysis patients, the association of serum albumin and CRP is not precise, and the reported correlation coefficients are usually less than 0.50; hence, other factor(s) possibly unrelated to inflammation must affect albumin [104, 105]. (3) Serum albumin concentrations usually do not fluctuate on a month-to-month basis, whereas serum CRP and other inflammatory markers do [107]. (4) In some but not all controlled trials involving patients with acute or chronic illnesses, the provision of nutritional support without management of inflammation improves hypoalbuminaemia and clinical outcome [108–111]. (5) Malnourished CKD patients may be deficient in antioxidants, such as vitamin C or carotenoids, which may lead to increased oxidative stress and thus to inflammation [60]. A study using food frequency questionnaires to compare food intake of dialysis patients with that of normal individuals detected such dietary inadequacies, which could be attributed to nutritional restrictions such as low-potassium, low-phosphorus diets [60]. Studies in malnourished children have shown that protein-energy malnutrition may lead to oxidative stress, which can lead to increased activity of pro-inflammatory cytokines [52]. Moreover, in dialysis patients a reverse association has been reported between serum vitamin C (ascorbate) and serum CRP levels [112]. (6) There is evidence that certain nutrients, such as arginine and glutamine, enhance the immune response [113]. Moreover, preliminary data suggest that levocarnitine protects against endotoxins and also suppresses elaboration of TNF-α from monocytes [114]. Thus, protein-energy malnutrition may decrease host resistance and predispose to latent or overt infection, which is an inflammatory disorder. In summary, given the fact that mortality is still very high in dialysis patients

(approximately 10–20% per year in Westernised countries), inflammation, independent of clinically evident comorbid conditions or malnutrition, cannot fully explain this extremely poor clinical outcome, especially since in otherwise healthy individuals inflammation has been found to be associated with an annual mortality rate that is only at 2–3% [115].

The foregoing considerations indicate that there is a lack of conclusive consensus with regard to the nature and direction of the association between protein-energy malnutrition and inflammation in renal cachexia. Hypoalbuminaemia, a strong and reliable predictor of cardiovascular disease and mortality in patients with renal insufficiency, is probably caused by both inflammation and protein-energy malnutrition, and it is not clear which one of these two conditions has a larger influence on serum albumin concentration [22, 104, 116].

## Consequences of the Wasting Syndrome in CKD

The renal wasting syndrome, be it due to inflammation, malnutrition, or both as MICS, has been found to be associated with cardiovascular diseases and atherosclerosis in the CKD population, overwhelming and even *reversing* the effect of traditional cardiovascular risk factors especially in maintenance dialysis patients (Table 4) [117]. MICS is associated with adverse relevant clinical consequences, including refractory anaemia, increased rate of atherosclerotic cardiovascular disease, and poor outcome, including low quality of life and increased hospitalisation and mortality, and may be the cause of reverse epidemiology in patients with renal failure (Fig. 3).

### Refractory Anaemia

Elements of MICS and subsequent cachexia may blunt the responsiveness of anaemia to recombinant human erythropoietin (EPO) in CKD patients. Refractory anaemia appears to be more common in those dialysis patients who suffer from protein-energy malnutrition and/or inflammation [68, 118, 119]. Several previous studies

**Table 4.** Reverse epidemiology of cardiovascular (*CV*) risk factors in dialysis patients: the effect of CV risk factors in maintenance dialysis patients is the opposite of the general population. (Data from [123])

| Risk factors of cardio-vascular disease | Direction of the associations between risk factors and outcomes | |
|---|---|---|
| | General population | Maintenance dialysis patients |
| BMI | High BMI and obesity are generally deleterious. | High BMI, or weight for height, and moderate obesity are protective. Underweight is deleterious |
| Serum cholesterol | Hypercholesterolemia, high LDL and low HDL are deleterious. | Hypercholesterolaemia (and maybe high LDL) is protective. Low serum cholesterol is deleterious |
| BP | Hypertension and even borderline high BP are deleterious. | Pre-dialysis low BP may indicate a deleterious state |
| Serum creatinine | A mild to moderate increase in serum creatinine is an independent risk factor of CVD. | An increased pre-dialysis serum creatinine level is associated with a better survival |
| Total plasma homocysteine | A high level is a risk factor for increased CVD in the general population and likely in dialysis patients | Several recent studies have found that a low level is associated with increased risk of cardiovascular disease and mortality |
| Serum iron | A high serum iron level is associated with haemochromatosis and poor outcome. | A low iron and transferrin saturation level has been recently found to be associated with higher mortality and hospitalisation in dialysis patients |
| AGEs | Patients with higher AGE levels, such as diabetic patients, have a poor outcome. | A recent report indicates a paradoxically reverse association between lower AGE levels and higher mortality in dialysis patients |
| Energy (calorie) and/or protein intake | A high energy and food intake may be associated with risk of obesity and increased mortality. | Increased protein intake is associated with better survival |

*CVD*, cardiovascular disease; *MD*, maintenance dialysis; *LDL*, low-density lipoprotein; *HDL*, high-density lipoprotein; *BMI*, body mass index; *BP*, blood pressure; *AGEs*, advanced glycation end-products

report an association between anaemia and inflammation, such as occurs in dialysis patients, which is reflected by a high serum concentration of CRP [118, 120] or of pro-inflammatory cytokines such as IL-6 and TNF-$\alpha$ [121, 122]. We recently reported that serum IL-6 levels had the strongest correlation with administered EPO dose in 339 haemodialysis patients, and that the association remained statistically significant in different statistical analyses and after multivariate adjustments [124]. Both serum CRP and TNF-$\alpha$ showed similar trends and their associations with EPO dose remained significant in some but not all analysis modalities conducted in that study [124].

An inverse association was reported between markers of nutritional status or inflammation, e.g. serum prealbumin, TIBC, and total cholesterol concentration, and blood lymphocyte count, and the EPO dose [124]. Such associations are less well-described than the association between EPO dose and inflammation. Improving nutritional status in CKD patients may improve anaemia and lead to a lower required EPO dose. A cross-sectional study of 59 dialysis patients showed that the required EPO dose was higher in the poorly nourished patients as per SGA scoring [68]. In a meta-analysis by Hurot et al., L-carnitine administration, which is used to improve nutritional state, was associated with improved haemoglobin and a decreased EPO dose and EPO resistance in

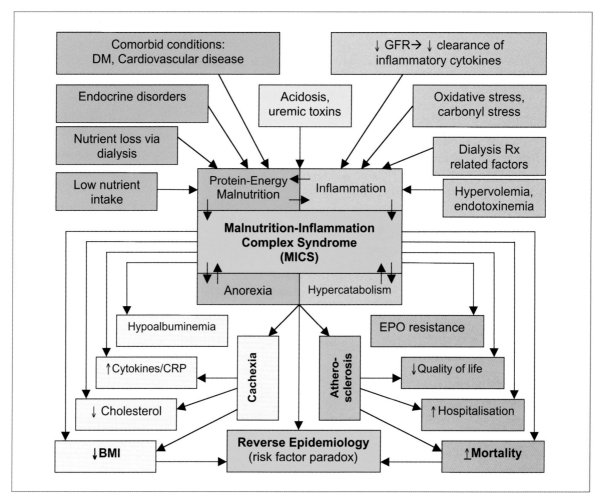

**Fig. 3.** The causes and consequences of malnutrition-inflammation complex syndrome (MICS). Modified from [123]
*BMI*, body mass index; *DM*, diabetes mellitus; *GFR*, glomerular filtration rate; *EPO*, erythropoietin

anaemic dialysis patients [125]. Moreover, anabolic steroids have also been used successfully to simultaneously improve both nutritional status and anaemia in dialysis patients [126]. Insulin-like growth factor (IGF)-1 is reported to enhance bone marrow progenitor cell proliferation in uraemic mice [127]. Hence, CKD-associated anaemia may represent both an EPO and a functional IGF-1 deficient state [127].

It is still not completely clear how MICS is related to CKD-associated refractory anaemia pathophysiologically. It has long been known that anaemia is frequently observed in patients suffering from chronic inflammatory disorders even with a normal kidney function [128]. Several mechanisms for cytokine-induced anaemia have been proposed, including impaired iron metabolism,

suppression of endogenous EPO production, and reduced erythropoiesis [129, 130]. Serum ferritin, a measure of iron stores and a positive acute-phase reactant, has been shown to be paradoxically high in ESRD patients with refractory anaemia [131, 132]. Increased ferritin production may prevent iron delivery to erythrocyte precursors [131]. Moreover, the uptake of iron from the intestine is reduced in inflammatory states [129]. Patients with inflammatory diseases have inappropriately low levels of blood endogenous erythropoietin [133]. IL-1 and TNF-$\alpha$ have been shown to inhibit endogenous erythropoietin production in vitro [134]. Furthermore, increased release or activation of inflammatory cytokines, such as IL-6 or TNF-$\alpha$, has been shown to have a suppressive effect on erythropoiesis [135]. IL-6 and IL-1 have been found to antagonise EPO's ability to stimulate bone marrow proliferation in culture [136]. Finally, patients with inflammation may be more prone to gastrointestinal bleeding [129, 130].

## Atherosclerotic Cardiovascular Disease

Cachexia, by virtue of MICS, may predispose CKD patients to atherosclerotic cardiovascular disease [24, 49, 51]. Dialysis patients with coronary heart disease often have hypoalbuminaemia and elevated levels of acute-phase reactants [24]. Moreover, progression of carotid atherosclerosis during dialysis may be related to IL-6 levels [137]. It should be noted that the cascade of inflammatory factors leading to an acute-phase reaction is counter-regulated by various anti-inflammatory cytokines, such as IL-10. Recently, Girndt et al., in a study of 300 haemodialysis patients [138], showed that the –1082A allele, which is associated with low production of IL-10, is associated with an increased risk of cardiovascular events. Inflammatory processes may promote proliferation and infiltration of inflammatory cells into the tunica intima of small arteries, including the coronary arteries; these processes lead to atherosclerosis and stenosis of blood vessels and consequent coronary and other vascular diseases [137, 139]. Epidemiological evidence suggests that inflammation may be linked to cardiovascular disease via specific low-grade infections, such as caused by *Chlamydia pneumoniae* [137, 139]. *C. pneumoniae* infection is shown to predict adverse outcome in dialysis patients [140], and elevated *C. pneumoniae* IgA titres predict progression of carotid atherosclerosis in these individuals [141]. Myeloperoxidase, an abundant enzyme secreted by neutrophils, may also link inflammation to oxidative stress and atherosclerosis in dialysis patients [142]. Indeed, recent data have shown that a functional variant of the myeloperoxidase gene is associated with cardiovascular disease in CKD patients [143]. Inflammation might also directly cause endothelial dysfunction via stimulation of intercellular adhesion molecules in CKD patients [144]. The association between elements of MICS and atherosclerosis has been under-

scored by some investigators, who have chosen the term 'malnutrition-inflammation-atherosclerosis' (MIA) syndrome for this entity [29, 145].

## Clinical Outcome and Reverse Epidemiology

Many recent studies have suggested that protein-energy malnutrition and inflammation in maintenance dialysis patients are associated with a decreased quality of life and increased hospitalisation and mortality, especially from cardiovascular diseases [10, 27, 28, 123]. Epidemiological studies indicate that hypoalbuminaemia and increased serum CRP are strong predictors of poor clinical outcome in the CKD population [36, 37]. Compared to traditional risk factors, such as obesity, hypercholesterolaemia, and hypertension, hypoalbuminaemia per se, which is generally considered an indicator of MICS, has one of the most striking and consistent associations with the prediction of clinical outcome in these individuals [146].

In highly industrialised, affluent countries, protein-energy malnutrition is an uncommon cause of poor outcome in the general population, whereas over-nutrition is associated with a greater risk of cardiovascular disease and has an immense epidemiological impact on the burden of this disease and on shortened survival. In contrast, in maintenance dialysis patients, under-nutrition is one of the most common risk factors for adverse cardiovascular events [22, 117, 147]. Hence, certain markers that predict a low likelihood of cardiovascular events and an improved survival in the general population, such as decreased body mass index (BMI) [73–75, 148, 149] (Fig. 4) or lower serum cholesterol levels [49, 87], are risk factors for increased cardiovascular morbidity and death in dialysis patients [117]. Obesity, hypercholesterolaemia, and hypertension appear paradoxically to be protective features that are associated with greater survival of dialysis patients. A similar protective role has been described for high serum creatinine and total homocysteine levels in these patients [150].

The association between under-nutrition and adverse cardiovascular outcome in dialysis

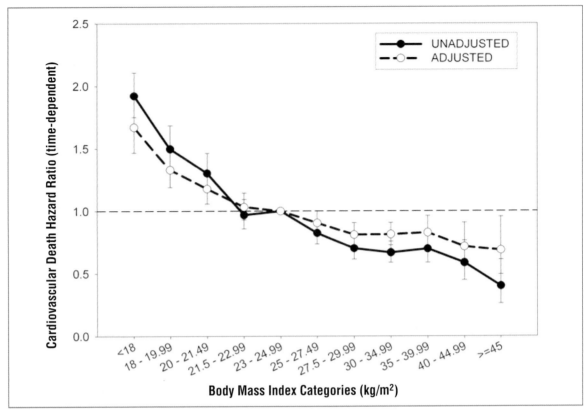

**Fig. 4.** Reverse epidemiology of obesity in maintenance haemodialysis patients. Association between changes in BMI over time and cardiovascular mortality in a 2-year cohort of 51 841 maintenance haemodialysis patients [149]

patients, in contrast to the case in non-dialysis individuals, has been referred to as 'reverse epidemiology' [117]. The aetiology of this inverse association between conventional risk factors and clinical outcome in dialysis patients is not clear. Several possible causes have been hypothesised, including survival bias and time discrepancy between competing risk factors (under-nutrition vs over-nutrition). However, the presence of MICS in dialysis patients offers the most plausible explanation for the existence of reverse epidemiology. Protein-energy malnutrition, inflammation, or the combination of the two are much more common in dialysis patients than in the general population, and many elements of MICS, such as low weight-for-height or BMI, hypocholesterolaemia, or hypocreatininaemia, are known risk factors of poor outcome in dialysis patients [117]. The existence of reverse epidemiology may have a bearing on the management of dialysis patients. It is possible that new standards or goals for such

traditional risk factors as BMI, serum cholesterol, and blood pressure should be considered for these individuals.

The phenomenon of risk-factor paradox is caused or at least accentuated by MICS in several ways. First, patients who are underweight or who have a low serum cholesterol, creatinine, or homocysteine, may be suffering from the MICS and its poor outcome. Thus, MICS may both cause these alterations and also be associated with increased mortality, either caused by the illnesses that engender MICS or by atherosclerotic cardiovascular disease that seems to be promoted by MICS [27, 151, 152]. Second, the above paradoxical factors may indicate a state of under-nutrition, which may predispose to infection or other inflammatory processes [22]. Finally, it has been argued that when individuals are malnourished, they are more susceptible to the ravages of inflammatory diseases [153]. Hence, any condition that potentially attenuates the magnitude of protein-energy malnutrition or inflammation should be favourable to dialysis patients. Suliman et al. reported a more specific example of the contribution of MICS to risk-factor reversal concerning hyperhomocysteinaemia in dialysis patients [154–156]. In their study, plasma total homocysteine levels were shown to be dependent on nutritional status, protein intake, and serum albumin in haemodialysis patients. Dialysis patients with cardiovascular disease had lower plasma homocysteine levels as well as a higher prevalence of malnutrition and hypoalbuminaemia than those without cardiovascular disease. Furthermore, in another study, plasma total homocysteine was shown to rise during treatment of malnourished peritoneal dialysis patients who were given a daily exchange of an amino-acid-containing peritoneal dialysate (containing 1.7 g methionine) [157]. The puzzling inverse relationship between low blood pressure and poor outcome in the dialysis population might also be accounted for by nutritional status and/or inflammation. Iseki et al. [158] showed a significant association between a low diastolic blood pressure, hypoalbuminaemia, and risk of death in a cohort of 1243 haemodialysis patients who were followed for up to 5 years. The death rate was inversely correlated with diastolic blood pressure, which per se was positively correlated with serum albumin and negatively correlated with age. Hence, hypotension may in some cases be a manifestation of MICS in dialysis patients.

## Diagnosis and Management of MICS and Wasting Syndrome in CKD

Since various markers of nutritional state and inflammation may independently predict outcome and assess different aspects of nutritional status, several researchers have tried to develop composite scores to identify the wasting syndrome and MICS in CKD. Ideally, such a scoring system would not only reflect the overall nutritional and inflammatory status of a chronic dialysis patient but would predict outcome. Wolfson et al. [81] introduced a composite score based on body weight, mid-arm muscle circumference, and serum albumin and found that 70% of haemodial-

ysis patients were malnourished. Marckman et al. [159] developed a nutritional scoring system based on serum transferrin, relative body weight, triceps skinfold, and mid-arm muscle circumference. The SGA of nutritional status was designed primarily to evaluate surgical patients with gastrointestinal diseases [68]. It has since been employed in a number of epidemiological studies and clinical trials in dialysis patients [69]. SGA is significantly correlated with morbidity and mortality among dialysis patients [160, 161]. The K/DOQI has recommended SGA as an appropriate nutritional assessment tool for dialysis patients [162]. CANUSA (Canada-USA) [163] and other studies [164] have led to improved, more quantitative versions of the SGA. The recently developed MIS is based on the SGA, but also includes BMI and serum albumin and transferrin concentrations in an incremental fashion [28]. In two independently conducted longitudinal studies in haemodialysis patients, the MIS was strongly correlated with 12-month hospitalisation rates and mortality [28, 70] and had superior outcome-predictability compared to measurements of serum albumin [70]. MIS is believed to reflect the degree of severity of MICS in dialysis patients.

Protein-energy malnutrition and inflammation lead to wasting syndrome and cachexia and are powerful predictors of death risk for CKD patients; thus, if they are treatable, it is possible that nutritional and anti-inflammatory interventions will improve poor outcome in the CKD population. Experience with nutritional support of sick or malnourished individuals who do not have CKD may provide some insight into the independent role of protein-energy malnutrition on clinical outcome in dialysis patients. Ample evidence suggests that maintaining an adequate nutritional intake in patients with a number of acute or chronic catabolic illnesses improves their nutritional status irrespective of its aetiology [165, 166]. In some of these studies, such improvement was associated with reduced morbidity and mortality and improved quality of life [167]. However, evidence as to whether nutritional treatment improves morbidity and mortality in dialysis patients is quite limited. There are no large-scale, randomised, prospective interventional studies that have examined these issues. Among studies based on the nutritional response to such interventions, Kuhlmann et al. reported that prescription of 45 Kcal/kg/day and 1.5 g protein/kg/day, as compared to no such prescription, induced weight gain and improved serum albumin and other measures of nutritional status in malnourished haemodialysis patients [109]. Leon et al. reported that tailored nutritional intervention increased serum albumin levels in 52 haemodialysis patients, and this effect was observed even among patients with high serum CRP levels [108]. Several retrospective studies demonstrated a beneficial effect of intradialytic parenteral nutrition (IDPN) on clinical outcome [168–171]. Recently, Pupim et al. [110] demonstrated that IDPN promoted a large increase in whole-body protein synthesis and a significant decrease in whole-body proteolysis in seven haemodialysis patients without signs of inflammation. However, a number of other studies of IDPN failed to show improvement in nutritional status or clinical outcome in dialysis patients [172, 173]. Many of these studies used small sample sizes, failed to restrict study subjects to those with protein-energy malnutrition, did not control for concurrent food intake, did not define or adjust appropriately for comorbid conditions, performed nutritional interventions for only short periods of time, or had only a short period of follow-up. Thus, until large-scale, prospective, randomised interventional studies are conducted, it will be difficult to ascertain the potential benefits of increasing nutritional intake in malnourished dialysis patients [173].

A number of other techniques have been employed for the prevention or treatment of protein-energy malnutrition in dialysis patients. Routine methods include preventing protein-energy malnutrition before the onset of dialysis therapy, dietary counselling, maintenance of an adequate dose of dialysis, avoidance of acidaemia, and aggressive treatment of superimposed catabolic illnesses [56]. More novel, non-dietary interventions in addition to IDPN include an appetite stimulant such as megestrol acetate [174], L-carnitine [175, 176], and growth factors including recombinant human growth hormone (rhGH) [177], IGF-1 [178], and anabolic steroids [179]. Nonetheless, although

L-carnitine and these hormones may cause increased nitrogen retention, with the exception of the probable effects of L-carnitine administration on quality of life, none of these treatments have yet been shown to improve quality of life, morbidity, or mortality in dialysis patients.

Although epidemiological evidence strongly links inflammation to poor outcome in individuals with renal insufficiency, it must be recognised that as yet there are no randomised clinical trials to indicate improvement of cachexia and its outcome by inflammation-reducing approaches. However, some treatment modalities may target inflammation directly, or they may focus on oxidative and carbonyl stress or endothelial dysfunction. The following approaches may be considered: (1) Statins (HMG-CoA reductase inhibitors) have been shown to decrease CRP levels independently of their lipid-lowering effects and may be associated with reduced mortality in CKD patients [180, 181]. (2) Angiotensin-converting enzyme inhibitors may have anti-inflammatory properties in both the general population and in CKD patients [182], and are associated with delayed progression of chronic renal failure and improved outcome in these individuals [18]. (3) Vitamin E may have anti-inflammatory effects, and its administration may be associated with a decreased risk for cardiovascular mortality in chronic dialysis patients [183]. In the general population, some epidemiological studies indicate that a vitamin-E-rich diet is associated with a better cardiovascular outcome [184], but large clinical trials, such as the HOPE study, did not confirm such results [185, 186]. There are several forms of vitamin E, and it is possible that purified supplements, particularly the commonly used DL α-tocopherol (tocopheral) form, may not show the benefits of natural (national) dietary vitamin E or γ-tocopherol (tocopheral) components. A number of preliminary studies indicate that vitamin-E-coated dialysers may have favourable effects and anti-oxidant properties [187]. 4) Optimisation of dialysis treatment may improve inflammatory status in dialysis patients, and the type of dialysis membrane may have a bearing [188]. Ultra-pure dialysate and biocompatible membranes have been shown to decrease serum CRP [189, 190].

## Conclusions and Future Steps

Both chronic inflammation and protein-energy malnutrition, together also referred to as MICS, are involved in engendering the commonly encountered wasting syndrome in CKD population. Hypoalbuminaemia is a marker of MICS and a strong outcome-predictor in these patients. The wasting syndrome in CKD patients per se is a chronic and slowly progressive condition that worsens over time in both pre-dialysis [54, 55] and dialysis patients [191]. Hence, a state of 'cachexia in slow motion' can be described in these individuals. The effect of MICS on overall clinical and psychosocial aspects of CKD patients is so overwhelming that it even reverses the conventional associations between risk factors and outcome, leading to a counter-intuitive state of reverse epidemiology. However, dialysis patients are not the only population with a reverse epidemiology. Individuals with chronic heart failure (CHF) and geriatric populations have risk-factor reversal as well [192]. Hence, a better understanding of the role of chronic cachexia in CKD patients may help improve clinical management of not only these patients but also CHF, geriatric, and other vulnerable populations. According to an epidemiological study of over 55 000 haemodialysis patients, if an intervention could increase serum albumin above 3.8 g/dl and by doing so improve survival in dialysis patients, almost one-third of all deaths among these patients could be hypothetically prevented or delayed. Since approximately 60 000 patients out of over 300 000 haemodialysis patients in the USA die every year, a hypoalbuminaemia-correcting intervention might theoretically prevent 15 000–20 000 deaths every year [25]. If this is correct, there is a great need to develop effective nutritional and/or anti-inflammatory interventions and to carry out randomised, prospective, controlled clinical trials to demonstrate the benefits of such interventions.

## References

1. National Kidney Foundation (2002) K/DOQI clinical practice guidelines for chronic kidney disease: evaluation, classification, and stratification. Am J Kidney Dis 39:S1-S266
2. Keith DS, Nichols GA, Gullion CM et al (2004) Longitudinal follow-up and outcomes among a population with chronic kidney disease in a large managed care organization. Arch Intern Med 164:659–663
3. Jones CA, McQuillan GM, Kusek JW et al (1998) Serum creatinine levels in the US population: third National Health and Nutrition Examination Survey. Am J Kidney Dis 32:992–999
4. Anonymous (2003) System USRD: USRD 2003 Annual Data Report; Atlas of End Stage Renal Diseases in the United States. National Institute of Health, National Institute of Diabetes and Digestive and Kidney Diseases, Bethesda
5. Hirth RA, Held PJ, Orzol SM, Dor A (1999) Practice patterns, case mix, Medicare payment policy, and dialysis facility costs. Health Serv Res 33:1567–1592
6. Garella S (1997) The costs of dialysis in the USA. Nephrol Dial Transplant 12(Suppl 1):10–21
7. Anonymous (2002) United States Renal Data System: US Department of Public Health and Human Services, Public Health Service, National Institutes of Health, Bethesda, Maryland
8. Devereaux PJ, Schunemann HJ, Ravindran N et al (2002) Comparison of mortality between private for-profit and private not-for-profit hemodialysis centers: a systematic review and meta-analysis. JAMA 288:2449–2457
9. Eggers PW, Frankenfield DL, Greer JW et al (2002) Comparison of mortality and intermediate outcomes between medicare dialysis patients in HMO and fee for service. Am J Kidney Dis 39:796–804
10. Kalantar-Zadeh K, Kopple JD, Block G, Humphreys MH (2001) Association among SF36 quality of life measures and nutrition, hospitalization, and mortality in hemodialysis. J Am Soc Nephrol 12:2797–2806
11. Carlson DM, Duncan DA, Naessens JM, Johnson WJ (1984) Hospitalization in dialysis patients. Mayo Clin Proc 59:769–775
12. Fried L, Abidi S, Bernardini J et al (1999) Hospitalization in peritoneal dialysis patients. Am J Kidney Dis 33:927–933
13. Habach G, Bloembergen WE, Mauger EA et al (1995) Hospitalization among United States dialysis patients: hemodialysis versus peritoneal dialysis. J Am Soc Nephrol 5:1940–1948
14. Foley RN, Parfrey PS, Sarnak MJ (1998) Epidemiology of cardiovascular disease in chronic renal disease. J Am Soc Nephrol 9:S16–S23
15. Foley RN, Parfrey PS, Sarnak MJ (1998) Clinical epidemiology of cardiovascular disease in chronic renal disease. Am J Kidney Dis 32:S112–S119
16. Shlipak MG, Heidenreich PA, Noguchi H et al (2002) Association of renal insufficiency with treatment and outcomes after myocardial infarction in elderly patients. Ann Intern Med 137:555–562

17. Shlipak MG, Simon JA, Grady D et al (2001) Renal insufficiency and cardiovascular events in postmenopausal women with coronary heart disease. J Am Coll Cardiol 38:705–711

18. Mann JF, Gerstein HC, Pogue J et al (2001) Renal insufficiency as a predictor of cardiovascular outcomes and the impact of ramipril: the HOPE randomized trial. Ann Intern Med 134:629–636

19. Fung F, Sherrard DJ, Gillen DL et al (2002) Increased risk for cardiovascular mortality among malnourished end-stage renal disease patients. Am J Kidney Dis 40:307–314

20. Kalantar-Zadeh K, Supasyndh O, Lehn RS et al (2003) Normalized protein nitrogen appearance is correlated with hospitalization and mortality in hemodialysis patients with Kt/V greater than 1.20. J Ren Nutr 13:15–25

21. Bergstrom J, Lindholm B (1999) Malnutrition, cardiac disease, and mortality. Perit Dial Int 19:S309–S314

22. Kalantar-Zadeh K, Kopple JD (2001) Relative contributions of nutrition and inflammation to clinical outcome in dialysis patients. Am J Kidney Dis 38:1343–1350

23. Qureshi AR, Alvestrand A, Divino-Filho JC et al (2002) Inflammation, malnutrition, and cardiac disease as predictors of mortality in hemodialysis patients. J Am Soc Nephrol 13(Suppl 1):S28-S36

24. Zimmermann J, Herrlinger S, Pruy A et al (1999) Inflammation enhances cardiovascular risk and mortality in hemodialysis patients. Kidney Int 55:648–658

25. Kalantar-Zadeh K, Kilpatrick RD, Kuwae K et al (2004) Population attributable mortality risk for albumin <3.8 g/dL: how many lives can be saved if hypoalbuminemia can be corrected in hemodialysis patients? 37th annual conference of the American Society of Nephrology; J Am Soc Neph

26. Stenvinkel P, Heimburger O, Paultre F et al (1999) Strong association between malnutrition, inflammation, and atherosclerosis in chronic renal failure. Kidney Int 55:1899–1911

27. Bergstrom J (2000) Inflammation, malnutrition, cardiovascular disease and mortality in end-stage renal disease. Pol Arch Med Wewn 104:641–643

28. Kalantar-Zadeh K, Kopple JD, Block G, Humphreys MH (2001) A malnutrition-inflammation score is correlated with morbidity and mortality in maintenance hemodialysis patients. Am J Kidney Dis 38:1251–1263

29. Pecoits-Filho R, Lindholm B, Stenvinkel P (2002) The malnutrition, inflammation, and atherosclerosis (MIA) syndrome — the heart of the matter. Nephrol Dial Transplant 17(Suppl 11):28–31

30. Newman Dorland W, Anderson D (2000) Dorland's illustrated medical dictionary, WB Saunders, Philadeplhia

31. Kalantar-Zadeh K, Ikizler TA, Block G et al (2003) Malnutrition-inflammation complex syndrome in dialysis patients: causes and consequences. Am J Kidney Dis 42:864–881

32. Gabay C, Kushner I (1999) Acute-phase proteins and other systemic responses to inflammation. N Engl J Med 340:448–454

33. Kushner I (2003) Acute phase proteins, in UpToDate, edited by Rose B, Wellesley, MA, UpToDate, Inc

34. Streetz KL, Wustefeld T, Klein C et al (2001) Mediators of inflammation and acute phase response in the liver. Cell Mol Biol (Noisy-le-grand) 47:661–673

35. Suffredini AF, Fantuzzi G, Badolato R et al (1999) New insights into the biology of the acute phase response. J Clin Immunol 19:203–214

36. Owen WF, Lowrie EG (1998) C-reactive protein as an outcome predictor for maintenance hemodialysis patients. Kidney Int 54:627–63

37. Yeun JY, Levine RA, Mantadilok V, Kaysen GA (2000) C-reactive protein predicts all-cause and cardiovascular mortality in hemodialysis patients. Am J Kidney Dis 35:469–476

38. Zoccali C, Benedetto FA, Mallamaci F et al (2000) Inflammation is associated with carotid atherosclerosis in dialysis patients. Creed Investigators. Cardiovascular Risk Extended Evaluation in Dialysis Patients. J Hypertens 18:1207–1213

39. Iseki K, Tozawa M, Yoshi S, Fukiyama K (1999) Serum C-reactive protein (CRP) and risk of death in chronic dialysis patients. Nephrol Dial Transplant 14:1956–1960

40. Noh H, Lee SW, Kang SW et al (1998) Serum C-reactive protein: a predictor of mortality in continuous ambulatory peritoneal dialysis patients. Perit Dial Int 18:387–394

41. Kalantar-Zadeh K, Block G, McAllister CJ et al (2004) Appetite and inflammation, nutrition, anemia and clinical outcome in hemodialysis patients. Am J Clin Nutr 80:299-307

42. Shlipak MG, Chertow GC, Massie BM (2003) Beware the rising creatinine level. J Card Fail 9:26–28

43. Lowbeer C, Stenvinkel P, Pecoits-Filho R et al (2003) Elevated cardiac troponin T in predialysis patients is associated with inflammation and predicts mortality. J Intern Med 253:153–160

44. Kalantar-Zadeh K, Kopple J (2006) Inflammation in renal failure, in UpToDate (vol 10.2), Boston, UpToDate, Inc

45. Kalantar-Zadeh K, Stenvinkel P, Barba L et al (2003) Nutrition and Inflammation in Renal Insufficiency. Advances in Renal Replacement Therapy

46. Kaysen GA (2001) The microinflammatory state in uremia: causes and potential consequences. J Am Soc Nephrol 12:1549–1557

47. Kalantar-Zadeh K, Kopple J (2003) Inflammation in renal failure, in UpToDate (since Oct 2002), edited by Rose B, Wellesley, MA, UpToDate, Inc

48. Kimmel PL, Phillips TM, Simmens SJ et al (1998) Immunologic function and survival in hemodialysis patients. Kidney Int 54:236–244

49. Bologa RM, Levine DM, Parker TS et al (1998) Interleukin-6 predicts hypoalbuminemia, hypocholesterolemia, and mortality in hemodialysis patients. Am J Kidney Dis 32:107–114

50. Pecoits-Filho R, Barany P, Lindholm B et al (2002) Interleukin-6 is an independent predictor of mortality in patients starting dialysis treatment. Nephrol Dial Transplant 17:1684–1688

51. Stenvinkel P, Barany P, Heimburger O et al (2002) Mortality, malnutrition, and atherosclerosis in ESRD: what is the role of interleukin-6? Kidney Int Suppl:103–108

52. Tatli MM, Vural H, Koc A et al (2000) Altered antioxidant status and increased lipid peroxidation in marasmic children. Pediatr Int 42:289–292

53. Torun B, Chew F (1999) Protein-energy malnutrition. In: Shils M, Olson J, Shike M, Ross A (eds) Modern nutrition in health and disease, 9th ed. William & Wilkins, Baltimore, pp 963–988

54. Kopple JD, Levey AS, Greene T et al (1997) Effect of dietary protein restriction on nutritional status in the Modification of Diet in Renal Disease Study. Kidney Int 52:778–791

55. Kopple JD, Greene T, Chumlea WC et al (2000) Relationship between nutritional status and the glomerular filtration rate: results from the MDRD study. Kidney Int 57:1688–1703

56. Kopple JD (1997) Nutritional status as a predictor of morbidity and mortality in maintenance dialysis patients. ASAIO J 43:246–250

57. Kopple JD, Zhu X, Lew NL, Lowrie EG (1999) Body weight-for-height relationships predict mortality in maintenance hemodialysis patients. Kidney Int 56:1136–1148

58. Mehrotra R, Kopple JD (2001) Nutritional management of maintenance dialysis patients: why aren't we doing better? Annu Rev Nutr 21:343–379

59. Kalantar-Zadeh K, Kopple JD (2003) Nutritional management of hemodialysis patients. In: Kopple JD, Massry S (eds) Nutritional management of renal disease, 2nd edn. Lippincott Williams & Wilkins, Philadelphia

60. Kalantar-Zadeh K, Kopple JD, Deepak S et al (2002) Food intake characteristics of hemodialysis patients as obtained by food frequency questionnaire. J Ren Nutr 12:17–31

61. Kalantar-Zadeh K, Kopple JD (2003) Trace elements and vitamins in maintenance dialysis patients. Adv Ren Replace Ther 10:170–182

62. Kopple JD (1997) McCollum Award Lecture 1996: protein-energy malnutrition in maintenance dialysis patients. Am J Clin Nutr 65:1544–1557

63. Kopple JD (1999) Pathophysiology of protein-energy wasting in chronic renal failure. J Nutr 129:247S–251S

64. Mehrotra R, Kopple JD (2003) Causes of protein-energy malnutrition in chronic renal failure. In: Kopple JD, Massry S (eds) Nutritional management of renal disease, 2nd edn. Lippincott Williams &

65. Qureshi AR, Alvestrand A, Danielsson A et al (1998) Factors predicting malnutrition in hemodialysis patients: a cross-sectional study. Kidney Int 53:773–782

66. Bergstrom J (1995) Why are dialysis patients malnourished? Am J Kidney Dis 26:229–241

67. Ikizler TA, Greene JH, Wingard RL et al (1995) Spontaneous dietary protein intake during progression of chronic renal failure. J Am Soc Nephrol 6:1386–1391

68. Kalantar-Zadeh K, Kleiner M, Dunne E et al (1998) Total iron-binding capacity-estimated transferrin correlates with the nutritional subjective global assessment in hemodialysis patients. Am J Kidney Dis 31:263–272

69. Enia G, Sicuso C, Alati G, Zoccali C (1993) Subjective global assessment of nutrition in dialysis patients. Nephrol Dial Transplant 8:1094–1098

70. Kalantar-Zadeh K, Kopple JD, Humphreys MH, Block G (2004) Comparing outcome predictability of markers of malnutrition-inflammation complex syndrome in haemodialysis patients. Nephrol Dial Transplant 19:1507–1519

71. Kalantar-Zadeh K, Kopple JD (2003) Malnutrition as a cause of morbidity and mortality in dialysis patients. In: Kopple JD, Massry S (eds) Nutritional management of renal disease, 2nd edn. Lippincott Williams & Wilkins, Philadelphia

72. Kalantar-Zadeh K, Block G, McAllister CJ et al (2003) Association between self-reported appetite and markers of inflammation, nutrition, anemia and quality of life in hemodialysis patients. Am J Clin Nutrition

73. Culp K, Flanigan M, Dudley J et al (1998) Using the Quetelet body mass index as a mortality indicator for patients starting renal replacement therapy. ANNA J 25:321–330; discussion 331–322

74. Leavey SF, McCullough K, Hecking E et al (2001) Body mass index and mortality in 'healthier' as compared with 'sicker' haemodialysis patients: results from the Dialysis Outcomes and Practice Patterns Study (DOPPS). Nephrol Dial Transplant 16:2386–2394

75. Port FK, Ashby VB, Dhingra RK et al (2002) Dialysis dose and body mass index are strongly associated with survival in hemodialysis patients. J Am Soc Nephrol 13:1061–1066

76. Kalantar-Zadeh K, Block G, Kelly MP et al (2001) Near infra-red interactance for longitudinal assessment of nutrition in dialysis patients. J Ren Nutr 11:23–31

77. Blumenkrantz MJ, Kopple JD, Gutman RA et al (1980) Methods for assessing nutritional status of patients with renal failure. Am J Clin Nutr 33:1567–1585

78. Pollock CA, Ibels LS, Allen BJ et al (1995) Total body nitrogen as a prognostic marker in maintenance dialysis. J Am Soc Nephrol 6:82–88

79. Arora P, Strauss BJ, Borovnicar D et al (1998) Total body nitrogen predicts long-term mortality in haemodialysis patients - a single-centre experience. Nephrol Dial Transplant 13:1731–1736

80. Boddy K, King PC, Lindsay RM et al (1972) Total body potassium in non-dialysed and dialysed patients with chronic renal failure. Br Med J 1:771–775

81. Wolfson M, Strong CJ, Minturn D et al (1984) Nutritional status and lymphocyte function in maintenance hemodialysis patients. Am J Clin Nutr 39:547–555

82. Kaysen GA, Levin N (2002) Why measure serum albumin levels? J Ren Nutr 12:148–150

83. Sreedhara R, Avram MM, Blanco M et al (1996) Prealbumin is the best nutritional predictor of survival in hemodialysis and peritoneal dialysis. Am J Kidney Dis 28:937–942

84. Kopple JD, Mehrotra R, Suppasyndh O et al (2002) Observations with regard to the National Kidney Foundation K/DOQI clinical practice guidelines concerning serum transthyretin in chronic renal failure. Clin Chem Lab Med 40:1308–1312

85. Neyra NR, Hakim RM, Shyr Y, Ikizler TA (2000) Serum transferrin and serum prealbumin are early predictors of serum albumin in chronic hemodialysis patients. J Ren Nutr 10:184–190

86. Avram MM, Fein PA, Antignani A et al (1989) Cholesterol and lipid disturbances in renal disease: the natural history of uremic dyslipidemia and the impact of hemodialysis and continuous ambulatory peritoneal dialysis. Am J Med 87:55N-60N

87. Iseki K, Yamazato M, Tozawa M, Takishita S (2002) Hypocholesterolemia is a significant predictor of death in a cohort of chronic hemodialysis patients. Kidney Int 61:1887–1893

88. Lowrie EG, Lew NL (1990) Death risk in hemodialysis patients: the predictive value of commonly measured variables and an evaluation of death rate differences between facilities. Am J Kidney Dis 15:458–482

89. Cooper BA, Bartlett LH, Aslani A et al (2002) Validity of subjective global assessment as a nutritional marker in end-stage renal disease. Am J Kidney Dis 40:126–132

90. Visser R, Dekker FW, Boeschoten EW et al (1999) Reliability of the 7-point subjective global assessment scale in assessing nutritional status of dialysis patients. Adv Perit Dial 15:222–225

91. Kaysen GA, Dubin JA, Muller HG et al (2002) Relationships among inflammation nutrition and physiologic mechanisms establishing albumin levels in hemodialysis patients. Kidney Int 61:2240–2249

92. Grodstein GP, Blumenkrantz MJ, Kopple JD (1980) Nutritional and metabolic response to catabolic stress in uremia. Am J Clin Nutr 33:1411–1416

93. Chertow GM (1999) Estimates of body composition as intermediate outcome variables: are DEXA and BIA ready for prime time? J Ren Nutr 9:138–141

94. Dumler F (1997) Use of bioelectric impedance analysis and dual-energy X-ray absorptiometry for monitoring the nutritional status of dialysis patients. ASAIO J 43:256–260

95. Pollock CA, Allen BJ, Warden RA et al (1990) Total body nitrogen by neutron activation analysis in maintenance dialysis patients. Am J Kidney Dis 16:38–45

96. Ikizler TA, Hakim RM (1996) Nutrition in end-stage renal disease. Kidney Int 50:343–357

97. Kalantar-Zadeh K, Dunne E, Nixon K et al (1999) Near infra-red interactance for nutritional assessment of dialysis patients. Nephrol Dial Transplant 14:169–175

98. Yeun JY, Kaysen GA (1998) Factors influencing serum albumin in dialysis patients. Am J Kidney Dis 32:S118–S125

99. Stenvinkel P, Barany P, Chung SH et al (2002) A comparative analysis of nutritional parameters as predictors of outcome in male and female ESRD patients. Nephrol Dial Transplant 17:1266–1274

100. Kaizu Y, Kimura M, Yoneyama T et al (1998) Interleukin-6 may mediate malnutrition in chronic hemodialysis patients. Am J Kidney Dis 31:93–100

101. Flores EA, Bistrian BR, Pomposelli JJ et al (1989) Infusion of tumor necrosis factor/cachectin promotes muscle catabolism in the rat. A synergistic effect with interleukin 1. J Clin Invest 83:1614–1622

102. Espat NJ, Copeland EM, Moldawr LL (1994) Tumor necrosis factor and cachexia: a current perspective. Surg Onc 3:255–262

103. McCarthy DO (2000) Tumor necrosis factor alpha and interleukin-6 have differential effects on food intake and gastric emptying in fasted rats. Res Nurs Health 23:222–228

104. Kaysen GA, Chertow GM, Adhikarla R et al (2001) Inflammation and dietary protein intake exert competing effects on serum albumin and creatinine in hemodialysis patients. Kidney Int 60:333–340

105. Kaysen GA, Stevenson FT, Depner TA (1997) Determinants of albumin concentration in hemodialysis patients. Am J Kidney Dis 29:658–668

106. Ginn HE, Frost A, Lacy WW (1968) Nitrogen balance in hemodialysis patients. Am J Clin Nutr 21:385–393

107. Kaysen GA, Dubin JA, Muller HG et al (2000) The acute-phase response varies with time and predicts serum albumin levels in hemodialysis patients. The HEMO Study Group. Kidney Int 58:346–352

108. Leon JB, Majerle AD, Soinski JA et al (2001) Can a nutrition intervention improve albumin levels among hemodialysis patients? A pilot study. J Ren Nutr 11:9–15

109. Kuhlmann MK, Schmidt F, Kohler H (1999) High protein/energy vs. standard protein/energy nutritional regimen in the treatment of malnourished hemodialysis patients. Miner Electrolyte Metab 25:306–310

110. Pupim LB, Flakoll PJ, Brouillette JR et al (2002) Intradialytic parenteral nutrition improves protein

and energy homeostasis in chronic hemodialysis patients. J Clin Invest 110:483–492

111. Caglar K, Fedje L, Dimmitt R et al (2002) Therapeutic effects of oral nutritional supplementation during hemodialysis. Kidney Int 62:1054–1059

112. Stenvinkel P, Holmberg I, Heimburger O, Diczfalusy U (1998) A study of plasmalogen as an index of oxidative stress in patients with chronic renal failure. Evidence of increased oxidative stress in malnourished patients. Nephrol Dial Transplant 13:2594–2600

113. Hulsewe KW, van Acker BA, von Meyenfeldt MF, Soeters PB (1999) Nutritional depletion and dietary manipulation: effects on the immune response. World J Surg 23:536–544

114. De Simone C, Famularo G, Tzantzoglou S et al (1994) Carnitine depletion in peripheral blood mononuclear cells from patients with AIDS: effect of oral L-carnitine. AIDS 8:655–660

115. Ridker PM, Rifai N, Rose L et al (2002) Comparison of C-reactive protein and low-density lipoprotein cholesterol levels in the prediction of first cardiovascular events. N Engl J Med 347:1557–1565

116. Kaysen GA (2000) Malnutrition and the acute-phase reaction in dialysis patients-how to measure and how to distinguish. Nephrol Dial Transplant 15:1521–1524

117. Kalantar-Zadeh K, Block G, Humphreys MH, Kopple JD (2003) Reverse epidemiology of cardiovascular risk factors in maintenance dialysis patients. Kidney Int 63:793–808

118. Barany P, Divino Filho JC, Bergstrom J (1997) High C-reactive protein is a strong predictor of resistance to erythropoietin in hemodialysis patients. Am J Kidney Dis 29:565–568

119. Stenvinkel P, Alvestrand A (2002) Inflammation in end-stage renal disease: sources, consequences, and therapy. Semin Dial 15:329–337

120. Gunnell J, Yeun JY, Depner TA, Kaysen GA (1999) Acute-phase response predicts erythropoietin resistance in hemodialysis and peritoneal dialysis patients. Am J Kidney Dis 33:63–72

121. Goicoechea M, Martin J, de Sequera P et al (1998) Role of cytokines in the response to erythropoietin in hemodialysis patients. Kidney Int 54:1337–1343

122. Sitter T, Bergner A, Schiffl H (2000) Dialysate related cytokine induction and response to recombinant human erythropoietin in haemodialysis patients. Nephrol Dial Transplant 15:1207–1211

123. Kalantar-Zadeh K, Fouque D, Kopple JD (2004) Outcome research, nutrition, and reverse epidemiology in maintenance dialysis patients. J Ren Nutr 14:64–71

124. Kalantar-Zadeh K, McAllister CJ, Lehn RS et al (2003) Effect of malnutrition-inflammation complex syndrome on EPO hyporesponsiveness in maintenance hemodialysis patients. Am J Kidney Dis 42:761–773

125. Hurot JM, Cucherat M, Haugh M, Fouque D (2002) Effects of L-carnitine supplementation in maintenance hemodialysis patients: a systematic review. J Am Soc Nephrol 13:708–714

126. Navarro JF, Mora C (2001) In-depth review effect of androgens on anemia and malnutrition in renal failure: implications for patients on peritoneal dialysis. Perit Dial Int 21:14–24

127. Brox AG, Zhang F, Guyda H, Gagnon RF (1996) Subtherapeutic erythropoietin and insulin-like growth factor-1 correct the anemia of chronic renal failure in the mouse. Kidney Int 50:937–943

128. Voulgari PV, Kolios G, Papadopoulos GK et al (1999) Role of cytokines in the pathogenesis of anemia of chronic disease in rheumatoid arthritis. Clin Immunol 92:153–160

129. Stenvinkel P (2001) The role of inflammation in the anaemia of end-stage renal disease. Nephrol Dial Transplant 16(Suppl 7):36–40

130. Stenvinkel P, Barany P (2002) Anaemia, rHuEPO resistance, and cardiovascular disease in end-stage renal failure; links to inflammation and oxidative stress. Nephrol Dial Transplant 17(Suppl 5):32–37

131. Kalantar-Zadeh K, Don BR, Rodriguez RA, Humphreys MH (2001) Serum ferritin is a marker of morbidity and mortality in hemodialysis patients. Am J Kidney Dis 37:564–572

132. Kalantar-Zadeh K, Luft FC, Humphreys MH (1999) Moderately high serum ferritin concentration is not a sign of iron overload in dialysis patients. Kidney Int 56:758–759

133. Miller CB, Jones RJ, Piantadosi S et al (1990) Decreased erythropoietin response in patients with the anemia of cancer. N Engl J Med 322:1689–1692

134. Jelkmann W, Pagel H, Wolff M, Fandrey J (1992) Monokines inhibiting erythropoietin production in human hepatoma cultures and in isolated perfused rat kidneys. Life Sci 50:301–308

135. Means RT Jr, Krantz SB (1992) Progress in understanding the pathogenesis of the anemia of chronic disease. Blood 80:1639–1647

136. Schooley JC, Kullgren B, Allison AC (1987) Inhibition by interleukin-1 of the action of erythropoietin on erythroid precursors and its possible role in the pathogenesis of hypoplastic anaemias. Br J Haematol 67:11–17

137. Becker AE, de Boer OJ, van Der Wal AC (2001) The role of inflammation and infection in coronary artery disease. Annu Rev Med 52:289–297

138. Girndt M, Kaul H, Sester U et al (2002) Anti-inflammatory interleukin-10 genotype protects dialysis patients from cardiovascular events. Kidney Int 62:949–955

139. Kaplan N (2001) Risk factor for atherosclerotic disease. In: Braunwald E ZD Libby P (eds) Heart disease: a textbook of cardiovascular medicine Saunders WB, Philadelphia, PA, pp 1010–1039

140. Haubitz M, Brunkhorst R (2001) C-reactive protein and chronic Chlamydia pneumoniae infection—long-term predictors for cardiovascular disease and survival in patients on peritoneal dialysis. Nephrol

Dial Transplant 16:809–815

141. Stenvinkel P, Heimburger O, Jogestrand T (2002) Elevated interleukin-6 predicts progressive carotid artery atherosclerosis in dialysis patients: association with Chlamydia pneumoniae seropositivity. Am J Kidney Dis 39:274–282

142. Daugherty A, Dunn JL, Rateri DL, Heinecke JW (1994) Myeloperoxidase, a catalyst for lipoprotein oxidation, is expressed in human atherosclerotic lesions. J Clin Invest 94:437–444

143. Pecoits-Filho R, Stenvinkel P, Marchlewska A et al (2003) A functional variant of the myeloperoxidase gene is associated with cardiovascular disease in end-stage renal disease patients. Kidney Int Suppl:172–176

144. Mezzano D, Pais EO, Aranda E et al (2001) Inflammation, not hyperhomocysteinemia, is related to oxidative stress and hemostatic and endothelial dysfunction in uremia. Kidney Int 60:1844–1850

145. Chung SH, Stenvinkel P, Heimburger O et al (2000) Prevention and treatment of the malnutrition, inflammation and atherosclerosis (MIA) syndrome in uremic patients. Pol Arch Med Wewn 104:645–654

146. Foley RN, Parfrey PS, Harnett JD et al (1996) Hypoalbuminemia, cardiac morbidity, and mortality in end-stage renal disease. J Am Soc Nephrol 7:728–736

147. Fleischmann E, Teal N, Dudley J et al (1999) Influence of excess weight on mortality and hospital stay in 1346 hemodialysis patients. Kidney Int 55:1560–1567

148. Iseki K, Ikemiya Y, Fukiyama K (1997) Predictors of end-stage renal disease and body mass index in a screened cohort. Kidney Int Suppl 63:S169-S170

149. Kalantar-Zadeh K, Kilpatrick RD, McAllister CJ et al (2004) Time-dependant association between body mass index and cardiovascular mortality in hemodialysis patients. J Am Soc Nephrol 15:126A

150. Kalantar-Zadeh K, Block G, Humphreys MH et al (2004) A low, rather than a high, total plasma homocysteine is an indicator of poor outcome in hemodialysis patients. J Am Soc Nephrol 15:442–453

151. Lowrie EG (1983) History and organization of the National Cooperative Dialysis Study. Kidney Int Suppl 13:S1-S7

152. Ritz E (1996) Why are lipids not predictive of cardiovascular death in the dialysis patient? Miner Electrolyte Metab 22:9–12

153. Lowrie EG (1997) Conceptual model for a core pathobiology of uremia with special reference to anemia, malnourishment, and mortality among dialysis patients. Semin Dial 9:115–129

154. Suliman ME, Lindholm B, Barany P, Bergstrom J (2001) Hyperhomocysteinemia in chronic renal failure patients: relation to nutritional status and cardiovascular disease. Clin Chem Lab Med 39:734–738

155. Suliman ME, Qureshi AR, Barany P et al (2000) Hyperhomocysteinemia, nutritional status, and cardiovascular disease in hemodialysis patients. Kidney Int 57:1727–1735

156. Suliman ME, Stenvinkel P, Barany P et al (2003) Hyperhomocysteinemia and its relationship to cardiovascular disease in ESRD: influence of hypoalbuminemia, malnutrition, inflammation, and diabetes mellitus. Am J Kidney Dis 41:S89–S95

157. Bostom A, Brosnan JT, Hall B et al (1995) Net uptake of plasma homocysteine by the rat kidney in vivo. Atherosclerosis 116:59–62

158. Iseki K, Miyasato F, Tokuyama K et al (1997) Low diastolic blood pressure, hypoalbuminemia, and risk of death in a cohort of chronic hemodialysis patients. Kidney Int 51:1212–1217

159. Marckmann P (1989) Nutritional status and mortality of patients in regular dialysis therapy. J Intern Med 226:429–432

160. Lawson JA, Lazarus R, Kelly JJ (2001) Prevalence and prognostic significance of malnutrition in chronic renal insufficiency. J Ren Nutr 11:16–22

161. Anonymous (1996) Adequacy of dialysis and nutrition in continuous peritoneal dialysis: association with clinical outcomes. Canada-USA (CANUSA) Peritoneal Dialysis Study Group. J Am Soc Nephrol 7:198–207

162. Anonymous (2000) National Kidney Foundation, Kidney Disease-Dialysis Outcome Quality Initiative: K/DOQI Clinical Practice Guidelines for nutrition in chronic renal failure. Am J Kidney Dis 35:S1–S140

163. Anonymous (1996) Adequacy of dialysis and nutrition in continuous peritoneal dialysis: association with clinical outcomes. Canada-USA (CANUSA) Peritoneal Dialysis Study Group. J Am Soc Nephrol 7:198–207

164. Kalantar-Zadeh K, Kleiner M, Dunne E et al (1999) A modified quantitative subjective global assessment of nutrition for dialysis patients. Nephrol Dial Transplant 14:1732–1738

165. Kopple JD, Massry SG (1996) Nutritional management of renal disease. In: Kopple JD (ed) Nutritional management of nondialyzed patients with chronic renal failure, edited by JD K, William and Wilkins, Baltimore, pp 479–531

166. Mortelmans AK, Duym P, Vandenbroucke J et al (1999) Intradialytic parenteral nutrition in malnourished hemodialysis patients: a prospective long-term study. JPEN J Parenter Enteral Nutr 23:90–95

167. Koretz RL (1999) Does nutritional intervention in protein-energy malnutrition improve morbidity or mortality? J Ren Nutr 9:119–121

168. Foulks CJ (1994) The effect of intradialytic parenteral nutrition on hospitalization rate and mortality in malnourished hemodialysis patients. J Renal Nutr 4:5–10

169. Chertow GM, Owen WF, Lazarus JM (1994) Outcomes of older patients receiving chronic dialysis. JAMA 272:274

170. Capelli JP, Kushner H, Camiscioli TC et al (1994) Effect of intradialytic parenteral nutrition on mortality rates in end-stage renal disease care. Am J Kidney Dis 23:808–816

171. Siskind MS, Lien YH (1993) Effect of intradialytic parenteral nutrition on quality of life in hemodialysis patients. Int J Artif Organs 16:599–603

172. Pupim LB, Kent P, Hakim R (1999) The potential of intradialytic parenteral nutrition: a review. Miner Electrolyte Metab 25:317–323

173. Foulks CJ (1999) An evidence-based evaluation of intradialytic parenteral nutrition. Am J Kidney Dis 33:186–192

174. Boccanfuso JA, Hutton M, McAllister B (2000) The effects of megestrol acetate on nutritional parameters in a dialysis population. J Ren Nutr 10:36–43

175. Semeniuk J, Shalansky KF, Taylor N et al (2000) Evaluation of the effect of intravenous l-carnitine on quality of life in chronic hemodialysis patients. Clin Nephrol 54:470–477

176. Chazot C, Laurent G, Charra B et al (2001) Malnutrition in long-term haemodialysis survivors. Nephrol Dial Transplant 16:61–69

177. Johannsson G, Bengtsson BA, Ahlmen J (1999) Double-blind, placebo-controlled study of growth hormone treatment in elderly patients undergoing chronic hemodialysis: anabolic effect and functional improvement. Am J Kidney Dis 33:709–717

178. Fouque D, Peng SC, Shamir E, Kopple JD (2000) Recombinant human insulin-like growth factor-1 induces an anabolic response in malnourished CAPD patients. Kidney Int 57:646–654

179. Johnson CA (2000) Use of androgens in patients with renal failure. Semin Dial 13:36–39

180. Chang JW, Yang WS, Min WK et al (2002) Effects of simvastatin on high-sensitivity C-reactive protein and serum albumin in hemodialysis patients. Am J Kidney Dis 39:1213–1217

181. Seliger SL, Weiss NS, Gillen DL et al (2002) HMG-CoA reductase inhibitors are associated with reduced mortality in ESRD patients. Kidney Int 61:297–304

182. Stenvinkel P, Andersson P, Wang T et al (1999) Do ACE-inhibitors suppress tumour necrosis factor-alpha production in advanced chronic renal failure? J Intern Med 246:503–507

183. Boaz M, Smetana S, Weinstein T et al (2000) Secondary prevention with antioxidants of cardiovascular disease in endstage renal disease (SPACE): randomised placebo-controlled trial. Lancet 356:1213–1218

184. Abbey M (1995) The importance of vitamin E in reducing cardiovascular risk. Nutr Rev 53:S28–S32

185. Hoogwerf BJ, Young JB (2000) The HOPE study. Ramipril lowered cardiovascular risk, but vitamin E did not. Cleve Clin J Med 67:287–293

186. Lonn E, Yusuf S, Hoogwerf B et al (2002) Effects of vitamin E on cardiovascular and microvascular outcomes in high-risk patients with diabetes: results of the HOPE study and MICRO-HOPE substudy. Diabetes Care 25:1919–1927

187. Clermont G, Lecour S, Cabanne JF et al (2001) Vitamin E-coated dialyzer reduces oxidative stress in hemodialysis patients. Free Radic Biol Med 31:233–241

188. Bloembergen WE, Hakim RM, Stannard DC et al (1999) Relationship of dialysis membrane and cause-specific mortality. Am J Kidney Dis 33:1–10

189. Schindler R, Boenisch O, Fischer C, Frei U (2000) Effect of the hemodialysis membrane on the inflammatory reaction in vivo. Clin Nephrol 53:452–459

190. Memoli B, Minutolo R, Bisesti V et al (2002) Changes of serum albumin and C-reactive protein are related to changes of interleukin-6 release by peripheral blood mononuclear cells in hemodialysis patients treated with different membranes. Am J Kidney Dis 39:266–273

191. Chertow GM, Johansen KL, Lew N et al (2000) Vintage, nutritional status, and survival in hemodialysis patients. Kidney Int 57:1176–1181

192. Kalantar-Zadeh K, Block G, Horwich T, Fonarow GC (2004) Reverse epidemiology of conventional cardiovascular risk factors in patients with chronic heart failure. J Am Coll Cardiol 43:1439–1444

# Gastrointestinal Diseases

Hiroyuki Okano

## Introduction

The pathophysiology, evaluation, and treatment of malnutrition have been extensively investigated in recent years, and knowledge has accumulated gradually. As a result, it is now well-known that several benign digestive diseases may cause malnutrition. This chapter reviews recent clinical aspects of malnutrition related to common digestive diseases, such as Crohn's disease, short bowel syndrome, chronic liver diseases, and chronic pancreatitis. In addition, recent progress in nutritional support in the treatment of these diseases is discussed.

## Crohn's Disease

The incidence of Crohn's disease has been rising steadily. Crohn's disease is a chronic transmural inflammation that may involve any portion of the gastrointestinal tract but most commonly involves the ileum. Malnutrition, due to reduced dietary intake, malabsorption, enteric loss of nutrients, increased caloric needs, and drug-nutrient interactions, accompanies Crohn's disease in 25–80% of cases [1, 2].

The nutritional status of patients with Crohn's disease is already affected negatively at the time of diagnosis [3]. Considering that malnutrition has a negative effect on morbidity and mortality of hospitalised patients [2, 4], an early diagnosis is of great importance to improve the prognosis of these patients.

In the following sections, malnutrition in Crohn's disease is discussed according to the deficiency of macronutrients (protein and energy) and micronutrients (vitamins, minerals and electrolytes) (Table 1).

### Protein-Energy Malnutrition

The main cause of protein-energy malnutrition in Crohn's disease patients is anorexia, probably resulting from postprandial abdominal pain, diarrhoea, dietary restriction, and the side effects of medications [5, 6]. In addition, animal studies have shown that anorexia can result from increased levels of tumour necrosis factor (TNF)-$\alpha$, interleukin (IL)-1, and other cytokines [7, 8]. These weight-loss-inducing cytokines increase the expression of leptin mRNA in adipose tissue as well as plasma

**Table 1.** Nutritional problems of patients with Crohn's disease. (Data from [9])

| Deficiency | Assessment |
| --- | --- |
| Protein-energy | Subjective global assessment, serum albumin and total protein (reduced) |
| Vitamin | Erythrocyte, folate, vitamin B12, INR (will often be high because of reduced vitamin K-dependent coagulation factors), vitamin D, parathyroid hormone (increased secondary to low serum calcium levels) |
| Minerals and electrolytes | Calcium, magnesium, phosphorus, sodium, potassium, chloride, phosphate, ferritin, iron, serum electrolytes |

*INR*, International Normalised Ratio

levels of leptin, despite the decrease in food intake that normally suppresses leptin expression [10-11]. Thus, leptin may also be involved in anorexia accompanying Crohn's disease. In contrast, Lanfranchi and Geerling showed that energy intake was not decreased, but tended to increase in patients with Crohn's disease in the stage of remission or low activity [13, 14]. These results suggest that the amount of dietary intake in patients with Crohn's disease depends on the activity of the disease.

It has also been proposed that weight loss in patients with Crohn's disease is caused by increased resting caloric needs [15]. Actually, active inflammation, infection, sepsis, and accelerated mucosal turnover may result in increased nutritional requirements; however, Chan and Stokes showed that total energy expenditure was not high in patients with Crohn's disease [16, 17]. Thus, there is a lack of consensus as to whether the basal metabolic rate is increased in these patients.

Macronutrient status can be assessed using the subjective global assessment (SGA), in addition to measurements of serum albumin and total protein [18, 19]. The SGA is a qualitative assessment of the severity of a patient's malnutrition, based on weight loss, dietary intake, gastrointestinal symptoms, functional capacity, disease activity, muscle mass, subcutaneous fat, oedema, and ascites. The SGA has been shown to be reproducible among observers, with better than 80% agreement when two independent observers assessed the same patient [18, 19].

## Vitamins, Minerals, and Electrolytes

A wide array of vitamin, mineral, and electrolyte deficiencies frequently occurs in Crohn's disease patients and with variable clinical significance. These deficiencies may result from extensive inflammation, surgical resection of small bowel, or both, and require haematological and biochemical examination. The prevalence of decreased nutrient levels among patients with Crohn's disease is summarised in Table 2. Of particular clinical relevance is the deficiency in iron, vitamin B12, folate, calcium, vitamin D, and zinc.

**Table 2.** Prevalence of nutritional deficiencies among patients with Crohn's disease. (Data from [20])

| Deficiency | Prevalence (%) |
| --- | --- |
| Weight loss | 65–76 |
| Growth retardation | 40 |
| Hypoalbuminaemia | 25–80 |
| Anaemia | 60–80 |
| Iron | 39 |
| Folate | 54 |
| Vitamin B12 | 48 |
| Calcium | 13 |
| Magnesium | 14–88 |
| Potassium | 6–20 |
| Zinc | 40–50 |

## Iron

Anaemia is very common in patients with Crohn's disease and its cause is multifactorial. Since the serum iron level is low in both iron-deficient anaemia and anaemia resulting from chronic disease, the total iron-binding capacity, or transferrin level, can be useful in distinguishing between them. However, it may also be necessary to evaluate the effect of iron therapy or to measure iron levels in bone marrow.

## Vitamin B12

Since Crohn's disease frequently involves the terminal ileum, where the vitamin B12-intrinsic factor complex is absorbed, serious impairment of the enterohepatic circulation of vitamin B12 is commonly observed in Crohn's disease patients. Moreover, because vitamin B12 stores in the liver must decrease before serum concentrations become low, the incidence of decreased vitamin B12 stores is probably quite high [21]. Megaloblastic anaemia is commonly seen with vitamin B12 deficiency; however, the patient seldom manifests symptoms of deficiency, such as paresthaesia, numbness, gait ataxia, anosmia, faecal incontinence, leg weakness, impaired manual dexterity, urinary incontinence, or personality changes.

## Folate

Folate supplementation is also frequently required, because patients with Crohn's disease have poor dietary intake and enhanced intestinal loss. In addition, sulfasalazine, which is used for therapy of Crohn's disease, competitively inhibits the jejunal folate-conjugating enzyme, often producing folate malabsorption [22], leading to folate deficiency and subsequent megaloblastic anaemia.

## Calcium and Vitamin D

Osteoporosis is increasingly being recognised as a leading extra-intestinal complication of inflammatory bowel disease. Calcium is absorbed in the proximal small intestine by a vitamin D-dependent $Ca^{2+}$-binding protein, and vitamin D is absorbed in the duodenum and jejunum. Therefore, in Crohn's disease patients with extended inflammation or resection of the small intestine, osteoporosis results from impaired absorption of calcium and vitamin D.

However, there are also some conflicting data suggesting that many factors, other than calcium or vitamin D deficiency, contribute to the pathogenesis of osteoporosis in Crohn's disease [23, 24]. These factors include cytokines, such as TNF-α, that disproportionately stimulate osteoclast activity, or corticosteroid usage [25, 26]. Overt vitamin D deficiency disease may occur in Crohn's disease patients and patients often present with bone pain and mild myopathy. Other symptoms at presentation include bone pain and mild myopathy.

## Zinc

Acute inflammation and hypoalbuminaemia may decrease serum zinc concentrations, despite normal total-body zinc content [27]. Zinc deficiency is associated with altered taste sensation, decreased oral intake causing further malnutrition [27, 28], and delayed wound healing.

## Others

The precise mechanism involved in the development of Crohn's disease is unknown: however, the effects of oxidative stress on the bowels of patients with active Crohn's disease are thought to play a role [29, 30].

Unlike normal conditions in the intestine, an imbalance between endogenous anti-oxidant defences and free-radical production is seen in Crohn's disease [31]. Circulating nutritional anti-oxidants, such as β-carotene, vitamin C, vitamin E, selenium, and zinc, are important factors in the prevention of free-radical-mediated tissue injury; however, serum concentrations of these anti-oxidants were reported to be low in patients with Crohn's disease [32], whereas no clinical signs of deficiency were seen.

## Nutritional Support

The indications for nutritional support of patients with Crohn's disease are largely based on clinical experience, although the role of enteral diets for inducing remission continues to be debated. Three meta-analyses on enteral nutrition as primary therapy in Crohn's disease have been published [33–35]. These reports similarly demonstrate that clinical remission is more often successfully induced with corticosteroids than enteral diets, although enteral nutrition remains an important therapeutic tool. The precise mechanism by which an enteral diet induces remission in Crohn's disease is not understood, although several mechanisms of action have been proposed, including reduction of immune stimuli in the gut [36], nutritional improvement [37], bowel rest, a trophic effect of glutamine [38], and reduction of intestinal permeability [39]. In any event, more randomised, controlled trial data subjected to meta-analyses are required to confirm the clinical effect of enteral nutrition in the treatment of Crohn's disease.

## Short Bowel Syndrome

Short bowel syndrome is a malabsorptive state of the small intestine resulting from intestinal resection. When more than 75% of the small intestine is resected, a clinical syndrome usually occurs. Its major features are diarrhoea, malabsorption, and malnutrition. The severity of this disease depends on the length and site of residual intestine, as well as other factors. In addition, adaptation of the residual intestine following resection may compensate the impaired absorbing function to some extent.

## Adaptation

The adaptation capacity of the proximal small bowel following resection is greater than that of the distal one. Compensatory changes, such as slight lengthening and increases in diameter and villus height have been observed [40–44], although the precise mechanism of adaptation has not been determined. Several factors, including gut hormones, have been proposed to play a role in adaptation [45]. Recently, glucagon-like peptide 1 (GLP-1) and glucagon-like peptide 2 (GLP-2) were suggested to be involved in the adaptation of the small bowel. Jeppesen et al. observed a significant rise of GLP-1 and GLP-2 levels in patients with less than 140 cm of remnant small bowel, which provided initial data supporting a trophic hormone associated with adaptation in short bowel patients [46]. In addition, it was reported that parenteral administration of GLP-2 resulted in a significant improvement in intestinal absorption of energy, body weight, lean body mass, wet weight, and fat mass [47]. The growth-associated polyamines, putrescine, spermidine, and spermine, which increase RNA and DNA synthesis, and ornithine decarboxylase, which is the rate-limiting enzyme in polyamine synthesis, have also attracted attention as possible candidates for growth- and adaptation-inducing factors [48, 49].

## Clinical Syndrome

The clinical consequences of extensive small bowel resection are listed in Table 3. The conditions of organs that secrete digestive enzymes, the degree of adaptation, the presence or absence of an ileocoecal valve or colon influence the clinical state.

**Table 3.** Clinical consequences of short bowel syndrome. (Data from [50])

Diarrhoea/steatorrhoea

Vitamin/mineral/nutrient deficiency

Gastric acid hypersecretion

Hyperoxaluria/nephrolithiasis

Cholelithiasis

Bacterial overgrowth

## Nutrients Deficiency and Diarrhoea

Under physiological conditions, each nutrient is absorbed at a specific site of the small intestine. The majority of carbohydrates, proteins, and fats are normally absorbed within the first 150 cm of small bowel. Folic acid, calcium, magnesium, iron, vitamin C, and fat-soluble vitamins (A, D, E, and K) are also absorbed in the proximal intestine. Thus, resection of the proximal intestine means a reduction in the absorption area for these nutrients. In addition, the loss of intestinal lactase, sucrase-isomaltase, and $\alpha$-dextrinase, resulting from resection of the proximal bowel, induces carbohydrates malabsorption. Of the disaccharidases, lactase levels are the most prone to decrease, resulting in luminal hyperosmolarity. Bacterial fermentation of lactose leads to large amounts of lactic acid, which further induce osmotic diarrhoea [51].

In the terminal ileum, specialized cells are responsible for the absorption of bile salts and vitamin B12. Resection of this site cannot be compensated by adaptation and results in diarrhoea or anaemia. Indeed, following resection of less than 50 cm of ileum induces an increased concentration of bile acid delivered into the colon, leading to a watery diarrhoea [49], while resection of > 100 cm of ileum results in bile-salt depletion, leading to steatorrhaea [52]. The development of bacterial overgrowth in short bowel syndrome as a result of excluded loop, shortened intestine, loss of the ileocoecal valve, and dysmotility may further reduce the absorption of fat and vitamin B12 [53].

Carbohydrate and protein, which are not metabolised by the small bowel, are converted by colonic bacteria to short-chain fatty acids, which are readily absorbed across the colonic mucosa. Mid-chain fatty acids, which are water-soluble, are also absorbed in the colon. Therefore, the capacity for fatty acid absorption in patients with short bowel syndrome depends on the presence of colon.

## Management of Short Bowel Syndrome

Comprehensive management of patients with short bowel syndrome involves meticulous attention to meeting their metabolic and nutritional needs. Medical therapies, enteral or parenteral nutritional support, and, in some cases, consideration of surgical intervention are necessary.

Patients with short bowel syndrome should receive adequate macronutrients and micronutrients to prevent energy malnutrition and specific nutrient deficiencies, and should be provided with sufficient fluids to prevent dehydration. Most patients will require total parenteral nutrition while post-operative complications are addressed and until metabolic issues stabilise. This period is marked by significant fluid and electrolyte loss due to severe diarrhoea (stage I). Subsequently, there is stabilisation of the diarrhoea as adaptation progresses. Maximal adaptation may require up to 2 years to occur (stage II). During the long-term management period, many patients will be able to achieve nutritional and metabolic stability solely with oral intake. Nonetheless, lifelong supplementation or complete parenteral support is needed (stage III) (Table 4).

Special pharmacologic enhancement of intestinal adaptation has been discussed. Since GLP-2 may promote adaptation of the small intestine, as previously described [47], investigational studies of a longer-acting, genetically engineered analogue of GLP-2 are underway. Details of the dietary macronutrients and micronutrients required for patients with short bowel syndrome were provided in the AGA Technical Review [54].

## Chronic Liver Disease

In patients with chronic liver disease, malnutrition is commonly seen regardless of whether its aetiology is alcohol or not [55, 56], and it is known that the severity of liver disease correlates with the severity of malnutrition [57]. Mechanisms of malnutrition in chronic liver disease are multifactorial and include inadequate diet, impaired digestion or absorption of nutrients, metabolic disorders, and altered energy metabolism (Table 5). One of the most important factors of malnutrition in chronic liver diseases is poor dietary intake, especially in advanced stages. Dietary restriction of sodium, liquid, and/or protein, recommended in order to prevent ascites, oedema, and encephalopathy, often results in malnutrition.

Malabsorption and maldigestion of nutrients

**Table 4.** Clinical stages of short bowel syndrome. (Data from [58])

| Stage I | Stage II | Stage III |
| --- | --- | --- |
| Immediate postoperative period (0–2 months)[a] | Bowel adaptation period (2–24 mo)[a] | Long-term management period (> 2 years)[a] |
| Careful fluid and electrolyte monitoring and replacement | Progression of oral diet Parenteral supplementation | Maximize enteral absorption with tailored regimen |
| Antisecretory therapy | Antisecretory therapy | Parenteral supplementation? |
| Antimotility therapy | Antimotility therapy | Antimotility therapy as needed |
| Total parenteral nutrition | | Vitamin and mineral supplementation as needed Surgical intervention? |

[a]Estimates

should also be noted in patients with chronic liver disease and are due to a direct ethanol effect, low intraluminal bile salt concentration, gastrointestinal bleeding, mucosal congestion, insufficiency of digestive enzymes, bacterial overgrowth, etc. In addition, lactulose or kanamycin, which is prescribed for encephalopathy, promotes malabsorption.

**Table 5.** Aetiologic factors for protein-calorie malnutrition in liver cirrhosis. (Data from [59])

Inadequate diet
   Anorexia, nausea, and vomiting
   Alteration in taste perception
   Salt-protein-restricted diets
Impaired digestion or absorption of nutrients
   Altered pancreatic or biliary secretion
   Drugs (non-absorbable disaccharides)
Metabolic disorders
   Diminished glycogen stores and glycogenolysis
   Enhanced gluconeogenesis and lipolysis
   Increased protein catabolism
Altered energy metabolism
   Hypermetabolism during complications of the disease (ascites, infections, etc)
   Decreased glucose use
   Increased lipid oxidation

## Protein-Energy Malnutrition

Patients with chronic liver disease exhibit a progressive loss of fat and muscle mass, which leads to mixed protein-energy malnutrition. When investigating whole-body protein metabolism, protein synthesis, degradation, and amino acid oxidation have to be estimated in a specific manner. McCullough and Glamour reported that there appear to be few differences in protein turnover in stable cirrhosis patients and in healthy controls, while oxidation of amino acids in these patients was generally normal or reduced [60]. However, increased protein catabolism is thought to be an important contributing factor to malnutrition because a 'normal' measurement of protein breakdown may be too high in a patient suffering from wasting. Indeed, protein turnover and catabolism can increase in this condition as well as in metabolic stress.

It continues to be debated whether body wasting in patients with liver cirrhosis is related to hypermetabolism or not. Resting energy expenditure (REE), estimated by use of indirect calorimetry, in stable cirrhotic patients is usually not significantly different from that in normal controls. However, Shanbhogue et al. reported that REE per g creatinine in 24-h urine in end-stage liver disease patients was significantly higher than that in the normal population [61]. Muller et al. also found hypermetabolic patients, as judged by adjusted REE, had greater losses of muscle mass, fat-free mass, and body cell mass [62].

Recently, leptin has been considered one of the main markers of nutritional status. Leptin is a cytokine-type peptide hormone that is produced mainly by adipocytes; it decreases appetite and increases energy expenditure [63]. The effect of liver disease on leptin status is a controversial issue, although some studies have shown that serum leptin increases in cirrhosis of alcoholic aetiology [64, 65]. Currently, a high serum leptin concentration in cirrhotic patients is thought to result from the increased protein-bound fraction, which is directly related to energy expenditure [66]. Since ghrelin, which is a novel endogenous ligand for the growth hormone (GH) secretagogue receptor, competes with leptin, it was also investigated in cirrhotic patients [67]. Tacke et al. reported that ghrelin increased in liver cirrhosis independent of its aetiology; however, the precise mechanisms remain unclear [68]. Ghrelin might increase to counteract metabolic decompensation in liver cirrhosis by its various metabolic functions. In a recent study, it was shown that long-term administration of leptin increases ghrelin mRNA expression in the stomach, with a concomitant decrease in food intake and body weight in rats [69]: therefore, increased leptin may play a role in liver cirrhosis.

Most patients with cirrhosis have impaired glucose tolerance due to insulin resistance, which results in impaired glucose utilisation [70]. Defects in peripheral receptor binding of insulin and nonoxidative glucose disposal in the form of muscle glycogen appear to be responsible for peripheral insulin insensitivity, characteristic of nearly all cirrhotic patients independent of clinical or nutritional status. Metabolic changes are obvious in the fasting state because the liver of cirrhotic patients is unable to store enough glycogen to supply an adequate amount of glucose through glycogenolysis [71]. Therefore, gluconeogenesis is activated, leading to a premature protein catabolism to supply amino acids for glucose synthesis. The preferential use of lipid substrates as alternative energy sources is activated in liver cirrhosis as a consequence of impaired glucose metabolism. Lipolysis is enhanced and lipid oxidation is increased, resulting in the loss of fat tissue [70].

## Micronutrient Metabolism

Deficiencies of water-soluble vitamins, including vitamin C, and the B complex compounds, are particularly common in cirrhotic patients with active alcoholism. Similarly, low plasma concentration of fat-soluble vitamins (A, E, D, and K) may occur in patients with cirrhosis of any aetiology [72]. Abnormalities in vitamin activation, conversion, release, and transport by carrier molecules all result from hepatocellular injury. Low serum levels of some trace elements, such as zinc and selenium, have also been detected in cirrhotic patients [73]. In most patients with liver cirrhosis, while micronutrient deficiencies are clinically silent, the biological antioxidant effects of micronutrients are notably impaired.

In liver cirrhosis, one of the most important micronutrients is zinc. Zinc deficiency can alter cognitive function, appetite and taste, immune function, and protein metabolism, and has been claimed to be a precipitating factor for hepatic encephalopathy [74]. Vitamin A and other retinoids are known to have antineoplastic properties. Cirrhotic patients with hepatocellular carcinoma (HCC) had significantly lower retinol levels than patients with cirrhosis alone, and it suggested that decreased serum retinol may be a risk factor for the development of HCC [75]. Although many other studies have shown a relationship between retinol and HCC, further research is needed to confirm it.

## Nutritional Support

The objective of nutritional support in patients with liver cirrhosis is to provide adequate calories, protein, and other nutrients to ensure the availability of synthetic and energy substrates to hepatocytes without inducing hepatic encephalopathy (Table 6) [76, 77]. In general, cirrhotic patients without encephalopathy require no restriction of protein, but a diet high in complex carbohydrates and calories and supplemented with multivitamins, calcium,

**Table 6.** Nutritional support for liver failure with cirrhosis. (Data from [77])

| |
|---|
| Cirrhosis without encephalopathy |
| No protein restriction (1.0–1.2 g/kg per day) |
| High complex carbohydrate, high-calorie diet (30–35 Kcal/kg per day) |
| Frequent small meals and bedtime snack |
| Water restriction only with hyponatraemia |
| Sodium restriction only with ascites or oedema |
| Supplemental multivitamins, calcium, zinc, and magnesium |
| |
| Cirrhosis with acute encephalopathy |
| Temporary protein restriction (0.6–0.8 g/kg per day) until encephalopathy is ameliorated or resolved |
| Substitute or supplement with BCAA for refractory encephalopathy or negative nitrogen balance |
| Normal protein intake (1.0–1.2 g/kg per day) as encephalopathy resolves |
| High-calorie diet (30–35 Kcal/kg per day) enterally or with TPN |
| Water restriction with hyponatraemia |
| Sodium restriction with ascites or oedema |
| |
| Cirrhosis with chronic encephalopathy |
| Restrict standard protein (0.6–0.8 g/kg per day) |
| Initiate vegetarian diet or high-fiber diet with low animal protein |
| Frequent carbohydrate-rich meals and a bedtime snack |
| Sodium restriction with severe ascites or oedema |
| Water restriction only with severe hyponatraemia |
| Supplemental vitamins and minerals as needed |

zinc, and magnesium is essential. In case of hyponatraemia, water restriction should be imposed, and in case of ascites or oedema, sodium restriction is needed. Cirrhosis patients with encephalopathy require protein restriction and solutions enriched in branched-chain amino acids (BCAAs) [78]. Because BCAAs compete with tryptophan, which is the precursor of brain serotonin, across the blood-brain barrier, they block the increased hypothalamic activity of serotonin that strongly decreases appetite; therefore, BCAAs may also serve to counteract anorexia and cachexia [79].

Nutritional support for patients with liver cirrhosis is a great challenge and continues to be controversial. Based on the results of a limited number of trials, there is no apparent beneficial effect of parenteral nutrition or protein-sparing therapy on the mortality of patients with liver cirrhosis. Only intravenous BCAA solutions have been confirmed by meta-analysis to be valuable in treating hepatic encephalopathy [80].

## Chronic Pancreatitis

Chronic pancreatitis refers to permanent damage to the exocrine pancreas with or without significant changes in function. Several forms of chronic pancreatitis exist, including alcoholic, tropical, hereditary, autoimmune, and idiopathic [81]; however, in developed countries, almost 70 % of chronic pancreatitis is caused by alcohol use. One large-scale study revealed that almost half of patients with alcoholic chronic pancreatitis developed exocrine insufficiency over a mean follow-up of 14.6 years [82], leading to marked weight loss. Thus, patients with chronic pancreatitis are at high risk for poor nutritional status.

### Mechanisms of Malnutrition in Chronic Pancreatitis

Malnutrition and weight loss in patients with chronic pancreatitis mainly result from maldigestion and abdominal pain (Fig. 1). The loss of aci-

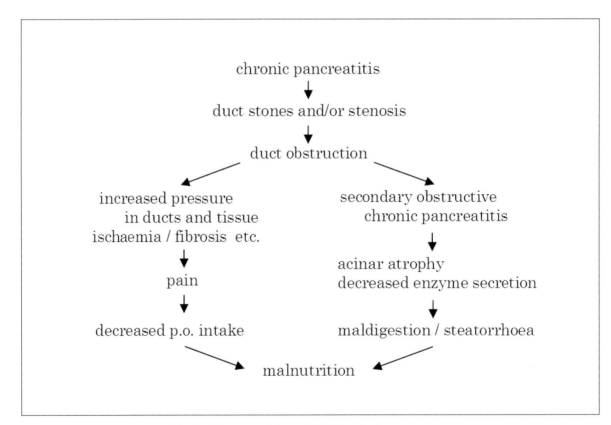

**Fig. 1.** Malnutrition in patients with chronic pancreatitis. Modified from [83]

nar cells causes insufficient secretion of lipase, colipase, amylase, and proteases, which results in maldigestion of lipid, carbohydrates, and protein. Of these nutrients, fat maldigestion is the most clinically apparent. However, because the pancreas secretes a large surplus of enzymes, pancreatic enzyme output must be reduced to less than 10% of normal before fat absorption is appreciably impaired. Fat digestion depends not only on the amount of pancreatic lipase and colipase, but also on the activity of these enzymes. Since lipase has maximal enzymatic activity in the range of pH 6.5–8, decreased bicarbonate delivery to the duodenum leads to inactivation of lipase through a pH drop. In addition, since duodenal acidification precipitates bile salts, mixed micelle formation is impaired, resulting in the malabsorption of fat. All these pathophysiological events contribute to massive steatorrhoea, leading to malnutrition and weight loss in chronic pancreatitis patients.

Moreover, abdominal pain induced by food ingestion is common in these patients and results in decreased oral intake leading to weight loss. Inadequate food intake owing to recurrent or near continuous pain usually accounts for the initial 10–20% loss of body weight. However, the pathophysiology of this abdominal pain is poorly understood. Pancreatic hypertension, elevated interstitial fluid pressure, pancreatic ischaemia, damage to pancreatic nerves, tissue necrosis, pseudocyst formation, and common bile duct and/or duodenal obstruction may cause the abdominal pain [84].

Other factors may contribute to malnutrition in patients with chronic pancreatitis. Increased resting energy expenditure, small-bowel bacterial overgrowth, severe alcoholism, and poor control of associated diabetes may have a role. Hebuterne et al. reported that the measured REE was significantly higher than the predicted energy expenditure in underweight patients with chronic pancreatitis but not in control groups [85]. Therefore, weight loss accompanied by hypermetabolism should be taken into consideration in patients with chronic pancreatitis. Small-bowel bacterial overgrowth deconjugates bile salt, impairing micelle formation. Almost 40% of patients with chronic pancreatitis have co-existent small-bowel

bacterial overgrowth [86]. The mechanisms for this association are not clear but may include small-bowel dysmotility induced by narcotics, shifts in hormone levels (especially cholecystokinin) induced by chronic pancreatitis, or previous surgery. In addition, in the majority of patients suffering from chronic pancreatitis, pancreatic endocrine insufficiency is correlated with exocrine dysfunction. The prevalence of impaired or diabetic glucose tolerance is 40–70%, and half of these patients suffer from an insulin-dependent diabetes mellitus. The aetiology of diabetes mellitus that results from chronic pancreatitis includes a loss of β-cells secreting insulin, impaired β-cell responsiveness to glucose, and disturbances of the enteroinsular axis via diminished levels of incretins. The susceptibility to severe hypoglycaemia in patients with diabetes mellitus secondary to chronic pancreatitis is higher than in type I diabetics. This is mainly caused by impaired glucagon secretion and also influenced by malnutrition and concomitant hepatic dysfunction due to the alcoholic toxicity [87].

Although abnormalities can be identified on small-bowel function tests and deficiencies of fat-soluble vitamins, calcium, zinc, selenium, etc. may be demonstrated, the presence of clinical syndromes are rare, as with demonstrable low B12 uptake in some 10–15% of patients [88].

The absorption of fat-soluble vitamins (A, E, and K) is usually preserved [84, 88, 89] in patients with chronic pancreatitis, and, although vitamin D is not significantly reduced, osteopaenia and osteoporosis are much more common than previously thought [90]. Deficiencies of water-soluble vitamin are often seen in chronic alcoholics, and impairment of copper, selenium, and zinc metabolism is particularly pronounced in patients with combined chronic pancreatitis and diabetes mellitus [91].

## Management of Enzyme Insufficiency

Nutritional support of patients with chronic pancreatitis has created a challenge for clinicians. The reduced ingestion of food, which results from abdominal pain, together with the increased metabolic demands of this disease often cause a negative energy balance, and occasionally undernutrition or malnutrition. There are limited data on the nutritional assessment of outpatients with chronic pancreatitis, and the efficacy of enzyme therapy remains controversial. Trolli et al. demonstrated that patients undergoing enzyme therapy had better nutritional status, as based on serum albumin levels and percent of ideal body weight [92]. Therefore, enzyme therapy that is simple and has few side effects should be used in patients with chronic pancreatitis [93]. The pancreatic enzyme supplements currently on the market have high enzymatic activity; however, their efficacy depends on many factors, including enzyme formulation, dosage, and scheduling. This is especially the case for lipase, which is easily denatured by gastric acid; therefore, acid-suppressing medications and enteric-release enzyme formulations should be used in the treatment of chronic pancreatitis patients.

## References

1. Lewis JD, Fisher RL (1994) Nutrition support in inflammatory bowel disease. Med Clin North Am 78:1443–1456
2. Zurita VF, Rawls DE, Dyck WP (1995) Nutritional support in inflammatory bowel disease. Dig Dis 13:92–107
3. Geerling BJ, Badart-Smook A, Stockbrugger RW, Brummer RJ (2000) Comprehensive nutritional status in recently diagnosed patients with inflammatory bowel disease compared with population controls. Eur J Clin Nutr 54:514–521
4. Charney P (1995) Nutrition assessment in the 1990s: where are we now? Nutr Clin Pract 10:131–139
5. Schneeweiss B, Lochs H, Zauner C et al (1999) Energy and substrate metabolism in patients with active Crohn's disease. J Nutr 129:844–848
6. Rigaud D, Angel LA, Cerf M et al (1994) Mechanisms of decreased food intake during weight loss in adult Crohn's disease patients without obvious malabsorption. Am J Clin Nutr 60:775–781
7. Bodnar RJ, Pasternak GW, Mann PE et al (1989) Mediation of anorexia by human recombinant tumor necrosis factor through a peripheral action in the rat. Cancer Res 49:6280–6284
8. Hellerstein MK, Meydani SN, Meydani M et al (1989) Interleukin-1-induced anorexia in the rat. Influence of prostaglandins. J Clin Invest 84:228–235
9. Jeejeebhoy KN (2002) Clinical nutrition: 6. Management of nutritional problems of patients with Crohn's disease. CMAJ 166:913–918
10. Sarraf P, Frederich RC, Turner EM et al (1997) Multiple cytokines and acute inflammation raise mouse leptin levels: potential role in inflammatory anorexia. J Exp Med 185:171–175
11. Grunfeld C, Zhao C, Fuller J et al (1996) Endotoxin and cytokines induce expression of leptin, the ob gene product, in hamsters. J Clin Invest 97:2152–2157
12. Finck BN, Kelley KW, Dantzer R et al (1998) In vivo and in vitro evidence for the involvement of tumor necrosis factor-alpha in the induction of leptin by lipopolysaccharide. Endocrinology 139:2278–2283
13. Lanfranchi GA, Brignola C, Campieri M et al (1984) Assessment of nutritional status in Crohn's disease in remission or low activity. Hepatogastroenterology 31:129–132
14. Geerling BJ, Badart-Smook A, Stockbrugger RW, Brummer RJ (1998) Comprehensive nutritional status in patients with long-standing Crohn disease currently in remission. Am J Clin Nutr 67:919–926
15. Royall D, Greenberg GR, Allard JP et al (1995) Total enteral nutrition support improves body composition of patients with active Crohn's disease. JPEN 19:95–99
16. Chan AT, Fleming CR, O'Fallon WM, Huizenga KA (1986) Estimated versus measured basal energy requirements in patients with Crohn's disease. Gastroenterology 91:75–78
17. Stokes MA, Hill GL (1993) Total energy expenditure in patients with Crohn's disease: measurement by the combined body scan technique. JPEN 17: 3–7
18. Baker JP, Detsky AS, Wesson DE et al (1982) Nutritional assessment: a comparison of clinical judgement and objective measurements. N Engl J Med 306:969–972
19. Detsky AS, McLaughlin JR, Baker JP et al (1987) What is subjective global assessment of nutritional status? JPEN 11:8–13
20. Song HK, Buzby GP (2001) Nutritional support for Crohn's disease. Surg Clin North Am 81:103–115
21. Loew D, Wanitschke R, Schroedter A (1999) Studies on vitamin B12 status in the elderly-prophylactic and therapeutic consequences. Int J Vitam Nutr Res 69:228–233
22. Hoffbrand AV, Stewart JS, Booth CC, Mollin DL (1968) Folate deficiency in Crohn's disease: incidence, pathogenesis, and treatment. Br Med J 2:71–75
23. Silvennoinen J (1996) Relationships between vitamin D, parathyroid hormone and bone mineral density in inflammatory bowel disease. J Intern Med 239:131–137
24. Scharla SH, Minne HW, Lempert UG et al (1994) Bone mineral density and calcium regulating hormones in patients with inflammatory bowel disease (Crohn's disease and ulcerative colitis). Exp Clin Endocrinol 102:44–49

25. Murch SH, Lamkin VA, Savage MO et al (1991) Serum concentrations of tumour necrosis factor alpha in childhood chronic inflammatory bowel disease. Gut 32:913–917

26. Bernstein CN, Seeger LL, Sayre JW et al (1995) Decreased bone density in inflammatory bowel disease is related to corticosteroid use and not disease diagnosis. J Bone Miner Res 10:250–256

27. Hendricks KM, Walker WA (1988) Zinc deficiency in inflammatory bowel disease. Nutr Rev 46:401–408

28. Tiomny E, Horwitz C, Graff E et al (1982) Serum zinc and taste acuity in Tel-Aviv patients with inflammatory bowel disease. Am J Gastroenterol 77:101–104

29. Nielsen OH, Ahnfelt-Ronne I (1991) Involvement of oxygen-derived free radicals in the pathogenesis of chronic inflammatory bowel disease. Klin Wochenschr 69:995–1000

30. McKenzie SJ, Baker MS, Buffinton GD, Doe WF (1996) Evidence of oxidant-induced injury to epithelial cells during inflammatory bowel disease. J Clin Invest 98:136–141

31. Grisham MB (1994) Oxidants and free radicals in inflammatory bowel disease. Lancet 344:859–861

32. Di Mascio P, Murphy ME, Sies H (1991) Antioxidant defense systems: the role of carotenoids, tocopherols, and thiols. Am J Clin Nutr 53:194S–200S

33. Fernandez-Banares F, Cabre E, Esteve-Comas M, Gassull MA (1995) How effective is enteral nutrition in inducing clinical remission in active Crohn's disease? A meta-analysis of the randomized clinical trials. JPEN 19:356–364

34. Griffiths AM, Ohlsson A, Sherman PM, Sutherland LR (1995) Meta-analysis of enteral nutrition as a primary treatment of active Crohn's disease. Gastroenterology 108:1056–1067

35. Silk DB, Payne-James J (1989) Inflammatory bowel disease: nutritional implications and treatment. Proc Nutr Soc 48:355–361

36. O'Morain C, Segal AW, Levi AJ (1984) Elemental diet as primary treatment of acute Crohn's disease: a controlled trial. Br Med J (Clin Res Ed) 288:1859–1862

37. Harries AD, Jones LA, Danis V et al (1983) Controlled trial of supplemented oral nutrition in Crohn's disease. Lancet 1:887–890

38. Souba WW, Smith RJ, Wilmore DW (1985) Glutamine metabolism by the intestinal tract. JPEN J Parenter Enteral Nutr 9:608–617

39. Wyatt J, Vogelsang H, Hubl W et al (1993) Intestinal permeability and the prediction of relapse in Crohn's disease. Lancet 341:1437–1439

40. Vanderhoof JA, Langnas AN (1997) Short-bowel syndrome in children and adults. Gastroenterology 113:1767–1778

41. Solhaug JH, Tvete S (1978) Adaptive changes in the small intestine following bypass operation for obesity. Scand J Gastroenterol 13:401–408

42. Doldi SB (1991) Intestinal adaptation following jeju-no-ileal bypass. Clin Nutr 10:138–145

43. Dowling RH, Booth CC (1966) Functional compensation after small-bowel resection in man. Lancet 2:146–147

44. Weinstein LD, Shoemaker CP, Hersh T, Wright HK (1968) Enhanced intestinal absorption after small bowel resection in man. Arch Surg 99:560–561

45. Sham J, Martin G, Meddings JB, Sigalet DL (2002) Epidermal growth factor improves nutritional outcome in a rat model of short bowel syndrome. J Pediatr Surg 37:765–769

46. Jeppesen PB, Hartmann B, Thulesen J et al (2000) Elevated plasma glucagon-like peptide 1 and 2 concentrations in ileum resected short bowel patients with a preserved colon. Gut 47:370–376

47. Jeppesen PB, Hartmann B, Thulesen J et al (2001) Glucagon-like peptide 2 improves nutrient absorption and nutritional status in short-bowel patients with no colon. Gastroenterology 120:806–815

48. Welters CF, Dejong CH, Deutz NE, Heineman E (2001) Intestinal function and metabolism in the early adaptive phase after massive small bowel resection in the rat. J Pediatr Surg 36:1746–1751

49. Schiller LR (2001) Diarrhea following small bowel resection. In: Bayless TM, Hanauer SB (ed) Advanced Therapy of Inflammatory Bowel Disease. BC Decker, Hamilton, pp 471–474

50. Stollman NH, Neustater BR, Rogers AI (1996) Short-bowel syndrome. Gastroenterologist 4:118–128

51. Shanbhogue LK, Molenaar JC (1994) Short bowel syndrome: metabolic and surgical management. Br J Surg 81:486–499

52. Weser E (1976) The management of patients after small bowel resection. Gastroenterology 71:146–150

53. Edes TE (1990) Clinical management of short-bowel syndrome. Enhancing the patient's quality of life. Postgrad Med 88:91–95

54. Buchman AL, Scolapio J, Fryer J (2003) AGA technical review on short bowel syndrome and intestinal transplantation. Gastroenterology 124:1111–1134

55. Thuluvath PJ, Triger DR (1994) Evaluation of nutritional status by using anthropometry in adults with alcoholic and nonalcoholic liver disease. Am J Clin Nutr 60:269–273

56. Caregaro L, Alberino F, Amodio P et al (1996) Malnutrition in alcoholic and virus-related cirrhosis. Am J Clin Nutr 63:602–609

57. Mendenhall C, Roselle GA, Gartside P, Moritz T (1995) Relationship of protein calorie malnutrition to alcoholic liver disease: a reexamination of data from two Veterans Administration Cooperative Studies. Alcohol Clin Exp Res 19:635–641

58. Dudrick SJ, Latifi R, Fosnoch De (1991) Management of the short-bowel syndrome. Surg Clin North Am 71:625–643

59. Merli M, Nicolini G, Angeloni S, Riggio O (2002) Malnutrition is a risk factor in cirrhotic patients undergoing surgery. Nutrition 18:978–986

60. McCullough AJ, Glamour T (1993) Differences in

amino acid kinetics in cirrhosis. Gastroenterology 104:1858–1865

61. Shanbhogue RL, Bistrian BR, Jenkins RL et al (1987) Resting energy expenditure in patients with end-stage liver disease and in normal population. JPEN 113: 305–308

62. Muller MJ, Lautz HU, Plogmann B et al (1992) Energy expenditure and substrate oxidation in patients with cirrhosis: the impact of cause, clinical staging and nutritional state. Hepatology 15:782–794

63. Trayhurn P, Hoggard N, Mercer JG, Rayner DV (1999) Leptin: fundamental aspects. Int J Obes Relat Metab Disord 23:22–28

64. McCullough AJ, Bugianesi E, Marchesini G, Kalhan SC (1998) Gender-dependent alterations in serum leptin in alcoholic cirrhosis. Gastroenterology 115:947–953

65. Henriksen JH, Holst JJ, Moller S et al (1999) Increased circulating leptin in alcoholic cirrhosis: relation to release and disposal. Hepatology 29:1818–1824

66. Ockenga J, Bischoff SC, Tillmann HL et al (2000) Elevated bound leptin correlates with energy expenditure in cirrhotics. Gastroenterology 119:1656–1662

67. Kojima M, Hosoda H, Date Y et al (1999) Ghrelin is a growth-hormone-releasing acylated peptide from stomach. Nature 402:656–660

68. Tacke F, Brabant G, Kruck E et al (2003) Ghrelin in chronic liver disease. J Hepatol 38:447–454

69. Toshinai K, Mondal MS, Nakazato M et al (2001) Upregulation of Ghrelin expression in the stomach upon fasting, insulin-induced hypoglycemia, and leptin administration. Biochem Biophys Res Commun 281:1220–1225

70. Merli M, Eriksson LS, Hagenfeldt L, Wahren J (1986) Splanchnic and leg exchange of free fatty acids in patients with liver cirrhosis. J Hepatol 3:348–355

71. Riggio O, Merli M, Leonetti F et al (1997) Impaired nonoxidative glucose metabolism in patients with liver cirrhosis: effects of two insulin doses. Metabolism 46:840–843

72. Cabre E, Gassull MA (1993) Nutritional aspects of chronic liver disease. Clin Nutr 12:S52–S63

73. McClain CJ, Marsano L, Burk RF, Bacon B (1991) Trace metals in liver disease. Semin Liver Dis 11:321–339

74. Van der Rijt CC, Schalm SW, Schat H et al (1991) Overt hepatic encephalopathy precipitated by zinc deficiency. Gastroenterology 100:1114–1118

75. Newsome PN, Beldon I, Moussa Y et al (2000) Low serum retinol levels are associated with hepatocellular carcinoma in patients with chronic liver disease. Aliment Pharmacol Ther 14:1295–1301

76. Latifi R, Killam RW, Dudrick SJ (1991) Nutritional support in liver failure. Surg Clin North Am 71:567–578

77. Dudrick SJ, Kavic SM (2002) Hepatobiliary nutrition: history and future. J Hepatobiliary Pancreat Surg 9:459–468

78. Teran JC, McCullough AJ (2001) Nutrition in liver diseases. In: Gottschlich MM (ed) The science and practice of nutrition support. A case-based core curriculum. Kendall/Hunt, Dubuque, pp 539–552

79. Inui A (2002) Cancer anorexia-cachexia syndrome: current issues in research and management. CA Cancer J Clin 52:72–91

80. Koretz RL, Lipman TO, Klein S (2001) American Gastroenterological Association. AGA technical review on parenteral nutrition. Gastroenterology 121:970–1001

81. Etemad B, Whitcomb DC (2001) Chronic pancreatitis: diagnosis, classification, and new genetic developments. Gastroenterology 120:682–707

82. Layer P, Yamamoto H, Kalthoff L et al (1994) The different courses of early- and late-onset idiopathic and alcoholic chronic pancreatitis. Gastroenterology 107:1481–1487

83. Testoni PA, Tittobello A (1997) Endoscopy in pancreatic disease: diagnosis and therapy. Mosby, Chicago, p 100

84. Apte MV, Keogh GW, Wilson JS (1999) Chronic pancreatitis: complications and management. J Clin Gastroenterol 29:225–240

85. Hebuterne X, Hastier P, Peroux JL et al (1996) Resting energy expenditure in patients with alcoholic chronic pancreatitis. Dig Dis Sci 41:533–539

86. Kumar A, Forsmark CE, Toskes PP (1996 ) Small bowel bacterial overgrowth: The changing face of an old disease. Gastroenterology 110:A340 (abs)

87. Raue G, Keim V (1999) Secondary diabetes in chronic pancreatitis. Z Gastroenterol. 1:4–9

88. Twersky Y, Bank S (1989) Nutritional deficiencies in chronic pancreatitis. Gastroenterol Clin North Am. 18:543–565

89. Scolapio JS, Malhi-Chowla N, Ukleja A (1999) Nutrition supplementation in patients with acute and chronic pancreatitis. Gastroenterol Clin North Am 28:695–707

90. Haaber AB, Rosenfalck AM, Hansen B et al (2000) Bone mineral metabolism, bone mineral density, and body composition in patients with chronic pancreatitis and pancreatic exocrine insufficiency. Int J Pancreatol 27:21–27

91. Quilliot D, Dousset B, Guerci B et al (2001) Evidence that diabetes mellitus favors impaired metabolism of zinc, copper, and selenium in chronic pancreatitis. Pancreas 22:299–306

92. Trolli PA, Conwell DL, Zuccaro G Jr (2001) Pancreatic enzyme therapy and nutritional status of outpatients with chronic pancreatitis. Gastroenterol Nurs 24:84–87

93. Pitchumoni CS (1998) Chronic pancreatitis: pathogenesis and management of pain. J Clin Gastroenterol 27:101–107

# Chronic Obstructive Pulmonary Disease (COPD) and Treatment of COPD-Related Cachexia

Emiel F.M. Wouters

## Introduction

The association between weight loss and severe chronic obstructive pulmonary disease (COPD) has long been recognised. Fowler and Godlee [1] first described the association of weight loss and emphysema in the late nineteenth century. Attempts to establish different COPD classifications led to the realisation that body weight might be an important disease determinant [2]. This led to the classical description of the pink puffer (emphysematous type) and the blue bloater (bronchitic type). The pink puffing patient is characteristically thin, breathless, and with marked hyperinflation of the chest. The blue and bloated patient may not be particularly breathless, at least when at rest, but has severe central cyanosis. In the 1960s, several studies reported that low body weight and weight loss are negatively associated with survival in COPD [3]. Nevertheless, therapeutic management of weight loss and muscle wasting in patients with COPD has become of interest only recently, since these features were generally considered as terminal progression in the disease process and therefore inevitable and irreversible. Furthermore, it was even suggested that weight loss is an adaptive mechanism to decreased oxygen consumption. Recent studies have challenged this conclusion and showed that weight loss and low body weight are associated with poor prognosis, independent of, or at least not closely correlated with, the degree of lung function impairment [4, 5]. Moreover, weight gain after nutritional support was associated with decreased mortality [6].

The renewed interest in therapeutic nutritional support in COPD runs parallel to changing concepts in the management of the disease, predominantly aiming treatment not only at primary organ failure but also at the systemic consequences of the disease, including nutritional depletion. Depletion in this context refers both to weight loss and, more specifically, to a decrease in body cell mass, defined as the actively metabolising (organs) and contracting (muscle) tissue. The term depletion is introduced since the decrease in body cell mass in acute and chronic disease is caused not only by decreased food intake, as suggested by the term 'malnutrition,' but also by metabolic alterations. Fat-free mass can be considered as a good estimate of body cell mass [7].

In clinically stable patients with moderate to severe COPD, depletion of fat-free mass has been reported in 20% of COPD out-patients [8] and in 35% of those eligible for pulmonary rehabilitation [9]. Limited data are available regarding the prevalence of nutritional depletion in representative groups of patients with mild COPD and in patients suffering from acute respiratory failure, although in the latter values up to 50% have been reported [10]. There is no clear relationship between measures of nutritional status and airflow obstruction, but weight loss and underweight are associated with decreased diffusing capacity and are observed more frequently in emphysematous patients than in patients with chronic bronchitis [11]. The difference in body weight between the two COPD subtypes is merely a difference in fat mass. Depletion of fat-free mass, despite a relative preservation of fat mass, also occurs in chronic bronchitis [11].

## Rationale for Nutritional Support

Despite the fact that COPD is characterised by an irreversible airflow obstruction, current medical treatment is aimed at reaching the personal best value of lung function and prevention of a rapid decline. This treatment has had only limited success, particularly when considering improvement of daily functioning and quality of life. The most prominent symptoms of COPD are dyspnoea and impaired exercise capacity. During the past 10 years, research has shown that, besides airflow obstruction and loss of alveolar structure, skeletal muscle weakness is an important determinant of these symptoms [12]. In addition, recent studies have shown that skeletal muscle dysfunction is predominantly determined by skeletal muscle mass in COPD [11, 13].

Several groups have also reported that, besides peripheral muscle strength, body weight and whole body fat-free mass are significant determinants of exercise capacity and exercise response [14–16]. Patients with a depleted fat-free mass had lower peak oxygen consumption, peak work rate, and an early onset of lactic acid production compared to non-depleted patients. These findings suggest that the functional consequences of nutritional depletion not only relate to muscle wasting per se, but also to alterations in muscle morphology and metabolism. Indeed, experimental studies and studies of other wasting conditions have shown that nutritional depletion causes generalised fibre atrophy and specifically decreases the cross-sectional area of type II muscle fibres [17]. Furthermore, altered levels of glycolytic and oxidative enzymes have been described [17, 18] as well as depletion of energy-rich substrates, such as phosphocreatine and glycogen [19, 20].

The functional consequences of underweight and particularly of depletion of fat-free mass are also reflected in a decreased health status as measured by a disease-specific questionnaire [21].

Examination of several different COPD populations have now convincingly shown that a low body mass index (BMI) and weight loss are associated with an increased mortality risk [4, 6]. Remarkably, overweight patients with moderate to severe COPD even have a lower mortality risk than normal-weight patients [4, 6]. After adjustment for the effect of age, gender, lung function, smoking, and resting lung function, an increased mortality risk was found in patients with a BMI < 25 kg/m$^2$ [6]. This could be related to the functional consequences of an abnormal body composition in

some of the patients as well as to adverse effects of recent weight loss on other outcome measures. In this context, it is of interest to note that recent weight loss is an important factor for outcome of acute exacerbations, as indicated by non-elective hospital readmission [22] and the need for and outcome of mechanical ventilation [23]. These effects could be related to the specific effects of (acute) nutritional depletion on respiratory muscle function or on immune function, but limited data are available for COPD patients.

Based on the relationship between nutritional status and outcome, the following screening measures of nutritional status are recommended.

Underweight is normally defined as a BMI < 21 kg/m$^2$. In Caucasians, this value is comparable to 90% of ideal body weight, based on the Metropolitan Life Insurance tables. However, according to recent recommendations the cut-off point in elderly patients should be extended to 24 kg/m$^2$ [24]. Interestingly, this value strikingly corresponds to the increased mortality risks in patients with COPD, i.e. a BMI < 25 kg/m$^2$.

## Causes of Weight Loss and Muscle Wasting

To be able to judge the need for and the effectiveness of nutritional therapy as well as the optimal nutritional support strategy, insight is needed into the underlying mechanisms and contributing factors of overall weight loss and specific tissue wasting in COPD. Weight loss, especially loss of fat mass, occurs if energy expenditure exceeds dietary intake. More specifically, muscle wasting is a consequence of an imbalance between protein synthesis and protein breakdown. Alterations in both parts of the energy balance have been reported in patients with COPD, and increasing evidence points towards the involvement of altered anabolic and catabolic mediators in the regulation of either protein synthesis, protein breakdown, or both.

### Energy Metabolism

Much research during the last decade has been focussed on energy expenditure in COPD. Total energy expenditure (TEE) can be divided into different components, with the basal metabolic rate usually being the largest component. Physical-activity-induced thermogenesis can vary substantially between different individuals. Other components of TEE are diet-induced thermogenesis (DIT), drug-induced thermogenesis, and the thermoregulatory component. Gas-exchange measurements made in patients in the awake-relaxed condition after an overnight fast allow determination of the so-called resting energy expenditure (REE). Under those conditions, the thermic effect of food is considered insignificant and it is assumed that the ambient temperature is within the thermoneutral zone for the individual. REE thus comprises the sleeping basal metabolic rate and the energy cost of arousal.

Based on the assumption that REE is the major component of TEE in sedentary persons, several studies have measured REE in COPD patients. After adjustment for the metabolically active fat-free mass, REE was found to be elevated in COPD [25]. While in healthy control subjects fat-free mass could explain up to 84% of the individual variation in REE, this was only 43% in COPD patients [25]. Other factors have therefore been considered, including the work of breathing, hormone levels, drug therapy, and inflammation. A likely cause of the increased metabolic rate in COPD patients is increasing respiratory muscle work, since the energy cost of increasing ventilation is higher in patients with advanced disease than in healthy controls of comparable age and gender. REE, however, correlates only weakly if at all, to individual lung function tests and blood gas values, or to combinations thereof [25]. Thus, patients with the worst lung function, in whom the work of breathing should be the highest, are not necessarily hypermetabolic. Nasal intermittent positive-pressure ventilation, which eliminates diaphragmatic and intercostal activity, did not reduce REE to normal in a group of hypermetabolic patients [26]. Furthermore, in COPD and in chest-wall disease, airflow obstruction and oxygen cost of breathing (OCB) were mutually related, but no correlation was found between OCB and REE [27]. Differences in hormone levels have been suggested as an explanation for the increase in REE. However, despite raised circulating levels of nora-

drenaline, other hormones, e.g. adrenaline, cortisol, and thyroxine, were found to be normal in COPD patients [28]. It is not yet known whether sympathetic hormones cause any change in skeletal muscle β-receptor density or sensitivity, and further studies are needed to investigate the effects of high catecholamines on hypermetabolism.

Maintenance bronchodilating treatment for many patients consists of inhaled β-agonists. Two weeks of salbutamol increased REE by less than 8% in healthy males [29]. Acute inhalations of clinical doses of salbutamol, in contrast, have been shown to dose-dependently increase REE in healthy subjects by up to 20% [30]. High doses of nebulised salbutamol are commonly administered during acute disease exacerbations. Nevertheless, no significant acute metabolic effects of this treatment were shown in elderly COPD patients in comparison with an age-matched control group [31].

Another contributing factor to hypermetabolism may be related to inflammation. The polypeptide cytokine tumour necrosis factor (TNF) is a pro-inflammatory mediator produced by different cell types. TNF also triggers the release of other cytokines, which themselves mediate an increase in energy expenditure, and the mobilisation of amino acids and muscle protein catabolism. Using different markers, several studies have provided clear evidence for the involvement of TNF-related systemic inflammation in the pathogenesis of tissue depletion. Elevated levels of TNF in plasma and of soluble TNF-receptors were found in patients with COPD [32–34], particularly those suffering from weight loss. Some studies showed a direct relationship between TNF and resting metabolic rate whereas according to others this was mediated by elevated levels of acute-phase proteins [35]. Since DIT accounts only for 10% of total daily energy expenditure, the influence of a possibly increased DIT on total daily energy expenditure will be small. Normal and increased DIT have been described in COPD patients [36]. Despite the methodological difficulties in measuring total daily energy expenditure, recent studies have focused attention on activity-related energy expenditure in COPD patients. Using the doubly labelled water ($^2H_2O^{18}$) technique to measure TEE it was demonstrated that COPD patients had a significantly higher TEE than healthy subjects [37]. Remarkably, the non-resting component of total daily energy expenditure was significantly higher in COPD patients than in healthy subjects, resulting in a TEE/REE ratio of 1.7 in COPD patients and 1.4 in normal subjects. Otherwise, when TEE was measured in patients with COPD and healthy persons in a respiration chamber, no differences were found between the two groups, possibly due to limitations of activities in the respiration chamber [38]. No difference in TEE between hypermetabolic and normometabolic COPD patients was found and REE did not correlate significantly with total daily energy expenditure, when fat-free mass was taken into account [39]. These data are in line with studies of TEE in other chronic wasting diseases, like cystic fibrosis and human immunodeficiency virus infections, in which the disease-related increase in REE was not reflected in the TEE.

The increased activity-related energy expenditure could be explained by the observed decreased mechanical efficiency of leg exercise [40]. Part of the increase in oxygen consumption during exercise can be related to inefficient ventilation in case of increased ventilatory demand, especially under conditions of dynamic hyperinflation. Furthermore, studies indicate severely impaired oxidative phosphorylation during exercise in COPD patients, accompanied by an increased and highly anaerobic metabolism involving both energy-release from high energy phosphate compounds and enhanced glycolysis [41]. It is generally known that anaerobic metabolism is inefficient compared to aerobic metabolism.

Besides an impaired oxidative phosphorylation during exercise, recent studies have shown alterations in resting cellular energy metabolism in peripheral muscle. A decrease in the activity of citrate synthase [42], an increase in the glycolytic enzyme phosphofructokinase [43], and (in hypoxaemic patients) an increase in the activity and expression of cytochrome oxidase have been reported [44]. These enzymatic adaptations could indicate a shift towards a more glycolytic metabolism. The functional consequences of these changes were reflected in alterations in adenosine nucleotide metabolism as evidenced by a decreased PCr/Cr and detectable levels of inosine

monophosphate, indicative of an imbalance between the utilisation and resynthesis of ATP in resting muscle of patients with COPD [45]. It could be speculated that the observed changes in intracellular metabolites result in an increased overall energy metabolism. Limited data are available regarding possible alterations in substrate metabolism in COPD related to the overall and cellular energy metabolic state. On the muscular level, in addition to an altered energy state, alterations in the profile of muscle amino acids have recently been described [46]. In contrast to the increased fat oxidation seen in other catabolic states, an increased utilisation of carbohydrate was shown in depleted COPD patients compared to depleted patients without underlying lung disorders [47]. Severely hypoxaemic COPD patients were found to have an altered glucose metabolism that could not readily be explained by changes in glucoregulatory hormones or short-term alterations in oxygenation [48]. No evidence for insulin resistance is yet available [49]. Clearly more data are needed, however, regarding substrate metabolism in well defined sub-groups of COPD based on the pattern and degree of tissue depletion and on the presence of tissue hypoxia and perhaps also of systemic inflammation.

## Dietary Intake

Hypermetabolism can explain why some COPD patients lose weight despite an apparent normal to even high dietary intake. Nevertheless, it has been shown that dietary intake in weight-losing patients is lower than in weight-stable patients both in absolute terms and in relation to measured REE [50]. This is quite remarkable because the normal adaptation to an increase in energy requirements in healthy men is an increase in dietary intake. The reasons for a relatively low dietary intake in COPD patients are not completely understood. It has been suggested that they eat suboptimally because chewing and swallowing change the breathing pattern and decrease arterial oxygen saturation. Furthermore, gastric filling in these patients may reduce the functional residual capacity and lead to an increase in dyspnoea. Very intriguing is the role of leptin in energy homeostasis. This adipocyte-derived hormone represents the afferent hormonal signal to the brain in a feedback mechanism regulating fat mass. In addition, leptin has a regulating role in lipid metabolism and glucose homeostasis, increases thermogenesis, and has effects on T-cell-mediated immunity. There are few data on leptin metabolism in COPD. Circulating leptin levels correlate well with BMI and fat percentage in COPD patients, as expected, but the values were significantly lower than in healthy subjects [34]. In experimental studies, the administration of endotoxins or cytokines produced a prompt increase in serum leptin levels [51]. One study also observed a relationship between leptin and soluble TNF-receptor 55 in COPD patients, in particular those with the emphysematous sub-type. Leptin levels as well as those of soluble TNF-receptor 55 were, in turn, inversely related to dietary intake in absolute terms as well as adjusted for REE [52]. The exact regulation of leptin in COPD needs further exploration. Another factor of interest in evaluating dietary intake is the influence of psychological dysfunctioning, such as anxiety, depression, and appetite. Although no systematic studies have been reported thus far, limited physical abilities, financial constraints and lack of supportive care of COPD patients should also be considered as factors that may interfere with dietary intake.

## Outcome of Nutritional Intervention

### Oral Nutritional Supplements

The first trials of nutritional supplementation in patients with COPD included short-term in-patient nutritional intervention programmes. In two studies [53, 54], a significant increase in body weight and respiratory muscle function was reported after 2–3 weeks of oral or enteral nutritional support. It was suggested that the effect of this short period of nutritional repletion may have been related more to repletion of muscle water and potassium than to constitution of muscle protein nitrogen. Besides, it is likely that increased cellular energy levels contribute more to improving muscle strength over the short-term than increased nitrogen retention [55]. Only one study, consisting of nine patients with advanced COPD, has addressed

the immune response to short-term nutritional intervention [56]. Refeeding and weight gain were associated with a significant increase in absolute lymphocyte count and with an increase in reactivity to skin test antigens after 21 days of refeeding.

Since then several studies have investigated the effectiveness of nutritional therapy over a more prolonged intervention period, ranging from 1–3 months. One in-patient study [57] and one out-patient study [58] showed significant improvement in respiratory and peripheral skeletal-muscle function, exercise capacity, and health-related quality of life after 3 months of oral supplementation of about 1000 Kcal daily. In three other out-patient studies, however, despite a similar nutritional supplementation regimen, the average weight gain was less than 1.5 kg in 8 weeks [59–61]. Besides noncompliance, the poor treatment response may be attributed, at least partly, to inadequate assessment of energy requirements and to the fact that the patients were consuming supplements instead of their regular meals.

## Nutrition and Exercise

From a functional point of view, it is obvious that nutritional support should be combined with exercise, if possible. A daily nutritional supplement as an integrated part of a pulmonary rehabilitation program indeed resulted in significant weight gain (0.4 kg/week), despite a daily supplementation that was much less than in most previous out-patient studies [62]. The combination of nutritional support and exercise not only increased body weight but also resulted in a significant improvement of fat-free mass and respiratory muscle strength. The clinical relevance of treatment response was shown in a post-hoc survival analysis of this study, which demonstrated that weight gain and increased respiratory muscle strength were associated with significantly increased survival rates [63]. On Cox regression analysis, weight gain during the rehabilitation period remained a significant predictor of mortality independent of baseline lung function and other risk factors, including age, sex, smoking, and resting arterial blood gases. In view of the ventilatory limitation and disease symptoms, exercise in most rehabilitation settings consists of general physical training, with emphasis on endurance exercise.

Increases in body weight, fat-free mass, and improvements in ventilatory muscle function, handgrip strength, peak work capacity, and health status have also been reported in depleted patients following nutritional supplementation therapy incorporated into a pulmonary rehabilitation programme [63, 64].

## Timing of Nutritional Support

Most studies have investigated the effects of nutritional supplementation in clinically stable patients. Anamnestic data, however, indicate that in some patients weight loss follows a stepwise pattern, associated with acute (infectious) exacerbations. During an acute exacerbation, energy balance is often negative due to a further increase in REE, but particularly due to a temporarily dramatic decrease in dietary intake [65]. Furthermore, these patients may have an increased risk for protein breakdown, which may limit the effectiveness of nutritional supplementation [66]. Factors contributing to weight loss and muscle wasting during an acute exacerbation include an increase in symptoms, more pronounced systemic inflammation, alterations in leptin metabolism, and the use of high doses of glucocorticoids [64, 65]. One study showed a positive effect of nutritional support during hospitalisation for an acute exacerbation, but clearly more research is needed to evaluate the relative effectiveness of nutritional support during or immediately after such episodes [66].

## Practical Implementation of Nutritional Support

Based on current insights into the relationship between nutritional depletion and outcome in COPD patients, a flow chart for nutritional screening and therapy is presented in Fig. 1. Simple screening can be performed based on repeated measurements of body weight. Patients are characterised by BMI (BMI = weight/height in m²) and the presence or absence of involuntary weight loss.

Nutritional supplementation is indicated for underweight patients (BMI < 21 kg/m²). Involuntary weight loss in patients with a BMI < 25 kg/m² should be treated to prevent further deterioration, whereas in patients with a BMI > 25 kg/m² involuntary weight loss should be monitored to assess whether it is progressive. If possible, measurement of fat-free mass as an indirect measure of muscle mass provides a more detailed screening of patients, since it allows identification of normal-weight patients with a depleted fat-free mass, who, despite a normal body weight, should nonetheless be considered as candidates for dietary therapy.

Depending on the underlying cause of energy imbalance (decreased dietary intake or increased nutritional requirements), initial nutritional therapy may range from adaptations of the dietary behaviour and food pattern to implementation of nutritional supplements. Nutritional support should be given as energy-dense supplements well-divided during the day to avoid loss of appetite and adverse metabolic and ventilatory effects resulting from a high caloric load. When feasible, patients should be encouraged to follow an exercise program. For severely disabled cachectic patients unable to perform exercise training, even simple strength manoeuvres combined with ADL training and energy conservation techniques may be effective. Exercise not only improves the effectiveness of nutritional therapy, but also stimulates appetite. After 4–8 weeks, the response to therapy can be determined. If weight gain and functional improvement are noted, the caregiver and the patient have to decide whether further improvement by a similar strategy is feasible or whether maintenance is the aim. If the desired response is not obtained, it may be necessary to consider compliance issues. If compliance is not the problem, more calories may be needed either by supplements or by enteral routes. A patient's nutritional status in relation to functional status can be screened during hospitalisation for an acute exacerbation or during out-patient follow up. The pulmonologist can consult the dietician for insight into the cause and treatment of an impaired energy balance in weight-losing subjects and the physiotherapist for the type and intensity

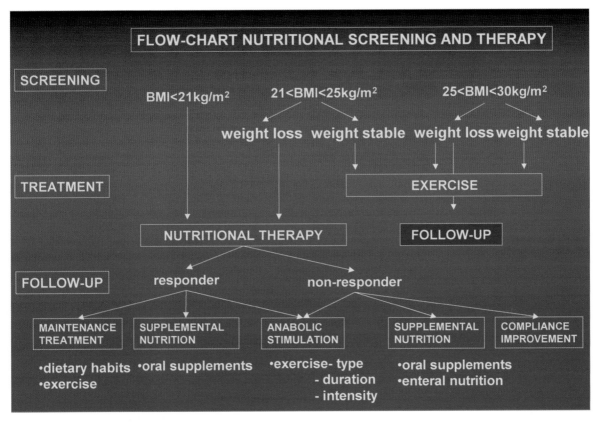

**Fig. 1.** COPD and treatment

of exercise program. Despite optimal implementation of nutritional therapy as part of an integrated treatment approach to COPD, it should be recognised that a sub-group of patients may not respond, due to an underlying mechanism of weight loss that cannot be reversed merely by caloric supplementation. Potential reversibility by means of specific nutrients (nutriceuticals) or pharmaceuticals will be a major focus of future research in this field.

# References

1. Fowler JS, Volkow ND, Wang GJ et al (1996) Inhibition of monoamine oxidase B in the brains of smokers. Nature 379:733–736
2. Filley GF, Beckwitt HJ, Reever JT, Mitchelli RS (1968) Chronic obstructive bronchopulmonary disease. 2. oxygen transport in two clinical types. Am J Med 44:26–38
3. Vandenbergh E, van der Woestijne KP, Gyselen A (1967) Weight changes in the terminal stages of chronic obstructive pulmonary disease. Am Rev Respir Dis 95:556–566
4. Wilson DO, Rogers RM, Wright EC, Anthonisen NR (1989) Body weight in chronic obstructive pulmonary disease. The National Institutes of Health Intermittent Positive-Pressure Breathing Trial. Am Rev Respir Dis 139:1435–1438
5. Gray Donald K, Gibbons L, Shapiro SH et al (1996) Nutritional status and mortality in chronic obstructive pulmonary disease. Am J Respir Crit Care Med 153:961–966
6. Schols A, Slangen J, Volovics L, Wouters EFM (1998) Weight loss is a reversible factor in the prognosis of chronic obstructive pulmonary disease. Am J Resp Crit Care Med 157:1791–1797
7. Schols AM, Wouters EF, Soeters PB, Westerterp KR (1991) Body composition by bioelectrical-impedance analysis compared with deuterium dilution and skinfold anthropometry in patients with chronic obstructive pulmonary disease. Am J Clin Nutr 53:421–424
8. Engelen MP, Schols AM, Baken WC et al (1994) Nutritional depletion in relation to respiratory and

peripheral skeletal muscle function in out-patients with COPD. Eur Respir J 7:1793–1797

9. Bissonnette DJ, Madapallimatam A, Jeejeebhoy KN (1997) Effect of hypoenergetic feeding and high-carbohydrate refeeding on muscle tetanic tension, relaxation rate, and fatigue in slow- and fast-twitch muscles in rats. Am J Clin Nutr 66:293–303

10. Fiaccadori E, Del Canale S, Coffrini E et al (1988) Hypercapnic-hypoxemic chronic obstructive pulmonary disease (COPD): influence of severity of COPD on nutritional status. Am J Clin Nutr 48:680–685

11. Anonymous (1999) Skeletal muscle dysfunction in chronic obstructive pulmonary disease. A statement of the American Thoracic Society and European Respiratory Society. Am J Respir Crit Care Med 159:S1–S40

12. Engelen MP, Schols AM, Lamers RJ, Wouters EF (1999) Different patterns of chronic tissue wasting among patients with chronic obstructive pulmonary disease. Clin Nutr 18:275–280

13. Bernard S, LeBlanc P, Whittom F et al (1998) Peripheral muscle weakness in patients with chronic obstructive pulmonary disease. Am J Respir Crit Care Med 158:629–634

14. Palange P, Forte S, Felli A et al (1995) Nutritional state and exercise tolerance in patients with COPD. Chest 107:1206–1212

15. Palange P, Forte S, Onorati P et al (1998) Effect of reduced body weight on muscle aerobic capacity in patients with COPD. Chest 114:12–18

16. Baarends EM, Schols AM, Mostert R, Wouters EF (1997) Peak exercise response in relation to tissue depletion in patients with chronic obstructive pulmonary disease. Eur Respir J 10:2807–2813

17. Russell DM, Walker PM, Leiter LA et al (1984) Metabolic and structural changes in skeletal muscle during hypocaloric dieting. Am J Clin Nutr 39:503–513

18. Layman DK, Merdian Bender M, Hegarty PV, Swan PB (1981) Changes in aerobic and anaerobic metabolism in rat cardiac and skeletal muscles after total or partial dietary restrictions. J Nutr 111:994–1000

19. Pichard C, Vaughan C, Struk R et al (1988) Effect of dietary manipulations (fasting, hypocaloric feeding, and subsequent refeeding) on rat muscle energetics as assessed by nuclear magnetic resonance spectroscopy. J Clin Invest 82:895–901

20. Shoup R, Dalsky G, Warner S et al (1997) Body composition and health-related quality of life in patients with obstructive airways disease. Eur Respir J 10:1576–1580

21. Schols AM, Soeters PB, Dingemans AM et al (1993) Prevalence and characteristics of nutritional depletion in patients with stable COPD eligible for pulmonary rehabilitation. Am Rev Respir Dis 147:1151–1156

22. Pouw E, Ten Velde G, Croonen B et al (2000) Early nonelective readmission for chronic obstructive pulmonary disease is associated with weight loss. Clin Nutr 19:95–99

23. Vitacca M, Clini E, Porta R et al (1996) Acute exacerbations in patients with COPD: predictors of need for mechanical ventilation. Eur Respir J 9:1487–1493

24. Beck AM, Ovesen L (1998) At which body mass index and degree of weight loss should hospitalized elderly patients be considered at nutritional risk? Clin Nutr 17:195–198

25. Schols AM, Fredrix EW, Soeters PB et al (1991) Resting energy expenditure in patients with chronic obstructive pulmonary disease. Am J Clin Nutr 54:983–987

26. Hugli O, Schutz Y, Fitting JW (1995) The cost of breathing in stable chronic obstructive pulmonary disease. Clin Sci (Lond) 89:625–632

27. Sridhar MK, Carter R, Lean MEJ, Banham SW (1994) Resting energy expenditure and nutritional state of patients with increased oxygen cost of breathing due to emphysema, scoliosis and thoracoplasty. Thorax 49:781–785

28. Hofford JM, Milakofsky L, Vogel WH et al (1990) The nutritional status in advanced emphysema associated with chronic bronchitis. A study of amino acid and catecholamine levels. Am Rev Respir Dis 141:902–908

29. Wilson SR, Amoroso P, Moxham J, Ponte J (1993) Modification of the thermogenic effect of acutely inhaled salbutamol by chronic inhalation in normal subjects. Thorax 48:886–889

30. Amoroso P, Wilson SR, Moxham J, Ponte J (1993) Acute effects of inhaled salbutamol on the metabolic rate of normal subjects. Thorax 48:882–885

31. Creutzberg EC, Schols AM, Bothmer-Quaedvlieg FC et al (1998) Acute effects of nebulized salbutamol on resting energy expenditure in patients with chronic obstructive pulmonary disease and in healthy subjects. Respiration 65:375–380

32. De Godoy I, Donahoe M, Calhoun WJ et al (1996) Elevated TNF-alpha production by peripheral blood monocytes of weight-losing COPD patients. Am J Respir Crit Care Med 153:633–637

33. Di Francia M, Barbier D, Mege JL, Orehek J (1994) Tumor necrosis factor-alpha levels and weight loss in chronic obstructive pulmonary disease. Am J Respir Crit Care Med 150:1453–1455

34. Takabatake N, Nakamura H, Abe S et al (1999) Circulating leptin in patients with chronic obstructive pulmonary disease. Am J Resp CritCare Med 159:1215–1219

35. Schols AM, Buurman WA, Staal van den Brekel AJ et al (1996) Evidence for a relation between metabolic derangements and elevated inflammatory mediators in a subgroup of patients with chronic obstructive pulmonary disease. Thorax 51:819–824

36. Hugli O, Frascarolo P, Schutz Y et al (1993) Diet-induced thermogenesis in chronic obstructive pulmonary disease. Am Rev Respir Dis 148:1479–1483

37. Baarends EM, Schols AM, Pannemans DL et al

(1997) Total free living energy expenditure in patients with severe chronic obstructive pulmonary disease. Am J Respir Crit Care Med 155:549–554

38. Hugli O, Schutz Y, Fitting JW (1996) The daily energy expenditure in stable chronic obstructive pulmonary disease. Am J Respir Crit Care Med 153:294–300

39. Baarends EM, Schols AM, Westerterp KR, Wouters EF (1997) Total daily energy expenditure relative to resting energy expenditure in clinically stable patients with COPD. Thorax 52:780–785

40. Baarends EM, Schols A, Akkermans MA, Wouters EF (1997) Decreased mechanical efficiency in clinically stable patients with COPD. Thorax 52:981–986

41. Wuyam B, Payen JF, Levy P et al (1992) Metabolism and aerobic capacity of skeletal muscle in chronic respiratory failure related to chronic obstructive pulmonary disease. Eur Respir J 5:157–162

42. Maltais F, Simard AA, Simard C et al (1996) Oxidative capacity of the skeletal muscle and lactic acid kinetics during exercise in normal subjects and in patients with COPD. Am J Respir Crit Care Med 153:288–293

43. Jakobsson P, Jorfeldt L, Henriksson J (1995) Metabolic enzyme activity in the quadriceps femoris muscle in patients with severe chronic obstructive pulmonary disease. Am J Respir Crit Care Med 151:374–377

44. Sauleda J, Garcia-Palmer F, Wiesner RJ et al (1998) Cytochrome oxidase activity and mitochondrial gene expression in skeletal muscle of patients with chronic obstructive pulmonary disease. Am J Respir Crit Care Med 157:1413–1417

45. Pouw EM, Schols AMWJ, Vusse GJ, Wouters EF (1998) Elevated inosine monophosphate levels in resting muscle of patients with stable COPD. Am J Respir Crit Care Med 157:453–457

46. Pouw EM, Schols AM, Deutz NE, Wouters EF (1998) Plasma and muscle amino acid levels in relation to resting energy expenditure and inflammation in stable chronic obstructive pulmonary disease. Am J Respir Crit Care Med 158:797–801

47. Goldstein SA, Thomashow BM, Kvetan V et al (1988) Nitrogen and energy relationships in malnourished patients with emphysema. Am Rev Respir Dis 138:636–644

48. Hjalmarsen A, Aasebo U, Birkeland K et al (1996) Impaired glucose tolerance in patients with chronic hypoxic pulmonary disease. Diab Metab 22:37–42

49. Jakobsson P, Jorfeldt L, von Schenck H (1995) Insulin resistance is not exhibited by advanced chronic obstructive pulmonary disease patients. Clin Physiol 15:547–555

50. Schols AM, Soeters PB, Mostert R et al (1991) Energy balance in chronic obstructive pulmonary disease. Am Rev Respir Dis 143:1248–1252

51. Grunfeld C, Zhao C, Fuller J et al (1996) Endotoxin and cytokines induce expression of leptin, the ob gene product, in hamsters. J Clin Invest 97:2152–2157

52. Schols A, Creutzberg E, Buurman W et al (1999) Plasma leptin is related to pro-inflammatory status and dietary intake in patients with COPD. Am J Respir Crit Care Med 160:1220–1226

53. Vermeeren MA, Schols AM, Quaedvlieg FC, Wouters EF (1994) The influence of an acute disease exacerbation on the metabolic profile of patients with chronic obstructive pulmonary disease. Clin Nutr 13 (suppl. 1):38–39

54. Wilson DO, Rogers RM, Sanders MH et al (1986) Nutritional intervention in malnourished patients with emphysema. Am Rev Respir Dis 134:672–677

55. Whittaker JS, Ryan CF, Buckley PA, Road JD (1990) The effects of refeeding on peripheral and respiratory muscle function in malnourished chronic pulmonary disease patients. Am Rev Respir Dis 142:283–288

56. Russell DM, Prendergast PJ, Darby PL et al (1983) A comparison between muscle function and body composition in anorexia nervosa: the effect of refeeding. Am J Clin Nutr 38:229–237

57. Fuenzalida CE, Petty TL, Jones ML et al (1990) The immune response to short-term nutritional intervention in advanced chronic obstructive pulmonary disease. Am Rev Respir Dis 142:49–56

58. Rogers RM, Donahoe M, Constatino J (1992) Physiologic effects of oral supplemental feeding in malnourished patients with chronic obstructive pulmonary diseases, a randomized control study. Am Rev Respir Dis 146:1511–1517

59. Efthimiou J, Fleming J, Gomes C, Spiro SG (1988) The effect of supplementary oral nutrition in poorly nourished patients with chronic obstructive pulmonary disease. Am Rev Respir Dis 137:1075–1082

60. Otte KE, Ahlburg P, D'Amore F, Stellfeld M (1989) Nutritional repletion in malnourished patients with emphysema. JPEN J Parenter Enteral Nutr 13:152–156

61. Knowles JB, Fairbarn MS, Wiggs BJ et al (1988) Dietary supplementation and respiratory muscle performance in patients with COPD. Chest 93:977–983

62. Lewis MI, Belman MJ, Dorr Uyemura L (1987) Nutritional supplementation in ambulatory patients with chronic obstructive pulmonary disease. Am Rev Respir Dis 135:1062–1067

63. Schols AM, Soeters PB, Mostert R et al (1995) Physiologic effects of nutritional support and anabolic steroids in patients with chronic obstructive pulmonary disease. A placebo-controlled randomized trial. Am J Respir Crit Care Med 152:1268–1274

64. Creutzberg EC, Wouters EF, Mostert R et al (2003) Efficacy of nutritional supplementation therapy in depleted patients with chronic obstructive pulmonary disease. Nutrition 19:120–127

65. Creutzberg EC, Wouters EFM, Vanderhoven-Augustin IM et al (2000) Disturbances in leptin metabolism are related to energy imbalance during

acute exacerbations of chronic obstructive pulmonary disease. Am J Respir Crit Care Med 162:1239–1245

66.  Saudny Unterberger H, Martin JG, Gray Donald K (1997) Impact of nutritional support on functional status during an acute exacerbation of chronic obstructive pulmonary disease. Am J Respir Crit Care Med 156:794–799

# Cachexia in Cardiovascular Illness

Sabine Strassburg, Stefan D. Anker

## Introduction

Cachexia (body wasting) in patients with cardiovascular illness usually develops when patients have chronic heart failure (CHF). As an increasing public health problem and a leading cause of morbidity and mortality worldwide, CHF is associated with a poor prognosis [1]. The onset of cachexia in CHF patients (cardiac cachexia) is a serious complication of their disease and even worsens the prognosis of the underlying disease [2]. This connection between advanced heart failure and significant weight loss has long been recognised. The earliest report dates back to the school of medicine of Hippocrates some 2300 years ago. The term 'cachexia' is of Greek origin and derives from the words *kakos* (bad) and *hexis* (condition). The term 'cardiac cachexia' was first used in 1860 by Mauriac [3].

## Definition and Diagnosis

Cachectic heart-failure patients are weaker and fatigue earlier, which is due to both reduced skeletal muscle mass and impaired muscle quality. A simple and fast applicable definition of 'clinical cardiac cachexia' is the following: in CHF patients without signs of other primary cachectic states (e.g. cancer, thyroid disease, or severe liver disease), cardiac cachexia can be diagnosed when weight loss of > 6% of the previous normal weight is observed over a period of > 6 months [4]. The previous normal weight of a heart-failure patient would be the average weight prior to the onset of heart disease (before the diagnosis). It is important to document dry weight loss measured in a non-oedematous state to prove the diagnosis.

However, different definitions have been used by the various research groups that have investigated the wasting process in heart failure and other conditions. For example, in heart-failure studies, patients have also been classified as 'malnourished' when the percentage of ideal weight was < 90% or body fat content was < 15% for men and < 22% for women [5]. Further possible definitions are a body fat content of < 27% (men) or < 29% (women) [6], or when body weight is < 85% of the ideal one [7] or even < 80% [8]. Also, a documented weight loss of at least 10% of lean tissue [9] has been proposed. Several of these definitions are based on body composition variables. These can be measured by bioelectrical impedance measurement, dual energy x-ray absorptiometry (DEXA) scanning, computed tomography (CT), or nuclear magnetic resonance (NMR). However, these techniques are expensive and not available everywhere.

Primarily, it is important to recognise changes in weight as early as possible in CHF patients. This can easily be done by a carefully documented weight history (taken from the non-oedematous patient) for all in- and out-patients with CHF. Moreover, obtaining this information is neither time-consuming nor expensive.

## Incidence, Prevalence, and Prognosis

Heart failure is a common disorder, with a prevalence of approximately 0.3–2% in the general population [10]. The incidence is > 10% in subjects older than 80 years and then doubles every decade [11]. However, the incidence of heart failure is expected to grow because of the increasing age of the population, improved diagnostic techniques for the detection of heart failure, and improved treatment and survival of patients with coronary artery disease.

Also, cachexia in heart failure is not as rare as previously thought and ranges between 10–15%, but data vary dependent on the definition. Up to 50% of CHF patients are malnourished to some degree [5]. With a definition of cachexia as oedema-free weight loss > 7.5%, the incidence of cachexia in the Studies of Left Ventricular Dysfunction (SOLVD) treatment trial was 35% over 3 years, with a cross-sectional prevalence of this degree of weight loss between 12 and 14% [10]. A prospective study on the frequency and prognostic importance of cachexia in CHF outpatients demonstrated that 16% of the patients were cachectic [12]. The observed weight loss amounted to 6–30 kg and the 18-month mortality was 50% in cachectic patients. Therefore, in patients with CHF, increasing BMI is not an adverse prognostic feature. Thinner patients appear to have a poorer prognosis [13] (Fig. 1). This is independent of functional disease severity, age, measures of exercise capacity, and cardiac function.

## Pathogenesis

A complex imbalance of different body systems may cause the development of body wasting, with alterations in the body composition. Available evidence suggests that metabolic, neurohormonal, and immune abnormalities play an important role in the pathophysiology of cardiac cachexia. Pittman and Cohen, in 1964, proposed increased catabolism (protein loss) and reduced anabolism due to cellular hypoxia as the principal pathogenic factor [14]. Currently, several further mechanisms are thought to be responsible for the development of cardiac cachexia. These include dietary deficiency, malabsorption/metabolic dysfunction, and loss of nutrients, e.g. via the urinary or digestive tracts [15]. While several recent studies on the metabolic and immunologic changes have provided interesting results in the last few years, the mechanisms behind the transition from heart failure to cardiac cachexia have yet to be clarified completely.

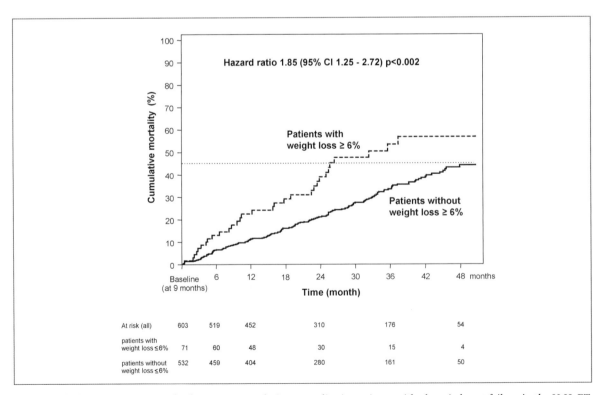

**Fig. 1.** Weight loss 6% or more and subsequent cumulative mortality in patients with chronic heart failure in the V-HeFT II study. Data from [4]

## Alterations in Body Composition

Patients with cardiac cachexia suffer from a general loss of fat, lean, and bone tissues. Loss of lean tissue, e.g. skeletal muscle, causes early fatigue and muscle weakness in CHF patients. This mainly occurs in patients with NYHA class III and IV [16] disease and in cachectic subjects [17]. It is known that muscle atrophy [18] is present in up to 68% of patients with CHF [19]. Pathophysiologically, ultrastructural abnormalities, such as fibre-type distribution and reduced capillary length and density in the skeletal muscle of CHF patients [20], have been shown in heart-failure patients, reflecting a decreased oxidative capacity of skeletal muscle.

Besides this significant loss of lean tissue, CHF patients also have a lower fat tissue mass (i.e. energy reserves) and decreased bone mineral density (i.e. osteoporosis) [21, 22] (Table 1). Other studies confirmed these findings and found significantly correlated plasma levels of inflammatory cytokines and catabolic hormones [23], which might represent a mechanism for these changes in body composition.

**Table 1.** Body composition (whole body analysis) in healthy controls compared with non-cachectic and cachectic patients with chronic heart failure (*CHF*) as determined by DEXA (dual x-ray absorptiometry). All results mean ± SEM (ranges given in brackets). The derived measures were indented. Adapted from [17]

| | Controls $n = 15$ | Non-cachectic CHF patients $n = 36$ | Cachectic CHF patients $n = 18$ |
|---|---|---|---|
| *Total body results* | | | |
| Fat tissue (kg) | 20.3 ± 1.9 (11.3 - 37.6) | 21.6 ± 1.2 (11.2 - 36.6) | 13.6 ± 0.8 •••• **** (7.4 - 19.7) |
| - Body fat tissue content (%) | 23.9 ± 1.5 (16.2 - 36.7) | 25.3 ± 1.0 (15.5 - 37.8) | 21.6 ± 1.1 (13.8 - 116.3) |
| - Body fat tissue / height (g/cm) | 116 ± 11 (63.3 - 225.0) | 124 ± 7 (63.9 - 212.9) | 80 ± 5 •• *** (43.7 - 116.3) |
| Lean tissue (kg) | 58.2 ± 1.4 (50.4 - 72.0) | 57.4 ± 1.0 (45.8 - 74.9) | 46.0 ± 1.2 •••• **** (37.9 - 53.1) |
| - Body lean tissue content (%) | 70.8 ± 1.5 (57.5 - 78.8) | 69.0 ± 0.9 (56.9 - 79.4) | 73.6 ± 1.3 ** (66.7 - 88.9) |
| - Body lean tissue / height (g/cm) | 331 ± 7 (292.1 - 389.2) | 331 ± 5 (283.3 - 423.0) | 269 ± 6 •••• **** (226.9 - 305.1) |
| Bone mineral density (g/cm$^2$) | 1.22 ± 0.02 (1.055 - 1.380) | 1.23 ± 0.01 (1.065 - 1.509) | 1.16 ± 0.02 • ** (1.033 - 1.286) |
| Bone mineral content (g) | 3184 ± 107 (2563 - 3915) | 3126 ± 56 (2503 - 4059) | 2628 ± 58 •••• **** (2240 - 3020) |
| - Bone mineral content / height (g/cm) | 18.1 ± 0.6 (14.6 - 21.2) | 18.0 ± 0.3 (14.7 - 23.1) | 15.4 ± 0.3 •••• **** (13.0 - 23.1) |

•, $p < 0.05$ vs controls; ••, $p < 0.01$ vs controls; ••••, $p < 0.0001$ vs controls; **, $p < 0.01$ vs non-cachectic CHF patients; ***, $p < 0.001$ vs non-cachectic CHF patients; ****, $p < 0.0001$ vs non-cachectic CHF patients; $n$, number of patients

## Immune Activation

There is evidence that neurohormonal changes and immune activation in CHF patients play a major role in the pathogenesis of cardiac cachexia. While tumour necrosis factor-α (TNF-α) is increased in cardiac cachexia as a sign of immune activation [6, 7, 24], the levels of this cytokine are not increased in all CHF patients [25]. Keeping the definition of cardiac cachexia as > 7.5% weight loss in 6 months, the TNF-α plasma level is higher in cachectic (Fig. 2), than in non-cachectic CHF patients. TNF-α level is also the strongest predictor of the degree of previous weight loss [26]. In animal experiments, TNF-α-producing cells implanted in the brain caused profound anorexia [27]. When TNF-α-producing cells were implanted in skeletal muscle, cachexia occurred, which proves a causative role for increased levels of TNF-α in the genesis of cachexia. Other important

cytokines in CHF are interleukin (IL)-1, IL-6, interferon (IFN)-γ, and transforming growth factor (TGF)-β. Besides cytokines, there are other elevated inflammatory markers, e.g. erythrocyte sedimentation rate, which also relate adversely to the prognosis [28].

The exact mechanism for the activation of the immune system is not clear and several possibilities have been discussed, including a role for TNF-α since it is a validated marker for immune activation in cardiac cachexia. Hypoxia has been suggested as the main stimulus for increased TNF-α production in CHF patients [29]. As the failing myocardium is capable of producing TNF-α [30], another hypothesis assumes that the heart itself is the main source of inflammatory cytokines [31]. Nevertheless, treatment of patients with ventricular assistance devices failed to provide long-term beneficial anti-inflammatory effects [32]. Also,

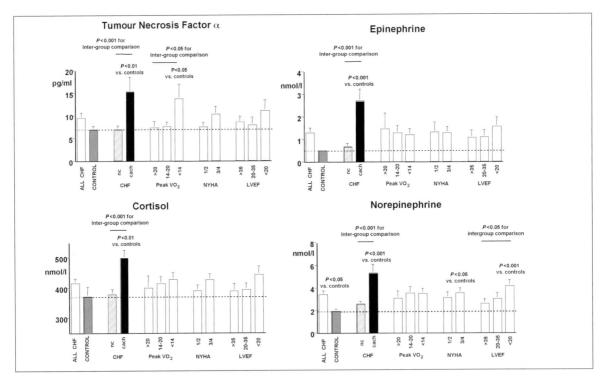

**Fig. 2.** Tumour necrosis factor alpha (TNF-α), epinephrine, norepinephrine and cortisol plasma levels in 53 chronic heart failure (CHF) patients and 16 healthy controls. Patients are sub-grouped according to: (1) cachectic state (*nc*, non-cachectic [n = 37]; *cach*, cachectic [n = 16]): (2) maximal oxygen consumption (peak $VO_2$) (< 14 [n = 17] vs 14-20 [n = 24] vs >20 ml/kg per min [n = 12]); (3) New York Association class (NYHA) (class 1/2 [n = 16] vs class 3/4 [n = 37]); (4) left ventricular ejection fraction (LVEF) (< 20% vs 20-35% [n = 17] vs > 35% [n = 12]). Data presented as mean ± SEM $P$-values for Fisher's test are given if ANOVA showed significant inter-group variation. Adapted from [26]

endotoxin stimulates inflammatory cytokine production [33]. Therefore, bacterial translocation due to bowel-wall oedema in CHF with subsequent endotoxin release represents a possible mechanism to activate the immune reaction (endotoxin hypothesis) [34]. There is evidence that endotoxin-mediated inflammation is important in cardiogenic shock [35]. Furthermore, an increased sensitivity of peripheral monocytes to lipopolysaccharides (LPS) and high levels of neopterin (a marker of monocyte activation) indicate monocyte activation in CHF patients [36]. In contrast, lipids play a beneficial role in patients with CHF by binding to and detoxifying the effects of endotoxin [37]. High lipoprotein levels were found to be inversely related to low plasma levels of TNF and other inflammatory cytokine variables [38]. Furthermore, it may explain why low, but not high serum lipoprotein levels are associated with a poor prognosis in CHF patients [39, 40].

Another aspect is anaemia, which can be the cause of heart failure, but also its consequence (Fig. 3) [41]. Reduced haemoglobin is frequently seen in inflammatory conditions, and pro-inflammatory cytokines may be pivotal triggers of anaemia in CHF. Studies also document that lower plasma haemoglobin levels in CHF are related to female gender, older age, poor kidney function, lower body weight, greater inflammation, and advanced disease status (based on left ventricular ejection fraction, exercise capacity, and mortality analyses) [41].

### Neurohormonal Abnormalities

Besides activation of the immune system, neurohormonal abnormalities are also important in the pathophysiology of the development of cardiac cachexia. Attributed to impaired cardiac function, a general neurohormonal activation, in which the sympathetic nervous system, the renin-angiotensin-aldosterone axis, and the natriuretic peptide system are stimulated, occurs when heart failure deteriorates to a chronic disease state.

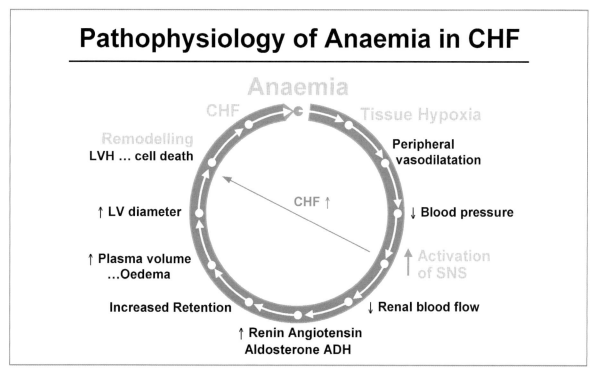

**Fig. 3.** The cardiorenal anaemia syndrome - anaemia as a cause and consequence of heart failure: anaemia, plasma volume and haemodynamic changes, sympathetic activation, vasoconstriction, tissue ischaemia, and tissue injury are components of a vicious circle. *ADH*, antidiuretic hormone; *LV*, left ventricular; *LVH*, left ventricular hyperthrophy; *SNS*, sympathetic neervous system. Adapted from [41]

Initially, these changes have a beneficial effect; however, later they contribute to increased vascular resistance, afterload, ventricular enlargement, and remodelling.

The overall sympathetic activity is demonstrated by an increased plasma norepinephrine level [42]. Norepinephrine and epinephrine levels were markedly increased in a cachectic group of 53 CHF patients, who were stratified for LVEF, NYHA class, and presence of cachexia, compared to non-cachectic CHF patients and healthy subjects [26] (Fig. 2). Both of norepinephrine and epinephrine can cause a catabolic metabolic shift [25, 26] and lead to an increase in resting energy expenditure in CHF patients [43].

The importance of neuroendocrine activation in the development of cachexia in CHF is also reflected in increased aldosterone plasma levels and increased plasma renin activity [26]. Adult patients with congenital heart disease have significantly higher levels of the neurohormones ANP, BNP, ET-1 (all $p < 0.0001$), norepinephrine, renin ($p = 0.003$), and aldosterone ($p = 0.024$) [44]. Interestingly, there was a highly significant stepwise increase in the concentrations of ANP, BNP, ET-1, and norepinephrine with increasing disease severity. Angiotensin II- and aldosterone-activity explain the fibrosis of smooth muscle cells as well as the reduction of circulating insulin-like growth factor (IGF)-1 [45]. Renin again stimulates the production of angiotensin II and norepinephrine (renin-angiotensin-system) [46].

Furthermore, the growth hormone (GH)/IGF-1 axis is involved in the pathogenesis of the wasting process [47, 48]. Abnormal GH/IGF-1 ratios and low testosterone levels correlate with the degree of weight loss in cachectic CHF patients [26].

The hormone cortisol is also considered to be part of the general stress response and exerts a catabolic effect. Increased cortisol was demonstrated in untreated patients with severe CHF (Fig. 2) [49], which was probably due to an elevated release of adrenocorticotropic hormone [50]. This catabolic/anabolic imbalance was confirmed by a study in which the anabolic steroid dehydroepiandrosterone was lowest in cachectic CHF patients and cortisol levels were particularly increased in cachectic CHF patients [26].

The protein leptin is involved in the regulation of food intake and energy balance [51], and it serves as an important signal from fat to brain. Raised levels of leptin can decrease food intake and increase resting energy expenditure [52]. The role of leptin in the development of cardiac cachexia has not yet been elucidated, but it was reported that plasma leptin levels are increased in CHF [53] and higher leptin levels are associated with increased sympathetic activity [52]. However, there are some contradictory reports on this issue [54, 55].

## Therapeutic Options

Cardiac cachexia is characterised by an imbalance of the catabolic and anabolic body system (Fig. 4) [56]. So far, there is no validated world-wide accepted therapy, but possible starting points for the therapy can be discussed. Due to the various changes in different physiological systems, e.g. immunological and neurohormonal, that contribute to cachexia, it appears unlikely that a single agent will be completely effective in treating this condition.

### Drugs

Prevention of the deterioration of CHF, such as occurs with the onset of cachexia, is one of the main goals of therapy. Increasing knowledge about the pathophysiology of CHF and its sequelae has led to an increasing number of therapeutic options. However, there is no specific drug therapy for cachexia associated with CHF. Most of the drugs currently in use, particularly ACE inhibitors, β-blockers, and aldosterone antagonists, have an effect on the neurohormonal system. For instance, ACE inhibitors reduce circulating levels of atrial and brain natriuretic peptides (ANP, BNP) [57, 58], TNF-$\alpha$ [59], and IL-6 [60]. The effects on catecholamines, other neurohormones, and endothelial function mediated by ACE inhibitors are thought to improve the nutritional status of tissues and reduce ischaemia and oxidative stress. Thus, these drugs prevent tissue damage and apoptosis in patients with heart failure [4]. It was demon-

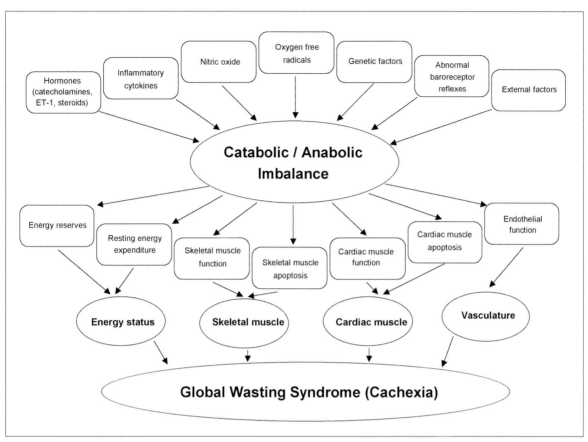

**Fig. 4.** The development of cachexia due to a complex interaction of different body systems and an imbalance of catabolic and anabolic systems. *ET-1*, endothelin-1. (Adapted from [56])

strated that treatment with the ACE inhibitor enalapril reduced the risk of over 6% weight loss by 19% [4]. Also, it has been shown that ACE inhibitors can restore depressed levels of circulating IGF-1 in CHF patients by reducing angiotensin II activity [61]. A further option is therapy with an angiotensin II type-1 receptor antagonist itself, which resulted in reduced plasma levels of TNF-α, IL-6, and BNP [62]. Angiotensin II is a potent stimulator of the immune and neurohormonal axis.

Recently, β-blockers were found to act beneficially in CHF and to prevent or even partially reverse cachexia [63]. In a study with CHF patients, after therapy with carvedilol or metoprolol for 6 months, subjects with baseline cachexia gained significantly more weight gain than subjects in the non-cachectic group [64]. The β-blocker carvedilol is thought to have an inhibitory effect on reactive oxygen species and apoptosis [65]. All-cause mortality was lower in the metoprolol group in a study

enrolling 3991 patients [66]. Also, carvedilol therapy led to a reduced overall mortality rate of 3.2% ($n = 696$) vs 7.8% in the placebo group ($n = 398$) [67]. However, there was no difference between cachectic and non-cachectic patients in this study.

The importance of high levels of cytokines favours implementation of an anti-cytokine therapy. Although anti-cytokine treatment is established in other diseases [68–70], its value in the management of CHF remains controversial [71]. The effects of two drugs, etanercept, which reduces the bioactivity of TNF-α, and infliximab, an anti-TNF-α antibody, have been studied. Contradictory to the initial favourable effects in early pilot studies [72, 73], larger studies failed to show a benefit for either drug [74–76].

Interestingly, phosphodiesterase inhibitors (e.g. amrinone, vesnarinone, pimobendan), which have short-term haemodynamic benefits in heart failure, can inhibit the production of TNF-α and other cytokines from stimulated human lymphocytes [77]. Furthermore, it has been suggested that another phosphodiesterase inhibitor, pentoxiphylline, reduces TNF-α plasma concentrations [78], but in a well-controlled study pentoxifylline therapy did not reduce TNF-α levels in CHF patients [79].

Blocking the inflammatory activation is also possible with the anti-cytokine anti-IL-6. It was shown that proteolysis, muscle atrophy, and weight loss were prevented by anti-IL-6 antibody therapy in animal models [80].

Recombinant human GH can be considered as another option for the treatment of cardiac cachexia. Since normal doses had no significant clinical benefits compared to placebo [81], high doses of GH may be necessary to overcome GH resistance, which is present in patients with cardiac cachexia [82]. In fact, case reports involving three cachectic patients showed an increase of muscle mass and strength and an improvement of exercise capacity with high dose (about 6–8 times higher than normal) GH therapy [83, 84]. The use of anabolic steroids to increase muscle mass in cardiac cachexia is limited due to negative side effects on other organs, e.g. kidney function [15, 85]. Recently, ghrelin was found to improve ventricular function and increase body weight in animal studies [86]. Therefore, the GH-releasing peptide ghrelin, which has been isolated from the stomach, presents another option for the treatment of cardiac cachexia and therefore merits further research. Ghrelin causes a positive energy balance by stimulating food intake, and it also exhibits cardiovascular effects, e.g. inhibition of apoptosis by cardiomyocytes and endothelial cells [87].

The above-mentioned endotoxin hypothesis implies further therapeutic strategies. Drugs directed against endotoxin-producing bacteria in the bowel or endotoxin itself, or its binding to cells could prevent the effect of cytokine release due to endotoxin. However, further research on the benefits of this approach is needed.

## Nutritional Support

Nutritional support seems to be an easy way of improving the nutritional status in cachectic heart-failure patients. However, non-surgical studies with such patients are rare, and perioperative studies evaluating the effect of nutritional support on mortality have yielded contradictory results [8, 88]. In a non-surgical study, intensive nutritional support led to an increase in the amount of lean tissue [89]. Another study demonstrated no significant effect on the clinical status of heart failure in stable CHF patients without any signs of severe malnutrition [90]. However, only small numbers of patients were involved and cachexia was not assessed. Other studies of heart failure have failed to quantify nutrient and caloric intake [5], and most studies are limited by the poor compliance of patients with nutritional regimens. Therefore, nutritional-support studies in cardiac cachexia patients are still needed.

It is noteworthy that studies in healthy older people demonstrated a high incidence of inadequate nutritional intake [91], and non-intentional weight loss was also shown to be an independent predictor of mortality in the elderly [4].

Catecholamines and cytokines, which are elevated in heart failure, are stimuli for free-radical production. Therefore, antioxidants and free radical scavengers, such as vitamins C and E, are therapeutic options in cardiac cachexia. This was proven by a study showing that muscle wasting in mice was prevented by an antioxidant [92]. Additionally, it was shown that antioxidants suppress the production of free radicals in leucocytes [93]. The presence of elevated levels of markers of oxidative stress in heart-failure patients correlates with functional class, reduced exercise tolerance, lower antioxidant levels, and worse prognosis, including cachexia [94, 95]. These patients also tend to have micronutrient deficiency through, e.g. urinary losses or therapy with diuretics. Deficiencies of specific micronutrients, such as selenium, copper, calcium, zinc, or thiamine, can also cause heart failure [96]. Thus, it is important to keep CHF patients on a diet with sufficient calories and with sufficient micronutrients and vitamins to replace early losses. Interestingly, statins have also been shown to possess anti-inflammatory characteristics and counterbalance increased levels of oxygen free-radicals in CHF [39, 97].

Fish oil (n-3 polyunsaturated fatty acids) is a

supplement that has been shown to improve cachexia symptoms in dogs with CHF [98]. Accordingly, an oral nutritional supplement enriched with fish oil reversed cachexia in patients with pancreatic cancer [99]. In healthy volunteers [100] and patients with rheumatic disease [101], fish oil reduced TNF-$\alpha$ and IL-1 concentrations; thus, it might exert an anti-inflammatory effect. Further supplements or therapy with appetite-stimulating drugs, like megestrol acetate, are being studied.

## Exercise

Exercise training is a therapeutic option that has been probably underevaluated so far. Moderate exercise training improves exercise capacity by reversing muscular metabolic abnormalities and atrophy as well as impaired blood flow and neurohormonal abnormalities [102]. Pathophysiologically, skeletal-muscle cytochrome *c* oxidase activity is increased with long-term training, and this is associated with reduced local expression of pro-inflammatory cytokines [103]. Exercise training may therefore help to retard the catabolic process in CHF, and it has been suggested that moderate exercise training could safely be performed by cachectic CHF patients with NYHA class I–III disease [104]. However, exercise training is not possible in every patient due to a decreased exercise capacity.

## Conclusions

The onset of cardiac cachexia is a serious complication in heart failure and is associated with a poor prognosis. Despite declining trends in overall cardiovascular mortality, mortality and morbidity from heart failure are increasing. The results of the studies described herein support the importance of a specific evaluation of the cachectic status in CHF patients. Cachexia is easily detectable by weight documentation in the non-oedematous patient. Immune and neurohormonal abnormalities play significant roles in the pathogenesis of the wasting process, although further research is needed to elucidate the pathophysiology. Interestingly, the degree of body wasting is correlated with the level of these neurohormonal and immune abnormalities. As knowledge about the pathophysiology of cardiac cachexia has increased, a growing number of treatment strategies for the prevention and therapy of cardiac cachexia are becoming available. Individualised management will have an important influence on the quality of life of heart-failure patients with cachexia and may improve their long-term prognosis.

## References

1. McMurray JJ, Stewart J (2000) Epidemiology, aetiology, and prognosis of heart failure. Heart 833:596–602
2. Anker SD, Coats AJ (1999) Cardiac cachexia: a syndrome with impaired survival and immune and neuroendocrine activation. Chest 115:836–847
3. Doehner W, Anker SD (2002) Cardiac cachexia in early literature: a review of research prior to Medline. Int J Cardiol 85:7–14
4. Anker SD, Negassa A, Coats AJ et al (2003) Prognostic importance of weight loss in chronic heart failure and the effect of treatment with angiotensin-converting-enzyme inhibitors: an observational study. Lancet 361:1077–1083
5. Carr JG, Stevenson LW, Walden JA, Heber D (1989) Prevalence and haemodynamic correlates of malnutrition in severe congestive heart failure secondary to ischemic or idiopathic dilated cardiomyopathy. Am J Cardiol 63:709–713
6. McMurray J, Abdullah I, Dargie HJ, Shapiro D (1991) Increased concentrations of tumor necrosis factor in 'cachectic' patients with severe chronic heart failure. Br Heart J 66:356–358
7. Levine B, Kalman J, Mayer L et al (1990) Elevated circulating levels of tumor necrosis factor in severe chronic heart failure. N Engl J Med 323:236–241
8. Otaki M (1994) Surgical treatment of patients with cardiac cachexia. An analysis of factors affecting operative mortality. Chest 105:1347–1351
9. Freeman LM, Roubenoff R (1994) The nutrition implications of cardiac cachexia. Nutr Rev 52:340–347
10. Cowie MR, Mosterd A, Wood DA et al (1997) The epidemiology of heart failure. Eur Heart J 18:208–225
11. Kannel WB, Ho K, Thom T (1994) Changing epidemiological features of cardiac failure. Br Heart J 72(Suppl):S3–S9

12. Anker SD, Ponikowski P, Varney S et al (1997) Wasting as independent risk factor for mortality in chronic heart failure. Lancet 349:1050–1053

13. Davos CH, Doehner W, Rauchhaus M et al (2003) Body mass and survival in patients with chronic heart failure without cachexia: the importance of obesity. J Card Fail 9:29–35

14. Pittman JG, Cohen P (1964) The pathogenesis of cardiac cachexia. N Engl J Med 271:403–409

15. Anker SD, Sharma R (2002) The syndrome of cardiac cachexia. Int J Cardiol 85:51–66

16. Harrington D, Anker SD, Chua TP et al (1997) Skeletal muscle function and its relation to exercise tolerance in chronic heart failure. J Am Coll Cardiol 30:1758–1764

17. Anker SD, Swan JW, Volterrani M et al (1997) The influence of muscle mass, strength, fatigability and blood flow on exercise capacity in cachectic and non-cachectic patients with chronic heart failure. Eur Heart J 18:259–269

18. Lipkin DP, Jones DA, Round JM, Poole-Wilson PA (1988) Abnormalities of skeletal muscle in patients with chronic heart failure. Int J Cardiol 18:187–195

19. Mancini DM, Walter G, Reichek N et al (1992) Contribution of skeletal muscle atrophy to exercise intolerance and altered muscle metabolism in heart failure. Circulation 85:1364–1373

20. Drexler H, Riede U, Münzel T et al (1992) Alterations of skeletal muscle in chronic heart failure. Circulation 85:1751–1759

21. Anker SD, Clark AL, Teixeira MM et al (1998) Loss of bone mineral in patients with cachexia due to chronic heart failure. Am J Cardiol 83:612–615

22. Anker SD, Ponikowski PP, Clark Al et al (1999) Cytokines and neurohormones relating to body composition alterations in the wasting syndrome of chronic heart failure. Eur Heart J 20:683–693

23. Doehner W, Rauchhaus M, Florea VG et al (2001) Uric acid in cachectic and noncachectic patients with chronic heart failure: relationship to leg vascular resistance. Am Heart J 141:792–799

24. Dutka DP, Elborn JS, Delamere F et al (1993) Tumor necrosis factor alpha in severe congestive heart failure. Br Heart J 70:141–143

25. Anker SD, Clark AL, Kemp M et al (1997) Tumor necrosis factor and steroid metabolism in chronic heart failure: possible relation to muscle wasting. J Am Coll Cardiol 30:997–1001

26. Anker SD, Chua TP, Ponikowski P et al (1997) Hormonal changes and catabolic/anabolic imbalance in chronic heart failure and their importance for cardiac cachexia. Circulation 96:526–534

27. Tracey KJ, Morgello S, Koplin B et al (1990) Metabolic effects of cachectin/tumor necrosis factor are modified by site of production: cachectin/tumor necrosis factor-secreting tumor in skeletal muscle induces chronic cachexia, while implantation in brain induces predominantly acute cachexia. J Clin Invest 86:2014–2024

28. Sharma R, Rauchhaus M, Ponikowski PP et al (2000) The relationship of erythrocyte sedimentation rate to inflammatory cytokines and survival in patients with chronic heart failure treated with angiotensin-converting enzyme inhibitors. J Am Coll Cardiol 36:523–528

29. Hasper D, Hummel M, Kleber FX et al (1998) Systemic inflammation in patients with heart failure. Eur Heart J 19:761–765

30. Torre-Amione G, Kapadia S, Lee J et al (1996) Tumor necrosis factor-alpha and tumor necrosis factor receptors in the failing human heart. Circulation 93:704–711

31. Seta Y, Shan K, Bozkurt B et al (1996) Basic mechanisms in heart failure: the cytokine hypothesis. J Card Fail 3:243–249

32. Clark AL, Loebe M, Potapov EV et al (2001) Ventricular assist device in severe heart failure: effects on cytokines, complement and body weight. Eur Heart J 22:2275–2283

33. Genth-Zotz S, von Haehling S, Bolger AP et al (2002) Pathophysiological quantities of endotoxin induce tumor necrosis factor release in whole blood from patients with chronic heart failure. Am J Cardiol 90:1226–1230

34. Anker SD, Egerer KR, Volk HD et al (1997) Elevated soluble CD14 receptors and altered cytokines in chronic heart failure. Am J Cardiol 79:1426–1430

35. Brunkhorst FM, Clark AL, Forycki ZF, Anker SD (1999) Pyrexia, procalcitonin, immune activation and survival in cardiogenic shock: the potential importance of bacterial translocation. Int J Cardiol 72:3–10

36. Vonhof S, Brost B, Stille-Siegener M et al (1998) Monocyte activation in congestive heart failure due to coronary artery disease and idiopathic dilated cardiomyopathy. Int J Cardiol 63:237–244

37. Rauchhaus M, Coats AJ, Anker SD (2000) The endotoxin-lipoprotein hypothesis. Lancet 356:930–933

38. Rauchhaus M, Koloczek V, Volk H et al (2000) Inflammatory cytokines and the possible immunological role for lipoproteins in chronic heart failure. Int J Cardiol 76:125–133

39. Horwich TB, Hamilton MA, Maclellan WR, Fonarow GC (2002) Low serum total cholesterol is associated with marked increase in mortality in advanced heart failure. J Card Fail 8:216–224

40. Rauchhaus M, Clark AL, Doehner W et al (2003) The relationship between cholesterol and survival in patients with chronic heart failure. J Am Coll Cardiol 42:1933–1940

41. Okonko DO, Anker SD (2004) Anemia in chronic heart failure: pathogenetic mechanisms. J Card Fail 10 (1 Suppl):S5–S9

42. Goldstein DS (1981) Plasma norepinephrine as an indicator of sympathetic neural activity in clinical cardiology. Am J Cardiol 48:1147–1154

43. Lommi J, Kupari M, Yki-Jarvinen H (1998) Free fatty acid kinetics and oxidation in congestive heart failu-

re. Am J Cardiol 81:45–50

44. Bolger AP, Sharma R, Li W et al (2002) Neurohormonal activation and the chronic heart failure syndrome in adults with congenital heart disease. Circulation 106:92–99

45. Brink M, Wellen J, Delafontaine P (1996) Angiotensin II causes weight loss and decreases circulating insulin-like growth factor I in rats through a pressor-independent mechanism. J Clin Invest 97:2509–2516

46. Staroukine M, Devriendt J, Decoodt P, Verniory A (1984) Relationships between plasma epinephrine, norepinephrine, dopamine and angiotensin II concentrations, renin activity, hemodynamic state and prognosis in acute heart failure. Acta Cardiol 39:131–138

47. Niebauer J, Pflaum CD, Clark AL et al (1998) Deficient insulin-like growth factor I in chronic heart failure predicts altered body composition, anabolic deficiency, cytokine and neurohormonal activation. J Am Coll Cardiol 32:393–397

48. Anker SD, Volterrani M, Pflaum CD et al (2001) Acquired growth hormone resistance in patients with chronic heart failure: implications for therapy with growth hormone. J Am Coll Cardiol 38:443–452

49. Anand IS, Ferrari R, Kalra GS et al (1989) Edema of cardiac origin. Studies of body water and sodium renal function, hemodynamic indexes, and plasma hormones in untreated congestive cardiac failure. Circulation 80:299–305

50. Nicholls MG, Espiner EA, Donald RA, Hughes H (1974) Aldosterone and its regulation during diuresis in patients with gross congestive heart failure. Clin Sci Mol Med 47:301–315

51. Flier JS (2004) Obesity wars: molecular progress confronts an expanding epidemic. Cell 116:337–350

52. Witte KK, Clark AL (2002) Nutritional abnormalities contributing to cachexia in chronic illness. Int J Cardiol 85:23–31

53. Leyva F, Anker SD, Egerer K et al (1998) Hyperleptinaemia in chronic heart failure. Relationships with insulin. Eur Heart J 19:1547–1551

54. Filippatos GS, Tsilias K, Venetsanou K et al (2000) Leptin serum levels in cachectic heart failure patients. Relationship with tumor necrosis factor-alpha system. Int J Cardiol 76:117–122

55. Doehner W, Pflaum CD, Rauchhaus M et al (2001) Leptin, insulin sensitivity and growth hormone binding protein in chronic heart failure with and without cardiac cachexia. Eur J Endocrinol 145:727–735

56. Sharma R, Coats AJS, Anker SD (2000) The role of inflammatory mediators in chronic heart failure: cytokines nitric oxide, and endothelin-1. Int J Cardiol 72:175–186

57. Sigurdsson A, Swedberg K, Ullmann B (1994) Effects of ramipril on the neurohormonal response to exercise in patients with mild or moderate congestive heart failure. Eur Heart J 15:247–254

58. Van Veldhuisen DJ, Genth-Zotz S, Brouwer J et al (1998) High- versus low-dose ACE inhibition in chronic heart failure: a double-blind, placebo-controlled study of imidapril. J Am Coll Cardiol 32:1811–1818

59. Liu L, Zhao SP (1999) The changes in circulating tumor necrosis factor levels in patients with congestive heart failure influenced by therapy. Int J Cardiol 69:77–82

60. Gullestad L, Aukrust P, Ueland T et al (1999) Effect of high- versus low-dose angiotensin converting enzyme inhibition on cytokine levels in chronic heart failure. J Am Coll Cardiol 34:2061–2067

61. Corbalan R, Acevedo M, Godoy I et al (1998) Enalapril restores depressed circulating insulin-like growth factor 1 in patients with chronic heart failure. J Card Fail 4:115–119

62. Tsutamoto T, Wada A, Maeda K et al (2000) Angiotensin II type 1 receptor antagonist decreases plasma levels of tumor necrosis factor alpha, interleukin-6 and soluble adhesion molecules in patients with chronic heart failure. J Am Coll Cardiol 35:714–721

63. Coats AJS, Anker SD, Roecker EB et al (2001) Prevention and reversal of cardiac cachexia in patients with severe heart failure by carvedilol: results of the COPERNICUS study. Circulation 104:II-437 (abs)

64. Hryniewicz K, Androne AS, Hudaihed A, Katz SD (2003) Partial reversal of cachexia by beta-adrenergic receptor blocker therapy in patients with chronic heart failure. J Card Fail 9:464–468

65. Feuerstein G, Yue TL, Ma X, Ruffulo RR (1998) Novel mechanisms in the treatment of heart failure: inhibition of oxygen radicals and apoptosis by carvedilol. Prog Cardiovasc Dis 41:17–24

66. Anonymous (1999) Effect of metoprolol CR/XL in chronic heart failure: Metoprolol CR/XL Randomized Intervention Trial in Congestive Heart Failure (MERIT-HF). Lancet 353:2001–2007

67. Packer M, Bristow MR, Cohn JN et al (1996) The effect of carvedilol on morbidity and mortality in patients with chronic heart failure. N Engl J Med 334:1349–1355

68. Goldenburg MM (1999) Etanercept, a novel drug for the treatment of patients with severe, active rheumatoid arthritis. Clin Ther 21:75–87

69. Moreland LW (1999) Inhibitors of tumor necrosis factor for rheumatoid arthritis. J Rheumatol 26:7–15

70. Present DH, Rutgeerts P, Targan S et al (1999) Infliximab for the treatment of fistulas in patients with Crohn's disease. N Engl J Med 340:1398–1405

71. Sharma R, Anker SD (2002) Cytokines, apoptosis and cachexia: the potential for TNF antagonism. Int J Cardiol 85:161–171

72. Deswal A, Bozkurt B, Seta Y et al (1999) Safety and efficacy of a soluble P75 tumor necrosis factor receptor (enbrel, etanercept) in patients with advanced heart failure. Circulation 99: 3224–3226

73. Fichtlscherer S, Rössig L, Breuer S et al (2001) Tumor necrosis factor antagonism with etanercept improves systemic endothelial vasoreactivity in patients with advanced heart failure. Circulation 104: 3023–3025

74. Mann DL, McMurray JJ, Packer M et al (2004) Targeted anticytokine therapy in patients with chronic heart failure. Circulation 109:1594–1602

75. Chung ES, Packer M, Lo KH et al (2003) Randomized, double-blind, placebo-controlled, pilot trial of infliximab, a chimeric monoclonal antibody to tumor necrosis factor-alpha, in patients with moderate-to-severe heart failure: results of the Anti-TNF Therapy Against Congestive Heart Failure (ATTACH) trial. Circulation 107: 3133–3140

76. Anker SD, Coats AJS (2002) How to RECOVER from RENAISSANCE? The significance of the results of RECOVER; RENAISSANCE; RENEWAL and ATTACH. Int J Cardiol 86:123–130

77. Matsumori A, Shioi T, Yamada T et al (1994) Vesnarinone, a new inotropic agent, inhibits cytokine production by stimulated human blood from patients with heart failure. Circulation 89:955–958

78. Sliwa K, Skudicky D, Candy G et al (1998) Randomised investigation of effects of pentoxiphylline on left-ventricular performance in idiopathic dilated cardiomyopathy. Lancet 351:1091–1093

79. Skudicky D, Bergmann A, Sliwa K et al (2001) Beneficial effects of pentoxifylline in patients with idiopathic dilated cardiomyopathy treated with angiotensin-converting enzyme inhibitors and carvedilol: results of a randomized study. Circulation 103:1083–1088

80. Tsujinaka T, Fujita J, Ebisui C et al (1996) Interleukin 6 receptor antibody inhibits muscle atrophy and modulates proteolytic systems in interleukin 6 transgenic mice. J Clin Invest 97:244–249

81. Osterziel KJ, Strohm O, Schuler J et al (1998) Randomised, double-blind, placebo-controlled trial of human recombinant growth hormone in patients with chronic heart failure due to dilated cardiomyopathy. Lancet 351:1233–1237

82. Cicoira M, Kalra PR, Anker SD (2003) Growth hormone resistance in chronic heart failure and its therapeutic implications. J Card Fail 9:219–226

83. Cuneo RC, Wilmshurst P, Lowy C et al (1989) Cardiac failure responding to growth hormone. Lancet 1:838–839

84. O'Driscoll JG, Green DJ, Ireland M et al (1997) Treatment of end-stage cardiac failure with growth hormone. Lancet 349:1068

85. Sharma R, Anker SD (2002) Immune and neurohormonal pathways in chronic heart failure. Congest Heart Fail 8:23–28

86. Nagaya N, Kangawa K (2003) Ghrelin improves left ventricular dysfunction and cardiac cachexia in heart failure. Curr Opin Pharmacol 3:146–151

87. Nagaya N, Kangawa K (2003) Ghrelin, a novel growth hormone-releasing peptide, in the treatment of chronic heart failure. Regul Peptides 114:71–77

88. Abel RM, Fischer JE, Buckley MJ et al (1976) Malnutrition in cardiac surgical patients: results of a early postoperative parenteral nutrition. Arch Surg 111: 45–50

89. Heymsfield SB, Casper K (1989) Congestive heart failure: clinical management by use of continuous nasoenteric feeding. Am J Clin Nutr 50:539–544

90. Broquist M, Arnquist H, Dahlström U et al (1994) Nutritional assessment and muscle energy metabolism in severe chronic congestive heart failure-effects of longterm dietary supplementation. Eur Heart J 15:1641–1650

91. McGandy RB, Russel RM, Hartz SC et al (1986) Nutritional status survey of healthy non-institutionalized elderly: energy and nutrient intake from three-day diet records and nutrient supplements. Nutr Res 6:785–798

92. Buck M, Chojkier M (1996) Muscle wasting and dedifferentiation induced by oxidative stress in a murine model of cachexia is prevented by inhibitors of nitric oxide synthesis and antioxidants. EMBO J 15(8):1753–1765

93. Herbaczynska-Cedro K, Kosiewicz-Wasek B, Cedro K (1995) Supplementation with vitamins C and E suppresses leukocyte oxygen free radical production in patients with myocardial infarction. Eur Heart J 16:1044–1049

94. Belch JJ, Bridges AB, Scott N, Chopra M (1991) Oxygen free radicals and congestive heart failure. Br Heart J 65:245–248

95. Nishiyama Y, Ikeda H, Haramaki N et al (1998) Oxidative stress is related to exercise intolerance in patients with heart failure. Am Heart J 135:115–120

96. Witte KKA, Clark AL, Cleland JGF (2001) Chronic heart failure and micronutrients. J Am Coll Cardiol 37:1765–74

97. Von Haehling S, Anker SD, Bassenge E (2003) Statins and the role of nitric oxide in chronic heart failure. Heart Fail Rev 8:99–106

98. Freeman LM, Rush JE, Kehayias JJ et al (1998) Nutritional alterations and the effect of fish oil supplementation in dogs with heart failure. J Vet Intern Med 12:440–448

99. Barber MD, Ross JA, Voss AC et al (1999) The effect of an oral nutritional supplement enriched with fish oil on weigth loss in patients with pancreatic cancer. Br J Cancer 81:80–86

100. Endres S, Ghorbani R, Kelly VE et al (1989) The effect of dietary supplementation with n-3 polyunsaturated fatty acids on the synthesis of IL-1 and tumor necrosis factor by mononuclear cells. N Engl J Med 320:265–271

101. Kremer JM, Jubiz W, Michalek A et al (1987) Fish-oil fatty acid supplementation in active rheumatoid arthritis: a double-blinded, controlled, crossover study. Ann Intern Med 106:497–503

102. Coats AJ, Adamopoulos S, Meyer TE et al (1990) Effects of physical training in chronic heart failure. Lancet 335:63–66

103. Schulze PC, Gielen S, Schuler G, Hambrecht R (2002) Chronic heart failure and skeletal muscle catabolism: effects of exercise training. Int J Cardiol 85:141–149

104. Coats AJ, Adamopoulos S, Radaelli A et al (1992) Controlled trial of physical training in chronic heart failure. Exercise performance, hemodynamics, ventilation, and autonomic function. Circulation 85:2119–2131

# SECTION 7
# CACHEXIA AND AGEING

# Epidemiology of Malnutrition in the Elderly

Shing-Shing Yeh, Michael W. Schuster

## Epidemiology

Weight loss among geriatric patients is not unusual. In fact, 30–50% of nursing-home residents have substandard body weight, substandard mid-arm muscle circumference, and low serum albumin levels [1–8]. The incidence of weight loss has been reported to be 5–15% in the elderly community overall [9]. Morley and Kraenzle [10] found that among 156 nursing home residents, 15–21% had weight loss of 5 lbs. or more over 3–6 months.

Wallace and Schwartz reported that involuntary weight loss in the geriatric population exceeds 13% (in a group of 247 community-residing male veterans, 65 years of age or older) [11]. The prevalence of malnutrition in the hospitalised elderly can be as high as 32% [12, 13], and 54% of newly admitted residents to long-term-care facilities were found to be malnourished [14]. Malnutrition is a major problem among residents in such facilities [15, 16]. Thomas and associates found that 29% of acutely hospitalised patients admitted to rehabilitation were malnourished [17], and 63% of the admissions were at risk for malnutrition; thus, more than 91% of the patients admitted to a subacute care facility were either malnourished or at risk of malnutrition [17]. This may reflect the high prevalence of acute illness that results, at least in part, from malnutrition in the elderly.

## Definition of Malnutrition

The criteria used to define malnutrition vary. Body weight, body mass index (BMI), triceps skin-fold thickness, and arm circumference are the most commonly used anthropometric methods to define malnutrition [14]. A broad panel of biochemical variables has been advocated to define nutritional status, such as serum albumin, lymphocyte count, pre-albumin, transferrin, and retinol-binding protein [18, 19], but no single biological parameter is satisfactory as the sole predictor of malnutrition [19–22].

## Consequence of Malnutrition

Wasting and cachexia [23–25] are associated with severe physiological, psychological, and immunological consequences, regardless of the underlying causes, and they have been associated with increased infections, decubiti, and even death [26–30]. Goodwin [31], Braun [32], and Morley [33] found that malnutrition may also cause or exacerbate cognitive and mood disorders. Marton [6], Rabinovitz [4], and Yamashita (The Gain Registry) [34] found that weight loss and cachexia are even predictive of morbidity and mortality. Ho et al. found a two-fold increase in mortality in those elderly who lost over 2 kg in 2 years [35], and Newman et al. reported a two-fold increase in mortality in elderly subjects who had a weight loss of 5% over 3 years [36]. In addition, Reynolds et al. found a three-fold increase in mortality in older women who had weight loss of over 4.5% in 2 years [37]. Wallace et al. found that involuntary weight loss greater than 4% of body weight over a 1-year period was the most sensitive and important independent predictor of increased mortality [9, 11]. It is also interesting to note that even intentional weight loss in the elderly is associated with increased mortality [11, 36].

## Causes of Malnutrition in the Elderly

The major causes of weight loss, as determined by several large studies, are summarised in Table 1. In

**Table 1.** Diagnostic spectrum of involuntary weight loss. (Modified from [3])

| Population (n) | 70% In-patient (n = 91) | In-patient (n = 154) | In-patient (n = 50) | In-patient (n = 158) | Out-patient (n = 107) | Out-patient (n = 45) |
|---|---|---|---|---|---|---|
| Age (mean) | 59 | 64 | 59 | 68 | 62 | 72 |
| Neoplasm | 19% | 36% | 10% | 24% | 6% | 16% |
| Gastrointestinal | 14% | 17% | 18% | 19% | 6% | 11% |
| Psychiatric | 9% | 10% | 42% | 11% | 22% | 18% |
| Endocrine | 4% | 4% | 10% | 11% | 5% | 9% |
| Cardiopulmonary | 14% | | 2% | 10% | 9% | |
| Other diagnosis[a] | 18% | 9% | 8% | 8% | 16% | 22% |
| Unknown | 26% | 23% | 10% | 16% | 36% | 24% |

[a]Other medical diagnoses: neurologic, infectious, alcohol, medication, renal, inflammatory disease; n, number of patients

these studies, most diagnoses were made from standard evaluations that included a careful history, physical examination, and basic screening lab tests (complete blood count, electrolyte, renal, liver and thyroid function test, stool haemoccult, chest radiograph, and urinalysis) [4–8]. The most interesting findings indicated that 10–36% of weight loss was due to an unknown aetiology [5, 6, 8], 6–36% was due to neoplasm [4–6, 8], 9–42% to depression and related psychiatric problems [4–6, 8], and 14–19% to gastrointestinal and swallowing-related problems [4–6, 8]. Although it may be informative, from a clinical standpoint, to review all of the aetiologies that have been noted in case series and respective studies of weight loss in the elderly, Morley et al. [38] have devised a simple mnemonic for remembering the major causes of weight loss (Table 2).

Blaum et al. carried out a cross-sectional, minimum-data-set assessment, data analysis of 6832 residents of a community nursing home (sampled from 202 nursing homes in seven American states). They found that poor oral intake, eating dependency, decubiti, and chewing problems increased the likelihood of low BMI (< 19.4) and weight loss (a 5% weight loss, or 10% weight loss in 180 days) [39]. In females age 85 or older, being bed-bound (bedfast) and having suffered a hip fracture increased the odds of low BMI, while depressed behaviours and two or more chronic

**Table 2.** Treatable causes of malnutrition (meals on wheels) (Adapted from [38])

M Medication effect
E Emotional problems (depression)
A Anorexia tardive (nervosa, alcoholism)
L Late-life paranoia
S Swallowing disorders

O Oral factors (e.g., poorly fitting dentures, caries)
N No money

W Wandering and other dementia-related behaviours
H Hyperthyroidism, hypothyroidism, hyperparathyroidism, hypoadrenalism
E Enteric problems (malabsorption)
E Eating problems (inability to feed oneself)
L Low-salt, low-cholesterol diets
S Stones, social problems (e.g., isolation, inability to obtain preferred foods)

diseases increase the odds of weight loss [39] (Tables 3, 4).

Studies have revealed that dietary intervention and nutritional supplements improve malnutrition. By this approach, weight gain occurred in 50% of admitted malnourished patients, although 37% of patients remained malnourished despite the intervention [14]. Increased awareness of the importance of malnutrition may decrease the prevalence of malnutrition over time [40].

**Table 3.** Logistic regression: multivariate association of resident characteristics with low BMI. (Modified from [39])

| Independent variable | Coefficient | Odds ratio point estimate | Odds ratio 95% confidence limits |
|---|---|---|---|
| Poor intake | 0.80 | 2.23 | 1.95–2.56 |
| Eating dependency | 0.60 | 1.83 | 1.59–2.56 |
| Bedfast | 0.50 | 1.64 | 1.38–1.95 |
| Fracture of femur | 0.49 | 1.64 | 1.22–2.19 |
| Presence of decubiti | 0.36 | 1.44 | 1.20–1.72 |

**Table 4.** Logistic regression: multivariate association of resident characteristics with weight loss. (Modified from [39])

| Independent Variable | Coefficient | Odds ratio point estimate | Odds ratio 95% confidence limits |
|---|---|---|---|
| Poor intake | 1.37 | 3.93 | 3.32–4.66 |
| Eating dependency | 0.53 | 1.70 | 1.42–2.04 |
| Presence of decubiti | 0.45 | 1.57 | 1.26–1.96 |
| Depressed behaviours | 0.41 | 1.51 | 1.20–1.90 |
| Chewing problems | 0.37 | 1.44 | 1.19–1.74 |
| Two or more chronic diseases | 0.35 | 1.41 | 1.18–1.70 |

# References

1. Abbasi AA, Rudman D (1993) Observations on the prevalence of protein-calorie undernutrition in VA nursing homes. J Am Geriat Soc 41:117–121
2. Abbasi AA, Rudman D (1994) Undernutrition in the nursing home: prevalence, consequences, causes and prevention. Nutr Rev 52:113–122
3. Wallace JI, Schwartz RS (2002) Epidemiology of weight loss in humans with special reference to wasting in the elderly. Int J Cardiol 85:15–21
4. Rabinovitz M, Pitlik SD, Leifer M et al (1986) Unintentional weight loss: an analysis of 154 cases. Arch Int Med 146:186–187
5. Huerta G, Viniegra L (1989) Involuntary weight loss as a clinical problem. Rev Invest Clin 41:5–9 [Spanish]
6. Marton KI, Sox HC Jr, Krupp JR (1981) Involuntary weight loss: diagnostic and prognostic significance. Ann Intern Med 95:568–574
7. Lankisch P, Gerzmann M, Gerzmann JF, Lehnick D (2001) Unintentional weight loss: diagnosis and prognosis. The first prospective follow-up study from a secondary referral centre. J Intern Med 249:41–46
8. Thompson M, Morris L (1991) Unexplained weight loss in ambulatory elderly. J Am Geriatr Soc 39:497–500
9. Wallace JI, Schwartz RS (1997) Involuntary weight loss in elderly outpatients: recognition, etiologies, and treatment. Clin Geriatr Med 13:717–735
10. Morley J, Kraenzle D (1994) Causes of weight loss in a community nursing home. J Am Geriatr Soc 42: 583–585
11. Wallace JI, Schwartz RS, LaCroix AZ et al (1995) Involuntary weight loss in older outpatients: incidence and clinical significance. J Am Geriatr Soc 43:329–337
12. Incalzi RA, Gemma A, Capparella O et al (1996) Energy intake and in-hospital starvation. A clinically relevant relationship. Arch Intern Med 156:425–429
13. Willard MD, Gilsdorf RB, Price RA (1980) Protein-calorie malnutrition in a community hospital. JAMA 243:1720–1722
14. Thomas DR, Verdery RB, Gardner L et al (1991) A prospective study of outcome from protein-energy malnutrition in nursing home residents. JPEN J Parenter Enteral Nutr 15:400–404
15. Lipschitz DA (1982) Protein calorie malnutrition in the hospitalized elderly. Prim Care 9:531–543
16. Rudman D, Feller AG (1989) Protein-calorie under-nutrition in the nursing home. J Am Geriatr Soc 37:173–183
17. Thomas DR, Zdrowski CD, Wilson MM et al (2002) Malnutrition in subacute care. Am J Clin Nutr 75:308–313

18. Dionigi R, Dominioni L, Jemos V et al (1986) Diagnosing malnutrition. Gut 27 (Suppl 1):5–8

19. Morley JE (2003) Anorexia and weight loss in older persons. J Gerontol A Biol Sci Med Sci 58:131–137

20. Kergoat MJ, Leclerc BS, Petitclerc C, Imbach A (1987) Discriminant biochemical markers for evaluating the nutritional status of elderly patients in long-term care. Am J Clin Nutr 46:849–861

21. Morgan DB, Newton HM, Schorah CJ et al (1986) Abnormal indices of nutrition in the elderly: a study of different clinical groups. Age Ageing 15:65–76

22. Bastow MD (1982) Anthropometrics revisited. Proc Nutr Soc 41:381–388

23. Chandra RK (1983) Nutrition, immunity and infection present knowledge and future directions. Lancet 1:688–691

24. Haydock D, Hill G (1987) Improved wound healing in surgical patients receiving intravenous nutrition. B J Surg 4:320–323

25. Lennmarken C, Larson J (1986) Skeletal muscle function and energy metabolites in malnourished surgical patients. Acta Chir Scand 152:169–173

26. Pinchcofsky-Devin GD, Kaminski MV Jr (1986) Correlation of pressure sores and nutritional status. J Am Geriatr Soc 34:435–440

27. Silver AJ, Morley JE, Strome LS et al (1988) Nutritional status in an academic nursing home. J Am Geriatr Soc 36:487–491

28. Rudman D, Mattson DE, Nagraj HS et al (1987) Antecedents of death in the men of a Veterans Administration nursing home. J Am Geriatr Soc 35:496–502

29. Rudman D, Feller AG, Nagraj HS et al (1987) Relation of serum albumin concentration to death rate in nursing home men. JPEN J Parenter Enteral Nutr 11:360–363

30. Rudman D, Feller AG (1989) Protein-calorie undernutrition in the nursing home. J Am Geriatr Soc 37:173–183

31. Goodwin JS, Goodwin JM, Garry PJ (1983) Association between nutritional status and cognition in a healthy elderly population. JAMA 249:2917–2921

32. Braun JV, Wykle MH, Cowling WR 3rd (1988) Failure to thrive in older persons: a concept derived. Gerontologist 28:809–812

33. Morley J (1996) Anorexia in older persons: epidemiology and optimal treatment. Drugs Aging 8:134–156

34. Yamashita BD, Sullivan DH, Morley JE et al (2002) The GAIN (Geriatric Anorexia Nutrition) Registry: the impact of appetite and weight on mortality in a long-term care population. J Nutr Health Aging 6:275–281

35. Ho SC, Woo J, Sham A (1994) Risk factor change in older persons, a perspective from Hong Kong: weight change and mortality. J Gerontol 49:M269–M272

36. Newman AB, Yanez D, Harris T et al (2001) Weight change in old age and its association with mortality. J Am Geriatr Soc 49:1309–1318

37. Reynolds MW, Fredman L, Langenberg P, Magaziner J (1999) Weight, weight change, mortality in a random sample of older community-dwelling women. J Am Geriatr Soc 47:1409–1414

38. Morley JE (1997) Anorexia of aging: physiologic and pathologic. Am J Clin Nutr 66:760–773

39. Blaum CS, Fries BE, Fiatarone MA (1995) Factors associated with low body mass index and weight loss in nursing home residents. J Gerontol A Biol Sci Med Sci 50:M162–M168

40. Coats KG, Morgan SL, Bartolucci AA, Weinsier RL (1993) Hospital-associated malnutrition: a reevaluation 12 years later. J Am Diet Assoc 93:27–33

# Pathophysiology of Body Composition Changes in Elderly People

Alessandra Coin, Giuseppe Sergi, Emine M. Inelmen, Giuliano Enzi

## Body Composition in the Elderly

Aging is associated with changes in body composition that have important consequences on health and physical function. Thus, studying body composition changes is of increasing interest in geriatric research, and measures are being developed to favourably influence body composition in old age, in addition to exercise and diet.

With advancing age, the lean components, such as total body water, skeletal muscle, organ mass, and bone mineral, tend to decrease, while total body fat increases and becomes redistributed more in the abdominal than in the peripheral adipose tissues [1–6] (Fig. 1). These changes seem to be associated primarily with a small positive imbalance between energy intake and expenditure due to an increasingly sedentary life style [7]. Some changes could depend on age-related endocrine and metabolic alterations, however [5, 8], and may occur relatively rapidly.

Increased body fat and centralised fat distribution have been shown to be associated in the elderly with risk factors for non-insulin-dependent diabetes and heart disease [9]. Bone mineral loss is a major risk factor for bone fractures, which are a significant cause of morbidity, institutionalization in nursing homes, and mortality among the elderly [10]. Sarcopenia, defined as a decrease in muscle mass and function, may be associated with impaired immunocompetence and physical functional status [11].

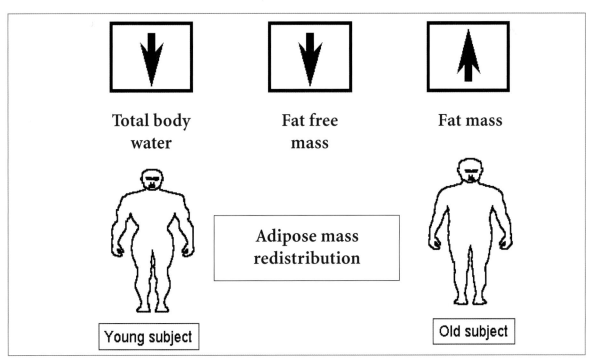

**Fig. 1.** Body composition changes with advancing age

Accurate body composition information is considered to be more difficult to obtain in the elderly than in younger age groups for a variety of reasons [12]. Several methods are available for assessing body composition, but it is questionable whether some of them can be used in an older population. In clinical practice, anthropometry cannot adequately estimate nutritional status, and measuring fat mass (FM) and fat-free mass (FFM) is recommended. Among the various methods, dual-energy X-ray absorptiometry (DEXA) is the most suitable for evaluating FFM and FM, regardless of FFM hydration. Bioelectrical impedance analysis (BIA) accurately estimates body fluids (total body water and extracellular water), but its reliability in assessing FFM depends on hydration status.

## Fat Mass and Distribution Changes

### Total Adipose Tissue

Little is known about age-related changes in body fatness in elderly adults. Most studies have documented increases up to 50–60 years of age, after which body fatness appears to stabilise [13–16]. In a cross-sectional survey, Baumgartner et al. [6] suggest that body fatness (in terms of both absolute FM and percent body fat) may be relatively stable in elderly men, but may decrease with age in elderly women. In their study, the distribution of body fat, as assessed by DEXA, did not appear to change with age beyond 65 years, leading to the conclusion that the accumulation of abdominal and visceral fat with age (in both men and women) occurs primarily in middle age, while FM remains constant or increases slightly in subsequent decades. In a longitudinal observation of body composition in older adults, as determined using hydrodensitometry, Hughes et al. [17] found an overall increase in adipose tissue in an older cohort, but this increase was attenuated with advancing age in women, whereas there was no apparent age-related effect in men. Younger women, especially those who were premenopausal at the baseline assessment, gained fat, whereas women > 70 years old lost fat as they grew older. Visser et al. [18] recently measured body composition changes by DEXA during a 1- and 2-year fol-

low-up in 2040 men and women 70–79 years old taking part in the Health, Aging, and Body Composition Study. The investigators observed a 2% increase in total FM in the men, while no changes were seen in the women, thus confirming previous reports. In contrast, a recent 2-year longitudinal survey recorded an increase in total and percent body fat in women, but not in men [19].

In conclusion, an increase in body fatness up to 50–60 years of age is well-documented, while the occurrence of further changes in body fat in subsequent years remains unclear; however, fatness appears to be stable in the elderly body [13–16].

It has been claimed that increased body fat in elderly individuals plays an important part in the increase in proinflammatory cytokines. Several studies have demonstrated that adipose tissue secretes interleukin (IL)-6 [20, 21] as well as tumour necrosis factor (TNF)-α [22–25]. A recent study using univariate and multivariate linear regression analysis demonstrated that the relative amount of truncal fat, measured by DEXA, correlates with the levels of plasma TNF-α and IL-6, after adjusting for age group and gender [26].

### Intra-Abdominal Fat

The age-related redistribution of adipose tissue within the body is perhaps more important than the total body fat gain. As shown in Fig. 2, the visceral/subcutaneous fat ratio at the abdominal level, as detected by computed tomography, increases with age in both normal-weight and overweight subjects [27]. Intra-abdominal fat (IAF) increases with age both quantitatively and proportionally more than peripheral fat mass [28–30], even in the absence of obesity. IAF gain apparently starts before the age of 20 years both in men and women, but the accumulation of IAF accelerates at the age of menopause in women [28–30]. DEXA in healthy subjects confirms that the ratio of upper- to lower-body fat increases linearly after 20 years of age in both genders [30]. Between the 20 and 70 years, it increases from 1.07 to 1.67 in men and from 0.81 to 1.21 in women [30]. Similarly, IAF area, measured at the L4 level by CT, increases linearly in obese subjects with advancing age, even without significant changes in

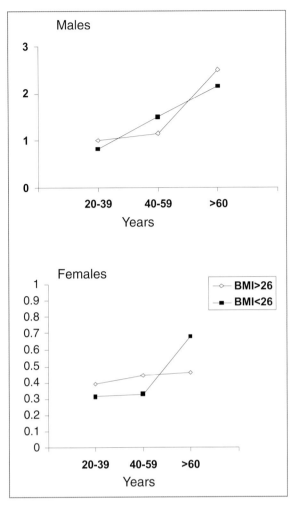

**Fig. 2.** Changes of the visceral/subcutaneous (V/S) fat ratio at the abdominal level by sex, age, and overweight, as detected by computed tomography

whole FM [29]. The cause of this centralisation of body fat is a combination of several age-related factors, such as changes in hormone levels and fatty-acid utilisation, less physical activity, and leptin resistance [31, 32].

It is this increase in IAF that seems to cause insulin resistance, rather than aging per se [31, 33]. Studies on patients with type II diabetes suggest that the metabolic link between increased IAF and insulin resistance is the greater availability and/or oxidation of free fatty acids [34–37]. Physical inactivity certainly enhances IAF accumulation and, more directly, insulin resistance [38, 39]. However, the significant independent effects of menopause and sarcopenia on insulin resistance remain to be established [31].

# Lean Mass Changes

## Fat-Free Mass

As people grow older, their FFM seems to decrease, particularly bone and muscle mass, while central lean body mass seems relatively preserved [40, 41]. Lean mass peaks in the third to fourth decade of life, followed by a steady decline with advancing age [2,3]. Recent methodologically accurate longitudinal studies have confirmed the decline in muscle mass suggested by earlier cross-sectional studies. A 14.7% decline in muscle cross-sectional area, measured using CT, was observed in older men over a period of 12 years [42]. In addition, a 2–3% decline in appendicular skeletal muscle mass, as determined by DEXA measurements, was recorded in healthy older men and women over a period of 4.7 years [43]. Studies on total body potassium content (TBK) and body cell mass (BCM) suggest that the composition, or 'quality,' of FFM changes with age, possibly due to an insufficient cell replacement [44]. Active cell mass may be replaced by inert extracellular solids and fluids to a greater extent in women than in men, but there is no obvious explanation for this apparent gender difference.

## Muscle Mass Changes: Sarcopenia

The loss of muscle mass with aging is increasingly recognised as having important consequences in old age because it may be associated with weakness, disability, and morbidity [45–47]. In 1989, Rosenberg focused renewed attention on this phenomenon by giving it a name, *sarcopenia* [48]. *Sarco,* from the Greek, denotes flesh (muscle), and *penia* indicates a deficiency; thus, sarcopenia translates loosely as muscle deficiency. It is now used to refer specifically to the gradual loss of skeletal muscle mass and strength that takes place with advancing age. It is distinct from muscle loss (cachexia) caused by inflammatory diseases, or from the weight loss and muscle wasting caused by starvation or advanced disease [49]. Of course, superimposed illnesses will accelerate the loss of muscle mass, and thus increase the risk of disability, frailty, and death.

Despite acceptance of the term sarcopenia, precise criteria have not been agreed upon. DEXA has been used to explore changes in total and regional body composition, including appendicular skeletal muscle mass (ASMM), which is the sum of the lean mass of legs and arms (also defined as appendicular lean mass, ALM).

Similar to body mass index (BMI), a common definition of sarcopenia accounts for body size by dividing the ASMM by the height squared [44, 50, 51]. In the New Mexico Aging Process Study [45], sex-specific cut-off points for $kg/m^2$ in the ASMM index were set as two standard deviations below the mean for a healthy young-adult population, similar to the definition of osteoporosis. These cut-off points were 7.26 $kg/m^2$ in men and 5.45 $kg/m^2$ in women. According to this definition, the prevalence of sarcopenia increases from 13–24% among people under 70 to more than 50% among those over 80 (Table 1). Other authors classified their patients as sarcopenic if their ASMM index fell into the sex-specific lowest 20% of the distribution of the index; this definition resulted in very similar cut-off values (7.23 $kg/m^2$ in men and 5.67 $kg/m^2$ in women) [52]. The same authors also measured sarcopenia using the ALM, adjusted for FM and height [52]. The prevalence of sarcopenia according to the first method was 50.4% in men and 51.9% in women with a normal BMI (< 25), while based on the second method it was lower (32.8% in men and 23% in women) and different individuals were defined as sarcopenic.

Janssen et al. [53] used BIA to measure skeletal muscle (SM) mass in large cohorts of individuals. The BIA equation for calculating SM mass was developed and cross-validated by comparing BIA measurements with the whole-body SM mass, as determined by magnetic resonance [54]. Absolute SM mass (kg) was converted to percentage SM mass (SM mass/body mass x 100) and termed as the skeletal muscle index (SMI). The classification criteria were developed using the NHANES III data set. Subjects were considered as having a normal SMI even if it was more than one standard deviation above the sex-specific mean for young adults (aged 18–39). Class I sarcopenia corresponded to an SMI between one and two standard deviations below young-adult values, and class II

sarcopenia coincided with an SMI more than two standard deviations below the mean. Using this approach, the prevalence of class I (59% vs 45%) and class II (10% vs 7%) sarcopenia was greater among older (≥ 60 years) women than among older men ($p < 0.001$) (Table 1).

Sarcopenia has been attributed to a reduction in muscle fibre number and size [55]. Type II (fast-twitch, white) fibres are more susceptible than type I (slow-twitch, red) to age-related fibre atrophy and loss [55]. The extent of sarcopenia is muscle-specific, with some muscles exhibiting substantial weight reductions with age (e.g. vastus lateralis, rectus femoris, soleus, plantaris, gastrocnemius, and extensor digitorum longus). Other muscles show no such weight loss (adductor longus, epitrochlearis, and flexor digitorum longus).

A number of mechanisms are thought to cause sarcopenia, including selective decline and changes in motor-unit organisation, contraction-induced injuries, deficient satellite-cell recruitment, increased free radicals and oxidative stress, and age-related accumulation of mitochondrial abnormalities (mitochondrial DNA mutations and electron transport system abnormalities) [55]. More generally, sarcopenia may be considered partly the result of the withdrawal of anabolic stimuli (sex steroids, growth hormones, physical activity, dietary proteins, insulin action), which are prevalent in men, and possibly an increase in catabolic stimuli (subclinical inflammation, production of catabolic cytokines such as TNF-$\alpha$, IL-6, IL-1$\beta$), which are prevalent in women [56]. According to a recent theory on aging, the increase in body fat may have an important role in the increase of pro-inflammatory cytokines. In fact, several studies have demonstrated that adipose tissue secretes IL-6 and TNF-$\alpha$ [26]. The latter may have a role in the onset of muscle wasting, indicating a link between age-related FM redistribution and sarcopenia [26, 57].

Sarcopenia is independently associated with important health outcomes and disabilities, and is therefore considered a public health problem. In advanced sarcopenia, muscle weakness is clearly the limiting factor determining functional capacity and performance, whereas in milder sarcopenia the relationship between structure and function

**Table 1.** Sarcopenia: criteria of classification

| Author [reference] | Method of measurement | Index | Cut-off and classes | Prevalence of sarcopenia |
|---|---|---|---|---|
| Baumgartner RN et al. [12] | Dual-energy X-ray absorptiometry | ASMI[a, b] | 2 SD below the mean value for young adults (Rosetta Study): Males (M): < 7.26 Females (F) : < 5.45 | Non-Hispanic whites (New Mexico Elder Health Survey) |
| Janssen I et al. [53] | BIA[d] | SMI[e] | Class I sarcopenia: 1 SD below the mean value for young adults (NHANES III): men 37–31%; women 28–22% Class II sarcopenia: 2 SD below the mean value for young adults: men < 31%; women < 22% | NHANES III |

Prevalence of sarcopenia — Non-Hispanic whites (New Mexico Elder Health Survey) [Baumgartner RN et al. [12]]

|   | <70 years | 70–74 years | 75–80 years | > 80 years |
|---|---|---|---|---|
| M | 13.5 | 19.8 | 26.7 | 52.6 |
| F | 32.1 | 33.3 | 35.9 | 43.2 |

Prevalence of sarcopenia — NHANES III [Janssen I et al. [53]]

|   | 60–69 years | | 70–79 years | | >80 years | |
|---|---|---|---|---|---|---|
|   | Cl. I | Cl. II | Cl. I | Cl. II | Cl. I | Cl. II |
| M | 47% | 6% | 42% | 7% | 43% | 7% |
| F | 59% | 9% | 57% | 11% | 61% | 11% |

[a] ASM: appendicular skeletal muscle mass measured as the sum of the lean soft-tissue masses for the arms and legs as described in [62]
[b] ASM/height$^2$
[c] SMI mass index = SM mass/body mass × 100
[d] Bioelectrical impedance analysis
[e] SM mass calculated using the BIA equation of Janssen et al (53): [(height/BIA resistance × 0.401) + (gender × 3.825) + (age × -0.071)] + 5.102, where height is in cm; resistance is in ohms; for gender, men = 1 and women =0; age is in years

may be more complex. As seen in young adults, changes in muscle strength and size in response to resistance training or inactivity are not always related [59, 60]. Resistance exercise can lead to major improvements in function with little or no change in muscle mass, or even in strength [60]. It is generally agreed that the loss of SM mass and function can be prevented by specific intervention strategies, starting from the fifth decade of life [61].

Another measure to fight sarcopenia is to ensure an adequate intake of energy and proteins. Further research is needed both to identify treatments based on a better understanding of the pathophysiology of sarcopenia and to make better use of treatments that are already available.

# References

1. Borkan GA, Norris AH (1977) Fat redistribution and the changing body dimensions of the adult male. Hum Biol 49:495–514
2. Schoeller DA (1989) Changes in total body water with age. Am J Clin Nutr 50 (Suppl):1176–1181
3. Forbes GB, Reina JC (1970) Adult lean body mass declines with age: some longitudinal observations. Metabolism 19:653–663
4. Calloway NO, Foley CF, Lagerbloom P (1965) Uncertainties in geriatric data. II. Organ size. J Am Geriatr Soc 13:20–28
5. Mazess RB (1982) On aging bone loss. Clin Orthop Relat Res 165:239–249
6. Baungartner RN, Stauber PM, McHugh D et al (1995) Cross-sectional age differences in body composition in persons 60+ years of age. J Gerontol Med Sci 50:M307–M316
7. Bortz WM (1982) Disuse and aging. JAMA 248:1203–1208
8. Ley CJ, Lees B, Stevenson JC (1992) Sex- and menopause-associated changes in body fat distribution. Am J Clin Nutr 55:950–954
9. Chumlea WC, Baumgartner RN, Garry PJ et al (1992) Fat distribution and blood lipids in a sample of healthy elderly people. Int J Obesity 16:125–133
10. Anonymous (1992) Health data on older Americans. National Center for Health Statistics, United States. Series 3, no 27. Government Printing Office, Washington DC
11. Roche AF (1994) Sarcopenia: a critical review of its measurement and health-related significance in the middle-aged and elderly. Am J Hum Biol 6:33–42
12. Baumgartner RN (1993) Body composition in elderly persons: a critical review of needs and methods. Prog Food Nutr Sci 17:223–260
13. Norris AH, Lundy T, Shock NW (1963) Trends in selected indices of body composition in men between the ages of 30 and 80 years. Ann NY Acad Sci 110:623–639
14. Novak LP (1972) Aging, total body potassium, fat-free mass, and cell mass in males and females between age 18 and 85 years. J Gerontol 27:438–443
15. Cohn SH, Vaswani A, Zanzi I et al (1976) Changes in body chemical composition with age measured by total body neutron activation. Metabolism 25:85–95
16. Bruce A, Andersson M, Arvidsson B, Isaksson B (1980) Body composition. Prediction of normal body potassium, body water and body fat in adults on the basis of body height, body weight and age. Scand J Clin Lab Invest 40:461–473
17. Huges VA, Frontera WR, Roubenoff R et al (2002) Longitudinal changes in body composition in older men and women: role of body weight change and physical activity. Am J Clin Nutr 76:473–481
18. Visser M, Pahor M, Tylavsky F et al (2003) One- and two-year change in body composition as measured by DXA in a population-based cohort of older men and women. J Appl Physiol 94:2368–2374
19. Zamboni M, Zoico E, Scartezzini T et al (2003) Body composition changes in stable weight elderly subjects: the effects of sex. Aging Clin Exp Res 15:321–327
20. Fried SK, Bunkin DA, Greenberg AS (1998) Omental and subcutaneous adipose tissues of obese subjects release interleukin-6: depot difference and regulation by glucocorticoid. J Clin Endocr Metab 83:847–850
21. Kern PA, Ranganathan S, Li C et al (2001) Adipose tissue tumor necrosis factor and interleukin-6 expression in human obesity and insulin resistance. Am J Physiol Endocr Metab 280:E745–E751
22. Dandona P, Weinstock R, Thusu K et al (1998) Tumor necrosis factor-alpha in sera of obese patients: fall with loss. J Clin Endocrinol Metab 83:2907–2910
23. Katsuki A, Sumida Y, Murashima S et al (1998) Serum levels of tumor necrosis factor-alpha are increased in obese patients with noninsulin-dependent diabetes mellitus. J Clin Endocrinol Metab 83:859–862
24. Garaulet M, Pere-Llamas F, Fuente T et al (2000) Anthropometric, computed tomography and fat cell data in an obese population: relationship with insulin, leptin, tumor necrosis factor-alpha, sex hormone-binding globulin and sex hormones. Eur J Endocrinol 143:657–666
25. Bertin E, Nguyen P, Guenounou M et al (2000) Plasma levels of tumor necrosis factor-alpha (TNF-alpha) are essentially dependent on visceral fat amount in type 2 diabetic patients. Diabetes Metab 26:178–182
26. Pedersen M, Bruunsgaard H, Weis N et al (2003) Circulating levels of TNF-alpha and IL-6 in relation to truncal fat mass and muscle mass in healthy elderly individuals and in patients with type-2 diabetes. Mech Ageing Dev 124:495–502
27. Enzi G, Gasparo M, Biondetti PR et al (1986) Subcutaneous and visceral fat distribution according

to sex, age, and overweight, evaluated by computed tomography. Am J Clin Nutr 44:739–746

28. Wang Q, Hassager C, Ravn P et al (1994) Total and regional body-composition changes in early post-menopausal women: age-related or menopause-related? Am J Clin Nutr 60:843–848

29. Zamboni M, Armellini F, Harris T et al (1997) Effects of age on body fat distribution and cardiovascular risk factors in women. Am J Clin Nutr 66:111–115

30. Horber FF, Gruber B, Thomi F et al (1997) Effect of sex and age on bone mass, body composition and fuel metabolism in humans. Nutrition. 13:524–534

31. Beaufrère B, Morio B (2000) Fat and protein redistribution with ageing: metabolic considerations. Eur J Clin Nutr 54:S48–53

32. Ma XH, Muzumdar R, Yang XM et al (2002) Aging is associated with resistance to effects of leptin on fat distribution and insulin action. J Gerontol A Biol Sci Med Sci 57:B225–B231

33. Ferrannini E, Vichi S, Beck-Nielsen H et al (1996) European group for the study of insulin resistance (EGIR). Insulin action and age. Diabetes 45:947–953

34. Boden G (1997) Role of fatty acids in the pathogenesis of insulin resistance and NIDDM. Diabetes 46:3–10

35. Girard J (1995) Role of free fatty acids in insulin resistance of subjects with non-insulin-dependent diabetes. Diabetes Metab 21:79–88

36. Laville M, Rigalleau V, Riou J, Beylot M (1995) Respective role of plasma nonesterified fatty acid oxidation and total lipid oxidation in lipid-induced insulin resistance. Metabolism 44:639–644

37. Bjorntop P (1997) Body fat distribution, insulin resistance, and metabolic diseases. Nutrition 13:795–803

38. Hunter GR, Kekes-Szabo T, Treuth MS et al (1996) Intra-abdominal adipose tissue, physical activity and cardio-vascular risk in pre- and post-menopausal women. Int J Obes Relat Metab Disord 20:860–865

39. Yamanouchi K, Nakajima H (1992) Effects of daily physical activity on insulin action in the elderly. J Appl Physiol 73:2241–2245

40. Cohn SH, Vaswani AN, Yasumura S et al (1985) Assessment of cellular mass and lean body mass by noninvasive nuclear techniques. J Lab Clin Med 105:305–311

41. Kyle UG, Genton L, Hans D et al (2001) Total body mass, fat mass, fat-free mass, and skeletal muscle in older people: cross-sectional differences in 60-year-old persons. J Am Geriatr Soc 49:1633–1640

42. Frontera WR, Hughes VA, Fielding RA et al (2000) Aging of skeletal muscle: a 12 year longitudinal study. J Appl Physiol 88:1321–1326

43. Gallagher D, Ruts E, Visser M et al (2000) Weight stability masks sarcopenia in elderly men and women. Am J Physiol Endocrinol Metab 279:E366–E375

44. Kehayas JJ, Fiatarone MA, Zhuang H et al (1997) Total body potassium and body fat: relevance to aging. Am J Clin Nutr 66:904–910

45. Baumgartner RN, Koehler KM, Gallagher D et al (1998) Epidemiology of sarcopenia among the elderly in New Mexico. Am J Epidemiol 147:755–763

46. Frontera WR, Hughes VA, Lutz KJ et al (1991) A cross-sectional study of muscle strength and mass in 45- to 78-yr-old men and women. J Appl Physiol 71:644–650

47. Hughes VA, Frontera WR, Wood M et al (2001) Longitudinal muscle strength changes in older adults: influence of muscle mass, physical activity, and health. J Gerontol A Biol Sci Med Sci 56:B209–B217

48. Rosenberg IH (1989) Summary comments. Am J Clin Nutr 50:1231–1233

49. Rubenoff R, Heymsfield SB, Kehayias JJ et al (1997) Standardization of nomenclature of body composition in weight loss. Am J Clin Nutr 66:192–196

50. Melton LJ 3rd, Khosla S, Riggs BL (2000) Epidemiology of sarcopenia. Mayo Clin Proc 75:S10–S12

51. Tanko LB, Movsesyan L, Mouritzen U et al (2000) Appendicular lean tissue mass and the prevalence of sarcopenia among healthy women. Metabolism 5:69–74

52. Newman AB, Kupelian V, Visser M et al (2003) Health ABC Study Investigators Sarcopenia: alternative definitions and associations with lower extremity function. J Am Geriatr Soc 51:1602–1609

53. Janssen I, Heymsfield SB, Ross R (2002) Low relative skeletal muscle mass (sarcopenia) in older persons is associated with functional impairment and physical disability. J Am Geriatr Soc 50:889–896

54. Janssen I, Heymsfield SB, Baumgartner RN, Ross R (2000) Estimation of skeletal muscle mass by bioelectrical impedance analysis. J Appl Physiol 89:465–471

55. Bua EA, McKiernan SH, Wanagat J et al (2002) Mitochondrial abnormalities are more frequent in muscles undergoing sarcopenia. J Appl Physiol 92:2617–2624

56. Payette H, Roubenoff R, Jacques PF et al (2003) Insulin-like growth factor-1 and interleukin 6 predict sarcopenia in very old community-living men and women: the Framingham Heart Study. J Am Geriatr Soc 51:1237–1243

57. Reid MB, Li YP (2001) Tumor necrosis factor-alpha and muscle wasting: a cellular perspective. Respir Res 2:269–272

58. Hakkinen K, Kallinem M, Linnamo V et al (1996) Neuromuscular adaptations during bilateral versus unilateral strength training in middle-aged and elderly men and women. Acta Physiol Scand 158:77–88

59. Suzuki Y, Murakami T, Haruna Y et al (1994) Effects of 10 and 20 days bed rest on leg muscle mass and strength in young subjects. Acta Physiol Scand Suppl 616:5–18

60. Nelson ME, Layne JE, Neurenberger A et al (1999) The effect of a home-based exercise program on functional performance in the frail elderly: an update. Med Sci Sports Exerc 31:S377 (abs)

61. Roubenoff R, Hughes VA (2000) Sarcopenia: current concepts. J Gerontol Med Sci 55:M716–M724

# The Pharmacokinetics and Pharmacodynamics of Drugs in Elderly Cachectic (Cancer) Patients

Dario Cova, Vito Lorusso, Nicola Silvestris

The word *cachexia* is derived from the Greek words *kakòs*, meaning 'bad,' and *hexis*, meaning 'condition' [1]. From an epidemiological point of view, while patients with haematological malignancies and breast cancer seldom have this syndrome, most other solid tumours are associated with a high frequency of cachexia [2]. Indeed, its prevalence increases from 50% to more than 80% before death, and in more than 20% of patients cachexia is the main cause of death [3].

The older population includes the majority of cancer patients. In fact, increasing age is directly associated with increasing rates of cancer, corresponding to an 11-fold greater incidence in persons over the age of 65 vs those under 65 [4]. Older persons, compared to younger populations, typically have more diseases, take more medications, experience more adverse effects and drug interactions, and have more variability in their nutritional status and underlying health status, all of which contribute to pharmacokinetic (drug absorption, distribution, metabolism, and excretion) and pharmacodynamic (the effect of a drug on its target site) differences [5]. Thus, in this scenario, the study of cancer cachexia in the geriatric population requires a series of pathophysiological and clinical considerations that are essential for a therapeutic approach mainly aimed at the quality of residual life in this subset of patients.

## Metabolic Changes

Enhanced lipid mobilisation, decreased lipogenesis, and decreased activity of lipoprotein lipase, the enzyme responsible for triglyceride clearance from plasma, in favour of an increased gluconeogenesis and hepatic protido-synthesis are the main biochemical events associated to neoplastic cachexia

[6]. The study of body composition in neoplastic patients, carried out with several techniques, shows a loss of fat mass with sparing of the visceral organs and an increase in extracellular mass, mainly in more serious cases. Correspondingly, from a clinical point of view, it is possible to observe a large decrease in muscle mass, the absence of the adipose panniculus, an increased resistance to insulin, an increase of acute-phase proteins, and a great loss of weight compared to the patient's basal weight. Indeed, the metabolic adjustment in cachectic patients is different from that observed in simple malnutrition. In the latter, there is a decrease in oxygen consumption in order to reduce energetic expense, whereas in cachectic cancer patients this compensation mechanism does not occur [7]. The main metabolic alterations in neoplastic cachexia, which lead to alterations in the pharmacokinetic and pharmacodynamic parameters of drugs are shown in Table 1.

## Pharmacokinetics

Age can affect most pharmacokinetic parameters, including gastrointestinal absorption, volume of distribution ($V_d$), hepatic drug metabolism, and excretion (Table 2) [8].

### Gastrointestinal Absorption

In cancer patients, atrophic gastritis, hypotony of gastric muscle, decreased gastric secretion, and reduced intraluminal surface area may cause diminished absorption of oral agents, possibly resulting in their reduced effectiveness [9]. Moreover, some studies have shown a close relation between cachexia and the absorption of drugs such as tetracycline, rifampicin, and anticonvulsants [8, 10].

**Table 1.** Main metabolic alterations in patients with neoplastic cachexia

| Glucose-related | Glucose turnover | Increased | Lipid | Lipoprotein lipase | Decreased |
|---|---|---|---|---|---|
| | Resistance to insulin | Increased | | Fatty acid turnover | Increased |
| | Glycogenic deposits | Decreased | | Lipid deposits | Decreased |
| Protein-related | Muscle catabolism | Increased | Basal metabolism | | Increased |
| | Synthesis of muscle proteins | Decreased | Oxidative metabolism (Cytochrome-P450-associated) | | Decreased |

**Table 2.** Variation of pharmacokinetic parameters in elderly cachectic cancer patients

| Parameter | Variations | Pathogenetic mechanisms |
|---|---|---|
| Gastrointestinal absorption | Decreased | Decreased mucous surface Decreased splanchnic circulation Decreased gastric motility Decreased enzymatic secretion |
| Volume of distribution ($V_d$) | Decreased for lipid-soluble drugs Increased for water-soluble drugs | Increased water content, decreased adipose content Reduced circulation of plasma proteins Reduced haemoglobin concentration |
| Hepatic metabolism of drugs | Decreased activation and deactivation of drugs (phase I) | Reduced concentration of enzymes of the P-450 cytochrome system Pharmacological interaction Decreased hepatic circulation |
| Excretion | Renal: decreased | Reduction of glomerular filtrate rate |

## Volume of Distribution

Modifications of body composition, plasma protein profile, and blood cells (e.g. erythrocytes) alter the $V_d$ of several drugs in cachectic cancer patients. A progressive increase in body fat and a decline in body water, occurring up to age 85, tend to reduce the $V_d$ of water-soluble drugs, such as anthracyclines, and increase those of fat-soluble compounds, such as carmustine [11]. Indeed, the age-related decrease in plasma albumin of up to 15–20% influences the concentration of free fraction of drugs in the plasma, mostly those that are highly protein bound [12].

The relation between $V_d$ and haemoglobin con-

centration is also of considerable interest. Since the prevalence of anaemia increases with age, the relationship between anaemia and $V_d$ of antitumoural substances is of particular interest with respect to elderly patients. In fact, the close binding to erythrocytes of many drugs, such as anthracyclines, taxanes, epipodophyllotoxins, and vinca alkaloids, as well as decreased concentration of haemoglobin can be associated with both an increase in the plasma concentration of the drug and an increase in its toxicity. This effect is reversible after the normalisation of haemoglobin concentration, generally obtainable with the use of erythropoietin [13]. Dose modification according to haemoglobin level seems important for several anticancer drugs, but, so far, there is no standard approach.

## Hepatic Function

The hepatic metabolism of drugs involves two kinds of reactions: *Phase I reactions* are mediated by the cytochrome P-450 system and include oxi-doreductions, which can both activate and deactivate drugs. With aging, the activity of such reactions progressively decreases due to a decrease in enzyme concentrations and competitive interaction with other drugs (polypharmacotherapy) commonly taken by elderly people with poly-pathologies [14, 15]. Antineoplastic drugs metabolised with phase I reactions include oxyphosphorins (cyclophosphamide and iphosphamide), anthracyclines (idarubicin and daunorubicin), capecitabine, and nitrosoureas.

Conjugation mechanisms responsible for the formation of glucuronides and other water-soluble compounds are associated with *phase II reactions,* which do not seem to change significantly with aging [16].

Elderly cachectic patients generally show a significant prolongation of the effects of drugs metabolised at the hepatic level. Observations in animal models have shown that the metabolic activity of cytochrome P-450 is remarkably reduced with a low-protein diet. Similar results were obtained in patients suffering from caloric-proteic malnutrition. In addition, the hepatic metabolism of drugs is affected by the hepatic circulation, the progressive reduction of which is a constant characteristic of cachexia. This, in turn, is associated with a reduced capacity of the liver to remove drugs from the circulation and thus with a consequent reduction in drug clearance [17]. Accordingly, studies carried out in cachectic patients showed a reduced phenobarbital clearance associated with an increase in its steady-state plasma concentration. Also, paracetamol, one of the drugs most frequently used by cachectic patients, is mainly discarded through conjugation mechanisms. Trials in cachectic subjects showed a substantial reduction in urinary metabolites conjugated with glucuronic acid and with sulfate. In such patients, formation of the toxic intermediate N-acetyl-parabenzoquinine can be responsible for toxic effects. Similarly, research carried out with sulfamides demonstrated a correlation between malnutrition and an increase of both half-life and drug bioavailability [18].

## Excretion

The glomerular filtration rate (GFR) declines consistently with age by approximately 1 ml/min per year from the age of 40, as a consequence of reduction in nephrons [19]. Nevertheless, the decline in GFR is not associated with a concomitant increase in plasma creatinine because of the age-related loss of muscle mass. Therefore, creatinine is not a reliable indicator of GFR in the elderly.

GFR, plasma flow, tubular secretion, and changes in urinary pH are modified in cachectic cancer patients (Table 3). All these factors can contribute to a decrease in the renal excretion of drugs and their metabolites in these subjects. For example, clinical observations showed a higher toxicity of methotrexate 24–28 h after their administration and of anthracyclines. In contrast, the clearance of 5-fluorouracil was found to be independent of patients' nutritional state [20].

## Pharmacodynamics

In elderly cancer patients, cachexia can affect pharmacodynamic properties of a specific drug in terms of its toxicity and activity, as demonstrated by a reduction of the ability to repair DNA damage caused by chemotherapy and to catabolise the metabolites of such drugs. For example, DNA adducts induced by cisplatinum are cleared within 24 h by circulating monocytes in subjects ≤ 50 years old but in > 90 h in subjects age 70 and older. Similarly, the reduced concentration of dihydropyrimidine dehydrogenase, an enzyme involved in fluorinate pyrimidine catabolism, may cause an increase incidence of mucositis. Finally, in elderly subjects, pharmacodynamic alterations may result in resistance to cytotoxic chemotherapy. The four main mechanisms of *multiple drug resistance* (MDR) in elderly patients are: expression of the MDR-1 gene, resistance to apoptosis, reduced fraction of tumour growth, and anoxia of tumour cells [12, 21].

**Table 3.** Variation of pharmacokinetics parameters of some drugs in elderly cachectic cancer patients

| Drug | Pharmacokinetic parameters | | Bioavailability | Volume of distribution |
|---|---|---|---|---|
| | Half-life | Clearance | | |
| Chloramphenicol | = | = | ↓ | = |
| Tetracycline | = | = | ↓ | = |
| Rifampicin | = | = | ↓ | = |
| Anticonvulsant | = | = | ↓ | = |
| Antipyrine | ↑ | ↓ | = | ↓ |
| Phenazone | ↑ | ↓ | = | ↓ |
| Phenobarbital | ↑ | ↓ | = | ↓ |
| Phenitoin | ↑ | ↓ | ↑ | ↑ |
| Sulfadiazide | ↑ | ↓ | = | ↓ |
| Theophylline | ↑ | ↓ | = | ↓ |
| Paracetamol | ↑ | ↓ | ↑ | ↓ |
| Salicylate | ↑ | ↓ | ↑ | ↓ |
| Penicillin | ↑ | ↓ | = | ↓ |
| Cefoxitin | ↑ | ↓ | = | ↓ |
| Gentamicin | ↑ | ↓ | = | ↓ |
| Methotrexate | ↑ | ↓ | = | ↓ |
| Bleomycin | ↑ | ↓ | = | ↑ |
| Etoposide | ↑ | ↓ | = | ↑ |
| Topotecan | ↑ | ↓ | = | ↑ |
| Adriamycin | ↑ | ↓ | = | ↓ |
| Epirubicin | ↑ | ↓ | = | ↓ |
| Cyclophosphamide | ↑ | ↓ | = | ↑ |
| 5-Fluorouracil | ↑ | = | = | ↑ |
| Tegafur | ↑ | ↓ | ↓ | ↑ |
| Melphalan | ↑ | ↓ | ↓ | ↑ |
| Vinorelbine | ↑ | ↓ | = | ↑ |

**Table 4.** Criteria to evaluate hepatic function and drug dose in elderly cachectic patients

| Hepatic function | Thrombotest (%) | AST (U/l) | Albuminaemia (g/l) | Bilirubin (mg/dl) | Drug dose (%) |
|---|---|---|---|---|---|
| Good | > 40 | < 51 | > 34 | < 1.2 | 100 |
| Moderate | 25–39 | 51–200 | 28–34 | 1.2–3.0 | 50–75 |
| Poor | < 25 | > 200 | < 28 | > 3.0 | 25–50 |

## Guidelines for Dose Adjustment

Evidence regarding the success of dose reduction strategies in the elderly population is scarce. The main reason includes the previous exclusion of these patients from clinical trials. Nevertheless, studies on the altered efficacy and toxicity of anti-cancer drugs used to treat elderly patients are a useful aid for clinicians. The three main principles to follow in adjusting the dose of a specific drug in the presence of toxicity, or with the aim of pre-venting it, are: (1) monitoring of plasma levels of a specific drug and/or its active metabolites, (2) dose adjustment related to the functionality of emunctory systems, and (3) dose reduction in relation to toxicity level, which can be evaluated clinically or by using laboratory parameters [20]. Dose adjustment related to the functionality of emunctory systems represents a very commonly used way to minimise toxic effects of drugs, as this approach compensates for the decline of emunctory functions associated with age, under either physiological conditions or associated with organ pathologies, particularly renal and hepatic ones. It is therefore crucial to know the clearance pathway of the administered drug. Drugs with predominantly renal excretion can be particularly toxic in the presence of a reduced GFR. As a consequence, the dose of such drugs needs to be reduced when creatinine clearance is below 60 ml/min. Any dose variations, even initial ones, of the drug must be correlated with the GFR of the subject, using the Cockcroft-Gault formula to evaluate creatinine clearance or the Kintzel-Dorr formula for correction of the standard dose [22, 23].

The doses of drugs with predominantly hepatic clearance should also be correspondingly reduced [24]. Biohumoral parameters of hepatic function are shown in Table 4 according to serum AST values, albumin, bilirubin, and thrombotest (Owen's test).

## Conclusions

Neoplastic cachexia is a complex and multifactorial syndrome that can affect drug efficacy, mainly in elderly cancer patients, due to organ insufficiencies and comorbidities.

The use of antitumoural drugs in this phase of disease, particularly in elderly patients, is extremely cumbersome because of the clear implications on the quality of residual life. Furthermore, in such patients, problems related to obtaining an accurate clinical picture make it difficult to elaborate guidelines for treatments that often remain empirical. In this context, the knowledge of the pharmacokinetic and pharmacodynamic characteristics of the drugs to be administered is important in the therapeutic decision-making procedure [25].

## References

1. Tisdale MJ (1997) Biology of cachexia. J Natl Cancer Inst 89:1763–1773
2. Inui A (2002) Cancer anorexia-cachexia syndrome: current issues in research and management. CA Cancer J Clin 52:72–91
3. Bruera E (1997) Anorexia, cachexia and nutrition. BMJ 315:1219–1222
4. Yancik R (1997) Cancer burden in the aged: an epidemiological and demographic overview. Cancer 80:1273–1283
5. Wildiers H, Highley MS, dei Bruijn EA et al (2003) Pharmacology of anticancer drugs in the elderly population. Clin Pharmacokinet 42:1–30
6. Tisdale MJ (2000) Metabolic abnormalities in cachexia and anorexia. Nutrition 16:1013–1014
7. Kotler DP (2000) Cachexia. Ann Intern Med 133:622–634
8. Vestal RE (1997) Aging and pharmacology. Cancer 80:1302–1310
9. Skirvin JA, Lichtman SM (2002) Pharmacokinetic considerations of oral chemotherapy in elderly patients with cancer. Drugs Aging 19:25–42
10. Raghuram TC, Krishnasvamy K (1981) Tetracycline absorption in malnutrition. Drug Nutr Interact 1:23–29
11. Lichtman SM, Skirvin JA (2000) Pharmacology of antineoplastic agents in older cancer patients. Oncology 14:1743–1763
12. Mangoni AA, Jackson SH (2004) Age-related changes in pharmacokinetics and pharmacodynamics: basic principles and practical applications. Br J Clin Pharmacol 57:6–14
13. Schrijvers D, Highley M, De Bruyn E et al (1999) Role of red blood cells in pharmacokinetics of chemotherapeutic agents. Anticancer Drugs 10:147–153
14. Sotaniemi EA, Arranto AJ, Pelkonen O et al (1997) Age and cytochrome P450-linked drug metabolism in humans: an analysis of 226 subjects with equal histopathologic conditions. Clin Pharm Ther 61:331–339
15. Corcoran MB (1998) Polypharmacy in the older patient. In: Balducci L, Lyman GH, Ershler WB Comprehensive geriatric oncology. Harwood Academic Publishers, London, pp 525–532
16. John V, Mashru S, Lichtman J (2003) Pharmacological factors influencing anticancer drug selection in the elderly. Drugs Aging 20:737–759
17. Jorquera F, Culebras DM, Gonzalezgallego J (1996) Influence of nutrition on liver oxidative metabolism. Nutrition 12:442–447
18. Sadean MR, Glass PS (2003) Pharmacokinetics in the elderly. Best Pract Res Clin Anaesthesiol 17:191–205
19. Kintzel PE, Dorr RT (1995) Anticancer drug renal toxicity and elimination: dosing guidelines for altered renal function. Cancer Treat Rev 21:33–64
20. Gurney H (1996) Dose calculation of anticancer drugs: a review of the current practice and introduction of an alternative. J Clin Oncol 14:2590–2611
21. Vuyk J (2003) Pharmacodynamics in the elderly. Best Pract Res Clin Anaesthesiol 17:207–218
22. Cockcroft DW, Gault MH (1976) Prediction of creatinine clearance from serum creatinine. Nephron 16:31–41
23. Kinzel PE, Dorr RT (1995) Anticancer drug renal toxicity and elimination: dosing guidelines for altered renal function. Cancer Treat Rev 21:33–64

24. Koren G, Beatty K, Seto A et al (1992) The effects of impaired liver function on the elimination of antineoplastic agents. Ann Pharmacother 26:363–371

25. Balducci L, Extermann M (1997) Cancer chemotherapy in the older patient: what the medical oncologist needs to know. Cancer 80:1317–1322

# Pathophysiology of Cachexia in the Elderly

Osama QuBaiah, John E. Morley

## Introduction

The physiological decline in food intake that occurs with aging is an appropriate response to the reduced physical activity of this population. This physiological decline is termed the 'anorexia of aging' [1]; however, cachexia in the elderly seems to be reaching epidemic levels, with 30–40% of men and women over age 75 being 10% underweight or more [2]. There is no agreed upon definition for cachexia, which means 'poor condition' in Greek [3]. While it has traditionally been thought that chronic illness fully explains the pathogenesis of cachexia, this concept is proving inadequate [4]. In general, cachexia is characterised by weight loss due to loss of fat and skeletal muscle mass [5].

Many chronic illnesses can be associated with cachexia, although the condition may develop in older people without obvious disease [3]. Starvation is different from cachexia in the sense that macronutrient changes can be reversed by feeding in starvation but not in cachexia. There are four major causes of weight loss in older persons: starvation, sarcopenia, cachexia and dehydration (Table 1).

## Regulation of Appetite in the Elderly

Regulation of appetite is a sophisticated process that involves feedback from peripheral sensory endings and the interaction of a variety of neurotransmitters in the central nervous system [1]. Numerous studies have shown that food intake declines over the human lifespan, with males having a greater decrease in food intake than females. A large part of the anorexia of aging seems to be related to the changes in gastrointestinal activity that occurs with aging [1].

During a meal, the fundus distends to accommodate food, a process termed adaptive relaxation. Food is then passed to the antrum after mixing with stomach secretions. Antral distension is the major signal for termination of a meal [1]. With aging, there appears to be impaired gastric fundal accommodation [6] due to impaired adaptive relaxation, which is caused by a decline in the local release of nitric oxide. Older mice have decreased nitric oxide synthase activity in their fundus [7]. The decline in adaptive relaxation that occurs with aging leads to more rapid antral filling. In addition, some studies suggested that large-

**Table 1.** Comparison of the major features of starvation, sarcopenia, cachexia and dehydration

|  | Starvation (Anorexia of aging) | Sarcopenia | Cachexia | Dehydration |
|---|---|---|---|---|
| Weight loss | ++ | + | +++ | ++ |
| Loss of lean mass | + | + | +++ | 0 |
| Loss of fat mass | ++ | 0 | ++ | 0 |
| Cytokine excess | +/- | + | +++ | 0 |
| Albumin | – | 0 | — | 0 |
| Anaemia | +/- | 0 | ++ | 0 |
| Hypogonadism | +/- | + | ++ | 0 |

volume solid meals delay the rate of gastric emptying in the elderly [8–11]. This will eventually lead to prolongation of antral distension, which results in satiety (Fig. 1).

Infusion of lipid into the duodenum leads to the release of the peptide hormone cholecystokinin (CCK), which, in turn, leads to satiety. Evidence from animal studies indicates that CCK suppresses appetite in older animals more than in younger animals [12, 13]. This finding was also confirmed in humans. In addition, the basal circulating concentration of CCK and its response to lipids increases with aging, mainly due to a decline in the CCK clearance rate. CCK exerts its effects by increasing contractile activity in the pylorus, leading to slowing of gastric emptying and increasing the antral response to gastric distension [14]. CCK also directly stimulates the ascending vagal fibres that carry satiating signals to the nucleus tractus solitarii and to the hypothalamus [15].

Glucagon-like peptide is another gastrointestinal hormone involved with satiation, but its levels do not change with aging [16]. In contrast, amylin levels, which in mice decreases food intake in young and old mice, increase from middle age to old age [17].

The hormone leptin is released from adipose tissue [18] and exerts its effects by decreasing food intake and increasing the metabolic rate. Circulating leptin levels increase in older men and decrease in older women [19]. The increase in leptin levels in men is related to the decrease in testosterone that occurs with aging [1], which, in turn, is associated with muscle loss [20] and an increase in body fat [21]. Testosterone replacement in older men leads to a decline in leptin levels [1]. The increase in leptin with aging in men is considered a major factor in the increased anorexia of aging that occurs in males compared to females.

Although animal studies suggest that a decline

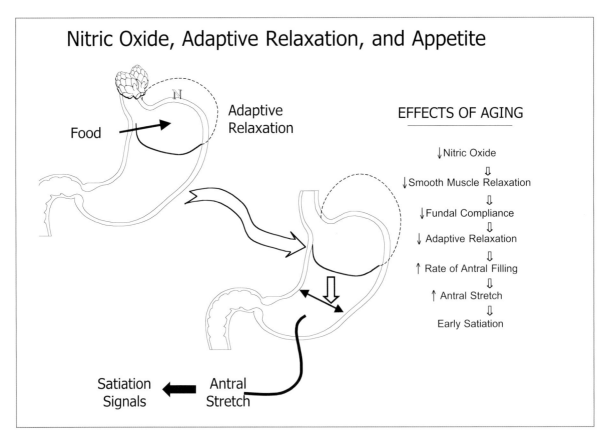

**Fig. 1.** Alterations in stomach motility that lead to the anorexia of aging

in opioid activity in the central nervous system may be associated with anorexia in older animals [22, 23], a study in humans did not show any difference in the effect of naloxone on food intake [12]. In humans, alteration in the thirst drive, which is modulated by μ-opioid receptors, appears to play a role in the development of age-related hypodipsia. Similarly, numerous neurotransmitters, such as neuropeptide Y, norepinephrine, and serotonin are involved in appetite regulation, although their role in the pathogenesis of the anorexia of the aging has been poorly investigated. An excess of corticotropin releasing factor is thought to be involved in the pathogenesis of the severe anorexia associated with depression in older persons.

## Factors Leading to Reduced Food Intake in the Elderly

### Hedonic Qualities of Food

As a general rule, aging is associated with decreased appreciation of the hedonic qualities of food [24]. This change seems to be caused more by alterations in olfaction than in taste. There is a marked decline in odour detection and taste thresholds increase with aging. However, these changes are minor unless the person smokes, is on medications, or has zinc deficiency. Older persons tend to prefer more intense flavours than do younger persons [25]. For example, it was shown that elderly persons had an increase in food intake when the flavour was enhanced with monosodium glutamate [26].

### Social Factors

Studies have shown that elderly persons consume more food when eating a meal in the company of others [27, 28]. The explanation for this, in part, is that eating in company results in spending a longer time eating the meal. In nursing homes, several factors can lead to malnutrition and cachexia in the elderly, including the reduced variability of food, the complicated process of food preparation and distribution, and inadequate attention by caretakers to the individual needs of each of the patients [24]. Retirement can lead to reduced household income and thus to insecurity about buying food and then to weight loss [29]. Moreover, retirement can also lead to social isolation, changes in life style, and loss of contacts. All of these add up to the risk of weight loss and cachexia following retirement. Simple changes, such as the expansion of commercial shopping areas, the erection of high-rise apartments, or the increasing diversity of the neighbourhood, may elicit a strong sense of insecurity within an environment the older adult previously perceived as safe [29].

### Psychological Factors

Depression and dementia interact to accelerate weight loss [24]. Depression has been shown to be the major cause of weight loss in community and institutional settings [30], while demented patients lose weight due to failure to eat – although some demented patients may increase their energy expenditure by wandering. Some persons with cognitive impairment develop apraxia of eating. Other factors that may contribute to the development of weight loss in demented patients are difficulty swallowing, dental diseases, lack of concern about eating, and memory loss. In demented patients, disturbance of the mechanisms for appetite regulation may lead to hypo- or hyperphagia. The latter usually occurs early in the course of the dementing process.

### Medical Factors

Although dentition was always mentioned as a factor leading to reduced food intake, studies did not confirm that poor dental health makes older patients prefer food of softer consistency [31]. However, poor dentition does lead to a slight decrease in daily food intake. Chronic diseases, some of which are common in older people, have been shown to produce anorexia and cachexia: these include cancers, AIDS, rheumatologic diseases, end-stage renal disease, chronic obstructive pulmonary disease, and heart failure. The most common reversible causes of weight loss are given in Table 2.

Drugs have also been implicated to cause reduced food intake and cachexia, by causing either a taste complaint or nausea and vomiting. Among the drugs with these possible complications are antihypertensives, diuretics, sleeping pills, and nonsteroidal anti-inflammatory agents.

**Table 2.** Reversible causes of weight loss

Social:
    Loneliness
    Problems in shopping
    Problems in food preparation
    Poverty
    Elderly abuse

Psychological:
    Depression
    Late-life paranoia
    'Cholesterol' phobia
    Alcoholism
    Anorexia tardive

Medical:
    Decreased food intake:
      - Iatrogenic
      - Medications
      - Therapeutic diets
      - Altered food consistency
    Dysphagia
    Dentition problems
    Addison's disease
    Hypercalcaemia
    Some cancers

Malabsorption

Diarrhoea, e.g. caused by *Clostridium difficile*

Gluten enteropathy

Bacterial overgrowth

Pancreatic insufficiency

Hypermetabolism

Hyperthyroidism

Phaeochromocytoma

Essential tremor

Diabetes mellitus

## Sarcopenia

Sarcopenia is severe age-associated loss of muscle mass that causes limitations in activities of daily living and an increased mortality in affected persons, especially those who have obese sarcopenia (the 'fat frail').

The causes of sarcopenia are multifactorial (Table 3). Aging itself is associated with a decline in physical activity. Small increases in cytokines, especially interleukin (IL)-6, have been implicated in the proteolysis of muscle involved in the pathophysiology of sarcopenia [32]. Decreased food intake can lead to loss of muscle protein, as it is broken down for use in more essential proteins. The amino acid creatine is found only in meat and is essential for muscle function. Older persons who are anorectic or vegetarian have inadequate creatine intake for muscle maintenance.

With aging, testosterone levels decrease because of failure of the hypothalamic-pituitary-gonadal axis [33]. The decline in testosterone occurs at the rate of about 1% per year, beginning at 30 years of age. Loss of testosterone leads to an increase in adipocyte precursors and a decrease in satellite precursors. In addition, it is associated with a decline in muscle-protein synthesis. Testosterone replacement in older persons increases muscle mass and, to a lesser degree, muscle strength [34].

Myostatin is a protein that blocks muscle synthesis. Mice made transgenic for myostatin have a marked decrease in muscle mass, mimicking cachexia [35]. Recently, a human with a double deletion of the myostatin gene was reported to have muscle hypertrophy [36].

**Table 3.** Causes of sarcopenia

Aging

Physical inactivity

Anorexia

Decreased creatine intake

Peripheral vascular disease

Hypogonadism

Cytokine excess

Myostatin excess

A final cause of sarcopenia is atherosclerosis, which causes peripheral vascular disease. This is associated with decreased muscle mass and strength in the lower extremities, as well as decreased mobility.

## Cachexia Pathophysiology

Cachexia in the elderly cannot be completely explained by reduced food intake; rather, several social and psychological factors, disease conditions, and medications can aggravate the physiological anorexia of aging and lead to weight loss [1]. Furthermore, a person eats less when he or she eats alone compared to when eating in a group. The pleasurable qualities of food are determined by taste, smell, and vision [1], with olfaction being the most important determinant [1].

The decreased sense of smell and the changes in taste that occur with aging (taste threshold, difficulty in recognising taste mixtures, and increased perception of irritating tastes) contribute to anorexia [1]. Other factors that contribute to the development of cachexia are detailed in the following sections.

## Cytokines

The immune system, particularly inflammatory cytokines, has a crucial role in cachexia (Fig. 2). Cytokines are the cause of inflammatory reactions in disease states, and the most important contributor to this process is tumour necrosis factor (TNF). TNF, together with IL-1, IL-6, and interferon (IFN)-γ regulate apoptosis, which may mediate cachexia associated with chronic disease states.

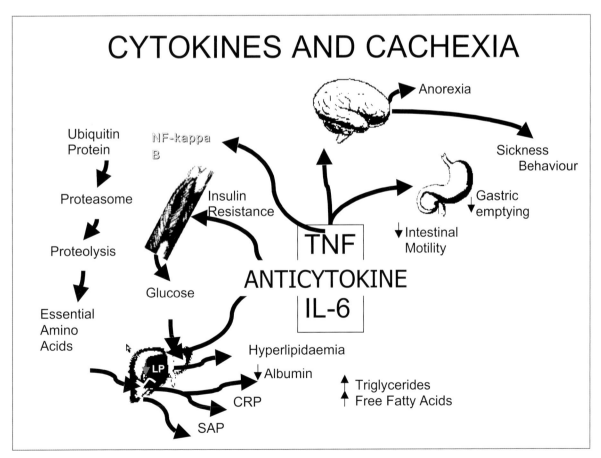

**Fig. 2.** Pathophysiology of cachexia. *IL-6*, interleukin-6; *TNF*, tumour necrosis factor; *CRP*, C-reactive protein; *SAP*, serum amyloid protein; *NF-kappaB*, nuclear factor–kappaB

Studies have shown an increased concentration of cytokines in the circulation of patients with cachexia. In cancer patients, for example, the patient's clinical status determines the serum level of TNF-α. In a study of 91 patients with B-cell chronic lymphocytic leukaemia, serum levels of TNF-α were high in all stages of the disease, with a progressive increase in relation to the stage [37]. It was also found that TNF-α levels were higher in patients with endometrial carcinoma than in healthy postmenopausal women or women with endometrial hyperplasia. In addition, TNF-α levels increased with advancing stage of the disease [38].

Other studies have shown that cytokines are able to induce the metabolic changes typically associated with cachexia, such as stimulating muscle proteolysis through the ubiquitin-proteasome pathway, or inhibiting lipoprotein lipase, which is responsible for mobilising triglycerides from the circulation into adipocytes [39]. Cytokines in general exert their effect by crossing the blood-brain barrier and stimulating ascending fibres in the vagus. Cytokines cause anorexia and muscle wasting, as well as decreased nitrogen retention, anaemia, decreased albumin synthesis, and extravasation of albumin from the intravascular space [1]. An excess of cytokines is commonly detected in frail older persons [1].

## Tumour Necrosis Factor

TNF-α is a 17-kDa peptide that is largely produced by the monocyte/macrophage cell line. Other cells, including T-cells, NK cells, mast cells, and adipocytes, also produce this cytokine. Production of TNF-α is synergistically regulated by other cytokines, such as IL-1 and IFN-γ [39], and TNF-α in turn stimulates leptin and IL-6 production [1]. Studies have shown that injecting rats with recombinant human TNF-α led to significant depletion of body protein. It was also demonstrated that injection of TNF-α directly into the cerebral ventricles of rats suppressed food and water intake, while peripheral administration of an equal or higher dose had no such effect [39]. While TNF-α failed to produce a sustained weight loss, the net metabolic alterations exerted by the cytokine may

depend on the site of production [40]. This was demonstrated by intracerebral injection of TNF-α-secreting cells, which resulted in body weight loss and anorexia, while TNF-α-producing cells inoculated into peripheral tissue triggered cachexia, including weight loss, depletion of lipid and protein stores, and anaemia but without significant anorexia [39, 40].

Short intravenous infusion of recombinant human TNF-α increased plasma triglyceride levels, and glycerol turnover by more than 80%, free fatty acid turnover by more than 60%, and protein turnover. Those changes resolved with continuous administration [5].

Some evidence suggests that treatment of patients who have tumours or infections with antibody directed against TNF-α attenuates the wasting syndrome [39]. In another study, administration of anti-murine-TNF-α antibody to rats carrying the Yoshida AH-130 ascites hepatoma slowed the rates of protein degradation in skeletal muscle and liver, but did not affect weight loss [5].

## Interleukin-6

Interleukin-6 has been called the 'geriatric cytokine,' and there is evidence from animal studies supporting a role for IL-6 in the development of cancer cachexia [5, 41–43]. Those studies, based on a murine colon-26 adenocarcinoma model [41–43], showed that administration of anti-mouse-IL-6 monoclonal antibody blocked the development in mice of weight loss and other parameters of cachexia [5, 41–43].

It seems that IL-6 is able to induce cachexia by several mechanisms, including triggering of the acute-phase response [5], inhibiting the activity of lipoprotein lipase in adipose tissue in mice [5], and inducing muscle atrophy in IL-6 transgenic mice [5]. Further evidence for the role of IL-6 in the development of cachexia comes from the findings of Strassman et al., who reported that IL-1-dependent IL-6 production was responsible for adenocarcinoma-associated cachexia [44]. Other studies used two subclones of the murine colon 26 adenocarcinoma cell line, clone 20, which is cachexigenic, and clone 5, which is non-cachexigenic. Possible involvement of IL-6 in the development of cachexia was suggested by the finding of increased serum levels of biologically active IL-6 in mice carrying clone 20, but not in those carrying clone 5 [42, 45, 46]. The injection of anti-IL-6 antibody partially inhibited the weight loss caused by inoculation of clone 20, suggesting that IL-6 is necessary, but not sufficient, for the development of cachexia [47].

Muscle atrophy in IL-6 transgenic mice was totally blocked by antibody to the mouse IL-6 receptor [48]. IL-6 administration to rats acutely activated total and myofibrillar protein degradation in skeletal muscles [49]. In another study, it was suggested that IL-6 up-regulates pathways of protein degradation [50]. It was also demonstrated that weight-losing patients with non-small-cell lung cancer had statistically significant increases in IL-6 and C-reactive protein, which was not the case in patients with the same tumour but without weight loss [5, 51].

## Interleukin-1

Interleukin-1 is an inflammatory cytokine that has biological activity similar to that of TNF-α. It is mainly produced by macrophages and endothelial cells, and is known to be a pyrogen and a potent trigger of the acute-phase response. IL-1 suppresses lipoprotein lipase and stimulates intracellular lipolysis. Administration of recombinant IL-1 induces anorexia, weight loss, hypoalbuminaemia, and elevated amyloid P levels in mice [52]. In one study, it was observed that IL-1 administration to rats led to accelerated peripheral protein loss with preservation of liver protein [53]. However, administration of an IL-1-receptor antagonist to rats bearing the Yoshida ascites hepatoma was ineffective in preventing tissue depletion and protein degradation [54], and transfection of a cachectic tumour cell line (colon 26) with the gene for IL-1 receptor antagonist failed to stop tumour-induced cachexia [46]. In general, the mechanism by which IL-1 can produce cachexia is thought to be either an effect on hepatocytes, with a subsequent effect on the hypothalamic appetite centre [55], or a direct effect on the central nervous system [46, 57–60].

## Interferon-γ

IFN-γ is secreted by activated T-cells and NK cells. Immunologically, it is the most potent monocyte-macrophage activating factor [39]. The metabolic effects of IFN-γ include inhibition of lipoprotein lipase, both in an adipocyte cell line and in vivo [61]. IFN-γ also inhibits the production of lipoprotein lipase and glycerol-phosphate dehydrogenase, both of which are involved in lipogenesis in primary cultures of rat adipocytes [62]. In addition, IFN-γ stimulates lipolysis in vitro and in vivo [63].

It was shown that a potentially lethal cachexia developed in nude mice inoculated with Chinese hamster ovary (CHO) cells overexpressing the mouse IFN-γ gene [64]. The mice developed weight loss, fat-store atrophy, and reduced food intake [39], which were predominantly due to effects not related to a decline in food intake. In addition, the degree of cachexia was proportional to the number of IFN-γ-producing cells and was blocked by pretreatment of the mice with anti-IFN-γ antibodies [39]. Mice bearing Lewis lung tumours developed a similar condition [65]. In that model, treatment with anti-IFN-γ antibody exerted anti-cachectic effects, partially through antagonising tumour growth. In addition, even after its effect on tumour growth had diminished, the antibody continued to have anti-cachectic properties.

Another study supporting the role of IFN-γ in cachexia compared the effects of anti-IFN-γ and anti-TNF-α antibodies on cachexia in rats bearing methylcholantrene-induced tumours [66]. The conclusion was that endogenous IFN-γ production is more crucial than that of TNF-α in the development of cachexia.

## Leukaemia Inhibitory Factor

A role was suggested for LIF in the development of cancer cachexia, due to its ability to decrease lipoprotein lipase activity. LIF mRNA was shown to be present in two types of melanoma xenografts that induced weight loss in transplanted animals, whereas none was detected in non-cachexia-inducing xenografts [5, 67]. It seems unlikely that inhibition of lipoprotein lipase alone could account for fat-cell depletion, and there is no mechanism to explain the catabolism of skeletal muscle.

## Lipid Mobilising Factors

Almost all of the evidence behind a role for lipid mobilising factors (LMFs) in cachexia is derived from tumour studies. LMFs exert their effects on adipose tissue, leading to the release of free fatty acids and glycerol. There is evidence that tumours produce an LMF, as demonstrated in a study in which nonviable preparations of Krebs-2 carcinoma, when injected into mice, were able to induce the early, rapid stage of fat depletion [5]. More evidence for the presence of an LMF was provided by the finding that ascites serum from rats transplanted with the Walker 256 carcinoma stimulated lipolysis in an in vitro assay [68]. In addition, injecting serum from mice bearing a thymic lymphoma into controls produced fat loss [69]. The factor presumed to induce fat loss was found in tumour extracts, in the sera of patients with adenocarcinomas of the cervix and stomach, and in tissue-culture medium [5]. Together, those results led to the proposal that LMF was tumour-derived and released into the circulation. Other studies showed that the concentration of LMF in the sera of cancer patients was proportional to the extent of weight loss [70], and was reduced in patients responding to chemotherapy [71]. In general, LMF is absent or present in small amounts in tumours that do not induce cachexia [72], and is absent from normal serum, even during starvation [73].

## Protein Mobilising Factors

There is evidence for the existence of protein mobilising factors (PMFs) in the sera of animals [74] and humans [75] with cancer cachexia, but not in the sera of healthy controls. In addition, PMFs could not be detected in the urine of healthy individuals, in the urine of patients who developed weight loss due to reasons other than cancer, or in the urine of cancer patients with no cachexia. Injecting PMF into non-tumour bearing-mice

resulted in rapid weight loss with no change in food and water intake [5], while an analysis of body composition showed selective depletion of lean body mass [5].

## Role of Ghrelin in Cachexia

Many aspects of appetite regulation that involve peripheral signalling to hypothalamic pathways remain poorly understood. Growth hormone (GH) secretion from the anterior pituitary is regulated by GH-releasing hormone (GHRH), which stimulates the release of GH as well as its inhibitor somatostatin [76]. GH secretagogues are synthetic compounds able to stimulate secretion of the hormone [77] but which act through a receptor different from that for GHRH receptor. Instead, ghrelin was discovered to be the natural ligand for that receptor. Ghrelin is mainly secreted by gastric endocrine cells in the fundus into the systemic circulation [78]. Fasting increases, while feeding decreases circulating ghrelin concentrations [78]. These changes are negatively correlated with the serum concentrations of leptin and insulin.

The infusion of ghrelin stimulates eating and produces obesity in rats [79], and a study in humans showed that ghrelin infusion led to short-term increase in hunger [80]. Maintenance of weight reduction after gastric bypass surgery was suggested to be due to markedly low levels of ghrelin [76]. It has also been shown that ghrelin levels are elevated in cachectic patients with chronic heart failure or anorexia nervosa [78]. Several studies are currently underway to explore the effects of ghrelin and its agonists on cachexia.

## Role of the Central Melanocortin System in Cachexia

The melanocortin system can be defined as the hypothalamic and brain-stem neurons expressing pro-opiomelanocortin (POMC), hypothalamic neurons expressing neuropeptide Y (NPY) and melanocortin antagonist agouti-related protein (AgRP), and the neurons downstream of these systems [81]. POMC is a propeptide precursor synthesised in neurons in the hypothalamic arcuate nucleus. There are two central melanocortin receptors, melanocortin-3 receptor (MC3-R) and melanocortin-4 receptor (MC4-R) [81]. Evidence that melanocortin plays a role in energy home-ostasis in humans stems from the presence of obesity syndromes involving defects in two different steps in the melanocortin pathway [81].

Some studies have led to the assumption that melanocortin neurons mediate the anorexic effects of elevated leptin, while others have shown that the melanocortin system exerts its effects independent of leptin [81]. POMC neurons mediate the inhibition of food intake and energy storage through the production of α-melanocyte-stimulating hormone (MSH) from a POMC precursor [81]. Central administration of MC4-R agonist can lead to inhibition of food intake, increasing energy expenditure, lower serum insulin, and reduced body weight [81], whereas inhibition of the melanocortin system with an antagonist, or deletion of MC4-R, leads to hyperphagia and obesity [82, 83].

## Diagnosis and Screening for Cachexia

The rate of detection of cachexia is low among physicians. Even after diagnosis was made, appropriate intervention was instituted in only one-third of the patients, according to one study [84]. The low rates of detection and intervention are most often due to the inability to make the diagnosis [85]; thus, there is a need for improved screening for cachexia [85]. The Mini Nutritional Assessment (MNA) is a well-validated tool that was specifically designed for use with community-dwelling elderly [85]. The positive predictive value of the MNA for detecting cachexia is 97%, while its sensitivity is 96% and its specificity is 98%. The MNA incorporates several domains, including functional status, lifestyle, diet, self-evaluation of health, and anthropometric indices [86], and does not require laboratory tests. Another screening tool for undernutrition is the DETERMINE questionnaire, which was designed for community-dwelling elderly, and is self-administered [87]; however, it still needs to be validated. The SCREEN questionnaire has been validated and successfully used in Canada [88]. The mini-CNAQ was developed to pick up early changes in appetite in older persons [89]. The SCALES assessment is a useful,

sensitive screening tool (Table 4) that is simple to use and easy to administer [88]. The inclusion of data on cholesterol and albumin levels make SCALES sensitive enough to allow the physician to accurately diagnose cachexia. Table 5 provides an overview of the different laboratory tests for deter-

**Table 4.** Examples of geriatric nutritional assessment tools

---

A.  *Mini-CNAQ (pronounced 'snack')*
    *(Council of Nutrition Appetite Questionnaire)*

1.  My appetite is
    A. Very poor
    B. Poor
    C. Average
    D. Good
    E. Very good

2.  When I eat
    A. I feel full after eating only a few mouthfuls
    B. I feel full after eating about a third of a meal
    C. I feel full after eating over half a meal
    D. I feel full after eating most of the meal
    E. I hardly ever feel full

3.  Food tastes
    A. Very bad
    B. Bad
    C. Average
    D. Good
    E. Very good

4.  Normally I eat
    A. Less than one meal a day
    B. One meal a day
    C. Two meals a day
    D. Three meals a day
    E. More than 3 meals a day

Instructions: Complete the questionnaire by circling the correct answers and then tally the results based upon the following numerical scale: A = 1, B = 2, C = 3, D = 4, E = 5
Scoring: If the mini-CNAQ is less than 14, there is a significant risk of weight loss

B.  *SCALES*
    Sadness
    Cholesterol
    Albumin
    Loss of weight
    Eating problems
    Shopping problems

---

**Table 5.** Laboratory tests for determining cachexia in older persons

| Test | Comment |
| --- | --- |
| Weight loss | Best test; < 5% in 3 months or 10% in 6 months |
| Body mass index (BMI) | < 21 is highly suggestive |
| Midarm muscle or calf | Good indicators of loss of muscle mass muscle circumference |
| Albumin/prealbumin | Very low levels suggest cachexia or nephrotic syndrome or liver disease |
| Cholesterol | Low levels in cachexia |
| Haemoglobin | Anaemia usually coexists with cachexia |
| CD4 T-cells | Decreased in severe cachexia and starvation |
| C-reactive protein | Elevated in cachexia |
| Interleukin-2 receptors | Elevated in cachexia |
| Uric acid | Elevated in cachexia |

mining cachexia in older persons.

In addition to using a screening tool for malnutrition, it is also important to look for risk factors. Identifying risk factors of malnutrition helps the physician to develop strategies that allow the patient to be well-nourished at all times. The risk factors of malnutrition can be grouped by the mnemonic 'MEALS ON WHEELS' (Table 6).

In the clinical setting, weight measurement and calculation of body mass index are the most widely used indices for nutritional assessment. The use of biochemical markers to assess and treat nutritional risk is discouraged because they have poor predictive value [89, 90]. The most cost-effective parameter of proven clinical usefulness in monitoring nutritional status is body weight measurement [91]. The hallmark of a well-designed nutritional surveillance program is the ability to detect impending nutritional compromise long before laboratory indices become abnormal.

**Table 6.** The risk factors of malnutrition grouped by the mnemonic 'MEALS ON WHEELS'

Medications (polypharmacy, herbal preparations)
Emotional risk factors (dysphoria, depression, psychosis)
Appetite disorders (anorexia tardive, abnormal eating attitudes)
Late-life paranoia (social isolation)
Swallowing disorders

Oral factors (tooth loss, periodontal infections, gingivitis, poorly fitting dentures)
No money (poverty)

Wandering (dementia)
Hyperactivity/hypermetabolism (tremors, movement disorders, thyrotoxicosis)
Enteral problems (chronic diarrhoea, malabsorption syndromes)
Eating problems (altered food preferences, decreased taste and flavor perception)
Low-nutrient diets (low-salt, low-cholesterol, antidiabetic diets)
Shopping and food preparation problems (impaired mobility, unsafe environment, inadequate transportation)

# References

1. Morley JE (2002) Pathophysiology of anorexia. Clin Geriatr Med 18:661–673
2. Thomas D (2002) Undernutrition in the elderly. Clin Geriatr Med 18:xiii-xiv
3. Kotler D (2000) Cachexia. Ann Intern Med 133:622–634
4. Anker S (2002) Cachexia: time to receive more attention. Int J Cardiol 85:5–6
5. Tisdale M (1997) Biology of cachexia. J Natl Cancer Inst 89:1763–1773
6. Rayner CK, MacIntosh CG, Chapman IM et al (2000) Effects of age on proximal gastric motor and sensory function. Scand J Gastroenterol 35:1041–1047
7. Morley JE, Kumar VB, Mattammal MB et al (1996) Inhibition of feeding by nitric oxide synthase inhibitor: effects of aging. Eur J Pharmacol 31:15–19
8. Clarkston WK, Pantano MM, Morley JE et al (1997) Evidence for the anorexia of aging: gastrointestinal transit and hunger in healthy elderly vs. young adults. Am J Physiol 272:R243–R248
9. Horowitz M, Maddern G, Chatterton BE et al (1984) Changes in gastric emptying rates with age. Clin Sci (Colch) 67:213–218
10. Horowitz M, Wishart JM, Jones KL, Hebbard GS (1996) Gastric emptying in diabetes: an overview. Diabet Med 13:S16–S22
11. Wegener M, Borsch G, Schaffstein J et al (1988) Effect of acing on the gastrointestinal transit of a lactulose-supplemented mixed solid-liquid meal in humans. Digestion 39:40–46
12. MacIntosh CG, Sheehan J, Davani N et al (2001) Effects of aging on the opioid modulation of feeding in humans. J Am Geriatr Soc 49:1518–1524
13. Silver AJ, Flood JF, Morley JE (1988) Effects of gastrointestinal peptides on ingestion in old and young mice. Peptides 9:221–225
14. MacIntoshCG, Morley JE, Wishart J et al (2001) Effect of exogenous cholecystokinin (CCK)-8 on food intake and plasma CCK, leptin, and insulin concentration in older and young adults: evidence for increase CCK activity as a cause of the anorexia of aging. J Clin Endocrinol Metab 86:5830–5837
15. Levine AS, Morley JE, Wishart J et al (1986) Neuropeptides as regulators of consummatory behavior. J Nutr 116:2067–2077
16. MacIntosh CG, Andrews JM, Jones KL et al (1999) Effects of age on concentrations of plasma cholecystokinin, glucagons-like peptide 1, and peptide YY and their relation to appetite and pyloric motility. Am J Clin Nutr 69:999–1006
17. Morley JE, Flood JF, Horwitz M et al (1994) Modulation of food intake by peripherally administered amylin. Am J Physiol 267:R178–R184
18. Morley JE, Perry MH, Baumgartner RP et al (1999) Leptin, adipose tissue and aging is there a role for testosterone? J Gerontol A Biol Sci Med Sci 54:B108–B109
19. Baumgartner RN, Waters DL, Morley JE et al (1999) Age related changes in sex hormones affect the sex difference in serum leptin independently of changes in body fat. Metabolism 48:378–384
20. Baumgartner RN, Waters DL, Gallagher D et al (1999) Predictors of skeletal muscle mass in elderly men and women. Mech Ageing Dev 107:123–136
21. Morley JE, Farr SA, Suarez MD et al (1995) Nitric oxide synthase inhibition and food intake: effects on motivation to eat in female mice. Pharmacol Biochem Behav 50:369–373
22. Gosnell BA, Levin AS, Morley JE (1983) The effects of aging on opioid modulation of feeding in rats. Life Sci 32:2793–2799
23. Kavaliers M, Hirst M (1985) The influence of opiate agonists on day-night feeding rhythms in young and old mice. Brain Res 326:160–167
24. van Staveren WA, de Graaf C, de Groot LCPGM (2002) Regulation of appetite in frail persons. Clin Geriatr Med 18: 675–684
25. De Graaf C, Polet P, van Staveren WA (1994) Sensory perception and pleasantness of food flavors in elderly subjects. J Gerontol A Biol Sci Med Sci 49:P93–P99
26. Griep MI, Mets TF, Massart DL (1997) Different effects of flavor amplification of nutrient dense foods on preference and consumption in young and elderly subjects. Food Quality and Preference 8:151–156
27. De Castro JM (1995) Social facilitation of food intake in humans. Appetite 24:260
28. Feunekes GI, de Graaf C, van Staveren WA (1995) Social facilitation of food intake is mediated by meal duration. Physiol Behav 58:551–558
29. Morley JE, Morley PMK (1995) Psychological and social factors in the pathogenesis of weight loss. Annu Rev Gerontol Geriatr 15:83–109
30. Morley JE (1997) Anorexia of aging: physiologic and pathologic. Am J Clin Nutr 66:760–773
31. De Groot CP, van Staveren WA, de Graaf C (2000) Determinants of macronutrient intake in elderly people. Eur J Clin Nutr 54(Suppl 3):S70-S76
32. Morley JE, Baumgartner RN, Roubenoff R et al (2001) Sarcopenia. J Lab Clin Med 137:231–243
33. Morley JE, Perry HM (2003) Androgen treatment of male hypogonadism in older males. J Steroid Biochem Mol Biol 85:367–373
34. Wittert GA, Chapman IM, Haren MT et al (2003) Oral testosterone supplementation increases muscle and decreases fat mass in healthy elderly males with low-normal gonadal status. J Gerontol Med Sci 58:618–625
35. McNally EM (2004) Powerful genes – myostatin regulation of human muscle mass. N Engl J Med 350:2642–2644
36. Schuelke M, Wagner KR, Stolz LE et al (2004) Brief report – myostatin mutation associated with gross

muscle hypertrophy in a child. N Engl J Med 350:2682–2688

37. Adami F, Guarini A, Pini M et al (1994) Serum levels of TNF alpha in patients with B-cell chronic lymphocytic leukemia. Eur J Cancer 30A:1259–1263

38. Shaarawy M, Abdel-Aziz O (1992) Serum TNF alpha levels in benign and malignant lesions of the endometrium in postmenopausal women, a preliminary study. Acta Oncol 31:417–420

39. Matthys P, Billiau A (1997) Cytokines and cachexia. Nutrition 13:763–769

40. Tracey KJ, Morgello S, Koplin B et al (1990) Metabolic effects of cachectin/tumor necrosis factor are modified by site of production. J Clin Invest 86:2014–2024

41. Strassmann G, Fong M, Kenney JS, Jacob CO (1992) Evidence for the involvement of interleukin 6 in experimental cancer cachexia. J Clin Invest 89:1681–1684

42. Soda K, Kawakami M, Kashii K, Miyata M (1995) Manifestations of cancer cachexia induced by colon 26 adenocarcinoma are not fully ascribable to Interleukin-6. Int J Cancer 62:332–336

43. Strassmann G, Fong M, Freter CE et al (1993) Suramin interferes with interleukin-6 receptor binding in vitro and inhibits colon-25 mediated experimental cancer cachexia in vivo. J Clin Invest 92:2152–2159

44. Strassmann G, Masui Y, Chizzonite R et al (1993) Mechanisms of experimental cancer cachexia. Local involvement of IL-1 in colon-26 tumor. J Immunol 150:2341–2345

45. Fujimoto-Ouchi K, Tamura S, Mori K et al (1995) Establishment and characterization of cachexia-inducing and non-inducing clones of murine colon 26 carcinoma. Int J Cancer 61:522–528

46. Yasumoto K, Mukaida N, Harada A et al (1995) Molecular analysis of the cytokine network involved in cachexia in colon 26 adenocarcinoma-bearing mice. Cancer Res 55:921–927

47. Mori K, Fujimoto-Ouchi K, Ishikawa T et al (1996) Murine interleukin-12 prevents the development of cancer cachexia in a murine model. Int J Cancer 67:849–855

48. Tsujinaka T, Fujita J, Ebisui C et al (1996) Interleukin 6 receptor antibody inhibits muscle atrophy and modulates proteolytic systems in interleukin 6 transgenic mice. J Clin Invest 97:244–249

49. Goodman MN (1994) Interleukin-6 induces skeletal muscle protein breakdown in rats. Proc Soc Exp Biol Med 205:182–185

50. Ebisui C, Tsujinaka T, Morimoto T et al (1995) Interleukin-6 induces proteolysis by activating intracellular proteases (cathepsins B and L, proteasome) in C2C12 myotubes. Clin Sci (Colch) 89:431–439

51. Scott HR, McMillan DC, Crilly A et al (1996) The relationship between weight loss and interleukin 6 in non-small-cell-lung cancer. Br J Cancer 73:1560–1562

52. Moldawer LL, Andersson C, Gelin J, Lundholm KG (1988) Regulation of food intake and hepatic protein synthesis by recombinanant-derived cytokines. Am J Physiol 254:G450–G456

53. Fong Y, Moldawer LL, Marano M et al (1989) Cachectin/TNF or IL-1 alpha induces cachexia with redistribution of body proteins. Am J Phsiol 256:R659–R665

54. Costelli P, Llovera M, Carbo N et al (1991) Interleukin-1 receptor antagonist (IL-1ra) is unable to reverse cachexia in rats bearing an ascites hepatoma (Yoshida AH-130). Cancer Res 51:415–421

55. Nixon DW, Heymsfield SB, Cohen AE et al (1980) Protein caloric undernutrition in hospitalized cancer patients. Am J Med 68:683–690

56. Shapot VS, Blinov VA (1974) Blood glucose levels and gluconeogenesis in animals bearing transplantable tumors. Cancer Res 34:1827–1832

57. Lundholm K, Bylund AC, Holm J, Schersten T (1976) Skeletal muscle metabolism in patients with malignant tumor. Eur J Cancer 12:465–473

58. Emery PW, Edwards RH, Rennie MJ et al (1984) Protein synthesis measured in vivo in cachectic patients with cancer. Br Med J (Clin Res Ed) 289:584–586

59. Fearon KC, Hansell DT, Preston T et al (1988) Influence of whole body protein turnover rate on resting energy expenditure in patients with cancer. Cancer Res 48:2590–2595

60. Holm E, Hagmuller E, Staedt U et al (1995) Substrate balances across colonic carcinomas in humans. Cancer Res 55:1373–1378

61. Kurzrock R, Rohde MF, Quesada JR et al (1986) Recombinant gamma-interferon induces hypertriglyceridemia and inhibits postheparin lipase activity in cancer patients. J Exp Med 164:1093–1101

62. Gregoire F, Broux N, Hauser N et al (1992) Interferon- gamma and interleukin-1 beta inhibit adipoconversion in cultured rodent preadipocytes. J Cell Physiol 151:300–309

63. Memon RA, Feingold KR, Moser AH et al (1992) In vivo effects of interferon-alpha and interferon-gamma on lipolysis and ketogenesis. Endocrinology 131:1695–1702

64. Matthys P, Dijkmans R, Proost P et al (1991) Severe cachexia in mice inoculated with interferon-gamma-producing tumor cells. Int J Cancer 49:77–82

65. Matthys P, Heremans H, Opdenakker G et al (1991) Anti-interferon-gamma antibody treatment, growth of Lewis lung tumors in mice and tumor-associated cachexia. Eur J Cancer 27:182–187

66. Langstein HN, Doherty GM, Fraker DL et al (1991) The roles of gamma-interferon and tumor necrosis factor alpha in an experimental rat model of cancer cachexia. Cancer Res 51:2302–2306

67. Mori M, Yamaguchi K, Honda S et al (1991) Cancer cachexia syndrome developed in nude mice bearing melanoma cells producing leukemia-inhibiting fac-

tor. Cancer Res 51:6656–6659

68. Kralovic RC, Zepp FA, Cenedella RJ (1977) Study of the mechanism of carcass fat depletion in experimental cancer. Eur J Cancer 13:1071–1079

69. Kitada S, Hays EF, Mead JF (1980) A lipid mobilizing factor in serum of tumor-bearing mice. Lipids 15:168–174

70. Groundwater P, Beck SA, Barton C et al (1990) Alteration of serum and urinary lipoltytic activity with weight loss in cachectic cancer patients. Br J Cancer 62:816–821

71. Beck SA, Groundwater P, Barton C, Tisdale MJ (1990) Alterations in serum lipolytic activity of cancer patients with response to therapy. Br J cancer 62:822–825

72. Beck SA, Tisdale MJ (1987) Production of lipolytic and proteolytic factors by a murine tumor-producing cachexia in the host. Cancer Res 47:5919–5923

73. Beck SA, Mulligan HD, Tisdale MJ (1990) Lipolytic factors associated with murine and human cancer cachexia. J Natl Cancer Inst 82:1922–1926

74. Smith KL, Tisdale MJ (1993) Mechanism of muscle degradation in cancer cachexia. Br J Cancer 68:314–318

75. Belizario JE, Katz M, Chenker E, Raw I (1991) Bioactivity of skeletal muscle proteolysis-inducing factors in the plasma proteins from cancer patients with weight loss. Br J Cancer 63:705–710

76. Flier JS, Maratos-Flier E (2002) The stomach speaks-ghrelin and weight regulation. N Engl J Med 346:1662–1663

77. Bowers CY (2001) Unnatural growth hormone-releasing peptide begets natural ghrelin. J Clin Edocrinol Metab 86:1464–1469

78. Inui A, Meguid MM (2002) Ghrelin and cachexia. Diabetes Obes Metab 4:431

79. Tschop M, Smiley DL, Heiman ML (2000) Ghrelin induces adiposity in rodents. Nature 407:908–913

80. Wren AM, Seal LJ, Cohen MA et al (2001) Ghrelin enhances appetite and increases food intake in humans. J Clin Endocrinol Metab 86:5992

81. Marks DL, Cone RD (2001) Central melanocortins and the regulation of weight during acute and chronic disease. Program Abstr Endocr Soc Annu Meet 56:359–375

82. Jacobowitz DM, O'Donohue TL (1978) Alpha-melanocyte-stimulating hormone: immunohisto-chemical identification and mapping in neurons of rat brain. Proc Natl Academic Science 75:6300–6304

83. Huszar D, Lynch CA, Fairchild-Huntress V et al (1997) Targeted disruption of the melanocortin-4 receptor results in obesity in mice. Cell 88:131–141

84. Wilson MG, Vaswani S, Liu D et al (1998) Prevalence and causes of undernutrition in medical outpatients. Am J Med 104:56–63

85. Wilson MG (2002) Undernutrition in medical outpatients. Clin Geriatr Med 18:759–771

86. Guigoz Y, Vellas B (1997) The mini nutritional assessment for grading the nutritional state of elderly patients, presentation of the MNA, history and validation. Facts, Research, and Intervention Geriatrics Newsletter. Nutrition 6:2

87. Anonymous (2000) Position of the American Dietetic Association. Nutrition, aging and continuum of care. J Am Diet Assoc 100:580–595

88. Morley JE (1994) Nutritional assessment is a key component of geriatric assessment. Facts and Research in Gerontology 2:5

89. Ballmer-Weber BK, Drummer R, Kung E et al (1995) Interleukin-2 induced increase of vascular permeability without decrease of the intravascular albumin pool. Br J Cancer 71:78

90. Courtney ME, Greene HL, Folk CC et al (1982) Rapidly declining serum albumin values in newly hospitalized patients: porevalence, severity and contributory factors. J Parenter Enter Nutr 6:143–145

91. Blaum CS, O'Neill EF, Clements KM et al (1997) The validity of the minimum data set for assessing nutritional status in nursing home residents. Am J Clin Nutr 66:787–794

# Cytokines and Disability in Older Adults

David R. Thomas

## Introduction

A decline in functional status is a profound predictor of morbidity and mortality [1]. The mortality rate increases from 15% in individuals with only one impairment in an instrumental activity of daily living (IADL) to 21% in persons with one or two IADL impairments. In subjects with five or six IADL impairments, the mortality rate reaches 37% [2]. Disabled older adults are four to six times more likely to die than the nondisabled [3]. Up to half of the geriatric patients admitted to a hospital have either loss of or a diminished performance in at least one ADL during admission. This decline in functional status occurs as early as the second day of hospital admission [4, 5].

A decline in functional status is a major predictor of risk for nursing home placement [6, 7], subsequent acute illness [8], and declining quality of life [9]. An estimated 59% of adults with five or more ADL impairments will be admitted to nursing homes [10]. Among those older adults with substantial functional disability who are in nursing homes, disability declines faster at the end of 6 months compared to individuals with greater function [11]. Older adults with disability have a shorter life expectancy in the nursing home than institutionalised adults of the same age who are less impaired [12].

Among community-dwelling older adults, impairment in functional status itself predicts a further decline in disability [2]. For example, performance-based measures of lower-body function predict subsequent disability [13, 14]. Impaired functional status also correlates with an increased risk for falls, fear of falling, and disability [15–17]. Loss of both IADL and sarcopenia (loss of muscle mass) are strongly related to functional decline [18, 19]. Impaired functional status is often associated with subclinical cardiovascular disease [20]. Thus, disability in functional status represents a marker for poor outcome in older persons [21, 22].

Impaired functional status places burdens not only on the individual patient, but also on the healthcare system as a whole. Almost half (46.3%) of U.S. Medicare-reimbursed expenditures occur in the 20% of older persons who have functional dependence. More than 40% of nursing-home and home-health expenditures occur in the 10% of functionally dependent patients. Altogether, a decline in functional status accounts for more than 20% of nursing home, hospital, and outpatient expenditures [23].

## Functional Decline and Aging

The most important functional change that occurs with aging is a reduction in active skeletal muscle; however, this decline in muscle mass occurs in both sedentary and active aging adults [24–26]. Dynamic, static, and isokinetic muscle strength decreases with age [27], so that a substantial proportion (65%) of older men and women report that they cannot lift 10 pounds using their arms [28]. This decline in strength has been hypothesised to explain some of the functional decline that occurs with aging [29]. Accordingly, a research agenda has been developed to ascertain whether this decline in strength and function is inevitable or related to habitual inactivity.

Maximal oxygen consumption ($VO_{2max}$) declines with age at a rate of 3–8% per decade beginning at 30 years of age [30, 31]. While the major contributor to $VO_{2max}$ is lean muscle mass, after correction for muscle mass, there is no important decline in $VO_{2max}$ with aging [32]. Physically active older men have a higher $VO_{2max}$

than inactive younger men [33]. Thus, although there is a decline in exercise capacity with aging, there is reason to believe that this trend is reversible.

Studies in younger adults consistently show that muscle strength and muscle mass increase with high-intensity training (70–90% of one repetition maximum). In older men, upper-arm strength can increased by 23–48% [34, 35] and lower-extremity strength by 107–226% with exercise [36]. Similar increases, in the range of 28–115%, have been reported in older women [37]. Aniansson demonstrated a 9–22% increase in lower-extremity strength at 12 weeks in healthy men age 69–74 years [38]. Results were similar in men age 56–65 years after 15 weeks of exercise [39].

The muscle loss that occurs with aging is thought to result from either disease (hypogonadism, thyroid disease, growth hormone deficiency), medications (diuretics, corticosteroids), disuse, or malnutrition [40].

## Interaction of Cytokines and Functional Status

Recently, a body of evidence has emerged suggesting that functional decline is associated with an excess production of cytokines. Cytokines are cell-associated proteins produced and secreted by inflammatory cells. They have the capacity to act at low concentrations on other cells, both locally and systematically, via specific cell receptors. Cytokines act principally in a paracrine fashion, and their concentrations in tissues are often several times higher than those found in the peripheral circulation.

Aging is characterised by a progressive increase in the concentrations of glucocorticoids and catecholamines and a decrease in the production of growth and sex hormones – a pattern reminiscent of that seen in chronic stress. Plasma levels of interleukin (IL)-6 increase with age, probably as the result of catecholamine hypersecretion and sex-steroid hyposecretion. However, age-associated changes in cytokine production are inconsistent [41].

Cohen and Pieper found that IL-6 levels correlate with the functional disability of the communi-

ty-dwelling elderly [42]. Therefore, IL-6 may contribute to the increased morbidity and mortality seen in chronically stressed or physiologically aged persons. Interleukin-6 and D-dimer levels have been associated with subsequent mortality and a decline in functional status. The relative risk of mortality increases to 1.28 (95% confidence interval [CI]: 0.98–1.69) for individuals with only IL-6 levels in the highest quartile, 1.53 (95% CI: 1.18–1.97) for those with only D-dimer levels in the highest quartile, and 2.00 (95% CI: 1.53–2.62) for those with levels of both in the highest quartile. Subjects with both high IL-6 and high D-dimer levels had the greatest declines in all measures of functional status [43].

In highly functioning, healthy, nondisabled older persons, a baseline measurement of serum albumin and plasma IL-6 was associated with 4-year mortality. In those subjects without evidence of IL-6-mediated inflammation, a lower albumin was associated with an adjusted relative risk of 2.1 for mortality, compared with subjects with higher albumin. In the presence of elevated IL-6 levels, both higher and lower serum albumin levels had similar risks (adjusted relative risks 4.0 and 3.8, respectively) compared with persons having a higher albumin and low IL-6. Higher serum albumin levels may have a protective effect in healthy older persons who do not have evidence of cytokine-mediated inflammation. This protective effect is not apparent in the presence of inflammation [44].

Older women with high IL-6 serum levels have a higher risk of developing physical disability and experience a steeper decline in walking ability than those with lower levels [45]. Older women in the highest IL-6 tertile were 1.76 (95% CI: 1.17–2.64) times more likely to develop disability due to mobility impairment and 1.62 (95% CI: 1.02–2.60) times more likely to develop mobility impairment and disability with respect to ADL . The increased risk of disability associated with IL-6 concentration was nonlinear, with the risk rising rapidly beyond plasma levels of 2.5 pg/ml. The effect of IL-6 on muscle atrophy may be a direct effect on muscles and/or due to the pathophysiologic role played by IL-6 in specific diseases [46].

In congestive heart failure (CHF) patients, elevated plasma cytokine levels are associated with worse functional status and adverse prognosis. Among 732 elderly Framingham Study subjects (mean age 78 years, 67% women), who were free of prior myocardial infarction and CHF, serum IL-6, C-reactive protein (CRP), and spontaneous production of tumour necrosis factor (TNF)-α were obtained at baseline and then after 5 years. After adjustment for established risk factors, including the occurrence of myocardial infarction on follow-up, there was an increased risk of CHF per tertile increment in cytokine concentration (60% for TNF-α and 68% for serum IL-6, respectively). A serum CRP level greater than 5 mg/dl was associated with a 2.8-fold increased risk of CHF. Subjects with elevated levels of all three biomarkers (serum IL-6, TNF-α, and CRP), had a four-fold increased risk of CHF (95% CI 1.34–12.37). Thus, a single determination of serum inflammatory markers, particularly elevated IL-6, was associated with increased risk of CHF in people without prior myocardial infarction [47]. Other studies have also demonstrated that the highest levels of TNF-α are associated with the poorest functional status in CHF patients [48].

IL-1, IL-6, TNF-α (cachexin), interferon (IFN)-γ, leukaemia inhibitory factor (D-factor), and prostaglandin E2 have been associated with cancer cachexia. The possible transfer of these cytokines via the circulation has been demonstrated in non-tumour bearing rats, who developed cachexia after parabiotic anastomosis to sarcoma-bearing cachexia rats [49].

There is increasing evidence that cytokines can produce cognitive impairment [50, 51]. Cytokines, besides producing a direct effect on muscle function, may also impair functional status by altering central nervous system function. Cognitive impairment has been demonstrated to be associated with functional decline [52–56].

Cytokines are also related to a number of disease conditions, including cancer [57], end-stage renal disease [58], chronic pulmonary disease [59], CHF [60], rheumatoid arthritis [61], and AIDS [62]. These same conditions are frequently associated with a decline in functional status. Cytokines, especially IL-1, IL-6 and TNF-α, are potent causes of appetite suppression, weight loss, and hypoal-

buminaemia [63–65], and play a role in mortality, weight loss, and appetite suppression. Cytokines also decreased haemoglobin levels [66], which has been shown to be associated with disability [67].

Not all populations demonstrate a direct relationship between functional status and cytokine levels. In subjects on maintenance haemodialysis, the levels of inflammatory cytokines are uniformly high. No significant associations among inflammatory cytokines and physical activity, performance, or function has been shown in this population [68]. Whether functional status is directly related to the level of cytokines or independent of cytokine status in this population is unknown.

## Interventions To Improve Functional Status

The importance of identifying functional decline lies in the fact that it may be amenable to intervention. An inpatient geriatric evaluation unit has demonstrated substantial improvement in functional status and a better survival rate at 1-year of follow-up, compared with usual hospital care [69]. Geriatric hospital units have improved ability to transfer, dress, and bathe compared to usual care [70]. Improvement in ADL and fewer discharges to a nursing home was demonstrated in another study [71]. In patients with delirium, an intervention aimed at educating nurses, mobilising patients, assessing medications, and making environmental modifications improved functional status at discharge [72]. Persons with CHF have poor physical function but improve when they receive support from a geriatric team [73].

Improvement in the functional mobility score is directly related to the duration of physical therapy in patients with orthopaedic disorders [74]. In a meta-analysis of post-discharge interventions at home, both functional decline (RR: 0.76; 95% CI: 0.64–0.91) and mortality (RR: 0.76; 95% CI: 0.65–0.88) were reduced in older adults [75]. A tai-chi exercise program was shown to be effective in improving functional status in healthy, physically inactive older adults [76], but whether improvement can occur in impaired individuals is not known.

A number of studies have demonstrated a relationship between exercise and mortality. Older men who expend 500–3500 kcal per week in exercise had lower death rates than non-exercisers [77]. In a cohort study of twins (which removes genetic confounders), a twin who exercised at a level of vigorous walking at least six times monthly for 30 min had a lower risk for death (hazard ratio 0.66 vs 0.44, $p = 0.005$) compared to the twin who had no or less exercise [78].

Most studies demonstrating an improvement in muscle strength have shown its direct relationship to the intensity of the exercise intervention. The data suggest that exercise programs must be high-intensity (70–90% of one repetition maximum) rather than low-intensity (against gravity) in order to produce benefit. The benefit of strength training has been demonstrated to exist even in frail, institutionalized, elderly men and women. After 8 weeks of intensive training in volunteers age 90 years, muscle strength increased by $174 \pm 31\%$ and mid-thigh muscle size by $9 \pm 4.5\%$ (79). Muscle strength improved by $113 \pm 8\%$ following high-intensity exercise training by long-term care residents with a mean age of 87 years [80]. Exercise also improves muscle mass, as measured by computed tomography of the thigh in institutionalized older adults [81].

Cardiovascular function changes little at rest, but declines at maximal exercise stress with aging. Improvement in cardiovascular mortality has been shown over 4 months in older subjects who exercised by cycling at 70% of their age-adjusted maximal heart rate. After 2 years, new cardiovascular diagnoses were made in 2.5% of the home-exercise supervised group, 2% of the non-supervised group, and in 13% of the control group [82]. However, some controversy over the relationship of exercise to cardiovascular disease continues. The Canadian Health Survey found no relationship between physical activity and coronary mortality [83]. The data on the cardioprotective effect of activity in women is not conclusive [84, 85].

## Interventions To Reduce Cytokines

Physical training can reduce the plasma levels of proinflammatory cytokines in CHF patients. This immunomodulatory effect may be related to the training-induced improvement in functional status of these patients. Plasma levels of TNF-$\alpha$, soluble TNF receptors I and II (sTNF-RI and sTNF-RII, respectively), IL-6, and soluble IL-6 receptor (sIL-6R) were measured before and after a 12-week program of physical training by patients with stable CHF and a mean left ventricular ejection fraction of 23%. Physical training produced a significant reduction in plasma levels of the measured cytokines. An increase in VO$_{2max}$ was also seen. Good correlations were found between a training-induced increase in VO$_{2max}$ and a training-induced reduction in the levels of the proinflammatory cytokine TNF-$\alpha$ in patients with CHF. In contrast, no significant difference in circulating cytokines was found with physical training in normal subjects [86].

Testosterone levels decline with aging in both men [87] and women [88]. Testosterone replacement in men increases muscle mass [89–91] and strength [92, 93], and decreases fat mass [90, 94, 95]. Adipocytes are a potent source of cytokines, including TNF-$\alpha$ and leptin. The effect of testosterone on functional status may be mediated by reducing cytokine excess through an effect on adipocytes [96–98].

Recently, megestrol acetate, a potent orexigenic agent, has been shown to produce its effects by decreasing cytokine release [99, 100]. This suggests that one approach to preventing functional decline is to use a cytokine inhibitor [101]. A large number of other pharmacological agents have been tried, with varying success, with the aim of lowering excessive cytokines [102].

## Conclusions

Published studies demonstrate that functional status is an important marker for further decline, morbidity, and mortality in older persons. Exercise-based interventions have been shown to improve functional status and outcomes over time. The data further demonstrate that exercise regimens are safe and can be implemented in older adults, even into the ninth decade of life.

Pro-inflammatory cytokines appear to be associated with functional status in older adults. Measurement of these cytokines may be a predictor of performance on functional status tests. Furthermore, exercise-based interventions have been shown to modulate cytokine inflammatory markers. However, the final relationship of functional status limitation to pro-inflammatory cytokines remains to be determined.

The association of cytokines and functional status suggests that attempts to modulate the effect of cytokines on physical function may be promising. Several drugs are known to act as cytokine suppressors. Although much work remains to be done, continued research into the modulation of cytokines to improve physical function appears to be promising.

# References

1. Thomas DR (2002) Focus on functional decline in hospitalized older adults. J Gerontol A Biol Sci Med Sci 57:M567–M568

2. Manton KG (1988) A longitudinal study of functional change and mortality in the United States. National Long Term Care Survey. J Gerontol 43:S153–S161

3. Corti MC, Salive ME, Guralnik J (1996) Serum albumin and physical function as predictors of coronary heart disease mortality and incidence in older persons. J Clin Epidemiol 49:519–526

4. Hirsch CH, Sommers L, Olsen A et al (1990) The natural history of functional morbidity in hospitalized older patients. J Am Geriatr Soc 38:1296–1303

5. Warshaw GA, Sampson S, Matthias R et al (1982) Functional disability in the hospitalized elderly. J Am Med Assoc 248:847–850

6. Fortinsky RH, Covinsky KE, Palmer RM, Landefeld CS (1999) Effects of functional status changes before and during hospitalization on nursing home admission of older patients. J Gerontol A Biol Sci Med Sci 54:M521–M526

7. Foley DJ, Ostfeld AM, Branch LG et al (1992) The risk of nursing home admission in three communities. J Aging Health 4:155–173

8. Fried LP, Bush TL (1988) Morbidity as a focus of preventive health care in the elderly. Epidemiol Rev 10:48–64

9. Thomas DR (2001) The critical link between health-related quality of life and age-related changes in physical activity and nutrition. J Gerontol A Biol Sci Med Sci 56:M599–M602

10. Guralnik JM, Simonsick EM, Ferrucci L et al (1994) A short physical performance battery assessing lower extremity function: association with self-reported disability and prediction of mortality and nursing home admission. J Gerontol 49:M85–M94

11. Buttar A, Blaum C, Fries B (2001) Clinical characteristics and six-month outcomes of nursing home residents with low activities of daily living dependency. J Gerontol A Biol Sci Med Sci 56:M292–M297

12. Donaldson LJ, Clayton DG, Clarke M (1980) The elderly in residential care: Mortality in relation to functional capacity. J Epidemiol Community Health 34:96–101

13. Guralnik JM, Ferrucci L, Simonsick EM et al (1995) Lower-extremity function in persons over the age of 70 years as a predictor of subsequent disability. N Engl J Med 332:556–556

14. Markides KS, Black SA, Ostir GV et al (2001) Lower body function and mortality in Mexican American elderly people. J Gerontol A Biol Sci Med Sci 56:M243–M247

15. Rogers A, Rogers RG, Belanger A (1990) Longer life but worse health? Measurement and dynamics. Gerontologist 30:640–649

16. Tinnetti ME, Speechley M, Ginter SF (1990) Risk factors for falls among elderly persons living in the community. N Engl J Med 322:286–290

17. Nourhashemi F, Andrieu S, Gillette-Guyonnet S et al (2001) Instrumental activities of daily living as a potential marker of frailty: a study of 7364 community-dwelling elderly women (the EPIDOS Study). J Gerontol A Biol Sci Med Sci 56:M448-M453

18. Morley JE, Baumgartner RN, Roubenoff R et al (2001) Sarcopenia. J Lab Clin Med 137:231–243

19. Morley JE (2001) Anorexia, sarcopenia, and aging. Nutrition 17:660–663

20. Newman AB, Gottdiener JS, McBurnie MA et al (2001) Associations of subclinical cardiovascular disease with frailty. J Gerontol A Biol Sci Med Sci 56:M158–M166

21. Fried LP, Tangen CM, Walston J et al (2001) Frailty in older adults: evidence for a phenotype. J Gerontol A Biol Sci Med Sci 56:M146-M156

22. Gillick M (2001) Pinning down frailty. J Gerontol A Biol Sci Med Sci 56:M134–M135

23. Fried TR, Bradley EH, Williams CS, Tinetti ME (2001) Functional disability and health care expenditures for older persons. Arch Intern Med 161:2602–2607

24. Aniansson A, Sperling L, Rundgren A, Lehnberg E (1983) Muscle function in 75 year old men and women: a longitudinal study. Scand J Rehabil Med 9:92–102

25. Davies C, Thomas D, White M (1986) Mechanical properties of young and elderly human muscle. Acta Med Scand Suppl 711:219–226

26. Larron L, Grimby G, Karlsson J (1979) Muscle strength and speed of movement in relation to age and muscle morphology. J Appl Physiol 46:451–456

27. Aniansson A, Grimby G, Rundgren A (1980)

Isometric and isokinetic quadriceps muscle strength in 70-year-old men and women. Scand J Rehabil Med 12:161–168

28. Jette AM, Branch LG (1985) Impairment and disability in the aged. J Chronic Dis 38:59–65

29. Jette AM, Branch LG (1981) The Framingham Disability Study. II Physical disability among the aging. Am J Public Health 71:1211–1216

30. Astrand I (1960) Aerobic work capacity in men and women with special reference to age. Acta Physiol Scand 49:1–92

31. Astrand I, Astrand P-O, Hallback I et al (1973) Reduction in maximal oxygen uptake with age. J Appl Physiol 35:649

32. Fleg JL, Lakatta EG (1985) Loss of muscle mass is a major determinant of the age-related decline in maximal aerobic capacity. Circulation 72:S464

33. Steinhaus LA, Dustman RE, Rubling RO et al (1988) Cardiorespiratory fitness of young and older active and sedentary men. Br J Sports Med 22:163–166

34. Moritani T, DeVries H (1980) Potential for gross muscle hypertrophy in older men. J Gerontol 35:672–682

35. Brown AB, McCartney N, Sale DG (1990) Positive adaptations to weightlifting training in the elderly. J Appl Physiol 69:1725–1733

36. Frontera WR, Meredith CN, O'Reilly KP et al (1988) Strength conditioning in older men: skeletal muscle hypertrophy and improved function. J Appl Physiol 64:1038–1044

37. Charette SL, McEvoy L, Pyka G et al (1991) Muscle hypertrophy response to resistance training in older women. J Appl Physiol 70:1912–1916

38. Anniansson A, Gustafsson E (1981) Physical training in elderly men. Clin Physiol 1:87–98

39. Larsson L (1982) Physical training effects on muscle morphology in sedentary males of different ages. Med Sci Sports Exerc 14:203–206

40. Fiatarone MA, Evans WJ (1993) The etiology and reversibility of muscle dysfuntion in the aged. J Gerontol 48:77–83

41. Gardner EM, Murasko DM (2002) Age-related changes in Type 1 and Type 2 cytokine production in humans. Biogerontology 3:271–290

42. Cohen HJ, Pieper CF, Harris T et al (1997) The association of plasma IL-6 levels with functional disability in community-dwelling elderly. J Gerontol 52:M201–M208

43. Cohen HJ, Harris T, Pieper CF (2003) Coagulation and activation of inflammatory pathways in the development of functional decline and mortality in the elderly. Am J Med 114:180–187

44. Reuben DB, Ferrucci L, Wallace R et al (2000) The prognostic value of serum albumin in healthy older persons with low and high serum interleukin-6 (IL-6) levels. J Am Geriatr Soc 48:1404–1407

45. Ferrucci L, Penninx BW, Volpato S et al (2002) Change in muscle strength explains accelerated decline of physical function in older women with high interleukin-6 serum levels. J Am Geriatr Soc 50:1947–1954

46. Ferrucci L, Harris TB, Guralnik JM et al (1999) Serum IL-6 level and the development of disability in older persons. J Am Geriatr Soc 47:639–646

47. Vasan RS, Sullivan LM, Roubenoff R et al (2003) Inflammatory markers and risk of heart failure in elderly subjects without prior myocardial infarction: the Framingham Heart Study. Circulation 107:1486–1491

48. Cicoira M, Bolger AP, Doehner W et al (2001) High tumor necrosis factor-alpha levels are associated with exercise intolerance and neurohormonal activation in chronic heart failure patients. Cytokine 15:80–86

49. Tisdale MJ (1997) Biology of cachexia. J Natl Cancer Inst 89:1763–1773

50. Banks WA, Farr SA, La Scola ME, Morley JE (2001) Intravenous human interleukin-1 alpha impairs memory processing in mice: dependence of blood-brain barrier transport in posterior division of the septum. J Pharmacol Exp Ther 299:536–541

51. Banks WA, Morley JE (2003) Memories of made of this: recent advances in understanding cognitive impairments and dementia. J Gerontol A Biol Sci Med Sci 58:314–321

52. Chan DC, Kasper JD, Black BS, Rabins PV (2003) Presence of behavioral and psychological symptoms predicts nursing home placement in conmmunity-dwelling elders with cognitive impairment in univariate but not multivariate analysis. J Gerontol A Biol Sci Med Sci 58:548–554

53. Sands LP, Yaffe K, Covinsky K et al (2003) Cognitive screening predicts magnitued of functional recovery from admission to 3 months after discharge in hospitalized elders. J Gerontol A Biol Sci Med Sci58:37–45

54. Blaum CS, Ofstedal MB, Liang J (2002) Low cognitive performance, comorbid disease, and task-specific disability: findings from a nationally representative survery. J Gerontol A Biol Sci Med Sci 57:523–531

55. Njegovan V, Man-Son-Hing M, Mitchell SL, Molnar FJ (2001) The hierarchy of functional loss associated with cognitive decline in older persons. J Gerontol A Biol Sci Med Sci 56:638–643

56. Royall DR, Chiodo LK, Polk MJ (2000) Correlates of disability among elderly retirees with 'subclinical' cognitive impairment. J Gerontol A Biol Sci Med Sci 55:541–546

57. Shike M, Russell DM, Detsky AS et al (1984) Changes in body composition in patients with small-cell cancer. The effect of total parenteral nutrition as an adjunct to chemotherapy. Ann Intern Med 101:303–309

58. Mitch WE (1998) Mechanisms causing loss of lean body mass in kidney disease. Am J Clin Nutr 67:359–366

59. Hedlund J, Hansson LO, Ortqvist A (1995) Short- and long-term prognosis for middle-aged and elder-

ly patients hospitalized with community-acquired pneumonia: impact of nutritional and inflammatory factors. Scand J Infect Dis 27:32–37

60. Toth MJ, Gottlieb SS, Goran MI et al (1997) Daily energy expenditure in free-living heart failure patients. Am J Physiol 272:469–475

61. Roubenoff R, Roubenoff RA, Cannon JG et al (1994) Rheumatoid cachexia: cytokine-driven hypermetabolism accompanying reduced body cell mass in chronic inflammation. J Clin Invest 93:2379–2386

62. Kotler DP, Wang J, Pierson RN (1985) Body composition studies in patients with the acquired immunodeficiency syndrome. Am J Clin Nutr 42:1255–1265

63. Baez-Franceschi D, Morley JE (1999) Physio-pathology of the catabolism associated with malnutrition in the elderly. Z Gerontol Geriatr 32:12–19

64. Thomas DR (2002) Distinguishing starvation from cachexia. Clin Geriatr Med 18:883–891

65. Thomas DR (2002) Dietary prescription for chronic obstructive pulmonary disease. Clin Geriatr Med 18:835–839

66. Ershler WB (2003) Biological interactions of aging and anemia: a focus on cytokines. J Am Geriatr Soc 51:S18–S21

67. Wilkinson TJ, Warren MR (2003) What is the prognosis of mild normocytic anemia in older people? Intern Med J 33:14–17

68. Hung AM, Chertow GM, Young BS et al (2002) Inflammatory markers are unrelated to physical activity, performance, and functioning in hemodialysis. J Ren Nutr 12:170–176

69. Rubenstein LZ, Josephson KR, Wieland GD et al (1987) Geriatric assessment on a subacute hospital ward. Clin Geriatr Med 3:131–143

70. Applegate WB, Akins D, Vander Zwaag R et al (1983) A geriatric rehabilitation and assessment unit in a community hospital. J Am Geriatr Soc 31:206–210

71. Landefeld CS, Palmer RM, Kresevic DM et al (1995) A randomized trial of care in a hospital medical unit especially designed to improve the functional outcomes of acutely ill older patients. N Engl J Med 332:1338–1344

72. Wanich CK, Sullivan-Marx EM, Gottlieb GL, Johnson JC (1992) Functional status outcomes of nursing intervention in hospitalized elderly. Image J Nurs Sch 24:201–207

73. Rich MW (2001) Heart failure in the 21st century: a cardiogeriatric syndrome. J Gerontol A Biol Sci Med Sci 56:M88–M96

74. Kirk-Sanchez NJ, Roach KE (2001) Relationship between duration of therapy services in a comprehensive rehabilitation program and mobility at discharge in patients with orthopedic problems. Phys Ther 81:888–895

75. Stuck AE, Egger M, Hammer A et al (2000) Home visits to prevent nursing home admission and functional decline in elderly people. Systematic review and meta-regression analysis. JAMA 287:1022–1028

76. Li FZ, Harmer P, McAuley E et al (2001) An evalua-tion of the effects of Tai Chi exercise on physical function among older persons: a randomized controlled trial. Ann Behav Med 23:139–146

77. Paffenbarger RS Jr, Hyde RT, Wing AL, Hsieh CC (1986) Physical activity, all-cause mortality, and longevity of college alumni. N Engl J Med 314:605–613

78. Kujala UM, Kaprio J, Sarna S, Koskenvuo M (1998) Relationship of leisure-time physical activity and mortality: the Finnish twin cohort. JAMA 279:440–444

79. Fiatarone MA, Marks EC, Ryan ND et al (1990) High-intensity strength training in nonagenarians. Effects on skeletal muscle. JAMA 263:3029–3034

80. Fiatarone MA, O'Neill EF, Ryan ND et al (1994) Exercise training and nutritional supplementation for physical frailty in very elderly people. N Engl J Med 330:1769–1775

81. Meredith CN, Frontera WR, O'Reilly KP, Evans WJ (1992) Body composition in elderly men: effect of dietary modification during strength training. J Am Geriatr Soc 40:155–162

82. Posner JD, Gorman KM, Gitlin LN et al (1990) Effects of exercise training in the elderly on the occurrence and time to onset of cardiovascular diagnoses. J Am Geriatr Soc 38:205–210

83. Arraiz GA, Wigle DT, Mao Y (1992) Risk assessment of physical activity and physical fitness in the Canada Health Survey Mortality follow-up Study. J Clin Epidemiol 45:419–428

84. Kannel WB, Sorlie P (1979) Some health benefits of physical activity: the Framingham Study. J Clin Epidemiol 139:857–861

85. Lapidus L, Bengtsson C (1986) Socioeconomic factors and physical activity in relation to cardiovascular disease and death: a 12-year follow-up of participants in a population study of women in Gothenburg, Sweden. Br Heart J 55:295–301

86. Adamopoulos S, Parissis J, Karatzas D et al (2002) Physical training modulates proinflammatory cytokines and the soluble Fas/soluble Fas ligand system in patients with chronic heart failure. J Am Coll Cardiol 39:653–663

87. Matsumoto AM (2002) Andropause: clinical implications of the decline in serum testosterone levels with aging in men. J Gerontol A Biol Sci Med Sci 57:M76–M79

88. Morley JE, Perry HM (2003) Androgens and women at the menopause and beyond. J Gerontol A Biol Sci Med Sci 58:409–416

89. Wittert GA, Chapman IM, Haren MT et al (2003) Oral testosterone supplementation increases muscle and decreases fat mass in healthy elderly males with low-normal gonadal status. J Gerontol A Biol Sci Med Sci 2003;58:618–625

90. Kenny AM, Dawson L, Kleppinger A et al (2003) Prevalence of sarcopenia and predictors of skeletal muscle mass in nonobese women who are long-term users of estrogen-replacement therapy. J Gerontol A Biol Sci Med Sci 58:M436–M440

91. Iannuzzi-Sucich M, Prestwood KM, Kenny AM (2002) Prevalence of sarcopenia and predictors of skeletal muscle mass in healthy, older men and women. J Gerontol A Biol Sci Med Sci 57:772–777

92. Kenny AM, Prestwood KM, Gruman CA et al (2001) Effects of transdermal testosterone on bone and muscle in older men with low bioavailable testosterone levels. J Gerontol A Biol Sci Med Sci 56:266–272

93. Morley JE (2001) Andropause: is it time for the geriatrician to treat it? J Gerontol A Biol Sci Med Sci 56:263–265

94. Wittert GA, Chapman IM, Haren MT et al (2003) Oral testosterone supplementation increases muscle and decreases fat mass in healthy elderly males with low-normal gonadal status. J Gerontol A Biol Sci Med Sci 58:618–625

95. Morley JE (2003) The need for a men's health initiative. J Gerontol A Biol Sci Med Sci 58:614–617

96. Bhasin S (2003) Testosterone supplementation for aging-associated sarcopenia. J Gerontol A Biol Sci Med Sci 58:1002–1008

97. Morley JE, Kaiser FE, Sih R et al (1997) Testosterone and frailty. Clin Geriatr Med 13:685–695

98. Perry HM, Miller DK, Patrick P, Morley JE (2000) Testosterone and leptin in older African-American men: relationship to age, strength, function and season. Metabolism 49:1085–1091

99. Yeh SS, Wu SY, Levine DM et al (2001) The correlation of cytokine levels with body weight after megestrol acetate treatment in geriatric patients. J Gerontol A Biol Sci Med Sci 56:48–54

100. Lambert CP, Sullivan DH, Evans WJ (2003) Effects of testosterone replacement and/or resistance training on interleukin-6, tumor necrosis factor alpha, and leptin in elderly men ingesting megastrol acetate: a randomized controlled trial. J Gerontol A Biol Sci Med Sci 58:165–170

101. Mantovani G, Macciò A, Lai P et al (1998) Cytokine involvement in cancer anorexia/cachexia: role of megestrol acetate and medroxyprogesterone acetate on cytokine downregulation and improvement of clinical symptoms. Crit Rev Oncog 9:99–106

102. Mantovani G, Macciò A, Massa E, Madeddu C (2001) Managing cancer related anorexia/cachexia. Drugs 61:499–514

# SECTION 8
# CACHEXIA AND HIV INFECTION/AIDS

# HIV Infection-Related Cachexia and Lipodystrophy

Daniele Scevola, Angela Di Matteo, Omar Giglio, Filippo Uberti

## Introduction

### Cachexia in the World

Protein energy malnutrition (PEM) is, alone or associated with other diseases, the first step in the development of cachexia [1–3]. An insufficient amount of food is the leading cause of malnutrition and infectious diseases are the second. In developing countries, 20% of the population – more than 800 million people – eats a quantity of food only sufficient to supply energy for a sedentary life, i.e. 1.2–1.4 times the resting energy expenditure (REE). More than 192 million children suffer from PEM and 2 billion people lack different micronutrients (vitamins, minerals, essential fatty and amino-acids) [4–7]. Even in Western countries, where an enormous surplus of food is produced, many groups of people, especially the poor, the elderly, drug addicts, pregnant women, patients with liver, kidney and gastro-intestinal (GI)-tract diseases, cancer, AIDS , show nutritional defects. In general, 60% of the world's population (41% in developing countries) consumes less than 2600 Kcal/person/day, an amount of energy considered barely sufficient for limited activity. In 15 countries, inhabitants have < 3000 Kcal/per day at their disposal, and the dietary energy supply (DES) is < 2000 Kcal/person in 11 countries. The development of severe nutritional defects is therefore inevitable [4–7].

Malnutrition reaches cachexia, its extreme limit, during the course of cancer and infectious diseases [2, 8]. In 1987, the Center for Disease Control (CDC) included wasting syndrome (a form of cachexia) in its list of diseases indicative of AIDS [9]. Deriving from the Greek *kakos,* which means bad, and *hexis,* which means disposition, cachexia defines a state of general wasting associated with individual, social, or medical causes (Table 1). It is caused by a series of factors, such as anorexia, sickness, dysgeusia, poor alimentary habits, and digestive and absorption disturbances linked to digestive tract infections.

All these factors cause a progressive loss of weight, loss of lipid stores and muscular body mass, negative nitrogen balance, and thus depletion of circulating and visceral proteins [10–19], resulting in extreme cases, African 'slim disease' [20, 21].

Many anthropometric studies [14, 16, 22–27] have pointed out that, before the introduction of highly active anti-retroviral therapy (HAART), weight loss was present in 59–84% of HIV-positive subjects, both hospitalised and out-patients. This weight loss was in some cases considerable (30% and more) compared to the patients' usual or ideal weight or to the percentiles of a normal reference population.

Table 1. General causes of cachexia

| |
| --- |
| Voluntary or induced starvation |
| *Social causes:* |
|    Old age |
|    Poverty |
|    Inability to prepare food |
| *Medical causes:* |
|    Diabetes mellitus |
|    Other endocrine diseases |
|    Psychiatric diseases |
|    Kidney diseases |
|    Digestive tract diseases |
|    Infectious diseases |
|    Tumours |

# Pathophysiology of Cachexia

## Mechanisms of Cachexia

There is no general agreement about the reference standards for evaluating human body weight [28], but the most frequently used in the study of nutritional status is still Blackburn's method, which is based on the anthropometric tables of the Metropolitan Life Insurance Company [29].

According to this method, the indicative signs of malnutrition and cachexia are either a weight loss > 10% of the ideal or usual body weight or a percentile value lower by at least 15% than the corresponding age group for weight/height.

The reference to the ideal weight, although valid for healthy subjects, cannot be translated to sick people, for whom it is more rational to refer to the usual weight or the weight before the onset of illness [30] or the weight/age/height percentiles of the general population in that particular country [29].

With reference to the criteria used (ideal weight, usual weight, height/weight ratio) and the standards of reference, the classification of the nutritional status of a patient changes, with a slight deviation (3%) between ideal weight and usual weight, but with significant deviation (22–25%) among these and the percentiles of the general population [31]. Accordingly, a loss of weight > 10% of the ideal or usual weight or a percentile value lower by at least 15% than the corresponding age group for weight/height is considered diagnostic of malnutrition and cachexia.

The study of body compartments (thin mass, fat mass, bone tissue, total water), potassium and total nitrogen, muscular and circulating proteins, and bioimpedance discriminates between the body's content of water and fat, considered functionally inert, and the biologically active cellular mass, represented by the muscles and viscera [13–18, 22, 24–27].

The differences found between body weight and cellular mass are due either to an excess of extracellular water or to fat deposits. Fat is subject to variations not synchronous with those of the cellular mass, related to genetic factors (initial number and size of fat cells) and to hormonal causes, i.e. leptin, lipoprotein lipase (LPL), estradi-ol, progesterone, glucagon, insulin, corticosteroids, growth hormone. In non-complicated starvation, fat reserves are depleted first, followed by protein reserves [32]. In AIDS, depletion of cellular mass can start in the presence of preserved fat deposits [33, 34].

Lack of protein-caloric nutrients due to famine, voluntary refusal, nervous anorexia, or poor diets, causes slimming. Infectious diseases, cancer, burns, traumas, or surgery induce hypercatabolism, which, by means of very similar metabolic responses (e.g. acute-phase response [APR]) leads to self-cannibalism and to cachexia [35, 36]. Self-cannibalism is, in the short-term, the physiological strategy for coping with a pathogenic noxa. It can be advantageous because it immediately supplies amino acids to repair tissue damage and for the synthesis of acute-phase proteins in the liver [32, 37].

Under physiological conditions, the central nervous system balances the quantity of assumed and consumed calories through hunger and satiety, and body weight is maintained. The human body consumes energy in three ways: (1) calories burnt for basal metabolism (REE); (2) calories for the absorption of nutrients (dynamic-specific action, DSA); and (3) calories for physical activity. A rapid weight loss (in days) reflects a predominant reduction of the hydric mass of the body, while a reduction of tissue mass takes longer, i.e. weeks or months.

# Biochemical Phases of Cachexia

The organism has to supply 150–180 g glucose/day for oxidative phosphorylation in the brain and bone marrow.

In the normal fast, hypoglycaemia stimulates the production of glucagon, which induces glycogenolysis in the liver and in the muscle to produce glucose. But if glycogen stores can supply glucose only for 12–18 h, then hypoglycaemia stimulates the production of epinephrine, which in turn starts lipolysis in fat stores. About 160 g fat (triglycerides, FFA, glycerol)/day can be transformed into glucose to maintain vital processes. But, if the requirement for energy is prolonged, then lipids alone are not sufficient to maintain glucose levels, as their use is limited by the accumulation of ketones (ketoacidosis) and by the decrease of insulin. At this point, the organism, which has depleted glycogen stores and is self-limited in using lipids, goes on to use muscular and visceral proteins to produce glucose. About 75 grams of proteins/day are used for gluconeogenesis during normal starvation, with urinary loss of about 12 grams nitrogen/day. If the fast is prolonged, the organism adapts itself to utilise more ketone bodies and to reduce nitrogen loss to between 8 and 3 g/day. Differently from normal starvation, in stressed starvation it is not hypoglycaemia that starts catabolic events, but the increase of hormonal factors, including cortisol, glucagon, epinephrine, leptin, cytokines (tumour necrosis factor [TNF], interleukin [IL]-1, IL-2, IL-6, IL-10, interferons [IFNs], and prostaglandins [PGs]). These hormones may not increase in the blood; rather, in metabolically active tissues. Consumption of lean mass of up to 500 g/day, with a urinary loss of nitrogen of 20 g/day, may be reached.

The calorie balance represents an equation in which the energy introduced by food can be used for muscular work and metabolic activity, or it can be saved and stored in the tissues. If the consumption of energy exceeds the intake, the system goes into a condition of caloric deficit and the organism tries to maintain the homeostasis by burning its reserves. The caloric balance can be overturned by causes that alter the availability of nourishment, its absorption, and its metabolism (Table 2).

**Table 2.** Causes of energetic imbalance

*Reduced oral intake*:
    Lack of foods, old age
    Anorexia, depression, dementia
    Cerebral disturbances
    Functional or organic obstacles to the passing of food

*Reduced caloric absorption*:
    Digestive disturbances
    Malabsorption
    Diarrhoea

*Metabolic disturbances:*
    Protein-synthesis defects
    Hypermetabolism
    Futile metabolic cycle
    Cytokine action
    Enzymatic or endocrine disturbances
    Fever

During serious illness, a normal type of nourishment is not sufficient to balance the intense catabolism and nitrogen loss caused by the pathologic process, in which glucose, lipid, and protein reserves are burnt in order to cover energy needs (self-cannibalism). If self-cannibalism persists, the effect is fatal: the loss of a third of body proteins (= 2 kg proteins or 8 kg cellular mass) in a person of average weight causes death in less than one month. The degree of cachexia itself, independent from its cause, is a mortality factor. If the depletion of cellular mass and total body potassium is examined with reference to the survival time, a linear correlation (Fig. 1) is observed in AIDS and in cancer patients [22–24, 34, 38]. At the time of

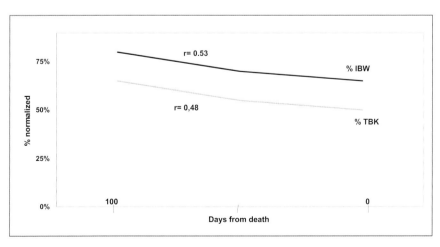

**Fig. 1.** Relationship of ideal body weight (*IBW*) and total body potassium (*TBK*) to the timing of death. Death occurs when body weight is about one third below ideal values and TBK just above 50% of normal

death, cellular mass is reduced, on average, to 54% of normal, corresponding to 66% of ideal weight. In voluntary or forced starvation, death occurs when the body weight is reduced to almost a third of the ideal weight [22].

## Cachexia in AIDS

The control of HIV infection remains elusive: during the 1990s, 10–20 million new cases among adults and 5–10 million among children were registered, with an estimated cumulative total of 30–40 million cases of HIV infection in 2005 and more than 10 million of cases of AIDS [7, 39] (Fig. 2).

While AIDS is still a fatal disease, new, highly active and more effective therapies have improved patient survival and quality of life. Among these, dietary therapy and palliative care have played an important role [2, 40–42]. Many of the symptoms of AIDS, such as slimming, anorexia, asthaenia, sickness, and nutritional deficits, seem to be reversible if properly treated by administration of proteins, calories, vitamins, minerals, and specific drugs [43–46].

Malnutrition in all its forms is one of the most common and striking phenomena of AIDS [22, 47]. Multiple factors, such as anorexia, sickness, dysgeusia, poor alimentary habits, as well as digestive and absorption disturbances linked to digestive tract infections, cause a progressive weight loss, depletion of lipid stores and lean body mass, and negative nitrogen balance with depletion of circulating and visceral proteins [10, 12, 14–18, 48–53]. The extreme manifestation of this condition is referred to as 'slim disease' [1, 20]. In the 1987 revision of clinical and laboratory criteria defining AIDS, a new condition, wasting syndrome, was included in the list of indicative diseases [9]. HIV wasting syndrome is defined as emaciation and weight loss (predominantly loss of body cell mass) > 10 % of baseline body weight, plus either chronic diarrhoea (at least two loose stools per day for more than 30 days) or chronic weakness and documented fever (for over 30 days) in the absence of concurrent illness.

Since 1988, thousands of AIDS cases have been registered worldwide on the basis of detection of the wasting syndrome, but the real prevalence of cachexia in HIV-positive patients is underestimat-

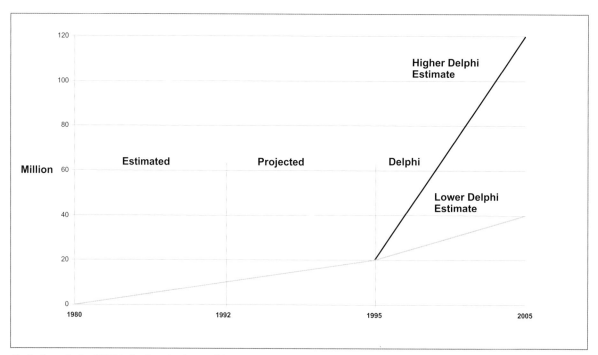

**Fig. 2.** Cumulative HIV infections in the world, 1980-2005

ed, because an associated opportunistic disease (infection or neoplasia) is frequently the greater focus of attention. While cachexia, better than wasting syndrome, defines the severe weight loss that occurs in HIV infection, in the past few years, wasting syndrome has been the third most common indicative condition of AIDS in the USA [54] and the fourth in Italy. Many studies [2, 13–18, 23, 40–42, 47] have pointed out that, as determined by anthropometric methods, the AIDS-related loss of weight, compared to the usual or ideal weight or to normal population reference percentiles (Fig. 3), is often considerable (30% and more) and is seen in 59–84% of HIV-positive subjects, both hospitalised and out-patients.

Intense anorexia and progressive slimming have a dramatic psychological impact on AIDS patients and their families, and cause a deterioration in the quality of life, an increased susceptibility to infections, and intolerance to drugs [11, 47]. Slimming is due to many factors: the direct cytopathic effect of HIV on intestinal cells [55], opportunistic infections [56, 57], cytokines [58, 59], drugs, and neoplasms. There is a reduced intake and assimilation of nutrients, with increased protein-calorie consumption and a condition of cellular hypercatabolism [60], which, if not treated, very quickly leads to death. However, from a macroscopic point of view, weight loss is the most striking event. Terminal cachexia manifests itself clinically, but less evident alterations of the nutritional status must be diagnosed very early on, so that treatment can be administered in time to avoid malnutrition becoming the cause of the disease. For example, such patients exhibit a decrease in body temperature and basal metabolism, which can, however, be high compared with the caloric intake calculated for normal subjects [60]. In addition, there are abnormalities of the skin, muscular and skeletal systems, digestive tract, liver, and respiratory function [24]. Neurological signs may also be present.

Malnutrition also compromises nonspecific factors, including resistance to pathogens and reduced activity of the bone marrow, lymphatic tissues, and reticuloendothelial system. Other, less evident disturbances involve chemical-haematological nutritional parameters, i.e. the development of anaemia and hypoalbuminaemia, reduced plasma titres of vitamins B6 and B12, folic acid,

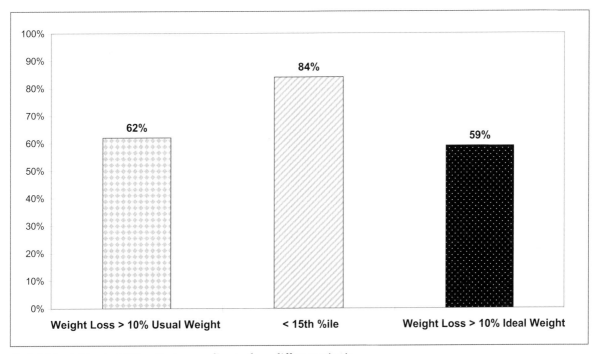

**Fig. 3.** Malnutrition in AIDS patients according to three different criteria

selenium, zinc, copper, calcium, and potassium [61–65]. Cell-body mass also progressively decreases (Fig. 4), so that cachexia becomes a disease within a disease and may be included among the various cofactors that have been hypothesised to affect progression of HIV infection to AIDS [66]. In 60% of HIV-positive subjects, PEM is present along with and vitamin and mineral deficits, which together cause progressive physical-metabolic wastage and increased susceptibility to opportunistic infections and drug toxicity. In 80% of deaths due to AIDS, malnutrition is a concurrent cause, and thus must be identified very early by anthropometric and nutritional methods [2, 14–18, 26, 41, 42, 66].

The presence or absence of nutritional cofactors accelerates or retards the progression of HIV by influencing immune functions. It is well-known that PEM reduces phagocytosis [67–69] and IgA secretion, enhancing bacterial adhesion to respiratory epithelial cells. AIDS is not a food- or drink-borne disease but adequate nutrition may improve the clinical condition of the patient and his or her quality of life. Consequently, evaluation of the nutritional status is a fundamental component of the multidimensional approach to treating HIV-positive patients, both because there is an evident correlation between malnutrition, morbidity, and lethality [70, 71] and because a relatively large number of subjects live in socio-economic conditions that favour the onset of multiple nutritional defects. Study schemes are available that are specific enough to allow definition of the compartmental composition of the body, visceral protein endowment, and structure of the fat deposits [2]. These schemes can be used to demonstrate that malnutrition presents a mosaic of alterations arising from caloric-protein and food shortage as well as from infections of the gastrointestinal tract. These conditions may be specifically treated.

Among the multiple aetiologies of cachexia (Table 2), the most likely causes of wasting in HIV infection are reduced oral intake, hypermetabolism, endocrine abnormalities, especially due to cytokines [34, 72], and futile metabolic cycles of lipids.

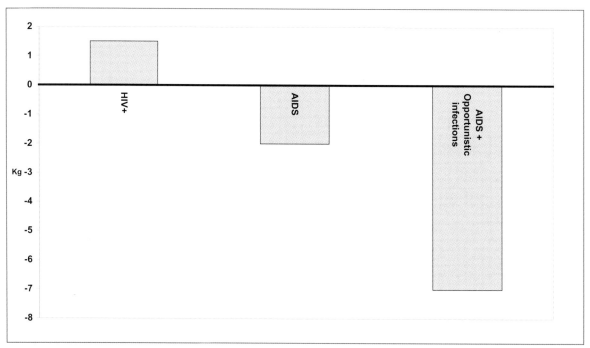

**Fig. 4.** Body weight loss and HIV disease progression

## Reduced Oral Intake

A common feature in HIV-infected patients is the reduced oral intake of macro- and micro-nutrients, mainly due to extensive disease involvement of the GI tract. Thus, 'enteropathogenic AIDS' [17, 52, 53] is the best example of a condition in which chronic weight loss is caused by many different agents affecting gastrointestinal functions, from the oral cavity to the rectum. The loss of appetite (anorexia) and the consequent reduced caloric intake are mainly due to TNF, which inhibits gastric motility and gastrointestinal evacuation, IL-1 and IFN-γ.

## Hypermetabolism and Protein Catabolism

The progression of disease in HIV patients is associated with an increased REE [60]; however, weight loss is better correlated with calorie intake than with REE [73]. While opportunistic infections, malignancies, and high levels of cytokines and hormones in tissues may explain hypermetabo-

lism, it is not clear whether increased REE alone (Fig. 5) can cause wasting, in the absence of other processes [74, 75].

Depending on the type of cachexia, the body's protein compartment undergoes several modifications, which are, in some cases, not related to fat changes [22]. New insights regarding muscle atrophy occurring in aging, AIDS, diabetes, immobility, and space flight have been gained in the last few years. For example, it is now known that ubiquitin ligases are involved in the breakdown of muscle proteins [76]. An acute calorie defect, e.g. a total 24-h fast, forces the organism to use energy reserves, so that approximately 150 g of fat and 60 g of protein are burned. Subsequently, energy-saving mechanisms become involved. These reduce protein breakdown by as much as three-fold, whereas the energy withdrawal from adipose tissue remains unchanged [34]. Basal metabolism accounts for about a fifth of the calories normally consumed at rest. In contrast, serious infection induces acute protein loss (which may be > 120 g/day) [32]. During the septic period, starvation

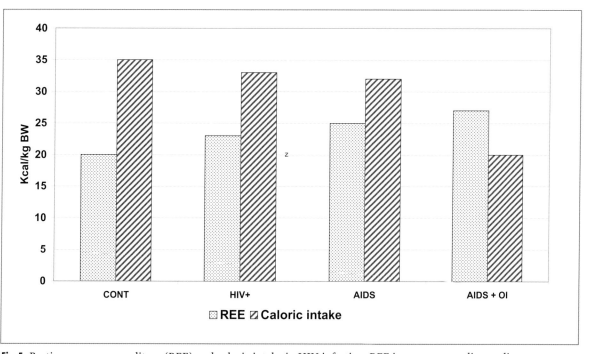

**Fig. 5.** Resting energy expenditure (REE) and caloric intake in HIV infection. REE increases according to disease progression, while caloric intake becomes insufficient to maintain basal needs. *OI*, opportunistic infection

does not activate the energy-saving mechanism that occurs in the absence of infection, so that calorie withdrawal causes a further protein loss that can reach 90 g/day [32, 34]. In sepsis, the basal energy requirement increases because of the hyperthermia [77] induced by cytokines and futile cycles [78].

### Endocrine Abnormalities and Cytokines

Several endocrine abnormalities, such as low levels of testosterone and growth hormone and increased production of cytokines, have been correlated with weight loss in AIDS, while adrenal and thyroid hormones show conflicting patterns [63]. The synergic action of TNF and other cytokines is considered the most probable mechanism causing cachexia [8, 79, 80] (Fig. 6, 7).

The clinical symptoms of anorexia, nausea, fever, asthenia, fatigue, lethargy, myalgia, sickness, diarrhoea, anaemia, leucocytopaenia, tachycardia, headache, neurovegetative disturbances, etc., can be attributed to the release of cytokines by macrophages and activated inflammatory cells.

Lipid metabolism disturbances, anorexia, and weight loss together lead to cachexia and are caused by the combined action of TNF, IL-1, IL-6, and IFN-γ, the production of each being stimulated by infections and cancer [82, 83]. We demonstrated [84] high levels of TNF-α in HIV patients who had lost more than 10% of their ideal weight (Table 3).

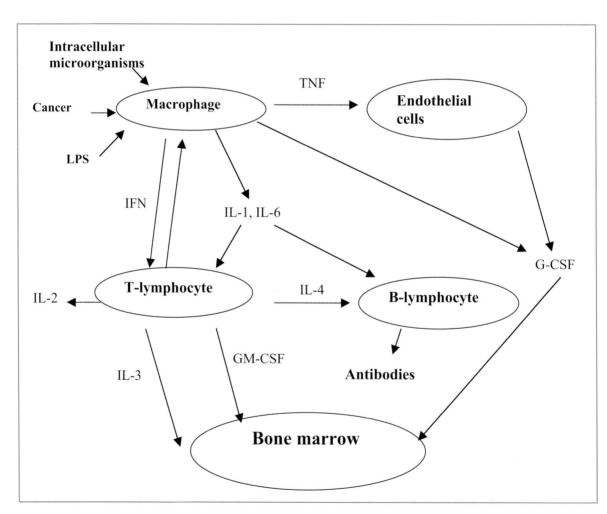

**Fig. 6.** Pattern of cytokine production. *LPS*, lipopolysaccharide; *G-CSF* granulocyte colony-stimulating factor; *GM-CSF* granulocyte/macrophage colony-stimulating factor. For other abbreviations, see text

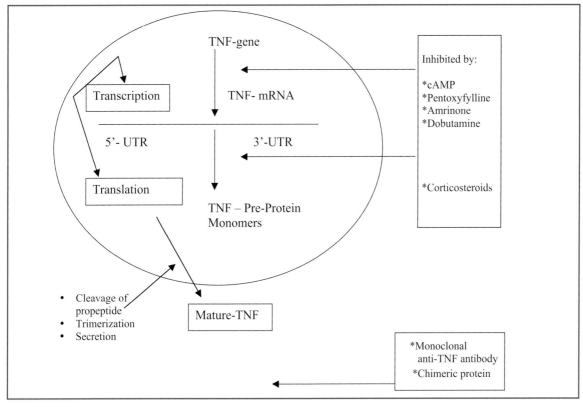

**Fig. 7.** Regulation of tumour necrosis factor (TNF) synthesis in macrophages

**Table 3.** TNF blood levels in 50 AIDS patients

| > 400 pg/ml | 400–201 pg/ml | 200–100 pg/ml | < 100 pg/ml |
|---|---|---|---|
| Disease ($n = 13$) | Disease ($n = 14$) | Disease ($n = 6$) | Disease ($n = 17$) |
| Toxo (2) | Toxo (1) | Crypto (1) | Toxo (3) |
| PCP (6) | PCP (4) | Lymphoma (1) | PCP (3) |
| HIV (2) | Toxo + KS (1) | TBC (1) | Salm (1) |
| MAC (2) | PCP + HSV (1) | CMV (1) | TBC (1) |
| PCP + Toxo (1) | MAC (2) | HIV (2) | Crypto (2) |
| | Toxo + MAC(2) | | Candida (1) |
| | HIV (2) | | VZV (1) |
| | Toxo + PCP(1) | | HIV (5) |

*Toxo*, neurotoxoplasmosis; *PCP*, *Pneumocystis carinii* pneumonia; *MAC*, *Mycobacterium avium* complex; *HSV*, herpes simplex virus; *KS*, Kaposi's sarcoma; *Crypto*, cryptosporidiosis; *TBC*, tuberculosis; *CMV*, cytomegalovirus; *Salm*, salmonellosis; *VZV*, varicella zoster virus

## Futile Metabolic Cycles of Lipids

Lipid metabolism seems to be particularly involved with and affected by cytokines. Early studies [85, 86] pointed out the cachexia-promoting effects of TNF, IL-1, and IFNs.

Initially, the cachexia seen in different extreme clinical situations was thought to be due to TNF, which for that reason was also called cachectin. The injection of TNF into animals, while causing hypertriglyceridaemia and reduction of appetite and water intake, does not cause cachexia if the correct amount of calories is given [87]. Many studies have shown, instead, that disturbances in lipid metabolism, anorexia, and weight loss, all of which lead to cachexia, are due to the combined action of TNF, IL-1, IL-6, and IFN-γ [85, 86], whose production is stimulated by infection and neoplasms [78, 82].

Hypertriglyceridaemia starts mainly through the inhibition of LPL, which regulates the clearance of plasma triglycerides (Fig. 8) and energy production from lipids (Table 4).

LPL is inhibited by TNF and estradiol, and is stimulated by progestins. An increase in liver lipogenesis is associated with increased production of very-low-density lipoprotein (VLDL). In the fat

cell, LPL inhibition causes a reduction of lipogenesis with consequent lipolysis. These effects can be avoided by the administration of inhibitors of prostaglandin synthesis [38].

The increase in plasma triglycerides observed in cachexia is due not only to LPL inhibition and clearance, but also to increased VLDL synthesis from free fatty acids (FFA), resulting from the lipolysis of peripheral fat [78]. By blocking lipolysis in the fat cell, for example with phenyl-isopropyl-adenosine, FFA and plasma triglycerides can be reduced [83, 89]. This indicates that liver synthesis of VLDL starts from FFA mobilised from peripheral fat, re-esterified to triglycerides by the liver, and secreted as VLDL [78] – a typical exam-

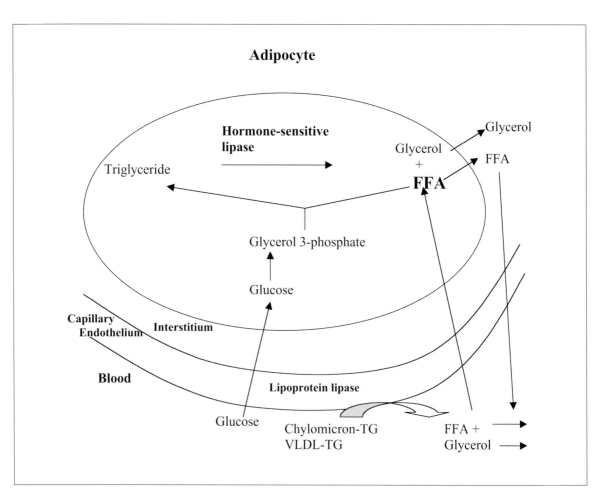

**Fig. 8.** Role of lipoprotein lipase (LPL) in lipid metabolism. *FFA*, Free fatty acids; *TG*, triglyceride; *VLDL*, very-low-density lipoprotein

**Table 4.** Role of LPL in tissues

| Tissue | Role |
| --- | --- |
| Muscle (cardiac, skeletal) | Energy provision |
| White adipose tissue | Triglyceride storage |
| Brown adipose tissue | Thermogenesis |
| Lactating breast | Milk triglyceride synthesis |
| Lung | Surfactant synthesis[a] |
| Brain | Phospholipid and glycolipid synthesis[a] |
| Adrenal, kidney, spleen, foetal liver | Unknown |

[a]Putative

ple of the energy-wasting 'futile' metabolic cycle (Fig. 9). Fatty acids mobilised from peripheral fat reach the liver, where they escape oxidation, are then re-esterified to triglycerides, and pass into blood circulation as VLDL. These lipoproteins return in the adipose tissue to be hydrolysed again to fatty acids by LPL and are stored in fat cells as triglycerides [58]. This vicious cycle, caused by

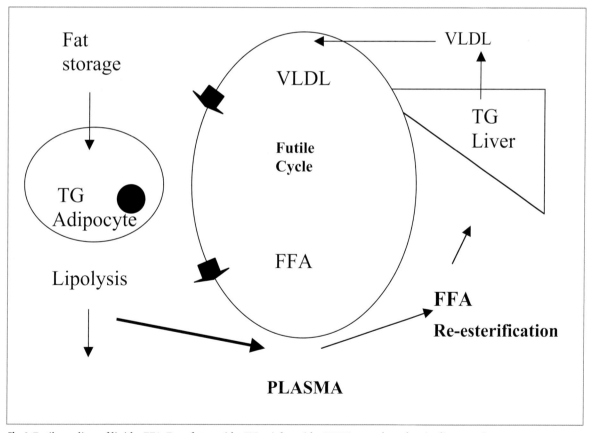

**Fig. 9.** Futile cycling of lipids. *FFA*, Free fatty acids; *TG*, triglyceride; *VLDL*, very-low-density lipoprotein

TNF, IL-1, IL-6, and IFN-γ, does not produce energy (ATP), but rather consumes it, thereby contributing to weight loss.

## Lipid Mobilisation Factor

Lipid mobilisation factor, like many other hormones and β-adrenergic stimuli, carries out its catabolic function by increasing intracellular cyclic AMP (cAMP). In fat cells, the cAMP increase activates a protein kinase, which, in turn, activates, by phosphorylation, a triglyceride lipase. The effects seem therefore to be mediated by guanine-nucleotide-binding proteins (G-proteins), which are important molecules regulating membrane transduction signals. These proteins are controlled by protein products of the gene *ras 21* and are inhibited by fish oil [90].

# Fat Tissue

To better understand the role played by lipids in disturbances associated with HIV infection and with new antiretroviral therapies, it is necessary to review several concepts regarding fat tissue in humans. Actually, fat tissue seems to be both the main player in and the victim of such disorders. Fat tissue not only stores and mobilises rapidly available energy (~ 9 Kcal/g), but also produces hormone-like substances, such as leptin and adiponectin [91], and, especially, cytokines, such as TNF-α [92] and IL-6 [93]. For these reasons, fat tissue is an important metabolic organ. Leptin regulates hypothalamic centres of hunger and satiety [94, 95]; adiponectin reduces plasma levels of glucose, fatty acids, and triglycerides, thereby preventing fat accumulation in muscles and liver [96, 97]. Some 60% of adipose tissue is composed of adipocytes, the rest being blood cells, pericytes, preadipocytes, and fibroblasts [98]. In the human embryo, fat tissue is observed beginning at the second trimester of pregnancy, and its body distribution remains constant throughout foetal and adult life. At birth, the fatty mass is 14% of body weight, with changes depending on the mother's general condition. During the first year of life, adipocytes undergo hypertrophy, and then replicate until full body development is completed. Only 2% of mature adipocytes undergo mitosis, under appropriate stimulation. Therefore, adipocyte hypertrophy, rather than an increase in their number, seems responsible for the diffuse or localised increases in fatty masses [99]. There is, however, a pool of quiescent or immature adipocytes that can differentiate into mature adipocytes under hormonal and vitamin stimulation [98, 100]. During differentiation, markers such as LPL mRNA, glycerol triphosphate dehydrogenase (GPDH), hormone-susceptible lipase (HSL), perilipin, a glucose carrier (GLUT4), and β-3 receptors are acquired. Triglycerides comprise 90% of the mature adipocyte and provide a source of easily available energy through their hydrolysis to fatty acids and glycerol. Mature adipocyte expresses α-2 -adrenergic receptors (α2AR) and adipsin [98]. Adipose tissue secretes LPL, adipsin, complement C3 and B fractions, P450 aromatase, leptin, and growth factors [94, 101]. Its main metabolic functions are lipid hydrolysis and synthesis. Lipolysis is initiated via the activation of β-adrenergic receptors, which in turn activates adenyl cyclase, with subsequent cAMP production via ATP hydrolysis. cAMP activates a protein kinase that, in turn, activates HSL and the hydrolysis of triglyceride to fatty acids and glycerol. The β-1 receptors are epinephrine- and norepinephrine-specific, β-2 receptors are isoprenaline-specific, and β-3 receptors are activated by high doses of catecholamines. α-1 and α-2 receptor activation terminates lipolysis by inhibiting adenyl cyclase. Liposynthesis is driven by LPL, a 55-kDa glycoprotein activated by apoprotein C-II. It hydrolyses circulating triglycerides of chylomicrons and VLDLs. The distribution of adipose tissue throughout the body depends on genetic and hormonal factors [102]. In females, fat tissue is mainly localised to the thighs, with a central redistribution occurring after menopause. In males, fat tissue has mainly a visceral distribution [103, 104]. Excess visceral fat storage is associated with hyperinsulinaemia, diabetes, hyperlipaemia, hypertension, decreased glucose tolerance, and increased cardiovascular disease risk [105]. The metabolic activity of adipose tissue varies according to its anatomic distribution. Epiploic fat is more susceptible to catecholamines than epigastric fat, because its adipocytes are larger and contain more β-3 receptors. Since there is increased lipolytic hydrolysis in visceral fat, the flow of FFA is directly conveyed to the liver. Hepatic VLDL synthesis increases, whereas the uptake of insulin by the liver decreases. Chronic hyperinsulinaemia induces a peripheral insulin resistance [103], increasing diabetes risk. Subcutaneous thigh fat is less susceptible to catecholamines and has a higher LPL index, implying a greater liposynthetic activity. The number of cortisol and androgen receptors is higher in visceral than in subcutaneous fat [102]; as a consequence, LPL stimulation is stronger. Androgen stimulation of β-receptors increases HSL lipolytic activity. The function of brown adipose tissue (BAT) in humans is still not clear. In many animal species, 25% of body weight consists of BAT, which is involved in thermal homeostasis and heat dispersion when the animal is exposed to low/high temperature or hyper-/hypo-feeding. Heat is produced by uncoupling fatty acid oxidation and ATP production in mitochondria through an uncoupling protein (UCP) [106]. In humans, adipocytes identical to those of BAT are observed only in pathological conditions, such as Cushing's syndrome, pheocromocytoma, and multiple symmetric lipomatosis. This last syndrome is characterised by the distribution of multiple, non-encapsulated lipomas to the nape, neck, and supraclavicular and mediastinal regions, along with high LPL activity and decreased lipolysis [107–110]. It has also been suggested that BAT plays a role also in diet-induced thermogenesis.

## Changing Patterns of Cachexia in the HAART Era

A familiarity with the information on adipose tissue provided in the previous section is necessary to understand the complex nutritional changes related to HIV infection and its treatments. It has long been known that during the progression of HIV infection, as well as of other chronic infections and tumours, patients may undergo progressive weight loss and changes in body composition, particularly in fat and muscle masses, and in metabolic pathways, particularly lipid metabolism [62,

111]. This is known as wasting syndrome [9] or cachexia [2, 112].

From 1987 to 1993, wasting syndrome was the AIDS-defining disease in 20% of patients and in up to 70% of patients at the time of death. The incidence of wasting syndrome per 1000 person-years increased from 7.5 in the period 1988–1990 to 14.4 in 1991–1993 and 22.1 in 1994–1995. The incidence decreased to 13.4 in 1996–1999 [113]. Dworkin et al. [19], in a large study, obtained similar results; they found that the incidence of wasting syndrome decreased from 30.2 cases per 1000 person-years in 1992 to 11.9 cases in 1999, with the most significant rate of decline occurring after 1995.

With the introduction of potent antiretroviral combination treatments, including nucleoside and non-nucleoside reverse transcriptase inhibitors (NRTI, NNRTI) and protease inhibitors (PIs), which have prolonged patient survival, the incidence of the previously described changes has been dramatically reduced. Since 1996, when HAART was introduced, the number of patients who died of AIDS and opportunistic infections has decreased by two-thirds, although wasting remains a clinical problem for patients [114, 115]. In addition, new disorders involving lipids, glucose metabolism, and body fat have acquired greater clinical importance [116–120]. The changes are characterised by hyperlipidaemia, generalised, central, or peripheral fat redistribution, and hormonal disturbances [116, 120–124], and have been named lipodystrophy syndrome, HIV-associated adipose redistribution syndrome (HARS) [125], or metabolic syndrome-X (Tables 5, 6, 7).

Prior to 1996, only a small percentage (3%) of patients developed hypercholesterolaemia, hypertriglyceridaemia, and diabetes. The main fat disturbances in cachexia are a decrease in cholesterol levels, an increase of triglycerides, and a global loss of fat together with lean tissue in any body region. These patterns can be clearly distinguished from lipodystrophy (Table 6).

Some of the symptoms and signs of lipodystrophy were already known before the introduction of PIs, as they occur with d4T-containing regimens without PIs at an incidence of 20% compared to 0% in AZT-containing regimens [126]. After 1996, it was possible to demonstrate a clear time correla-

**Table 5.** Changes in body shape following protease inhibitor therapy

|  | No change | Mild | Moderate | Severe |
|---|---|---|---|---|
| Body shape | 17% | 42% | 30% | 11% |
| Loss of subcutaneous fat | 32% | 31% | 27% | 10% |
| Crix belly | 35% | 30% | 22% | 13% |
| Buffalo hump | 80% | 10% | 7% | 3% |

**Table 6.** Differences between cachexia and lipodystrophy syndromes

|  | Cachexia | Lipodystrophy | | |
|---|---|---|---|---|
| Body weight | ⇓ | ⇑ | or | ⇓ |
| Body fat | ⇓ All districts | Peripheral ⇓ | | Central ⇑ |
| Lean body mass | ⇓ | Unchanged ⇓ | | |
| Total cholesterol | ⇓ | ⇑ | | |
| VLDL cholesterol | ⇓ | ⇑ | | |
| LDL cholesterol | ⇓ | ⇑ | | |
| HDL cholesterol | ⇓ | ⇓ | | |
| Triglycerides | ⇑ | ⇑ ⇑ | | |
| Diabetes/insulin resistance | No | Yes | | |
| Coronary artery disease | No | Yes | | |

tion between changes in fat and glucose metabolism and the introduction of PIs. A significant portion, ranging from 5 to 75%, of HIV patients receiving PIs noted changes in lipid metabolism and body fat distribution [127] after an average time of 10 months with Ritonavir/Saquinavir and more than 1 year with Indinavir. These alterations were seen primarily in 32% of patients treated with Indinavir (Crixivan, MSD; this is the origin of the term 'crix belly') [128]. However, more evident abnormalities, referred to as 'protease paunch' [129], are caused by other PIs, such as Nelfinavir (Viracept, Agouron; in 39% of patients), and the dual combination of Ritonavir (Norvir, Abbott) [130] plus Saquinavir (Invirase/Fortovase, Roche; in 66% of patients) [116]. Amprenavir (Agenerase, Glaxo Wellcome/Vertex) seems to have fewer side effects. No data are available for Tipranavir (Texega, Pharmacia Upjohn), DMP-450 (Triangle Pharmaceuticals), and ABT-378 (Abbott).

Abnormal fat accumulation may be visceral (omentum, mesentery, retroperitoneum, pelvic areas), associated with abdominal fullness and bloating (syntomatic fat deposition) [128], or peripheral [116], ranging from benign bilateral symmetric lipomatosis [131] to multiple symmetric lipomatosis and to a dorsal ('buffalo hump') and/or cervical fat pad ('bull neck') [118]. More recently, lipodystrophy syndrome has been better characterised [132–134] with case-definition signs. Fat redistribution (HARS) may have the aspect of either *peripheral lipoatrophy/dystrophy*, involving the face (loss of buccal, parotid, Bichat's, and preauricular pads, sunken cheeks and eyes, prominent zygomatic arches); buttocks; pronounced thinning of the arms and legs with prominence of subcutaneous veins, muscles, and bones; loss of normal skin texture, folds and trophism; or *central lipohypertrophy*, with accumulation of fat in the trunk, breast, and/or dorso-cervix, leading to bull

**Table 7.** Diagnostic criteria for HIV lipodystrophy syndrome

*Main criteria*
- HIV infection
- HAART
- Loss of peripheral fat tissue
- Increased central fat tissue (abdominal girth)

*Minor criteria*
- Visible subcutaneous veins
- Loss of temple, nasolabial, and cheek fat pads
- Buffalo hump or bull neck
- Breast hypertrophy
- Enlarged supraclavicular fat pads
- Bilateral symmetric lipomatosis (enlarged axillary fat pads)
- Decreased thighs size
- Hyperlipidaemia (cholesterol, triglycerides)

*Adjunctive criteria*
- Diabetes
- Peripheral insulin resistance
- Hyperinsulinism
- Hyperuricaemia
- Low serum testosterone
- Increased C-peptide
- Increased free fatty acids
- Coronary artery disease, ischaemic heart disease
- Hypertension

neck, buffalo hump, and enlargement of abdominal girth and the breasts in women (Fig. 10, 11).

The changes in body shape negatively affect the patient's self perception, with negative consequences on compliance. Female patients especially are psychologically distressed by the changes in their body shape. For this reason, many patients stop PI treatment, with the subsequent risk of progression of HIV infection. Lipodystrophy syndrome also affects HIV-infected children, with a prevalence of 26% for any fat redistribution, 8.81% for central lipohypertrophy, 7.55% for peripheral lipoatrophy, and 9.64% for a combined type [135].

Simple measurement of skin folds, hips, and the waist [136, 137] is important to monitor and compare self-reporting symptoms and real changes in body fat redistribution. A finer assessment may be done using bioelectrical impedance assay [138, 139], dual-energy X-ray absorptiometry [119, 140, 141], magnetic resonance imaging [142, 143], computed tomography [144, 145], or ultrasonography [146].

## Pathophysiology of Lipodystrophy

### Mechanisms of Lipodystrophy

#### The Effects of Protease Inhibitors

Different hypotheses have been put forward to explain the putative mechanism of HAART drugs in the development of lipodystrophy syndrome [116–120, 122–124, 126, 134, 141, 147–152]. The first postulates that PIs primarily block cytochrome P450, which is involved in fat metabolism. The second postulates an interaction between PIs and human proteins. HIV protease has a sequence homology of 12 amino acids with two human proteins playing an important role in fat metabolism, namely, LDL-receptor-related protein (LRP) and cytoplasmic retinoic-acid-binding protein type-1 (CRABP-1). PIs inhibit both HIV protease and these two proteins. Inhibition of LRP leads to a reduction in the absorption of fatty acids by capillary endothelium and liver cells. This causes elevated serum triglycerides, visceral fat accumulation, buffalo humps, bull neck, insulin resistance, type II diabetes, breast hypertrophy, etc. Inhibition of CRABP-1 and cytochrome P450 3A isoform results in decreased cell differentiation and cell death (apoptosis), with reduced triglyceride storage and release. Under normal conditions retinoic acid in peripheral adipocytes binds to CRABP-1 and is then transformed, by a catalysed reaction with cytochrome P450 3A isoform, into cis-9-retinoic-acid, which activates the retinoic X receptor (RXR). Another suggested mechanism is alteration of the expression of steroid regulatory element-binding protein-1 (SREBP-1) in adipocytes and in the liver by PIs [153].

Several other PI-related disturbances have been proposed to explain dyslipidaemia and lipodystrophy, such as inhibition of LPL [154] and defects of lamin A/C (LMNA) and PPARG genes, which are associated with autosomal dominant familial partial lipodystrophies [148].

In capillary vessel endothelium, exposure of hepatocytes and adipocytes to PIs can result in the

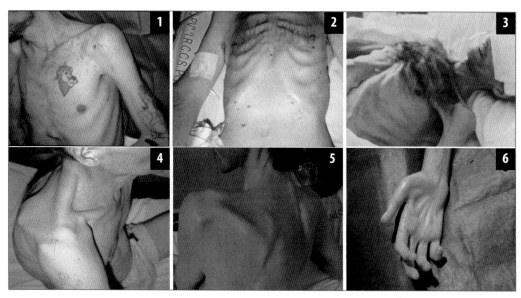

**Fig. 10.** Some clinical examples of AIDS related cachexia: **1, 2, 3** Three cases of massive loss of subcutanoeus fat and muscles in torax, arms, abdomen and prescalenic regions (*frontal view*). **4, 5** Patients having lost dorso-cervical muscular mass and fat, with evidence of scapular and clavicular bones (*lateral and dorsal view*). **6** Example of extreme cachexia with disappearance of tenar and ipotenar pads and hypotrophy of metacarpal muscles

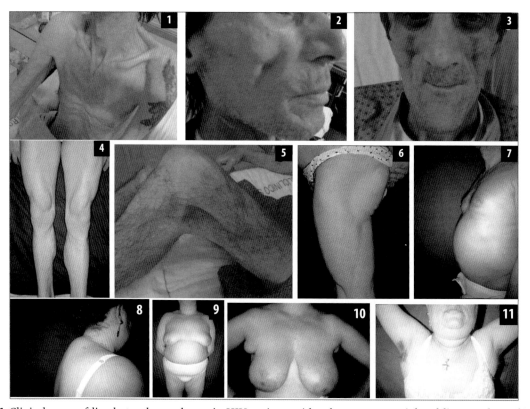

**Fig. 11.** Clinical cases of lipodystrophy syndrome in HIV patients with subcutaneous peripheral lipoatrophy and/or localised fat accumulation. **1** Patient with generalised peripheral lipoatrophy. **2, 3** Example of atrophy of fat pads of the face (Bichat pads loss). **4** Loss of subcutaneous fat and prominence of veins and muscles in the legs. **5** Atrophy of fat and muscles in the knee region. **6** Regional fat atrophy in the buttock region. **7** Increased abdominal fat in a patient with associated peripheral lipoatrophy. **8** Typical buffalo hump and increase of neck fat. **9** Enlargement of the breast due to accumulation of subcutaneous and mammary fat. **10, 11** Bilateral benign symmetric lipomatosis with enlargement of breast and bullneck

disturbed absorption of fatty acids through LPL inhibition [155]. All these alterations increase plasma triglycerides, resulting in central/visceral adiposity, insulin resistance leading to type II diabetes, and breast hypertrophy. We have been working on this hypothesis since our early studies on the mechanisms of cachexia, in which TNF was found to inhibit and progestin derivatives to stimulate LPL, the key enzyme of lipid metabolism [2, 156, 157].

### Effects of Nucleoside Reverse Transcriptase Inhibitors

The DNA polymerase hypothesis explains the mitochondrial toxicity of NRTIs as an effect of the inhibition of mtDNA polymerase-γ [121, 158, 159, 150]. Mitochondrial structure and function are altered and energy production impaired with intracellular lipid accumulation, hepatic steatosis, lactic acidosis, myopathy, pancreatitis, peripheral neuropathy, nephrotoxicity, and lipodystrophy.

In addition to HIV reverse transcriptase inhibition, NRTIs block many cellular polymerases and other enzymes in the following scale of potency: zalcitabine ≥ didanosine ≥ stavudine > lamivudine > zidovudine > abacavir. Stavudine treatment may induce lipodystrophy, thereby also reducing plasma levels of adiponectin [160, 161].

## Conclusions

Infectious diseases and drugs, with separate mechanisms, induce fat loss in people infected with HIV. The natural course of HIV infection finally leads to cachexia (slim disease). The combined actions of HIV, opportunistic infections, and HAART (including NRTIs, NNRTIs, and PIs) result in the redistribution of fat throughout the body (lipodystrophy), with simultaneous fat gain and fat loss in peripheral and central sites (lipohypertrophy and lipoatrophy). This clinical condition, therefore reflects the unstable balance between forces driving progression or resolution of the disease. For this reason, a study of regional and total body-fat modifications during the course of HIV infection must be included in any program of control and treatment of the disease.

## References

1. Torun B, Viteri FE (1988) Protein-energy malnutrition. In: Shils ME, Young VR (eds) Modern nutrition in health and disease, 7th edn. Lea & Febiger, Philadelphia, pp 746–773
2. Scevola D (1993) La cachessia nelle malattie infettive e neoplastiche. Edizioni Medico Scientifiche, Pavia
3. Watson RR (1994) Nutrition and AIDS. CRC Press, Boca Raton
4. Anonymous (1986) WHO: Working group on the use and interpretation of anthropometric indicators of nutritional status. Bull World Health Organ 64:929–941
5. Anonymous (1991) World population prospects 1990. United Nations, New York
6. Anonymous (1992) Health and health-related problems. WHO, Geneva
7. Anonymous (1992) Scope and dimension of nutrition problems. WHO, Geneva
8. Bruera E, Higginson I (1996) Cachexia–anorexia in cancer patients. Oxford University Press, Oxford
9. Center for the Disease Control (1987) CDC. Revision of the CDC surveillance case definition for acquired immunodeficiency syndrome. MMWR Morb Mortal Wkly Rep 36 (Suppl 1):3S–15S
10. Dworkin B, Wormser GP, Rosenthal WS et al (1985) Gastrointestinal manifestations of the acquired immunodeficiency syndrome: a review of 22 cases. Am J Gastr 8:774–778
11. Anonymous (1989) Malnutrition and weight loss in patients with AIDS. Nutr Rev 11:354–356
12. Anonymous (1989) HIV-associated enteropathy. Lancet 2:777–778
13. Scevola D (1989) Malattie infettive nel paziente neoplastico: aspetti clinici e terapeutici. Upjohn, Caponago, Milano
14. Scevola D, Barbarini G, Zambelli A et al (1989) Nutritional status in AIDS patients, 5th edn. Int Conf AIDS, Abs Book, Montreal, p 465
15. Scevola D, Zambelli A, Bottari G et al (1990) Problemi nutrizionali nella infezione-malattia da HIV. Alim Nutr Metab 11:159–170
16. Scevola D, Barbarini G, Zambelli A et al (1990) Evaluation and therapy of malnutrition in enteropathogenic AIDS, 6th edn. Int Conf AIDS, Abs Book, San Francisco, p 168
17. Scevola D, Zambelli A, Franchini A et al (1990) AIDS enteropatico: quadri endoscopici. Giorn Ital End Dig 13:93–103
18. Scevola D, Barbarini G, Bottari G et al (1990) Nutritional management of enteropathogenic

human immunodeficiency virus infection. Eur J Gastroent Hepat 2:S100–S101

19. Dworkin MS, Williamson JM (2003) Adult/Adolescent spectrum of HIV disease project. AIDS wasting syndrome: trends, influence on opportunistic infections, and survival. J Acquir Immune Defic Syndrome 33:267–273

20. Marquart KH, Muller HA, Sailer J, Moser R (1985) Slim disease (AIDS). Lancet 2:186–187

21. Serwadda D, Mugerwa RD, Sevankambo NK et al (1985) Slim disease: a new disease in Uganda and its association with HTLV-III infection. Lancet 2:849–852

22. Kotler DP, Tierney AR, Francisco A et al (1989) The magnitude of body cell mass depletion determines the timing of death from wasting in AIDS. Am J Clin Nutr 50:444–447

23. Chlebowski RT, Grosvenor MB, Bernhard NH et al (1989) Nutritional status, gastrointestinal dysfunction, and survival in patients with AIDS. Am J Gastroenterol 84:1288–1293

24. Kotler DP, Tierney AR, Dilmanian FA et al (1991) Correlation between total body potassium and total body nitrogen in patients with acquired immunodeficiency syndrome. Clin Res 39:649A

25. Scevola D, Barbarini G, Bottari G et al (1991) Prevalence, etiology and management of AIDS malnutrition, 7th edn. Int Conf AIDS, WB 2169, Florence

26. Kotler DP, Rosenbaum KB, Wang J et al (1998) Alterations in body fat distribution in HIV-infected men and women, 12th edn. World AIDS Conference, Geneva, Switzerland, June-July, Abs 32173

27. Kotler DP, Rosenbaum K, Wang J, Pierson R (1999) Studies of body composition and fat distribution in HIV-infected and control subjects. J Acquir Immune Defic Syndr Human Retrovirol 20:228–237

28. Gray GE, Gray LK (1980) Anthropometric measurements and their interpretations: principles, practice and problems. J Am Diet Assoc 77:534–539

29. Blackburn GC, Bistrian BR, Maini BS et al (1977) Nutritional and metabolic assessment of the hospital patient. J Parenter Enteral Nutr 31:11- 22

30. Clouse RE (1983) The role of body weight in nutritional evaluation. Clin Consult 3:1

31. O'Sullivan P, Linke RA, Dalton S (1985) Evaluation of body weight and nutritional status among AIDS patients. J Am Diet Ass 85:1483–1484

32. Brennan MF (1977) Uncomplicated starvation versus cancer cachexia. Cancer Res 37:2359–2364

33. Grunfeld C, Kotler D, Hamadeh R et al (1989) Hypertriglyceridemia in the acquired immunodeficiency syndrome. Am J Med 86:27–31

34. Grunfeld C, Kotler DP (1992) Wasting in the acquired immunodeficiency syndrome, seminars in liver disease. Thieme, New York

35. Douglas RG, Shaw JHF (1989) Metabolic response to sepsis and trauma. Br J Surg 76:115–122

36. Tisdale MJ (1991) Cancer cachexia. Br J Cancer 63:337–342

37. Beisel WR, Powanda MC (2003) Metabolic effects of infection on protein and energy status. J Nutr 133:3225–3275

38. Heymsfield SB, McManus C, Smith J et al (1982) Anthropometric measurement of muscle mass: revised equations for calculating bone-free arm musle area. Am J Clin Nutr 36:680–690

39. Anonymous (2004) WHO, 57th edn. World Health Assembly 22 May 2004 and Document A57/4

40. Scevola D, Bottari G, Faggi A et al (1994) Palliative care in infectious diseases. Eur J Pall Care 1:88–91

41. Scevola D, Bottari G, Oberto L, Faggi A (1996) AIDS cachexia: basics and treatment. In: Ruf B, Pohle HD, Goebel FD, L'age M (eds) HIV-Infektion, Pathogenese, Diagnostik und Therapie. Sociomedico Verlag, Graefelfing, pp 281–327

42. Scevola D, Bottari G, Oberto L et al (1996) Problemi nutrizionali del paziente AIDS e strategie terapeutiche. Quaderni di Cure Palliative (S1):51–64

43. Carrot Top Nutrition Resources (1988) Nutrition handbook for AIDS. Carrot Top Nutrition Resources, Aurora

44. Anonymous (1989) Task Force on Nutrition Support in AIDS. Guidelines for nutrition support in AIDS. Nutrition 5:39–46

45. Raiten DJ (1990) Nutrition and HIV infection. LSRO, FASEB, Bethesda

46. Anonymous (1994) ADA Reports. Position of the American Dietetic Association and the Canadian Dietetic Association: nutrition intervention in the care of persons with human immunodeficiency virus infection. J Am Diet Assoc 94:1042–1045

47. King AB (1990) Malnutrition in HIV infection: prevalence, etiology and management. PAAC Notes 2:122–159

48. Sharkey SJ, Sharkey KA, Sutherland LR et al (1992) Nutritional status and food intake in human immunodeficiency virus infection. J Acquir Immune Defic Syndrome 5:1091–1098

49. Scevola D, Grossi P, Zambelli A (1987) L'endoscopia nella diagnosi della patologia associata all'AIDS. In: Aiuti F, Moroni M, Pocchiari F (eds) AIDS e sindromi correlate. Monduzzi Editore, Bologna, pp 211–214

50. Scevola D (1992) La patologia anorettale nell'AIDS. In: Bianchi-Porro G, Parente F (eds) Le manifestazioni gastroenterologiche in corso di AIDS. Edizioni Libreria Cortina, Verona, pp 143–156

51. Scevola D, De Rysky C (1992) La patologia orofaringea nell'AIDS. In: Bianchi-Porro G, Parente F (eds), Le manifestazioni gastroenterologiche in corso di AIDS. Edizioni Libreria Cortina, Verona, pp 29–41

52. Scevola D (1994) Patologia d'organo. Apparato gastrointestinale. In: Dianzani F, Ippolito G, Moroni M (eds) Il libro italiano dell'AIDS. McGraw-Hill, Milano, pp 305–312

53. Scevola D (1998) Patologie del canale digerente, enterocoliti, e diarree infettive. In: Dianzani F, Ippolito G, Moroni M (eds). AIDS 1998. Il contributo italiano. Piccin Nuova Libraria, Padova, pp 345–354

54. Nahler BL, Chu SY, Nwanyanwu C et al (1993) HIV wasting syndrome in the United States. AIDS 7:183–188

55. Ullrich R, Zeitz M, Heise W et al (1989) Small intestinal structure and function in patients infected with human immunodeficiency virus (HIV): evidence for HIV-induced enteropathy. Ann Intern Med 111:15–21

56. Rondanelli EG (1989) AIDS: clinical and laboratory Atlas. EMP, Pavia

57. Gorbach SL, Knox TA, Roubenoff R (1993) Interactions between nutrition and infection with human immunodeficiency virus. Nutr Rev 8:226–234

58. Grunfeld C (1991) Mechanisms of wasting in infection and cancer: an approach to cachexia in AIDS. In: Kotler DP (ed) Gastrointestinal and nutritional manifestations of AIDS. Raven Press, New York, pp 207–229

59. Matsuyama T, Kobayashi N, Yamamoto N (1991) Cytokines and HIV infection: is AIDS a tumor necrosis factor disease? AIDS 5:1405–1417

60. Melchior JC, Salmon D, Rigaud D et al (1991) Resting energy expenditure is increased in stable, malnourished HIV-infected patients. Am J Clin Nutr 53:437–441

61. Bogden JD, Baker H, Frank O et al (1990) Micronutrient status and HIV infection. Ann NY Acad Sci 587:189–195

62. Coodley G (1990) Nutritional deficiency and AIDS. Ann Int Med 113:807

63. Coodley GO, Loveless MO, Nelson HD, Coodley MK (1994) Endocrine dysfunction in the HIV wasting syndrome. J Acquir Immune Defic Syndr 7:46–51

64. Timbo BB, Tollefson L (1994) Nutrition: a cofactor in HIV disease. J Am Diet Assoc 94:1019–1022

65. Baum MK, Shor-Posner G (1997) Nutritional status and survival in HIV-1 disease. AIDS 11:689–690

66. Scevola D, Bottari G, Zambelli A et al (1992) Trattamento dietetico ed ormonale dei deficit nutrizionali nell'AIDS. Clin Dietol 19:127–140

67. McMurray DN, Loomis SA, Casazza LJ et al (1981) Development of impaired cell-mediated immunity in mild and moderate malnutrition. Am J Clin Nutr 34:68–77

68. Bistrian BR, Blackburn GL, Scrimshaw NS, Fatt JP (1975) Cellular immunity in semistarved states in hospitalized adults. Am J Clin Nutr 28:1148–1155

69. Chandra RK (1988) Nutritional regulation of immunity. In: Chandra RK (ed) Nutrition and immunology. Alan R Liss, New York, pp 1–7

70. Moseson M, Zelenivnch-Jacquotte A, Belsito DV et al (1989) The potential role of nutritional factors in the induction of immunologic abnormalities in HIV-positive homosexual men. J Acquir Immune Defic Syndrome 2:235–247

71. Prasad C, Chandra RK (1991) Nutrition and immunity. In: Kotler DP (ed) Gastro intestinal and nutritional manifestations of AIDS. Raven Press, New York, pp 35–49

72. Heber D (1995) Pathophysiology of cancer/HIV malnutrition. In: Nutrition in cancer and HIV infection. Symp. N 8, 19th ed. Clinical Congress ASPEN, Miami Beach, Florida, pp 200–205

73. Grunfeld C, Pang M, Shimizu L et al (1992) Resting energy expenditure, caloric intake and short-term weight change in human immunodeficiency virus infection and the acquired immunodeficiency syndrome. Am J Clin Nutr 55:455–460

74. Hellerstein MK, Meydani SN, Meydani M et al (1989) Interleukin-1 induced anorexia in the rat. J Clin Invest 84:228–235

75. Hellerstein MK, Kahn J, Mudie H, Viteri F (1990) Current approach to the treatment of human immunodeficiency virus-associated weight loss: pathophysiologic considerations and emerging management strategies. Semin Oncol 17:17–33

76. Hoffman EP, Nader GA (2004) Balancing muscle hypertrophy and atrophy. Nat Med 6:584–585

77. Grunfeld C, Feingold KR (1992) Metabolic disturbances and wasting in the acquired immunodeficiency syndrome. N Engl J Med 5:329–337

78. Wolfe RR, Shaw JHF, Durkot MJ (1985) Effect of sepsis on VLDL kinetics: responses in basal state and during glucose infusion. Am Physiol 248:E732–E740

79. Tabibzadeh SS, Poubouridis D, May LT, Sehgal PB (1989) Interleukin-6 immunoreactivity in human tumors. Am J Pathol 135:427–433

80. Singer P, Katz DP, Dillon L et al (1992) Nutritional aspects of the acquired immunodeficiency syndrome. Am J Gastroenterol 87:265–273

81. Nerad JL, Gorbach SL (1994) Nutritional aspects of HIV infection. Infect Dis Clin North Am 8:499–515

82. Feingold KR, Soued M, Serio MK et al (1989) Multiple cytokines stimulate hepatic lipid synthesis in vivo. Endocrinology 125:267–274

83. Feingold KR, Adi S, Staprans I et al (1990) Diet affects the mechanisms by which TNF stimulates hepatic triglyceride production. Am J Physiol 259:E177–E184

84. Scevola D, Zambelli A, Bottari G et al (1991) Appetite stimulation and body weight gain with medroxyprogesterone acetate in AIDS anorexia and cachexia. Farmaci e Terapia 3:77–83

85. Beutler B, Cerami A (1986) Cachectin and tumor necrosis factor as two sides of the same biological coin. Nature 320:584–588

86. Beutler B, Cerami A (1986) Recombinant interleukin-1 suppresses lipoprotein lipase activity in 3T3- L1 cells. J Immunol 135:3969–3971

87. Mullen BJ, Harris RBS, Patton JS, Martin RJ (1990) Recombinant tumor necrosis factor-alfa chronically

administered in rats: lack of cachectic effect. Proc Soc Exp Biol Med 193:318–325

88. Feingold KR, Doerrler W, Dinarello CA et al (1992) Stimulation of lipolysis in cultured fat cells by TNF, IL-1 and the interferons is blocked by inhibition of prostaglandin synthesis. Endocrinology 130:10–16

89. Feingold KR, Soued M, Serio MK et al (1990) The effect of diet on tumor necrosis factor timulation of hepatic lipogenesis. Metabolism 39:623–632

90. Karmali RA, Chao CC, Basu A, Modak M (1989) Effect of n-3 and n-6 fatty acids on mammary H ras expression and PGE2 levels in DMBA-treated rats. Anticancer Res 9:1169–1174

91. Mora S, Pessin JE (2002) An adipocentric view of signaling and intracellular trafficking. Diabetes Metab Res Rev 18:345–356

92. Hotamisligil GS, Shargill NS, Spiegelman BM (1993) Adipose expression of tumor necrosis factor-alfa: direct role in obesity-linked insulin resistance. Science 259:87–91

93. Fried SK, Bunkin DA, Greenberg AS (1998) Omental and subcutaneous adipose tissues of obese subjects release interleukine-6: depot difference and regulation by glucocorticoid. J Clin Endocrinol Metab 83:847–850

94. Zhang Y, Proenca R, Maffei M et al (1994) Positional cloning of the mouse obese gene and its human homologue. Nature 372:425–432

95. Faggioni R, Feingold KR, Grunfeld C (2001) Leptin regulation of the immune response and the immunodeficiency of malnutrition. FASEB J 15:2565–2571

96. Yamauchi T, Kamon J, Waki TH et al (2001) The fat-derived hormone adiponectin reverses insulin resistance associated with both lipoatrophy and obesity. Nat Med 7:941–946

97. Tsao TS, Lodish HF, Fruebis J (2002) ACRP30, a new hormone controlling fat and glucose metabolism. Eur J Pharmacol 440:213–221

98. Ailhaud G, Grimaldi P, Nègrel R (1992) Cellular and molecular aspects of adipose tissue development. Ann Rev Nutr 12:207–233

99. Sugihara H, Yonemitsu N, Toda S et al (1988) Unilocular fat cells in three-dimensional collagen gel matrix culture. J Lipid Res 29:691–698

100. Ailhaud G, Amri EZ, Grimaldi P (1996) Fatty acids and expression of lipid-related genes in adipose cells. Proc Nutr Soc 55:151–154

101. Digito M, D'Incau F et al (1996) Release of mitogenic factors by cultured preadipocytes from patients with multiple symmetric lipomatosis. Intern J Obes Relat Metab Disord 20:38

102. Bjorntorp P (1996) The regulation of adipose tissue distribution in humans. Intern J Obes Relat Metab Disord 20:291–302

103. Bjorntorp P (1993) Visceral obesity: a 'Civilisation syndrome.' Obes Res 1:206–222

104. Xu X, De Pergola G, Bjorntorp P (1990) The effects of androgens on the regulation of lipolysis in adi-pose precursor cells. Endocrinology 126:1229–1234

105. Enzi G, Pavan M, Digito M et al (1993) Clustering of metabolic abnolmalities and other risk factors for cardiovascular disease in visceral obesity. Diab Nutr Metab 6:47–55

106. Cannon B, Jacobsson A, Rehnmark S, Nedergaard J (1996) Signal transduction in brown adipose tissue recruitment: noradrenaline and beyond. Intern J Obes Relat Metab Disord 3:S36–S42

107. Enzi G, Biondetti PR, Fiore D, Mazzoleni F (1982) Computed tomography of deep fat masses in multiple symmetric lipomatosis. Radiology 144:121–124

108. Enzi G, Favaretto L, Martini R et al (1983) Metabolic abnormalities in multiple symmetric lipomatosis. Elevated lipoprotein lipase activity in adipose tissue with hyperalfalipo- proteinemia. J Lipid Res 24:566–574

109. Enzi G (1984) Multiple symmetric lipomatosis: an update clinical report. Medicine 63:56–64

110. Zancanaro C, Sbarbati A, Morroni M et al (1990) Multiple symmetric lipomatosis. Ultrastructural investigation of the tissue and preadipocytes in primary culture. Lab Invest 63:253–258

111. Melchior JC, Niyongabo T, Henzel D et al (1999) Malnutrition and wasting, immunodepression, and chronic inflammation as independent predictors of survival in HIV-infected patients. Nutrition 15:865–869

112. Wheeler DA, Gibert CL, Launer CA et al (1998) Weight loss as a predictor of survival and disease progression in HIV infection. Terry Beirn Community programs for Clinical Research on AIDS. J Acquir Immune Defic Syndr Hum Retrovirol 18:80–85

113. Smit E, Skolasky RL, Dobs AS et al (2002) Changes in the incidence and predictors of wasting syndrome related to human immunodeficiency virus infection, 1987–1999. Am J Epidemiol 156:211–218

114. Wanke CA, Silva M, Knox TA et al (2000) Weight loss and wasting remain common complications in individuals infected with human immunodeficiency virus in the era of highly active antiretroviral therapy. Clin Infect Dis 31:803–805

115. Wanke CA, Silva M, Ganda A et al (2003) Role of acquired immune deficiency syndrome - defining conditions in human immunodeficiency virus-associated wasting. Clin Infect Dis 37 (Suppl 2):S81–S84

116. Carr A, Samaras K, Burton S et al (1998) A syndrome of peripheral lipodystrophy, hyperlipidaemia and insulin resistance in patients receiving HIV protease inhibitors. AIDS 12:F51–F58

117. Carr A, Samaras K, Chisholm DJ, Cooper DA (1998) Pathogenesis of HIV-1-protease inhibitor-associated peripheral liopdystrophy, hyperlipidemia, and insulin resistance. Lancet 352:1881–1883

118. Lo JC, Mulligan K, Tai VW et al (1998) 'Buffalo hump' in men with HIV-infection. Lancet 351:867–870

119. Carr A, Samaras K, Thorisdottir A et al (1999) Diagnosis, prediction, and natural course of HIV-1 protease-inhibitor-associated lipodystrophy, hyperlipidaemia, and diabetes mellitus; a cohort study. Lancet 353:2093–2099

120. Carr A, Miller J, Law M, Cooper DA (2000) A syndrome of lipoatrophy, lactic acidaemia and live dysfunction associated with HIV nucleoside analogue therapy: contribution to protease inhibitor-related lipodystrophy syndrome. AIDS 14:F25–F32

121. Chen D, Misra A, Garg A (2002) Lipodystrophy in human immunodeficiency virus-infected patients. J Clin Endocrinol Metab 87:4845–4856

122. Bernasconi E (1999) Metabolic effects of protease inhibitor therapy. AIDS Read 9:254–269

123. Bernasconi E, Boubaker K, Junghans C et al (2002) Abnormalities of body fat distribution in HIV-infected persons treated with antiretroviral drugs. J Acquir Immune Defic Syndrome 31:50–55

124. Galli M, Cozzi-Lepri A, Ridolfo AL et al (2002) Incidence of adipose tissue alterations in first-line antiretroviral therapy. Arch Intern Med 162:2621–2628

125. Salomon J, de Truchis P, Melchior JC (2002) Body composition and nutritional parameters in HIV and AIDS patients. Clin Chem Lab Med 40:1329–1333

126. Jain RG, Furfine ES, Pedneault et al (2001) Metabolic complications associated with antiretroviral therapy. Antiviral Res 51:151–177

127. Dubè MP, Sattler FR (1998) Metabolic complications of antiretroviral therapies. AIDS Clin Care 10:41–44

128. Miller KD, Jones E, Yanovski JA et al (1998) Visceral abdominal-fat accumulation associated with use of indinavir. Lancet 351:871–875

129. Rosenberg HE, Mulder J, Sepkowitz K et al (1998) 'Protease-paunch' in HIV+ persons receiving protease inhibitor therapy: incidence, risks and endocrinologic evaluation, 5th ed. Conference on Retroviruses and Opportunistic Infections, Chicago, February 1998, Abstract 408

130. Sullivan AK, Nelson MR (1997) Marked hyperlipidaemia on ritonavir. AIDS 11:938–939

131. Hengel RL, Watts NB, Lennox JL (1997) Benign symmetric lipomatosis associated with protease inhibitors. Lancet 350:1596

132. Carr A, Emery S, Law M et al (2003) An objective case definition of lipodystrophy in HIV- infected adults: a case-control study. Lancet 361:726–735

133. Carr A, Law M (2003) An objective lipodystrophy severity grading scale derived from lipodystropy case definition score. J Acquir Immune Defic Syndr 33:571–576

134. Tien PC, Grunfeld C (2004) What is HIV-associated lipodystrophy? Defining fat distribution changes in HIV infection. Curr Opin Infect Dis 17:27–32

135. European Paediatric Lipodystrophy Group (2004) Antiretroviral therapy, fat redistribution and hyperlipidaemia in HIV-infected children in Europe. AIDS 18:1443–1451

136. Durnin JV, Womersley J (1974) Body fat assessed from total body density and its estimation from skinfold thickness: measurements on 481 men and women aged from 16 to 72 years. Br J Nutr 37:77–97

137. Scevola D, Marinelli M (1991) Dietetica medica. Edizioni Medico Scientifiche, Pavia

138. Boulier A, Fricker J, Thomasset AL et al (1990) Fat-free mass estimation by the two-electrode impedance method. Am J Clin Nutr 52:581–585

139. Ott M, Fischer H, Polat H et al (1995) Bioelectrical impedance analysis as a predictor of survival in patients with human immunodeficiency virus infection. J Acquir Immune Defic Syndr Hum Retrovirol 9:20–25

140. Mallon P, Miller J, Cooper D, Carr A (2003) Prospective evaluation of the effects of antiretroviral therapy on body composition in HIV-1 infected men starting therapy. AIDS 17:971–979

141. Nolan D, Hammond E, James I et al (2003) Contribution of nucleoside-analogue reverse transcriptase inhibitor therapy to lipoatrophy from the population to the cellular level. Antivir Ther 8:617–626

142. Engelson ES, Kotler DP, Tan YX et al (1999) Fat distribution in HIV-infected patients reporting truncal enlargement quantified by whole-body magnetic resonance imaging. Am J Clin Nutr 69:1162–1169

143. Saag M, Tien P, Gripshover B et al (2003) Body composition in HIV infected men with and without peripheral lipoatrophy is different than controls. In: Conference on retroviruses and opportunistic infections, 10th ed. CCO, Boston, p 320

144. Enzi G, Gasparo M, Biondetti PR et al (1986) Subcutaneous and visceral fat distribution accordino to sex, age, and overweight, evaluated by computer tomography. Am J Clin Nutr 44:739–746

145. Saint-Marc T, Partisani M, Poizot-Martin I et al (2000) Fat distribution evaluated by computed tomography and metabolic abnormalities in patients undergoing antiretroviral therapy: preliminary results of the LIPOCO study. AIDS 14:37–49

146. Martinez E, Bianchi L, Garcia-Viejo MA et al (2000) Sonographic assessment of regional fat in HIV-1-infected people. Lancet 356:1412–1413

147. Behrens GMN, Stoll M, Schmidt RE (2000) Lipodystrophy syndrome in HIV infection. Drug Saf 1:57–76

148. Garg A (2004) Acquired and inherited lipodystrophies. N Engl J Med 350:1220–1234

149. Gervasoni C, Ridolfo AL, Trifirò G et al (1999) Redistribution of body fat in HIV-infected women undergoing combined antiretroviral therapy. AIDS 13:465–471

150. Kakuda TN (2000) Pharmacology of nucleoside and nucleotide reverse transcriptase inhibitor-induced mitochondrial toxicity. Clin Ther 22:685–708

151. Boyle BA (1999) Lipodystrophy: a new phenome-

neon? AIDS Reader 9:15–17

152. Nolan D, John M, Mallal S (2001) Antiretroviral therapy and the lipodystrophy syndrome. Part 2: Concepts in aetiopathogenesis. Antivir Ther 6:145–160

153. Bastard JP, Caron M, Vidal H et al (2002) Association between altered expression of adipogenic factor SREBP-1 in lipoatrophic adipose tissue from HIV-1-infected patients and abnormal adipocyte differentiation and insulin resistance. Lancet 359:1026–1031

154. Ranganathan S, Kern PA (2002) The HIV protease inhibitor saquinavir impairs lipid metabolism and glucose transport in cultured adipocytes. J Endocrinol 172:155–162

155. Baril L, Idhammou A, Beucler I et al (1999) Are the decreased lipolytic enzyme activities responsible for the hypertriglyceridemia in PI-treated patients. 6th Conference on retroviruses and opportunistic infections, Chicago, III/1999, Abs 664

156. Solerte SB, Rondanelli M, Fioravanti M et al (1995) Impaired regulation of GH-IGF-1-IGFBP3 axis and ACTH-adrenal function in AIDS patients (CDC IVC) with wasting syndrome. A possible defensive mechanism. J Endocrinol Invest 18:43

157. Scevola D, Oberto L, Bottari G, Faggi A (1995) Lipidi e malattie infettive. Abs Book XII Congresso Nazionale ADI, Torino 16–18/11/1995, p 187

158. Lewis W, Dalakas MC (1995) Mitochondrial toxicity of antiviral drugs. Nat Med 1:417–422

159. Brinkman K, Smeitink JA, Reiss P (1999) Mitochondria toxicity induced by nucleoside-analogue reverse-transcriptase inhibitors is a key factor in the pathogenesis of antiretroviral-therapy-related lipodystrophy. Lancet 354:1112–1115

160. Mynarcik DC, Combs T, McNurlan MA et al (2002) Adiponectin and leptin levels in HIV-infected subjects with insulin resistance and body fat redistribution. J Acquir Immune Defic Syndr 31:514–520

161. Lindegaard B, Keller P, Bruunsgaard H et al (2004) Low plasma level of adiponectin is associated with stavudine treatment and lipodystrophy in HIV-infected patients. Clin Exp Immunol 135:273–279

# Treatment of AIDS Anorexia-Cachexia Syndrome and Lipodystrophy

Daniele Scevola, Omar Giglio, Silvia Scevola

## Introduction

Anorexia-cachexia syndrome [1] and lipodystrophy [2–6] are two conditions frequently associated with the course of HIV infection. Under many circumstances, they can be included as components of a single disease, multifactorial in origin, leading to alterations of energetic metabolism and to body fat tissue modifications. The risk for the clinician is of only partially considering the two diseases, for which, until recently, a true definition [3] was lacking. The approach to therapy, due to the multifactorial origin, must be multidisciplinary, involving experts in nutrition, infectious diseases, physiology, gastroenterology, etc.

*Anorexia-cachexia syndrome* is a condition also associated with cancer [1] and chronic infections, such as tuberculosis. It is characterised clinically by the loss of appetite and body weight, and biochemically by a series of metabolic abnormalities, e.g. elevation of blood levels of triglycerides (TGs) and very-low-density lipoproteins (VLDL), and a reduction of cholesterol. Cachexia associated with hypertriglyceridaemia is an intriguing medical problem because usually an excess of caloric intake and obesity are the main causes of elevated TG levels. Hypothyroidism, alcohol excess, oestrogen, β-blockers, thiazide therapy, lipoprotein lipase deficiency, diabetes, renal diseases, and genetic disorders are the other causes of hypertriglyceridaemia. In AIDS cachexia, by contrast , caloric and fat intake are reduced, and hypertriglyceridaemia is associated with low cholesterol levels, suggesting different causative mechanisms. Firstly a strong positive relationship exists between hypertriglyceridaemia and tumour necrosis factor (TNF) levels [7]. Since TNF inhibits lipoprotein lipase, TGs are not utilised for energy production or liposynthesis and their level therefore increases in the blood.

Secondly lethargy, another cause of decreased cholesterol and increased plasma TGs, is frequent in AIDS patients.

Malnutrition, in all its forms, but mainly protein-energy malnutrition (PEM), was and remains one of the most common and striking phenomena of AIDS [8–11]. Many factors contribute to PEM, such as anorexia, nausea, dysgeusia, dysphagia, poor alimentary choices, digestive and assimilation disorders, opportunistic infections, direct cytopathic effect of HIV on intestinal cells [12], cytokines [13, 14], drugs and neoplasias, and each of them can cause progressive weight loss. Since 1987 [15], 'slim disease,' or 'wasting syndrome,' has been included in the list of illnesses indicative of AIDS. Wasting syndrome is a common indicative condition of AIDS in many countries [16, 17]; nonetheless, its predominance is probably underestimated because, when associated with an opportunistic disease, the latter is usually reported [18]. A number of studies [8, 19–26] have shown that significant weight loss, measured with respect to the normal or ideal weight or to reference percentiles used for the normal population, is found in 59–84% of HIV-positive subjects, and in many of them it is considerable (30% and over). The intense anorexia and progressive weight loss have a dramatic psychological impact on patients and their families, causing a decline in the quality of life, an increased susceptibility to infections, and intolerance of many drugs [8, 27]. Body temperature and basal metabolism decrease, but remain elevated compared to normal subjects with normal caloric intake [28]. Skin, musculoskeletal system, gastrointestinal, hepatic, and respiratory functions [29] are compromised. Neurological signs may appear. In addition, malnutrition reduces the amounts of nonspecific factors conferring resistance to pathogenic agents, as well as the activity of the bone marrow, lymphatic tissues, and the reticular-endothelial system. Other, more subtle disorders involve haematological functions, including the development of anaemia, hypoalbuminaemia, and a reduction in the plasma levels of vitamins B6, B12, folic acid, selenium, zinc, copper, calcium and potassium [30–33]. Body weight decreases progressively as the malnutrition worsens being correlated with a more unfavourable prognosis. Thus, cachexia becomes an illness within an illness, a possible co-factor in the evolution from simple HIV carriage to full blown AIDS, and it should be studied and treated specifically in each patient [34–48]. More recently in Western countries, as a consequence of the introduction of highly active antiretroviral therapy (HAART), the wasting/cachexia syndrome as depicted above has changed into another syndrome, characterised [2, 3, 49] by fat redistribution, insulin resistance, and atherogenic dyslipidaemia. Fat redistribution changes, defined as lipoatrophy (loss of subcutaneous adipose tissue, SAT) and central fat (visceral adipose tissue, VAT) accumulation or lipomatosis, have been reported in HIV patients taking protease inhibitors (PIs), nucleoside analogue reverse-transcriptase inhibitors (NRI), or both [2, 49]. These body fat changes and metabolic disturbances have been termed *lipodystrophy* [2–5, 49], which since the introduction of HAART is encountered more frequently than the previous wasting, wasting syndrome, or cachexia. There are many differences between these conditions. In wasting syndrome, weight loss is prevalent and includes both fat mass and free fat mass, especially muscle mass. In lipodystrophy, malnutrition signs are absent, muscle mass is preserved, and peripheral fat loss is associated with increased central fat. The numerous methods to assess lipodystrophy explain the large variability in the reported prevalence, ranging from 20 to 80% [2, 6, 49, 50]. Since 2003, a definition of lipodystrophy has been in use that takes into consideration age, gender, stage and duration of HIV infection, waist to hip ratio, trunk to peripheral fat ratio, percent leg fat, intra-abdominal to extra-abdominal fat ratio, anion gap, serum HDL cholesterol concentration. This approach results in a sensitivity of 79% and a specificity of 80% [3]. Direct measures of fat,

including anthropometry, CT scan, DEXA and MRI, must be used to assess the prevalence and incidence of lipodystrophy in order to define the best mode of treatment and its efficacy. HAART has decreased by two-thirds [8] the lethality of AIDS and opportunistic infections, but patients receiving HAART suffer from several lipid abnormalities [9, 12–17, 19–24] that increase cardiovascular morbidity, compromising the quality of life and efficacy of the therapy. In conclusion, AIDS is changing from a 'slim disease' to a 'lipodystrophic disease' as a consequence of prolonged survival and direct effect of HAART. Fat metabolism disturbances increase by two- to three-fold the risk of cardiovascular disease in HIV patients. New strategies addressed at preventing and managing these emerging disorders of fat metabolism and redistribution [25, 26] are therefore urgently needed.

## Therapy of Cachexia

The energetic basis of wasting in HIV infection may help to explain the pathogenesis of AIDS cachexia and the elements of therapy. Energy balance results from calories introduced and calories expended or not absorbed: resting energy expenditure (REE) is reduced accordingly during weight-loss episodes, but the reduction in energy intake exceeds that of REE because of anorexia and other GI symptoms (Fig. 1).

The parameters most frequently used at the start of nutritional therapy are: weight loss > 10%; albumin value < 3.5 g/dl; reduction of transferrin, creatinine/weight index, vitamins, and microelements; and changes in other indicative indices of nutrition (see Chp. 3.4).

Treatment of identified and reversible causes of body weight loss is essential for the maintenance and/or repletion of weight, but only a combined nutritional-pharmacological approach increasing energy and protein intake can successfully reverse the anorexia-cachexia syndrome of AIDS. In addition, treatment of the malnutrition is a primary medical objective, along with specific therapies aimed at the basic pathology [51]. Among the palliative treatments, besides pain relief, treatment of malnutrition and weight loss perhaps represents

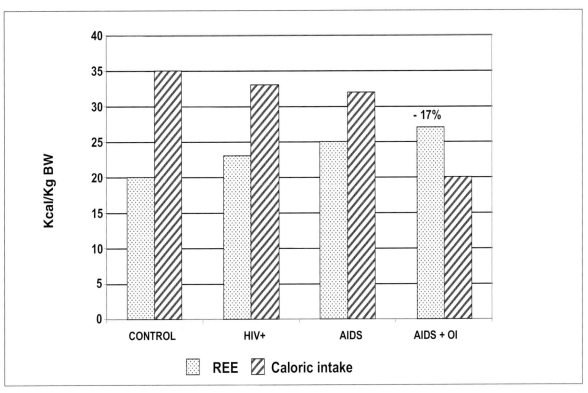

**Fig. 1.** Resting energy expenditure (REE) and caloric intake in HIV infection. REE increases according to disease progression, while caloric intake becomes insufficient (-17%) to maintain basal needs. *OI*, opportunistic infections; *BW*, body weight. (Modified from [52, 53])

the most gratifying therapeutic aspect for the patient, giving him or her a tangible feeling of improvement – as anthropometric, biochemical and immunological nutritional parameters normalise – that is immediately visible in the mirror, on the weight scale, and in response to improved physical capabilities [26].

The therapy of cachexia is primarily based on a correct administration of nutrients and drugs. When the first signs of malnutrition appear, prompt nutritional treatment, based on the prescription of a balanced diet containing adequate proteic-caloric, vitamin, and mineral quantities, is highly advisable [54]. As long as the patient is autonomous, the doctor's task is to prescribe a diet that covers the caloric-proteic requirement with respect to ideal weight, basal metabolism, and physical activity, and which attempts to compensate for previous losses. The number of calories that must be supplied can be calculated using the Harris-Benedict formula [55] (Table 1).

**Table 1.** The Harris-Benedict equation for calculating the number of supplemental calories needed to treat weight loss due to different conditions

Male: $66 + (13.7 \times W) + (5 \times H) - (6.8 \times A)$
Female: $655 + (9.6 \times W) + (1.7 \times H) - (4.7 \times A)$

**Adjunctive calories for different pathologies**

| | |
|---|---|
| Surgical operation | + 5% |
| Trauma | +10–15% |
| Complicated trauma | +20–50% |
| Peritonitis | +15–20% |
| Minor infections | + 5–20% |
| Severe infections | +40–60% |

$W$, actual weight (kg); $H$, height (cm); $A$, age (years)

Hypercaloric-hyperproteic diets represent the simplest way to increase body weight. Nevertheless, the patient must be able to take in and assimilate a sufficient quantity of nutrients. This is not always possible by natural ways, and in many cases, the patient will require enteral and/or parenteral nutrition, both in hospital and at home [24, 54, 56]. By means of special formulations, this type of nutrition can guarantee the necessary supply of energy, nutrients, vitamins, mineral salts, and enzymes, and thereby normalise the catabolic pathways of metabolism.

## Carbohydrates

Bearing in mind that dextrose infusion inhibits protein breakdown, the administration of 150–200 g of dextrose (e.g. 3 l at 5%) reduces the urinary loss of nitrogen by half. Hepatic neoglycogenesis is blocked, but not oxidative deamination. At least 600 g of dextrose are necessary to block the latter and to reduce the urinary loss of nitrogen to 25%. In order to maintain glycaemia < 150 g/dl, insulin administration must be associated with the insulin clamp technique (8-fold the baseline value).

## Protein

In order to block protein loss, it is necessary to administrate amino acids in quantities of 1.5–2 g/kg/day, as well as a sufficient amount (< 0.7 g/kg) of essential amino acids. Selective mixtures of branched-chain amino acids are useful in treating patients with associated liver diseases and a tendency to encephalopathy.

The administration of nutritional supplements reduces the length of hospitalisation and rehabilitation, as well as the mortality rate. Early and aggressive nutritional treatment improves the prognosis of various pathological conditions [57].

## Lipids

Lipid administration has little influence on nitrogen loss if it is not supplemented with glucose and proteins. Lipids must be prescribed to avoid deficits in essential fatty acids. New, energetic substrates, such as polyunsaturated omega-3 fatty acids (PUFAs), ornithine-ketoglutarate acid (OKGA), medium-chain triglycerides (MCT), short-chain fatty acids (SCFAs), and glutamine are suggested in order to modulate the different stages of cachexia (Fig. 2).

Hypocholesterolaemia and hypertriglyceridaemia are frequently observed in wasting syndrome and are associated with a poor prognosis. Derangement of serum lipids and a reduction of body fat deposits are consequences of impaired food intake and reflect a series of metabolic disturbances, mainly due to alterations in TNF, interleukin (IL)-1, IL-2, IL-6, interferons (IFNs), and other cytokines.

A reduced supply of n-6 PUFAs and an increased supply of omega-3 fatty acids (ω-3FAs) may reduce the inflammatory cascade of cytokine production. This effect seems to be due to eicosapentaenoic acid (EPA), C20:5, n-3 and docosahexaenoic acid (DHA), C22:6, n-3, the main component of fish oil that decreases plasma triglycerides and VLDL while increases levels of LDL-cholesterol. In contrast to other fatty acids of the n-3 and n-6 series, EPA is a direct suppressant of lipid mobilisation factor in both in vitro and in vivo studies; it also counteracts weight loss, lipolysis, and protein catabolism as well as tumour growth [58].

Plasma levels of ω-3FAs are inversely associated with the risk of coronary heart disease (CHD), blood pressure, renal $PGE_2$ production, as well as IL-1, IL-2, IL-6, and TNF production by mononuclear cells. Fish oil also protects the liver from reperfusion injury by reducing the synthesis of vasoconstrictive eicosanoids (from arachidonic acid). Weight gain has been reported in rats fed with fish oil.

Since ω-3FAs are precursors for eicosanoids and any increase in the amount of n-3 family compounds in the diet produces some biological effects, with clinical implications in anorexia-cachexia syndrome, we studied [59] the effect of 10 g of fish-oil ω-3FAs/day in AIDS patients who lost > 10% of their usual weight and who had elevated TGs and TNF, and hypocholesterolaemia. The study was a pilot, unblinded, randomised comparison between a dietary regimen containing 10 g of fish oil daily for 30 days and an equivalent dietary regimen without fish oil.

The study included 20 cachectic AIDS patients (stage IV C) who had lost > 10% of their usual weight in the 3 months prior to the beginning of the

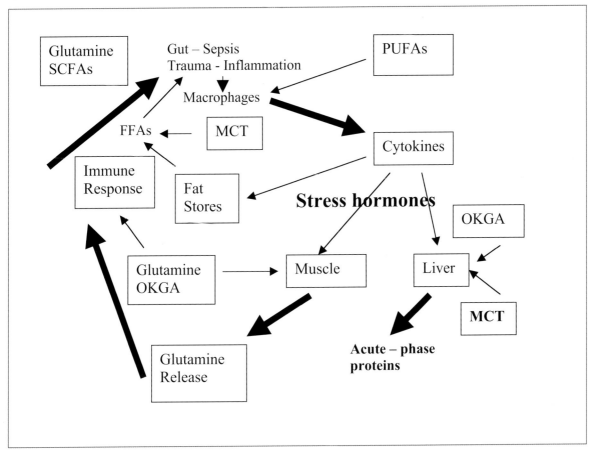

**Fig. 2.** New substrates in the therapy of cachexia. *PUFA*, poly-unsaturated fatty acid; *OKGA*, ornithine ketoglutaric acid; *FFA*, free fatty acid; *SCFA*, short-chain fatty acid; *MCT*, medium-chain triglyceride

study and who had hypertriglyceridaemia, hypocholesterolaemia, and elevated plasma TNF levels. The subjects (12 men and 8 women, age 30–37 years, mean 33.6 years) were weighed, measured (body circumferences and skinfold thickness) and randomly allocated to receive a personalised hypercaloric-hyperproteic diet with or without fish oil.

All patients were under antiretroviral treatment and secondary prophylaxis for opportunistic infections (6 for MACD, 3 for neurotoxoplasmosis, 5 for PCP, 3 for CMV, 3 for candida). Patients with intractable diarrhoea, acute opportunistic infections, and/or a Karnofsky score < 50 were excluded. The caloric needs were calculated for each patient according to a modified Harris-Benedict equation, and extra calories were prescribed in relation to the patient's clinical condition. Caloric

intakes was registered by means of a dietary questionnaire. TNF levels, anthropometric parameters, and clinical and laboratory data were determined at baseline and after 30 days.

One gram fish oil pills containing 18% EPA and 12% DHA as their ethyl esters, with 3 mg vitamin E per gram as antioxidant were provided by Novartis, Italy.

In our patients FO reduced the high levels of TNF, which allowed utilisation of TGs for liposynthesis and thus as energy for physical activity. It may well be that the entire cytokine network, the dysregulation of which may be involved in AIDS progression, responds to FO administration.

PUFAs serve as substrates within inflammatory cells for the formation of eicosanoid mediators. Eicosanoids derived from 20:omega-3 PUFAs (EPA,

DHA) are less proinflammatory and vasoactive than those derived from arachidonic acid (20:4 omega-6) and linoleic acid (18:2 omega-6) via the cyclooxygenase and lipooxygenase pathways.

Dietary FO inhibits δ-6-desaturase and cyclooxygenase, thereby reducing the metabolism of linoleic and arachidonic acid and the production of their derivatives eicosanoids, $PGE_2$, $TXA_2$, and $TXB_2$. The addition to FO of vitamin E as antioxidant may be beneficial, because vitamin E supplementation per se reduces TNF and IL-6, which are well-known enhancers of HIV replication in macrophages/monocytes.

The clinical conditions of the subjects in the two groups were comparable at entry but, at the end, only those who received fish oil showed statistically significant improvements in the studied parameters. The mean weight gain was 2.4 kg; lean and fatty body masses, respectively, increased 1.4 and 0.67 kg; TGs decreased from 230 to 149 mg/dl; and cholesterol increased from 169 to 200 mg/dl. TNF levels decreased from 360 to 88 pg/ml. Caloric intake went from < 1550 Kcal/day to > 2200 Kcal/day.

The subset of AIDS patients affected by wasting syndrome with high levels of triglycerides and TNF and low cholesterol may benefit from a diet supplemented with adequate amounts of fish oil containing n-3 PUFA, which decrease the production of inflammatory cytokines and of futile metabolic cycles.

## Medium-Chain Triglycerides

In MAC-16 tumours, an anti-cachectic effect can be obtained, together with a reduction of tumour mass, by administration of amount of MCT > 80% of the required energy [58, 60]. Cachexia and tumour growth rate [61] can be reduced by replacing a portion of dietary carbohydrates with lipid derivatives of fish oil at 50% of the total calories in the animal diet. Even those neoplastic patients with a weight loss > 32%, can recover their weight with isocaloric diets in which energy is supplied by MCT at 70% [62].

In conclusion, while enteral and/or parenteral nutritional therapy is effective in the short-term, there are long-term disadvantages regarding practicality and cost. Hyperproteic-hypercaloric diets administered by the natural oral alimentary route compensate for weight losses and maintain weight gains. Moreover, such diets can be designed according to the metabolic requirements of the individual patient and supplemented with food concentrates, mineral salts, and vitamins. Malnourished patients under such diets autonomously and rapidly regain close to their ideal body weight. Unfortunately, nutritional therapy programs with the addition of special nourishment and oral supplements are not – or are only partially – paid for by national health services.

## Drugs

It is important that every underweight patient at risk for malnutrition undergoes intense nutritional support in order to improve the prognosis of the underlying disease as well as the quality of life. The patient's ability to maintain his or her weight at close to ideal or normal levels may be aided by the prescription of appetite-stimulating drugs (Table 2), such as cyproheptadine [63, 64], medroxyprogesterone acetate (MPA) [65, 66], megestrol acetate (MA) [67–69], insulin-like growth factor-1 (IGF-1) [70], corticosteroids, and growth hormone [71, 72].

### Medroxyprogesterone Acetate and Megestrol Acetate: Clinical Experiences

The progestin derivatives MPA and MA have been widely used in the treatment of cancer cachexia, which shows clinical features and, probably, pathological mechanisms similar to those of AIDS wasting syndrome [73, 74]. In anorectic and cachectic AIDS patients, MPA and MA have proved to be particularly effective [65–69, 75–80].

### Medroxyprogesterone Acetate

In two clinical studies [22, 66], we used MPA(1 g/day, os) and a hypercaloric diet to correct anorexia and cachexia occurring in HIV-infected patients. In the first study [22], MAP was administered to 74 AIDS patients. The control group of 96

**Table 2.** Drugs for the treatment of cachexia

*Hormones*
  Insulin, insulin-like growth factor-1
  Growth hormone
  Steroids: nandrolone decanoate, oxandrolone, dexamethasone, prednisone, metilprednisolone, progestin derivatives (medroxyprogesterone acetate, megestrol acetate)

*Anti-cytokines*
  Hydralazine sulfate (reduces PEP-carboxykinase)
  Pentoxyfylline (increases cAMP)
  Amrinone (reduces phosphodiesterase)
  Dobutamine (β-agonist; increases cAMP)
  Thalidomide (reduces TNF)
  FANS(indomethacin, ibuprofen, aspirin; reduce cytokines synthesis)
  Antibodies against TNF, LPS, IL-1, etc. (reduce cytokine effects)

*Anti-serotonin*
  Cyproheptadine (reduces serotonin)

malnourished but not anorectic patients received only the hypercaloric diet. In all patients, nutritional status and body composition were evaluated. By means of traditional anthropometry, and a monopolar bioelectrical impedance analyser, we determined at baseline, weekly for the first month and fortnightly thereafter: actual (W) and ideal (IBW) body weight; body surface area (S); body mass index (BMI); midarm (MAC) and midarm muscle circumference (MAMC); arm muscle area (AMA); triceps (TSF), biceps (BSF), subscapular (SSF), and iliac (ISF) skinfold thickness; lean(LBM) and fat (FBM) body mass; total body water (TBW), and body impedance (BIA). Basal energy expenditure (BEE) for each patient was calculated with an adapted Harris-Benedict formula. Food intake (Kcal/day), appetite(scale: 0 = very poor to 3 = very good), sense of well-being (Karnofsky scale), muscle power and endurance (Cyclette); and routine clinical and laboratory data. TNF levels were measured before and after MPA treatment. Any specific and necessary therapy was prescribed. At the end of the study, there were 50 patients (67.6%) in the MPA group and 80 (83.3%) in the diet-only group. At the beginning of the study, median weight loss was 11.3 kg (= at

least 10% of IBW) in the first group and 5.1 kg (= at least 10 % of baseline weight) in the second. In a mean time of 52.3 days, MPA-treated patients had increased caloric intake (+1322 kcal), W (+6.2 kg), %IBW (+9.2), increases in four skinfold thicknesses (+10.8 mm) [TSF (+3 mm), BSF (+1 mm), SSF (+2.7 mm), ISF(+4.1 mm)], MAC (+2.1 cm), MAMC (+1.1 cm), AMA (+4.1 cm$^2$), S (+0.9 m$^2$), BMI (+2.1), LBM (+2.6 kg), FBM (+3.6 kg), % body fat (+5), %TBW (+0.1)]. Patients treated only with diet had increased daily caloric intake (+900 kcal), gaining W (+2.4 kg), increases in four skinfold thicknesses (+5.8 mm) [TSF (+1.1 mm), BSF (+1.4 mm), SSF (+1.2 mm), ISF (+2.1 mm), MAC (+0.7 cm), MAMC (+0.3 cm), AMA (+1.1 cm$^2$), S(+0.02 m$^2$), BMI (+0.51), LBM (+0.9 kg), FBM (+1.1 kg), % body fat (+0.7), % TBW(+0.6), in a mean time of 100.1 days. Thus, 93% of patients responded to MPA and 73% to diet. Weight gain in MPA patients was significantly greater and obtained more quickly than in diet patients; it was also prevalently associated with increases in fat and lean tissue. TBW remained constant during treatment, as confirmed by anthropometry and a mild reduction of BIA (-31.3 ohm), compared with the value of the patient's diet (-13.5 ohm). Appetite, muscle power and endurance, and sense of well-being significantly improved in the MPA group. No adverse changes in routine haematological or biochemical profiles attributable to MPA were reported. We also were able to demonstrate a reduction of high initial levels (> 100 pg/ml) of TNF-α after MPA treatment. In conclusion, our experience provides evidence that MPA improves appetite, nutritional status, and quality of life in AIDS anorectic and cachectic patients, counteracting disturbances of fat and protein metabolism induced by high levels of cytokines produced during chronic infection.

In another study [66], 151 subjects, 74 in the placebo and 77 in the MPA group, were enrolled at ten teaching and general Departments of Infectious Diseases to evaluate the efficacy of MPA (flavoured granules formulation 1 g/day) in promoting weight gain in AIDS cachectic patients. The study was a 12-week randomised, double blind, placebo-controlled, multicentre clinical study. The eligibility excluded pregnancy, steroid contraindications, renal and liver diseases, and intractable diarrhoea. The 151 patients (109 men and 42 women), who ranged in age from 22 to 61 years (mean 33.6 ± 7.4) and had lost ≥ 10% of their usual body weight, were randomly assigned to orally receive either 1 g MPA or placebo once daily for 12 weeks. Baseline and monthly, appetite, caloric intake, body weight, body composition, and quality of life (Karnofsky scale) were assessed.

Adequate nutritional support was personalised for each patient according to a Harris-Benedict modified equation.

Of the 77 patients receiving MPA and of the 74 placebo recipients 52 and 49, respectively, could be evaluated at the end of the study.

Most patients receiving MPA had increased caloric intake, resulting in a mean weight gain of 5.5 kg, compared with 1.9 kg for the placebo group ($p < 0.05$). From baseline to week 12, patients in the MPA group significantly increased their daily caloric intake.

Significantly ($p < 0.001$) more MPA subjects than placebo gained ≥ 10% of baseline body weight. The mean difference in percentage from baseline to 12 weeks between the two groups for skinfold thickness of the triceps and iliac, and lean and body fat was statistically significant ($p < 0.05$). The values of appetite scale and Karnofsky scores increased. No serious adverse effects were observed. The study therefore shows that 1 g of MPA, given orally once a day, is safe, well-tolerated, and effective in controlling AIDS cachexia during a period of 12 weeks.

## Megestrol Acetate

The progestogenic synthesised derivative MA has been successfully used in the treatment of neoplastic cachexia, anorexia, and in AIDS patients [24, 56, 81–83], but the optimal dosage of the drug remains to be defined. Also, the mechanism of action of MA is many-sided and not yet completely understood. It is thought that the stimulation of appetite by progestogens takes place at the hypothalamic level [84–86]. A second effect of MA, which has been demonstrated in vitro, is the promotion of fibroblast transformation into adipocyte. Finally, evidence has emerged showing anti-TNF and anti-IL-1 action [83].

A dose-response and cost-benefit compromise may be achieved with a dose of 320 mg/day. We designed a controlled study to evaluate the safety and efficacy of MA at this dosage in the treatment of anorexia and cachexia in AIDS patients [68]. The trial had a total duration of 60 days divided into two 30-day periods: the first was a double-blind randomised versus placebo study; while in the second all patients received MA. Inclusion criteria were AIDS and body weight loss > 10% of usual weight.

## Results

*Patients.* Of the 56 AIDS patients (45 men and 11 women) enrolled in the study, 12 were assigned to subgroup 4A (MA: 7; placebo: 5), 39 into subgroup 4C1 (MA: 19; placebo: 20), and five into subgroup 4C2 (MA: 2; placebo: 3). The 82.1% of the patients who were drug addicts were divided equally into the MA group ($n = 23$) and the placebo group ($n = 23$). The average age (± SD) of the patients was 32.68 ± 5.21 years and was comparable between men and women and in the two groups: MA men 32.17 ± 4.88 years, MA women 33.20 ± 5.36 years; placebo men 33.36 ± 5.93 years, placebo women 31.67 ± 4.32 years. The average height for the entire sample was 171.23 ± 7.82 cm. The average current weight was 55.22 ± 8.35 kg (MA men 59.04 ± 5.84 kg, MA women 44.30 ± 5.29 kg; placebo men 56.82 ± 8.64 kg, placebo women 47.67 ± 6.74 kg). The usual weight was 67.26 ± 9.97 kg (MA men 70.17 ± 6.34 kg, MA women 51.70 ± 7.41 kg; placebo men 70.50 ± 9.31 kg; placebo women 56.17 ± 7.60 kg). The difference compared to the actual weight of 12.04 kg was equal to a weight loss of 18%. The ideal weight was 64.21 ± 6.25 kg (MA men 66.38 ± 4.80 kg, MA women 54.88 ± 3.87 kg; placebo men 65.57 ± 5.78; placebo women 58.65 ± 4.79 kg). The difference compared to the actual weight of 8.99 kg was equal to 11.62%.

*Weight.* In the double-blind phase, the initial weight of subjects in the two groups was comparable: MA 55.24 ± 8.32 kg; placebo 55.65 ± 9.21 kg. However, after 30 days of treatment, the increase for the MA subgroup was +3.87 ± 2.24 kg vs a decrease of -0.32 ± 2.36 kg for the placebo subgroup.

The differences between usual weight and actual weight at the start and after 30 days decreased in subjects treated with MA, from -11.37 ± 4.72 kg to -7.50 ± 4.60 kg, while they remained unchanged in the placebo group, from 10.06 ± 2.86 kg to 10.38 ± 4.30 kg. In the 'open' phase, the patients who were already receiving MA showed a modest weight gain, from 59.10 ± 8.61 kg to 59.11 ± 9.1 kg, while those who went from placebo to MA had a more significant increase in weight, from 55.32 ± 9.26 kg to 58.47 ± 9.69 kg. These data show that, 30 days after the start of MA administration, a peak is reached that remains mostly stable during the following 30 days of treatment.

*Body Mass Index.* A BMI index < 20 kg/m$^2$ is significant when evaluating weight loss: all patients enrolled in our trial had baseline values < 20 (MA 18.82 ± 2.09 kg/m$^2$, placebo 18.70 ± 1.84 kg/m$^2$), but after 30 days of treatment the MA group re-entered the normal range (20.06 ± 2.00 kg/m$^2$) whereas in the placebo group the BMI value fell further (18.48 ± 2.03 kg/m$^2$).

*Body Circumferences*
*Circumference of the wrist:* MA, from 15.70 ± 1.22 cm to 15.70 ± 1.22 cm; placebo, from 15.50 ± 0.95 cm to 15.33 ± 0.93 cm.
*Circumference of the arm:* MA, from 23.72 ± 3.13 cm to 24.63 ± 3.12 cm; placebo, from 23.29 ± 2.57 cm to 23.21 ± 2.88 cm.
*Circumference of the waist:* MA, from 73.70 ± 7.49 cm to 76.48 ± 7.65 cm; placebo, from 73.41 ± 6.36 cm to 73.29 ± 6.06 cm.
*Circumference of the buttocks:* MA, from 84.26 ± 4.48 cm to 86.61 ± 4.95 cm; placebo, from 83.47 ± 4.64 cm to 82.71 ± 4.82 cm.
*Circumference of the thigh:* MA, from 44.43 ± 4.13 cm to 46.57 ± 4.57 cm; placebo, from 44.18 ± 3.32 cm to 43.47 ± 3.56 cm.
*Circumference of the arm muscles (MAMC):* The measurements were significantly different in the two groups. In subjects treated with MA, MAMC increased from 204.40 ± 65.22 mm to 213.52 ± 50.61 mm, while in subjects receiving placebo MAMC decreased from 215.26 ± 29.58 mm to 202.78 ± 56.41 mm.

*Skinfolds.* Skinfolds are a measure of subcutaneous fat, which represents about half of all body fat. In those MA-treated patients, skinfold thickness increased significantly, while there was a modest increase in placebo-treated subjects that was a result of the hypercaloric-hyperproteic diet.
*TSF:* MA, from 5.15 ± 1.63 mm to 7.23 ± 2.11 mm; placebo, from 5.95 ± 2.76 mm to 6.00 ± 2.54 mm.
*SSF:* MA, from 8.70 ± 2.95 mm to 11.00 ± 3.85 mm; placebo, from 10.50 ± 4.29 mm to 10.65 ± 4.54 mm.
*ISF:* MA, from 5.33 ± 2.54 mm to 8.03 ± 3.67 mm; placebo, from 7.29 ± 6.93 mm to 7.35 ± 6.86 mm.

*Body Impedance.* Cutaneous BIA values decreased in both groups, dropping in the MA group from 497.57 ± 83.40 ohms to 456.17 ± 90.75 ohms, and in the placebo group from 507.47 ± 91.97 ohms to 505.35 ± 98.45 ohms.
*Fat-free mass:* BIA measurements confirmed those obtained from body circumference measurements, with an increase in the MA group from 52.94 ± 8.29 kg to 56.50 ± 8.61 kg and a reduction in the placebo group from 53.41 ± 7.89 Kg to 52.64 ± 7.96 Kg.
*Fat mass:* In the MA group, there was an increase from 2.30 ± 2.43 kg to 2.39 ± 3.01 kg and in the placebo group from 2.24 ± 3.42 kg to 2.65 ± 4.48 kg.
*TBW:* TBW determination is important in a study involving progestogenic derivatives, which are believed to cause water retention. Our data exclude significant action of this type, in that the values for MA subjects went from 73.44 ± 2.00% to 73.51 ± 2.45%, and for the placebo from 72.83 ± 2.20% to 73.26 ± 2.15%.
*Basal metabolism (REE):* The caloric consumption necessary for maintaining vital functions and thermoregulation with respect to sex, age, weight, and body surface comprise the REE. For MA subjects, this increased from 1594.75 ± 167.41 Kcal to 1674.67 ± 183.99 Kcal and for subjects receiving placebo dropped from 1606.93 ± 201.31 Kcal to 1601.52 ± 201.06 Kcal.

In the open phase of the study, a slight further increase for MA subjects during the second month of treatment and a significant increase in patients who went onto MA after placebo period were observed.

*Caloric Intake.* MA patients had an actual basal caloric intake of 1415.49 ± 435.30 Kcal and a theoretical intake of 2096.52 ± 476/68 Kcal, with a difference of 681.03 Kcal. After 30 days of therapy, the actual intake increased to 2872.43 ± 539.84 Kcal as opposed to a theoretical intake of 2268.70 ± 468.45 Kcal, with a positive difference of + 603.73 Kcal. Patients in the placebo group showed an actual basal intake of 1390.12 ± 423.27 Kcal as opposed to a theoretical intake of 2000 ± 525.36 Kcal, with a difference of -609.99 Kcal. After 30 days of placebo and dietetic counselling the actual intake increased to 1850 ± 815.13 Kcal as opposed to a theoretical intake of 2015.29 ± 513.88 Kcal, with a difference of -165.29 Kcal. It should be noted that, under basal conditions, all patients consumed fewer calories than were necessary to maintain weight, whereas after 30 days both the MA and the placebo group increased their caloric intake albeit differently. In the open phase of the study, the actual caloric intake increased further, from 2872.43 ± 539.84 Kcal to 3158.93 ± 464.55 Kcal, with a difference of +908.93 Kcal after 60 days of MA, and from 2015.29 ± 513.88 Kcal to 2557 ± 756.84 Kcal, with a difference of +418.33 Kcal after 30 days of MA following placebo. The difference between the final and basal intake was 1456.95 ± 565.96 Kcal for MA and 459.88 ± 820.26 Kcal for placebo, with high statistical significance ($p < 0.0001$).

*Appetite.* At the time of enrolment the amount of appetite as measured with the visual analogue scale (VAS) was very poor in ten patients (4 MA, 6 placebo) and poor in 30 (19 MA, 11 placebo). At the second and third examination, only two placebo patients had a very poor appetite, eight placebo patients had a poor appetite; in 11 (7 MA, 4 placebo) appetite was fair, in 15 (13 MA, 2 placebo) good, and in 4 (3 MA, 1 placebo) very good. Clinically and statistically, the results were highly significant ($p < 0.0001$). In the open phase, appetite stabilised in the MA group (2 fair, 8 good, 4 very good) and there was clear improvement in patients who went onto MA after placebo, with none having a very poor appetite, 3 with poor appetite, 3 fair, 7 good, and 2 very good.

*Performance Status.* The Karnofsky index showed that MA improved the score by 66.52 ± 8.85 to 70.43 ± 9.28, whereas placebo failed to modify these values, 64.71 ± 8.74 to 64.71 ± 10.07. In the open phase, the scores of the MA group increased further (from 70.43 ± 9.28 to 75.00 ± 6.50) and those of the placebo group who switched to MA also increased (from 64.71 ± 10.07 to 68.67 ± 10.60).

*Tumour Necrosis Factor.* The TNF levels of the MA group decreased by 302.90 ± 355.44 pg/ml to 107.57 ± 166.28 pg/ml. In the placebo group, they increased from 243.52 ± 288.55 pg/ml to 364.65 ± 380.01 pg/ml.

*Adverse Events.* No adverse events occurred that were serious enough to lead to a suspension in drug administration or to a change in treatment. Minor intolerances were, however, reported by 40 patients, 25/27 (92.59%) in the MA group and 15/20 (75%) in the placebo group, with a difference in the incidence of 17.59%; this is a very low percentage and indicative of the good tolerability of the drug. For MA subjects, a reduction in libido was recorded (40% vs placebo 5%), gastrointestinal discomfort (29.63% vs placebo 15%), pruritus (22.22% vs placebo 10%), amenorrhoea (11.11% vs placebo 0%), sleep disorders (14.81% vs placebo 35%), and nausea and vomiting (0% vs placebo 10%).

*Biochemical Parameters.* No significant changes were observed in the biochemical or virological parameters in the two groups of patients.

*Compliance.* The degree of compliance was calculated only for the double-blind phase as the ratio between the difference in tablets given to the patient and those returned and the number of days of treatment. Overall, compliance for all the patients (ITT) was 94.67% ± 5.78 (MA) and 92.16% ± 10.44 (placebo); for patients evaluated for the efficacy of the drug, the percentage was 95.43% ± 4.49 (MA) and 94.88% ± 6.68 (placebo).

*Completion of the Study.* Of the 56 patients enrolled, 43 (76.8%) completed the double-blind phase: 24/28 (85.7%) in the MA group and 19/28 (67.9%) in the placebo group. The difference emphasises the subjective perception of the efficacy of the placebo.

*Conclusions.* The results obtained in this randomised study demonstrate the efficacy of MA treatment in rectifying loss of weight and appetite in AIDS patients.

The main variable studied was Δ-weight, in which, after 30 days of therapy, there was a significant, important difference between the MA (+3.87 ± 2.24 kg) and the placebo (-0.2 ± 2.36 kg) groups. The statistical significance of these values is evident both in terms of analysis for protocol ($t$ = 5.7161, d.o.f. = 38, $p$ < 0.00001) and for analysis of intention to treat ($t$ = 5.5234, d.o.f.=45, $p$ < 0.00001). The positive data for weight are also strengthened by results obtained for caloric intake and appetite – variables closely connected with body weight increase – since these were also significantly modified by MA. In fact, the increase in caloric intake was 1456.94 Kcal compared to 459.88 Kcal in the placebo group ($t$ = 4.5532, d.o.f.+38, $p$ < 0.0001). At the third examination, in the MA group, appetite was fair in 7 patients, good in 13, and very good in 3, as opposed to the placebo group in which appetite was very poor in 2 patients, poor in 8, good in 2 and very good in 1; the degree of significance was high ($p$ < 0.0001).

Data relating to the open phase of the study, when all patients were taking MA, irrefutably confirms the efficacy of this drug; in fact, patients who were already under this treatment further increased their weight by 0.01 kg and their caloric intake by 908.93 Kcal. Appetite improved to fair in 2 patients, good in 8, and very good in 8. Subjects who were initially in the placebo group increased their weight by 3.15 kg, their caloric intake by 418.33 Kcal, and their appetite, which improved to poor in 3 patients, fair in 3, good in 7, and very good in 2. Only a few undesirable effects were recorded, by two out of 27 patients in the MA

group and 5 out of 20 in the placebo group, with no requests to stop treatment. Unwanted side effects consisted of a reduction in libido, amenorrhoea, intestinal discomfort, and pruritus. No negative effects on the CD4+/CD4+ lymphocyte population or on β2-microglobulin were recorded, while a reduction in TNF levels was noted.

In conclusion, it can be stated that, at a dose of 320 mg/day, MA is an effective and safe drug in the treatment of AIDS cachexia.

*Megestrol Acetate and rhGH*
The metabolic effects of growth hormone (GH) and progestin derivatives, i.e. MPA and MA, are well-documented in humans. GH predominantly promotes positive nitrogen balance, increasing lean body mass (LBM) but simultaneously reducing fat body mass (FBM) [87–89]; MA prevalently increases FBM, body water, and appetite [90, 91]. In AIDS-cachexia syndrome, there are important losses in LBM, FBM, and appetite [92–95], but the administration of GH alone may be insufficient to correct metabolism disturbances that lead to this condition. We therefore tested whether improved results could be obtained with the combined use of GH and MA [71].

Five AIDS (stage IV C) cachectic and anorectic patients (4 men, 1 woman, 25–56 years, mean 35.2 ± 13 years), who lost a mean 19.4% of their IBW, were treated with rhGH (Humatrope, Lilly France SA, Fegersheim, France) 0.63 mg/m² subcutaneously/day for 30 days. Eight comparable patients (7 men, 1 woman, 25–56 years, mean 33.7 ±10 years), who lost a mean 23.6 % of IBW, received the same dose of rhGH for 15 days together with MA (Megestil, Boheringer Mannheim, Milan, Italy) 320 mg orally/day for 30 days.

Anthropometric [(W, IBW, body circumferences (MAC, MAMC), BMI, skinfold thickness (biceps, triceps, sub-scapular, iliac), body compartments (LBM, FBM, TBW)], biochemical, hormonal and immunological assessments were carried out at baseline and after 1, 2, and 4 weeks. Selected measurements were also made before and after the therapies. Blood samples were collected for determination of IGF-1, insulin, cortisol, GH, aldosterone, T3, T4, dehydroepiandrosterone sulfate (DHEA-S), insulin-like-growth-factor binding protein-3 (IGFBP-3), and TNF. Body composition was determined by BIA. Individual caloric needs were calculated by means of a corrected Harris-Benedict equation, as previously described [95]. Appetite, quality of life, and food and caloric intake were recorded at the same times by means of an appetite scale, Karnofsky index, and a dietary diary. Written informed consent was obtained from each patient. All values were expressed as mean ± SD and compared by Student's $t$ test and analysis of variance (ANOVA). Significance was designated at the 95% confidence level.

*Results.* The five patients receiving rhGH completed treatment, whereas three subjects in the rhGH + MA group were excluded from the study when treatment was suspended due to opportunistic infections (1 after 3 days, 1 after 7 days, 1 after 15 days).

Patients treated with rhGH alone continued to lose weight from baseline value (55.1 kg) to 53.2 kg (-1.9 kg) after 30 days of therapy, while patients receiving combined therapy gained 0.5 kg after 15 days and 0.1 kg in the next 15 days on MA alone (Table 3). In both groups, but significantly in MA patients, there was an increase in body fat and a decrease in lean tissue after 30 days. Combined treatment of 15 days produced a gain in LBM (+ 0.1 kg) and in FBM (+ 0.7 kg). Caloric intake increased from 1848 to 3605 Kcal/day after 15 days, doubling (+ 52.6 %) the baseline value after 30 days of MA treatment (from 1848 to 3898 Kcal/day). MA alone maintained fat and food intake gains from 15th to 30th day. Caloric intake in rhGH-treated patients increased from 2194 to 2768 Kcal/day. During rhGH treatment, IGF-1, aldosterone, and insulin levels significantly increased ($p < 0.05$) in both groups but more in MA subjects; T4 and T3 increased but not statistically significantly. GH levels decreased more in rhGH- than in rhGH + MA-treated patients. Cortisol levels significantly decreased ($p < 0.05$) only in rhGH + MA subjects (Table 4). No significant changes were observed in DHEA-S and IGFBP-3 levels and routine haematological or biochemical parameters in either group. TNF levels decreased in patients in

whom secondary infections were successfully treated.

*Conclusions.* This is one of the first studies investigating the effects of rhGH administered together with MA in AIDS cachectic patients who lost > 10% of their usual body weight. In contrast with previous studies [96, 97] of rhGH administered to AIDS patients, we did not document weight gain after 30 days of rhGH treatment (0.63 mg/m², sc/day). Even when our patients had increased caloric intake, they continued to lose weight. However, rhGH + MA (320 mg, orally/day) resulted in significant increase of appetite, caloric intake, body weight, and fat.

Our data give rise to doubt about the rationale of rhGH use in treating AIDS cachexia. AIDS patients have reduced LBM, fat body mass, and cholesterol, while normal adults with GH deficiency have reduced LBM and increased body fat, cholesterol, and TGs [88, 89, 98]. Baseline GH levels in our patients were higher than normal, and exogenous rhGH may modestly contribute to reversing the metabolic alterations due to cytokines and secondary infections. Nonetheless, appetite is scarcely influenced by rhGH. There may be other reasons for rhGH treatment of AIDS patients, such as to restore a GH deficiency in children or in selected adults. Our results confirm the efficacy of MA in improving appetite, caloric intake, and weight gain but further work is necessary to define which patients might benefit from single or combined use of GH and progestin derivatives.

## Therapy of Lipodystrophy Syndrome

No accepted guidelines for the treatment of lipodystrophy syndrome exist, rather, only anecdotal approaches. There is also no validated drug therapy to ameliorate or correct lipodystrophy-associated abnormalities [99]. Instead, treatment must be directed at reducing fat accumulation in visceral adipose tissue (VAT), and dorsocervical fat (buffalo hump), and/or increasing SAT in conditions of lipoatrophy. Thus, prevention is by far the best approach to reverse lipodystrophy.

**Table 3.** Anthropometric data of patients treated with rhGH (0.63 mg/m², sc/day) alone (*n* = 5) or with rhGH + MA (320 mg, orally/day) (*n* = 5), means ± SD

| | rhGH | | rhGH + MA | | MA |
| | Baseline | 30 days | Baseline | 15 days | 30 days |
|---|---|---|---|---|---|
| W: | 55.1 ± 8.6 | 53.2 ± 7.7 | 47.7 ± 6.8 | 48.2 ± 6.7 | 48.3 ± 7.1 |
| % IBW: | 19.4 | 22.2 | 23.6 | 24.6 | 19.6 |
| BMI : | 17.4 ± 1.2 | 16.8 ± 1.1 | 15.7 ± 1.9 | 16.1 ± 2.2 | 16.7 ± 2.4 |
| SUM: | 17.5 ± 2.5 | 16.3 ± 2.0 | 21.2 ± 3.8 | 21.3 ± 5.2 | 23.5 ± 6.0 |
| LBM | 54.3 ± 6.7 | 52.0 ± 8.4 | 45.1 ± 10.3 | 45.2 ± 9.0 | 44.8 ± 9.8 |
| FBM: | 0.77 ± 1.0 | 1.3 ± 2.2 | 1.9 ± 2.8 | 2.6 ± 4.1 | 4.2 ± 4.8 |
| BIA: | 482 ± 110 | 536+-129 | 643 ± 116 | 638 ± 92 | 656+-87 |
| TBW: | 72.7 ± 2 | 72.4 ± 0.5 | 73.6 ± 2.3 | 73.7 ± 1.2 | 73.4 ± 1.3 |
| Caloric intake: | 2194 ± 600 | 2768 ± 1611 | 1848 ± 480 | 3605 ± 915 | 3898 ± 634 |

*W*, body weight (kg); *% IBW*, percentage of W loss with respect to ideal body weight; *BMI*, body mass index [weight (kg)/height (m²)]; *SUM*, sum (mm) of four skinfold thicknesses (biceps; triceps; subscapular; iliac); *LBM*, lean body mass (kg). *FBM*, fat body mass (kg); *BIA*, bioelectrical impedance analysis (ohms); *TBW*, total body water (%); caloric intake, Kcal/day

**Table 4.** Hormonal profile of patients treated with rhGH (0.63 mg/m²/day) alone (*n* = 5) or with rhGH + MA (320 mg/orally/day; *n* = 5), means ± SD

| rhGH | rhGH + MA | | MA | | |
| | Baseline | 30 days | Baseline | 15 days | 30 days |
|---|---|---|---|---|---|
| W | 55.1 ± 8.6 | 53.2 ± 7.7 | 48.2 ± 6.7 | 47.7 ± 6.8 | 48.3 ± 7.1 |
| % IBW | 19.4 | 22.2 | 23.6 | 24.6 | 19.6 |
| BMI | 17.4 ± 1.2 | 16.8 ± 1.1 | 15.7 ± 1.9 | 16.1 ± -2.2 | 16.7 ± 2.4 |
| SUM | 17.5 ± 2.5 | 16.3 ± 2.0 | 21.2 ± 3.8 | 21.3 ± 5.2 | 23.5 ± 6.0 |
| LBM | 54.3 ± 6.7 | 52.0 ± 8.4 | 45.1 ± 10.3 | 45.2 ± 9.0 | 44.8 ± 9.8 |
| FBM | 0.77 ± 1.0 | 1.3 ± 2.2 | 1.9 ± 2.8 | 2.6 ± 4.1 | 4.2 ± 4.8 |
| BIA | 482 ± 110 | 536 ± 129 | 643 ± 116 | 638 ± 92 | 656 ± 87 |
| TBW | 72.7 ± 2 | 72.4 ± 0.5 | 73.6 ± 2.3 | 73.7 ± 1.2 | 73.4 ± 1.3 |
| Caloric intake | 2194 ± 600 | 2768 ± 1611 | 1848 ± 480 | 3605 ± 915 | 3898 ± 634 |

*IGF-1*, insulin-like growth factor-1; *IGFBP-3*, insulin-like-growth-factor binding protein-3; *DHEA-S*, dehydroepiandrosterone sulfate

## Prevention of Lipodystrophy

Strategies for preventing or reducing the risk of lipodystrophy are:
- Avoid combination of PIs and NRTIs
- Early antiretroviral treatment
- Early intervention for metabolic changes
- Dietary advice, dietary supplementation and physical exercise.

## Management of Lipodystrophy

In established lipodystrophy, there are four categories of intervention:
- Lifestyle changes regarding diet, physical activity, and smoking
- Changes in the treatment regimen
- Use of specific drug therapies to correct specific abnormalities
- Cosmetic surgery.

## Management of Fat Accumulation

### Diet and Exercise

Specific dietary and exercise intervention, as extrapolated from subjects not infected with HIV [100], seems to be also effective in lipodystrophy for preventing hyperlipidaemia as well as reducing lipid levels and abnormal fat distribution, especially VAT [101–106]. A Mediterranean low-fat diet, rich in vegetables, fresh fruits, fibre, and fish, is recommended for its high content of omega-3 fatty acids. Diets very low in fat [107], i.e. containing < 15% fat calories, are recommended for persons with high cholesterol and TG levels.

A beneficial role of antioxidants, B vitamins, and carnitine in reversing mitochondrial damage induced by NRTI [108], and related to lipodystrophy and lactic acidosis, has been reported by many authors [108–116]. Vitamins $B_1$ (thiamine) and $B_2$ (riboflavin) are given at a dose of 100 mg and 50 mg, respectively, in addition to dietary intervention. Improved β-oxidation of long-chain fatty acids is achieved with 100 mg levocarnitine (Sigma-tau, Italy)/kg/day in children and 2–4 g/day in adults. Independent of other specific therapies, we usually administer fish oil or/and vegetable-derived PUFAs [117–119] together with L-carnitine, in order to increase β-oxidation of long-chain fatty acids, and replace saturated fats with polyunsaturated fats (data available on line). Consumption of purified and concentrated preparations of fish-oil derivatives (Enerzona Omega-3Rx, New Vitality, Italy) and adherence to insulin-sparing diets are highly effective in controlling metabolic pathways that can lead to fat disorders (data available on line).

Physical exercise is also prescribed to partly compensate for the reduction of peripheral fat tissue with muscle-mass hypertrophy (body building) [105, 106]. Intensive aerobic and anaerobic exercise can decrease VAT in normal and HIV subjects by 17–20% [106, 120]. Exercise increases the production of the adrenergic hormone epinephrine, the lipolytic effect of which is more evident for visceral fat than for peripheral fat. Physical exercise associated with a high-fibre, moderate-fat, low-glycaemic-index diet ameliorates lipodystrophy patterns [103]. Progressive resistance training decreases truncal fat and improves LBM [106, 121, 122].

### Androgens

Testosterone and other synthetic androgens at low or replacement doses in males with testosterone levels < 250 ng/dl can be used to reduce intra-abdominal fat, but a reduction of peripheral fat is also observed [123].

### Insulin-Sensitising Agents (Metformin)

Metformin is a drug that reduces glucose production in the liver. At a dosage of 500–850 mg 2–3 times a day, it decreases VAT, TGs, and LDL, and improves fasting insulin levels and the insulin response in an oral glucose tolerance test [124, 125]; however, serious lactic acidosis can occur during metformin therapy.

### Growth Hormone and GH-Releasing Hormone

Prior to the availability of HAART for use in treating AIDS-related wasting, GH had been shown to promote gains in lean mass and loss of fat mass [126, 127]. We demonstrated favourable effects of GH in association with MA [71] in the treatment of wasting syndrome, and the data suggested a role for GH in reducing central fat accumulation and increasing muscle mass. Since the introduction of HAART, studies have pointed out that rhGH improves fat redistribution, reducing waist circumference (VAT) and breast size, while increasing fat-free mass [128, 129]. GH improves fat metabolism and reduces both fat accumulation and lipoatrophy, including loss of facial fat pads. The optimal dose for treating lipodystrophy is not yet established but is less than the 4–6 mg/day administered to patients with wasting [130]. Adverse effects, however, at the doses employed are common and include arthralgias, myalgias, diabetes, and hypertriglyceridaemia. In addition, there is reversion of truncal adiposity after drug discontinuation, suggesting the need to establish a maintenance dose. In order to maintain physiological levels of GH, which appear to be reduced in lipodystrophic HIV patients, the effect of GHRH in the treatment of lipodystrophy was studied [131]. GHRH, at the dose of 1 mg subcutaneously twice daily, increases LBM and subcutaneous fat, reduces truncal and visceral fat, and increases the concentration of IGF-1.

### Leptin

The discovery of leptin, in 1994 [132], and the identification of its role in body weight homeostasis, food intake, energy expenditure, and adipose tissue metabolism represent an enormous progress in understanding and treating lipodystrophy [133–137]. As a result, lipodystrophy may be considered as a localised form of obesity, with associated typical changes in the neuroendocrine system as well as in metabolism and immune functions [137–139]. Low leptin levels or non-functional leptin receptors have been shown in lipodystrophy [140]. Leptin replacement ameliorated hormonal and fat-tissue abnormalities characteristic of the syndrome [141, 142] after 4 months of therapy.

## Management of Lipoatrophy

### Switch Therapy

Switch therapy consists of replacing a drug causing fat loss or fat redistribution with another drug that has fewer or none of these effects. The majority of switch studies have focused on replacing a combination of NRTIs and PIs with a PI-sparing regimen [143]; changing from one PI to another does not seem to be useful. The replacement of PIs by NRTIs or NNRTIs leads to significant improvement of metabolic and fat abnormalities [144, 145]. In HAART, NRTIs inhibit DNA polymerase, which ultimately induces lipodystrophic changes [124, 144–147], in the following decreasing hierarchic order; zalcitabine > didanosine > stavudine > lamivudine > zidovudine > abacavir. Thus, some studies have demonstrated an improvement in lipoatrophy in response to switching from stavudine or zidovudine to abacavir [148], and from stavudine to abacavir or zidovudine [149, 150]. In the TARHEEL study (Trial to Assess the Regression of Hyperlactataemia and to Evaluate the Regression of Established Lipodystrophy) of HIV-1-positive subjects, replacing stavudine with abacavir or zidovudine resulted in a median increase in arm fat of 35%, in leg fat of 12%, and in trunk fat of 18%, after 48 weeks of therapy [149].

New antiretroviral drugs with less effects on fat metabolism are expected.

### Cosmetic Surgery

Cosmetic surgery for lipodystrophy was introduced to correct both fat accumulation and lipoatrophy. Anomalous dorsal and abdominal fat accumulations can be reduced with ultrasound-assisted liposuction and endermology, and facial shape can be restored by lipofilling the temple, nasolabial, and cheek areas with fat cells taken from the patient's abdomen [151, 152] or by injecting new fill. These cells remain in place even during lipodystrophy progression.

Traditional plastic surgery approaches have also been used for cosmetic results, mainly for facial changes affecting the nasolabial folds and buccal and temporal fat-pad areas. Implants usually consist of fat transfer and collagen injections, but loss of the implanted fat is a not uncommon risk. Satisfactory results were reported with polylactic acid (New-Fill) injections every 15 days for treating facial lipoatrophy [153]. Polylactic acid and similar compounds (e.g. hyaluronic acid), however, are not approved for this type of use in the USA. Success, as judged by evaluating on 3D photos, is around 48% and additional injections are needed within 1–2 years. Side effects include pain in 80%, the development of non-inflammatory small nodules, bleeding, and malaise. New-Fill is not a true filler, like collagen or transferred fat, but stimulates fibroblasts to produce collagen in the injection sites. The product is hypoallergenic and biodegradable over 2 years [154]. Suction-assisted lipotomy has been used to remove 'buffalo hump' but fat deposits can reappear [152, 155, 156]. Malar atrophy can benefit from surgical correction, with dermafat grafts transferred from the abdominal wall to malar pockets through a transoral approach. The aesthetic results were judged to be satisfactory and persisting during 2 years of follow-up [151].

### Correction of Metabolic Abnormalities Associated with Lipodystrophy

Persons infected with HIV could represent an emerging population at higher risk of coronary heart disease (CHD), due to their prolonged life expectancy despite metabolic disturbances induced by therapy [157–160]. Elevated TGs, LDL cholesterol, and VLDL cholesterol, and reduced levels of high-density lipoprotein (HDL) cholesterol are associated with visceral fat accumulation, peripheral lipodystrophy, lipoatrophy, and CHD. In 5–75% of HIV patients receiving HAART, lipid metabolism and body fat distribution worsen after 10–12 months of therapy.

Patients on HAART at risk of heart disease (CAD, IHD), because of high levels of cholesterol and/or TGs, may benefit from special diet, changes in life style, and drugs. The risk of increases in total cholesterol (> 0.6 mmol/l) is 19.6% for Ritonavir, 8.5% for Nelfinavir, and 3.8% for Indinavir.

Increased lipid concentrations in HIV-infected patients on HAART can be managed following the American National Cholesterol Education Program (NCEP), but new strategies addressed to prevent and manage such emerging disorders [161, 162] are still needed. Our guidelines, based on our own and experience and that of others [163–168] meet the intervention criteria defined by NCEP [169], including evaluation criteria, diet prescription, drugs, exercise, and were preliminarily discussed in The Pavia Consensus Statement, October 2001 [170, 171], together with recommendations of the HIV Medicine Association of the Infectious Disease Society of America and the Adult AIDS Clinical Trials Group [172].

### Patient Evaluation Criteria

Patients at risk of CHD must be routinely evaluated for risk factors, such as family history, smoking, hypertension, hormonal status, obesity, physical activity, alcohol abuse, hypogonadism, hypothyroidism, diabetes, and renal or hepatic disease. The guidelines include measurement of total cholesterol, HDL, LDL and VLDL cholesterol, TG, lactate [170–172], body compartments, body circumferences and skinfolds [160], and resting metabolic rate (RMR). The RMR is a measure of the energy expended for maintenance of physiological functions and generally represents the largest portion of daily energy expenditure (60–75%) [163–165]. We use the WHO equations for determining body weights and heights [166], and BIA and indirect calorimetry to predict the RMR and energy expenditure for different age and sex groups [167, 168].

Energy production is estimated by measuring $O_2$ consumption and $CO_2$ production using a special calorimeter (e.g. type MBM-200–23–01, Datex-Engstron Division Instrumentarium Corp. Helsinki, Finland). RMR values normally range between 0.7 and 1.6 Kcal/min according to the subject's body composition, gender, and level of training.

### Intervention Criteria

#### Nutritional and Pharmacological Approach

There are no universally accepted guidelines for the nutritional treatment of disturbances in lipid metabolism in HIV patients: however, according to NCEP [157, 169] and our studies as well as those of other authors [161, 160, 168, 170–173] in patients with preexisting CHD dietary intervention is recommended at LDL cholesterol level between 100 and 130 mg/dl, adding drug therapy if LDL cholesterol exceeds 130 mg/dl. Among patients without CHD, but presenting with two or more risk factors, dietary intervention is strongly indicated when LDL cholesterol is between 130 and 160mg/dl. Drug therapy must be added at LDL levels > 160 mg/dl. With less than two risk factors, dietary modifications should be recommended at LDL levels between 160 and 190 mg/dl; and drug therapy should be considered at LDL > 190 mg/dl. For patients with very high TG levels (> 400 mg/dl) the Adult AIDS Clinical Trials Group (AACTG) [172] suggests dietary intervention at a total cholesterol >240 mg/dl or HDL cholesterol < 35 mg/dl. Patients with isolated hypertriglyceridaemia (fasting serum levels > 200mg/dl) should follow an appropriate diet and a program of physical exercise. If levels exceed 1000 mg/dl, pharmacological therapy is strongly suggested because of the risk of pancreatitis. The same indication is mandatory for patients with a history of pancreatitis and TGs > 500mg/dl.

Diet and exercise in order to reduce hypercholesterolaemia are recommended before and during pharmacological intervention. In patients suffering from wasting and from lipid disturbances, it is preferable to treat the wasting first [168, 174, 175]. In patients without other risk factors, such as smoking, preexisting cardiovascular diseases, and lipid problems, 'wait and see' may be an appropriate strategy [176].

Nutritional intervention must be tailored to the needs of each patient, considering RMR, gut functions, concomitant diseases, hormonal status, appetite, and social conditions [160, 170, 175]. At the first signs of malnutrition, suitable nutritional treatment is advised [168] due to the positive effect on reducing infection and improving the quality of life. A balanced supply of n-6 and n-3 PUFAs, including EPA and DHA (the main components of fish oil) in a ratio of 0.9;1.5, may modulate cytokine production and reduce TGs. EPA, as a direct suppressant of lipid mobilisation factor, counteracts weight loss, lipolysis, and protein catabolism [177]. Amino acids (1.5–2 g/kg per day), of which a portion (< 0.7 g/kg) should be essential, must be administered to block protein loss. Branched-chain amino acids are important when patients present with associated hepatic encephalopathy. Early and aggressive nutritional treatment of wasting and lipid metabolism disturbances improves the general clinical status, thus reducing the length of hospital stay. Unfortunately, national health services do not completely support nutritional therapy programs.

Pharmacological intervention on appetite and on metabolic pathways, by administering drugs, such as cyproheptadine [178], progestin derivatives [174, 179–181], insulin-like growth factor-1 [182], steroids, and GH [160, 183, 184], may contribute to the success of any nutritional program.

### Drugs Lowering Lipids

Since diet and physical exercise reduce lipid levels in only 40% of patients, therapy with statins and/or fibrates for hypercholesterolaemia and/or hypertriglyceridaemia is almost always necessary [170, 172].

In our opinion, an isolated increase of TGs in a patient with normal HDL values should be treated only when levels of 1000 mg/dl are reached, and the consequent risk of pancreatitis becomes high [105]. In this situation, we also recommend replacement of saturated fats with unsaturated fats and the addition of statin or fibrate drugs, if diet alone fails. In combined disorders (high cholesterol, high TGs), statins and fibrates together may control lipid metabolism, but they also cause muscle damage (rhabdomyolysis). In some subjects, Gemfibrozil (600 mg BID), Atorvastatin (10 mg QD), or a combination thereof reduces total cholesterol by, respectively, 32, 19, and 30%, with a TG reduction of 59, 21, and 60%. Interactions between antiretroviral compounds, lipid-lowering agents, and anti-diabetic drugs are not well-described. What is known is that these drugs carry a risk of toxicity, because the majority of them (Atorvastatin, Lovastatin, Simvastatin, Bezafibrate, Ciprofibrate, Fenofibrate, Gemfibrozil) are metabolised by the same CYP3A liver enzymes as protease inhibitors and other drugs taken by HIV patients. Pravastatin, Cerivastatin, and Fluvastatin in contrast, are mainly excreted by the kidney. PIs, macrolides, and imidazole derivatives inhibit CYP3A and can raise statin levels 10- to 20-fold, leading to increased muscle and liver toxicity with elevation of CPK and ALT. CAD/IHD, due to elevated lipids or diabetes, require 5–10 years to develop, whereas myocardial infarctions are seen after a few weeks or months of PI therapy and have been attributed to thrombosis rather than to atherosclerosis. Metformin can reduce central fat and insulin resistance [186] but it also reduces general fat and muscle mass. Troglitazone (400 mg/day), Rosiglitazone, and Pioglitazone may normalise glucose levels but no effects on lipids and body fat have been observed [187–189]. GH [71, 190] reduces abdominal fat without influencing peripheral fat loss and lipids. Androgenic anabolic steroids (AAS), e.g. oxandrolone, nandrolone, and decanoate, increase muscular body mass without changes in lipids and body fat [191].

### Physical Exercise

The effects of exercise have been extensively studied in patients with known coronary artery disease. Exercise induces beneficial adaptation of the cardiovascular system as well as in peripheral muscle mass [168, 192–197] (Table 5, Fig. 3).

Aerobic exercise and resistance exercise are the most popular methods to prevent or treat sarcopenia and increase muscular performance [198]. In our experience, both forms of exercise, together with a personalised training diet, improves muscle endurance and body composition in HIV patients, as reported by Stringer [199] and Smith [193]. For developing complete muscle strength, three exercise methods are commonly used: weight training, isometric training, and isokinetic training. The neck, arms, and shoulders; the chest, abdomen and back; the buttocks and the legs can be conditioned separately by specific exercises. All our exercise programs include progressive resistance training of the major muscle groups.

HDL levels may increase in sedentary people who engage in aerobic training. Concurrently, LDL is lowered so the net result is a considerably improved ratio of HDL to LDL or HDL to total cholesterol. This exercise effect appears to be independent of whether or not the diet is low in fat or whether or not the exerciser is overweight. The effect of regular endurance-type exercise on blood lipid profile is certainly a strong argument for incorporating vigorous physical activity into a total program of health maintenance in HIV

**Table 5.** Beneficial effects of muscle exercise

| | |
|---|---|
| Resistance to fatigue | ↑ |
| Elasticity and flexibility | ↑ |
| Muscle mass and strength | ↑ |
| Respiratory capacity | ↑ |
| Appetite | ↑ |
| Intestinal functions | ↑ |
| Stress and insomnia | ↓ |

patients receiving HAART. It is well-known that exercise improves myocardial circulation and metabolism and enhances vascularisation, cardiac glycogen stores, and glycolytic capacity, which protect the heart from hypoxic stress [196]. Moreover, the mechanical and contractile properties of the myocardium are improved, enabling the conditioned heart to maintain or increase contractility during specific challenge. Heart rate and blood pressure are reduced, so that the work of the myocardium is significantly reduced at rest and during exercise.

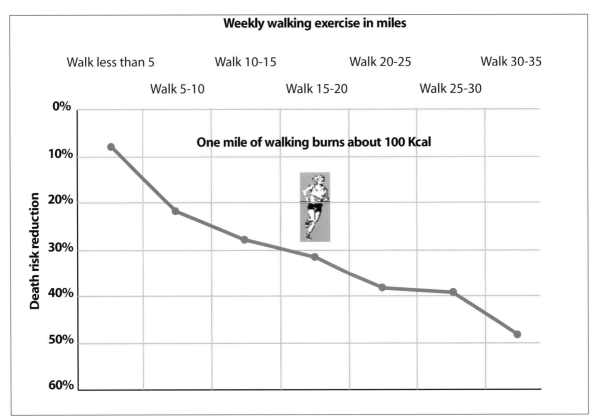

**Fig. 3.** Regularly walking/jogging more than 3 miles a day proportionally reduces the risk of death. No additional benefits are obtained with energy expenditure beyond 3500 kcal per week (reproduced from [197])

Exercise reduces symptoms and the amount of medication needed; it corrects nutritional imbalance, reduces the side effects of many drugs and of an altered diet. Many clinical signs and symptoms are responsive to exercise: atrophy of muscle and bone, postural hypotension, joint stiffness, reflexes, cardiovascular deconditioning, anorexia, gastrointestinal motility, insomnia, and depression. Exercise stimulates the muscles, which not only improves movement of the body in space but also increases biochemical reactions devoted to produce energy. The predominant energy pathways required for physical activities are the ATP-CP system, the lactic acid system, and the oxygen or aerobic system. These pathways often operate simultaneously (Fig. 4); however, there are marked differences in their relative contributions during exercise to the total energy requirement, which is related directly to the length of time and intensity that a specific activity is performed.

*Anaerobic Conditioning.* During intense, maximal bursts of energy lasting no more than 6 s, energy is provided anaerobically, almost exclusively by stored high-energy molecules of phosphates, ATP, and CP. Overload of the ATP-CP pool can be achieved by engaging specific muscles in maximum bursts of effort for 5 or 10 s. In physical activities chosen to enhance the ATP-CP energy capacity of specific muscles, a person must perform numerous bouts of intense, short-duration exercise. The energy for a performance lasting between 10 and 90 s is still supplied predominantly by anaerobic reactions, but lactic acid becomes a more important source of energy. To improve the lactic acid energy system, training must be of sufficient intensity and duration to stimulate lactic acid production as well as to overload the ATP-CP energy system. An effective way to increase the latter to near-maximum levels and overload the lactic acid system is repeated bouts of up to 1 min

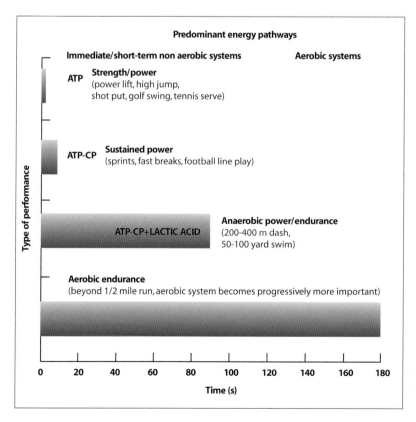

**Fig. 4.** The three energy systems (ATP-CP system, lactic acid system, aerobic system) involved in physical activities. In exercises requiring an intense, short burst of energy, the energy is provided anaerobically, almost exclusively by stored reserves of ATP and CP. In performances lasting between 10 and 90 s, energy from lactic acid production becomes an important source. After 2–4 min of continuous activity, the energy is released almost exclusively from aerobic reactions (reproduced from [197])

of extreme running, swimming, or cycling stopped 30–40 s before exhaustion. The exercise bout should be repeated several times after 1–2 min of recovery. The recovery time from such forms of exercise can be considerable when large amounts of lactic acid are produced (Fig. 2).

*Aerobic Conditioning.* After 2–4 min of continuous exercise, any physical activity becomes progressively more dependent on aerobic energy for the resynthesis of phosphates. Under aerobic conditions, pyruvic acid from carbohydrate metabolism and molecules from fat and protein are transformed into various intermediate substances, with the final formation of $CO_2$, $H_2O$, and large amounts of energy. If the $O_2$ supply and $O_2$ utilisation are adequate, lactic acid will not accumulate and fatigue will be absent. It is possible to reach a condition of endurance or aerobic fitness in which the body's ability to generate ATP aerobically exceeds the energy produced from anaerobic reactions. To have a practical measure of a person's cardiovascular capacity, we use the step-up shown in Fig. 5. This system measures the heart rate in response to

aerobic exercise: a low heart rate during exercise and a small increment with more intense exercise reflect a high level of cardiovascular fitness. A simple method to recover heart rates for evaluation of relative fitness for aerobic exercise is the Tecumseh step test [193].

The stepping cadence must be 22 steps/min for women and 24 for men, with a stepping height of 20 cm. After 3 min of stepping, the subject, in a standing position and exactly after 30 s after stopping, must measure his or her pulse for 30 s. The number of pulse beats, from 30 s to the 1-min post-exercise phase, is the heart rate score. By means of special equations and taking into account recovery heart rate, maximal $O_2$ consumption can be calculated [194].

*Determination of Frequency, Duration, and Intensity of Training.* The intensity of training is the most critical factor influencing successful aerobic conditioning. It can be expressed in different ways: as calories consumed, as a percentage of maximal $O_2$ consumption, as heart rate or percentage of maximum heart rate, or as multiples of

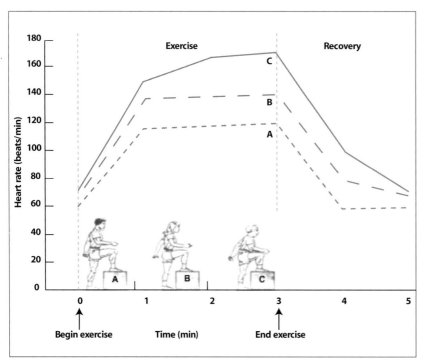

**Fig. 5.** Step-up exercise to evaluate cardiovascular capacity: the heart rate responses of three individuals during 3 min of regular stepping. The subjects have different degrees of condition: **A** is a professional football player, and at the end of 3 min his heart rate is 115 beats per min; **B** works out at a gym; her heart rate is 140 beats per min. **C** is a sedentary young person, his heart rate reaches 170 beats per min. Heart-rate recovery is complete 2 min after the end of exercise (reproduced from [197])

resting metabolic rate required to perform the work. The amount of exercise must be sufficient to produce an increase in heart rate to at least 130–140 beats/min, equivalent to about 50–55% of the maximum aerobic capacity or about 70% of the maximum exercise heart rate (Fig. 6).

Both continuous as well as intermittent overload are effective in improving aerobic capacity. As little as 3–5 min of vigorous exercise performed three times a week improves aerobic capacity and is less exhausting than steady-state exercise performed for 20 min. Our aerobic training program is conducted 3 days a week and includes 20–30 min of continuous exercise of sufficient intensity to expend about 300 kcal. For example, subjects trained on a bicycle ergometer 20–30 min a day (~ 300 kcal), three times a week for 8 weeks, with a training intensity of 85% of maximum heart rate improved maximal $O_2$ uptake by 7.8% [170, 195].

## The Future

Clinical experience suggests introduction of the routine control of lipid metabolism in the clinical treatment of HIV patients. This will protect patients from side effects of therapies that compromise their quality of life and the functions of organs, such as the pancreas and heart, that are targets in lipid disorders. Guidelines must be proposed in which the clinical examination of HIV patients includes assessment of body shape and body composition, and laboratory evaluation of blood lipids and hormones.

Clinical, anthropometric, impedenzometric, DEXA, MRI, and CT methods should be adopted for the evaluation of total adipose tissue, VAT, regional body-fat deposits, and other body compartments (TBW, FFM). REE and total energy expenditure should be assessed by means of indirect calorimetry and control of physical activity [200].

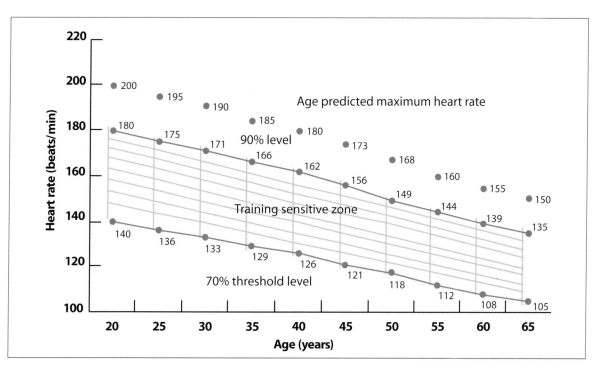

**Fig. 6.** Percentages (70–90%) of maximal heart rate (in the depicted training zone) required to train aerobic systems of energy production in individuals of different age groups. The subject must perform exercise for 3–5 min to obtain a desired pulse rate, counting for 10 s after stop. For example, a training heart rate equal to 70% of the age-related maximal value for a man of 40 years can be calculated by the formula (0.70 x 180 = 126 beats per minute). Exercise must be performed at least for 20 min. A training response occurs if an exercise is performed two, or preferably three times each week for at least 6 weeks (reproduced from [197])

# References

1. Bruera E, Higginson I (1996) Cachexia-anorexia in cancer patients. Oxford University Press
2. Carr A, Samaras K, Burton S et al (1998) A syndrome of peripheral lipodystrophy, hyperlipidaemia and insulin resistance in patients receiving HIV protease inhibitors. AIDS 12:51–58
3. Carr A, Emery S, Law M et al (2003) HIV lipodystrophy case definition study group. An objective case definition of lipodystrophy in HIV-infected adults. Lancet 361:726–735
4. Garg A, Misra A (2004) Lipodystrophies: rare disorders causing metabolic syndromes. Endocrinol Metab Clin North Am 33:305–331
5. Garg A (2004) Acquired and inherited lipodystrophies. N Engl J Med 350:1220–1234
6. Tien PC, Grunfeld C (2004) What is HIV-associated lipodystrophy? Defining fat distribution changes in HIV infection. Curr Opin Infect Dis 17:27–32
7. Ledru E, Christeff N, Patey O et al (2000) Alteration of tumor necrosis factor-alpha T-cell homeostasis following potent antiretroviral therapy: contribution to the development of immunodeficiency virus-associated lipodystrophy syndrome. Blood 95:3191–3198
8. King AB (1990) Malnutrition in HIV infection: prevalence, etiology and management. PAACnotes 2:122–159
9. Kotler DP, Tierney AR, Francisco A et al (1989) The magnitude of body cell mass depletion determines the timing of death from wasting in AIDS. Am J Clin Nutr 50:444–447
10. Watson RR (1994) Nutrition and AIDS. CRC Press, Boca Raton
11. Wanke CA, Silva M, Knox TA et al (2000) Weight loss and wasting remain common complications in individuals infected with human immunodeficiency virus in the era of highly active antiretroviral therapy. Clin Infect Dis 31:803–805
12. Ullrich R, Zeitz M, Heise W et al (1989) Small intestinal structure and function in patients infected with human immunodeficiency virus (HIV): evidence for HIV-induced enteropathy. Ann Intern Med 111:15–21
13. Matsuyama T, Kobayashi N, Yamamoto N (1991) Cytokines and HIV infection: is AIDS a tumor necrosis factor disease? AIDS 5:1405–1417
14. Grunfeld C, Kotler DP (1992) Wasting in the Acquired Immunodeficiency Syndrome, Seminars in Liver Disease. Thieme Inc, New York
15. Center for Disease Control (1987) Revision of the CDC surveillance case definition for acquired immunodeficiency syndrome. MMWR Morb Mortal Wkly Rep 36(Suppl 1):3S–15S
16. Nahler BL, Chu SY, Newanyanwu C et al (1993) HIV wasting syndrome in the United States. AIDS 7:183–188
17. Denning P, Chu SY, Hanson D et al (1994) The adult/adolescent spectrum disease (ASD) project group: HIV wasting syndrome in adults and adolescents with AIDS. 34th ICAAC, 4–7/10/1994, Orlando, Florida, p 114, abs 1135
18. Dworkin MS, Williamson JM; Adult/Adolescent Spectrum of HIV Disease Project (2003) Related AIDS wasting syndrome: trends, influence on opportunistic infections, and survival. J Acquir Immune Defic Syndr 33:267–273
19. Chlebowski RT, Grosvenor MB, Bernhard NH et al (1989) Nutritional status, gastrointestinal dysfunction, and survival in patients with AIDS. Am J Gastroenterol 84:1288–1293
20. Scevola D, Barbarini G, Zambelli A et al (1989) Nutritional status in AIDS patients. 5th International Conference on AIDS, Montreal, Abstracts Book, p 465
21. Scevola D, Barbarini G, Zambelli A et al (1990) Evaluation and therapy of malnutrition in enteropathogenic AIDS. 6th International Conference on AIDS, San Francisco, California, Abstracts Book, p 168
22. Scevola D, Zambelli A, Bottari G et al (1991) Appetite stimulation and body weight gain with medroxyprogesterone acetate in AIDS anorexia and cachexia. Farmaci e Terapia 3:77–83
23. Scevola D, Barbarini G, Bottari G et al (1991) Prevalence, etiology and management of AIDS malnutrition. 7th International Conference on AIDS, Florence, Abstracts Book, WB 2169
24. Scevola D, Bottari G, Zambelli A et al (1992) Trattamento dietetico ed ormonale dei deficits nutrizionali nell'AIDS. Clin Dietol 19:127–140
25. Scevola D (1993) La cachessia nelle malattie infettive e neoplastiche. Edizioni Medico Scientifiche, Pavia
26. Scevola D, Bottari G, Faggi A et al (1994) Palliative care in infectious diseases. Eur J Pall Care 1:88–91
27. Anonymous (1989) Malnutrition and weight loss in patients with AIDS. Nutr Rev 11:354–356
28. Melchior JC, Salmon D, Rigaud D et al (1991) Resting energy expenditure is increased in stable, malnourished HIV-infected patients. Am J Clin Nutr 53:437–441
29. Kotler DP, Tierney AR, Dilmanian FA et al (1991) Correlation between total body potassium and total body nitrogen in patients with acquired immunodeficiency syndrome. Clin Res 39:649A
30. Bogden JD, Baker H, Frank O et al (1990) Micronutrient status and HIV infection. Ann NY Acad Sci 587:189–195
31. Coodley G (1990) Nutritional deficiency and AIDS. Ann Intern Med 113:807
32. Coodley GO, Loveless MO, Merrill TM (1994) The HIV wasting syndrome: a review. J Acquir Immune Defic Syndr 7:681–694
33. Baum M, Cassetti L, Bonvehi P et al (1994) Inadequate dietary intake and altered nutrition sta-

tus in early HIV-1 infection. Nutrition 10:16–20

34. Timbo BB, Tollefson L (1994) Nutrition: a cofactor in HIV disease. J Am Diet Assoc 94:1019–1022

35. Macallan DC, Noble C, Baldwin C et al (1995) Energy expenditure and wasting in human immunodeficiency virus infection. N Engl J Med 333:83–88

36. Kotler DP, Wang J, Pierson R (1985) Studies of body composition in patients with the acquired immunodeficiency syndrome. Am J Clin Nutr 42:1255–1265

37. Cahill GF (1979) Starvation in man. N Engl J Med 282:668–675

38. Brennen MF (1977) Uncomplicated starvation versus cancer cachexia. Cancer Res 37:2359–2364

39. Grunfeld C, Feingold KR (1992) Metabolic disturbances and wasting in the acquired immunodeficiency syndrome. N Engl J Med 5:329–337

40. Wolfe RR, Shaw JH, Durkot MJ (1985) Effect of sepsis on VLDL kinetics: responses in basal state and during glucose infusion. Am J Physiol 248:E732–E740

41. Scevola D, Barbarini G, Bottari G et al (1990) Nutritional management of enteropathogenic human immunodeficiency virus infection. Eur J Gastroenterol Hepatol 2(S1):S100–S101

42. Sharkey SJ, Sharkey KA, Sutherland LR et al (1992) Nutritional status and food intake in human immunodeficiency virus infection. GI/HIV Study Group. J Acquir Immune Defic Syndr 5:1091–1098

43. Coodley GO, Loveless MO, Nelson HD, Coodley MK (1994) Endocrine dysfunction in the HIV wasting syndrome. J Acquir Immune Defic Syndr 7:46–51

44. Hellerstein MK, Khan J, Mudie H, Viteri F (1990) Current approach to the treatment of human immunodeficiency virus-associated weight loss: pathophysiologic considerations and emerging management strategies. Semin Oncol 17(Suppl 9):17–33

45. Tracey KJ, Morgello S, Koplin B et al (1990) Metabolic effects of cachectin/tumor necrosis factor are modified by site of production. J Clin Invest 86:2014–2024

46. Feingold KR, Soued M, Serio MK et al (1990) The effect of diet on tumor necrosis factor stimulation of hepatic lipogenesis. Metabolism 39:623–632

47. Hellerstein MK, Meydani SN et al (1989) Interleukin-1-induced anorexia in the rat. Influence of prostaglandins. J Clin Invest 84:228–235

48. Langstein HN, Doherty GM, Fraker DL et al (1991) The role of interferon gamma and tumor necrosis factor in an experimental rat model of cancer cachexia. Cancer Res 51:2302–2306

49. Carr A, Samaras K, Thorisdottir A et al (1999) Diagnosis, prediction and natural course of HIV protease inhibitor-associated lipodystrophy, hyperlipidaemia, and diabetes mellitus. Lancet 353:2093–2099

50. Safrin S, Grunfeld C (1999) Fat distribution and metabolic changes in patients with HIV infection. AIDS 13:2494–2505

51. Nemechek PM, Polsky B, Gottlieb MS (2000) Treatment guidelines for HIV-associated wasting. Mayo Clin Proc 75:386–394

52. Melchior JC, Salmon D, Rigaud D et al (1991) Resting energy expenditure is increased in stable, malnourished HIV-infected patients. Am J Clin Nutr 53:437–441

53. Melchior JC, Raguin G, Boulier A et al (1993) Resting energy expenditure in human immunodeficiency virus infected patients: comparison between patients with and without secondary infection. Am J Clin Nutr 57:614–619

54. Anonymous (1994) Position of The American Dietetic Association and the Canadian Dietetic Association: nutrition intervention in the care of persons with human immunodeficiency virus infection. J Am Diet Assoc 94:1042–1045

55. Harris JA, Benedict FG (1919) A biometric study of basal metabolism in man. Washington DC Carnegie Institution, Washington DC, p 227

56. Udine LM (1990) Home nutritional support and AIDS. In: Proceedings of the American Society for Parenteral and Enteral Nutrition. Fourteenth Clinical Congress, January 28–31 San Antonio, Texas, pp 311–314

57. Wilmore DW (1991) Catabolic illness: strategies for enancing recovery. N Engl J Med 325:695–702

58. Tisdale MJ, Beck SA (1991) Inhibition of tumour-induced lipolysis in vitro and cachexia and tumour growth in vivo by eicosapentaenoic acid. Biochem Pharmacol 41:103–107

59. Scevola D, Oberto L, Bottari G, Faggi A (1995) Lipidi e malattie infettive. XII Congresso Nazionale ADI, Torino 16–18/11/1995, Abstracts Book, p 187

60. Beck SA, Tisdale MJ (1989) Nitrogen excretion in cancer cachexia and its modification by a high fat diet in mice. Cancer Res 49:3800–3804

61. Tisdale MJ, Dhesi JK (1990) Inhibition of weight loss by omega-3 fatty acids in an experimental cachexia model. Cancer Res 50:5022–5026

62. Fearon KC, Borland W, Preston T et al (1988) Cancer cachexia: influence of systemic ketosis on substrate levels and nitrogen metabolism. Am J Clin Nutr 47:42–48

63. Kardinal CG, Loprinzi CL, Schaid DJ et al (1990) A controlled trial of cyproheptadine in cancer patients with anorexia and/or cachexia. Cancer 65:2657–2662

64. Nobel RE (1969) Effect of cyproheptadine on appetite and weight gain in adults. JAMA 209:2054–2055

65. Scevola D, Zambelli A, Bottari G et al (1991) Appetite stimulation and body weight gain with medroxyprogesterone acetate in AIDS anorexia and cachexia. Farmaci e Terapia 3:77–83

66. Scevola D, Parazzini F, Negri C, Moroni M (1995) Efficacy and safety of high-dose MPA treatment of AIDS cachexia: the Italian multicentre study. In: Proceedings of 4th Congress of the European Association for Palliative Care, Barcelona, December

6–9-1995, pp 443–447

67. Von Roenn JH (1994) Management of HIV-related body weight loss. Drugs 47:774–783

68. Scevola D, Bottari G, Oberto L et al (1995) A double-blind-placebo controlled trial of megestrol acetate on caloric intake and nutritional status in AIDS cachexia. In: Proceedings of 4th Congress of European Association for Palliative Care, Barcelona, December 6–9-1995, pp 427–437

69. Tchekmedyian NS, Hichman M, Heber D (1991) Treatment of anorexia and weight loss with megestrol acetate in patients with cancer and aquired Immunodeficiency Syndrome. Semin Oncol 18:35–42

70. Rondanelli M, Solerte SB, Fioravanti M et al (1997) Circadian secretory pattern of growth hormone, insulin-like growth factor type I, cortisol, adreno-corticotropic hormone, thyroid-stimulating hormone, and prolactin during HIV infection. AIDS Res Hum Retroviruses 14:1243–1249

71. Scevola D, Bottari G, Oberto L et al (1995) Megestrol acetate (MA) and growth hormone (rhGH) as combined therapy for AIDS cachexia. In: Proceedings of 4th Congress of European Association for Palliative Care, Barcelona, December 6–9-1995, pp 438–442

72. Douglas RG, Humberstone DA, Haystead A, Shaw JH (1990) Metabolic effects of recombinant human growth hormone: isotopic studies in the postabsorptive state during total parenteral nutrition. Br J Surg 77:785–790

73. Haller DG, Glick JG (1986) Progestational agents in advanced breast cancer: an overview. Semin Oncol 13:2–8

74. Grunfeld C (1991) Mechanisms of wasting in infection and cancer: an approach to cachexia in AIDS. In: Kotler DP (ed) Gastrointestinal and nutritional manifestations of AIDS. Raven Press, New York, pp 207–229

75. Hellerstein MK, Kahn J, Mudie H, Viteri F (1990) Current approach to the treatment of human immunodeficiency virus-associated weight loss: pathophysiologic consideration and emerging management strategies. Semin Oncol 17:17–33

76. Von Roenn JH, Murphy RI, Weber KM et al (1988) Megestrol acetate for treatment of cachexia associated with human immunodeficiency virus (HIV) infection. Ann Intern Med 109:840–841

77. Von Roenn JH, Armstrong D, Kotler DP et al (1994) Megestral acetate in patients with AIDS. Ann Intern Med 121:393–399

78. Von Roenn JH, Murphy RL, Wegener N (1990) Megestrol acetate for treatment of anorexia and cachexia associated with human immunodeficiency virus infection. Semin Oncol 17:13–16

79. Oster MH, Enders SR, Samuels SJ et al (1994) Megestrol acetate in patients with AIDS and cachexia. Ann Intern Med 121:400–408

80. Scevola D, Zambelli A, Bottari G et al (1991) Appetite stimulation and body weight gain with medrox-yprogesterone acetate in AIDS anorexia and cachexia. Farmaci e Terapia 3:77–83

81. Vonn Roenn JH, Armstrong D, Kotler DP et al (1994) Megestrol acetate in patients with AIDS related cachexia. Ann Intern Med 121:393–399

82. Giacosa A, Fascio F, Sukkar SG et al (1993) Megestrolo e anoressia neoplastica. ADI Notiziario 11 Congresso Nazionale Nutrizione e Cancro, Suppl 2:68–69

83. Scevola D, Bottari G, Oberto L (1992) Changes in caloric intake, anthropometric parameters and TNF levels induced by megestrol acetate in AIDS patients. 8th International Conference on AIDS, Abstracts Book, p 133, PUB 7505

84. Lyons PM, Truswell AS, Mira M et al (1989) Reduction of food intake in the ovulatory phase of menstrual cycle. Am J Clin Nutr 49:1164–1168

85. Bruera E, MacMillan K, Kuehm N et al (1990) A controlled trial of megestrol acetate on appetite, caloric intake, nutritional status and other symptoms in patients with advanced cancer. Cancer 66:1279–1282

86. Oster MH, Enders SR, Samuels SJ et al (1994) Megestrol acetate in cachectic patients with AIDS. Ann Intern Med 121:400–408

87. Davidson MB (1987) Effect of growth hormone on carbohydrate and lipid metabolism. Endocr Rev 8:115–131

88. Salomon F, Cuneo RC, Hesp R, Sonksen PH (1989) The effects of treatment with recombinant human growth hormone on body composition and metabolism in adults with growth hormone deficiency. N Engl J Med 321:1797–1803

89. Bengtsson BA, Eden S, Lonn L et al (1993) Treatment of adults with growth hormone (GH) deficiency with recombinant human GH. J Clin Endocrinol Metab 76:309–317

90. Cruz JM, Muss HB, Brockschmidt JK, Evans GW (1990) Weight changes in women with metastatic breast cancer treated with megestrol acetate: a comparison of standard versus high dose therapy. Semin Oncol 17 (S9):63–67

91. Tchkmedyian NS, Hichman M, Herber D (1991) Treatment of anorexia and weight loss with megestrol acetate in patients with cancer and acquired immunodeficiency syndrome. Semin Oncol 18:35–42

92. Grunfeld C, Feingold KR (1992) Metabolic disturbances and wasting in the acquired immunodeficiency syndrome. N Engl J Med 327:329–337

93. Kotler DP, Wang J, Pierson Jr RN (1985) Body composition studies in patients with the acquired immunodeficiency syndrome. Am J Clin Nutr 42:1255–1265

94. Kotler DP, Tiernay AR, Wang J, Pierson Jr RN (1989) Magnitude of body cell mass depletion and the timing of death from wasting in AIDS. Am J Clin Nutr 50:444–447

95. Scevola D (1993) La cachessia nelle malattie infettive e neoplastiche. Tipografia Viscontea, Pavia, Italy

96. Mulligan K, Grunfeld C, Hellerstein MK et al (1993) Anabolic effects of recombinant human growth hormone in patients wiyh wasting associated with human immunodeficiency virus infection. J Clin Endocrinol Metab 77:956–962

97. Krentz AJ, Koster FT, Crist DM et al (1993) Anthropometric, metabolic and immunological effects of recombinant human growth hormone in AIDS and AIDS-related complex. J Acquir Immune Defic Syndr 19:245–251

98. Rudman D, Feller AG, Nagraj HS et al (1990) Effects of human growth hormone in men over 60 years. N Engl J Med 323:1–6

99. Benavides S, Nahata MC (2004) Pharmacologic therapy for HIV-associated lipodystrophy. Ann Pharmacother 38:448–457

100. Ross R, Dagnone D, Jones PJ et al (2000) Reduction in obesity and related comorbid conditions after diet-induced weight loss or exercise-induced weight loss in men. A randomized, controlled trial. Ann Intern Med 133:92–103

101. Moyle G, Baldwin C, Phillipot M (2001) Managing metabolic disturbances and lipodystrophy: diet, exercise, and smoking advice. AIDS Read 11:589–592

102. Hadigan C, Jeste S, Anderson EJ et al (2001) Modifiable dietary habitus and their relation to metabolic abnormalities in men and women with human immunodeficiency virus infection and fat redistribution. Clin Infect Dis 33:710–717

103. Roubenoff R, Schmitz H, Bairos L et al (2002) Reduction of abdominal obesity in lipodystrophy associated with immunodeficiency virus infection by means of diet and exercise: case report and proof of principle. Clin Infect Dis 34:390–393

104. Barrios A, Blanco F, Garcia-Benayas T et al (2002) Effect of dietary intervention on highly active antiretroviral therapy related dislipemia. AIDS 16:2079–2081

105. Scevola D, DiMatteo A, Lanzarini P et al (2003) Effect of exercise and strength training on cardiovascular status in HIV-infected patients receiving highly active antiretroviral therapy. AIDS 17(S1):123–129

106. Scevola D, DiMatteo A, Giglio O et al (2004) Guidelines for the prevention of cardiovascular risk in HIV-infected patients treated with antiretroviral drugs. HIV&AIDS Review 3:177–184

107. McCarty MF (2003) Iatrogenic lipodystrophy in HIV patients. The need for very low fat diets. Med Hypotheses 61:561–566

108. McComsey G, Lederman M (2002) High doses of riboflavin and thiamine may help secondary prevention of hyperlactatemia. AIDS Read 12:222–224

109. De la Asuncion J, Del Olmo M, Sastre J et al (1998) AZT treatment induces molecular and ultrastructural oxidative damage to muscle mitochondria. Prevention by antioxidant vitamins. J Clin Invest 102:4–9

110. Paulik M, Lancaster M, Croom D et al (2000) Antioxidant rescue NRTI-induced metabolic changes in AKR/J mice. Antivir Ther 5:6–7

111. Fouty B, Frerman F, Reves R (1998) Riboflavin to treat nucleoside analogue-induced lactic acidosis. Lancet 352:291–292

112. Brinkman K, Vrouenrats S, Kauffman R et al (2000) Treatment of nucleoside reverse transcriptase inhibitor-induced lactic acidosis. AIDS 14:2801–2802

113. Luzzati R, Del Bravo P, Di Perri G et al (1999) Riboflavin and severe lactic acidosis. Lancet 353:901–902

114. Schramm C, Wanitschke R, Galle P (1999) Thiamine for the treatment of nucleoside analogue- induced severe lactic acidosis. Eur J Anaesthesiol 16:733–735

115. Gold D, Cohen B (2001) Treatment of mitochondrial cytopathies. Semin Neurol 21:309–325

116. Claessens Y, Cariou A, Chiche J et al (2000) L-carnitine as a treatment of life-threatening lactic acidosis induced by nucleoside analogues. AIDS 14:472–473

117. Scevola D, Oberto L, Bottari G, Faggi A (1995) Lipidi e Malattie Infettive. XII Congresso Nazionale ADI. Torino 16–18/11/1995, Abstracts Book, p 187

118. Scevola D, Bottari G, Oberto L, Faggi A (1996) AIDS cachexia: basics and treatment. In: Ruf B, Pohle HD, Goebel FD, L'age M (eds) HIV-Infektion, Pathogenese, Diagnostik und Therapie. Sociomedico Verlag, Graefelfing, pp 281–327

119. Scevola D, Bottari G, Oberto L et al (1996) Problemi nutrizionali del paziente AIDS e strategie terapeutiche. Quaderni di Cure Palliative S1:51–64

120. Schwartz RS, Shuman WP, Larson V et al (1991) The effect of intensive endurance exercise training on body fat distribution in young and older men. Metabolism 40:545–551

121. Roubenoff R, McDermott A, Weiss L et al (1999) Short-term progressive resistance training increases strength and lean body mass in adults infected with human immunodeficiency virus. AIDS 13:231–239

122. Roubenoff R, Weiss L, McDermott A et al (1999) A pilot study of exercise training to reduce trunk fat in adults with HIV-associated fat redistribution. AIDS 13:1373–1375

123. Jaque S, Schroeder E, Azen S et al (2002) Regional body composition changes during anabolic therapy. Clin Exerc Physiol 4:50–59

124. Saint-Marc T, Touraine JL (1999) Effects of metformin on insulin resistence and central adiposity in patients receiving effective protease inhibitor therapy. AIDS 13:1000–1002

125. Hadigan C, Corcoran C, Basgoz N et al (2000) Metformin in the treatment of HIV lipodystrophy syndrome: a randomized controlled trial. JAMA 284:472–477

126. Mulligan K, Grunfeld C, Hellerstein MK et al (1993) Anabolic effects of recombinant growth hormone in patients with wasting associated with human immunodeficiency virus infection. J Clin

Endocrinol Metab 77:956–962

127. Schambelan M, Mulligan K, Grunfeld C et al (1996) Recombinant human growth hormone in patients with HIV-associated wasting: a randomized, placebo-controlled trial. Serostim Study Group. Ann Intern Med 125:873–882

128. Torres RA, Unger KW, Cadman JA, Kassous JY (1999) Recombinant human growth hormone improves truncal adiposity and 'buffalo humps' in HIV-positive patients on HAART. AIDS 13:2479–2481

129. Wanke C, Gerrior J, Kantaros J et al (1999) Recombinant human growth hormone improves the fat redistribution syndrome (lipodystrophy) in patients with HIV. AIDS 13:2099–2103

130. Schwarz JM, Mulligan K, Lee J et al (2002) Effects of recombinant human growth hormone on hepatic lipid and carbohydrate metabolism in HIV-infected patients with fat accumulation. J Clin Endocrinol Metab 87:942

131. Koutkia P, Canavan B, Breu J et al (2004) Growth hormone-releasing hormone in HIV-infected men with lipodystrophy: a randomized controlled trial. JAMA 292:210–218

132. Zhang Y, Proenca R, Maffei M et al (1994) Positional cloning of the mouse obese gene and human homologue. Nature 372:425–432

133. Halaas JL, Gajiwala KS, Maffei M et al (1995) Weight-reducing effects of the plasma protein encoded by the obese gene. Science 269:543–546

134. Ahima RS, Prabakaran D, Mantzoros C et al (1996) Role of leptin in the neuroendocrine response to fasting. Nature 382:250–252

135. Ahima RS, Flier JS (2000) Leptin. Annu Rev Physiol 62:413–437

136. Friedman JM, Halaas JL (1998) Leptin and the regulation of body weight in mammals. Nature 395:763–770

137. Friedman JM (2004) Modern science versus the stigma of obesity. Nat Med 10:563–569

138. Faggioni R, Feingold KR, Grunfeld C (2001) Leptin regulation of the immune response and the immunodeficiency of malnutrition. FASEB J 15:2565–2571

139. Spiegelman BM, Flier JS (2001) Obesity and the regulation of energy balance. Cell 104:531–543

140. Oral EA, Ruiz E, Andewelt A et al (2002) Effect of leptin replacement on pituitary hormone regulation in patients with severe lipodystrophy. J Clin Endocrinol Metab 87:3110–3117

141. McDuffie JR, Riggs PA, Calis K et al (2004) Effects of exogenous leptin on satiety and satiation in patients with lipodystrophy and leptin insufficiency. J Clin Endocrinol Metab 89:4258–4263

142. Moran SA, Patten N, Young JR et al (2004) Changes in body composition in patients with severe lipodystrophy after leptin replacement therapy. Metabolism 53:513–519

143. Moyle G, Baldwin C (2000) Switching from a PI-based to a PI-sparing regimen for management of metabolic or clinical fat redistribution. AIDS Read 10:479–485

144. Vigouroux C, Gharakhanian S, Salhi Y et al (1999) Adverse metabolic disorders during highly active antiretroviral treatments (HAART) of HIV disease. Diabetes Metab 25:383–392

145. Behrens GM, Stoll M, Schmidt RE (2000) Lipodystrophy syndrome in HIV infection: what is it, what causes it and how can it be managed? Drug Saf 23:57–76

146. Mallal SA, John M, Moore CB et al (2000) Contribution of nucleoside analogue revers transcriptase inhibitors to subcutaneous fat wasting in patients with HIV infection. AIDS 14:1309–1316

147. Kakuda TN (2000) Pharmacology of nucleoside and nucleotide reverse transcriptase inhibitor-induced mitochondrial toxicity. Clin Ther 22:685–708

148. Carr A, Workman C, Smith DE et al (2002) Abacavir substitution for nucleoside analogs in patients with lipoatrophy. JAMA 288:207–215

149. McComsey GA, Ward DJ, Hessenthaler SM et al (2004) Improvement in lipoatrophy associated with highly active antiretroviral therapy in human immunodefiency virus-infected patients switched from stavudine to abacavir or zidovudine: the results of the TARHEEL study. Clin Infect Dis 38:263–270

150. Martin A, Smith DE, Carr A et al (2004) Reversibility of lipoatrophy in HIV-infected patients 2 years after switching from a thymidine analogue to abacavir : the MITOS Extension Study. AIDS 18:1029–1036

151. Strauch B, Baum T, Robbins N (2004) Treatment of human immunodeficiency virus-associated lipodystrophy with dermafat graft transfer to the malar area. Plast Reconstr Surg 113:363–370

152. Connolly N, Manders E, Riddler S (2004) Suction-assisted lilectomy for lipodystrophy. AIDS Res Hum Retroviruses 20:813–815

153. Amerd P, Saint-Marc T, Katz P (2000) The effects of polylactic acid as therapy for lipodystrophy of the face. Antivir Ther 5 (Suppl 5):76

154. Moyle G, Baldwin C (2002) Management of morphologic changes during antiretroviral therapy: insights from etiology. HIV/AIDS Update 2002, iMedOptions, LLC

155. Ponce-de-Leon S, Iglesias M, Ceballos J et al (1999) Liposuction for protease-inhibitor associated lipodystrophy. Lancet 353:1244

156. Wolffort FG, Cetrulo CL, Nevarre DR (1999) Suction-assisted lipectomy for lipodystrophy syndromes attributed to HIV-protease inhibitor use. Plast Reconstr Surg 104:1814–1820

157. Henry K, Melroe H, Huebesh J et al (1999) Experience with the National Cholesterol Education Program (NCEP) guidelines for the identification and treatment of protease inhibitor related lipid abnormalities: results of a prospective study. 6th Conference on Retroviruses and Opportunistic Infections, Chicago, Abstract 671

158. Grunfeld C, Feingold KR (1992) Metabolic disturbances and wasting in the acquired immunodeficiency syndrome. N Engl J Med 5:329–337

159. Lonergan JT, Havlir D, Barber E, Mathews WC (2001) Incidence and outcome of hyperlactatemia associated with clinical manifestations in HIV-infected adults receiving NRTI-containing regimens. 8th Conference on Retroviruses and Opportunistic Infections, February 4–8–2001, Chicago, Abstract 624

160. Johnson JA, Albu JB, Engelson ES et al (2004) Increased systemic and adipose tissue cytokines in patients with HIV-associated lipodystrophy. Am J Physiol Endocrinol Metab 286:E261–E271

161. Scevola D, Di Matteo A, Uberti F et al (2000) Reversal of cachexia in patients treated with potent antiretroviral therapy. AIDS Read 10:365–375

162. Henry K, Zackin R, Dube M et al (2001) Metabolic status and cardiovascular disease risk for a cohort of HIV-1-infected persons durably suppressed on an indinavir-containing regimen (ACTG 372A). Program and abstracts of the 8th Conference on Retroviruses and Opportunistic Infections, February 4–8–2001, Chicago, Abstract 656

163. Melchior JC, Salmon D, Rigaud D et al (1991) Resting energy expenditure is increased in stable, malnourished HIV-infected patients. Am J Clin Nutr 53:437–441

164. Grunfeld C, Pang M, Shimizu L et al (1992) Resting energy expenditure, caloric intake and short-term weight change in human immunodeficiency virus infection and the acquired immuno-deficiency syndrome. Am J Clin Nutr 55:455–460

165. Shevitz AH (2000) Resting energy expenditure in the HAART era. AIDS Read 10:539–544

166. Anonymous (1986) Use and interpretation of anthropometric indicators of nutritional status. WHO Working Group. Bulletin of the WHO 64:929–941

167. Kotler DP, Rosenbaum K, Wang J, Pearson RN (1999) Studies of body composition and fat distribution in HIV-infected and control subjects. J Acquir Immune Defic Syndr Hum Retrovirol 20:228–237

168. Scevola D (1993) La cachessia nelle malattie infettive e neoplastiche. Edizioni Medico Scientifiche, Pavia

169. Expert Panel on Detection, Evaluation, and Treatment of High Blood Cholesterol in Adults (2001) Executive Summary of The Third Report of The National Cholesterol Education Program (NCEP) Expert Panel on Detection, Evaluation, and Treatment of High Blood Cholesterol in Adults (Adult Treatment Panel III). JAMA 285:2486–2497

170. Scevola D, Di Matteo A, Lanzarini P et al (2003) Effect of exercise and strength training on cardiovascular status in HIV-infected patients receiving highly active antiretroviral therapy. AIDS 17(Suppl 1):S123–S129

171. Volberding PA, Murphy RL, Barbaro G et al (2003) The Pavia consensus statement. AIDS 17(Suppl 1):S170–S179

172. Dubé MP, Stein JH, Aberg JA et al (2003) Guidelines for the evaluation and management of dyslipidemia in human immunodeficiency virus (HIV)-infected adults receiving antiretroviral therapy: recommendations of the HIV Medicine Association of the Infectious Disease Society of America and the Adult AIDS clinical trials group. Clin Infect Dis 37:613–627

173. Barrios A, Blanco F, Garcìa-Benayas T et al (2002) Effect of dietary intervention on highly active antiretroviral therapy-related dyslipemia. AIDS 16:2079–2081

174. Von Roenn JH (1994) Management of HIV-related body weight loss. Drugs 47:774–783

175. Scevola D, Bottari G, Zambelli A et al (1992) Trattamento dietetico ed ormonale dei deficit nutrizionali nell'AIDS. Clin Dietol 19:127–140

176. Bernasconi E (1999) Metabolic effects of protease inhibitor therapy. AIDS Read 9:254–269

177. Tisdale M, Beck SA (1991) Inhibition of tumour induced lipolysis in vitro and cachexia and tumour growth in vivo by eicosapentaenoic acid. Biochem Pharmacol 41:103–107

178. Kardinal CG, Loprinzi CL, Schaid DJ et al (1990) A controlled trial of cyproheptadine in cancer patients with anorexia and/or cachexia. Cancer 65:2657–2662

179. Scevola D, Zambelli A, Bottari G et al (1991) Appetite stimulation and body weight gain with medroxyprogesterone acetate in AIDS anorexia and cachexia. Farmaci e Terapia 3:77–83

180. Scevola D, Parazzini F, Negri C, Moroni M (1995) Efficacy and safety of high-dose MPA treatment of AIDS cachexia: the Italian multicentre study. 4th Congress of the European Association for Palliative Care, Barcelona, December 6–9–1995, Abstracts Book, pp 443–447

181. Scevola D, Bottari G, Oberto L et al (1995) A double-blind-placebo controlled trial of megestrol acetate on caloric intake and nutritional status in AIDS cachexia. 4th Congress of European Association for Palliative Care, Barcelona, December 6–9–1995, Abstracts Book, pp 427–437

182. Rondanelli M, Solerte SB, Fioravanti M et al (1997) Circadian secretory pattern of growth hormone, insulin-like growth factor type I, cortisol, adrenocorticotropic hormone, thyroid-stimulating hormone, and prolactin during HIV infection. AIDS Res Hum Retroviruses 14:1243–1249

183. Scevola D, Bottari G, Oberto L et al (1995) Megestrol acetate (MA) and growth hormone (rHGH) as combined therapy for AIDS cachexia. 4th Congress of European Association for Palliative Care, Barcelona, December 6–9–1995, Abstracts Book, pp 438–442

184. Wanke C, Gerrior J, Kantaros J et al (1999) Recombinant human growth hormone improves the fat redistribution syndrome (lipodystrophy) in patients with HIV. AIDS 13:2099–2103

185. Henry K, Melroe H, Huebesh J et al (1999) Experience with the National Cholesterol Education

Program (NCEP) guidelines for the identification and treatment of protease inhibitor related lipid abnormalities: results of a prospective study. 6th Conference on Retroviruses and Opportunistic Infections, Chicago, Abstract 671

186. Saint-Marc T, Touraine JL (1999) Effects of metformin on insulin resistance and central adiposity in patients receiving effective protease inhibitor (PI). 6th Conference on Retroviruses and Opportunistic Infections, Chicago, Abstract 672

187. Walli RK, Michl GM, Muhlbayer D et al (2000) Effects of troglitazone on insulin sensitivity in HIV-infected patients with protease inhibitor-associated diabetes mellitus. Res Exp Med (Ber) 199:253–262

188. Calmy A, Hirschel B, Hans D et al (2003) Glitazones in lipodystrophy syndrome induced highly active antiretroviral therapy. AIDS 17:770–772

189. Carr A, Workman C, Carey D et al (2004) No effect of rosiglitazone for treatment of HIV-1 lipoatrophy: randomised, double-blind, placebo-controlled trial. Lancet 363:429–438

190. Torres R, Unger K (1999) The effect of recombinant human growth hormone on protease-inhibitor associated fat maldistribution syndrome. 6th Conference on Retroviruses and Opportunistic Infections, Chicago, Abstract 675

191. Strawford A, Barbieri T, Parks E et al (1999) Resistance exercise and supraphysiologic androgen therapy in eugonadal men with HIV-related weight loss. JAMA 281:1282–1290

192. Amsterdam EA (1977) Exercise in cardiovascular health and disease. Yorke Medical Books, New York

193. Smith BA, Neidig JL, Nickel JT et al (2001) Aerobic exercise: effects on parameters related to fatigue, dyspnea, weight and body composition in HIV-infected adults. AIDS 15:693–701

194. Montoye HJ (1975) Physical activity and health: an epidemiologic study of an entire community. Englewood Cliffs, NJ Prentice-Hall

195. Katch FI, Freedson PS, Jones CA et al (1985) Evaluation of acute cardiorespiratory responses to hydraulic resistance exercise. Medicine and Science in Sports and Exercise 17:168–173

196. Crow RS, Rantahargiu PM, Prineas RJ et al (1986) Risk factors, exercise fitness and electrocardiographic response to exercise in 12,866 men at risk of symptomatic coronary heart disease. Am J Cardiol 57:1075–1082

197. Barbaro, Giuseppe; Boccara, Franck (eds) (2005) Cardiovascular disease in AIDS. Springer, Milan

198. Pollock M, Gaesser G, Butcher J et al (1998) The recommended quantity and quality of exercise for developing and maintaining cardiorespiratory and muscular fitness, and flexibility in healthy adults. Med Sci Sports Exerc 30:975–991

199. Stringer WW, Berezovskaya M, O'Brien WA et al (1998) The effect of exercise training on aerobic fitness, immune indices, and quality of life in HIV+ patients. Med Sci Sports Exerc 30:11–16

200. Grinspoon S, Carr A (2005) Cardiovascular risk and body-fat abnormalities in HIV-infected adults. N Engl J Med 352:48–62

# SECTION 9
# CANCER-RELATED CACHEXIA

# Cancer Cachexia and Fat Metabolism

Josep M. Argilés, Vanessa Almendro, Sílvia Busquets, Francisco J. López-Soriano

## Introduction

Cancer cachexia is one of the worst effects of malignancy, accounting for nearly a third of cancer deaths. It is a pathological state characterised by weight loss together with anorexia, weakness, anaemia, and asthaenia. The complications associated with the appearance of the cachectic syndrome affect both the physiological and biochemical balance of the patient and influence the efficiency of anticancer treatment, resulting in a considerably decreased survival time. At the metabolic level, cachexia is associated with loss of body lipid stores. Alterations in lipid metabolism are partially mediated by changes in circulating hormone concentrations (insulin, glucagon, and glucocorticoids, in particular) or in their effectiveness. However, a large number of observations point towards cytokines, polypeptides released mainly by immune cells, as the molecules responsible for the above-mentioned metabolic derangements. The role of humoral factors in fat metabolism in the cancer patient has been discussed; among cytokines, tumour necrosis factor-$\alpha$ (TNF-$\alpha$) seems to have a key role in the lipid metabolic changes associated with cancer cachexia.

## Adipose Tissue Dissolution and Hypertriglyceridaemia

Lipid metabolism in cancer has been extensively studied, the main features being an important reduction in body fat content (particularly white adipose tissue) and a significant hyperlipaemia. Dissolution of the fat mass is the result of three different altered processes. First, there is an increase in lipolytic activity [1], which results in the release of large amounts of glycerol and fatty acids. Glycerol is basically directed to the liver, where it provides a gluconeogenic substrate, while fatty acids are used by other tissues as an alternative substrate to glucose. Interestingly, the oxidation of fatty acids is not suppressed by glucose [2], as opposed to what is observed during starvation, in which the rate of fatty acid oxidation is normalised by glucose administration. Although fatty acids seem to be a very poor substrate for very undifferentiated, malignant tumour cells, some studies have demonstrated that polyunsaturated fatty acids (linoleic and arachidonic acids) are able to promote tumour growth by stimulating mitosis [3]. These compounds seem to inactivate the GTPase-activating protein of the ras-mediated signal transduction pathways, thus stimulating cell division [3]. Second, an important decrease in the activity of lipoprotein lipase (LPL), the enzyme responsible for the cleavage of both endogenous and exogenous triacylglycerols (present in lipoproteins) into glycerol and fatty acids, occurs in white adipose tissue [1, 4, 5]; consequently, lipid uptake is severely hampered. Finally, de novo lipogenesis in adipose tissue is also reduced in tumour-bearing states [1], resulting in decreased esterification and, consequently, decreased lipid deposition.

Hyperlipaemia in cancer-bearing states seems to be the result of an elevation in triacylglycerols and cholesterol. Hypertriglyceridaemia is the consequence of decreased LPL activity, which results in a decrease in the plasma clearance of both endogenous (transported as very-low-density lipoproteins, VLDL) and exogenous (transported as chylomicra) triacylglycerols. Muscaritoli et al. [6] clearly demonstrated that the fractional removal rate and the maximum clearing capacity (calculated at high infusion rates, when LPL activity is saturated) are significantly decreased after the administration of an exogenous triacylglycerol load to cancer patients. In tumour-bearing animals with a high degree of cachexia, there is also an important association between decreased LPL activity and hypertriglyceridaemia [7, 8] (Fig. 1). Another factor that could contribute to the elevation in circulating triacylglycerols is an increase in liver lipogenesis [9].

Hypercholesterolaemia is often seen in tumour-bearing animals and in humans with cancer [10–12]. Interestingly, most cancer cells show an altered regulation in cholesterol biosynthesis, with a lack of feedback control on HMG-CoA reductase (3-hydroxy-3-methyl glutaryl CoA reductase), the key enzyme in the regulation of cholesterol biosynthesis. Cholesterol perturbations during cancer include changes in lipoprotein profiles, in particular an important decrease in the amount of cholesterol transported in the high-density lipoprotein (HDL) fraction. This has been observed in both experimental animals and human subjects [10–12]. HDL plays an important role in the transport of excess cholesterol from extrahepatic tissues to the liver for reutilisation or excretion into bile (reverse cholesterol transport). It is thus conceivable that the observed low levels of HDL-cholesterol are related, at least in part, to a decreased cholesterol efflux to HDL, as a consequence of increased utilisation and/or storage in proliferating tissues, such as neoplasms. However, since precursor particles of HDL are thought to derive from lipolysis of triacylglycerol-rich lipoproteins, such as VLDL and chylomicra [13], and since a significant positive correlation between plasma HDL-cholesterol and LPL activity in adipose tissue has been reported [13], the possibility that the low HDL-cholesterol concentrations observed during tumour growth are secondary to the decreased triacylglycerol clearance from plasma, as a result of LPL inhibition, must also be considered.

The elevation of circulating lipid therefore seems to be a hallmark of cancer-bearing states, to the extent that some authors have suggested that plasma levels can be used to screen patients for cancer [14].

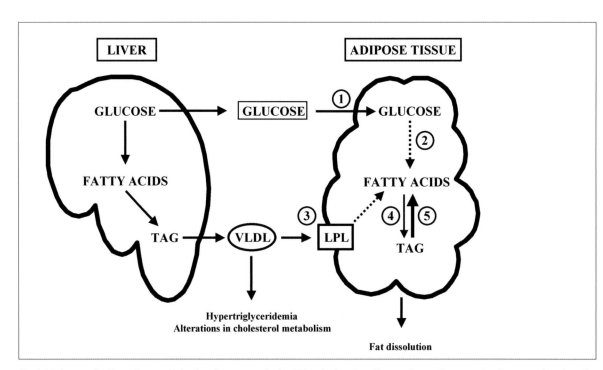

**Fig. 1.** Main metabolic pathways linked to fat accumulation/dissolution in adipose tissue. As a result of tumour burden, fat loss is accelerated due to: (1) decreased glucose uptake, (2) decreased fatty acid synthesis, (3) decreased triacylglycerol uptake through LPL, (4) decreased esterification, and (5) increased lipolysis. Enhanced hepatic production of VLDL, together with its reduced clearance contributes to the hypertriglyceridaemia of the cachectic patient, one of the hallmarks of wasting

# Cachexia, Cytokines, and Lipid Metabolism

As discussed above, during cachexia there is a dramatic loss of white adipose tissue, basically due a fall in the activity of LPL, and an increase in the activity of hormone-sensitive lipase (the rate-limiting enzyme of the lipolytic pathway). In addition to these metabolic events associated with cachectic states, there is an inhibition of glucose transport and de novo lipogenesis in adipose tissue.

TNF-α has been shown to decrease LPL activity in 3T3-L1 cells [15], associated with a decrease in LPL mRNA [16]. Fried and Zechner [17] reported that TNF-α produced a dose-dependent marked suppression of LPL activity in human adipose tissue maintained in organ culture. In vivo administration of TNF-α resulted in a decrease of adipose-tissue LPL activity in rat, mouse, and guinea pig [16, 18]. This decreased activity has been shown in rat to depress the uptake of exogenous [$^{14}$C]lipid by adipose tissue and to increase circulating triacylglycerols [19]. Such elevation may, in part, be the result of stimulation of lipolysis in adipose tissue, with subsequent increased secretion of VLDL from the liver [20, 21]. In contrast to these observations, in human primary cultures of isolated adipocytes, TNF-α was unable to decrease LPL [22]. Addition of the cytokine to 3T3-L1 cells increased lipolysis [23], a result confirmed by others using fully differentiated adipocytes [24]. TNF-α and interleukin (IL)-1 have both been shown to inhibit glucose transport in adipocytes [25] and, consequently, to decrease the availability of substrates for lipogenesis. Conversely, no direct action of TNF-α has been shown on de novo lipogenesis in adipose tissue of starved rats [20]. However, TNF-α decreased acetyl-CoA carboxylase (a key lipogenic enzyme) during preadipocyte differentiation by decreasing the mRNA levels of the enzyme [26]; this did not occur in fully differentiated adipocytes [26]. Using a polyclonal rat anti-TNF-α antibody, we demonstrated that TNF-α is involved in the abnormalities in lipid metabolism that occur in tumour-bearing rodents [27].

Interferon (IFN)-γ, like TNF-α, inhibits LPL activity in 3T3-L1 adipocytes and diminishes the rate of synthesis of long-chain lipids from smaller-chain fatty acids. This effect is similar to that observed in the inhibition of lipogenesis and LPL by TNF-α [28]. The ability of IFN-γ to mimic the effects of TNF-α on fat metabolism, and its apparent synergy with TNF-α suggest that IFN-γ plays a prominent role in cancer cachexia. In cultured adipocytes, IL-1, TNF-β (lymphotoxin), IFN-γ, and lipid mobilising factor (LIF) were all shown to decrease LPL activity [29]. Similarly, IL-1 and IFN-α, β, and γ increased lipolysis in adipocytes in culture [30].

Another important site that can account for hyperlipaemia is the de novo fatty-acid synthesis that takes place in the liver. Indeed, TNF-α has been shown to increase hepatic lipogenesis in vivo and subsequent VLDL production. In vivo administration of IL-1, IL-6, and IFN-γ to mice also produced a rapid increase in hepatic lipogenesis [31, 32]. IL-4 is a cytokine with marked inhibitory properties in regulating the immune response. By itself, IL-4 has no effect on hepatic fatty-acid synthesis, but it inhibits the stimulation of hepatic lipogenesis induced by TNF-α, IL-1, and IL-6 [33]. In addition, studies involving TNF p55 receptor-deficient mice have shown that the cytokine, via the p55 receptor, is involved in alterations in lipid metabolism associated with the implantation of a cachexia-inducing tumour. In conclusion, it may be suggested that TNF-α, and perturbations in hormonal homeostasis are likely to play important roles in forcing the metabolic balance of adipocytes towards the catabolic side (Fig. 2).

# Adipokines: Is Adipose Tissue an Endocrine Organ?

Although loss of fat tissue during cancer has not been considered as a very important alteration, compared to those affecting the quality of life or the prognosis of the cachectic cancer patient, we now know that adipose tissue is not just a fat reservoir. The concept of the adipocyte as an 'intelligent' cell that is able to communicate directly or indirectly with the brain is revolutionary compared to the previously held view of adipose tissue as a metabolically inactive fat deposit. Nowadays, we can go a step further and introduce the concept of the adipocyte as an 'intelligence' centre involved

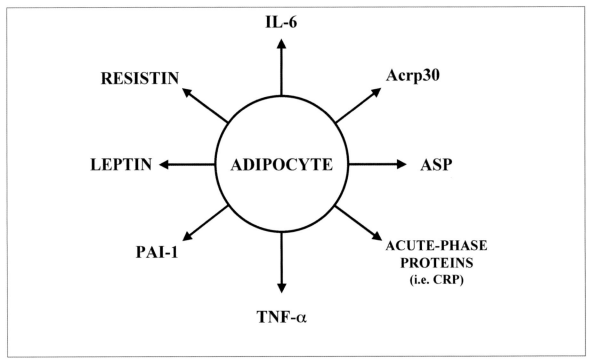

**Fig. 2.** The adipocyte as an endocrine organ. Recent work suggests that adipose tissue behaves as a true endocrine organ, releasing many active compounds involved in maintaining the homeostatic response and energy balance. These compounds include cytokines, such as TNF and IL-6; leptin (involved in food intake and thermogenesis); acute-phase reactants, such as CRP; resistin (involved in insulin resistance); ASP (involved in lipid synthesis), Acrp30 (probably involved in adipocyte differentiation); and PAI-1 (a haemostatic factor)

in the regulation of body weigh. But how is regulation accomplished?

Discovery of the hormone leptin [34] radically changed the field of body weight control. Leptin, a16-kDa protein synthesised in adipose tissue and secreted into the bloodstream, is the product of the *ob* gene. The protein travels to the brain, where it acts as a ponderostat or adipostat signal informing the brain about adipose tissue mass, and mediates a loss of appetite. Actually, the word leptin comes from the Greek *leptos,* which means thin. Mice that are *ob/ob* have a defect in leptin production, resulting in hyperphagia and, consequently, obesity. In other experimental models, such as the fatty rat, leptin production is normal but there seems to be a defect in the brain receptor [35]. Based on its amino-acid sequence, the receptor appears to be similar to the members of the class I cytokine receptor family [36]. Leptin production is correlated with an increase in fat mass and adipocyte size [37]. In addition to leptin, adipocytes synthesise and secrete many other mol-

ecules, especially cytokines. Thus, TNF-α is expressed and produced in adipose tissue, in particular in obesity conditions.

## The Intriguing Role of TNF: Is the Cytokine an 'Adipostat'?

TNF-α, which is expressed and secreted by adipose tissue, influences thermogenesis and, indirectly, via IL-1 or leptin [38], food intake. The cytokine also has a direct (possibly paracrine) function in adipose tissue, limiting its mass by stimulating lipolysis and decreasing LPL activity. Up to now, there have been no reports showing that leptin could have a similar function in lipid metabolism in adipose tissue. Conversely, TNF-α can also travel to the brain and influence hypothalamic function. One problem confronting such a hypothesis is the presence of the blood-brain barrier. However, a number of peripheral peptides, including angiotensin II, can rapidly affect the hypothalamus through nerve cells in the region of the circumventricular organs, which lie outside the blood-brain barrier [39]. Alternatively, signals could be brought to the hypothalamus through nerve cells in the region of vagal afferent axons. Indeed, the intracraneal administration of cytokines results in a more effective stimulation of thermogenesis [40]. TNF-$\alpha$ thus exerts central actions that are complementary to its peripheral effects on tissues. In addition, TNF-$\alpha$ administration results in an increase in circulating leptin concentrations [38].

It should be noted that it is not being suggested here that TNF-$\alpha$ is the sole adipostat; to the contrary, control of the fat mass is most likely accomplished by different molecules that signal the brain regarding fat mass. Among the molecules functioning as adipostats, TNF-$\alpha$ and leptin have fundamental roles, the former directly by influencing lipid metabolism and the latter probably only by being a satiation factor and an insulin-counterregulatory hormone [41]. Thus, TNF-$\alpha$ may be an important autocrine/paracrine regulator of fat-cell function that serves to limit adipose tissue expansion, probably by inducing insulin resistance, which may, in turn, cause metabolic disturbances.

It would be extremely naïve to point to TNF-$\alpha$ and leptin as the only modulatory signals that are involved in regulating adipose tissue mass. An extensive family of compounds synthesised by adipose tissue are thought to have a role in the entire process, interacting with both leptin and TNF-$\alpha$. An example of these compounds is plasminogen activator inhibitor-1 (PAI-1). PAI-1 is an important regulator fibrinolysis in that it binds to and rapidly inactivates tissue-type and urokinase-type plasminogen activators [42–44]. Interestingly, a number of investigations have established a significant correlation between elevated PAI-1 levels and obesity [45, 46], and thus to an increased risk of cardiovascular disease. Studies using animal models have found elevations in adipose tissue content and circulating PAI-1 concentrations. Furthermore, TNF-$\alpha$ treatment increases PAI-1 in adipose tissue [47]. It is difficult to speculate about the role of PAI-1 in adipose tissue. In several cell types, PAI-1 is deposited in the extracellular matrix, where it seems to protect matrix components by limiting plasmin generation. PAI-1 produced by adipocytes may preserve the integrity of the loose connective tissue elements that hold adipocytes together. This could be important in obese conditions, in which adipocytes tend to be more fragile due to their increased size.

Adipsin, which is identical to complement factor D and synthesised by fat cells, is profoundly deficient in mice with genetic and hypothalamic obesity [48]. In humans, circulating concentrations of adipsin tend to correlate positively with the degree of adiposity, being mildly elevated in obese individuals and mildly reduced in those with total lipoatrophy cachexia related to AIDS [49].

Acylation stimulating protein (ASP) is a small basic protein produced by adipocytes and isolated from human plasma. ASP has been shown to be the most potent stimulator of triacylglycerol synthesis in the adipocyte [50]. In addition, it is also a potent stimulator of glucose transport in muscle cells [51] and adipocytes [52]. Therefore, ASP is a potentially interesting factor in the pathophysiology of obesity. In fact, the adipsin-ASP system seems to have an important regulatory role in triacylglycerol clearance from plasma [53].

Another interesting peptide expressed in adipose tissue is adipoQ, also called Acrp-30 or adiponectin. The expression of adipoQ is reduced in adipose tissue of obese mice [54], in obese humans, and in type II diabetic patients [55, 56]. The protein is induced over 100-fold during adipocyte differentiation. Like adipsin, it is an abundant serum protein whose secretion is enhanced by insulin [57]. Very interestingly, adipoQ increases fatty acid oxidation in skeletal muscle, thus decreasing triacylglycerol content in this tissue [58]. The result is that adipoQ decreases insulin resistance and therefore may compensate for other molecules involved in promoting insulin resistance, such as TNF-$\alpha$ and IL-6.

The adipocyte is also able to synthesise and release IL-6 [59]. In fact, obese diabetic and nondiabetic patients have increased circulating IL-6 levels [60], and after weight loss, IL-6 levels (both in subcutaneous adipose tissue and in blood) are decreased [61], possibly due to the improved IL-6 sensitivity in these patients after weight reduction.

As one can easily realise, future studies will

reveal new compounds to be added to the list of molecules synthesised and released by adipose tissue cells and which may be involved in signalling fat mass. All of them may participate in the delicately balanced system of energy homeostasis, involving food intake and carbohydrate and lipid metabolism. Studying the interaction of TNF-$\alpha$ with these molecules may contribute to a better understanding of the cytokine's effects on the adipocyte.

## Concluding Remarks and Future Research

The weight-losing cancer patient suffers from a substantial loss of fat tissue. This is accompanied by profound changes in lipid metabolism, affecting almost all metabolic pathways involved in fat accretion/mobilisation in the adipocyte. Many of these changes are triggered by cytokines, TNF-$\alpha$ in particular. Until very recently, adipose tissue was considered exclusively as a fat reservoir; however, recent studies have demonstrated that the adipocyte is a key cell in the regulation of body weight, since it synthesizes and releases many active compounds, such as cytokines, which have very important effects in regulating energy balance. From this point of view, adipose tissue has to be considered an endocrine organ that releases compounds with important effects in other target tissues. Bearing this in mind, the loss of fat mass during cancer cachexia may be responsible for many of the metabolic changes observed in the cachectic cancer patient that ultimately lead to muscle-wasting and death.

In conclusion, taking into account fat metabolic changes during cancer and trying to counteract them may result in a reduction of the metabolic abnormalities of the cancer patient, and perhaps contribute to increasing survival time and improving the quality of life.

## References

1. Thompson MP, Koons JE, Tan ETH, Grigor MR (1981) Modified lipoprotein lipase activities, rates of lipogenesis, and lipolysis as factors leading to lipid depletion in C57BL mice bearing the preputial gland tumor, ESR-586. Cancer Res 41:3228–3232
2. Shaw JHF, Wolfe RR (1987) Fatty acid and glycerol kinetics in septic patients and in patients with gastrointestinal cancer. The response to glucose infusion and parenteral feeding. Ann Surg 205:368–376
3. Imagawa W, Bandyopadhyay G, Wallace D, Nadi S (1989) Phospholipids containing polyunsaturated acyl groups are mitogenic for normal mouse mammary epithelial cells in serum free primary culture. Proc Natl Acad Sci USA 86:4122–4126
4. Lanza-Jacoby S, Lansey SC, Miller EE, Cleary MP (1984) Sequential changes in the activities of lipoprotein lipase and lipogenic enzymes during tumor growth in rats. Cancer Res 44:5062–5067
5. Noguchi Y, Vydelingum NA, Younes RN et al (1991) Tumor-induced alterations in tissue lipoprotein lipase activity and mRNA levels. Cancer Res 51:863–869
6. Muscaritoli M, Cangiano C, Cascino A et al (1990) Plasma clearance of exogenous lipids in patients with malignant disease. Nutrition 6:147–151
7. López-Soriano J, Argilés JM, López-Soriano FJ (1996) Lipid metabolism in rats bearing the Yoshida AH-130 ascites hepatoma. Mol Cell Biochem 165:17–23
8. Evans RD, Williamson DH (1988) Tissue-specific effects of rapid tumour growth on lipid metabolism in the rat during lactation and on litter removal. Biochem J 252:65–72
9. Mulligan HD, Tisdale MJ (1991) Lipogenesis in tumour and host tissues in mice bearing colonic adenocarcinomas. Br J Cancer 63:719–722
10. Dessi S, Batetta B, Pulisci D et al (1991) Total and HDL cholesterol in human and hematologic neoplasms. Int J Hematol 54:483–486
11. Dessi S, Batetta B, Anchisi C et al (1992) Cholesterol metabolism during the growth of a rat ascites hepatoma (Yoshida AH-130). Br J Cancer 66:787–793
12. Dessi S, Batetta B, Spano O et al (1995) Perturbations of triglycerides but not of cholesterol metabolism are prevented by anti-tumour necrosis factor-$\alpha$ treatment in rats bearing an ascites hepatoma (Yoshida AH-130). Br J Cancer 72:1138–1143
13. Eisenberg S (1984) High density lipoprotein metabolism. J Lipid Res 25:1017–1058
14. Fanelli FR, Cangiano C, Muscaritoli M et al (1995) Tumor-induced changes in host metabolism: a possible marker of neoplastic disease. Nutrition 11:595–600
15. Price SR, Olivecrona T, Pekala PH (1986) Regulation of lipoprotein lipase synthesis by recombinant tumour necrosis factor: the primary regulatory role of the hormone in 3T3-L1 adipocytes. Arch Biochem Biophys 251:738–746
16. Cornelius P, Enerback S, Bjursell G et al (1988) Regulation of lipoprotein lipase mRNA content in

3T3-L1 cells by tumour necrosis factor. Biochem J 249:765–769

17. Fried SK, Zechner R (1989) Cachectin/tumour necrosis factor decreases human adipose tissue lipoprotein lipase mRNA levels, synthesis, and activity. J Lipid Res 30:1917–1923

18. Semb H, Peterson J, Tavernier J, Olivecrona T (1987) Multiple effects of tumour necrosis factor on lipoprotein lipase in vivo. J Biol Chem 262:8390–8394

19. Evans RD, Williamson DH (1988) Tumour necrosis factor-α (cachectin) mimics some of the effects of tumour growth on the disposal of α [$^{14}$C]lipid load in virgin, lactating and litter-removed rats. Biochem J 256:1055–1058

20. Feingold KR, Grunfeld C (1987) Tumour necrosis factor-a stimulates hepatic lipogenesis in the rat in vivo. J Clin Invest 80:1384–1389

21. Krauss RM, Grunfeld C, Doerrler WT, Feingold KR (1990) Tumor necrosis factor acutely increases plasma levels of very low density lipoproteins of normal size and composition. Endocrinology 127:1016–1021

22. Kern PA (1988) Recombinant human tumor necrosis factor does not inhibit lipoprotein lipase in primary cultures of isolated human adipocytes. J Lipid Res 29:909–914

23. Kawakami M, Murase T, Ogawa H et al (1987) Human recombinant TNF suppresses lipoprotein lipase activity and stimulates lipolysis in 3T3-L1 cells. J Biochem 101:331–338

24. Feingold KR, Doerrler W, Dinarello CA et al (1992) Stimulation of lipolysis in cultured fat cells by tumor necrosis factor, interleukin-1, and interferons is blocked by inhibition of prostaglandins synthesis. Endocrinology 130:10–16

25. Hauner H, Petruschke T, Russ M et al (1995) Effects of tumor necrosis factor-alpha (TNF-α) on glucose transport and lipid metabolism of newly-differentiated human fat cells in cell culture. Diabetologia 38:764–771

26. Pape ME, Kim KH (1988) Effect of tumor necrosis factor on acetyl-coenzyme A carboxylase gene expression and pre-adipocyte differentiation. Mol Endocrinol 2:395–403

27. Carbó N, Costelli P, Tessitore L et al (1994) Antitumor necrosis factor-α treatment interferes with changes in lipid metabolism in a cachectic tumor model. Clin Sci 87:349–355

28. Patton JS, Shepard HM, Wilking H et al (1986) Interferons and tumor necrosis factors have similar catabolic effects on 3T3 L1 cells. Proc Natl Acad Sci USA 83:8313–7

29. Tisdale MJ (1999) Wasting in cancer. J Nutr 129(1S Suppl):243S–246S

30. Gregoire F, De Broux N, Hauser N et al (1992) Interferon-gamma and interleukin-1 beta inhibit adipoconversion in cultured rodent preadipocytes. J Cell Physiol 151:300–309

31. Grunfeld C, Adi S, Soued M et al (1990) Search for

mediators of the lipogenic effects of tumor necrosis factor: potential role for interleukin 6. Cancer Res 50:4233–4238

32. Grunfeld C, Soued M, Adi S et al (1990) Evidence for two classes of cytokines that stimulate hepatic lipogenesis: relationships among tumor necrosis factor, interleukin-1 and interferon-alpha. Endocrinology 127:46–54

33. Grunfeld C, Soued M, Adi S et al (1991) Interleukin 4 inhibits stimulation of hepatic lipogenesis by tumor necrosis factor, interleukin 1, and interleukin 6 but not by interferon-alpha. Cancer Res 51:2803–2807

34. Zhang Y, Proenca R, Maffei M et al (1994) Positional cloning of the mouse obese gene and its human analogue. Nature 372:425–432

35. Phillips MS, Liu Q, Hammond HA et al (1996) Leptin receptor missense mutation in the fatty Zucker rat. Nat Genet 13:18–19

36. Madej T, Boguski MS, Bryant SH (1995) Threading analysis suggests that the obese gene product may be a helical cytokine. FEBS Lett 373:13–18

37. Hamann A, Matthaei S (1996) Regulation of energy balance by leptin. Exp Clin Endocrinol Diabetes 104:293–300

38. Grunfeld C, Zhao C, Fuller J et al (1996) Endotoxin and cytokines induce expression of leptin, the ob gene product, in hamsters. A role for leptin in the anorexia of infection. J Clin Invest 97:2152–2157

39. Tanaka J, Nomura M (1993) Involvement of neurons sensitive to angiotensin II in the median preoptic nucleus in the drinking response induced by angiotensin II activation of the subfornical organ in rats. Exp Neurol 119:235–239

40. Rothwell NJ (1993) Cytokines and thermogenesis. Int J Obesity 17:S98–S101

41. Remesar X, Rafecas I, Fernández-López JA, Alemany M (1997) Is leptin an insulin counter-regulatory hormone? FEBS Lett 402:9–11

42. Sprengers ED, Kluft C (1987) Plasminogen activator inhibitors. Blood 69:381–387

43. Astrup T (1978) Fibrinolysis: an overview. In: Davidson JF, Rowan RM, Samama MM, Desnoyers PC (eds) Progress in chemical fibrinolysis and thrombolysis. Raven Press, New York, pp 1–57

44. Vassalli JD, Sappini AP, Belin D (1991) The plasminogen activator/plasmin system. J Clin Invest 88:1067–1072

45. McGill JB, Schneider DJ, Arfken CL et al (1994) Factors responsible for impaired fibrinolysis in obese subjects and NIDDM patients. Diabetes 43:104–109

46. Vague P, Juhan-Vague I, Chabert V et al (1989) Fat distribution and plasminogen activator inhibitor activity in nondiabetic obese women. Metab Clin Exp 38:913–915

47. Samad F, Yamamoto K, Loskutoff DJ (1996) Distribution and regulation of plasminogen activator inhibitor-1 in murine adipose tissue in vivo. Induction by tumor necrosis factor-α and lipopoly-

saccharide. J Clin Invest 97:37–46

48. Flier JS, Cook KS, Usher P, Spiegelman BM (1987) Severely impaired adipsin expression in genetic and acquired obesity. Science 237:405–408

49. Napolitano A, Lowell BB, Damm D et al (1994) Concentrations of adipsin in blood and rates of adipsin secretion by adipose tissue in humans with normal, elevated and diminished adipose tissue mass. Int J Obesity 18:213–218

50. Cianflone K, Roncari DA, Maslowska M et al (1994) Adipsin/acylation stimulating protein system in human adipocytes: regulation of triacylglycerol synthesis. Biochemistry 33:9489–9495

51. Tao Y, Cianflone K, Sniderman AD et al (1997) Acylation-stimulating protein (ASP) regulates glucose transport in the rat L6 muscle cell line. Biochim Biophys Acta 1344:221–229

52. Maslowska M, Sniderman AD, Germinario R, Cianflone K (1997) ASP stimulates glucose transport in cultured human adipocytes. Int J Obesity 21:261–266

53. Cianflone K, Maslowska M, Sniderman AD (1995) The acylation stimulating protein-adipsin system. Int J Obesity 19:S34-S38

54. Hu E, Liang P, Spiegelman BM (1996) AdipoQ is a novel adipose-specific gene dysregulated in obesity. J Biol Chem 271:10697–10703

55. Arita Y, Kihara S, Ouchi N et al (1999) Paradoxical decrease of an adipose-specific protein, adiponectin, in obesity. Biochem Biophys Res Commun 257:79–83

56. Hotta K, Funahashi T, Arita Y et al (2000) Plasma concentration of a novel, adipose-specific protein, adiponectin, in type 2 diabetic patients. Arterioscler Thromb Vasc Biol 20:1595–1599

57. Scherer PE, Williams S, Fogliano M et al (1995) A novel serum protein similar to C1q, produced exclusively in adipocytes. J Biol Chem 270:26746–26749

58. Fruebis J, Tsao TS, Javorschi S et al (2001) Proteolytic cleavage product of 30-kDa adipocyte complement-related protein increases fatty acid oxidation in muscle and causes weight loss in mice. Proc Natl Acad Sci USA 98:2005–2010

59. Frübeck G, Gómez-Ambrosi J, Muruzábal FJ, Burrell MA (2001) The adipocyte: a model for integration of endocrine and metabolic signaling in energy metabolism regulation. Am J Physiol Endocrinol Metab 280:E827–E847

60. Raymond NC, Dysken M, Bettin K et al (2000) Cytokine production in patients with anorexia nervosa, bulimia nervosa, and obesity. Int J Eating Disord 28:293–302

61. Bastard JP, Jardel C, Bruckert E et al (2000) Elevated levels of interleukin 6 are reduced in serum and subcutaneous adipose tissue of obese women after weight loss. J Clin Endocrinol Metab 85:3338–3342

# The Role of Cytokines in Cancer Cachexia

Josep M. Argilés, Sílvia Busquets, Rodrigo Moore-Carrasco, Francisco J. López-Soriano

## Introduction

The cachectic syndrome, characterised by marked weight loss, anorexia, asthaenia, and anaemia, is invariably associated with the presence and growth of the tumour and leads to a malnutrition status due to the induction of anorexia or decreased food intake. In addition, the competition for nutrients between the tumour and the host leads to an accelerated starvation state that promotes severe metabolic disturbances in the host, including hypermetabolism, which leads to decreased energetic efficiency. Although the search for the cachectic factor(s) started a long time ago, and although many scientific and economic efforts have been devoted to its discovery, we are still far from a complete understanding of cancer cachex-

ia. The chapter discusses the different signalling pathways, particularly the role of transcriptional factors, involved in muscle wasting. The main aim is to summarise and evaluate the different molecular mechanisms and catabolic mediators (both humoral and tumoural) involved in cancer cachexia, since they may represent targets for promising future clinical investigations.

## Cytokines

Cytokines have a key role as the main humoural factors involved in cancer cachexia (Fig. 1), and a large number of them may be responsible for the metabolic changes associated with cancer wasting.

Anorexia may account for malnutrition, invari-

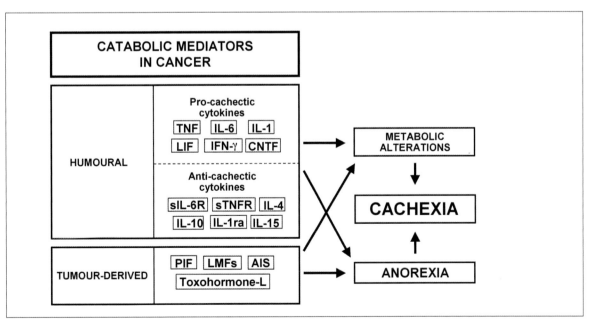

**Fig. 1.** Catabolic mediators in cancer. Both tumour-derived and humoural (cytokines) factors are involved in mediating the anorexia and metabolic changes characteristic of the cachectic state. For abbreviations, see text

ably associated with cancer cachexia; but, are cytokines involved in the induction of anorexia? Cytokines, such as interleukin (IL)-1 and tumour necrosis factor (TNF)-α have been suggested to be involved in cancer-related anorexia, possibly by increasing the levels of corticotropin-releasing hormone (CRH), a central nervous system neurotransmitter that suppresses food intake, and the firing of glucose-sensitive neurons, which would also decrease food intake. However, many other mediators may be involved in cancer-induced anorexia. Leptin (an adiposity signal to the hypothalamus that it is a member of the cytokine family) does not seem to play a role, at least in experimental models [1, 2], and in human subjects, cancer anorexia does not seem to be due to a dysregulation of leptin production [3]. Indeed, leptin concentrations are not elevated in weight-losing cancer patients [4, 5] and are inversely related to the intensity of the inflammatory response [6] and the levels of inflammatory cytokines [7, 8]. Concentrations of the peptide seem to be dependent only on the total amount of adipose tissue present in the patient. Cytokines have been implicated in cancer-induced anorexia since they modulate gastric motility and emptying, either directly in the gastrointestinal system or via the brain, by altering efferent signals that regulate satiety. IL-1, in particular, has been clearly associated with the induction of anorexia [9] in that it blocks neuropeptide Y (NPY)-induced feeding. The levels of this molecule (a feeding-stimulating peptide) are reduced in anorectic tumour-bearing rats [10], and a correlation between food intake and brain-IL-1 has been found in anorectic rats with cancer. The mechanism involved in the attenuation of NPY activity by cytokines may be related to an inhibition of cell firing rates or to an inhibition of NPY synthesis or an attenuation of its postsynaptic effects [11]. Other mediators have been proposed [12], including changes in the circulating levels of free tryptophan; these may induce changes in serotonin brain concentrations and, consequently, cause changes in food intake. Bing et al. [13] suggested that some tumour-derived compounds may mediate anorexia associated with tumour burden.

Different experimental approaches have demonstrated that cytokines are able to induce

weight loss. Nevertheless, the results obtained have to be carefully interpreted. Thus, episodic TNF-α administration has proved unsuccessful at inducing cachexia in experimental animals. Indeed, repetitive TNF-α administrations initially induce a cachectic effect, but tolerance to the cytokine soon develops and food intake and body weight return to normal. Other studies have shown that escalating doses of TNF-α are necessary to maintain the cachectic effects.

Strassman et al. [14] have shown that treatment with an anti-mouse IL-6 antibody reversed the key parameters of cachexia in murine colon adenocarcinoma tumour-bearing mice. These results seem to indicate that, at least in certain types of tumours, IL-6 has a more direct involvement than TNF-α in the cachectic state. Similar results were obtained in a mouse model that reproduced the cachexia associated with multiple myeloma [15, 16] and in a murine model of intracerebral injection of human tumours [17]. Conversely, other studies have shown in a very similar mouse tumour model that IL-6 is not involved in cachexia, and studies using incubated rat skeletal muscle have clearly demonstrated that IL-6 had no direct effect on muscle proteolysis.

Another interesting candidate for cachexia is interferon (IFN)-γ, which is produced by activated T and NK cells and possesses biological activities that overlap with those of TNF-α. Matthys et al. [18] used a monoclonal antibody against IFN-γ to reverse the wasting syndrome associated with growth of the Lewis lung carcinoma in mice, thus indicating that endogenous production of IFN-γ occurs in the tumour-bearing mice and is instrumental in bringing about some of the metabolic changes characteristic of cancer cachexia. The same group also demonstrated that severe cachexia develops rapidly in nude mice inoculated with CHO cells constitutively producing IFN-γ as a result of the transfection of the corresponding gene.

Other cytokines, such as leukaemia inhibitory factor (LIF), transforming growth factor (TGF)-β, or IL-1 have also been suggested as mediators of cachexia. Thus, mice engrafted with tumours secreting LIF developed severe cachexia. Concerning IL-1, although its anorectic and pyrogenic effects are well-known, administration of IL-

1 receptor antagonist (IL-1ra) to tumour-bearing rats did not result in any improvement in the degree of cachexia, so that the role of this cytokine in cancer cachexia may be secondary to the actions of other mediators. Interestingly, the levels of both IL-6 and LIF are increased in patients with different types of malignancies.

Ciliary neurotrophic factor (CNTF) is a member of the family of cytokines that includes IL-6 and LIF, and is produced predominantly by glial cells of the peripheral nervous system; however, this cytokine also seems to be expressed in skeletal muscle. Henderson et al. [19] demonstrated that CNTF induces potent cachectic effects and the production of acute-phase proteins (independent of the induction of other cytokine family members) in mice implanted with C6 glioma cells, genetically modified to secrete this cytokine. CNTF, however, exerted divergent direct effects dependent on the dose and exposure time of in vitro muscle preparations [20].

If anorexia is not the only factor involved in cancer cachexia, it becomes clear that metabolic abnormalities leading to a hypermetabolic state must have a very important role. Interestingly, injection of low doses of TNF-α, either peripherally or into the brain of laboratory animals, elicits rapid increases in the metabolic rate that are not associated with increased metabolic activity but rather with an increase in blood flow and thermogenic activity of brown adipose tissue (BAT), associated with uncoupling protein-1 (UCP1). During cachectic states, there is an increase in BAT thermogenesis, both in humans and experimental animals. Until recently, UCP1 (present only in BAT) was considered to be the only mitochondrial protein carrier that stimulated heat production, by dissipating the proton gradient generated during respiration across the inner mitochondrial membrane and therefore uncoupling respiration from ATP synthesis. However, two additional proteins sharing the same function, UCP2 and UCP3, have since been described. While UCP2 is expressed ubiquitously, UCP3 is expressed abundantly and specifically in skeletal muscle in humans and in BAT of rodents. Our research group has demonstrated that both UCP2 and UCP3 mRNAs are elevated in skeletal muscle during tumour growth

and that the effect of TNF-α mimics the increase in gene expression induced by these proteins [21]. In addition, TNF-α induces uncoupling of mitochondrial respiration, as recently shown in isolated mitochondria [22].

Several cytokines have been shown to mimic many of the metabolic abnormalities found in the cancer patient during cachexia. Among these metabolic disturbances, changes in lipid metabolism, skeletal muscle proteolysis and apoptosis, and acute-phase protein synthesis have been described [23]. Concerning muscle wasting, it seems that administration of TNF-α to rats results in increased proteolysis of skeletal muscle, associated with an increase in gene expression and higher levels of free and conjugated ubiquitin, both in experimental animals [24] and humans [25]. In addition, the in vivo action of TNF-α during cancer cachexia does not seem to be mediated by IL-1 or glucocorticoids. Other cytokines, such as IL-1 or IFN-γ, also activate ubiquitin gene expression. Therefore, TNF-α, alone or in combination with other cytokines [26], seems to mediate most of the changes concerning nitrogen metabolism associated with cachectic states. In addition to the massive muscle protein loss, and similar to that observed in skeletal muscle of patients with chronic heart failure who also suffer from cardiac cachexia [27], muscle DNA is also decreased during cancer cachexia, leading to DNA fragmentation and apoptosis [28, 29]. Moreover, TNF-α can mimic the apoptotic response in muscle of healthy animals [30].

## Factors Other Than Cytokines

In addition to humoural factors, tumour-derived molecules have also been suggested as mediators of cancer cachexia. Firstly, cancer cells are capable of constitutively producing cytokines. These may act on cancer cells in an autocrine manner or on supporting tissues, such as fibroblasts and blood vessels, to produce an environment conducive to cancer growth [31]. While tumour-produced cytokines may have a more important role in the anorexia-cachexia syndrome, several compounds produced by the host [32] are likely to have an important role in mimicking the metabolic changes associated with the cachectic state.

Perhaps the first evidence of tumour-derived catabolic factors came from studies with Krebs-2 carcinoma cells in mice; inactive extracts of these cells induced cachexia when injected into normal non-tumour-bearing mice [33]. Similarly, Kitada et al. [34] purified a low-molecular-mass (< 10 kDa) proteinaceous material from extract of thymic lymphoma in AKR mice that showed lipolytic activity in rat adipocyte suspensions. Thus, extracts of thymic lymphoma, conditioned medium from thymic lymphoma cell lines, and serum from lymphoma-bearing mice cause lipid mobilisation in experimental animals. Toxohormone L, a polypeptide of approximately 75 kDa, was isolated from the ascites fluid of hepatoma patients and sarcoma-bearing mice; it induces lipid mobilisation, immunosuppression, and involution of the thymus [35].

Tisdale's group at the University of Aston (UK) described and characterised a lipid-mobilising factor (LMF) that induces lipolysis in adipose tissue, in association with stimulation of adenylate cyclase activity [36]. Although this factor was originally purified from a cachexia-inducing mouse colon adenocarcinoma (MAC16). It has also been found in the urine of cancer patients, suggesting that it can induce lipid mobilisation and catabolism in cachectic cancer patients [37]. In fact, LMF is homologous to the plasma protease Zn-α2-glycoprotein (ZAG) in amino-acid sequence, electrophoretic mobility, and immunoreactivity. The 2.8 Å crystal structure of ZAG resembles a class I major histocompatibility complex (MHC) heavy chain, although it does not bind class I light chain β2-microglobulin. The ZAG structure includes a large groove analogous to class I MHC peptide binding grooves. Instead of a peptide, the ZAG groove contains a nonpeptidic compound implicated in lipid metabolism under pathological conditions. Hirai et al. [38] also suggested that LMF has a role in initiating hepatic glycogenolysis during experimental cancer cachexia through an increase in cyclic AMP in liver.

Anaemia-inducing factor (AIS), an approximately 50-kDa protein secreted by malignant tumour tissue, depresses erythrocyte and immunocompetent cell functions. AIS reduces food intake, body weight, and body fat in rabbits; it also shows an important lipolytic activity [39].

Todorov et al. [40] purified and characterised a 24-kDa proteoglycan, present in experimental animals [41] and in the urine of cachectic patients [42], that seems to account for increased muscle protein degradation and decreased protein synthesis [43]. This compound, known as PIF (proteolysis-inducing factor), activates protein degradation specifically through stimulation of the ATP-proteasome-dependent pathway. Injection of the compound into healthy animals results in muscle wasting, similar to that associated with experimental cancer cachexia. In vitro studies on C2C12 myoblasts have shown that eicosapentaenoic acid (EPA) blocks PIF action on proteolysis, in addition to suggesting that PIF acts intracellularly via the arachidonate metabolite 15-hydroxyeicosatetraenoic acid (15-HETE) [44]. PIF also increases NFκB expression in cultured cells (M. Tisdale, personal communication). Therefore, PIF may have a constitutive role in normal states and become altered or overproduced during cancer cachexia, with important effects on muscle protein catabolism and acute-phase protein (APP) synthesis in this pathological state (Fig. 2).

## Transcriptional Factors

At the moment there are few studies describing the involvement of different transcriptional factors in muscle wasting. Penner et al. [45] reported an increase in NFκB and AP-1 transcription factors during sepsis in experimental animals. Recent data from our laboratory do not support an involvement of NFκB in skeletal muscle during cancer cachexia (unpublished data). However, tumour burden results in a significant increase in the binding activity of AP-1. Interestingly, inhibition of NFκB is not able to revert muscle wasting in cachectic tumour-bearing animals [46]; however, inhibition of AP-1 results in a partial reversal of protein degradation in skeletal muscle associated with tumour growth (unpublished data). The increase in NFκB observed in skeletal muscle during sepsis can be mimicked by TNF-α. Indeed, TNF-α addition to C2C12 muscle cultures results

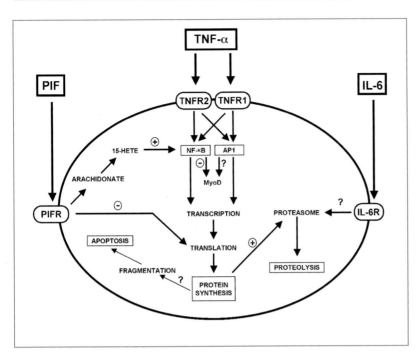

**Fig. 2.** Interactions between pro-inflammatory cytokines and PIF. Both humoural (TNF-α and IL-6) and tumoural (PIF) factors have been shown to activate intracellular muscle proteolysis by different mechanisms, but possibly sharing common pathways. For abbreviations, see text

in a short-term increase in NFκB [47, 48]; however, whether or not this increase in NFκB promoted by TNF-α is associated with increased proteolysis and/or increased apoptosis in skeletal muscle remains to be established. In relation to AP-1 activation, TNF-α has been shown to increase c-jun expression in C2C12 cells [49]; in turn, the effects of c-jun overexpression mimic those of TNF-α on differentiation, i.e. decreased myoblast differentiation [50]. Tumour mediators, PIF in particular, also seem to be able to increase NFκB expression in cultured muscle cells, this possibly being linked with increased proteolysis (M. Tisdale, personal communication). Other transcriptional factors reported to be involved in muscle changes associated with catabolic conditions include c/EBPβ and c/EBPδ, which are increased in skeletal muscle during sepsis [51], PW-1, and PGC-1. TNF-α decreases MyoD content in cultured myoblasts [52] and blocks differentiation by a mechanism that seems to be independent of NFκB and that involves PW-1, a transcriptional factor related to p53-induced apoptosis [53]. Cytokine action on muscle cells, therefore, seems to rely most likely on satellite cells blocking muscle differentiation or, in other words, regeneration.

Finally, the transcription factor PGC-1 has been associated with the activation of UCP2 and UCP3 and with increased oxygen consumption by cytokines in cultured myotubes [54]. This transcriptional factor is involved as an activator of PPAR-γ in the expression of uncoupling proteins.

## Strategies To Fight Cachexia Based on Cytokines and Transcriptional Factors

Since both anorexia and metabolic disturbances are involved in cancer cachexia, the development of different therapeutic strategies has focused on these two factors. Unfortunately, counteracting anorexia either pharmacologically or nutritionally has led to rather disappointing results in the treatment of cancer cachexia. It is basically for this reason that the strategies mentioned below rely on neutralising the metabolic changes induced by the tumour, which are ultimately responsible for the weight loss. Therefore, taking into account the involvement of cytokines in cachexia, therapeutic strategies have been aimed at blocking either their synthesis or their action.

For instance, TNF-α synthesis inhibitors have been used therapeutically. Pentoxifylline, a methylxantine derivative, was originally employed for the treatment of various types of vascular insufficiency, because of its haemorhoeological activity, thought to be based on its ability to reduce blood viscosity and increase the filterability of blood cells. While several studies in animal models have suggested that pentoxifylline is able to decrease the cytokine-induced toxicity of anti-neoplasic agents, while preserving anti-tumour treatment efficacy [55], clinical studies have shown that the drug failed to improve appetite or to increase the weight of cachectic patients [56]. Rolipram is a type IV phosphodiesterase inhibitor that decreases TNF-$\alpha$ production by lipopolysaccharide (LPS)-stimulated human monocytes. This compound was previously used in the treatment of endogenous depression in animals and humans, and it may have therapeutic activity in disease states in which TNF-$\alpha$ seems to play a role in the pathogenesis, such as in endotoxic shock. Thalidomide ($\alpha$-N-phthalimidoglutaramide) is a drug unfortunately associated with tragedy. Indeed, its use as a sedative in pregnant women caused over 10000 victims of severe malformations in newborn children. However, use of the drug has undergone a revival since it was demonstrated to suppress TNF-$\alpha$ production in monocytes in vitro and to normalise elevated TNF-$\alpha$ levels in vivo. Its use in cancer cachexia remains to be established but it may have a specific role in counteracting TNF-$\alpha$-mediated metabolic changes [57].

The use of anti-cytokine antibodies (either monoclonal or polyclonal) and cytokine receptor antagonists or soluble receptors has led to very interesting results. Thus, in rats bearing the Yoshida AH-130 ascites hepatoma (a highly cachectic tumour), anti-TNF-$\alpha$ therapy resulted in a partial reversal of the abnormalities associated with both lipid and protein metabolism [58]. In humans, however, clinical trials using anti-TNF-$\alpha$ treatment have led to poor results in reverting the protein wasting associated with sepsis [59]. Concerning IL-6, experimental models have proved that the use of antibodies is highly effective in preventing tumour-induced wasting. Strassman et al. [14] demonstrated that the experimental drug suramine (which prevents the binding of IL-6 to its cell-surface receptor, as demonstrated by radioreceptor binding assays and affinity binding

experiments) partially blocks the catabolic effects associated with the growth of colon-26 adenocarcinoma in mice. In humans, administration of an anti-IL-6 monoclonal antibody to patients with AIDS and suffering from an immunoblastic or a polymorphic large-cell cell lymphoma had a highly positive effect on fever and cachexia. Concerning other cytokines, anti-IFN-$\gamma$ therapy has also been effective in reverting cachexia in mice bearing the Lewis lung carcinoma [18], but clinical data are lacking. It has to be pointed out here that the routine use of anti-cytokine antibodies is, at present, too expensive, due to the fact that this type of therapy requires a very large number of antibody molecules in order to completely block cytokine action.

The appearance of the cachectic syndrome is dependent not only on the production of the above-mentioned cytokines, known as catabolic pro-inflammatory cytokines, but also on so-called anti-inflammatory cytokines (Fig. 1), such as IL-4 and IL-10. Mori et al. [60] demonstrated that administration of IL-12 to mice bearing colon-26 carcinoma alleviated the body weight loss and other abnormalities associated with cachexia, such as adipose tissue wasting and hypoglycaemia. The anti-cachectic properties were obtained at low doses of IL-12, insufficient to inhibit tumour growth. The effects of IL-12 seem to be dependent on an important decrease of IL-6, a cytokine responsible for cachexia associated with this tumour model. A similar action was described for INF-$\alpha$. Administration of this cytokine promoted a decrease in IL-6 mRNA expression in the tumour and in serum IL-6 levels, resulting in the amelioration of cachexia in a murine model of malignant mesothelioma. IL-15 has been reported to be an anabolic factor for skeletal muscle [61], and experiments carried out in our laboratory clearly demonstrate that the cytokine is able to reverse most of the abnormalities associated with cancer cachexia in a rat tumour model [62].

Additional anti-inflammatory strategies to influence cytokine levels during cachexia include the use of cyclooxygenase-2 inhibitors [63, 64]. These compounds, in addition to decreasing cytokine levels in cancer, result in an improvement in weight loss and cachexia.

Concerning therapeutic strategies based on events related to transcription factors in muscle wasting, several points can be raised. First, Kawamura et al. [65, 66] reported an oligonucleotide that competes with a NFκB-binding site reverts cachexia in a mouse experimental model, without affecting growth of the primary tumour. This treatment, however, reduces the metastatic capacity of colon-26 adenocarcinoma. In spite of this, administration of curcumine to tumour-bearing rats was unable to block muscle wasting, implying that NFκB is not involved in the cachectic response in this tumour model [48].

As noted above, AP-1 is clearly involved in muscle wasting during sepsis [45] and in cancer (unpublished data). Interestingly, administration of an inhibitor of NFκB and AP-1 resulted in a partial blockade of muscle wasting in rats bearing the AH-130 Yoshida ascites hepatoma, a highly cachectic rat tumour (unpublished data).

## Conclusions

Since metabolic alterations often appear soon after the onset of tumour growth, the scope of appropriate treatment, although not aimed at achieving immediate eradication of tumour mass, could influence the course of the patient's clinical state or, at least, prevent the steady erosion of dignity that the patient may feel in association with the syndrome. This would no doubt contribute to improving the patient's quality of life and, possibly, prolong survival. Although exploration of the role that cytokines play in the host response to invasive stimuli is an endeavour that has been underway for many years, considerable controversy still exists over the mechanisms of lean-tissue and body-fat dissolution that occur in the patient with either cancer or inflammation, and whether humoural factors regulate this process. A better understanding of the role of cytokines, both host and tumour-derived [32], in the molecular mechanisms of protein wasting in skeletal muscle, is essential for the design of effective therapeutic strategies. In any case, understanding the humoural response to cancer and modifying cytokine actions pharmacologically may prove very suitable, and no doubt future research will concentrate on this interesting field. Finally, understanding the intracellular signalling mechanisms, particularly those involving transcriptional factors, may also be very important for achieving effective therapeutic approaches.

## References

1. López-Soriano J, Carbó N, Tessitore L et al (1999) Leptin and tumour growth in the rat. Int J Cancer 81:726–729
2. Sato T, Meguid MM, Miyata G et al (2002) Does leptin really influence cancer anorexia? Nutrition 18:82–83
3. Kowalczuk A, Wiecek A, Franek E, Kokot F (2001) Plasma concentration of leptin, neuropeptide Y and tumour necrosis factor alpha in patients with cancers, before and after radio- and chemotherapy. Pol Arch Med Wewn 106:657–668
4. Tessitore L, Vizio B, Jenkins O et al (2000) Leptin expression in colorectal and breast cancer patients. Int J Mol Med 5:421–426
5. Brown DR, Berkowitz DF, Breslow MJ (2001) Weight loss is not associated with hyperleptinemia in humans with pancreatic cancer. J Clin Endocrinol Metab 86:162–166
6. Aleman MR, Santolaria F, Batista N et al (2002) Leptin role in advanced lung cancer. A mediator of the acute phase response or a marker of the status of nutrition? Cytokine 19:21–26
7. Mantovani G, Macciò A, Mura L et al (2000) Serum levels of leptin and proinflammatory cytokines in patients with advanced-stage cancer at different sites. J Mol Med 78:554–561
8. Mantovani G, Macciò A, Madeddu C et al (2001) Serum values of proinflammatory cytokines are inversely correlated with serum leptin levels in patients with advanced stage cancer at different sites. J Mol Med 79:406–414
9. Plata-Salaman CR (2000) Central nervous system mechanisms contributing to the cachexia-anorexia syndrome. Nutrition 16:1009–1012
10. Chance WT, Balasubramaniam A, Dayal R et al (1994) Hypothalamic concentration and release of neuropeptide Y into microdialysates is reduced in anorectic tumour-bearing rats. Life Sci 54:1869–1874
11. King PJ, Widdowson PS, Doods H, Williams G (2000) Effect of cytokines on hypothalamic neuropeptide Y release in vitro. Peptides 21:143–146
12. Laviano A, Russo M, Freda F, Rossi-Fanelli F (2002) Neurochemical mechanisms for cancer anorexia. Nutrition 18:100–105

13. Bing C, Taylor S, Tisdale MJ, Williams G (2001) Cachexia in MAC16 adenocarcinoma: suppression of hunger despite normal regulation of leptin, insulin and hypothalamic neuropeptide Y. J Neurochem 79:1004–1012

14. Strassmann G, Fong M, Freter CE et al (1993) Suramin interfers with interleukin-6 receptor binding in vitro and inhibits colon-26-mediated experimental cancer cachexia in vivo. J Clin Invest 92:2152–2159

15. Barton BE, Cullison J, Jackson J, Murphy T (2000) A model that reproduces syndromes associated with human multiple myeloma in nonirradiated SCID mice. Proc Soc Exp Biol Med 223:190–197

16. Barton BE, Murphy TF (2001) Cancer cachexia is mediated in part by the induction of IL-6-like cytokines from the spleen. Cytokine 16:251–257

17. Negri DR, Mezzanzanica D, Sacco S et al (2001) Role of cytokines in cancer cachexia in a murine model of intracerebral injection of human tumours. Cytokine 15:27–38

18. Matthys P, Heremans H, Opdenakker G, Billiau A (1991) Anti-interferon-γ antibody treatment, growth of Lewis lung tumours in mice and tumour-associated cachexia. Eur J Cancer 27:182–187

19. Henderson JT, Mullen BJ, Roder JC (1996) Physiological effects of CNTF-induced wasting. Cytokine 8:784–793

20. Wang MC, Forsberg NE (2000) Effects of ciliary neurotrophic factor (CNTF) on protein turnover in cultured muscle cells. Cytokine 12:41–48

21. Busquets S, Sanchés D, Alvarez B et al (1998) In the rat, TNF-α administration results in an increase in both UCP2 and UCP3 mRNAs in skeletal muscle: a possible mechanism for cytokine-induced thermogenesis? FEBS Lett 440:348–350

22. Busquets S, Aranda X, Ribas-Carbó M et al (2003) Tumour necrosis factor-alpha uncouples respiration in isolated rat mitochondria. Cytokine 22:1–4

23. Argilés JM, López-Soriano FJ (1998) Catabolic proinflammatory cytokines. Curr Opin Clin Nutr Metab Care 1:245–251

24. Bossola M, Muscaritoli M, Costelli P et al (2001) Increased muscle ubiquitin mRNA levels in gastric cancer patients. Am J Physiol 280:R1518–R1523

25. Baracos VE (2000) Regulation of skeletal-muscle-protein turnover in cancer-associated cachexia. Nutrition 16:1015–1018

26. Alvarez B, Quinn LS, Busquets S et al (2002) Tumour necrosis factor-alpha exerts interleukin-6-dependent and -independent effects on cultured skeletal muscle cells. Biochem Biophys Acta 1542:66–72

27. Sharma R, Anker SD (2002) Cytokines, apoptosis and cachexia: the potential for TNF-α antagonism. Int J Cardiol 85:161–171

28. Van Royen M, Carbó N, Busquets S et al (2000) DNA fragmentation occurs in skeletal muscle during tumour growth: a link with cancer cachexia? Biochem Biophys Res Commun 270:533–537

29. Belizario JE, Lorite MJ, Tisdale MJ (2001) Cleavage of caspases-1, -3, -6, -8 and -9 substrates by proteases in skeletal muscles from mice undergoing cancer cachexia. Br J Cancer 84:1135–1140

30. Carbó N, Busquets S, van Royen M et al (2002) TNF-α is involved in activating DNA fragmentation in murine skeletal muscle. Br J Cancer 86:1012–1016

31. Dunlop RJ, Campbell CW (2000) Cytokines and advanced cancer. J Pain Symptom Manage 20:214–232

32. Cahlin C, Korner A, Axelsson H et al (2000) Experimental cancer cachexia: the role of host-derived cytokines interleukin (IL)-6, IL-12, interferon-gamma, and tumor necrosis factor alpha evaluated in gene knockout, tumor-bearing mice on C57 Bl background and eicosanoid-dependent cachexia. Cancer Res 60:5488–5493

33. Costa G, Holland JF (1966) Effects of Krebs-2 carcinoma on the lipid metabolism of male Swiss mice. Cancer Res 22:1081–1083

34. Kitada S, Hays EF, Mead JF (1981) Characterization of a lipid mobilizing factor from tumors. Prog Lipid Res 20:823–826

35. Masuno H, Yamasaki N, Okuda H (1981) Purification and characterization of a lipolytic factor (toxohormone L) from cell free fluid of ascites sarcoma 180. Cancer Res 41:284–288

36. Khan S, Tisdale MJ (1999) Catabolism of adipose tissue by a tumour-produced lipid metabolising factor. Int J Cancer 80:444–447

37. Hirai K, Hussey HJ, Barber MD et al (1998) Biological evaluation of a lipid-mobilising factor isolated from the urine of cancer patients. Cancer Res 58:2359–2365

38. Hirai K, Ishiko O, Tisdale M (1997) Mechanism of depletion of liver glycogen in cancer cachexia. Biochem Biophys Res Commun 241:49–52

39. Ishiko O, Yasui T, Hirai K et al (1999) Lipolytic activity of anemia-inducing susbtance from tumor-bearing rabbits. Nutr Cancer 33:201–205

40. Todorov P, Cariuk P, McDevitt T et al (1996) Characterization of a cancer cachectic factor. Nature 22:739–742

41. Lorite MJ, Cariuk P, Tisdale MJ (1997) Induction of muscle protein degradation by a tumour factor. Br J Cancer 76:1035–1040

42. Wigmore SJ, Todorov PT, Ross JA et al (2000) Characteristics of patients with pancreatic cancer expressing a novel cancer cachexia factor. Br J Surgery 87:53–58

43. Lorite MJ, Thompson MG, Drake JL et al (1998) Mechanism of muscle protein degradation induced by a cancer cachectic factor. Br J Cancer 78:850–856

44. Smith HJ, Lorite MJ, Tisdale MJ (1999) Effects of a cancer cachectic factor on protein synthesis/degradation in murine C2C12 myoblasts: modulation by eicosapentaenoic acid. Cancer Res 59:5507–5513

45. Penner CG, Gang G, Wray C et al (2001) The transcription factors NF-kappaB and AP-1 are differen-

tially regulated in skeletal muscle during sepsis. Biochem Biophys Res Commun 281:1331–1336

46. Busquets S, Carbó N, Almendro V et al (2001) Curcumin, a natural product present in turmeric, decreases tumor growth but does not behave as an anticachectic compound in a rat model. Cancer Lett 167:33–38

47. Fernandez-Celemin L, Pasko N, Blomart V, Thissen JP (2002) Inhibition of muscle insulin-like growth factor I expression by tumor necrosis factor-alpha. Am J Physiol 283:E1279–E1290

48. Li YP, Schwartz RJ, Waddell ID et al (1998) Skeletal muscle myocytes undergo protein loss and reactive oxygen-mediated NF-kappaB activation in response to tumor necrosis factor alpha. FASEB J 12:871–880

49. Brenner DA, O'Hara M, Angel P et al (1989) Prolonged activation of jun and collagenase genes by tumor necrosis factor-alpha. Nature 337:661–663

50. Thinakaran G, Ojala J, Bag J (1993) Expression of c-jun/AP-1 during myogenic differentiation in mouse C2C12 myoblasts. FEBS Lett 319:271–276

51. Penner G, Gang G, Sun X et al (2002) C/EBP DNA-binding activity is upregulated by a glucocorticoid-dependent mechanism in septic muscle. Am J Physiol 282:R439–R444

52. Guttridge DC, Mayo MW, Madrid LV et al (2000) NF-kappaB-induced loss of MyoD messenger RNA: possible role in muscle decay and cachexia. Science 289:2363–2366

53. Coletti D, Yang E, Marazzi G, Sassoon D (2002) TNF-α inhibits skeletal myogenesis through a PW1-dependent pathway by recruitment of caspase pathways. EMBO J 21:631–642

54. Puigserver P, Rhee J, Lin J et al (2001) Cytokine stimulation of energy expenditure through p38 MAP kinase activation of PPARgamma coactivator-1. Mol Cell 8:971–982

55. Balazs C, Kiss E (1994) Immunological aspects of the effect of pentoxifylline. Acta Microbiol Immunol Hung 41:121–126

56. Goldberg RM, Loprinzi CL, Mailliard JA et al (1995) Pentoxifylline for treatment of cancer anorexia and cachexia? A randomized, double-blind, placebo-controlled trial. J Clin Oncol 13:2856–2859

57. Peuckmann V, Fisch M, Bruera E (2000) Potential novel uses of thalidomide: focus on palliative care. Drugs 60:273–292

58. Costelli P, Carbó N, Tessitore L et al (1993) Tumor necrosis factor-α mediates changes in tissue protein turnover in a rat cancer cachexia model. J Clin Invest 92:2783–2789

59. Reinhart K, Wiegand-Lohnert C, Grimminger F et al (1996) Assessment of the safety and efficacy of the monoclonal anti-tumor necrosis factor antibody fragment, MAK 195F, in patients with sepsis and septic shock: a multicenter, randomized, placebo-controlled, dose-ranging study. Crit Care Med 24:733–742

60. Mori K, Fujimoto-Ouchi K, Ishikawa T et al (1996) Murine interleukin-12 prevents the development of cancer cachexia in a murine model. Int J Cancer 67:849–855

61. Quinn LS, Haugk KL, Grabstein KH (1995) Interleukin-15: a novel anabolic cytokine for skeletal muscle. Endocrinology 136:3669–3672

62. Carbó N, López-Soriano J, Costelli P et al (2000) Interleukin-15 antagonizes muscle protein waste in tumour-bearing rats. Br J Cancer 83:526–531

63. Okamoto T (2002) NSAID zaltoprofen improves the decrease in body weight in rodent sickness behavior models: proposed new applications of NSAID. Int J Mol Med 9:369–372

64. Niu Q, Li T, Liu A (2001) Cytokines in experimental cancer cachexia. Zhonghua Zhong Liu Za Zhi 23:382–384

65. Kawamura I, Morishita R, Tomita N et al (1999) Intratumoral injection of oligonucleotides to the NF kappa B binding site inhibits cachexia in a mouse tumor model. Gene Ther 6:91–97

66. Kawamura I, Morishita R, Tsujimoto S et al (2001) Intravenous injection of oligodeoxynucleotides to the NF-kappaB binding site inhibits hepatic metastasis of M5076 reticulosarcoma in mice. Gene Ther 8:905–912

# Proinflammatory Cytokines: Their Role in Multifactorial Cancer Cachexia

Giovanni Mantovani, Clelia Madeddu

## Introduction

Cancer-related anorexia-cachexia syndrome (CACS) may result from circulating factors produced by the tumour or by the host immune system in response to the tumour, such as cytokines released by lymphocytes and/or monocyte/macrophages. A number of proinflammatory cytokines, including interleukin (IL)-1, IL-6, tumour necrosis factor (TNF)-α, interferon (IFN)-α and IFN-γ, have been implicated in the pathogenesis of cachexia associated with human cancer. TNF-α was first identified by Rouzer and Cerami [1] as a specific circulating mediator of the wasting resulting from a chronic experimental infectious disease. It was named cachectin and was subsequently found to be identical to TNF-α. However, data from numerous clinical and laboratory studies suggest that the action of cytokines, although important, may not alone explain the complex mechanism of CACS [2–5]. IL-1 and TNF-α have been proposed as mediators of the host's response to inflammation [6]. Human IL-1 and TNF-α administered to healthy animals produced a significant reduction in their food intake [7]. High serum levels of TNF-α, IL-2, and IFN-γ have been found in cancer patients or in experimental animals with cancer [8], and, although IL-6 levels appear to correlate with tumour progression in animal models [8], current evidence supports a role for IL-6 as a cachectic factor in the development of cancer cachexia in an animal model system [9]. Chronically elevated levels of these factors, either alone or in combination, are capable of reproducing the different features of CACS [9–12]. More direct evidence of cytokine involvement in CACS is provided by the observations that cachexia in experimental animal models [4, 13, 14] can be relieved by administration of specific cytokine antagonists. These studies showed that cachexia can rarely be attributed to any one cytokine but rather is associated with a set of cytokines that work in concert. These cytokines seem to play central roles in both cachexia-related inflammation and the acute-phase response [15].

Numerous evidence is provided in the literature on the role of cytokines in cancer cachexia. Balkwill et al. found that 50% of 226 fresh serum samples from cancer patients had a positive response for TNF when tested in an enzyme-linked immunoadsorbent assay [16]. More recently, TNF was detected in the serum of children with acute lymphoblastic leukaemia [17]. Similarly, considerable amounts of TNF have been found in the blood of tumour-bearing rats [18, 19]. Strassmann et al., using a murine colon adenocarcinoma, have shown that treatment with anti-mouse IL-6 antibody was successful in reversing the key parameters of cachexia in tumour-bearing mice [20]. In addition, in vitro studies of incubated rat skeletal muscle have clearly shown that IL-6 has no direct effect on muscle proteolysis.

Another interesting candidate for cachexia is IFN-γ, which is produced by activated T and NK cells and possesses biological activities that overlap with those of TNF. IFN-γ, is best known for its ability to activate mononuclear phagocytes and to enhance expression of class II MHC antigens. Matthys et al., using a monoclonal antibody against IFN-γ, were able to reverse the wasting syndrome associated with the growth of the Lewis lung carcinoma in mice [21], thus demonstrating that IFN-γ is produced endogenously in tumour-bearing mice and is instrumental in bringing about some of the generalised metabolic changes characteristic of cancer cachexia. Other cytokines, such as leukaemia inhibitory factor (LIF) [22] and transforming growth factor (TGF)-β [23], have also been proposed as mediators of cachexia. Interestingly, the levels of both IL-6 and LIF are increased in patients with different types of malignancies. Ciliary neurotrophic factor (CNTF) is a member of the family of cytokines that include IL-6 and LIF and is produced predominantly by glial cells of the peripheral nervous system [24]. Henderson et al. reported that CNTF induced potent cachectic effects and acute-phase protein synthesis in mice implanted with C6 glioma cells that had been genetically modified to secrete the cytokine [25]. Bearing these results in mind, it may be concluded that, although TNF has a very important role in the induction of cachexia, the metabolic derangement leading to this pathological state can also be influenced by other cytokines produced by immune cells in response to invasive stimuli [26].

## Proinflammatory Cytokines and the Acute-Phase Response

Among the specific causes of CACS, there is evidence of a chronic, low-grade, tumour-induced activation of the host immune system that shares numerous characteristics with the acute-phase response found after major traumatic events and septic shock. The latter is characterised by an increased production of cytokines [27, 28]; high levels of catecholamine, cortisol, and glucagon [27, 29–31]; increased peripheral amino-acid mobilisation and hepatic amino acid uptake [27, 32]; increased hepatic gluconeogenesis and acute-phase protein production [27, 33, 34]; and enhanced mobilisation of free fatty acids and increased metabolism [35]. The acute-phase response is a systemic reaction to tissue injury, typically observed during inflammation, infection or trauma. It consists of the release of hepatocyte-derived plasma proteins, known as acute-phase reactants, which include C-reactive protein, fibrinogen, complement factors B and C3, and of a reduced synthesis of albumin and transferrin. An acute-phase response is observed in patients with cancer. In fact, the cytokines IL-1, IL-6, and TNF-$\alpha$ are regarded as the major mediators of acute-phase protein induction in the liver. Unfortunately,

the role played by these proteins during cancer growth is still poorly understood.

## Proinflammatory Cytokines and Anorexia

Another cause of CACS which, due to its particular aspects and appearance, may be considered specific for the syndrome is decreased food intake. Malnutrition may be considered a hallmark of cancer cachexia and it is associated with anorexia – that is, loss of appetite and/or decreased food intake. Nutrition is a complex function resulting from the contribution of peripheral and central nervous afferents in the ventral hypothalamus. Stimulation of the medial hypothalamic nucleus inhibits feeding, while stimulation of the lateral nucleus promotes food intake. Among peripheral afferents, oral stimulation by pleasant tastes elicits eating, whereas gastric distension inhibits it.

There is evidence that while the proinflammatory cytokines IL-1, IL-6, and TNF-$\alpha$ are involved in cancer-related anorexia and decreased food intake (see below), they are probably not the only mediators of CACS. Since multiple factors are involved in the control of food intake, it is possible that there are also many factors contributing to tumour-associated anorexia. Indeed, anorexigenic compounds are either released by the tumour into the circulation or the tumour itself may induce metabolic changes resulting in the release of such substances by host tissues. Changes in tryptophan levels in patients with cancer result in increased brain serotonin synthesis and, thus, serotonergic activity, which leads to reduced food intake. Other factors could be involved in promoting inhibitory afferents to the hypothalamus by stimulating serotonergic and catecholaminergic fibres, such as increased lactate and fatty-acid blood levels, both of which are associated with tumour burden.

Few controlled clinical trials have investigated the incidence of cancer-related reduction of food intake: this may be because of the methodological difficulties associated with human diet analysis and the need for large patient and control groups.

A third potentially important cause of CACS may be the abnormal functioning of neuropeptides, leptin, ghrelin, and/or their reciprocal interactions. Body weight loss is a strong stimulus of food intake in humans. Therefore, the presence of CACS in patients with cancer suggests a failure of the adaptive feeding response. A large amount of evidence has accumulated in the last few years on the regulation of feeding and body weight. Leptin, a recently discovered hormone produced by the adipocyte *ob* gene, is an essential component of the homeostatic regulation of body weight. Leptin acts to control food intake and energy expenditure via neuropeptidergic effector molecules within the hypothalamus. Complex interactions take place among the nervous, endocrine, and immune systems inducing behavioural and metabolic responses. Proinflammatory cytokines, proposed as mediators of CACS, may have a central role in the long-term inhibition of feeding by mimicking the hypothalamic effect of excessive negative feedback signalling from leptin. This could be by continuous stimulation of anorexigenic neuropeptides, such as serotonin- and corticotropin-releasing factor; by inhibition of the neuropeptide Y orexigenic network, consisting of opioid peptides and galanin; and by the recently identified melanin-concentrating hormone, orexin and agouti-related peptide. Such abnormalities in the hypothalamic neuropeptide loop in tumour-bearing animals lead to the development of CACS. Although neuropeptide agonists/antagonists are currently used only in the treatment of obesity, they may also constitute an effective strategy for the treatment of CACS, particularly in combination with other agents with different mechanisms of action [36, 37]. A study by our group [38] demonstrated very low leptin levels associated with high levels of inflammatory cytokines in patients with advanced-stage cancer, several of whom had significant body weight loss.

## The Role of Proinflammatory Cytokines in Cancer Cachexia: Personal Studies

In a series of papers, we reported that the serum levels of proinflammatory cytokines (IL-1α and β, IL-6, and TNF-α) in cancer patients, especially in advanced-stage disease, are higher than those of healthy subjects [39–44]. In a study carried out on 29 advanced-stage cancer patients with tumours at different sites, we found that serum levels of proinflammatory cytokines, particularly IL-6, were significantly higher in cancer patients than in healthy individuals and that serum levels of proinflammatory cytokines inversely correlated with those of leptin [45]. In addition, there was a direct correlation between Eastern Cooperative Oncology Group performance status (ECOG PS) and serum levels of proinflammatory cytokines, i.e. IL-6 and TNF-α serum levels of patients with ECOG PS 0–1 were significantly lower than those of patients with ECOG PS 2–3. More interestingly, serum levels of proinflammatory cytokines correlated with patient survival. Very high levels of proinflammatory cytokines, particularly IL-6 (and low levels of leptin) correlated with a short survival time. Analysis of clinical response, survival, and serum levels of proinflammatory cytokines/leptin showed that: patients with very high levels of proinflammatory cytokines and very low serum levels of leptin died earlier of progressive disease and had very short survival (measured from the time of cytokines/leptin evaluation). Patients with intermediate serum levels of proinflammatory cytokines and leptin survived longer or are still alive with progressive disease. Patients with higher levels of leptin and lower levels of proinflammatory cytokines had the longest survival and are still alive and in a clinically objective response (complete response or partial response) or stable disease.

Whether tumour- or host-derived cytokines act by overruling the normal weight homeostasis in CACS or through a different pathway remains to be clarified. Since most authors, including us, have failed to find high leptin concentrations in cancer patients who lost body weight [46, 47], those with AIDS [48], or the elderly [49], an alternative explanation of CACS involves corticotropin-releasing hormone (CRH) pathways. Several cytokines, such as IL-1α, IL-6, and TNF-α, by increasing hypothalamic CRH gene expression, may activate the same CRH pathway as the leptin-catabolic effector system [50]. Considering that the leptin receptor is a member of the class I cytokine receptor family, and that leptin activates intracellular signal transduction pathways common to many cytokines, it is possible that some cytokines, such as the proinflammatory ones, act as leptin-like factors and mimic the effect of leptin, decreasing energy intake and increasing energy expenditure [50]. Putting into correlation the serum values of proinflammatory cytokines with the patient clinical features, we suggest that the former may offer a useful surrogate marker of patient nutritional and general performance status. Moreover, we consider them predictive of patient survival.

In another study [38], we investigated the presence of a correlation between cytokines (and other biological parameters such as CRP, leptin, and antioxidant enzyme) and the clinically most important indices, such as disease stage and ECOG PS. A direct correlation between stage/ECOG PS and serum levels of proinflammatory cytokines, particularly IL-6 and CRP, was observed such that the serum levels of IL-6 and CRP progressively increased from stage II/ECOG 0–1 to stage IV/ECOG 2–3. Patients at advanced stage and most compromised PS had the highest levels of IL-6/CRP and the lowest levels of leptin, IL-2, and antioxidant enzymes. Thus, it can be hypothesised that in this group of cancer patients the high levels of proinflammatory cytokines severely impaired the energetic and specific metabolic (i.e. glucose, proteic, and lipid) balance [42, 43], thereby preventing the physiological ability of the organism to maintain body redox equilibrium by synthesising the appropriate amount of antioxidant enzymes.

In one of our very recent papers we found that high levels of proinflammatory cytokines and increased oxidative stress may contribute to the development of cancer-related anemia. We assessed a population of previously untreated patients with advanced epithelial ovarian cancer to evaluate whether there was a correlation between hemoglobin (Hb) and parameters of inflammation and oxidative stress, stage of disease, and performance status (PS). In 91 patients with epithelial ovarian cancer and 95 healthy women matched for age, weight, and height, levels of Hb, C-reactive protein (CRP), fibrinogen (Fbg), proinflammatory cytokines, leptin, reactive oxygen species (ROS), and antioxidant enzymes were assessed at diagnosis before treatment.

The correlations between Hb, parameters of inflammation and oxidative stress, stage, and PS were evaluated. Hb levels were lower in patients with advanced epithelial ovarian cancer than in control subjects and inversely related to stage and PS. Hb negatively correlated with CRP, Fbg, interleukin 1β (IL-1β), IL-6, tumor necrosis factor α (TNF-α), and ROS, and positively correlated with leptin and glutathione peroxidase (GPx). Multivariate regression analysis showed that stage and IL-6 were independent factors determining Hb values. This evidence suggests that anemia in epithelial ovarian cancer is related to stage of disease and markers of inflammation [51].

# References

1. Rouzer CA, Cerami A (1980) Hypertryglyceridemia associated with Trypanosoma brucei brucei infection in rabbits: role of defective triglyceride removal. Mol Biochem Parasitol 2:31–38
2. McNamara MJ, Alexander HR, Norton JA (1992) Cytokines and their role in the pathophysiology of cancer cachexia. J Parenter Enteral Nutr 16:50S–55S
3. Tisdale MJ (1997) Biology of cachexia. J Natl Cancer Inst 89:1763–1773
4. Noguchi Y, Yoshikawa T, Matsumoto A et al (1996) Are cytokines possible mediators of cancer cachexia? Surg Today 26:467–475
5. Espat NJ, Copeland EM, Moldawer LL (1994) Tumor necrosis factor and cachexia: a current perspective. Surg Oncol 3:255–262
6. Moldawer LL, Gelin J, Schersten T et al (1987) Circulating interleukin 1 and tumor necrosis factor during inflammation. Am J Physiol 253:R922–R928
7. Moldawer LL, Andersson C, Gelin J (1988) Regulation of food intake and hepatic protein synthesis by recombinant-derived cytokines. Am J Physiol 254:6450–6456
8. Moldawer LL, Rogy MA, Lowry SF (1992) The role of cytokines in cancer cachexia. JPEN J Parenter Enteral Nutr 16:43S–49S
9. Strassmann G, Fong M, Kenney JS et al (1992) Evidence for the involvement of interleukin-6 in experimental cancer cachexia. J Clin Invest 89:1681–1684
10. Busbridge J, Dascombe MJ, Hoopkins S (1989) Acute central effects of interleukin-6 on body temperature, thermogenesis and food intake in the rat. Proc Nutr Soc 38:48A
11. Gelin J, Moldawer LL, Lonnroth C (1991) Role of endogenous tumor necrosis factor alfa and interleukin

1 for experimental tumor growth and the development of cancer cachexia. Cancer Res 51:415–421

12. McLaughlin CL, Rogan GJ, Ton J (1992) Food intake and body temperature responses of rat to recombinant interleukin 1 beta and a tripeptide interleukin 1 beta antagonist. Physiol Behav 52:1155–1160

13. Sherry BA, Gelin J, Fong Y (1991) Anticachectin/tumor necrosis factor alpha antibodies attenuate development of cancer cachexia. Cancer Res 51:415–421

14. Matthys P, Billiau A (1997) Cytokines and cachexia. Nutr 13:763–770

15. Moldawer LL, Copeland EM (1997) Proinflammatory cytokines, nutritional support, and the cachexia syndrome: interactions and therapeutic options. Cancer 79:1828–1839

16. Balkwill F, Burke F, Talbot D et al (1987) Evidence for tumour necrosis factro/cachectin production in cancer. Lancet 2:1229–1232

17. Saarinen UM, Koskelo EK, Teppo AM, Siimes MA (1990) Tumor necrosis factor in children with malignancies. Cancer Res 50:592–595

18. Costelli P, Carbò N, Tessitore L et al (1993) Tumor necrosis factor-alpha mediates changes in tissue protein turnover in a rat cancer cachexia model. J Clin Invest 92:2783–2789

19. Stovroff MC, Fraker DL, Norton JA (1989) Cachectin activity in the serum of cachectic, tumor-bearing rats. Arch Surg 124:94–99

20. Strassmann G, Fong M, Freter CE et al (1993) Suramin interferes with interleukin-6 receptor binding in vitro and inhibits colon-26-mediated experimental cancer cachexia in vivo. J Clin Invest 92:2152–2159

21. Matthys P, Heremans H, Opdenakker G, Billiau A (1991) Anti-interferon-gamma antibody treatment, growth of Lewis lung tumours in mice and tumour-associated cachexia. Eur J Cancer 27:182–187

22. Mori M, Yamaguchi K, Honda S et al (1991) Cancer cachexia syndrome developed in nude mice bearing melanoma cells producing leukemia-inhibitory factor. Cancer Res 51:6656–6659

23. Zugmaier G, Paik S, Wilding G et al (1991) Transforming growth factor beta 1 induces cachexia and systemic fibrosis without an antitumor effect in nude mice. Cancer Res 51:3590–3594

24. Mrosovsky N, Molony LA, Conn CA, Kluger MJ (1989) Anorexic effects of interleukin 1 in the rat. Am J Physiol 257:R1315–R1321

25. Henderson JT, Mullen BJ, Roder JC (1996) Physiological effects of CNTF-induced wasting. Cytokine 8:784–793

26. Argiles JM, Lopez-Soriano FJ (1999) The role of cytokines in cancer cachexia. Med Res Rev 19:223–248

27. Byerley LO, Alcock NW, Starnes HF (1992) Sepsis-induced cascade of cytokine mRNA expression: correlation with metabolic changes. Am J Physiol 261:E728–E735

28. Waage A, Brandtzaeg P, Halstensen A et al (1989) The complex pattern of cytokines in serum from patients with meningococcal septic shock. J Exp Med 169:333–338

29. Wilmore DW, Long JM, Mason AD et al (1974) Catecholamines: mediator of the hypermetabolic response to thermal injury. Ann Surg 180:653–668

30. Stoner HB, Barton RN, Little RA et al (1977) Measuring the severity of injury. BMJ 2:1247–1249

31. Wilmore DW, Moylan JA, Pruitt Bam Lindsey CA et al (1974) Hyperglucagonaemia after burns. Lancet 1:73–75

32. Rosenblatt S, Clowes GH Jr, George BC et al (1983) Exchange of amino acids by muscle and liver in sepsis. Arch Surg 118:167–175

33. Long CL (1977) Energy balance and carbohydrate metabolism in infection and sepsis. Am J Clin Nutr 30:1301–1310

34. Baumann H, Gauldie J (1994) The acute phase response. Immunol Today 15:74–80

35. Oliff A, Defeo-Jones D, Boyer M et al (1987) Tumor secreting human TNF/cachectin induce cachexia in mice. Cell 50:555–563

36. Inui A (1999) Cancer anorexia-cachexia syndrome: are neuropeptides the key? Cancer Res 15:4493–4501

37. Inui A (1999) Neuropeptide Y: a key molecule in anorexia and cachexia in wasting disorders? Mol Med Today 5:79–85

38. Mantovani G, Macciò A, Madeddu C et al (2002) Quantitative evaluation of oxidative stress, chronic inflammatory indices and leptin in cancer patients: correlation with stage and performance status. Int J Cancer 98:84–91

39. Mantovani G, Macciò A, Esu S et al (1994) Lack of correlation between defective cell-mediated immunity and levels of secreted or circulating cytokines in a study of 90 cancer patients. Int J Oncol 5:1211–1217

40. Mantovani G, Macciò A, Versace R et al (1995) Tumor-associated lymphocytes (TAL) are competent to produce higher levels of cytokines in neoplastic pleural and peritoneal effusions than those found in sera and are able to release into culture higher levels of IL-2 and IL-6 than those released by PBMC. J Mol Med 73:409–416

41. Mantovani G, Macciò A, Bianchi A et al (1995) Megestrol acetate in neoplastic anorexia/cachexia: clinical evaluation and comparison with cytokine levels in patients with head and neck carcinoma treated with neoadjuvant chemotherapy. Int J Clin Lab Res 25:135–141

42. Mantovani G, Macciò A, Lai P et al (1998) Cytokine activity in cancer-related anorexia/cachexia: role of megestrol acetate and medroxyprogesterone acetate. Semin Oncol 25:45–52

43. Mantovani G, Macciò A, Mura L et al (2000) Serum levels of leptin and proinflammatory cytokines in patients with advanced-stage cancer at different sites. J Mol Med 78:554–561

44. Mantovani G, Macciò A, Madeddu C et al (2003) Antioxidant agents are effective in inducing lymphocyte progression through cell cycle in advanced cancer

patients: assessment of the most important laboratory indexes of cachexia and oxidative stress. J Mol Med 81:664–673

45.  Mantovani G, Macciò A, Madeddu C et al (2001) Serum values of proinflammatory cytokines are inversely correlated with serum leptin levels in patients with advanced stage cancer at different sites. J Mol Med 79:406–414

46.  Wallace AM, Sattar N, McMillan DC (1998) Effect of weight loss and the inflammatory response on leptin concentrations in gastrointestinal cancer patients. Clin Cancer Res 4:2977–2979

47.  Simons JP, Schols AM, Campfield LA et al (1997) Plasma concentration of total leptin and human lung-cancer-associated cachexia. Clin Sci (Lond) 93:273–277

48.  Grunfeld C, Pang M, Shigenaga JK et al (1996) Serum leptin levels in the acquired immunodeficiency syndrome. J Clin Endocrinol Metab 81:4342–4346

49.  Yeh SS, Schuster MW (1999) Geriatric cachexia: the role of cytokines. Am J Clin Nutr 70:183–197

50.  Frühbeck G, Jebb SA, Prentice AM (1998) Leptin: physiology and pathophysiology. Clin Physiol 18:399–419

51.  Macciò A, Madeddu C, Massa D et al (2005) Hemoglobin levels correlate with interleukin-6 levels in patients with advanced untreated epithelial ovarian cancer: role of inflammation in cancer-related anemia. Blood 106:362–367

# Proteolysis-Inducing Factor in Cancer Cachexia

Michael J. Tisdale

## Introduction

Progressive atrophy of skeletal muscle in cancer cachexia leads to reduced power output and weakness (asthenia), resulting in reduced physical activity and a lower quality of life of the cancer patient. Eventually, loss of respiratory muscle becomes so extensive that function becomes significantly impaired, resulting in death through hypostatic pneumonia. Death normally occurs when patients have lost about 35% of their ideal body weight.

Certain cytokines, such as tumour necrosis factor (TNF)-$\alpha$, interleukins (IL)-1 and IL-6 and interferon (IFN)-$\gamma$ have been identified from experimental models of cancer cachexia as possible mediators of the loss of muscle mass. However, clinical studies in patients with advanced and terminal cancers of various types have found no correlation between circulating levels of these cytokines and weight loss and anorexia [1]. It has been suggested that increases in cytokines may be transient, but raised concentrations have been found in patients with other types of cachexia, such as in septicaemia [2] and in AIDS [3]. It has also been suggested that cytokines have a local effect, and that they are elevated in target tissues without an increase in overall serum levels. A characteristic of cytokines is that they inhibit the enzyme lipoprotein lipase (LPL) in adipose tissue, thus preventing triglyceride synthesis. However, in a study by Thompson et al. [4], not only were they unable to detect elevated serum levels of TNF-$\alpha$ in cancer patients, but the total LPL activity in adipose tissue, and the relative levels of mRNA for LPL and fatty acid synthase were not significantly different between cancer patients and controls. This suggests that, although cytokines have the potential to produce cachexia, and may well be important in tissue wasting in some conditions, such as sepsis and AIDS, they may not play a major role in cancer cachexia. This necessitated the search for alternative factors specific for cancer cachexia.

## Alternative Models of Cachexia

Most of the studies that have identified cytokines as important determinants in cancer cachexia have employed rat tumours. These tumours tend to grow rapidly, have a strong anorectic component, and may require large tumour masses before cachexia is apparent. However, most human tumours grow slowly, can produce cachexia in the absence of anorexia [5], and the tumour mass does not normally exceed 5% of the body weight. In human cachexia, there is also evidence for a circulatory factor capable of inducing protein degradation in skeletal muscle in patients with weight loss > 10% [6].

MAC16 is a chemically induced, transplantable adenocarcinoma of the colon, that is passaged in inbred NMRI mice [7]. In male animals, weight loss occurs when the tumour mass comprises more than 0.3% of body weight and reaches 30% when the tumour represents just 3% of body weight [8]. Weight loss involves a decrease in both carcass fat and skeletal muscle mass and is directly proportional to the weight of the tumour. Weight loss occurs in the absence of anorexia, and is associated with the presence of circulatory factors capable of directly inducing lipolysis in adipose tissue and protein degradation in skeletal muscle [8]. This tumour is, therefore, very similar to the metabolic component of human cancer cachexia, and has been used extensively for the isolation of tumour catabolic products, and for the evaluation of potential anti-cachectic agents.

## Isolation and Structure of Proteolysis-Inducing Factor

Initial attempts to purify a lipid mobilising factor (LMF) from the MAC16 tumour, using anion exchange chromatography, revealed the presence of a 24-kDa band on Western blotting, detected using serum from mice bearing the MAC16 tumour [9]. Antibodies to the 24-kDa material were not present in the serum of mice bearing the MAC13 tumour, which is histologically similar to the MAC16 tumour but which does not induce cachexia. A similar 24k-Da band on Western blots was detected using serum from MAC16-tumour-bearing mice, but not from those bearing the MAC13 tumour, in the urine of patients with cancer cachexia. This band was not present in Western blots of urine from normal subjects. These results suggested that the 24-kDa material was closely associated with the development of cachexia in mice and humans.

An antibody to the 24-kDa material was cloned from hybridomas produced by the fusion of splenocytes from mice bearing the MAC16 tumour and mouse myeloma cells [10]. The cloned antibody was used to isolate the 24-kDa factor by immunoaffinity chromatography and reverse-phase hydrophobic chromatography [11]. The purified material was found to be resistant to a range of proteolytic enzymes, but fragmentation was achieved using both peptide-$N$-glycosidase F and endo-$\alpha$-$N$-acetylgalactosaminidase, suggesting the presence of both $N$- and $O$-glycan chains. Lectin blotting suggested the presence of Gal $\beta$ (1→4) $N$-acetylglucosamine units [10]. Further structural studies revealed the 24-kDa material to be a sulphated glycoprotein with a central polypeptide core of $M_r$ 4000, one $O$-linked sulphated oligosaccharide chain of $M_r$ 6000 and one $N$-linked oligosaccharide chain of $M_r$ 10 000, both containing $N$-acetylglucosamine [12] (Fig. 1). The molecular mass of the 24-kDa material was subsequently confirmed by MALDI-TOF mass spectrometry, which showed a broad peak in this region, which may have been due to the presence of multiple species arising from the microheterogeneity normally associated with the presence of glycoforms [13].

Examination of the sequence of the human genome revealed that the gene for the polypeptide core of this proteolysis-inducing factor (PIF) is located on chromosome 12. Two peptides with 100% homology to PIF have been reported; an antimicrobial peptide, called dermicidin, secreted by sweat glands [14], and a neuronal survival peptide, called Y-P30 [15]. Neither of these peptides are glycosylated, and it is the oligosaccharide chains on PIF that are responsible for its biological activity [12]. Thus, neither of the homologous peptides would be expected to produce the same biological effects as PIF.

## Tumours as Source of PIF

The 24-kDa factor was initially isolated from the murine cachexia-inducing MAC16 tumour [11], but it was also found to be present in the urine of patients with carcinoma of the pancreas, breast, ovary, lung, colon, rectum, and liver in whom the rate of weight loss was ≥ to about 1 kg per month [16]. Patients who were weight-stable or in whom the rate of weight loss was < 1 kg month showed no evidence for excretion, even though they had the same tumour types. Subjects with weight loss associated with conditions other than cancer, such as sepsis, multiple injuries, major surgery, and sleeping sickness, showed no evidence for urinary secretion of the 24-kDa material, even though the rate of weight loss was higher than in cancer patients. Immunohistochemistry with the MAC16 monoclonal antibody showed that the 24-kDa material was present in the cytoplasm of tumours of the gastrointestinal tract, and a correlation was obtained between expression in tumours, detection in urine, and weight loss in cancer patients [17]. RT-PCR studies allowed the detection of PIF mRNA in prostate carcinoma cell lines, in primary prostate carcinoma tissue, and in its osseous metastasis [18]. In situ hybridisation showed that the mRNA was localised only in the epithelial cells of the tumour tissue, but not in the adjacent nonmalignant prostate epithelial cells or stromal cells. It was also present in the metastatic foci in bone, liver, and lymph node. The central core protein was detected in nine of 14 prostate carcinoma metastases, but not in normal prostate tissue or in patients with organ-confined tumours, and was present in nine of 19 urine specimens from prostatic carcinoma patients, but not in 19 urine samples of noncachectic patients, as previously observed [16, 17]. These results demonstrate that prostate carcinoma cells express the 24-kDa glycoprotein, that it is identical to the factor originally found in the murine MAC16 tumour [11], and that its expression is associated with disease progression and the development of cachexia.

The 24-kDa factor is not only associated with the development of cachexia in the MAC16 model, but may also play a major role in other cachexia models previously thought to involve cytokines. Thus, IL-6 has been suggested to be the mediator of cachexia in the murine colon 26 model, since serum levels of this cytokine appeared to correlate with the development of cachexia [19], and administration of anti-IL-6 monoclonal antibody, but not anti-TNF-α monoclonal antibody, attenuated the development of weight loss and other parameters of cachexia. However, other data [20, 21] raised doubts as to whether IL-6 alone is responsible for cachexia in this model. Two variants of the colon 26 tumour were developed [22]: cachexia-inducing (clone 20) and non-cachectic (clone 5). Serum IL-6 levels were found to be elevated in mice transplanted with either clone, suggesting that IL-6 alone is not responsible for the development of cachexia. However, mice transplanted with the clone 20 variant showed evidence for the 24-kDa factor in tumour, serum, and urine, while mice transplanted with the clone 5 variant showed no evidence for the factor in tumour, serum, and urine [23]. These results suggest that the 24-kDa factor acts together with IL-6 to induce cachexia in colon 26 adenocarcinoma. Further evidence for the importance of the 24-kDa factor in the development of cachexia in this model was the disappearance from tumour, serum, and urine in mice bearing the clone 20 variant, concomitant with attenuation of cachexia development after treatment with the fluorinated pyrimidine nucleoside 5$^\alpha$-deoxy-5-fluorouridine. This suggests that it should be possible to design anti-cachectic drugs targeted to interfere with biosynthesis of the 24-kDa factor.

## Biological Effects of PIF

Since the 24-kDa glycoprotein was originally purified with LMF, it was thought that it may be a lipolysis-inducing agent. However, it was found not to have an effect on adipose tissue, but instead induced protein degradation in isolated skeletal muscle [12]. It was therefore given the name proteolysis-inducing factor (PIF), and is likely to be the serum factor previously identified as inducing protein breakdown in skeletal muscle [6]. Biological activity was destroyed by preincubation with peptide N-glycosidase F and α-N-acetylgalactosaminidase, but not by neuraminidase or trypsin, suggesting that the N- and O-linked sulphated oligosaccharide chains are the biological determinants [12]. When administered intravenously to normal mice, PIF, isolated from either the MAC16 tumour [11] or from the urine of patients with cancer

cachexia [16], produced about 10% weight loss over a 24-h period without a reduction in food and water intake. The cachectic action of PIF was completely attenuated by pretreatment with the MAC16 monoclonal antibody, confirming that PIF from mice [11] and humans [16] is immunologically identical. Body composition analysis [16] showed that the majority of the weight loss was due to a loss of lean body mass. As in cancer cachexia, PIF produced a specific loss of skeletal muscle, while there was little effect on visceral protein reserves [24]. The decrease in lean body mass was accounted for by an increase (50%) in protein degradation, and a decrease (50%) in protein synthesis in gastrocnemius muscle [25]. Protein degradation was significantly decreased and protein synthesis increased to control values in mice pretreated with the monoclonal antibody.

A number of studies have shown that the predominant pathway mediating intracellular protein degradation in cancer cachexia is the ubiquitin-proteasome proteolytic pathway [24]. In mice bearing the MAC16 tumour, there are increased levels of ubiquitin-conjugated proteins and increased mRNA levels for proteasome subunits and the 14-kDa ubiquitin carrier protein E2 in skeletal muscle [24]. Administration of PIF to normal mice also caused increased expression of the ubiquitin-proteasome pathway in skeletal muscle, but not in visceral tissues [26]. These effects were also seen in tissue culture when murine myoblasts [26] or myotubes [27] were incubated with PIF for a 24-h period. The same concentrations of PIF as those inducing total protein degradation were also effective in inducing proteasome expression.

These results suggest that PIF plays a pivotal role in protein catabolism in cancer cachexia. Thus, PIF was detected in the urine of 80% of patients with pancreatic carcinoma, and these patients had a significantly greater total weight loss and rate of weight loss than patients whose urine did not contain PIF [28].

In addition to its effects on skeletal muscle, PIF is involved in hepatic gene expression [29]. Treatment of primary cultures of human hepatocytes and the human cell line Hep G2 with PIF activates the transcription factors nuclear factor-κB (NF-κB) and signal transducers and activators of transcription (STAT3), which result in the increased production of IL-6, IL-8, and C-reactive protein (CRP), and the decreased production of transferrin.

Thus, PIF is likely to be involved in the proinflammatory response observed in cachexia.

PIF may also play other roles in tumour pathogenesis outside the cachectic process. For example, it may contribute to tumour metastasis by inducing the expression of IL-8 and IL-6 in endothelial cells, as well as the cell-surface adhesion molecules intercellular adhesion molecule (ICAM)-1 and vascular cell adhesion molecule (VCAM), while reducing expression of the transmembrane proteoglycans syndecan-1 and syndecan-2 [30].

The normal role of PIF is unknown, but it is unlikely to be involved in normal cellular homeostasis, since mice transplanted with the MAC16 tumour produced antibodies to PIF [9]. Instead, the normal role of PIF may be in embryonic development, since PIF expression peaks in the mouse at embryonic day 8.5, a stage that is crucial in the development of skeletal muscle and liver [29]. In addition, vascular development, in particular umbilical arteries, also occurs at E8.5, and the organisation of endothelial cells into vessels requires cell-to-cell adhesion and thus cell-surface proteins, such as cadherin and ICAM. Syndecan-1 is also expressed at E8.5 and the decrease in its expression induced by PIF [30] suggests a role in development through the initiation of shedding of the functioning ectoderm portion of syndecan, allowing movement of the tissue to areas necessary for growth and development. It is likely that PIF production is shut off sometime before birth, but that certain tumours regain the ability to synthesise PIF through glycosyltransferases whose expression is normally restricted to the embryonic period. It is known that production of the polypeptide core of PIF continues into the adult [14, 15], so it is less likely that PIF expression is regulated through production of the protein.

## Mechanism of Muscle Protein Degradation by PIF

The transcription factor NF-$\kappa$B may also be important in PIF-induced expression of the ubiquitin-proteasome pathway in skeletal muscle, in addition to its role in liver and endothelial cells [31]. In murine myotubes that were used as a surrogate model of skeletal muscle, PIF produced a transient decrease in the cytosolic NF-$\kappa$B inhibitor protein

I$\kappa$B$\alpha$. This was accompanied by increased nuclear migration of NF-$\kappa$B, at the same concentrations of PIF as those inducing protein degradation, and increased expression of the regulatory components of the ubiquitin-proteasome proteolytic pathway. Moreover, the PIF-induced increase in proteasome activity was attenuated by the NF-$\kappa$B inhibitor peptide SN50, suggesting that NF-$\kappa$B is involved in increasing proteasome gene expression.

The mechanism for the activation of NF-$\kappa$B has not been fully delineated, but the first step appears to be the release of arachidonic acid from membrane phospholipids and its rapid metabolism to eicosanoids [32]. PIF was shown to increase the expression of calcium-independent cytosolic phospholipase $A_2$ (PLA$_2$) at the same concentrations as those inducing proteasome expression, and inhibitors of PLA$_2$ inhibited the induction of proteasome activity [33]. Of the eicosanoids formed in response to PIF, only one, 15-hydroxyeicosatetraenoic acid (15-HETE), a product of the action of 15-lipoxygenase (15-LOX) on arachidonic acid, was capable of inducing protein degradation in murine muscle cells [32]. An inhibitor of 15-LOX, 2, 3, 5-trimethyl-6-(3-pyridylmethyl)-1, 4-benzoquinone (CV-6504), was shown to be an effective inhibitor of cachexia in mice bearing the MAC16 tumour [34], reflecting the importance of this pathway in muscle atrophy. 15-HETE appears to be an important intracellular signal for the induction of the ubiquitin-proteasome proteolytic pathway by PIF [35]. 15-HETE acts like PIF to stimulate degradation of I$\kappa$B$\alpha$ and increase nuclear binding of NF-$\kappa$B. In addition, proteasome activity, increased by addition of exogenous 15-HETE to murine myotubes, is also attenuated by the NF-$\kappa$B inhibitor peptide SN50 [35].

The PIF-induced increase in protein degradation in muscle, but not the inhibition of protein synthesis, is effectively attenuated by the polyunsaturated fatty acid eicosapentaenoic acid (EPA) [32]. EPA has been shown to inhibit the onset of cachexia in mice bearing the MAC16 tumour, with a preservation of lean body mass through a reduction in protein degradation, but, as with PIF [32], without an effect on protein synthesis [36]. The effect is specific for EPA and is not seen with other polyunsaturated fatty acids. The action of EPA on muscle protein breakdown is achieved by down-regulation of the increased expression of the ubiquitin-proteasome pathway, with increased levels of the myofibrillar protein myosin [37]. EPA has been shown to be effective in attenuating further weight loss, and stabilising body weight in weight-losing patients with advanced pancreatic cancer [38]. This might be expected if EPA attenuated protein degradation. When EPA was administered together with a high-protein supplement to stimulate protein synthesis, patients with pancreatic cancer who were initially losing weight at a rate of 2.9 kg per month showed significant weight gain at both 3 (median 1 kg) and 7 weeks (median 2 kg) [39]. Moreover, body composition analysis showed that this weight gain was entirely lean body mass. Thus, while nutritional supplementation alone is ineffective in restoring lean body mass [40], it becomes effective when combined with an inhibitor of protein degradation.

EPA acts at several steps in the signalling cascade induced by PIF in skeletal muscle (Fig. 2), leading to increased expression of the ubiquitin-proteasome pathway. Thus, EPA reduces the release of arachidonic acid in response to PIF and the conversion to 15-HETE [32]. In addition, EPA blocks the action of 15-HETE added exogenously to muscle cells, suggesting that it acts at a further step in the pathway [35]. EPA was shown to attenuate binding of NF-κB in the nucleus by stabilisation of the NF-κB/IκB cytoplasmic complex. The mechanism behind this effect must involve the signalling steps by which 15-HETE induces degradation of IκBα, by inhibiting the phosphorylation process, which is critical for IκBα degradation by the ubiquitin-proteasome pathway.

The mechanism by which PIF induces expression of the ubiquitin-proteasome proteolytic pathway in cancer cachexia may be the same in other catabolic conditions. Thus, both EPA and the 15LOX inhibitor CV-6504 attenuated the increased protein degradation and expression of components of the ubiquitin-proteasome pathway in soleus muscle of mice after acute starvation [41]. These results suggest that protein catabolism in starvation and cancer cachexia is mediated through a common pathway, which is likely to involve a lipoxygenase metabolite as a signal transducer.

## Conclusions

PIF is a novel sulphated glycoprotein, secreted only by cachexia-inducing tumours, that may play a major role in muscle atrophy in cancer cachexia. PIF may serve as an appropriate target for the development of anticachectic agents.

## References

1. Maltoni M, Fabbri L, Nanni O et al (1997) Serum levels of tumour necrosis factor alpha and other cytokines do not correlate with weight loss and anorexia in cancer patients. Support Care Cancer 5:130–135
2. Waage A, Espevik T, Lamvik J (1986) Detection of tumour necrosis factor-like cytotoxicity in serum from patients with septicaemia but not from untreated cancer patients. Scand J Immunol 24:739–743
3. Horvath CJ, Desrosiers RD, Sehgal PK et al (1991) Effect of simian immunodeficiency virus infection on tumour necrosis factor-a production by alveolar macrophages. Lab Invest 65:280–286
4. Thompson MP, Cooper ST, Parry BR, Tuckey JA (1993) Increased expression of the mRNA for the hormone-sensitive lipase in adipose tissue of cancer patients. Biochem Biophys Acta 1180:236–241
5. Tisdale MJ (2001) Cancer anorexia and cachexia. Nutrition 17:438–442
6. Belizario JE, Katz M, Raw CI (1991) Bioactivity of skeletal muscle proteolysis-inducing factors in the plasma proteins from cancer patients with weight loss. Br J Cancer 63:705–710
7. Bibby MC, Double JA, Ali SA et al (1987) Characterization of a transplantable adenocarcinoma of the mouse colon producing cachexia in recipient animals. J Natl Cancer Inst 78:539–546
8. Beck SA, Tisdale MJ (1987) Production of lipolytic and proteolytic factors by a murine tumor-producing cachexia in the host. Cancer Res 47:5919–5923
9. McDevitt TM, Todorov PT, Beck SA et al (1995) Purification and characterization of a lipid-mobilizing factor associated with cachexia-inducing tumors in mice and humans. Cancer Res 55:1458–1463
10. Todorov PT, McDevitt TM, Cariuk P et al (1996) Induction of muscle protein degradation and weight loss by a tumor product. Cancer Res 56:1256–1261
11. Todorov P, Cariuk P, McDevitt T et al (1996) Characterization of a cancer cachectic factor. Nature 379:739–742
12. Todorov PT, Deacon M, Tisdale MJ (1997) Structural analysis of a tumor-produced sulfated glycoprotein capable of initiating muscle protein degradation. J Biol Chem 272:12279–12288
13. Choudhary G, Chakel J, Hancock W et al (1999) Investigation of the potential of capillary electrophoresis with off-line matrix-assisted laser desorption / ionization time-of-flight mass spectrometry for clinical analysis: examination of a glycoprotein

factor associated with cancer cachexia. Anal Chem 71:855–859

14. Schittek B, Hipfel R, Sauer B et al (2001) Dermicidin: a novel human antibiotic peptide secreted by sweat glands. Nat Immunol 2:1133–1137

15. Cunningham TJ, Jing H, Akerblom I et al (2002) Identification of the human cDNA for new survival / evasion peptide (DSEP): studies in vitro and in vivo of overexpression by neural cells. Exp Neurol 177:32–39

16. Cariuk P, Lorite MJ, Todorov PT et al (1997) Induction of cachexia in mice by a product isolated from the urine of cachectic cancer patients. Br J Cancer 76:606–613

17. Carbal Mazano R, Bhargava P, Torres-Duarte A et al (2001) roteolysis-inducing factor is expressed in tumours of patients with gastrointestinal cancers and correlates with weight loss. Br J Cancer 84:1599–1601

18. Wang Z, Corey E, Hass GM et al (2003) Expression of the human cachexia-associated protein (HCAP) in prostate cancer and in a prostate cancer animal model of cachexia. Int J Cancer 105:123–129

19. Strassman G, Fong M, Kenny JS, Jacob CO (1992) Evidence for the involvement of interleukin 6 in experimental cancer cachexia. J Clin Invest 89:1681–1684

20. Fujimoto-Ouchi K, Tamura S, Mori K et al (1995) Establishment and characterization of cachexia-inducing and non-inducing clones of murine colon 26 carcinoma. Int J Cancer 61: 522–528

21. Soda K, Kawakami M, Kashi K, Miyata M (1995) Manifestations of cancer cachexia induced by colon 26 adenocarcinoma are not fully ascribable to interleukin-6. Int J Cancer 62: 332–336

22. Yasumoto K, Nukaida N, Harada A et al (1995) Molecular analysis of the cytokine network involved in cachexia in colon 26 adenocarcinoma-bearing mice. Cancer Res 55:921–927

23. Hussey HJ, Todorov PT, Field WN et al (2000) Effect of a fluorinated pyrimidine on cachexia and tumour growth in murine cachexia models: relationship with a proteolysis inducing factor. Br J Cancer 83:56–62

24. Lorite MJ, Thompson MG, Drake JL et al (1998) Mechanism of muscle protein degradation induced by a cancer cachectic factor. Br J Cancer 78:850–856

25. Lorite MJ, Cariuk P, Tisdale MJ (1997) Induction of protein degradation by a tumour factor. Br J Cancer 76:1035–1040

26. Lorite MJ, Smith HJ, Arnold JA et al (2001) Activation of ATP-ubiquitin-dependent proteolysis in skeletal muscle in vivo and murine myoblasts in vitro by a proteolysis-inducing factor (PIF). Br J Cancer 85:297–302

27. Gomes-Marcondes MC, Smith HJ, Cooper JC, Tisdale MJ (2002) Development of an in vitro model system to investigate the mechanism of muscle protein catabolism induced by proteolysis-inducing factor. Br J Cancer 86:1628–1633

28. Wigmore SJ, Todorov PT, Barber MD et al (2000) Characteristics of patients with pancreatic cancer expressing a novel cachectic factor. Br J Surg 87:53–58

29. Watchorn TM, Waddell ID, Dowidar N, Ross JA (2001) Proteolysis-inducing factor regulates hepatic gene expression via the transcription factors NF-kB and STAT3. FASEB J 15:562–564

30. Watchorn TM, Waddell I, Ross JA (2002) Proteolysis-inducing factor differentially influences transcriptional regulation in endothelial subtypes. Am J Physiol 282:E763–E769

31. Whitehouse AS, Tisdale MJ (2003) Induced expression of the ubiquitin-proteasome pathway in murine myotubes by proteolysis-inducing factor (PIF) is associated with activation of the transcription factor NF-kB. Br J Cancer 89:1116–1122

32. Smith HJ, Lorite MJ, Tisdale MJ (1999) Effect of a cancer cachectic factor on protein synthesis / degradation in murine C2C12 myoblasts: modulation by eicosapentaenoic acid. Cancer Res 59:5507–5513

33. Smith HJ, Tisdale MJ (2003) Signal transduction pathways involved in proteolysis-inducing factor induced proteasome expression in murine myotubes. Br J Cancer 89:1783–1788

34. Hussey HJ, Bibby MC, Tisdale MJ (1996) Novel antitumour activity of 2, 3, 5-trimethyl-6-(3-pyridylmethyl)-1, 4-benzoquinone (CV-6504) against established murine adenocarcinomas (MAC). Br J Cancer 73:1187–1192

35. Whitehouse AS, Khal J, Tisdale MJ (2003) Induction of protein catabolism in myotubes by 15(S)-hydroxyeicosatetraenoic acid through increased expression of the ubiquitin-proteasome pathway. Br J Cancer 89:737–745

36. Beck SA, Smith KL, Tisdale MJ (1991) Anticachectic and antitumor effect of eicosapentaenoic acid and its effect on protein turnover. Cancer Res 51:6089–6093

37. Whitehouse AS, Smith HJ, Drake JL, Tisdale MJ (2001) Mechanism of attenuation of skeletal muscle protein catabolism in cancer cachexia by eicosapentaenoic acid. Cancer Res 61:3604–3609

38. Wigmore SJ, Barber MD, Ross JA et al (2000) Effect of oral eicosapentaenoic acid on weight loss in patients with pancreatic cancer. Nutr Cancer 36:177–184

39. Barber MD, Ross JA, Voss AC et al (1999) The effect of an oral nutritional supplement enriched with fish oil on weight-loss in patients with pancreatic cancer Br J Cancer 81:80–86

40. Evans WK, Makuch R, Clamon GH et al (1985) Limited impact of total parenteral nutrition on nutritional status during treatment for small cell lung cancer. Cancer Res 45:3347–3353

41. Whitehouse AS, Tisdale MJ (2001) Downregulation of ubiquitin-dependent proteolysis by eicosapentaenoic acid in acute starvation. Biochem Biophys Res Commun 285:598–602

# Lipid Mobilising Factor in Cancer Cachexia

Alessandro Laviano, Maurizio Muscaritoli, Filippo Rossi Fanelli

## Introduction

During disease, a formidable biological fight occurs between invading cells and the defending host. As a consequence, both sides use all the available weapons to succeed: invaders will try to shut off the host defence systems while the host will try to isolate and destroy the invaders. Metabolic perturbations inevitably develop and, if the challenge is prolonged over time, changes in body composition occur. Thus, cachexia could be considered as 'collateral damage' in the fight between invading cells and the defending host.

Cachexia involves weight loss, particularly from skeletal muscle and adipose tissue, anaemia, and fatigue, and is frequently accompanied by anorexia. It is pervasive among patients suffering from chronic diseases, but it has been particularly investigated during tumour growth. However, most of the mechanisms triggering cachexia in cancer appear to also be present in other catabolic states. Thus, this chapter will focus on the changes in lipid metabolism and the role of lipid mobilising factor (LMF) in cancer states, but the biochemical pathways described are reasonably the same as those leading to fat loss in other chronic diseases.

## Lipid Metabolism and Fat Loss in Cancer Patients

The pathophysiology of cancer cachexia is multifactorial and involves many different mediators producing various metabolic effects that could be categorised as metabolic effects of the tumour on the host, and metabolic effects of the host's response to the tumour [1]. As previously mentioned, cachexia is characterised by profound changes in intermediary metabolism, particularly in lipid metabolism. Fat loss is frequently observed in cancer cachexia as well as in starvation, since adipose tissue comprises 90% of adult fuel reserves. Cachectic cancer patients show increased glycerol and fatty-acid turnover compared to normal subjects [2]. Also, their fasting plasma glycerol concentrations are higher, suggesting increased lipolysis [3]. In healthy individuals, lipid mobilisation is suppressed by glucose administration. In cancer patients, glucose infusion does not suppress lipid mobilisation and fatty acid oxidation [4]. This phenomenon appears as an early event in cancer patients, occurring even before weight loss and cachexia develop [5].

## Lipid Mobilising Factor

A series of clinical and experimental data have indicated that the changes in lipid metabolism characterising tumour growth are mediated by a LMF produced by the tumour [6, 7]. This factor acts directly on adipocytes and stimulates lipolysis in a cyclic-AMP (cAMP)–dependent manner by a mechanism similar to that of lipolytic hormones [8]. This effect appears peculiar to LMF, since cytokines, which are known to influence lipid metabolism, inhibit the clearing enzyme lipoprotein lipase [9]. This, in turn, prevents adipocytes from extracting fatty acids from plasma lipoproteins for storage, resulting in a net flux of lipid into the circulation. However, the total lipoprotein lipase activity in the adipose tissue of cancer patients and the relative levels of the mRNA for lipase and fatty-acid synthase do not differ from those of controls [10]. There is, however, a twofold increase in the relative level of mRNA for hormone-sensitive lipase, suggesting that lipolysis is the major mechanism for lipid mobilisation in cancer cachexia.

Todorov et al. isolated a LMF from a cachexia-inducing murine tumour (MAC16) and from the urine of patients with nonresectable pancreatic carcinoma and weight loss [11]. The LMF was characterised as a protein of 43 kDa that was homologous with the plasma protein Zn-α2-glyco-protein (ZAG) with respect to amino acid sequence, electrophoretic mobility, and immunoreactivity. Both the 43-kDa protein and LMF stimulated adenylate cyclase in murine adipocyte plasma membranes in a GTP-dependent process and caused the release of glycerol from isolated adipocytes [12]. Mice treated with LMF decreased their body weight by losing carcass lipid, without any effect on food or water intake, but probably in relationship with increased energy expenditure, since an increase in oxygen uptake by interscapular brown adipose tissue (BAT) was also observed. This increase is likely to be related to changes in expression of uncoupling proteins because [13] increased thermogenesis in BAT can increase total energy expenditure and thus contribute to tissue wasting. Supporting this reasoning, it has been demonstrated that the resting energy expenditures of patients with lung and pancreatic carcinomas were higher than those of control subjects [14, 15].

In vitro studies showed that LMF-induced lipolysis is attenuated by the β-adrenergic receptor blocker propranolol [8], and propranolol was shown to reduce the basal metabolic rate of cancer patients [16]. These findings and the evidence showing that LMF stimulates BAT oxygen consumption indicates that a β3-adrenergic receptor is involved in this action. β3-Adrenergic agonists up-regulate uncoupling protein-1, leading to a net increase in energy utilisation [17]. Resting energy expenditure, whole-body oxygen uptake, and carbon dioxide production were found to be increased in cancer patients with progressive weight loss after β-adrenoreceptor blockage [18]. Therefore, it was concluded that wasting of body tissues can be explained in part by increased β-adrenoreceptor activity leading to elevated cardiovascular activity, and that production of LMF by cachectic tumours accounts for the loss of body fat and the increase in energy expenditure. This reasoning is supported by more recent evidence showing that induction of lipolysis in murine white adipocytes, and stimulation of adenylate cyclase in adipocyte plasma membranes, by a tumour-produced LMF, are attenuated by low concentrations of a specific β3-adrenoceptor antagonist [19]. Therefore, it appears that β3-adrenoreceptors are critical in mediating the metabolic effects of LMF.

The molecular mechanisms underlying the lipolytic effects of LMF have yet to be completely elucidated. However, it has been shown that the induction of lipolysis and formation of cyclic AMP by LMF are up-regulated in adipose tissue of cachectic mice bearing the MAC16 tumour. The up-regulated response is due to a modification of receptor number of guanine nucleotide-binding protein (G-protein) expression. The G-proteins involved in the adenylate cyclase pathway are members of the Gs and Gi families, which stimulate and inhibit adenylate cyclase, respectively. Adipocyte plasma membranes contain 2 Gs α-subunits and 2 Gi α-subunits, but not Go. A number of stimuli control G-protein expression in adipose tissue. LMF reduces membrane Gαi expression and increases expression of Gαs, changes that favour mobilisation of lipid stores from adipocytes and hence facilitate host tissue catabolism [20]. Thus, tumours secreting LMF maximise the catabolism of adipose tissue by continuous production of this lipolytic stimulus, together with increases in Gαs/Gαi, which sensitise adipocytes to a range of lipolytic stimuli. Very interesting, and promising on a therapeutic level, is the evidence that the polyunsaturated fatty acid eicosapentaenoic acid (EPA) inhibits both lipolysis and adenylate cyclase stimulation by LMF via direct attenuation of the action of LMF on G-protein expression in adipose tissue [20].

## LMF as Physiological Mediator of Lipolysis in Adipocytes

Recent data suggest that LMF is produced not only by tumour cells, but by adipose cells as well. As previously mentioned, LMF was first purified from a murine adenocarcinoma and from the urine of patients with cancer cachexia [11]. This factor has been shown to be identical to ZAG, a 43-kDa protein originally isolated from human plasma. Murine and human ZAG display 59% amino acid sequence homology, but share up to 100% identity in regions thought to be critical in lipid metabolism. The powerful lipid-mobilising effects of ZAG together with the secretory function of adipocytes have led to the hypothesis that ZAG is produced locally by adipose tissue and influences lipid breakdown within the tissue. In a study of ZAG gene expression and protein content in adipose tissue that was aimed at testing this hypothesis, Bing et al. found that ZAG is produced by murine and human white adipose tissue, traditionally considered as the major site of energy storage, and in BAT [21]. Furthermore, ZAG mRNA and protein levels were markedly increased in the adipose tissue of mice with cancer cachexia. It was therefore speculated that ZAG serves as a unique protein factor in the local modulation of lipid metabolism and contributes particularly to the substantial reduction of adiposity that occurs in cancer cachexia. Finally, ZAG may also influence the production of other adipokines since, according to a very recent report, the protein stimulates the expression of adiponectin in transfected 3T3-L1 cells [22].

## LMF as a Pleiotropic Mediator

In addition to its well-established effects on lipid metabolism, LMF appears to influence other metabolic pathways. In an elegant series of in vitro studies, it was shown that LMF increases muscle mass by an increase in protein synthesis and a decrease in protein catabolism [23]. The effect on protein synthesis appears to arise from increases in intracellular cAMP, possibly mediated through stimulation of a β3-adrenergic receptor. Since LMF was also found to stimulate protein synthesis in tumour cells, it could be speculated that it functions to increase overall tumour bulk without affecting cellular proliferation.

Energy metabolism is profoundly deranged during tumour growth. The mitochondrial uncoupling proteins (UCP)-1, -2, and –3 likely play essential roles in energy dissipation and disposal of excess lipid. As previously mentioned, in a murine model of cancer cachexia, the expression of uncoupling proteins is increased. Recent data indicate that LMF could be involved in inducing this up-regulation [24], and suggest that UCPs utilise excess lipid mobilised during fat catabolism in cancer cachexia.

Glucose metabolism is also affected by LMF. Treatment of ex-breeder male NMRI mice with LMF isolated from the urine of cachectic cancer patients caused a significant increase in glucose oxidation to $CO_2$, compared with control mice receiving phosphate-buffered saline [25]. Glucose utilisation was elevated in brain, heart, BAT, and gastrocnemius muscle. The tissue glucose metabolic rate was increased almost threefold in brain, accounting for the ability of LMF to decrease blood glucose levels. LMF also increased overall lipid oxidation. There was a significant increase in lipid accumulation in plasma, liver, and white and brown adipose tissue after administration of LMF. These results provide further evidence that changes in carbohydrate metabolism and loss of adipose tissue, together with increased whole-body fatty acid oxidation in cachectic cancer patients, may arise from tumour production of LMF.

An interesting question is whether there is any survival advantage to tumours that produce catabolic factors such as LMF. Tumours preferentially use glucose rather than lipids as an energy source due to the low oxygen tension. Since UCP-2 is thought to be involved in counteracting oxidative damage, if LMF induced UCP-2 expression in the tumour, this may be important in detoxifying free radicals, which are produced in excess during cachexia. Many anticancer drugs, such as adriamycin, bleomycin, and mitomycin C, exert their action through the generation of reactive oxygen radicals, and induction of UCP-2 by LMF may protect tumour cells from their cytotoxic action. This important issue was recently addressed experimentally, and the results showed that LMF antagonises the antiproliferative effect of agents working through a free-radical mechanism, which may partly explain the unresponsiveness to chemotherapy of cachexia-inducing tumours [26].

## Conclusions

There is a large bulk of evidence indicating that tumour-derived LMF is critical in mediating, in part, the changes in lipid, protein, glucose, and energy metabolisms that characterise tumour growth, and possibly other catabolic states, ultimately resulting in cachexia. Since these metabolic effects occur early during the disease, even before weight loss develops, there is an urgent need for early therapeutic intervention aimed at preventing/counteracting the detrimental consequences of LMF and other catabolic mediators on nutritional status. Interestingly, EPA appears to be effective in attenuating the metabolic alterations induced by LMF. Even more interesting is evidence showing that ZAG, an endogenous LMF, may act as modulator of lipolysis under physiological conditions, thus providing researchers in the obesity field with a novel and potentially highly effective therapeutic target.

## References

1. Tisdale MJ (2001) Cancer anorexia and cachexia. Nutrition 17:438–442
2. Shaw JH, Wolfe RR (1987) Fatty acid and glycerol kinetics in septic patients and in patients with gastrointestinal cancer. The response to glucose infusion and parenteral feeding. Ann Surg 205:368–376
3. Drott C, Persson H, Lundholm K (1989) Cardiovascular and metabolic response to adrenaline infusion in weight-losing patients with and without cancer. Clin Physiol 9:427–439
4. Edmonson JH (1966) Fatty acid mobilization and glucose metabolism in patients with cancer. Cancer 19:277–280
5. Costa G, Bewley P, Aragon M, Siebold J (1981) Anorexia and weight loss in cancer patients. Cancer Treat Rep 65(Suppl 5):3–7
6. Groundwater P, Beck SA, Barton C et al (1990) Alteration of serum and urinary lipolytic activity with weight loss in cachectic cancer patients. Br J Cancer 62:816–821
7. Beck SA, Tisdale MJ (1987) Production of lipolytic and proteolytic factors by a murine tumor producing cachexia in the host. Cancer Res 47:5919–5923
8. Khan S, Tisdale MJ (1999) Catabolism of adipose tissue by a tumour-produced lipid-mobilising factor. Int J Cancer 80:444–447
9. Berg M, Fraker DL, Alexander HR (1994) Characterization of differentiation factor/leukaemia inhibitory factor effect on lipoprotein lipase activity and mRNA in 3T3-LI adipocytes. Cytokine 6:425–432
10. Thompson MP, Cooper ST, Parry BR, Tuckey JA (1993) Increased expression of the mRNA for the hormone-sensitive lipase in adipose tissue of cancer patients. Biochim Biophys Acta 1180:236–242
11. Todorov PT, McDevitt TM, Meyer DJ et al (1998) Purification and characterization of a tumour lipid-mobilizing factor. Cancer Res 58:2353–2358
12. Hirai K, Hussey HJ, Barber MD et al (1998) Biological evaluation of a lipid-mobilizing factor isolated from the urine of cancer patients. Cancer Res 58:2359–2365
13. Bing C, Brown M, King P et al (2000) Increased gene expression of brown fat UCP1 and skeletal muscle UCP2 and UCP3 in MAC16-induced cancer cachexia. Cancer Res 60:2405–2410
14. Fredrix EW, Soeters PB, Wouters EF et al (1991) Effect of different tumor types on resting energy expenditure. Cancer Res 51:6138–6141
15. Falconer JS, Fearon KC, Plester CE et al (1994) Cytokines, the acute-phase response, and resting energy expenditure in cachectic patients with pancreatic cancer. Ann Surg 219:325–331
16. Gambardella A, Tortoriello R, Pesce L et al (1999) Intralipid infusion combined with propranolol administration has favourable metabolic effects in elderly malnourished cancer patients. Metabolism 48:291–297
17. Lowell BB, Flier JS (1997) Brown adipose tissue, beta 3-adrenergic receptors and obesity. Ann Rev Med Chem 48:307–316
18. Hyltander A, Daneryd P, Sandstrom R et al (2000) b-Adrenoceptor activity and resting energy metabolism in weight losing cancer patients. Eur J Cancer 36:330–334
19. Russell ST, Hirai K, Tisdale MJ (2002) Role of b3-adrenergic receptors in the action of a tumour lipid mobilizing factor. Br J Cancer 86:424–428
20. Islam-Ali B, Khan S, Price SA, Tisdale MJ (2001) Modulation of adipocyte G-protein expression in cancer cachexia by a lipid-mobilising factor (LMF). Br J Cancer 85:758–763
21. Bing C, Bao Y, Jenkins J et al (2004) Zinc-a2-glycoprotein, a lipid mobilizing factor, is expressed in adipocytes and is up-regulated in mice with cancer cachexia. Proc Natl Acad Sci USA 101:2500–2505
22. Gohda T, Makita Y, Shike T et al (2003) Identification of epistatic interaction involved in obesity using the KK/Ta mouse as a type 2 diabetes model: is Zn-alpha2 glycoprotein-1 a candidate gene for obesity? Diabetes 52: 2175–2181
23. Islam-Ali BS, Tisdale MJ (2001) Effect of a tumour-produced lipid-mobilizing factor on protein synthesis and degradation. Br J Cancer 84:1648–1655
24. Bing C, Russell ST, Beckett EE et al (2002) Expression of uncoupling proteins-1, -2 and -3

mRNA is induced by an adenocarcinoma-derived lipid-mobilizing factor. Br J Cancer 86:612–618

25. Russell ST, Tisdale MJ (2002) Effect of tumour-derived lipid-mobilising factor on glucose and lipid metabolism in vivo. Br J Cancer 87:580–584

26. Sanders PM, Tisdale MJ (2004) Role of lipid-mobilising factor (LMF) in protecting tumour cells from oxidative damage. Br J Cancer 90:1274–1278

# Dietary Intake, Resting Energy Expenditure, Weight Loss, and Survival in Cancer Patients

Kent Lundholm, Ingvar Bosaeus

## Introduction

Weight loss is frequently seen in patients with advanced cancer and has long been recognised to be associated with decreased survival [1]. Cancer cachexia is a complex syndrome depending on cytokines, eicosanoids, and classical hormones, and characterised by progressive weight loss with depletion of host reserves of skeletal muscle and adipose tissue. It is the net result of profound metabolic changes that appear in patients with advanced stages of cancer, and is characterised by net breakdown of skeletal muscle and alterations in fat and carbohydrate metabolism. Cachexia is the most common paraneoplastic syndrome, and is also referred to as the cancer anorexia-cachexia syndrome, with features of anorexia, early satiety, weakness, and fatigue.

Weight stability, or more precisely, stable body composition indicates energy balance, in which energy intake equals total energy expenditure. Energy intake is usually characterised by the macronutrient composition, i.e. the proportions of protein, fat, carbohydrate, and alcohol. Energy expenditure can be subdivided into components of resting energy expenditure (REE), the thermic effect of food (TEF), which represents the energy cost of postprandial metabolism of food, and activity-related energy expenditure (AEE) (Fig. 1). Negative energy balance, leading to progressive weight loss, can thus be attributed to changes in energy intake, components of energy expenditure, or both, and explained by metabolic alterations and different mediators (Fig. 2). Both anorexia and increased REE are common in progressive cancer, although a large span in REE, from hypo- to hypermetabolism, has been reported in malnourished cancer patients [2]. Sustained hypermetabolism over a long period of disease progression can

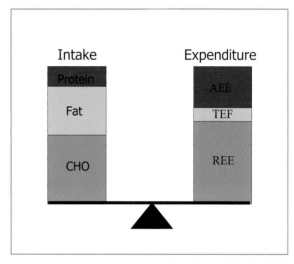

**Fig. 1.** Components of energy balance. *CHO*, Carbohydrate; *REE*, resting energy expenditure; *TEF*, thermic effect of food; *AEE*, activity-related energy expenditure

make a large contribution to negative energy balance and wasting if not compensated for by increased energy intake – which is, however, quite difficult in cancer patients. Hypermetabolism and diminished energy intake due to anorexia may thus constitute a vicious circle in the development of cancer cachexia [3]. In addition, a variety of metabolic derangements may contribute to the progressive wasting of cancer. Such metabolic changes may differ from those induced by voluntarily decreased energy intake or pure starvation. In simple starvation, muscle mass seems to be preserved at the expense of body fat depots, which are preferentially used to provide energy. In contrast, relatively more muscle tissue than body fat is assumed to be lost in the development of cancer cachexia [4]. Such changes in body composition may not be simply reversed by adequate energy and nutrient provision, as is usually the case for conditions of pure starvation.

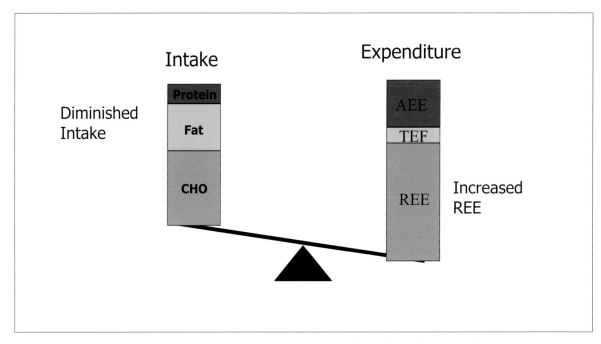

**Fig. 2.** Negative energy balance in cancer disease. Alterations in both intake and expenditure contribute

## Energy Intake

Several factors may contribute to the decreased intake of food in cancer patients. Anorexia, due to the disease itself or its treatment, is commonly recognised. Cancer patients may frequently suffer from symptoms affecting the gastrointestinal tract, for instance due to physical obstruction, constipation, or malabsorption. The effects or consequences of treatment by opiates, radiotherapy, or chemotherapy may all explain decreased food intake in the palliative care of cancer patients. However, reports on the degree of anorexia do not always indicate low intakes. Cohn et al. assessed energy and protein intake in relation to lean body mass in 22 oncology patients and found no difference from normal subjects, unless weight loss was present [4]. Parkinson et al., in a study of the effects of oral protein and energy supplements in 30 cancer patients, reported a mean intake of 1515 Kcal/day, corresponding to 25 Kcal/kg/day [5]. Simons et al. studied the effects of medroxyprogesterone acetate in 54 patients with advanced non-hormone-sensitive cancer, and reported a higher mean intake, about 2200 Kcal/day, corresponding to 34 Kcal/kg/day [6]. In contrast, in an analysis of

energy balance in 100 lung cancer patients, decreased intake was found in weight-losing patients with acute-phase response [7, 8]. Levine and Morgan studied food selection in 10 hospitalised cancer patients with weight loss and anorexia [9]. They found low energy intake (24 Kcal/kg/d), but the patients had maintained normal macronutrient composition despite cancer anorexia compared with hospitalised control subjects.

These results agree with our own observations of low intake in 297 patients with advanced cancer, mainly gastro-intestinal tumours [2]. Mean dietary intake was below maintenance requirements (26 Kcal/kg/day) but the patients' macronutrient composition was normal (Fig. 3). Weight loss of more than 10% was present in 43% of our patients, and elevated REE (> 110% of predicted) occurred in 48% of the patients. Dietary intake did, however, not differ significantly between normo- and hypermetabolic patients. Thus, weight loss was apparently not accounted for by diminished dietary intake, since absolute energy intake was not different; in fact, intake per kg body weight was higher in weight-losing patients than in weight-stable patients, although it is always diffi-

## Food intake and REE in weight losing cancer patients

| | |
|---|---|
| Age | 67 ± 1 kg |
| Weight loss | 9 ± 3 kg |
| REE | 23.9 ± 1 kcal/kg |
| Energy intake | 25.5 ± 1 kcal/kg |
| | |
| Carbohydrates | 46.2 ± 0.3% |
| Fat | 36.1 ± 0.5% |
| Protein | 15.6 ± 0.6% |

**Fig. 3.** Transectional information of daily caloric intake in cachectic weight-losing cancer patients in relationship to resting energy expenditure (REE) and caloric distribution among macronutrients (carbohydrates, fat, protein)

cult to normalise energy intake and expenditure in weight-losing subjects. Food preferences did not seem to be altered, since the proportion of dietary protein, carbohydrate, and fat was generally the same as in a general elderly population from the same geographic area (Fig. 3). Also, Fordy et al., in a study of 40 colorectal cancer patients with disseminated disease, did not find differences in diet composition between weight-stable and weight-losing patients [10]. Thus, reduced dietary intake has been repeatedly but not consistently reported of in weight-losing cancer patients, though long-term dietary intake may be difficult to assess precisely. The magnitude of reduced intake at the beginning of weight loss is, however, not clear, but diminished food intake cannot alone explain weight loss in all cancer patients. Accordingly, our own investigations indicated that REE was a more powerful predictor of weight loss than energy intake, based on multiple linear regression analysis. Thus, other components of the energy balance equation must be taken into consideration; dietary induced thermogenesis, AEE, and the energy cost of integrated metabolic and physiological homeostasis may all contribute to explain the variance in weight loss of cancer patients during disease progression, and thus the energy loss in substrate cycling [11].

## Energy Expenditure

Increased REE in cancer is frequent but not universally found in cancer patients with progressive weight loss [12–14] (Fig. 4). Also, in studies of malnourished cancer patients, a large span from hypo- to hypermetabolism has been reported [15, 16]. It would thus appear that cancer patients have a variable response to underfeeding, some being able to adapt appropriately to reduced REE for a period of time, while others show hypermetabolism or insufficient adaptation, accounting for low activity levels and anorexia. This would be in contrast to uncomplicated starvation, in which adaptation seems to occurs more effectively to reduced energy intake. Patients with cancer in some particular sites, such as lung and pancreas, may be more prone to develop hypermetabolism, although there are no clear-cut relationships to the type of tumor [17, 18]. Animal studies of cancer cachexia have suggested that there are changes in metabolic pattern over time, with initial hypermetabolism followed by hypometabolism preterminally [19]. Less is known about longitudinal changes in REE in cancer patients [17]. Jatoi et al. studied a small group of lung cancer patients and found decreased disease-free survival in eight hypometabolic compared to nine hypermetabolic patients [20]. In our

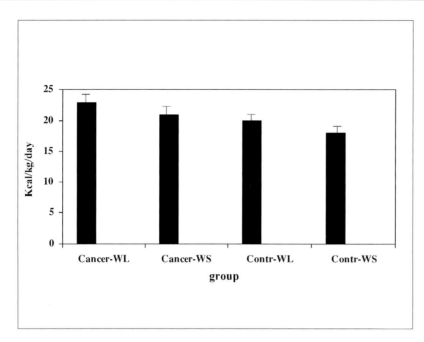

**Fig. 4.** REE in transectional analyses of weight-losing (*WL*) and weight-stable (*WS*) cancer patients compared to non-cancer patients with and without weight loss ($p < 0.01$ among all groups). (Data from [14])

own longitudinal observations, about half of the patients had elevated REE, defined as 110% or more of predicted REE [2]. Increased energy expenditure in cancer patients are significantly related to systemic inflammation, in which anaemia may attenuate the effectiveness of oxygen transportation and thereby increase the energy cost for circulatory homeostasis. However, anaemia may also correlate with increased energy consumption as a component of the acute-phase response, evident by an increased erythrocyte sedimentation rate or increased C-reactive protein levels [14]. In this context, it is noteworthy that pain does not seem to be a universal explanation to cancer cachexia in patients with solid gastrointestinal malignancy [21] (Fig. 5). Thus, it was possible to attenuate the increased REE in cancer patients by β-blockade to slow down hyperactive cardiovascular activity mediated in part by increased noradrenergic and adrenergic activity in combination with elevated production of glucocorticoids [22, 23]. Thus, the classical hormone system is activated during increased metabolism and diminished food intake, together with cytokines; this response is usually attenuated by anti-inflammatory treatment [24]. Accordingly, it is well-recognised that cyclooxygenase inhibitors decrease inflammation in cancer patients and

thereby improve energy balance by positive effects on both energy intake and production [24]. Another means to achieve this effect is to provide fish oils, which probably alter cell-membrane composition and thereby decrease production of powerful eicosanoids. Thus, it is conceptually possible to attenuate elevated REE in cancer patients on both the causative (cytokines, hormones, eicosanoids) and the effector (anaemia, hyperkinetic circulation, anorexia) sides. One simple way to improve energy balance would be to provide energy in excess of resting needs. This may, however, influence other components of total energy expenditure.

There have been few investigations of cancer cachexia and the other components of the total energy expenditure (TEE), i.e. TEF [25] and AEE [26]. Physical activity levels, as determined by questionnaires, was reported to predict chemotherapy toxicity in older lung cancer patients [27]. A study in 8 patients with advanced lung cancer found that TEE was not increased despite an increase in REE, indicating diminished activity [28]. A recent study made the same observation: TEE was assessed by doubly-labelled water in 24 patients with advanced pancreatic cancer. REE was increased but TEE was not changed, indicating decreased AEE [26]. During 8 weeks of

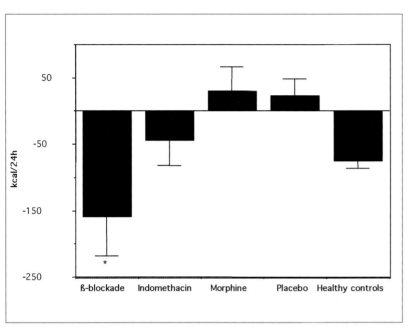

**Fig. 5.** REE in weight-losing cancer patients randomised to either β-blockade (propranolol), indomethacin, morphine, or placebo compared to healthy individuals on β-blockade (propranolol), as described by Hyltander et al. (Data from [21])

treatment with a control nutritional supplement, TEE, REE, and AEE were unchanged, but in patients receiving a supplement enriched with EPA, physical activity was increased [26]. Thus, low physical activity levels may be an important feature of energy balance in cancer patients, which may, in turn, affect functional performance and quality of life.

## Support of Energy Balance

The best way to improve energy balance is apparently to control tumour progression, which attenuates the metabolic abnormalities induced by the tumour and/or tumour-host interactions. When cure cannot be achieved, an obvious next option is to increase nutritional intake by oral nutritional support or artificial nutrition (Fig. 3). A number of studies have tried to achieve this, particularly on a short-term basis. However, few positive effects were reported in terms of anthropometric measures, response rate to therapy, survival, or quality of life. Parenteral nutrition is difficult to supply over extended periods of time and may be associated with a number of complications. A number of parenteral nutrition trials were carried out in the 1980s in cancer patients, who showed little benefit

but significant problems with infection complications. A position paper of the American College of Physicians in 1989 stated that 'parenteral nutritional support was associated with net harm, and no conditions could be defined in which such treatment appeared to be of benefit' [29]. This statement was based on studies that appeared to have design flaws and used nutritional regimens regarded as suboptimal by current standards. The disappointing results of stand-alone conventional nutritional supplementation to cancer patients led to a focus on the metabolic changes in cancer cachexia, and attempts to manipulate the metabolic alterations with a variety of pharmacological agents.

Megestrol acetate and medroxyprogesterone acetate have been extensively used and studied, primarily as appetite stimulants in weight-losing cancer patients. Several randomised trials in various groups of weight-losing cancer patients demonstrated increased appetite and also, less frequently, improved dietary intake [6, 30]. While weight loss may be attenuated or even reversed, gain of lean tissue was not demonstrated; instead, the weight gained tended to consist of fat and water. At best, these agents may improve negative energy balance but not reverse it. The metabolic alterations in advanced cancer have many parallels to those seen in the chronic systemic inflammatory response and appear, in some respects, to be different from the metabolic changes that occur in pure starvation. Thus, strategies to counteract the inflammatory response would seem to be optional. Steroids have been widely used and have been shown to improve appetite. However, steroids will not reverse ongoing weight loss and muscle wasting, and symptomatic benefits are often short-lived and associated with a number of adverse effects. Non-steroidal anti-inflammatory drugs (NSAIDs) have been shown to reduce the acute-phase protein response and REE and to preserve body fat by support of food intake in patients with advanced cancer on long-term treatment [24] (Fig. 6, 7). Thus, indomethacin stabilised performance status and prolonged survival in a number of cancer patients [31]. Therefore, anti-inflammatory

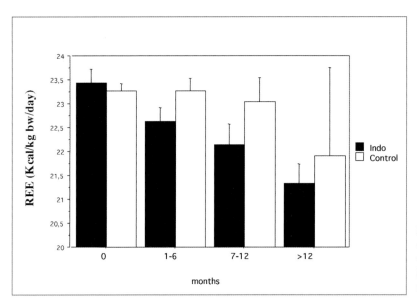

**Fig. 6.** Time-course changes of REE in unselected cancer patients treated with indomethacin (50 mg twice daily) compared to untreated cancer patients ($p < 0.003$). (Data from [32])

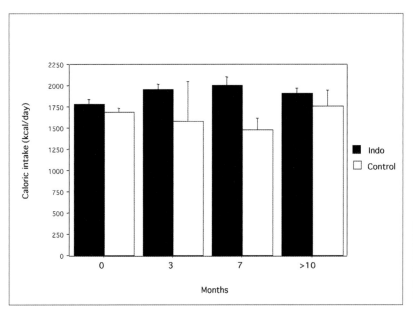

**Fig. 7.** Time-course changes of food intake in unselected cancer patients treated with indomethacin (50 mg twice daily) compared to untreated cancer patients ($p < 0.0006$). (Data from [32])

treatment seems to have a role in palliative care of cancer, although it is still difficult to predict responders and non-responders.

Based on current knowledge of metabolism and its control in weight-losing cancer patients, we evaluated the effect of nutritional support in combination with NSAID and erythropoietin treatment in 309 patients with progressive cachexia due to solid tumours, predominantly gastrointestinal malignancy [32]. As-treated analysis demonstrated that patients receiving nutritional support had prolonged survival, accompanied by improved energy balance, increasing body fat, and greater maximum exercise performance. The results support the conclusion that nutrition is a limiting factor for outcome in a majority of cancer patients with negative energy balance (Fig. 8), and treatments targeted towards both diminished nutritional intake and metabolic alterations are therefore effective. Accordingly, eicosapentaenoic acid (EPA), which is an essential polyunsaturated fatty acid of the n-3 class and present in relatively large amounts in fish oil, has been shown to have anti-inflammatory properties in doses of 2–6 g/day. Pilot studies of EPA supplements administered to pancreatic cancer patients have suggested promising results, with patients exhibiting improved appetite and partial reversal of weight loss. However, a larger controlled study could not entirely replicate the results of the pilot studies, although positive effects on weight, function, and quality of life were shown to be related to plasma concentrations of EPA [33]. Thus, the effect size and usefulness of nutritional supplements with EPA are still not clear, particularly regarding compliance and compared to anti-inflammatory treatment with conventional drugs.

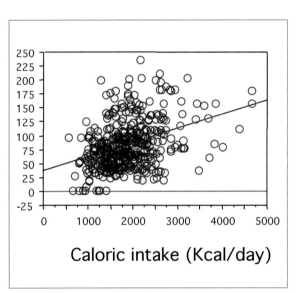

**Fig. 8.** The relationship between caloric intake and maximum exercise capacity in weight-losing cancer patients ($n = 419, p < 0.001$)

## Conclusions

The metabolic alterations in progressive cancer have many parallels to other conditions with chronic systemic inflammation, and differ in some respect to the metabolic changes in pure starvation. Artificial nutrition alone does not appear to affect overall survival in advanced cancer, but nutritional support in combination with treatment targeted to the inflammation and subsequent metabolic abnormalities seems to be of greater value. Appetite stimulants can improve anorexia and thereby also energy balance, but the duration of the therapeutic effects is less impressive so far. Thus, early-intervention therapeutic strategies aimed at modulating mediators of the catabolic response, such as cytokines and eicosanoids, in combination with maintaining an adequate supply of nutrients may be most rewarding.

## References

1.  Dewys WD, Begg C, Lavin PT et al (1980) Prognostic effect of weight loss prior to chemotherapy in cancer patients. Eastern Cooperative Oncology Group. Am J Med 69:491–497
2.  Bosaeus I, Daneryd P, Svanberg E et al (2001) Dietary intake and resting energy expenditure in relation to weight loss in cancer patients. Int J Cancer 93:380–383
3.  Baracos VE (2002) Hypercatabolism and hypermetabolism in wasting states. Curr Opin Clin Nutr Metab Care 5:237–239
4.  Cohn SH, Gartenhaus W, Vartsky D et al (1981) Body composition and dietary intake in neoplastic disease. Am J Clin Nutr 34:1997–2004
5.  Parkinson SA, Lewis J, Morris R et al (1987) Oral pro-

tein and energy supplements in cancer patients. Hum Nutr Appl Nutr 41:233–243

6. Simons JP, Schols AM, Hoefnagels JM et al (1998) Effects of medroxyprogesterone acetate on food intake, body composition, and resting energy expenditure in patients with advanced, nonhormone-sensitive cancer: a randomized, placebo-controlled trial. Cancer 82:553–560

7. Staal-van den Brekel AJ, Schols AM, ten Velde GP et al (1994) Analysis of the energy balance in lung cancer patients. Cancer Res 54:6430–6433

8. Wigmore SJ, Plester CE, Ross JA et al (1997) Contribution of anorexia and hypermetabolism to weight loss in anicteric patients with pancreatic cancer. Br J Surg 84:196–197

9. Levine JA, Morgan MY (1998) Preservation of macronutrient preferences in cancer anorexia. Br J Cancer 78:579–581

10. Fordy C, Glover C, Henderson DC et al (1999) Contribution of diet, tumour volume and patient-related factors to weight loss in patients with colorectal liver metastases. Br J Surg 86:639–644

11. Lundholm K, Edstrom S, Karlberg I et al (1982) Glucose turnover, gluconeogenesis from glycerol, and estimation of net glucose cycling in cancer patients. Cancer 50:1142–1150

12. Warnold I, Lundholm K, Schersten T (1978) Energy balance and body composition in cancer patients. Cancer Res 38:1801–1807

13. Bozzetti F, Pagnoni AM, Del Vecchio M (1980) Excessive caloric expenditure as a cause of malnutrition in patients with cancer. Surg Gynecol Obstet 150:229–234

14. Hyltander A, Drott C, Korner U et al (1991) Elevated energy expenditure in cancer patients with solid tumours. Eur J Cancer 27:9–15

15. Dempsey DT, Feurer ID, Knox LS et al (1984) Energy expenditure in malnourished gastrointestinal cancer patients. Cancer 53:1265–1273

16. Knox LS, Crosby LO, Feurer ID et al (1983) Energy expenditure in malnourished cancer patients. Ann Surg 197:152–162

17. Barber MD, Ross JA, Fearon KC (1999) Cancer cachexia. Surg Oncol 8:133–41

18. Tisdale MJ (2002) Cachexia in cancer patients. Nat Rev Cancer 2:862–871

19. Zylicz Z, Schwantje O, Wagener DJ et al (1990) Metabolic response to enteral food in different phases of cancer cachexia in rats. Oncology 47:87–91

20. Jatoi A, Daly BD, Hughes V et al (1999) The prognostic effect of increased resting energy expenditure prior to treatment for lung cancer. Lung Cancer 23:153–158

21. Hyltander A, Korner U, Lundholm KG (1993) Evaluation of mechanisms behind elevated energy expendi-

ture in cancer patients with solid tumours. Eur J Clin Invest 23:46–52

22. Drott C, Svaninger G, Lundholm K (1988) Increased urinary excretion of cortisol and catecholamines in malnourished cancer patients. Ann Surg 208:645–650

23. Drott C, Persson H, Lundholm K (1989) Cardiovascular and metabolic response to adrenaline infusion in weight- losing patients with and without cancer. Clin Physiol 9:427–439

24. Lundholm K, Daneryd P, Korner U et al (2004) Evidence that long-term COX-treatment improves energy homeostasis and body composition in cancer patients with progressive cachexia. Int J Oncol 24:505–512

25. Lindmark L, Bennegard K, Eden E et al (1986) Thermic effect and substrate oxidation in response to intravenous nutrition in cancer patients who lose weight. Ann Surg 204:628–636

26. Moses AW, Slater C, Preston T et al (2004) Reduced total energy expenditure and physical activity in cachectic patients with pancreatic cancer can be modulated by an energy and protein dense oral supplement enriched with n-3 fatty acids. Br J Cancer 90:996–1002

27. Jatoi A, Hillman S, Stella PJ et al (2003) Daily activities: exploring their spectrum and prognostic impact in older, chemotherapy-treated lung cancer patients. Support Care Cancer 11:460–464

28. Gibney E, Elia M, Jebb SA et al (1997) Total energy expenditure in patients with small-cell lung cancer: results of a validated study using the bicarbonate-urea method. Metabolism 46:1412–1417

29. Anonymous (1989) Parenteral nutrition in patients receiving cancer chemotherapy. American College of Physicians. Ann Intern Med 110:734–736

30. Bruera E, Macmillan K, Kuehn N et al (1990) A controlled trial of megestrol acetate on appetite, caloric intake, nutritional status, and other symptoms in patients with advanced cancer. Cancer 66:1279–1282

31. Lundholm K, Gelin J, Hyltander A et al (1994) Anti-inflammatory treatment may prolong survival in undernourished patients with metastatic solid tumors. Cancer Res 54:5602–5606

32. Lundholm K, Daneryd P, Bosaeus I et al (2004) Palliative nutritional intervention in addition to cyclooxygenase and erythropoietin treatment for patients with malignant disease: effects on survival, metabolism and function. A randomized prospective study. Cancer 100:1967–1977

33. Fearon KC, Von Meyenfeldt MF, Moses AG et al (2003) Effect of a protein and energy dense N-3 fatty acid enriched oral supplement on loss of weight and lean tissue in cancer cachexia: a randomised double blind trial. Gut 52:1479–1486

# The Ubiquitin/Proteasome System in Cancer Cachexia

Maurizio Muscaritoli, Maurizio Bossola, Giovanni Battista Doglietto, Filippo Rossi Fanelli

## Introduction

Cancer cachexia (CC) is probably the most debilitating and life-threatening paraneoplastic syndrome. It is characterised by weight loss, anorexia, asthaenia, loss of skeletal muscle protein, depletion of lipid stores, and severe metabolic alterations. CC syndrome is present in about 50% of cancer patients, especially those with tumours of the gastrointestinal tract and lung, and less frequently in those with haematological malignancies and other solid neoplasms, such as breast and thyroid cancer. The majority of terminally ill cancer patients experiences CC, which accounts for about 20% of cancer deaths. This figure translates into approximately 2000000 deaths per year worldwide [1].

The predominant phenotypic feature of CC is the steadily progressive depletion of muscle mass, which is not substantially reversible with any of the currently available nutritional, metabolic, or pharmacological approaches [2].

Muscle depletion reflects an imbalance between the rates of protein synthesis and breakdown. Studies carried out in experimental models as well as in human cancer have shown that muscle atrophy may result from increased degradation, reduced synthesis, or both. However, hypercatabolism of muscle protein, in particular of the myofibrillar proteins actin and myosin, is the most prominent feature, while changes in protein synthesis seem to occur less frequently. Intracellular protein degradation in skeletal muscle depends on several proteolytic systems, namely, the acidic lysosomal, the calcium-dependent, and the ATP-ubiquitin-dependent pathways [3–5].

This chapter will focus on the role played by the ATP-dependent ubiquitin/proteasome pathway in the pathogenesis of muscle wasting of CC.

## The Ubiquitin-Proteasome System

Proteins degraded by the ubiquitin/proteasome system are first conjugated to multiple molecules of ubiquitin, a 76-amino acid, 8.5-kDa residue that is highly conserved and present in the cytoplasm of all eukaryotic cells [6]. Ubiquitinated proteins are degraded by the proteolytic 26s proteasome, the catalytic core of which is the 20s proteasome, a barrel-shaped particle consisting of four stacked rings with seven subunits in each ring. This complex and tightly regulated process takes place through different steps (Fig. 1): (1) Ubiquitin is activated in the presence of ATP by ubiquitin-activating enzyme (E1). (2) Activated ubiquitin is transferred from E1 to ubiquitin-conjugating enzyme (E2). (3) The carboxyl group of the activated ubiquitin is coupled to the amino-groups of lysines in the protein substrates by ubiquitin-protein ligase (E3). Reiteration of the ubiquitin-conjugation reactions creates a chain of five or more ubiquitins linked to each other and then to the protein substrate. (4) The ubiquitinated proteins are unfolded by a 19s complex located on the end of the 20s core proteasome. (5) The unfolded proteins are transported into the central chamber of the 20s core proteasome, where the proteins are cleaved by proteolytic sites located on subunits in the inner rings. The proteins are cut progressively into small peptides of six to twelve amino acids that are subsequently released and rapidly hydrolysed to amino acids by cytosolic exopeptidases. (6) The release of ubiquitin from the substrate protein makes ubiquitin available for recycling in the proteolytic pathway [6].

Experiments using fluorogenic peptide substrates and inhibitors have defined five activities for the 20s proteasome: (1) a chymotrypsin-like (CTL) activity that cleaves after large hydrophobic

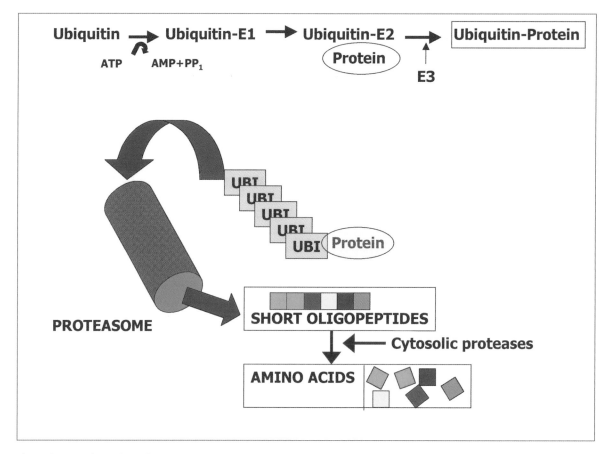

**Fig. 1.** The ATP-dependent ubiquitin-proteasome pathway. See text for details. *UBI*, ubiquitin molecule; *E1*, ubiquitin-activating enzyme; *E2*, ubiquitin-conjugating enzyme; *E3*, ubiquitin ligase

residues; (2) a trypsin-like (TL) activity that cleaves after basic residues; (3) a post-glutamyl hydrolase (PGP) activity that cleaves after acidic residues; (4) an activity that cleaves preferentially after branched-chain amino acids (BrAAP activity); (5) and an activity that cleaves after small neutral amino acids (SNAAP activity).

E3 ubiquitin-protein ligases are currently believed to be the key component of the conjugation apparatus that confers high specificity to the system. The several hundreds of intracytoplasmic ubiquitin-ligating enzymes, commonly designated as E3s, can be broadly divided into two categories: HECT (homologous to E6-AP C-terminus) domain-containing E3s, and RING (really important new gene)-finger-containing E3s [7]. A critical role in activating proteolysis during atrophy has been ascertained for only three of them, namely, E3[α] and ligases encoded by the genes muscle

ring-finger protein-1 (MuRF-1) and muscle atrophy F-box protein (MAFbx), also called atrogin-1 [7] (see below).

## The Role of the Ubiquitin/Proteasome Pathway in Experimental Cancer Cachexia

The first evidence that the ubiquitin/proteasome pathway plays a key role in muscle atrophy came from the observation that, while inhibition of calpain proteases and lysosomal proteases is responsible for the 10–20% reduction in intracellular proteolysis, ATP depletion produces much higher degrees of protein breakdown inhibition [8]. The availability of drugs specifically inhibiting proteasome proteolytic activities (i.e. proteasome inhibitors, such as lactacystin, peptide aldehydes, vinyl sulfones, and dipeptide boronic acid analogs) allowed for in vivo inhibition of proteolysis in experimental models of diabetes, acidosis, sepsis, and denervation atrophy. The results further confirmed the role of the ubiquitin/proteasome pathway in physiological and pathological muscle protein degradation [9–11].

Upregulation of components of the ATP-ubiquitin-dependent pathway has also been reported in experimental models of CC. In 1994, Llovera et al. [12] showed a 500% increase of ubiquitin gene expression in the muscle of rats bearing the fast-growing, cachexia-inducing AH-130 ascites hepatoma. Similarly, Temparis et al. [13] showed that mRNA levels for ubiquitin, 14-kDa E2, and proteasome subunits C8-C9 increased in the tibialis anterior muscles and correlated with the enhancement of energy-requiring proteolysis in Yoshida-sarcoma-bearing rats. Costelli et al. [14] described a 650% increase in the mRNA for 2.4-kb ubiquitin, and a 130% increase in the mRNA for 1.2-kb ubiquitin in the gastrocnemius muscles of rats bearing the Yoshida hepatoma.

Animal models have also shown that muscle proteasomal activity, as measured by the cleavage of specific fluorogenic substrates, is significantly increased in CC. Indeed, Costelli et al. [15] demonstrated that at least CTL activity is significantly increased ($+246 \pm 39\%$ with respect to controls) in the gastrocnemius muscle of AH-130 ascites-

hepatoma-bearing rats, giving the first demonstration that the previously documented modulations of mRNA expression [12–14] are indeed reflective of increased proteolytic activity. Those findings further confirmed the suggestion that muscle wasting in CC is, at least in part, a cytokine-driven phenomenon and that pro-inflammatory cytokines participate in the hyperactivation of intracellular systems involved in protein degradation. In fact, anticytokine treatment with pentoxifylline (a drug that inhibits TNF-$\alpha$ synthesis) and/or with suramin (an anti-protozoal drug blocking the peripheral actions of several cytokines, including interleukin-6 and TNF-$\alpha$) effectively reduced muscle protein loss by downregulating the activity of the ubiquitin/proteasome system (Fig. 2) and calpains [15].

More recently, much interest has been devoted to the role of two ubiquitin ligases specifically expressed in striated muscle, namely, atrogin-1/MAFbx and MuRF-1, in the pathogenesis of muscle atrophy [16]. Overexpression of these ligases was initially demonstrated in denervation/disuse-induced muscle atrophy [16], sepsis [17, 18], and during starvation. [19]. Subsequently, using cDNA microarrays, Lecker et al. [20] showed that a common set of genes, termed atrogins, were induced in muscles of fasted mice and in rats with cancer cachexia, streptozotocin-induced diabetes

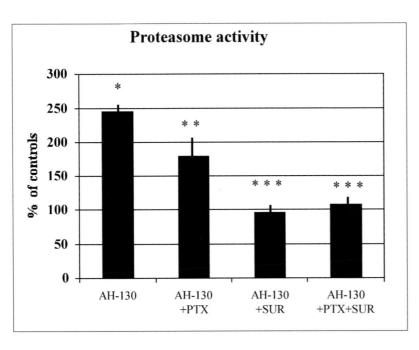

Fig. 2. Proteasome-specific activity in the gastrocnemius muscles of AH-130 ascites-hepatoma-bearing rats (*AH-130*) treated with pentoxyphilline (*PTX*), suramin (*SUR*), or both (*PTX+SUR*). Data are expressed as percent of controls ± SD. *, $p < 0.01$ vs controls; **, $p < 0.05$ vs AH-130; ***, $p < 0.01$ vs AH-130

mellitus, or uraemia. Among the strongly induced genes, some, such as ubiquitin fusion proteins, polyubiquitins, several proteasome subunits, and ubiquitin ligases, were related to protein degradation. The concept that ubiquitin ligases play a pivotal role in muscle atrophy was confirmed by the finding that mice knocked-out for atrogin genes do not develop denervation/disuse-induced muscle depletion [16].

## The Role of the Ubiquitin/Proteasome Pathway in Human Cancer Cachexia

Consistent with the observations in the experimental model, Williams et al. [21] demonstrated that mRNA levels for ubiquitin were approximately three times higher in rectus abdominis muscles from patients with miscellaneous cancers than in muscles from control patients. Moreover, the muscle mRNA levels for the 20s proteasome subunits were 300-400% higher than in healthy controls.

More recently, our group confirmed that the muscle ubiquitin/proteasome system is hyperactivated in humans bearing neoplastic diseases. Indeed, ubiquitin mRNA expression was markedly and significantly increased in muscle biopsies obtained preoperatively in 20 patients undergoing surgery for gastric cancer [22]. It is of interest that ubiquitin mRNA overexpression was observed even in patients reporting weight loss of < 5% of the usual body weight (Table 1). Moreover, patients with more advanced disease (i.e., in stage III–IV) had the highest ubiquitin mRNA values.

In a subsequent study [23], Bossola et al. evaluated proteasome-specific activities in intraoperative rectus abdominis muscle biopsies obtained from 23 patients undergoing laparotomy for gastric cancer and 14 controls undergoing laparotomy for benign abdominal diseases (Table 2). The authors showed that proteasome activity is significantly increased in the muscle of gastric cancer patients (five-fold increase in CTL activity, and a two-fold increase in PGP and TL activities). A concomitant, significant overexpression of muscle ubiquitin mRNA was also observed. Higher CTL activity was associated with advanced disease stage, weight loss, and hypoalbuminaemia, in keeping with the previous observation that muscle ubiquitin mRNA levels are influenced by tumour stage [22]. CTL activity was higher in cancer patients over 50 years old, though not in controls. This difference suggests that ageing may substantially alter the response to the catabolic stimuli

**Table 1.** Muscle ubiquitin m-RNA expression and weight loss in gastric cancer patients. (Data from [22])

| Group | Ubiquitin m-RNA (arbitrary units ± SD) |
| --- | --- |
| Controls | $1162 \pm 132$ |
| Gastric cancer (weight loss 0–5%) | $2338 \pm 929$[a] |
| Gastric cancer (weight loss 6–10%) | $2581 \pm 962$[a] |
| Gastric cancer (weight loss > 10%) | $2936 \pm 756$[a] |

[a] $p = 0.0005$ vs controls

**Table 2.** Muscle proteasome chymotrypsin-like (CTL) activity and weight loss in gastric cancer patients. (Data from [23])

| Group | Proteasome CTL activity (nkatal $\times 10^{-3}$/mg protein ± SD |
| --- | --- |
| Controls | $67.5 \pm 37.4$ |
| Gastric cancer (weight loss < 10%) | $185.3 \pm 112$[a] |
| Gastric cancer (weight loss >1 0%) | $621.6 \pm 499$[b] |

[a] $p < 0.0001$ vs controls
[b] $p < 0.003$ vs weight loss < 10%

evoked by the tumour.

Taken together, the results of the two latter clinical studies provide a number of interesting insights into the pathogenesis of muscle wasting in human cancer. First, they suggest a crucial involvement of the ATP-dependent ubiquitin/proteasome pathway in cancer-related muscle loss in humans. Second, the observation that both ubiquitin mRNA overexpression and increased proteasome proteolytic activities occur even in patients with insignificant or no weight loss strongly supports the concept that the pathogenic mechanisms ultimately leading to the phenotypic pattern of CC operate early during the clinical course of human neoplastic disease.

In 36 patients undergoing thoracothomy for lung cancer, Jagoe et al. [24] demonstrated an increase of skeletal muscle mRNA for cathepsin B with respect to healthy controls. mRNA levels for components of the ubiquitin/proteasome pathway were also higher in lung cancer patients than in controls, although the differences did not reach statistical significance. However, it should be noted that in Jagoe's study the majority of patients were in an early disease stage, while only nine out of 36 patients had advanced cancer.

## Conclusions

There is accumulating evidence, in both the experimental and clinical setting, suggesting an involvement of the ATP-dependent ubiquitin/proteasome system in the pathogenesis of muscle protein degradation in cancer-related cachexia, as well as in other types of muscle atrophy. Therefore, it is reasonable to hypothesise that single or multiple components of this finely regulated degradative pathway may provide the target of pharmacological, molecular or gene therapy.

Since hyperactivation of the ubiquitin/proteasome system has been demonstrated to be an early phenomenon, occurring even before the onset of weight loss and muscle wasting, preventive and therapeutic strategies for cancer cachexia must be adopted soon after a cancer has been diagnosed.

Based on currently available knowledge, however, it is likely that other proteolytic pathways, i.e. calpains and lysosomal proteases, also participate in the complex machinery responsible for muscle depletion in cancer - as well as in other acute and chronic diseases. The interrelationships between the ubiquitin/proteasome system and other cytosolic proteolytic pathways, however, remain to be fully elucidated.

**Table 3.** Ubiquitin (Ub)-proteasome pathway in human cancer cachexia

| Authors [reference] | Year | Type of cancer | No. of patients | Analysis | Results |
|---|---|---|---|---|---|
| Williams et al. [21] | 1999 | Miscellaneous | 6 | Ub mRNA 20s proteasome subunitsm-RNA | 300 increase 300-400% increase |
| Bossola et al. [22] | 2001 | Gastric | 20 | Ub mRNA | 200% increase related to disease stage |
| Jagoe et al. [24] | 2002 | Lung | 36 | Ub mRNA E1 mRNA E2 mRNA 20s proteasome C2 subunit | Increases were not statistically significant |
| Bossola et al. [23] | 2003 | Gastric | 23 | Ub mRNA Proteasome-specific activities | 130% increase 500% increase of CTL activity 200% increase of PGP activity 200% increase of TL activity CTL activity related to disease stage and nutritional status and age |

## References

1.  Inui A (2002) Cancer anorexia-cachexia syndrome: current issues in research and management CA Cancer J Clin 52:72–91
2.  Muscaritoli M, Bossola M, Bellantone R, Rossi Fanelli F (2004) Therapy of muscle wasting in cancer; what is the future? Curr Opin Clin Nutr Metab Care 7:459–466
3.  Hasselgren PO, Fischer JE (2001) Muscle cachexia: current concepts of intracellular mechanisms and molecular regulation. Ann Surg 233:9–17
4.  Costelli P, Baccino FM (2003) Mechanisms of skeletal muscle depletion in wasting syndromes: role of ATP-ubiquitin-dependent proteolysis. Curr Opin Clin Nutr Metab Care 6:407–412
5.  Langhans W (2002) Peripheral mechanisms involved with catabolism. Curr Opin Clin Nutr Metab Care 5:419–426
6.  Ciechanover A (1994) The ubiquitin-proteasome proteolytic pathway. Cell 79:13–21
7.  Lecker SH (2003) Ubiquitin-protein ligases in muscle wasting: multiple parallel pathways? Curr Opin Clin Nutr Metab Care 6:271–275
8.  Medina R, Wing SS, Haas A et al (1991) Activation of the ubiquitin-ATP-dependent proteolytic systems in skeletal muscle during fasting and denervation atrophy. Biomed Biochem Acta 50:347–356
9.  Bailey GL, Wang X, England BK et al (1996) The acidosis of chronic renal failure activates muscle proteolysis in rats by augmenting transcription of genes encoding proteins of the ATP-dependent ubiquitin proteasome pathway. J Clin Invest 97:1447–1453
10. Tawa NE, Odessey R, Goldberg AL (1997) Inhibitors of the proteasome reduce the accelerated proteolysis in atrophying rat skeletal muscle. J Clin Invest 100:197–203
11. Price SR, Bailey JL, Wang X et al (1996) Muscle wasting in insulinopenic rats results from activation of the ATP-dependent ubiquitin proteasome proteolytic pathway by a mechanism including gene transcription. J Clin Invest 98:1703–1708
12. Llovera M, Garcia-Martinez C, Agell N et al (1994) Ubiquitin gene expression is increased in skeletal muscle of tumour-bearing rats. FEBS Lett 338:311–318
13. Temparis S, Asensi M, Taillandier D et al (1994) Increased ATP-ubiquitin-dependent proteolysis in skeletal muscles of tumor-bearing rats. Cancer Res 54:5568–5573
14. Costelli P, Garcia-Martinez C, Llovera M et al (1995) Muscle protein wasting in tumor-bearing rats is effectively antagonized by a beta 2-adrenergic agonist (clenbuterol). Role of the ATP-ubiquitin-dependent proteolytic pathway. J Clin Invest 95:2367–2372
15. Costelli P, Bossola M, Muscaritoli M et al (2002) Anticytokine treatment prevents the increase in the activity of ATP-ubiquitin- and Ca(2+)-dependent proteolytic systems in the muscle of tumour-bearing rats. Cytokine 19:1–5
16. Bodine SC, Latres E, Baumhueter S et al (2001) Identification of ubiquitin ligases required for skeletal muscle atrophy. Science 294:1704–1708
17. Wray CJ, Mammen JM, Hershko DD et al (2003) Sepsis upregulates the gene expression of multiple ubiquitin ligases in skeletal muscle. Int J Biochem Cell Biol 35:698–705
18. Dehoux M, Van Beneden R, Fernandez-Celemin L et al (2003) Induction of MafBx and Murf ubiquitin ligase m-RNAs in rat skeletal muscles after LPS injection. FEBS Lett 544:214–217
19. Jagoe RT, Lecker SH, Gomez M et al (2002) Patterns of gene expression in atrophying skeletal muscle: response to food deprivation. FASEB J 16:1697–1712
20. Lecker SH, Jagoe RT, Gilbert A et al (2004) Multiple types of skeletal muscle atrophy involve a common program of changes in gene expression. FASEB J 18:39–51
21. Williams A, Sun X, Fischer JE et al (1999) The expression of genes in the ubiquitin proteasome proteolytic pathway is increased in skeletal muscle from patients with cancer. Surgery 126:744–750
22. Bossola M, Muscaritoli M, Costelli P et al (2001) Increased muscle ubiquitin mRNA levels in gastric cancer patients Am J Physiol Regul Integr Comp Physiol 280:R1518–R1523
23. Bossola M, Muscaritoli M, Costelli P et al (2003) Increased muscle proteasome activity correlates with disease severity in gastric cancer patients. Ann Surg 237:384–389
24. Jagoe RT, Redfern CP, Roberts RG et al (2002) Skeletal muscle m-RNA levels for cathepsin-B, but not components of the ubiquitin proteasome pathway are increased in patients with lung cancer referred for thoracotomy. Clin Sci 102:353–361

# Non-GI-Malignancy-Related Malabsorption Leads to Malnutrition and Weight Loss

Susumu Suzuki, Carolina G. Goncalves, Eduardo J.B. Ramos, Akihiro Asakawa, Akio Inui, Michael M. Meguid

## Introduction

Approximately 80% of patients with advanced-stage cancer have cancer anorexia-cachexia syndrome (CACS), in which one of the main manifestations is malnutrition [1]. CACS is characterised by anorexia, decreased food intake, tissue wasting, and body weight loss. It is also associated with changes in lipid, protein, and carbohydrate metabolism, leading to a decrease in fat and muscle mass, which independently influence mortality in cancer patients [2–5]. Anorexia and reduced food intake occur during growth of the tumour, thus compromising host defences which, in turn, detrimentally influences outcome [1]. Reduced food intake and malabsorption reduce energy intake, even though energy expenditure is increased [6–8].

Body weight is regulated by a feedback loop, involving peripheral signals from the gut, liver, and fat. These signals provide nutritional information via hormones and afferent vagal inputs to integrated centres in the brainstem and hypothalamus, where monoaminergic and peptidergic neurons integrate and transduce the information to modulate food intake [9, 10]. Direct involvement of the gastrointestinal (GI) tract or accessory digestive organs by the tumour causes profound abnormalities in GI structure and function, thus affecting nutrient digestion and absorption and leading to malnutrition [11]. However, it is not immediately obvious why a non-GI malignancy, such as lung cancer, affects GI structure and function thereby contributing to malnutrition. In this chapter, we review the relationship between non-GI malignancies and malabsorption that leads to malnutrition, weight loss, and cachexia.

## Changes in the Gastrointestinal Tract

Diseases involving the GI tract contribute to delayed gastric emptying (GE) and delayed small-bowel absorption. Such diseases include linitis plastica, pathologies of the small bowel, such as lymphomas, lymphangectasia, sarcoidosis, Whipple's disease, celiac disease, viral enteritis, and haemangiomas of the gut. These processes influence malabsorption by lymphatic infiltration of the mucosal and submucosal tissues. Less obvious aetiologies of delayed GE and malabsorption include cirrhosis, psoriasis, ileitis, and ulcerative colitis [12]. Human studies [13] document the association of gastroparesis and abnormal small-bowel function, which contribute to the malabsorption associated with non-GI tumours, which ultimately leads to malnutrition and cachexia. These GI processes are independent of tumour site, size, or overt constitutional changes [14], but are clinically manifested in advanced cancer, after weight loss, following chemotherapy or abdominal radiation [14].

As demonstrated schematically in Fig.1, changes induced by non-GI malignancies are mediated by several different mechanisms, including cytokine release in response to host-tumour interactions [1]. Cytokine release directly influences: (1) gut motility and absorptive function [15, 16]; (2) vagal-efferent innervation from the gut to nuclei in the hypothalamus that respond to signals generated by food intake and gastric motility [17, 18]; (3) GI hormones that regulate food intake, GE, and absorption in the small intestine [19–21]; and (4) immune function of the GI tract [22].

## Gastric Emptying

Gastric distension and delayed GE affect short-term regulation of food intake leading to early satiety without direct involvement of the GI tract [23]. This is related to gastric stasis [8, 24]. Bruera et al. reported prolonged GE in patients with advanced cancer, which was improved with the infusion of metoclopramide, which suggested the involvement of a dopaminergic pathway [25, 26]. Shivshanker reinforced these findings in a report describing significant delayed GE in cancer patients that was also improved with metoclopramide infusion [27]. GE was examined in our laboratory using a model of anorexia in a methyl-cholanthrene (MCA)-sarcoma-bearing rat. In these animals, it generally takes 18–20 days to develop anorexia and 28–30 days to develop profound cachexia, leading to death [28-30]. We showed a significant decrease in GE and small-bowel absorption at the onset of anorexia. The cancer-induced delay of GE may result from circulating factors produced by the tumour or by the host's response to the tumours, as outlined schematically in Fig. 1. GE is influenced by hormonal and nervous mechanisms [1, 31, 32], including cytokines, neurotransmitters, peptides, GI hormones, and nutrients. Interleukin (IL)-1, IL-6, tumour necrosis factor (TNF)-α, and interferon (IFN)-γ, concentrations are increased in cancer patients, and a role for these mediators, singularly or synergistically, has been proposed in this process [1, 3, 8]. These cytokines influence GE both directly and indirectly. Neuropeptides, such as corticotropin-releasing factor (CRF) [33], and GI hormones, such as cholecystokinin (CCK) [33, 34], are also possible mediators of delayed GE in cancer patients. Each mediator affects GE through a series of highly complex interactions. Given the correlation between malnutrition and poor clinical outcomes [1, 35], inhibition of cytokine activity may be an effective clinical approach to improve nutritional intake.

## Small Intestine

Creamer examined the structure of the mucosa of the small intestine in five patients with malignancy that arose outside the GI tract [36]. He concluded that 'weight loss and ill health' were associated

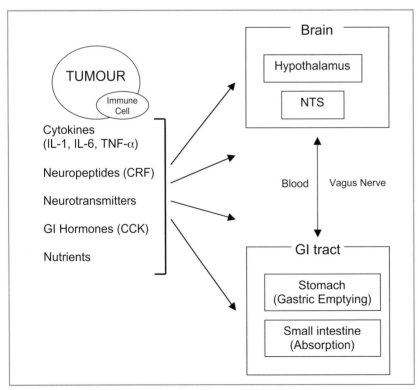

**Fig. 1.** The putative influence of non-gastrointestinal (GI) tumour on the regulation of brain and GI-tract activity, as these relate to gastric emptying and small bowel absorption. *NTS*, nucleus of the solitary tract

with an abnormal small-intestinal mucosa. As shown in Fig. 2, the changes were consistent with atrophy, hypoplasia, and flattening of the mucosa. Dymock et al., in1967, similarly reported atrophy of the jejunal mucosa in six patients who had a non-GI malignancy [13]. The mechanism for the structural changes in the small intestine was not clear and no definitive hypothesis was proposed. However, based on these early clinical observations, it is apparent that the small intestine, especially the jejunal mucosa, was affected by the presence of a non-GI malignancy.

The factors identified to date that cause CACS also induce cellular damage in the small intestine and influence cellular function of the mucosa, leading to malabsorption, loss of nutrient intake, and, consequently, to further cachexia, which affects the prognosis and quality of life. Intestinal function can be examined by evaluating urinary D-xylose excretion, vitamin B12 and folic acid absorption, and stool fat excretion. D-Xylose excretion reflects the absorption of monosaccharides and is an ATP-dependent process [13, 37]. Stool fat excretion reflects fat absorption, and folic acid excretion represents the absorption of water-soluble vitamins. D-Xylose is absorbed in the jejunum, whereas fat is absorbed farther along the jejunum and must first be emulsified by bile to render it absorbable. Vitamin B12 is absorbed over a relatively limited area of the terminal ileum [13, 37].

Figure 3 shows the data from 24 non-GI tract cancer patients who were studied by Klipstein and Smarth [38]. Other investigators [13, 14, 37] reported similar results, although the magnitude and range of the change varied widely in these uncontrolled observational studies, presumably influenced by the stage of each tumour and the duration of the patient's symptoms. Nevertheless, the data provide insight into the effects of non-GI tumours on gut mucosal function. These results can be sum-

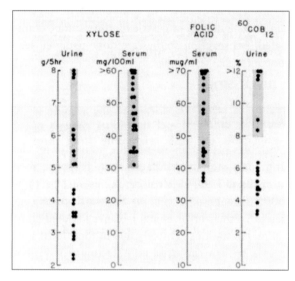

**Fig. 3.** Absorption studies. Range of normal values is indicated by *stippled areas.* (From [38])

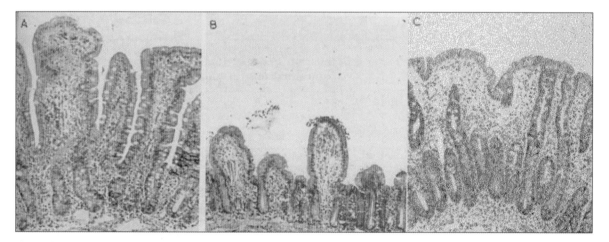

**Fig. 2.** Photomicrographs of jejunal mucosa showing **A** normal appearance, **B** hypoplastic appearance, and **C** a flat mucosa. (From [36])

marised as follows: D-Xylose absorption was decreased, as was folic acid absorption although to a lesser degree [38]; fat excretion was increased [13] and vitamin B12 absorption ranged from normal to decreased [37, 38]. Based on these data, one concludes that the jejunum is the critical area of the gut most affected by the influence of non-GI neoplasias. Tests to assess limitations of absorption that are done via the oral route or gavage may be adversely influenced by delayed gastric motility. Impaired GE delays the entrance of nutrients into the small intestine, thereby potentially decreasing the relative rate of absorption of different compounds for a given time. The influence of gastric motility can be eliminated if absorption studies are done using closed-loop intestinal techniques.

## Influencing Factors

Cytokines play a key role in the activation of the immune system and inflammatory response seen in anorexia [39, 40]. Most cytokines act predominantly through paracrine mechanisms, which suggests that their involvement in cancer-related clinical manifestations is mostly due to their local synthesis within the organs. As shown in Fig. 1, cytokines modulate gastric motility and GE, inhibiting food intake. Their effect on the GI system is mediated directly or indirectly via the brain through efferent signals from the autonomic nervous system [41]. Cytokines also induce the release of hormones that act as physiological satiety signals, such as CCK, glucagon, insulin, and leptin. In addition, cytokines activate cascades that induce the production and release of other cytokines, and their interaction with other peptides is also pivotal [42, 43], e.g. NPY blocks cytokine-induced anorexia, while cytokines block NPY-induced feeding [44]. There are also reciprocal interactions among cytokines, leptin, NPY, corticotropin-releasing factor (CRH), and glucocorticoids. Pro-inflammatory cytokines, including IL-1, IL-6, and TNF-α, play an important role in the aetiology of CACS [45-48]. These cytokines act directly on the hypothalamus [49] and indirectly on hypothalamic monoaminergic neurotransmitters [50] to reduce food intake [47, 51]. There are specific receptors for cytokines in the CNS and peripheral cytokines actively cross the blood brain-barrier to activate the central cytokine system [49]. Cytokines also act on several GI hormones, neuropeptides, and monoamines to delay gastrointestinal motility, and affect gastric motility and intestinal function to induce malabsorption. Cytokines can induce anorexia by producing early satiety, a phenomenon frequently observed during CACS. This has been extensively studied in our laboratory and, as shown in Fig. 7, early satiety initially involves a greater reduction in meal number than in meal size [52, 53].

Using our tumour-bearing-rat anorexia model, we demonstrated that increased IL-1 in the CSF inversely correlates with food intake [45] (Fig. 4), while administration of an IL-1β receptor antago-

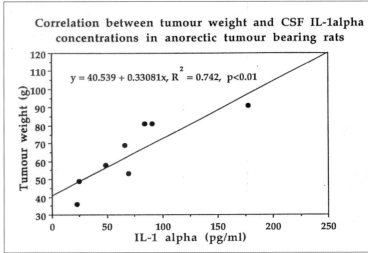

**Fig. 4.** Significant negative correlation between food intake and cerebrospinal fluid (CSF) interleukin (IL)-1α concentrations in anorectic tumour-bearing rats, suggesting a causal relationship between CSF IL-1α and anorexia during cancer. As the concentration of IL-1α in CSF increased, food intake significantly decreased. (From [45])

Correlation between tumour weight and CSF IL-1alpha concentrations in anorectic tumour bearing rats

$y = 40.539 + 0.33081x$, $R^2 = 0.742$, $p < 0.01$

nist (IL-1ra) ameliorates anorexia [54] (Fig. 5). Furthermore, we showed that administration of recombinant human soluble TNF receptor in anorectic tumour-bearing rats led to improvement of food intake with amelioration of anorexia [46] (Fig. 6). It has also been shown that the administration of cytokines to rodents mimics the neurological manifestations observed in cancer patients [49, 55, 56].

Elevated serum levels of IL-1 have been reported in cancer patients [8]. IL-1 is one of the cytokines produced by macrophages and lymphocytes during acute and chronic pathological processes [43, 49]. In an anorectic rat MCA sarcoma model, we demonstrated that IL-1 concentration in the CSF inversely correlates with food intake [45], and the injection of recombinant human interleukin-1α directly into the ventromedial nucleus (VMN), a food intake regulatory area, decreased food intake [47], while administration of an IL-1ra increased food intake [54] (Fig. 5). Furthermore, the administration of cytokines into rodents mimicked the neurological manifestations observed in cancer patients [45, ,49, 55, 56]. We

previously demonstrated that hepatic metabolism of cytokines contributes significantly to food inhibitory signals to the brain [49, 57] (Fig. 8).

Peripheral administration of IL-1β inhibits GE of a solid nutrient meal or a non-nutrient solution [58–60]. IL-1ra injected intravenously completely abolishes the delay in GE induced by intravenous IL-1β [15, 61]. Suto et al. [60, 61] also reported that IL-1β-induced inhibition of GE mediated by brain CRF pathways requires the prostaglandin pathways. Peripheral IL-1β induces $PGE_2$ release in the brain and activates the hypothalamic CRF pathways. CRF released endogenously by various stressors or central injection of CRF acts in the paraventricular nucleus (PVN) and the dorsal motor nucleus (DMN) of the vagus to inhibit gastric motor function through autonomic pathways [62]. The delay of GE induced by intravenous IL-1β was prevented by injection of ibuprofen, an inhibitor of prostaglandin synthesis [59], and by intracisternal injection of CRF antagonist, as shown in Fig. 9. IL-1α also slows down GE and decreases food intake [63] via significantly increased plasma CCK. Pretreatment with CCK-A (peripheral type) recep-

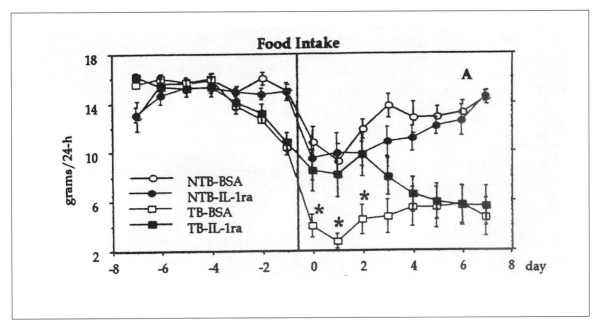

**Fig. 5.** Mean ± SE of food intake (g per 24 h) for each study group before and after IL-1 receptor antagonist (IL-1ra) injection. Data are presented as a function of ventromedial nucleus (VMN) microinjection day (day 0). *Vertical line* Approximate time of VMN microinjection during day 0. Following injection of IL-1ra into the VMN of anorectic tumour-bearing rats (*TB-IL-1ra*), food intake increased. *Asterisk* indicates significant differences between tumour-bearing rats injected with bovine serum albumin (*TB-BSA*) and TB-IL-1ra groups. (From [54])

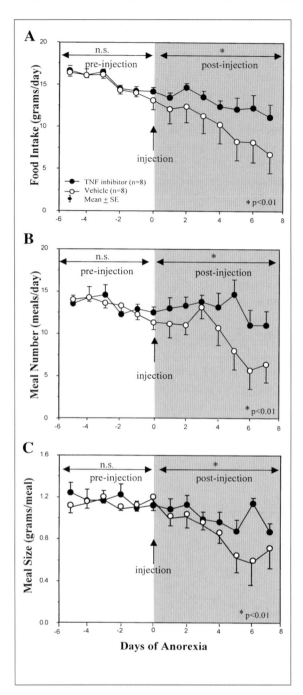

**Fig. 6.** Food intake in a tumour-bearing rat vs control. On infusing tumour necrosis-α (TNF) inhibitor, food intake improved by a significant increase with respect to meal number and size. Plot symbols show means ± SE of **A** food intake, **B** meal number, **C** meal size for the TNF inhibitor and control (vehicle) groups. *Asterisk* indicates significant differences ($p < 0.01$) between the two groups for the entire study period. (From [49])

tor antagonist partially blocked the decrease in food intake and slowed the GE rate by IL-1α [63]. However, there is a report that IL-1β directly blocks the absorption ability of the small intestine. Kreydiyyeh et al. [64] showed that IL-1β inhibited the mucosal uptake of [$^{14}$C] 3-$O$-methylglucose and the intestinal $Na^{+}$-$K^{+}$ ATPase. They concluded that the effect of IL-1β on hexose transport across the brush-border membrane could be attributed to its inhibitory effect on the $Na^{+}$-$K^{+}$ ATPase.

TNF-α is one of the representative cytokines that induce CACS, and is also the original 'cachectin' [17, 65]. TNF-α is produced by blood monocytes and tissue macrophages in response to the tumour as well as by the tumour itself [66] (see Fig. 4 in the chapter by Ramos et al.). TNF-α acts directly on the CNS to produce its anorectic effect by crossing the blood-brain barrier [67] and suppresses food intake in a dose-dependent manner [68]. By contrast, injection of the soluble pegylated analogue of TNF receptor increases food intake in cancer anorexic rats [47]. Intravenous administration of recombinant TNF-α to rats decreases the rate of intestinal glucose absorption [69], and delays the rate of GE [18, 69, 70]. The nucleus of the solitary tract (NST) in the medulla oblongata is possibly one locus for TNF-α action to control gastrointestinal function [70]. NST receives GI afferents via the vagus and these inhibit DMN stimulation of vagal input to the stomach. TNF-α induces persistent gastric stasis by functioning as a hormone that modulates intrinsic vago-vagal reflex, as shown in Fig. 9 [18].

As shown schematically in Fig. 1, CCK is involved in the functioning of the endocrine cells in the upper small intestine, principally acting to stimulate gallbladder contraction [71] and pancreatic secretion [72], and to delay GE after meals [73, 74]. CCK-induced anorexia is mediated via activation of afferent vagus nerve activity [75–77]. It has been shown that subdiaphragmatic vagotomy blocks the inhibitory effect of intraperitoneal injection of CCK on food intake [78]. Intraduodenal nutrients stimulate the release of CCK from the epithelial endocrine cells. CCK acts on the vagal afferent neurons through CCK-A

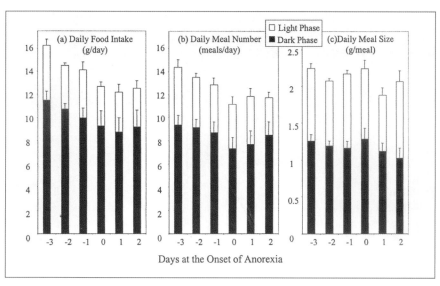

**Fig. 7.** With the onset of anorexia, total and day/night food intake decrease, primarily via a decrease in meal number. While there is an initial compensatory increase in meal size, this too eventually decreases, resulting in profound anorexia. These and similar data suggest that meal number and meal size are regulated independently and are influenced independently via cytokines. **a** Mean food intake, **b** meal number, **c** meal size on the last day of normal food intake (-3) and for the first 3 days (-2, -1, 0) of anorexia during the day and night. Data for days +1 and +2 are also shown. (From [53])

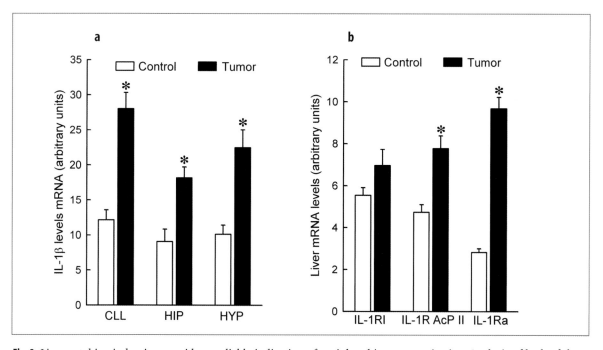

**Fig. 8.** Liver cytokine induction provides a reliable indication of peripheral immune activation. Analysis of both of these components and their comparison with changes in the hypothalamus shed light on cancer anorexia. **A** IL-1β mRNA levels in controls (*open bars*) or MCA tumour-bearing rats (*closed bars*). Values (means ± SE; n = 8 for each group) were standardised to arbitrary units. *CLL*, cerebellum; *HIP*, hippocampus; *HYP* hypothalamus. * $p \leq 0.05$ from pair-fed controls. **B** Liver mRNA levels of IL-1RI, IL-1R AcP II, and IL-1 Ra in controls (*open bars*) or MCA-tumour-bearing (*closed bars*) rats. Values (means ± SE; $n = 8$ for each group) were standardised to arbitrary units. * $p \leq 0.05$ from pair-fed controls. (From [49])

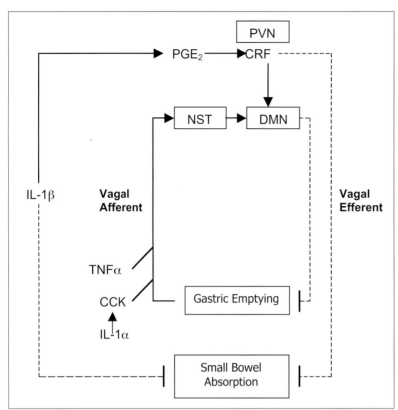

**Fig. 9.** Regulation of gastric emptying and small-intestinal absorption in cancer patients. *Solid line* Stimulation, *broken line* means inhibition. *PVN*, paraventricular nucleus; *NST*, nucleus of the solitary tract; *DMN*, dorsal motor nucleus

receptors and signals are transported to the dorsal vagal complex. The information is relayed to vagal efferent neurons to induce gastric relaxation [33]. CCK may act either locally or via the circulation to stimulate vagal afferent fibre discharge to regulate the emptying of gastric content [79]. Injection of IL-1 reduces food intake and GE in healthy animals via an increase in plasma CCK, and pretreatment with CCK receptor antagonist partially blocks this gastric stasis, suggesting that CCK mediates IL-$1\alpha$-induced anorexia (Fig. 9).

Convergent information suggests that CRF is involved in the changes observed in GI motility during stress exposure, which is a likely cause of CRF-induced delayed GE and gastric stasis in cancer patients (Fig. 1).

CRF can induce stress-related responses, including anorexia and anxiety-like behaviours [80]. Hypothalamic CRF levels are higher in tumour-bearing rats than in a pair-fed control group, suggesting that the CRF system is activated in cancer anorexia [81]. CRF injected into the cis-

terna magna or the lateral ventricle inhibits GE of liquid and solid meals in various experimental animals, including rats and mice [62, 82]. The responsive brain sites for CRF to influence gastric motor function are the PVN and the dorsoventral centre (DVC) [62]. CRF antagonists such as $\alpha$-helical CRF$_{9-41}$ and astressin, when injected into the CSF, blocked CRF-induced inhibition of GE, indicating specific interactions with CRF receptors in the brain [83].

Thus, IL-$1\beta$-induced inhibition of GR is mediated by brain CRF pathways. CRF acts in the PVN and the DMN of the vagus to inhibit gastric motor function through autonomic pathways [60, 61].

## Conclusions

Cancer anorexia-cachexia syndrome is a debilitating, life-threatening condition, and correlates with poor outcomes and compromised quality of life. Cachexia results from a functional inability to ingest sufficient amounts or to utilise nutrients, which can be related to obstruction or malabsorption. Direct involvement of the GI tract with cancer interferes with digestion and nutrient absorption, and leads to malnutrition. The occurrence of malabsorption in association with a cancer involving the GI tract is to be expected. But, as discussed in this chapter (Fig. 1), non-GI malignancies, including lung cancer, also affect GI structure and function. We have reviewed the relationships between cancer and malabsorption and referred to our ongoing research findings, as well as data in the literature, which provide a link between these two factors. Morphologically, there is significant atrophy affecting function so that malabsorption occurs. The main mediators of this process are cytokines. Elevated serum concentrations of IL-1, IL-6, and TNF-α have been found in some, but not all patients, and these cytokines seem to correlate with the progression of tumour burden [84–86]. Cytokines act on several GI hormones and neuropeptides, including CCK and CRF, acting via the vagus to inhibit GI motility. These cytokines delay GE but also act directly on the intestinal mucosa to induce malabsorption.

*Acknowledgements*

This work was supported in part, by DK/NCI 70239 awarded to Michael M. Meguid MD PhD and by a postdoctoral grant awarded to Carolina G. Goncalves MD, from SUNY Upstate Medical University Hendricks Fund #13230–52, and by grants to Akio Inui MD PhD from the Ministry of Education, Science, Sports and Culture of Japan.

# References

1. Laviano A, Meguid MM, Rossi Fanelli F (2003) Cancer anorexia: clinical implications, pathogenesis, and therapeutic strategies. Lancet Oncol 4:686–694
2. Mantovani G, Macciò A, Massa E, Madeddu C (2001) Managing cancer-related anorexia/cachexia. Drugs 61:499–514
3. Inui A (1999) Cancer anorexia-cachexia syndrome: are neuropeptides the key? Cancer Res 59:4493–4501
4. Warren S (1932) The immediate cause of death in cancer. Am J Med Sci 184:610–615
5. Lanzotti VJ, Thomas DR, Boyle LE et al (1977) Survival with inoperable lung cancer: an integration of prognostic variables based on simple clinical criteria. Cancer 39:303–313
6. Staal-van den Brekel AJ, Schols AM, ten Velde GP et al (1994) Analysis of the energy balance in lung cancer patients. Cancer Res 54:6430–6433
7. Wigmore SJ, Plester CE, Ross JA, Fearon KC (1997) Contribution of anorexia and hypermetabolism to weight loss in anicteric patients with pancreatic cancer. Br J Surg 84:196–197
8. Inui A (2002) Cancer anorexia-cachexia syndrome: current issues in research and management. CA Cancer J Clin 52:72–91
9. Prima V, Tennant M, Gorbatyuk OS et al (2004) Differential modulation of energy balance by leptin, ciliary neurotrophic factor, and leukemia inhibitory factor gene delivery: microarray deoxyribonucleic acid-chip analysis of gene expression. Endocrinology 145:2035–2045
10. Inui A (1999) Feeding and body-weight regulation by hypothalamic neuropeptides mediation of the actions of leptin. Trends Neurosci 22:62–67
11. Bruera E (1997) ABC of palliative care. Anorexia, cachexia, and nutrition. BMJ 315:1219–1222
12. Veerabagu MP, Meguid MM, Oler A, Levine RA (1996) Intravenous nucleosides and a nucleotide promote healing of small bowel ulcers in experimental enterocolitis. Dig Dis Sci 41:1452–1457
13. Dymock IW, MacKay N, Miller V et al (1967) Small intestinal function in neoplastic disease. Br J Cancer 21:505–511
14. Parrilli G, Iaffaioli RV, Martorano M et al (1989) Effects of anthracycline therapy on intestinal absorption in patients with advanced breast cancer. Cancer Res 49:3689–3691
15. Coimbra CR, Plourde V (1996) Abdominal surgery-induced inhibition of gastric emptying is mediated in part by interleukin-1 beta. Am J Physiol 270:R556–R560
16. Hardin J, Kroeker K, Chung B, Gall DG (2000) Effect of proinflammatory interleukins on jejunal nutrient transport. Gut 47:184–191
17. Wise BE, Schwartz MW, Cummings DE (2003) Melanocortin signaling and anorexia in chronic disease states. Ann N Y Acad Sci 994:275–281
18. Emch GS, Hermann GE, Rogers RC (2000) TNF-alpha activates solitary nucleus neurons responsive to gastric distension. Am J Physiol Gastrointest Liver Physiol 279:G582–G586
19. Cohen MA, Ellis SM, Le Roux CW et al (2003) Oxyntomodulin suppresses appetite and reduces food intake in humans. J Clin Endocrinol Metab 88:4696–4701
20. Asakawa A, Inui A, Yuzuriha H et al (2003) Characterization of the effects of pancreatic polypeptide in the regulation of energy balance. Gastroenterology 124:1325–1336

21. Tseng WW, Liu CD (2002) Peptide YY and cancer: current findings and potential clinical applications. Peptides 23:389–395

22. Niijima A, Meguid MM (1998) Influence of systemic arginine-lysine on immune organ function: an electrophysiological study. Brain Res Bull 45:437–441

23. Hunt JN (1980) A possible relation between the regulation of gastric emptying and food intake. Am J Physiol 239:G1–G4

24. Nelson KA, Walsh D, Sheehan FA (1994) The cancer anorexia-cachexia syndrome. J Clin Oncol 12:213–225

25. Bruera E, Catz Z, Hooper R et al (1987) Chronic nausea and anorexia in advanced cancer patients: a possible role for autonomic dysfunction. J Pain Symptom Manage 2:19–21

26. Bruera E, MacDonald N, Brenneis C et al (1986) Metoclopramide infusion with a disposable portable pump. Ann Intern Med 104:896

27. Shivshanker K, Bennett RW Jr, Haynie TP (1983) Tumor-associated gastroparesis: correction with metoclopramide. Am J Surg 145:221–225

28. Meguid M, Landel AM, Lo CC, Rivera D (1987) Effect of tumor and tumor removal on DNA, RNA, protein tissue content and survival of methylcholanthrene sarcoma-bearing rat. Surg Res Commun 1:261–271

29. Landel AM, Lo CC, Meguid MM, Rivera D (2005) Effect of methylcholanthrene-induced sarcoma and its removal on rat plasma and intracellular free amino acid content. Surg Res Commun 1:273–287

30. Suzuki S, Ramos EJ, Goncalves CG et al (2006) Effect of peripheral sarcoma on gastric emptying and small bowel absorption in tumor bearing rats. Clinical Nutrition (in press)

31. Wingate D (1976) The eupeptide system: A general theory of gastrointestinal hormones. Lancet 1:529–532

32. Mroz CT, Kelly KA (1977) The role of the extrinsic antral nerves in the regulation of gastric emptying. Surg Gynecol Obstet 145:369–377

33. Fujimiya M, Inui A (2000) Peptidergic regulation of gastrointestinal motility in rodents. Peptides 21:1565–1582

34. Daun JM, McCarthy DO (1993) The role of cholecystokinin in interleukin-1-induced anorexia. Physiol Behav 54:237–241

35. Giner M, Laviano A, Meguid MM, Gleason JR (1996) In 1995 a correlation between malnutrition and poor outcome in critically ill patients still exists. Nutrition 12:23–29

36. Creamer B (1964) Malignancy and the small-intestinal mucosa. Br Med J 5422:1435–1436

37. Somayaji BN, Nelson RS, McGregor RF (1972) Small intestinal function in malignant neoplasia. Cancer 29:1215–1222

38. Klipstein FA, Smarth G (1969) Intestinal structure and function in neoplastic disease. Am J Dig Dis 14:887–899

39. Rubin H (2003) Cancer cachexia: its correlations and causes. Proc Natl Acad Sci 100:5384–5389

40. Inui A (2001) Cytokines and sickness behavior: implications from knockout animal models. Trends Immunol 22:469–473

41. Plata-Salaman CR (2000) Central nervous system mechanisms contributing to the cachexia-anorexia syndrome. Nutrition 16:1009–1012

42. Meguid MM, Ramos EJ, Laviano A et al (2004) Tumor anorexia: effects on neuropeptide Y and monoamines in paraventricular nucleus. Peptides 25:261–266

43. Plata-Salaman CR (1996) Anorexia during acute and chronic disease. Nutrition 12:69–78

44. Sonti G, Ilyin SE, Plata-Salaman CR (1996) Neuropeptide Y blocks and reverses interleukin-1 beta-induced anorexia in rats. Peptides 17:517–520

45. Opara EI, Laviano A, Meguid MM, Yang ZJ (1995) Correlation between food intake and CSF IL-1 alpha in anorectic tumor bearing rats. Neuroreport 6:750–752

46. Torelli GF, Meguid MM, Moldawer LL et al (1999) Use of recombinant human soluble TNF receptor in anorectic tumor-bearing rats. Am J Physiol 277:R850–R855

47. Yang ZJ, Koseki M, Meguid MM et al (1994) Synergistic effect of rhTNF-a and rhIL-1a in inducing anorexia in rats. Am J Physiol 267:R1056–R1064

48. Tisdale MJ (1997) Biology of cachexia. J Natl Cancer Inst 89:1763–1773

49. Turrin NP, Ilyin SE, Gayle DA et al (2004) Interleukin-1beta system in anorectic catabolic tumor-bearing rats. Curr Opin Clin Nutr Metab Care 7:419–426

50. Yang ZJ, Blaha V, Meguid MM et al (1999) Interleukin-1a injection into ventromedial hypothalamic nucleus of normal rats depresses food intake and increases release of dopamine and serotonin. Pharmacol Biochem Behav 62:61–65

51. Debonis D, Meguid MM, Laviano A et al (1995) Temporal changes in meal number and meal size relationship in response to rHu IL-1a. Neuroreport 6:1752–1756

52. Muscaritoli M, Meguid MM, Beverly JL et al (1996) Mechanism of early tumor anorexia. J Surg Res 60:389–397

53. Meguid MM, Sato T, Torelli GF et al (2000) An analysis of temporal changes in meal number and meal size at onset of anorexia in male tumor-bearing rats. Nutrition 16:305–306

54. Laviano A, Gleason JR, Meguid MM et al (2000) Effects of intra-VMN mianserin and IL-1ra on meal number in anorectic tumor-bearing rats. J Investig Med 48:40–48

55. Strassmann G, Masui Y, Chizzonite R, Fong M (1993) Mechanisms of experimental cancer cachexia. Local involvement of IL-1 in colon-26 tumor. J Immunol 150:2341–2345

56. Laviano A, Renvyle T, Meguid MM et al (1995) Relationship between interleukin-1 and cancer anorexia. Nutrition 11:680–683

57. Turrin NP, Gayle D, Ilyin SE et al (2001) Pro-inflammatory and anti-inflammatory cytokine mRNA induction in the periphery and brain following intraperitoneal administration of bacterial lipopolysaccharide. Brain Res Bull 54:443–453

58. Robert A, Olafsson AS, Lancaster C, Zhang WR (1991) Interleukin-1 is cytoprotective, antisecretory, stimulates PGE2 synthesis by the stomach, and retards gastric emptying. Life Sci 48:123–134

59. McCarthy DO, Daun JM (1992) The role of prostaglandins in interleukin-1 induced gastroparesis. Physiol Behav 52:351–353

60. Suto G, Kiraly A, Tache Y (1994) Interleukin 1 beta inhibits gastric emptying in rats: mediation through prostaglandin and corticotropin-releasing factor. Gastroenterology 106:1568–1575

61. Suto G, Kiraly A, Plourde V, Tache Y (1996) Intravenous interleukin-1-beta-induced inhibition of gastric emptying: involvement of central corticotropin-releasing factor and prostaglandin pathways in rats. Digestion 57:135–140

62. Tache Y, Monnikes H, Bonaz B, Rivier J (1993) Role of CRF in stress-related alterations of gastric and colonic motor function. Ann N Y Acad Sci 697:233–243

63. Daun JM, McCarthy DO (1993) The role of cholecystokinin in interleukin-1-induced anorexia. Physiol Behav 54:237–241

64. Kreydiyyeh SI, Haddad JJ, Garabedian BS (1998) Interleukin-1 beta inhibits the intestinal transport of [$^{14}$C] 3-O-methylglucose in the rat. Life Sci 63:1913–1919

65. Cerami A, Tracey KJ, Lowry SF, Beutler B (1987) Cachectin: a pluripotent hormone released during the host response to invasion. Recent Prog Horm Res 43:99–112

66. Lonnroth C, Moldawer LL, Gelin J et al (1990) Tumor necrosis factor-alpha and interleukin-1 alpha production in cachectic, tumor-bearing mice. Int J Cancer 46:889–896

67. Gutierrez EG, Banks WA, Kastin AJ (1993) Murine tumor necrosis factor alpha is transported from blood to brain in the mouse. J Neuroimmunol 47:169–176

68. Katafuchi T, Motomura K, Baba S et al (1997) Differential effects of tumor necrosis factor-α and -β on rat ventromedial hypothalamic neurons in vitro. Am J Physiol 272:1966–1971

69. Arbos J, Lopez-Soriano FJ, Carbo N, Argiles JM (1992) Effects of tumour necrosis factor-alpha (cachectin) on glucose metabolism in the rat. Intestinal absorption and isolated enterocyte metabolism. Mol Cell Biochem 112:53–59

70. Hermann GE, Tovar CA, Rogers RC (1999) Induction of endogenous tumor necrosis factor-alpha: suppression of centrally stimulated gastric motility. Am J Physiol 276:R59–R68

71. Pendleton RG, Bendesky RJ, Schaffer L et al (1987) Roles of endogenous cholecystokinin in biliary, pancreatic and gastric function: studies with L-364,718, a specific cholecystokinin receptor antagonist. J Pharmacol Exp Ther 241:110–116

72. Ljung T, Hellstrom PM (1999) Vasoactive intestinal peptide suppresses migrating myoelectric complex of rat small intestine independent of nitric oxide. Acta Physiol Scand 165:225–231

73. Forster ER, Green T, Elliot M et al (1990) Gastric emptying in rats: role of afferent neurons and cholecystokinin. Am J Physiol 258:G552–G526

74. Raybould HE (1991) Capsaicin-sensitive vagal afferents and CCK in inhibition of gastric motor function induced by intestinal nutrients. Peptides 12:1279–1283

75. Zarbin MA, Wamsley JK, Innis RB, Kuhar MJ (1981) Cholecystokinin receptors: presence and axonal flow in the rat vagus nerve. Life Sci 29:697–705

76. Blackshaw LA, Grundy D (1990) Effects of cholecystokinin (CCK-8) on two classes of gastroduodenal vagal afferent fibre. J Auton Nerv Syst 31:191–201

77. Bucinskaite V, Kurosawa M, Miyasaka K et al (1997) Interleukin-1beta sensitizes the response of the gastric vagal afferent to cholecystokinin in rat. Neurosci Lett 229:33–36

78. Smith GP, Jerome C, Cushin BJ et al (1981) Abdominal vagotomy blocks the satiety effect of cholecystokinin in the rat. Science 213:1036–1037

79. Raybould HE, Lloyd KC (1994) Integration of postprandial function in the proximal gastrointestinal tract. Role of CCK and sensory pathways. Ann N Y Acad Sci 713:143–156

80. Smagin GN, Dunn AJ (2000) The role of CRF receptor subtypes in stress-induced behavioural responses. Eur J Pharmacol 405:199–206

81. McCarthy HD, McKibbin PE, Perkins AV et al (1993) Alterations in hypothalamic NPY and CRF in anorexic tumor-bearing rats. Am J Physiol 264:E638–E643

82. Tache Y, Garrick T, Raybould H (1990) Central nervous system action of peptides to influence gastrointestinal motor function. Gastroenterology 98:517–528

83. Martinez V, Rivier J, Wang L, Tache Y (1997) Central injection of a new corticotropin-releasing factor (CRF) antagonist, astressin, blocks CRF- and stress-related alterations of gastric and colonic motor function. J Pharmacol Exp Ther 280:754–760

84. Moldawer LL, Rogy MA, Lowry SF (1992) The role of cytokines in cancer cachexia. JPEN J Parenter Enteral Nutr 16:43–49

85. Noguchi Y, Yoshikawa T, Matsumoto A et al (1996) Are cytokines possible mediators of cancer cachexia? Surg Today 26:467–475

86. Matthys P, Billiau A (1997) Cytokines and cachexia. Nutrition 13:763–70

# Omega-3 Fatty Acids, Cancer Anorexia, and Hypothalamic Gene Expression

Eduardo J.B. Ramos, Carolina G. Goncalves, Susumu Suzuki, Akio Inui, Alessandro Laviano, Michael M. Meguid

## Introduction

A number of novel pathways and mediators controlling food intake, body weight, and energy expenditure have been identified using molecular and genetic techniques [1, 2]. It is now accepted that body weight is regulated by a feedback loop, in which peripheral signals from the gut, liver, and fat provide nutritional information via hormones and afferent vagal input to integrated centres in the brainstem and the hypothalamus. At these sites, monoaminergic and peptidergic neurons interact to integrate and transduce the incoming signals, thereby modulating food intake [2]. In this type of regulation, orexigenic and anorexigenic neuromediators are in a constant balance to maintain homeostasis. In several clinical diseases, ranging from inflammatory conditions such as obesity to cancer, an imbalance among these neuromediators occurs, leading, respectively, to either hyperphagia, with an increase in food intake, or to anorexia, with a decrease in food intake [3, 4].

Cancer anorexia represents a persistent and pathological form of satiety. Cancer anorexia-cachexia syndrome is observed in 80% of patients with advanced-stage cancer, and it is one of the most frequent causes of death [5]. The syndrome is characterised by anorexia, decreased food intake, tissue wasting, and body weight loss, associated with a decrease in muscle mass and adipose tissue [6]. The origin of this condition is multifactorial, and several mediators, including cytokines, neuropeptides, neurotransmitters, and tumour-derived factors, play important interactive roles [6–9].

In cancer anorexia, there is an initial reduction in meal number followed by a reduction in meal size (Fig. 1). This is similar to symptoms observed clinically and, as we have demonstrated, in anorectic tumour-bearing rats [10, 11]. This results in a profound decrease in food intake and progressive depletion of body stores and is among the major causes leading to malnutrition and, eventually, cachexia and death [5, 8]. The range of normal body mass index (BMI) is 20.1–24.9. A reduction in BMI in cancer patients to ≤ 18 causes a significant catabolic process that negatively impinges on: (1) quality of life, (2) the efficacy and benefits of antineoplastic therapy, and (3) patients' overall post-operative complications and outcomes [12, 13]. Thus, anorexia worsens outcome directly, because it is an independent negative prognostic factor [14], and indirectly, because it contributes to the development of malnutrition and cachexia. A number of drugs have been tested to treat anorexia; however, the results have been conflicting, mainly because these types of drugs were initially developed for other indications and then used, via lateral administration, to treat debilitating conditions. Thus, a strategic therapy based on data derived from a direct mechanistic understanding of the aetiology of cancer anorexia-cachexia is lacking. To date, the pathogenesis of anorexia and its onset remains a challenge awaiting full elucidation because of the significant impact on patient care and health care costs.

## The Brain–Gut–Brain Axis in the Regulation of Food Intake

The hypothalamic mechanisms regulating food intake and energy metabolism occur via interaction of the monoaminergic and the neuropeptidergic systems at various levels in the nervous system. The important components of these interactions include: (1) early satiety signals from the gut relayed via gastrointestinal afferent vagal fibres to

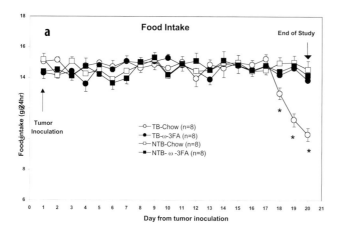

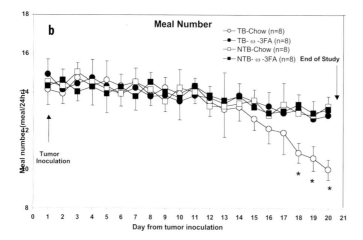

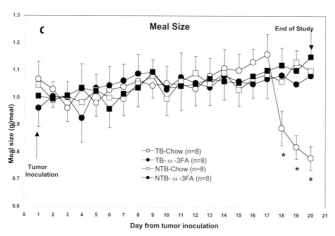

**Fig. 1.** Pattern of changes in (**a**) food intake (g per 24 h), (**b**) meal number (meals per 24 h), and (**c**) meal size (g/meal). Anorexia developed 18 days after tumour inoculation in tumour-bearing rats on chow (*TB-Chow*). * $p < 0.05$ vs. non-tumour-bearing chow-fed rats (*NTB-Chow*), non-tumour-bearing rats fed ω-3 fatty acids (NTB-ω-3 FA) and tumour-bearing rats fed ω-3 fatty acids (TB-ω-3 FA). (From [15])

the liver and the dorsovagal nuclei (visceral relay nuclei) in the brainstem that project onto the hypothalamus [16]; (2) effects of changing circulating glucose, amino acid, and fatty acid concentrations on the activity of nutrient-related neurons in vis-ceral relay nuclei and hypothalamus [17]; (3) hormone (ghrelin, cholecystokinin, polypeptide YY, insulin, and leptin) signals acting on the dorsal vagal complex and hypothalamus; hormones such as cholecystokinin (CCK) can also send messages to the brain via the gastric branch of the vagus nerve [18]; (4) changes in neurotransmitters and peptides in food-intake-related nuclei [19, 20], (5) control of the hypothalamic-pituitary-adrenal axis and sympathetic and parasympathetic output to immuno-endocrine organs, including the gastrointestinal tract, liver, adrenals, and pancreas; and (6) hypothalamic mechanisms regulating thyroid function, which is also important for energy expenditure [21].

Aspects of the gut-brain axis are discussed in Chap. 9.8. Gut hormones (Fig. 2) regulating food intake can be separated into short-term and long-term mediators. The former mediators are meal-related signals that act in accordance with the daily circadian rhythm of food intake and participate in a meal-to-meal control system. CCK and ghrelin have been implicated in the short-term and long-term (ghrelin) regulation of food intake, and have opposite actions on appetite. CCK is released from the gastrointestinal tract during eating and promotes a sense of fullness that encourages the end of

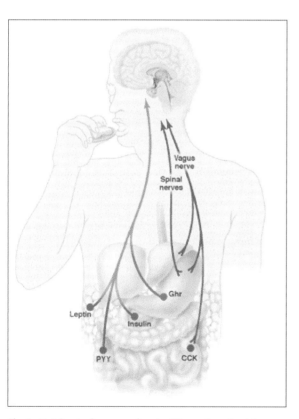

**Fig. 2.** Gut-brain hormonal axis. (Reproduced with permission from [22])

the meal [23]. Ghrelin is an appetite-stimulating hormone, blood concentrations of which rapidly increase just before a meal. At the end of the meal, ghrelin concentration falls rapidly, decreasing appetite [24]. Apart from insulin, whose role and actions are well defined, another long-term mediator of food intake is leptin, which is released into the blood by adipocytes. Leptin has sustained inhibitory effects on food intake and increases energy expenditure. When blood leptin concentrations decline, which occurs with a loss of adipose tissue, sensory neurons in the brain stimulate an increase in appetite [25]. Gut hormones, including pancreatic polypeptide and polypeptide $Y_{3-36}$ are also involved in the intermediate-term regulation of food intake. Pancreatic polypeptide (PP) produces a rapid and prolonged reduction in food intake when injected peripherally while central administration increase food intake in animal models. Polypeptide $Y_{3-36}$, which is secreted by endocrine cells of the small bowel and colon [26, 27], inhibits food intake for up to 12 h in humans and rodents [27]. Another well-known and well-characterised peptide is neuropeptide Y (NPY), which acts in the hypothalamus to increase food intake. PP, polypeptide Y, and NPY increase food intake when administered into the brain, while peripheral administration of PP produces inhibitory effects on feeding.

As shown in Fig. 3, the arcuate nucleus (ARC) synthesises NPY and agouti-related peptide (AgRP), which increase appetite. Adjacent neurons in the hypothalamus produce melanocortin peptides, which inhibit appetite. α-Melanocyte stimulating hormone (α-MSH) is a tridecapeptide melanocortin cleaved from pro-opiomelanocortin that acts to inhibit food intake [28]. This co-localisation has contributed to NPY, AgRP, and α-MSH currently being among the most-studied peptides. Immunohistochemical studies show a dense population of neurons producing α-MSH in the ARC, with projections to the dorsomedial nuclei, the medial preoptic area, and the anterior hypothalamus [29]. A moderately dense population of fibres also projects to the paraventricular nucleus (PVN), the lateral hypothalamic area (LHA), the posterior hypothalamus, and the central nucleus of the amygdala.

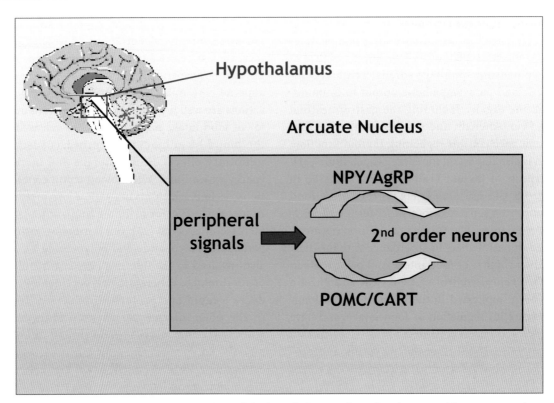

**Fig. 3.** Peripheral signals reach the arcuate nucleus of the hypothalamus, where they interact with two neuronal populations that project to second-order neuronal signalling pathways. NPY/Agouti-related peptide (*AgRP*) neurons stimulate food intake. Pro-opiomelanocortin (*POMC*)/cocaine and amphetamine-regulated transcript (*CART*) neurons inhibit food intake. (From [13])

## Cancer Anorexia

Cancer anorexia is defined as the loss of the desire to eat, and several factors are involved in its pathogenesis. Anorexia and reduced food intake are physiological responses prompted by the growing tumour, and persistent anorexia compromises host defences, which ultimately delays recovery. Anorexia contributes to the development of malnutrition and cachexia, since it reduces the oral intake of calories, thus promoting skeletal-muscle wasting [13].

In the methylcholanthrene-induced sarcoma (MCA)-bearing Fischer rat, anorexia develops with progression of tumour growth, so that a characteristic feeding pattern is observed with the onset of anorexia (Fig. 1, 11). A decrease in food intake occurs, first via a decrease in meal number associated with a simultaneous partial compensatory increase in meal size that lasts for approximately 24–48 h. Thereafter, meal size also decreases, and anorexia becomes apparent and profound [30–33], leading ultimately to the rats' demise [32]. The decrease in meal size and the resulting anorexia are mediated by the effects of cytokine on the hypothalamus, which in turn influences gastric emptying [34]. The same feeding-pattern changes are obtained in normal rats when interleukin (IL)-1, alone or together with tumour necrosis factor (TNF), is peripherally infused [35, 36]. This suggests a contributory role of cytokines in the pathogenesis of cancer anorexia. Furthermore, we demonstrated that IL-1α concentrations in CSF are inversely correlated with food intake in anorectic tumour-bearing rats [37], while we and others reported the presence of IL-1 receptors in both the ventromedial nucleus (VMN) and the LHA [7, 38] and demonstrated the occurrence of IL-1-receptor mRNA expression in the hypothalamus in tumour-bearing rats [7].

## Cytokines in Cancer Anorexia

Cytokines play a key role in the activation of the immune system and the inflammatory response typical of the catabolic state [39–41]. Different experimental approaches have demonstrated that cytokines are able to induce weight loss. They initiate a cascade of events that ultimately leads to a state of wasting, malnourishment, and eventually death. A number of pro-inflammatory cytokines, including IL-1, TNF-α, and interferon (IFN)-γ, have been isolated in tumours, as shown in Fig. 4 [7]. These cytokines together with IL-6, leukaemia inhibitory factor (LIF), and ciliary neurotrophic factor (CNTF) are also implicated in the aetiology of cancer anorexia-cachexia syndrome [6, 7].

A variety of tumours and peri-tumour cells release these cytokines into the circulation [42]. Elevated serum concentrations of IL-1, IL-6, and TNF- α occur in cancer patients and the concentrations of these cytokines correlate with tumour progression [4, 42, 43]. Furthermore, peripherally circulating cytokines stimulate receptors in the liver, and cytokine induction in this organ provides a reliable indication of peripheral immune activation [44]. At the same time, cytokines cross the blood–brain barrier to activate CNS cytokine systems via specific receptors in the brain (Fig. 5). Cytokines acts directly on the hypothalamus [45] and indirectly on hypothalamic monoaminergic [46] neurotransmitters to induce a variety of behavioural manifestations, including anorexia,

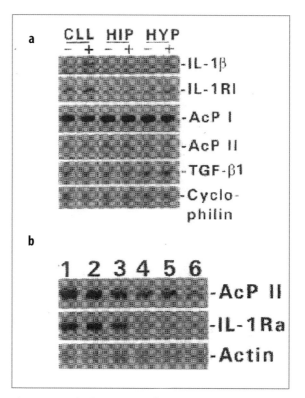

**Fig. 5. a** Interleukin-1β (*IL-1β*), IL-1 receptor type I (*IL-1RI*), IL-1 receptor accessory protein type I (*AcP I*), IL-1 receptor accessory protein type II (*AcP II*), transforming growth factor-β1 (*TGF-β1*), and cyclophilin mRNA levels in the cerebellum (*CLL*), hippocampus (*HIP*), and hypothalamus (*HYP*). Male Fischer MCA sarcoma rats (+) or controls (-). **b** AcP II, IL-1Ra, and actin mRNA levels in the liver of MCA sarcoma rats (*lanes 1–3*) or controls (*lanes 4–6*). Brain and liver tissue samples were collected 11 days after tumour-cell inoculation or in controls. Levels of AcP I (membrane-bound), and AcP II (soluble form) and IL-1Ra were not significantly changed in the hypothalamus, hippocampus, and cerebellum. In contrast, levels of AcP II and IL-1Ra mRNAs were significantly upregulated in the liver of TB rats compared to control. (From [7])

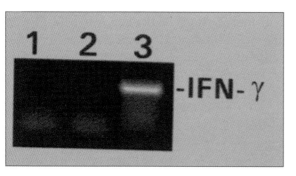

**Fig. 4.** Sample gel of RT-PCR product showing interferon (IFN)-γ mRNA expression in the hypothalamus of control (*lane 1*) and TB (*lane 2*) rats, as well as in the tumour tissue (*lane 3*). (From [7])

cognitive and motor deficits, decreased performance in verbal and visual-spatial memory tasks, and poor motor coordination. These behavioural manifestations are due to the effects of cytokines on the hypothalamus, hippocampus, and cerebellum (Fig. 6a, b) and are accompanied by whole-brain and hypothalamic immunohistochemically identifiable changes in monoaminergic and peptidergic systems [7, 36, 48, 49].

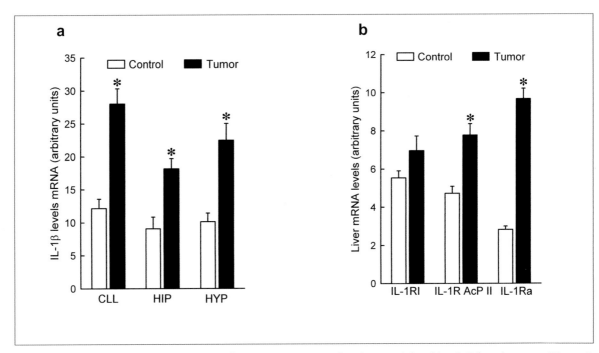

**Fig. 6. a** IL-1β mRNA levels in controls (*open bars*) or MCA tumour-bearing rats (*closed bars*). Values (means ± SE; $n = 8$ for each group) were standardised to arbitrary units. *CLL,* cerebellum, *HIP* hippocampus, *HYP* hypothalamus. * $p \leq 0.05$ from pair-fed controls. **b** Liver mRNA levels of IL-1RI, IL-1R AcP II, and IL-1 Ra in controls (*open bars*) or MCA tumour-bearing rats (*closed bars*). Values (means ± SE; $n = 8$ for each group) were standardised to arbitrary units. * $p \leq 0.05$ from pair-fed controls. (From [7])

Several hypothalamic nuclei working in an integrated function are involved in the control of food intake. Among the different brain nuclei and areas, the VMH appears to play a major role in both cancer and IL-1-induced anorexia. Evidence from our laboratory showed that the functional ablation of VMH, where mRNAs for both IL-1 and IL-1 receptors are detected, reverses established cancer anorexia [36]. More recent data indicated that the intra-VMH injection of IL-1-receptor antagonist (IL-Ra) significantly improves food intake in anorectic tumour-bearing rats [50]. These data strongly support the concept that cancer anorexia is primarily mediated by the direct action of IL-1 on the VMH.

Most cytokines act predominantly through paracrine mechanisms, which suggests that their involvement in cancer-related clinical manifestations is mostly due to their local synthesis within the organs, such as in the brain. In a rat methylcholanthrene (MCA)-induced tumour-bearing model, we demonstrated that the IL-1 concentration in the CSF inversely correlates with food

intake [37], while administration of an IL-1β antagonist alleviates anorexia [50]. We also measured specific components of the cytokine-induced anorectic reaction and found: (1) production of detectable levels of mRNA for the proinflammatory cytokines IL-1β, TNF-α, and IFN)-γ by the tumour tissue at the onset of anorexia; (2) significantly increased levels of IL-1β and IL-1-receptor type 1 (IL-1RI) mRNA in the hypothalamus, cerebellum, and hippocampus; (3) non-detectable changes in anti-inflammatory IL-1Ra and TGF-β1 mRNA in the regions of the brain studied; and (4) increased levels of IL-1Ra and IL-1-receptor accessory protein type II (IL-1RI AcP II) in the liver of TB rats (Fig. 5) [7]. These data are consistent with the suggestion that cytokines, particularly IL-1β, play a pivotal role in the inhibition of feeding by providing negative feedback on the hypothalamus [4, 7, 51]. It has been proposed that cytokines inhibit feeding by mimicking the hypothalamic effect of excessive negative feedback signalling via inhibition of the NPY/AgRP orexigenic network, as well as by persistent stimulation of the pro-opiomelanocortin (POMC) anorexigenic pathway [52]. Serotonin (5-HT) has also been demonstrated to inhibit food intake, since in normal rats peripherally infused IL-1 increases brain tryptophan concentrations, probably facilitating competitive crossing of the latter through the blood–brain barrier, consequently increasing 5-HT synthesis [42, 53]. But, more importantly, IL-1 increases 5-HT release by a physiological cascade, whereby the sum of its cytokine and tryptophan determinants amplifies 5-HT release [54]. Experimental data indicate 5-HT's influence via 5-HT$_{1B}$ receptors on magnocellular hypothalamic nuclei during cancer anorexia development, which may contribute to the decrease in food intake in cancer patients [55–57].

Recent data suggest that hypothalamic serotonergic neurotransmission is critical in linking cytokines and the melanocortin system. Fenfluramine is a 5-HT agonist that was once widely prescribed in the treatment of obesity to suppress appetite. Fenfluramine increases hypothalamic 5-HT concentrations, which in turn activate POMC neurons in the arcuate nucleus, thereby inducing anorexia and reducing food intake [55, 57]. In contrast, cytokines, particularly IL-1, stimulate the release of hypothalamic 5-HT [58]. Thus, it could be speculated that, during tumour growth, cytokines increase serotonergic activity, which, in turn, persistently activates POMC neurons, leading to the onset of anorexia and reduced food intake. Our studies in anorectic rats show that after the tumour is resected, food intake normalises (Fig. 7). When this occurred, normalisation of the 5-HT$_{1B}$ receptor and NPY expression in the hypothalamus after tumour resection in tumour-bearing rats was documented using immunocytochemical visualisation of antigens and semi-quantitative image analysis [59] (Fig. 8).

Since each anorexigenic cytokine family uses a different transducing system, cytokine-induced anorexia is a complex phenomenon that involves many signalling pathways [60]. It is unlikely that they represent separate and distinct pathogenic mechanisms; rather, it appears that close interrelationships exist among them.

## Neuropeptides and Cancer Anorexia

Several approaches have been used to study the role of neuropeptides in the regulation of eating behaviour, including various animal models (e.g. transgenic animals and gene-deletion models) and physiological studies evaluating the response of cannulated tumour-bearing animals to intracerebroventricular or hypothalamic intranuclear injection of peptides and monoamines. Although these studies provide further insight into the role of dif-

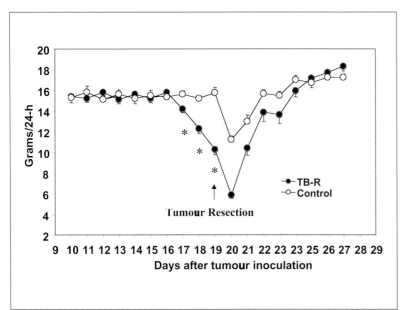

**Fig. 7.** Food intake in tumour-bearing rats (*TB-R*) and control groups before and after tumour resection and sham operation, respectively. In the TB-R group, food intake decreased with the onset of anorexia. When rats were defined as anorectic, tumours were resected, while their controls underwent sham operation. Food intake continued to be measured until it normalised in TB-R, at which time rats in both groups were killed to harvest their brains. (From [59])

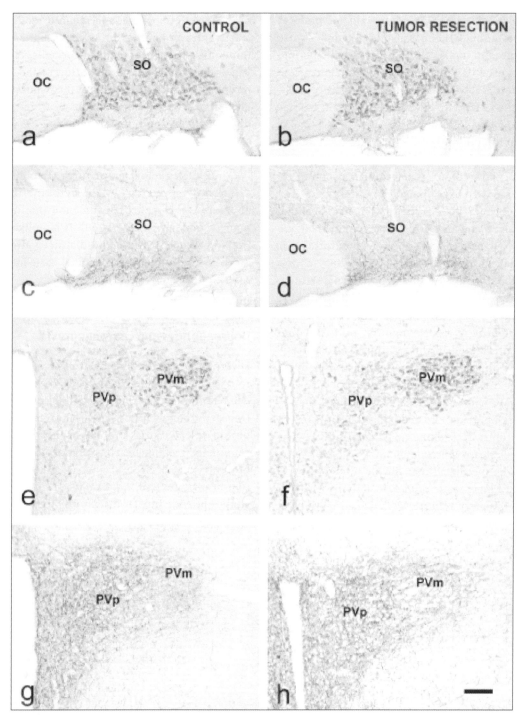

**Fig. 8.** Immunocytochemical visualisation of serotonin (5-HT)₁B receptors (**a, b, e, f**) and NPY immunoreactive fibers (**c, d, g, h**) in the hypothalamus of control and tumour-resected rats. *SO*, supraoptic; *PVm*, magnocellular part of paraventricular nucleus; *PVp*, parvocellular part of paraventricular nucleus; *OC*, optic chiasm; *Bar*, 100 μm. (From [59])

ferent neuropeptides in cancer anorexia-cachexia syndrome, our knowledge remains limited and fragmented, making difficult the development of targeted drug therapies for anorexia. Neuropeptides involved in cancer anorexia can be divided into orexigenic and anorexigenic. Among the anorexigenic peptides, hypothalamic α-MSH is thought to be of primary importance in the inhibition of feeding and body weight gain because it induces anorexia primarily via the type 4-melanocortin receptor (MC4-R). Stimulation of the hypothalamic MC4-R appears to integrate peripheral signals that lead to anorexia, weight loss,

hypodipsia, and decreased locomotion during illness [60]. Central administration of MC4-R agonists inhibits energy intake, increases energy expenditure, and reduces body weight [62, 63], whereas administration of MC4-R antagonists leads to an increase in food intake. It has been reported that weight loss and hypophagia induced by sarcoma growth can be reversed and prevented by the administration of the endogenous MC3/MC4 antagonist, AgRP. The prevention of tumour-induced hypophagia with early and repeated AgRP injections resulted in maintenance of normal food intake (Fig. 9) [61].

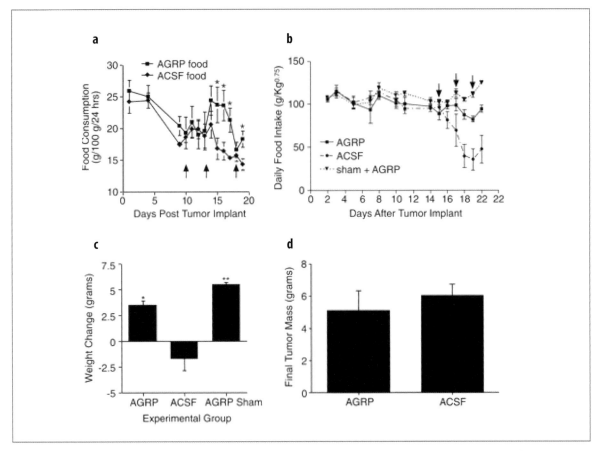

**Fig. 9.** Agouti-related peptide (AgRP) administration prevents cachexia in sarcoma-bearing mice. **a** Daily food consumption in sarcoma-bearing mice. Feeding can be restored in hypophagic mice, with the effect lasting for 2–3 days. *Arrows* Days of injection of AgRP (2.5 nmol; $^*p < 0.01$ vs wild-type control. **b** Daily food intake in sarcoma-bearing mice. Injections given earlier in the course of the disease prevents hypophagia in tumour-bearing animals and produces hyperphagia in sham-implanted controls. **c** Net weight change over 19 days. **d** Tumour burden showing that AgRP prevents tumour-induced carcass weight loss ($^*p < 0.0001$), without affecting final tumour mass. (From [61])

NPY, one of the most potent orexigenic neuropeptides, acts in the hypothalamus to stimulate food intake. NPY neurons in the ARC synthesise both NPY and AgRP, an endogenous melanocortin antagonist (Fig. 3). NPY/AgRP neurons are known to innervate and directly inhibit the function of POMC neurons. Thus, the activation of NPY/AgRP neurons inhibits melanocortin signalling at multiple levels, making them a logical target for the transduction of cachexigenic stimuli from the periphery. Previous data from in a tumour-bearing rat model indicated interactions between the monoamine system and NPY, thus pointing to a specific and integrated role for these neuromediators in the onset of cancer anorexia. The inhibition of NPY orexigenic effects is associated with specific changes in 5-HT and dopamine (DA) concentrations in the PVN, which, in turn, inhibits food intake and thus promotes the onset of cancer anorexia (Fig. 10a, b) [56]. Although the overall effect of these signals on NPY neuronal function remains controversial, studies have demonstrated that the NPY feeding system is dysfunctional in anorectic tumour-bearing rats [56].

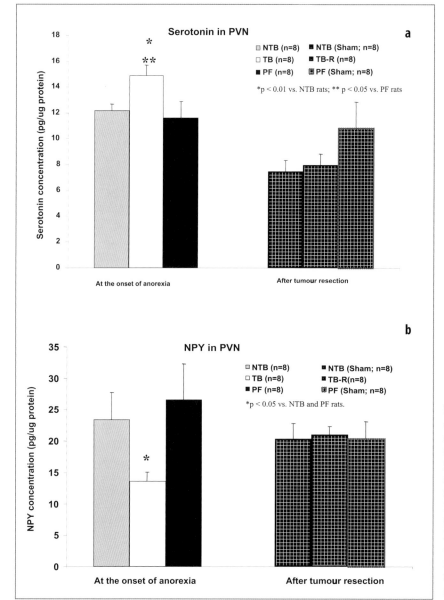

**Fig. 10. a** At the onset of anorexia in TB rats, a significant increase in 5-HT concentration was measured in the hypothalamic PVN. Values are mean ± standard error. *$p < 0.01$ vs NTB rats; **$p < 0.05$ vs. Pair-fed (PF) rats. **b** In contrast, a significant decrease in NPY concentration was measured in the PVN. Values are mean ± standard error. *$p < 0.05$ vs. NTB and PF rats. (From [56])

## Omega-3 Fatty-Acid Diet

Our current understanding of the mechanisms contributing to anorexia includes a critical role for the hypothalamic monoaminergic system. Its dysfunction during tumour growth appears to be initiated by: (1) increased supply to the brain of tryptophan, the amino acid precursor of 5-HT, resulting in an increase in hypothalamic 5-HT (Fig. 10a), and (2) the increased production of cytokines that exert their anorexic effect directly on the hypothalamus (Fig. 6). The cytokines also increase the uptake of tryptophan, further increasing the synthesis of 5-HT in the hypothalamus and thus contributing to anorexia. Since anorexia is mediated by cytokines and omega-3 fatty acids (ω-3 FAs) interfere with the synthesis of cytokines [64], the anti-anorectic therapeutic benefits of ω-3 FAs have been investigated.

Dietary factors modify the production and the activity of cytokines [65]. In healthy human volunteers, dietary fish oil (rich in long-chain ω-3 polyunsaturated fatty acids) supplementation inhibits in vitro production of IL-1 [65] and TNF-α [64, 65]. Dietary supplementation with ω-3 FAs also significantly reduces in vitro production of IL-1β and TNF-α in healthy women and decreases in vitro production of IL-1 from monocytes of rheumatoid arthritis patients [65]. The inhibition of cytokine production by ω-3 FAs is a long-lasting phenomenon, as the release of IL-1 α and IL-1β, and TNF- α remains inhibited 10 weeks after the end of the ω-3 FA supplementation [64]. The production of cytokines returned to the pre-supplementation level 20 weeks after the end of ω-3 FA supplementation. Long-chain ω-3 or (n-3) polyunsaturated fatty acids include eicosapentaenoic (EPA; C20: 5 n-3) and docosahexaenoic (DHA; C22:6 n-3) acids. These are derived from linolenic (C18:3 n-3) acid and undergo biological transformation to eicosanoids, which alter the production of inflammatory mediators, including cytokines. Suppression of cytokine production occurs by inhibiting the cyclo-oxygenase pathway, and hence prostaglandin and leukotriene synthesis [67]. In vitro, EPA is a potent suppressor of the secretion of several cytokines, including IL-1, IL-2, IL-6 and TNF-α, and it also inhibits T-cell proliferation [68]. EPA also competes for the incorporation of arachidonic acid into membrane phospholipids and inhibits its conversion to prostanoids.

In addition to inhibiting the production of cytokines, fish oil also diminishes the biological activities of cytokines including: (1) the direct anorexigenic effect induced by IL-1 [69] and TNF-α [70]; and (2) the indirect effect of enhanced amounts of tryptophan crossing the blood–brain barrier [44]. Furthermore, in rodents, dietary ω-3 FAs inhibit the pyrogenic and thermogenic responses to IL-1 [71]. Preliminary studies reported that a fish-oil-enriched diet significantly inhibits tumour induced weight loss in animal models and tumour-induced cachexia in humans [72, 73]. Thus, the use of ω-3 FAs as an exploratory tool helps to dissect the mechanism of the anticipated increase in food intake.

As mentioned above, we have shown that when the tumour grows, food intake decreases, initially by a decrease in meal number and then by a decrease in meal size, manifesting the characteristic-feeding pattern of cancer anorexia (Fig. 1A–C). These findings correspond with clinical observations in anorexic cancer patients, who initially decrease the number of meals they eat per day and then subsequently are unable to eat a full meal, i.e. they decrease their meal size. ω-3 FAs suppressed the appearance, growth, and progression of the tumour (Fig. 11) [73, 74], although the exact mechanism(s) by which this occurs is remains a subject of investigation. Possible mechanisms include: (1) reduced formation of eicosanoids derived from arachidonic acid; (2) incorporation of EPA and DHA into tumour membrane phospholipids, which may alter membrane function, the kinetic properties of enzymes responsive to receptor-cytokine or receptor-hormone interactions [15] and, in turn, cytokine activity; and (3) decreased concentrations of vascular endothelial growth factor and, consequently, decreased tumour vascular supply [75]. The inhibitory role of ω-3 FAs on vascular smooth muscle cell (VSMC) proliferation and therefore growth of blood vessels deserves consideration. ω-3 FAs have both anti-thrombotic and anti-atherogenic actions. These effects are mediated by endothelial cells, which influence vascular remodelling via modulating proliferation,

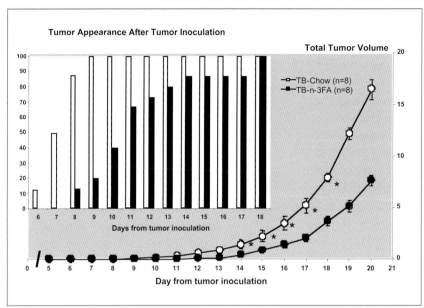

**Fig. 11.** Tumour appearance and changes of tumour volume in TB rats. Tumour appearance occurred 100% (8/8) within 9 days after tumour inoculation in TB-Chow rats; in TB-ω-3 FA rats, tumour appearance occurred 20% (2/8) within 9 days and 100% (8/8) on day 18 after tumour inoculation. *$p <$ 0.05 vs TB-ω-3 fatty acid rats. (From [15])

cell death, and structural alteration in blood vessels [76]. ω-3 FAs also influence vascular function and inhibit vessel proliferation via EPA and DHA. EPA inhibits VSMC proliferation [77], and DHA triggers VSMC apoptosis, implicating a role for these compounds in vascular remodelling [78]. Interestingly, the potency for this anti-proliferative action has been reported to be greater for EPA than for DHA [77]. Thus, that the ability of ω-3 FAs to suppress the appearance of the tumour and its progression might be explained by the inhibition of VSMC proliferation, consequently leading to a decrease in blood supply to the tumour.

Another interesting fact is that tω-3 FAs also act in the CNS. We have demonstrated that, besides an increase in food intake, the administration of ω-3 FAs to anorectic tumour-bearing rats leads to changes in the hypothalamic NPY, α-MSH, and 5-HT. Using immunohistochemical visualisation and semiquantitative image analysis, we demonstrated that tumour-bearing rats fed a diet rich in ω-3 FAs (TB-ω-3 FA) showed increased NPY immunoreactivity in many hypothalamic nuclei, (i.e. ARC, PVN, and supraoptic nuclei) and decreased α-MSH reactivity in the ARC and in the magnocellular part of PVN. Comparison of NPY immunostaining in different

hypothalamic nuclei of anorectic TB-ω-3 FA vs tumour-bearing chow-fed rats revealed a marked increase in some hypothalamic nuclei. Moreover, NPY immunostaining was not uniform or equal in different hypothalamic structures, and the most intense increase of NPY occurred in the ARC. Analysing the percent increase in staining associated with ω-3 FAs in the tumour-bearing condition, the greatest amount of change was observed in the hypothalamic PVN, where staining increased by 50% in magnocellular and 10% in parvocellular nuclei. The most intense decrease in α-MSH staining occurred in the ARC, with 64% less immunoreactivity than in the ARC of tumour-bearing rats on a chow diet. A similar decrease in 5-HT1B receptors occurred in supraoptic nuclei. These findings support the hypothesis that, in a sarcoma rat model of anorexia, ω-3 FAs lead to an increase in food intake and prevent the tumour-induced weight loss via hypothalamic up-regulation of the orexigenic NPY and down-regulation of anorexigenic α-MSH and 5-HT.

Studying the effects of ω-3 FAs on gene expression in the hypothalamus of tumour-bearing vs non-tumour-bearing chow-fed rats led to preliminary data showing that up-regulation of TNF-α and IL-1β occurs in the ARC of the former. This corresponds to our recent report showing that, in the brain, anorexia is associated with up-regulation of mRNAs for IL-1β and its receptor. This suggests that IL-1β and its receptor play a significant role in cancer-associated anorexia [7].

In TB-ω-3 FA, TNF-α and IL-1β expression in the ARC was lower than in tumour-bearing chow-fed rats (Table 1). These data, together with the data summarised in Fig. 6, showing increased mRNA in the hypothalamus, suggest that the effect of ω-3 FAs in the presence of tumour is to suppress

## Conclusions

The development of cachexia is a common feature in cancer patients, highly impinging on their quality of life and life expectancy. The anorexia-cachexia syndrome is a complex metabolic disorder and several hypotheses have been offered to explain its aetiology. Interaction between the growing tumour and the immune system leads to the release of cytokines, which act in the hypothalamus and cause an imbalance between the orexigenic and anorexigenic path-

**Table 1.** Gene expression profiles normalised to the baseline sample

|  | NTB-Chow | NTB-omega-3FA | TB-Chow | TB-omega-3FA |
|---|---|---|---|---|
| TNF-α |  |  |  |  |
| ARC | 1.00 | 0.28 | 1.19 | 1.15 |
| PVN | 1.00 | 0.58 | 0.92 | 0.82 |
|  |  |  |  |  |
| IL-1β |  |  |  |  |
| ARC | 1.00 | 1.06 | 2.04 | 1.19 |
| PVN | 1.00 | 1.25 | 0.79 | 0.97 |
|  |  |  |  |  |
| NPY |  |  |  |  |
| ARC | 1.00 | 0.09 | 0.33 | 0.71 |
| PVN | 1.00 | 29.85 | 2.06 | 7.77 |
|  |  |  |  |  |
| POMC |  |  |  |  |
| ARC | 1.00 | 0.03 | 0.09 | 1.36 |
| PVN | 1.00 | 16.27 | 0.79 | 1.00 |

*NTB-Chow*, non-tumour-bearing chow-fed rats; *FA*, fatty acids; *TB*, tumour-bearing; *TNF-α*, tumour necrosis factor-α; *ARC*, arcuate nucleus; *PVN*, paraventricular nucleus; *IL-1β*, interleukin-1β; *NPY*, neuropeptide Y; *POMC*, pro-opiomelanocortin

pro-inflammatory cytokines, as evidenced by decreased TNF-α and IL-1β in the ARC. As a result, food intake is improved. NPY expression is increased in the ARC by 215% and in PVN by 377%, preventing a decrease of food intake in this group compared to tumour-bearing chow-fed rats. These alterations in the hypothalamic pro-inflammatory cytokines and neuropeptides suggest that there are changes in food-intake regulatory pathways in the brain in response to cancer that ultimately result in anorexia.

ways. An understanding of the pathogenesis of the multifactorial syndrome of cancer anorexia and the effects on this syndrome of a diet supplemented with ω-3 FAs will provide insight into the mechanisms that regulate feeding activity. Currently, no effective pharmacological treatment exists to fully reverse anorexia. Thus, a better understanding of the detailed mechanisms underlying the complex pathogenesis of hypophagia and its metabolic dysregulation, which lead to cachexia, is needed to develop new therapeutic approaches.

## References

1. Inui A (1999) Feeding and body-weight regulation by hypothalamic neuropeptides- mediation of the actions of leptin. Trends Neurosci 22:62–67

2. Neary NM, Goldstone AP, Bloom SR (2004) Appetite regulation from gut to the hypothalamus. Clin Endocrinol 60:153–160

3. Ramos EJB, Xu Y, Middleton F et al (2003) Is obesity an inflammatory disease? Surgery 134:329–335

4. Inui A, Meguid MM (2003) Cachexia and obesity: two sides of the coin? Curr Opin Clin Nutr Metab Care 6:395–399

5. Warren S (1932) The immediate cause of death in cancer. Am J Med Sci 184:610–615

6. Mantovani G, Macciò A, Massa E, Madeddu C (2001) Managing cancer-related anorexia/cachexia. Drugs 61:499–514

7. Turrin NP, Ilyn SE, Gayle D et al (2004) Interleukin-1b system in anorectic catabolic tumor bearing rats. Cytokine, neuropeptide and G protein alpha-subunit mRNAs in anorectic MCA tumor bearing rats. Curr Opin Clin Nutri 7:419–426

8. Langstein HN, Norton JA (1991) Mechanisms of cancer cachexia. Hematol Oncol Clin North Am 5:103–123

9. Plata-Salaman CR (2000) Central nervous system mechanisms contributing to the cachexia-anorexia syndrome. Nutrition 16:1009–1012

10. Meguid MM, Laviano A, Rossi Fanelli F (1998) Food intake equals meal size x meal number. Appetite 31:404

11. Sato T, Meguid MM, Fetissov SO et al (2001) Hypothalamic dopaminergic receptor expressions in anorexia of tumor bearing rats. Am J Physiol Regul Integr Comp Physiol 281:R1907–R1916

12. Meguid MM, Laviano A (2001) Malnutrition, outcome and nutritional support: time to re-visit the issues. Ann Thorac Surg 71:766–768

13. Laviano A, Meguid MM, Rossi Fanelli F (2003) Cancer anorexia: clinical implications, pathogenesis, and therapeutic strategies. Lancet Oncol 4:686–694

14. Maltoni M, Pirovano M, Scarpi E et al (1995) Prediction of survival of patients terminally ill with cancer. Results of an Italian prospective multicentric study. Cancer 75:2613–2622

15. Ramos EJ, Middleton F, Laviano A et al (2004) Effects of ω-3 fatty acid supplementation on tumor bearing rats. J Am Coll Surg 199:716–723

16. Niijima A, Miyata G, Sato T, Meguid MM (2001) Hepato-vagal pathway associated with nicotine's anorectic effect in the rat. Auton Neurosc 93:48–55

17. Nandi J, Meguid MM, Inui A et al (2002) Central mechanisms involved with catabolism. Curr Opin Clin Nutr Metab Care 4: 407–418

18. Asakawa A, Inui A, Goto K et al (2002) Effects of agouti-related protein, orexin and melanin-concentrating hormone on oxygen consumption in mice. Int J Mol Med 10:523–525

19. Meguid MM, Fetissov SO, Varma M et al (2000) Hypothalamic dopamine and serotonin in the regulation of food intake. Nutrition 16:843–857

20. Meguid MM, Ramos EJ, Laviano A et al (2004) Tumor and anorexia: effects on neuropeptide Y and monoamines in paraventricular nucleus. Peptides 25:261–266

21. Niijima A, Meguid MM (1995) Effects of arginine-lysine mixture, glucose and ATP on the autonomic outflows to the thymus and spleen. Neurobiology 3:299–307

22. Marx J (2003) Cellular warriors at the battle of the bulge. Science 299:846–849

23. Costentin J (2004) Physiological and neurobiological elements of food intake. Ann Pharm Fr 62:92–102

24. Inui A, Asakawa A, Bowers CY et al (2004) Ghrelin, appetite, and gastric motility - the emerging role of the stomach as an endocrine organ. FASEB J 18:439–456

25. Ueno N, Dube MG, Inui A et al (2004) Leptin modulates orexigenic effects of ghrelin, attenuates adiponectin and insulin levels, and selectively the dark-phase feeding as revealed by central leptin gene therapy. Endocrinology 145:4176–4184

26. Asakawa A, Inui A, Yuzuriha H et al (2003) Characterization of the effects of pancreatic polypeptide in the regulation of energy balance. Gastroenterology 124:1325–1336

27. Batterham RL, Cowley MA, Small CJ et al (2002) Gut hormone PYY (3–36) physiologically inhibits food intake. Nature 418:650–654

28. O'Donohue TL, Dorsa DM (1982) The opiomelanotropinergic neuronal and endocrine systems. Peptides 3:353–395

29. Jacobowitz DM, O'Donohue TL (1978) Alpha-melanocyte stimulating hormone: immunohistochemical identification and mapping in neurons of rat brain. Proc Natl Acad Sci U S A 75:6300–6304

30. Meguid MM, Muscaritoli M, Beverly JL et al (1992) The early cancer anorexia paradigm: changes in plasma free tryptophan and feeding indexes. J Parenter Enteral Nutr 16:56S–59S

31. Meguid MM, Sato T, Torelli GF et al (2000) An analysis of temporal changes in meal number and meal size at onset of anorexia in male tumor-bearing rats. Nutrition 16:305–306

32. Meguid MM, Yang ZJ, Laviano A (1997) Meal size and number: relationship to dopamine levels in the ventromedial hypothalamic nucleus. Am J Physiol 272:R1925–R1930

33. Varma M, Torelli GF, Meguid MM et al (1999) Potential strategies for ameliorating early cancer anorexia. J Surg Res 81:69–76

34. Robert A, Olafsson AS, Lancaster C, Zhang WR (1991) Interleukin-1 is cytoprotective, antisecretory, stimulates PGE2 synthesis by the stomach, and

retards gastric emptying. Life Sci 48:123–134

35. Yang ZJ, Koseki M, Meguid MM et al (1994) Synergistic effect of rhTNF-alpha and rhIL-1 alpha in inducing anorexia in rats. Am J Physiol 267:R1056–R1064

36. Debonis D, Meguid MM, Laviano A et al (1995) Temporal changes in meal number and meal size relationship in response to rHu IL-1 alpha. Neuroreport 6:1752–1756

37. Opara EI, Laviano A, Meguid MM, Yang ZJ (1995) Correlation between food intake and CSF IL-1 alpha in anorectic tumor bearing rats. Neuroreport 6:750–752

38. Yabuchi K, Minami M, Katsumata S, Satoh M (1994) Localization of type I interleukin-1 receptor mRNA in the rat brain. Brain Res Mol Brain Res 27:27–36

39. Inui A (2001) Cytokines and sickness behavior: implications from knockout animal models. Trends Immunol 22:469–473

40. Meguid MM, Pichard C (2003) Cytokines: the mother of catabolic mediators! Curr Opin Clin Nutr Metab Care 6:383–386

41. Laviano A, Meguid MM, Rossi Fanelli F (2003) Improving food intake in anorectic cancer patients. Curr Opin Clin Nutr Metab Care 6:421–426

42. Langhans W, Hrupka B (1999) Interleukins and tumor necrosis factor as inhibitors of food intake. Neuropeptides 33:415–424

43. Mantovani G, Macciò A, Mura L et al (2000) Serum levels of leptin and proinflammatory cytokines in patients with advanced-stage cancer at different sites. J Mol Med 78:554–561

44. Sato T, Laviano A, Meguid MM et al (2003) Involvement of plasma leptin, insulin and free tryptophan in cytokine-induced anorexia. Clin Nutr 22:139–146

45. Turrin NP, Gayle D, Ilyin SE et al (2001) Pro-inflammatory and anti-inflammatory cytokine mRNA induction in the periphery and brain following intraperitoneal administration of bacterial lipopolysaccharide. Brain Res Bull 54:443–453

46. Plata-Salaman CR (1996) Anorexia during acute and chronic disease. Nutrition 12:69–78

47. Laviano A, Yang Z-J, Meguid MM et al (1995) Hepatic vagus does not mediate IL-1 alpha induced anorexia. Neuro Report 6:1266

48. Yang ZJ, Blaha V, Meguid MM et al (1999) Interleukin-1a injection into ventromedial hypothalamic nucleus of normal rats depresses food intake and increases release of dopamine and serotonin. Pharmacol Biochem Behav 62:61–65

49. Laviano A, Yang Z-J, Meguid MM et al (1994) A pilot study demonstrating reversal of cancer anorexia in the rat by the functional ablation of ventromedial nucleus of hypothalamus (VMH). Clin Nutr 13(S 1):22 (abs)

50. Laviano A, Gleason JR, Meguid MM et al (2000) Effects of intra-VMN mianserin and IL-1ra on meal number in anorectic tumor-bearing rats. J Investig Med 48:40–48

51. Inui A (2002) Cancer anorexia-cachexia syndrome: current issues in research and management. CA Cancer J Clin 52:72–91

52. Inui A (1999) Cancer anorexia-cachexia syndrome: are neuropeptides the Key? Cancer Res 59:4493–4501

53. Sato T, Laviano A, Meguid MM et al (2003) Involvement of plasma leptin, insulin and free tryptophan in cytokine-induced anorexia. Clin Nutr 22:139–146

54. Dunn AJ (1992) Endotoxin-induced activation of cerebral catecholamine and serotonin metabolism: comparison with interleukin-1. J Pharmacol Exp Therap 261:964–969

55. Makarenko IG, Meguid MM, Gatto L et al (2005) Hypothalamic 5-HT1B receptor changes in anoretic tumor bearing rats. Neurosci Lett 376:71–75

56. Meguid MM, Ramos EJ, Laviano A et al (2004) Tumor anorexia: effects on neuropeptide Y and monoamines in paraventricular nucleus. Peptides 25:261–266

57. Makarenko IG, Meguid MM, Ugrumov MV (2002) Distribution of serotonin 5HT 1B in the normal rat hypothalamus. Neurosci Lett 328:155–159

58. Mohankumar PS, Thyagarajan S, Quadri SK (1993) Interleukin-1beta increases 5-hydroxyindoleacetic acid release in the hypothalamus in vivo. Brain Res Bull 31:745–748

59. Makarenko IG, Meguid MM, Gatto L et al (2006) Cancer anorexia related changes of serotonin receptor (5-HT1B) and NPY using immunocytochemical visualization and semiquantitative image analysis in hypothalamus after tumor resection. Neurosci Lett 383:322–327

60. Heisler LK, Cowley MA, Tecott LH et al (2003) Central serotonin and melanocortin pathways regulating energy homeostasis. Ann N Y Acad Sci 994:169–174

61. Marks DL, Ling N, Cone RD (2001) Role of the central melanocortin system in cachexia. Cancer Research 61:1432–1438

62. Fan W, Boston BA, Kesterson RA et al (1997) Role of melanocortinergic neurons in feeding and the agouti obesity syndrome. Nature 385:165–168

63. Stair JN, Shu J, Camacho R et al (1999) Feeding behavior in rats chronically treated with melanocortin agonist, MTII. Soc Neurosci Abstr 25:619

64. Endres S, Ghorbani R, Kelley VE et al (1989) The effect of dietary supplementation with n-3 polyunsaturated fatty acids on the synthesis of interleukin-1 and tumor necrosis factor by mononuclear cells. N Engl J Med 320:265–271

65. Cooper AL, Gibbons L, Horan MA et al (1993) Effect of dietary fish oil supplementation on fever and cytokine production in human volunteers. Clin Nutr 12:321–328

66. Meydani SN, Endres S, Woods MM et al (1991) Oral

(n-3) fatty acid supplementation suppresses cytokine production and lymphocyte proliferation: comparison between young and older women. J Nutr 121:547–555

67. Zurier RB (1993) Fatty acids, inflammation and immune responses. Prostaglandins Leukot Essent Fatty Acids 48:57–62

68. Kumar GS, Das UN (1994) Effect of prostaglandins and their precursors on the proliferation of human lymphocytes and their secretion of tumor necrosis factor and various interleukin. Prostaglandins Leukot Essent Fatty Acids 50:331–334

69. Hellerstein MK, Meydani SN, Meydani M et al (1989) Interleukin-1-induced anorexia in the rat. Influence of prostaglandins. J Clin Invest 84:228–235

70. Mulrooney HM, Grimble RF (1993) Influence of butter and of corn, coconut and fish oils on the effects of recombinant human tumor necrosis factor-alpha in rats. Clin Sci (Colch) 84:105–112

71. Cooper AL, Rothwell NJ (1993) Inhibition of the thermogenic and pyrogenic responses to interleukin-1 beta in the rat by dietary N-3 fatty acid supplementation. Prostaglandins Leukot Essent Fatty Acids 49:615–626

72. Dagnelie PC, Bell JD, Williams SC et al (1994) Effect of fish oil on cancer cachexia and host liver metabolism in rats with prostate tumors. Lipids 29:195–203

73. Tisdale MJ (2000) Biomedicine. Protein loss in cancer cachexia. Science 289:2293–2294

74. Rose DP, Connolly JM, Meschter CL (1991) Effect of dietary fat on human breast cancer growth and lung metastasis in nude mice. J Nat Cancer Ins 83:1491–1495

75. Mukutmoni-Norris M, Hubbard NE, Erickson KL (2000) Modulation of murine mammary tumor vasculature by dietary n-3 fatty acids in fish oil. Cancer Lett 150:101–109

76. Abeywardena MY, Head RJ (2001) Long chain n-3 polyunsaturated fatty acids and blood vessel function. Cardiovasc Res 52:361–371

77. Terano T, Shiina T, Tamura Y (1996) Eicosapentaenoic acid suppressed the proliferation of vascular smooth muscle cells through modulation of various steps of growth signals. Lipids 31:S301–S304

78. Diep QN, Touyz RM, Schiffrin EL (2002) Docosahexaenoic acid, a peroxisome proliferator-activated receptor-a ligand, induces apoptosis in vascular smooth muscle cells by stimulation of p38 mitogen-activated protein kinase. Hypertension 36:851–855

# The Role of Pineal Hormone Melatonin in Cancer Cachexia

Paolo Lissoni, Luca A. Fumagalli, Fernando Brivio, Gianstefano Gardani, Angelo Nespoli

## Physiology

Melatonin (N-acetyl-5-methoxytriptamine) is the best-known among the indoles produced by the pineal gland (also called the epiphysis) according to a circadian rhythm. The pineal gland is the regulator of *photic* and *nonphotic* effects of the sun; indeed, it is the anatomical structure that coordinates the body's functions with the most important environmental rhythm, that is the light/dark rhythm. This fact may help us in understanding the history of the pineal gland: ancient myths and philosophic systems all over the world assigned a significant role to this gland, with respect to the health of the body and the spirit. Indeed, Cartesius (Reneé Descartes) described the pineal gland as the site of the soul. The Greek name given by Vesalius to the pineal gland, epiphysis (επι = above; φυσισ = nature), implies that it is the counterpart of the hypophysis (υπο = below φυσισ = nature), whereas effectively the physiological activity of the pineal gland counterbalances that of the hypothalamic-pituitary-adrenal (HPA) axis.

Melatonin targets are specific membrane receptors located in the brain and in other tissues. These receptors include the MT1 and MT2 receptors and the nuclear receptors RZR/ROR-α [1–3].

Melatonin membrane receptors are G-protein-coupled and thus regulated by cyclic-adenosine-monophosphate (cAMP) and phosphoinositide hydrolysis. MT1 receptors are mainly found in the hypothalamus and kidney, whereas MT2 receptors are expressed in the brain and retina. The two receptors are reported to have different affinities. Melatonin production occurs through the activation of enzymatic pathways and it peaks in the dark period of the day. Concerning its physiology, it is known that melatonin production starts in 1-month-old newborns, is abundant in infancy, and drops acutely in the puberty; it has therefore been proposed that melatonin is a clock marking the onset of puberty.

## Pineal Gland and Cancer

In cancer patients, the function of the pineal gland and the circadian secretion of pineal hormones are frequently disrupted [4–8]. Animal and in vitro models have shown that melatonin inhibits the growth of several tumours, such as breast cancer MCF7 [9, 10] and prostatic cancer [11, 12]. Chemical pinealectomy increased the growth of experimental tumours in animals. Recent experimental evidence in animal models of cancer showed that exposure to light during the dark phase of an alternating light–dark cycle suppresses the synthesis of melatonin, increases fatty acid metabolism, and promotes the growth of transplantable murine liver tumours and human breast cancer xenografts [13–15].

In humans, different authors have reported several findings: (1) the total 24-h amount of melatonin and its metabolites did not differ between healthy subjects and breast cancer patients [16]; (2) pineal gland function and the circadian secretion of pineal hormones in patients with solid tumours was found to be disrupted [4–7]; (3) accordingly, the risk of cancer was increased in subjects with melatonin night-shift [17–19].

From an endocrinological view, these apparently contradictory finding could be explained if the cancer-induced changes in the circadian pattern of melatonin availability were manifested over a period of time $> 24$ h, i.e. just as different patterns of cortisol incretion are characteristic of different adrenal-gland diseases.

In fact, studies have demonstrated an increased

cancer risk with alteration of melatonin incretion; however while a relationship between alterations of circadian amplitude or phase (time of melatonin upswing) and cancer was observed, the average amount of melatonin metabolites excreted in 24 h did not change [20].

Cancer patients suffer from an imbalance of several neurological and endocrine systems, including the pineal/opioid system [21, 22].

Another role of the pineal gland is the regulation of immune function [23]. Melatonin has been well-proven to influence both natural and adaptive immune activity; that is, cell-mediated immune function and phagocytosis. Melatonin modulates the response of immune cells to cytokines both in vitro and in vivo. The down-regulation of immune function in cancer is a major factor affecting the overall survival of patients with advanced-stage cancer. In this respect, although it is commonly underestimated in the daily clinical management of cancer patients, the role of melatonin in the restoration of normal immune function of cancer patients deserves further investigation. Melatonin acts on immune function by different pathways: through regulation of cytokine secretion by peripheral cells [24] and by central regulation of neurotransmitters [25]. As in HIV patients, the decrease in circulating lymphocytes is a poor prognostic factor in all major types of cancers, independent of better-known and ascertained prognostic factors, such as tumour stage, disease extension, and weight loss [26, 27]. Cancer-associated immunodeficiency, as in HIV, is mainly dependent on the inhibition of endogenous interleukin (IL)-2 production [28–32]. Pineal gland dysfunction has a role in cancer-associated immunodeficiency [33]. Based on our experience with cancer patients, the addition of melatonin to IL-2 immunotherapy increases the rebound lymphocytosis induced by IL-2 and exerts other effects on haematopoiesis [34–38].

The activity of pineal indoles on immune regulation suggests a major role for central nervous control of immune pathways [39–42]; for example, melatonin has been reported to have anti-inflammatory effects [43, 44]. Indeed, pineal gland function may act on several levels in the pathways leading to cancer-associated anorexia-cachexia syndrome.

## Cachexia and Melatonin

Cancer cachexia depends on derangements of metabolic, endocrine, and immune functions. Cachexia is a strong prognostic factor associated with a poor prognosis [26], due, in part, to its association with an increased rest energy expenditure (REE). The poor prognosis regarding overall survival induced by weight loss is the most important demonstration that the metabolic, immune, and endocrine alterations resulting from cancer cachexia warrant the most effective treatment to improve patient outcome.

Among the possible mediators involved in the pathophysiology of cancer anorexia-cachexia, the increased production of tumour necrosis factor (TNF)-$\alpha$ has long been implicated [45] as one of the major cytokines inducing wasting syndrome and enhancing REE. Melatonin was demonstrated to be able, both in vitro and in animals, to inhibit the lipopolysaccharide-induced TNF production in an endotoxic shock model [46]. In a preliminary study [47], we found evidence of feedback systems between the pineal release of melatonin and TNF secretion; other studies on the clinical use of melatonin in the palliation of symptoms suggested a role for melatonin activity in the improvement of the clinical conditions of patients with advanced-stage cancer [48].

## Dosing and Administration

Although a large number of pathophysiological studies on the role of melatonin in several models of disease have been published, our knowledge of the pharmacology of melatonin in clinical settings is still very poor. Earlier studies hypothesised or calculated that the replacement of endogenous hormone by synthetic melatonin would need dosing between 0.5 and 2 mg in human adults, although a clear-cut dosage has not yet been established [49].

Most clinical studies so far have consisted of the administration of empirical doses of melatonin, ranging from 5 mg to 20 or 40 mg, derived from extrapolations of data from animal studies. In any event, dose-activity studies in cancer patients are lacking as is a comparison of the different routes of administration. This knowledge gap may be due to the fact that melatonin receptors have only recently been clearly identified. An understanding of the function of these receptors is fundamental to gaining insight into melatonin action and the therapeutic administration of exogenous melatonin, e.g. identifying the optimal time-range of administration based on receptor exposure [50]. Detailed studies of MLT receptors will no doubt be critical for successful melatonin-based treatment, in order to reproduce a therapeutic physiological effect or to modify deranged pathways that occur in certain diseases (i.e. the decrease in REE).

Very recent studies on the use of melatonin as an hypnotic drug in animals and humans found that the pharmacological doses of melatonin that were needed were very different from those administered to improve sleep or for behaviour modulation in neurological disturbances [51]. An intravenous dose of 178 mg melatonin/kg was reported to have the same effects as propofol at 5.4 mg/kg and of thiopental at 12.5 mg/kg [52].

Taking into account all of the above-cited data,

it is clear that much work remains to be done to understand the activities, effectiveness, and the failures, reported in studies on melatonin thus far.

## Administration of Melatonin in Cancer-Associated Cachexia

To investigate the in vivo relationships between cancer cachexia, TNF, and melatonin, our Institution carried out a randomised clinical trial in 1994 in advanced-stage cancer patients with progressive disease after standard treatment [53].

This randomised, open-label study enrolled 100 patients with metastatic solid tumours who had not responded to previous conventional antitumour treatment and/or who were not eligible to receive other effective standard forms of treatment. Exclusion criteria were malnutrition due to difficult or impossible oral intake, i.e. intestinal occlusion, need of parenteral nutrition and/or prolonged i.v. fluid infusion, and a diagnosis of a tumours of the head and/or neck. Patients characteristics are listed in Table 1. Patients provided

**Table 1.** Clinical characteristics of metastatic untreatable patients receiving supportive care or supportive care and melatonin (MLT) 20 mg/day in the evening

|  | Supportive care | Supportive care + melatonin |
|---|---|---|
| Study patients no. | 51 | 49 |
| Died from rapid progression | 10 | 4 |
| Evaluable patient no. | 41 | 45 |
| Male/female | 27/14 | 29/16 |
| Median age (yrs) | 64 (39–74) | 66 (41–76) |
| Karnofsky performance status (median) | 60 (20–90) | 60 (20–90) |
| Previous chemotherapy | 39 | 43 |
| *Tumor types* | | |
| Non-small cell lung cancer | 13 | 14 |
| Breast cancer | 8 | 6 |
| Colorectal cancer | 6 | 7 |
| Gastric cancer | 4 | 6 |
| Hepatocarcinoma | 3 | 4 |
| Pancreatic cancer | 3 | 3 |
| Unknown primary tumor | 2 | 3 |
| Cervix carcinoma | 2 | 2 |
| *Dominant metastatic sites* | | |
| Soft tissues | 4 | 4 |
| Bone | 7 | 6 |
| Lung | 14 | 15 |
| Lung + liver | 3 | 4 |
| Brain | 2 | 3 |

informed consent and were stratified according to tumour type and disease site. They were then randomised to receive standard supportive care (control arm) or standard supportive care plus melatonin (treated arm). Patients were considered evaluable when observed for at least 2 months.

Standard supportive care included nonsteroidal anti inflammatory drugs and opioid drugs for pain palliation. Steroids (dexamethasone or methylprednisolone) were administered in case of dyspnoea or hypotension (i.e. lung infiltration). Melatonin was administered per os daily in the evening, at 20 mg/day. The dose was chosen empirically, based on the previous studies available at the time.

Serum TNF levels were measured by RIA using peripheral venous blood samples taken at baseline and at monthly intervals of 3 months. Normal values of serum TNF were determined in a group of 40 age-matched healthy subjects and were 2–10 pg/ml (95% confidence limit).

Initial respiratory distress, diagnosed as a rapid decline in arterial $PO_2$, the presence of lung infiltrates, but no congestive heart failure, as determined by ultrasound scan, occurred in 13 patients (6 treated and 7 controls). Respiratory distress was associated with lung lymphangitic metastases in ten of 13 patients. Fourteen patients died due to rapid disease progression (ten in the control arm, four in the treated arm) and were not evaluable. There were thus 86 evaluable patients, 41 in the control group and 45 in the treated group, and they were well-balanced regarding the main prognostic variables (tumour type, disease site, performance status, age).

## Clinical Findings

No adverse events associated with melatonin administration were observed. On the contrary, among patients with respiratory distress who received melatonin, five out of six had improved arterial $PO_2$ with disappearance of lung infiltrates. Rapid progression to death was observed in one of six melatonin-treated but in seven of seven control patients with respiratory distress ($p < 0.05$).

Weight loss > 10% vs baseline occurred in two of 45 patients in the treated arm (4%) and in 13 of 42 patients in the control group (32%) ($p < 0.01$). Mean ($\pm$ SE) weight loss in the control arm was 6 $\pm$ 2 kg vs 3 $\pm$ 1 kg in the treated arm ($p < 0.001$) (Fig. 1).

Concerning tumour progression, measured according to WHO criteria, progressive disease was observed in 37 of 41 control patients vs 24 of 45 patients in the melatonin group (90% vs 53%: $p < 0.05$); no objective response was observed.

## Serum TNF-$\alpha$ Levels

Cancer patients at baseline had serum levels of TNF-$\alpha$ (mean $\pm$ SE) that were higher than in healthy controls (41 $\pm$ 5 vs 6 $\pm$ 2 pg/ml: $p < 0.001$). At baseline, no difference in serum TNF-$\alpha$ levels was observed between the two study groups. In the control group, mean serum TNF-$\alpha$ levels showed a trend to increase compared to baseline (39 $\pm$ 3 vs 51 $\pm$ 5). Interestingly, TFN-$\alpha$ serum levels in the treated group, assessed after 2 and 3 months of melatonin administration, decreased significantly ($p < 0.05$ at 2 months; $p < 0.01$ at 3 months) vs baseline (Fig. 2).

## Study Conclusions

According to the results of this independent study, melatonin administration was effective in the inhibition of cancer-associated wasting syndrome. Noticeably, its clinical effect seems explainable by the inhibition of serum TNF-$\alpha$ release, which tends to increase in the natural course of advanced cancer. The ability of melatonin to modulate the inflammatory response in cancer patients seems to overcome TNF-$\alpha$-related activity; in other studies, even those of non-cancer diseases, melatonin inhibited the in vivo release of sIL-2R in serum and decreased the erythrocyte sedimentation rate (ESR). However, a larger, double-blinded, randomised study is needed to definitively confirm the effectiveness of melatonin in cancer cachexia; unfortunately, so far, neither public nor private sponsors have been interested in funding studies into the therapeutic benefit of a low-cost treatment involving a simple compound such as melatonin.

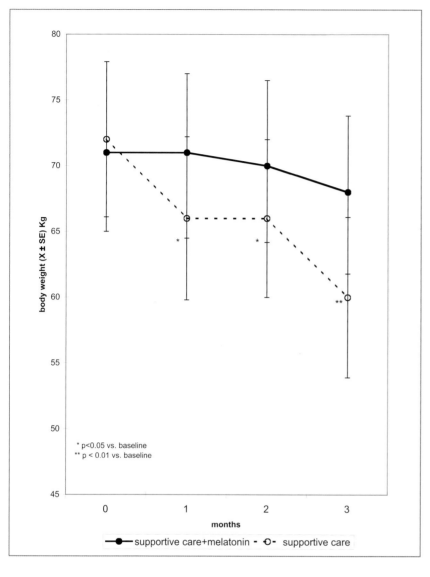

**Fig. 1.** Changes in body weight

## Overview of Supportive Cancer Care with Melatonin

The therapeutic potential of melatonin is wide-ranging [54]. Evidence derived from clinical and biological studies has supported our view that melatonin administration should be considered as hormone-replacement therapy aimed at the restoration of the physiological circadian rhythm in cancer patients. The cancer-associated disruption of circadian endocrine, immune, and neuro-logic systems is still far from being understood [55], although their prognostic impact on survival

has been well-demonstrated, as evidenced by studies showing that alterations of cortisol rhythm are predictive of overall survival [56].

In cancer patients, the addition of melatonin to standard treatments improved patient outcome in chemotherapy-treated patients [57, 58] and in those receiving hormone therapy [59, 60] or IL-2 immunotherapy [61, 62].

In chemotherapy-treated patients with advanced-stage cancer [63–65] the addition of melatonin decreased the rate of chemo-associated toxicity. In our above-reported study, 250 advanced cancer patients with poor clinical status (lung cancer: 104; breast cancer: 77; gastrointestinal tract

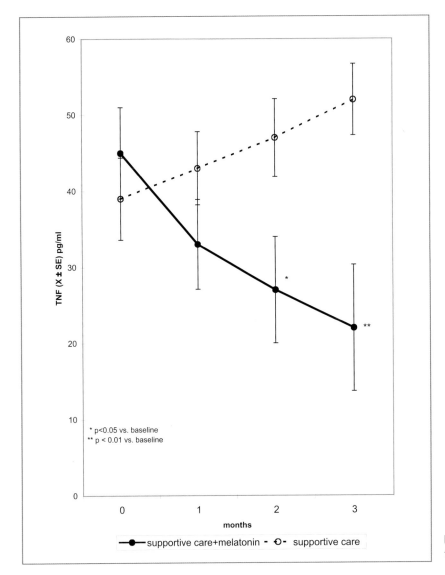

**Fig. 2.** Changes in serum levels of tumour necrosis factor (TNF)-α

neoplasms: 42; head and neck cancers: 27) received melatonin (20 mg/day, orally every day) plus chemotherapy, or chemotherapy alone. Chemotherapy consisted of standard cisplatin (CDDP) plus etoposide or gemcitabine alone for lung cancer; adriamycin alone, mitoxantrone alone, or paclitaxel alone for breast cancer; 5-FU plus folates for gastrointestinal tumours; and 5-FU plus CDDP for head and neck cancers. In the groups of patients receiving concomitant administration of melatonin, the frequency of chemo-associated toxicities was significantly reduced. In detail, the concomitant administration of melatonin significantly reduced the frequency of myelosuppression ($p < 0.001$), thrombocytopenia ($p < 0.05$), neurotoxicity ($p < 0.05$), cardiotoxicity ($p < 0.05$), stomatitis ($p < 0.05$), and asthaenia ($p < 0.001$). Leucopenia and anaemia were also less frequent in the melatonin group, without, however, statistically significant differences. While the incidence of nausea and vomiting, diarrhoea, and alopecia were not influenced by melatonin, both overall survival time and objective tumour regression rate were significantly higher in patients concomitantly treated with melatonin (tumour response rate: 42/124 vs 19/126: $p < 0.001$; 1-year survival: 63/124 vs 29/126: $p < 0.001$).

The ascertained influence of melatonin in

haematopoiesis through different pathways (direct receptor interaction, cytokine production, or monoaminergic stimulation of bone marrow) [66] might explain at least some of its clinical effects on the prevention of chemo-associated toxicities. Moreover, melatonin could also protect from chemo-associated toxicities by its proven anti-oxidant and free-radical scavenger activities [67, 68].

Among the different effects on haematopoiesis, the most relevant one seems the protective effect on platelet (toxicity). The ability of melatonin to increase platelet number is worth serious attention: noticeably, other pineal gland hormones such as 5-methoxytryptamine, also seem to be involved in thrombopoiesis [69, 70].

Other diseases, apart from cancer, are also characterised by severe disruption of circadian pineal rhythm, such as liver cirrhosis [71–74] and shock [75]. Thus, it should be kept in mind that other functions have been ascribed to the pineal gland besides melatonin release; several indoles are increted according to a circadian rhythm, but their functions are still largely unknown [76–88] and their therapeutic potential is far from being ascertained [88–90].

A wider vision and a deeper knowledge of the regulation by the pineal gland of immune, endocrine, and neurological systems will provide new insights into treating human diseases. The relationships between psychic status and immuno-endocrine functions should not be considered as immaterial and unmeasurable; the human conscience is neurochemically alive and active. As a result, higher functions can be affected by diseases but they can also be therapeutically restored, from their immune basis [21, 22, 91–93] up to mood modulation [21, 22, 55] and spiritual perception. Whereas today's clinical approach is mainly able to provide advanced cancer patients with palliative treatments, a further step in the evolution of science and of medicine is needed to achieve the promise of cancer cure. The application of our expanding knowledge of neuroimmunoendocrinology to clinical methodology and the clinical approach to treating cancer patients represents such a step.

## References

1. Garcia-Maurino S, Pozo D, Calvo JR, Guerrero JM (2000) Correlation between nuclear melatonin receptor expression and enhanced cytokine production in human lymphocytic and monocytic cell lines. J Pineal Res 29:129–137

2. Karasek M, Gruszka A, Lawnicka H et al (2003) Melatonin inhibits growth of diethylstilbestrol-induced prolactin-secreting pituitary tumor in vitro: possible involvement of nuclear RZR/ROR receptors. J Pineal Res 34:294–296

3. Carrillo-Vico A, Garcia-Maurino S, Calvo JR, Guerrero JM (2003) Melatonin counteracts the inhibitory effect of PGE2 on IL-2 production in human lymphocytes via its mt1 membrane receptor. FASEB J 17:755–757

4. Bartsch C, Bartsch H, Fuchs U et al (1989) Stage-dependent depression of melatonin in patients with primary breast cancer. Correlation with prolactin, thyroid stimulating hormone, and steroid receptors. Cancer 64:426–433

5. Tamarkin L, Danforth D, Lichter A et al (1982) Decreased nocturnal plasma melatonin peak in patients with estrogen receptor positive breast cancer. Science 216:1003–1005

6. Lissoni P, Viviani S, Bajetta E (1986) A clinical study of the pineal gland activity in oncologic patients. Cancer 57:837–842

7. Falkson G, Falkson HC, Steyn ME et al (1990) Plasma melatonin in patients with breast cancer. Oncology 47:401–405

8. Lissoni P, Crispino S, Barni S et al (1990) Pineal gland and tumor cell kinetics: serum levels of melatonin in relation to Ki-67 labeling rate in breast cancer. Oncology 47:275–277

9. Hill SM, Blask DE (1988) Effects of the pineal hormone melatonin on the proliferation and morphological characteristics of human breast cancer cells (MCF-7) in culture. Cancer Res 48:6121–6126

10. Cos S, Blask DE, Lemus-Wilson A, Hill AB (1991) Effects of melatonin on the cell cycle kinetics and 'estrogen-rescue' of MCF-7 human breast cancer cells in culture. J Pineal Res 10:36–42

11. Marelli MM, Limonta P, Maggi R et al (2000) Growth-inhibitory activity of melatonin on human androgen-independent DU 145 prostate cancer cells. Prostate 45:238–244

12. Bizzarri M, Cucina A, Valente MG et al (2003) Melatonin and vitamin D3 increase TGF-beta1 release and induce growth inhibition in breast cancer cell cultures. J Surg Res 110:332–337

13. Dauchy RT, Blask DE, Sauer LA et al (1999) Dim light during darkness stimulates tumor progression by enhancing tumor fatty acid uptake and metabolism. Cancer Lett 144:131–136

14. Blask DE, Dauchy RT, Sauer LA et al (2002) Light during darkness, melatonin suppression and cancer progression. Neuroendocrinol 23:52–56

15. Blask DE, Dauchy RT, Sauer LA et al (2003) Growth and fatty acid metabolism of human breast cancer (MCF-7) xenografts in nude rats: impact of constant light-induced nocturnal melatonin suppression. Breast Cancer Res Treat 79:313–320

16. Travis R, Allen D, Fentiman I, Key T (2004) Melatonin and breast cancer: a prospective study. J Natl Cancer Inst 96:475–482

17. Hansen J (2001) Increased breast cancer risk among women who work predominantly at night. Epidemiology 12:74–77

18. Davis S, Mirick DK, Stevens RG (2001) Night shift work, light at night, and risk of breast cancer. J Natl Cancer Inst 93:1557–1562

19. Shernhammer ES, Laden F, Speizer FE et al (2003) Night-shift work and risk of colorectal cancer in the nurses' health study. J Natl Cancer Inst 95:825–828

20. Hrushesky WJM, Blask DE (2004) Melatonin and breast cancer: a prospective study. J Natl Cancer 96:888–889

21. Esposti D, Lissoni P, Tancini G et al (1988) A study on the relationship between the pineal gland and the opioid system in patients with cancer. Preliminary considerations. Cancer 62:494–499

22. Lissoni P, Barni S, Tancini G (1994) Pineal-opioid system interactions in the control of immunoinflammatory responses. Ann N Y Acad Sci 741:191–196

23. Guerrero JM, Reiter RJ (2002) Melatonin-immune system relationships. Curr Top Med Chem 2:167–179

24. Lissoni P (1999) The pineal gland as a central regulator of cytokine network. Neuroendocrinol Lett 20:343–349

25. Esposti D, Lissoni P, Mauri R et al (1988) The pineal gland-opioid system relation: melatonin-naloxone interactions in regulating GH and LH releases in man J Endocrinol Invest 11:103–106

26. Stanley KE (1980) Prognostic factors for survival in patients with inoperable lung cancer. J Natl Cancer Inst 65:25–32

27. Lavin PT, Bruckner HW, Plaxe SC (1982) Studies in prognostic factors relating to chemotherapy for advanced gastric cancer. Cancer 50:2016–2023

28. Lissoni P, Barni S, Rovelli F, Tancini G (1991) Lower survival in metastatic cancer patients with reduced interleukin-2 blood concentrations. Oncology 48:125–127

29. Fischer JR, Schindel M, Stein N (1995) Selective suppression of cytokine secretion in patients with small cell lung cancer. Ann Oncol 6:921–926

30. Monson JRT, Ramsden C, Guillou PJ (1986) Decreased IL-2 production in patients with gastrointestinal cancer. Br J Surg 73:483–486

31. Rayman P, Uzzo RG, Kolenko V et al (2000) Tumor-induced dysfunction in Interleukin-2 production and Interleukin-2 receptor signaling: a mechanism of immune escape. Cancer J Sci Am 6 (S1):S81-S87

32. Dolan MJ, Clerici M, Blatt S et al (1995) In vitro T cell function, delayed-type hypersensitivity skin testing, and CD4+ T cell subset phenotyping independently predict survival time in patients infected with human immunodeficiency virus. J Infect Dis 172:79–87

33. Lissoni P, Tancini G, Barni S et al (1989) Alterations of pineal gland and of T lymphocyte subsets in metastatic cancer patients: preliminary results. J Biol Regul Homeost Agents 3:181–183

34. Lissoni P, Barni S, Ardizzoia A et al (1992) Immunological effects of a single evening subcutaneous injection of low-dose interleukin-2 in association with the pineal hormone melatonin in advanced cancer patients. J Biol Regul Homeost Agents 6:132–136

35. Lissoni P, Ardizzoia A, Tisi E et al (1993) Amplification of eosinophilia by melatonin during the immunotherapy of cancer with interleukin-2. J Biol Regul Homeost Agents 7:34–36

36. Lissoni P, Barni S, Tancini G et al (1993) A study of the mechanisms involved in the immunostimulatory action of the pineal hormone in cancer patients. Oncology 50:399–402

37. Lissoni P, Barni S, Brivio F et al (1995) Treatment of cancer-related thrombocytopenia by low-dose subcutaneous interleukin-2 plus the pineal hormone melatonin: a biological phase II study. J Biol Regul Homeost Agents 9:52–54

38. Lissoni P, Barni S, Brivio F et al (1995) A biological study on the efficacy of low-dose subcutaneous interleukin-2 plus melatonin in the treatment of cancer-related thrombocytopenia. Oncology 52:360–362

39. Carrillo-Vico A, Calvo JR, Abreu P et al (2004) Evidence of melatonin synthesis by human lymphocytes and its physiological significance: possible role as intracrine, autocrine, and/or paracrine substance. FASEB J 18:537–539

40. El-Sokkary GH, Reiter RJ, Abdel-Ghaffar Skh (2003) Melatonin supplementation restores cellular proliferation and DNA synthesis in the splenic and thymic lymphocytes of old rats. Neuroendocrinol Lett 24:215–223

41. Huang YS, Jiang JW, Cao XD, Wu GC (2003) Melatonin enhances lymphocyte proliferation and decreases the release of pituitary pro-opiomelanocortin-derived peptides in surgically traumatized rats. Neurosci Lett 343:109–112

42. Kuhlwein E, Irwin M (2001) Melatonin modulation of lymphocyte proliferation and Th1/Th2 cytokine expression. J Neuroimmunol 117:51–57

43. Lissoni P, Rovelli F, Meregalli S et al (1997) Melatonin as a new possible anti-inflammatory agent. J Biol Regul Homeost Agents 11:157–159

44. Cuzzocrea S, Reiter RJ (2002) Pharmacological actions of melatonin in acute and chronic inflammation. Curr Top Med Chem 2:153–165

45. Beutler B, Cerami A (1986) Cachectin and tumor-necrosis factor as two sides of the same biological coin. Nature 320:584–588

46. Sacco S, Aquilini L, Ghezzi P et al (1998) Mechanisms of the inhibitory effects of melatonin on tumor-necrosis factor production in vivo and in vitro. Eur J Pharmacol 343:249–255

47. Lissoni P, Barni S, Tancini G (1994) Role of the pineal gland in the control of the macrophage functions and its possible implication in cancer: a study of interactions between tumor-necrosis factor alpha and the pineal hormone melatonin. J Biol Regul Homeost Agents 8:126–129

48. Lissoni P, Barni S, Crispin S et al (1989) Endocrine and immune effects of melatonin therapy in metastatic cancer patients. Eur J Cancer Clin Oncol 25:789–795

49. Reiter RJ, Tan DX (2003) What constitutes a physiological concentration of melatonin? J Pineal Res 34:79–80

50. Akagi T, Ushinohama K, Ikesue S et al (2004) Chronopharmacology of melatonin in mice to maximize the antitumor effect and minimize the rhythm disturbance effect. J Pharmacol Exp Ther 308:378–384

51. Serfaty M, Kennell-Webb S, Warner J et al (2002) Double blind randomised placebo controlled trial of low dose melatonin for sleep disorders in dementia. Int J Geriatr Psychiatry 17:1120–1127

52. Naguib M, Hammond DL, Schmid PG 3rd et al (2003) Pharmacological effects of intravenous melatonin: comparative studies with thiopental and propofol. Br J Anaesth 90:504–507

53. Lissoni P, Paolorossi F, Tancini G et al (1996) Is there a role for melatonin in the treatment of neoplastic cachexia? Eur J Cancer 32A:1340–1343

54. Vijayalaxmi, Thomas CR Jr, Reiter RJ, Herman TS (2002) Melatonin: from basic research to cancer treatment clinics. J Clin Oncol 20:2575–2601

55. Lissoni P, Malugani F, Manganini V et al (2003) Psychooncology and cancer progression-related alterations of pleasure-associated neurochemical system: abnormal neuroendocrine response to apomorphine in advanced cancer patients. Neuroendocrinol Lett 24:50–53

56. Sephton SE, Sapolsky RM, Kraemer HC, Spiegel D (2000) Diurnal cortisol rhythm as a predictor of breast cancer survival. J Natl Cancer Inst 9:994–1000

57. Lissoni P, Chilelli M, Villa S et al (2003) Five years survival in metastatic non-small cell lung cancer patients treated with chemotherapy alone or chemotherapy and melatonin: a randomized trial. J Pineal Res 35:12–15

58. Cerea G, Vaghi M, Ardizzoia A et al (2003) Biomodulation of cancer chemotherapy for metastatic colorectal cancer: a randomized study of weekly low-dose irinotecan alone versus irinotecan plus the oncostatic pineal hormone melatonin in metastatic colorectal cancer patients progressing on 5-fluorouracil-containing combinations. Anticancer Res 23:1951–1954

59. Lissoni P, Barni S, Meregalli S et al (1995) Modulation of cancer endocrine therapy by melatonin: a phase II study of tamoxifen plus melatonin in metastatic breast cancer patients progressing under tamoxifen alone. Br J Cancer 71:854–856

60. Lissoni P, Cazzaniga M, Tancini G et al (1997) Reversal of clinical resistance to LHRH analogue in metastatic prostate cancer by the pineal hormone melatonin: efficacy of LHRH analogue plus melatonin in patients progressing on LHRH analogue alone. Eur Urol 31:178–181

61. Lissoni P, Barni S, Tancini G et al (1994) A randomised study with subcutaneous low-dose interleukin 2 alone vs interleukin 2 plus the pineal neurohormone melatonin in advanced solid neoplasms other than renal cancer and melanoma. Br J Cancer 69:196–199

62. Lissoni P, Barni S, Cazzaniga M et al (1994) Efficacy of the concomitant administration of the pineal hormone melatonin in cancer immunotherapy with low-dose IL-2 in patients with advanced solid tumors who had progressed on IL-2 alone. Oncology 51:344–347

63. Lissoni P, Barni S, Mandala M et al (1999) Decreased toxicity and increased efficacy of cancer chemotherapy using the pineal hormone melatonin in metastatic solid tumour patients with poor clinical status. Eur J Cancer 35:1688–1692

64. Lissoni P (2002) Is there a role for melatonin in supportive care? Support Care Cancer 10:110–116

65. Reiter RJ, Tan DX, Sainz RM et al (2002) Melatonin: reducing the toxicity and increasing the efficacy of drugs. J Pharm Pharmacol 54:1299–1321

66. Maestroni GJ (2000) Neurohormones and catecholamines as functional components of the bone marrow microenvironment. Ann N Y Acad Sci 917:29–37

67. Rodriguez C, Mayo JC, Sainz RM et al (2004) Regulation of antioxidant enzymes: a significant role for melatonin. J Pineal Res 36:1–9

68. Karasek M, Reiter RJ, Cardinali DP, Pawlikowski M (2002) Future of melatonin as a therapeutic agent. Neuro Endocrinol Lett 23(Suppl 1):118–121

69. Lissoni P, Mandala M, Rossini F et al (1999) Growth Factors: Thrombopoietic Property of the Pineal Hormone Melatonin. Hematology 4:335–343

70. Lissoni P, Bucovec R, Bonfanti A et al (2001) Thrombopoietic properties of 5-methoxytryptamine plus melatonin versus melatonin alone in the treatment of cancer-related thrombocytopenia. J Pineal Res 30:123–126

71. Steindl PE, Finn B, Bendok B et al (1995) Disruption of the diurnal rhythm of plasma melatonin in cirrhosis. Ann Intern Med 123:274–277

72. Reynolds FD, Dauchy R, Blask D et al (2003) The pineal gland hormone melatonin improves survival in a rat model of sepsis/shock induced by zymosan A. Surgery 134:474–479

73. Yerer MB, Aydogan S, Yapislar H et al (2003) Melatonin increases glutathione peroxidase activity and deformability of erythrocytes in septic rats. J Pineal Res 35:138–139

74. Mundigler G, Delle-Karth G, Koreny M et al (2002) Impaired circadian rhythm of melatonin secretion in sedated critically ill patients with severe sepsis. Crit Care Med 30:536–540

75. Wichmann MW, Haisken JM, Ayala A, Chaudry IH (1996) Melatonin administration following hemorrhagic shock decreases mortality from subsequent septic challenge. J Surg Res 65:109–114

76. Wurtman RJ, Larin F, Axelrod J et al (1968) Formation of melatonin and 5-hydroxyindole acetic acid from 14C-tryptophan by rat pineal glands in organ culture. Nature 217:953–954

77. Reiter RJ, Fraschini F (1969) Endocrine aspects of the mammalian pineal gland: a review. Neuroendocrinology 5:219–255

78. Axelrod J (1970) The pineal gland. Endeavour 29:144–148

79. Miller FP, Maickel RP (1970) Fluorometric determination of indole derivatives. Life Sci I 9:747–752

80. Ebels I, Balemans MG, Tommel DK (1972) Separation of pineal extracts on Sephadex G-10. 3. Isolation and comparison of extracted and synethetic melatonin. Anal Biochem 50:234–244

81. Koslow SH, Green AR (1973) Analysis of pineal and brain indole alkylamines by gas chromatography-mass spectrometry. Adv Biochem Psychopharmacol 7:33–43

82. Zurburg W, Ebels I (1975) Separation of pineal extracts by gelfiltration. II. Identification and isolation of two indoles from sheep pineal glands. J Neural Transm 36:59–69

83. Axelrod J (1974) The pineal gland: a neurochemical transducer. Science 184:1341–1348

84. Ebels I (1975) Pineal factors other than melatonin. Gen Comp Endocrinol 25:189–198

85. Ebels I, Horwitz-Bresser AE (1976) Separation of pineal extracts by gelfiltration. IV. Isolation, location and identification from sheep pineals of three indoles, identical with 5-hydroxytryptophol, 5-methoxytryptophol and melatonin. J Neural Transm 38:31–41

86. Reiter RJ, Vaughan MK (1977) Pineal antigonadotrophic substances: polypeptides and indoles. Life Sci 21:159–171

87. Pavel S (1978) Arginine vasotocin as a pineal hormone. J Neural Transm Suppl(13):135–155

88. Lissoni P, Fumagalli L, Paolorossi F et al (1997) Anticancer neuroimmunomodulation by pineal hormones other than melatonin:preliminary phase II study of the pineal indole 5-methoxytryptophol in association with low-dose IL-2 and melatonin. J Biol Regul Homeost Agents 11:119–122

89. Lissoni P (2000) Modulation of anticancer cytokines IL-2 and IL-12 by melatonin and the other pineal indoles 5-methoxytryptamine and 5-methoxytryptophol in the treatment of human neoplasms. Ann N Y Acad Sci 917:560–567

90. Lissoni P, Bucovec R, Bonfanti A et al (2001) Thrombopoietic properties of 5-methoxytryptamine plus melatonin versus melatonin alone in the treatment of cancer-related thrombocytopenia. J Pineal Res 30:123–126

91. Viviani S, Bidoli P, Spinazze S et al (1992) Normalization of the light/dark rhythm of melatonin after prolonged subcutaneous administration of interleukin-2 in advanced small cell lung cancer patients. J Pineal Res 12:114–117

92. Lissoni P, Mandala M, Brivio F (2000) Abrogation of the negative influence of opioids on IL-2 immunotherapy of renal cell cancer by melatonin. Eur Urol 38:115–118

93. Lissoni P, Malugani F, Malysheva O et al (2002) Neuroimmunotherapy of untreatable metastatic solid tumors with subcutaneous low-dose interleukin-2, melatonin and naltrexone: modulation of interleukin-2-induced antitumor immunity by blocking the opioid system. Neuro Endocrinol Lett 23:341–344

# Eating-Related Distress of Patients with Advanced, Incurable Cancer and of Their Partners

Florian Strasser

## Introduction

The mechanism of loss of weight (cachexia), appetite (anorexia), and strength (asthenia) of most patients with advanced, incurable cancer encompasses a complex combination of paraneo-plastic primary anorexia-cachexia syndromes (ACS). In addition, there are often secondary ACS due to other complications of advanced cancer, such as severe symptoms, disrupted function of the gastrointestinal tract, and reduced physical ability [1].

The complex [2], often contra-intuitive, multi-dimensional [3], and fluctuating mechanisms of ACS [4] may contribute to the distress [5]not only of patients but also their partners. Distress is not synonymous to the intensity of a certain symptom, but it may be described as the perceived impact of a health-related condition in the multidimensional context of a patient's life. The same symptom – its kind, intensity, and impact – may cause different forms of distress in different patients.

The palliation of distress becomes increasingly important in the palliative care context, which aims primarily at alleviating suffering caused by incurable illnesses rather than curing diseases [6]. Besides the traditional endpoints of nutritional interventions (such as body composition, body mass index, nutritional intake, physical function, eating-related symptoms, and survival), the assessment of eating-related distress is an emerging, additional endpoint of multidimensional nutritional intervention in the palliative care context. This chapter briefly reviews this new concept and discusses the implications on nutritional counselling.

## Nutrition in the Palliative Care Context

The goal of palliation is to alleviate the suffering of patients and their relatives that is caused by distressing symptoms and complications. Treatment is based on active assessments that take into account multidimensional (physical, psychological; emotional, social, spiritual; existential) aspects [6]. Palliative nutrition aims to primarily improve subjective well-being of patients and their relatives, rather than to improve weight or nutritional intake per se (for further discussion of this concept, see the chapter 'Palliative Management of Anorexia/Cachexia and Associated Symptoms' ).

## Symptom Assessment Close to the Patient's End-of-Life: Multidimensional Issues

Many symptoms related to nutrition can contribute to distress. Examples of such distressing symptoms include loss of appetite, chronic nausea, and taste alterations. However, these symptoms, when expressed by patients with advanced-stage cancer, may also have another meaning: the suffering associated with a progressive terminal disease. Multidimensional issues contribute to this form of suffering, including physical, psychological, emotional, social, spiritual, and existential issues. Patients may communicate this complex experience by a sensation of hurt or pain. Dame Cicely Saunders characterised this phenomenon as 'total pain' [7]. Patients may not directly articulate their suffering, but tend instead to use the 'open door' of pre-existing symptoms. This may cause an amplification (i.e. increased intensity of loss of appetite caused by suffering) [8] or masquerading (i.e. loss of appetite or fatigue stands for depressive symptoms or dyspnoea) [9] of symptoms. Since these and other symptom-specific phenomena complicate assessment of the patient's symptoms, attempts have been undertaken to identify risk factors for increased or altered symptom expression that result in refractory symptoms. For pain, the main risk factors include incident pain, neuropathic pain, psychosocial suffering, substance abuse, and impaired cognition [10]. A staging system for pain is currently in the multi-centre evaluation phase [11].

Eating-related symptoms may also carry a more multidimensional meaning, one that reflects the suffering. The concept of 'total anorexia' has not been defined, although attempts have been made to define 'total pain.' Likewise, a staging system for eating-related symptoms, in order to identify refractory eating-related symptoms, has not yet been developed.

Practically, assessments of eating-related symptoms in patients with progressive, terminal illness should take into account multidimensional issues. Examples of such distressing symptoms include loss of appetite, fatigue, weakness, early satiety (fullness), chronic nausea, taste alterations, and shortness of breath [12]. In addition, a wealth of other sensations and perceptions can contribute to distress: perceived change of body image, social withdraw from meals, feelings of guilt, helplessness and powerlessness to fulfil caloric requirements, 'terror' of the scales (patients feel terrorised by frequent weighing), perceived starving to death, uncertainty about healthy food, and tensions in relationship with partner(s). Finally, the consequences of malnutrition may contribute to distress, such as wound sores, infections, and shortness of breath.

## The Meaning of Eating in Terminally Ill Patients: Importance of Carers

In patients suffering from terminal disease, such as far-advanced and progressive cancer, the meaning of eating shifts as death becomes close. Gradual cessation of oral intake is part of the natural process of dying, and has been included as one

of the few key signs of diagnosing dying (in the Liverpool pathway) [13]. Assessing nutritional status in such patients concentrates increasingly on eating-related distress and on the distress of their carers. The research in this (difficult) field is still scarce, with few systematic research or focused review papers.

Mc Clement et al. observed three patterns of family interactions with patients and health-care providers around the issue of nutritional care in the Palliative Care Unit setting [14]. The authors used a qualitative systematic approach with repeated interviews until saturation. The first pattern was 'fighting back.' Family interactions were driven by expectations to reverse anorexia and cachexia, which were perceived as the cause, not as a consequence of the terminal illness. Substantial conflict between family members and health-care providers was reported. The second pattern, 'letting nature take its course,' was characterised by desire-driven care. Nutrition was understood not to stave off the inevitable and so family members found other ways to care ('being there,' 'simply be'). They appreciated the opportunities to say goodbye and to express feelings. In the third pattern, 'waffling,' family members were ambivalent, shifting between fighting back and letting nature take its course. This pattern was observed in family members with middle knowledge of the illness, and the other patterns in those with good (nature) and poor (fight) knowledge.

Meares et al. conducted semi-structured interviews with women primary caregivers of adult in-home hospice patients with terminal cancer [15]. This systematic qualitative study summarises as follows: 'Shift in thinking: "eating is best" to "not eating is best".' It reports seven elements related to gradual cessation of oral intake: (1) the meaning of food (cultural aspects, love, socialised role of food, social situations, dinner hour); (2) the caregiver as sustainer (knowledge of care-giving, difference of emotion and intellect, vigilance, balance of respect and concern in choice of action); (3) concurrent losses (lived experience enmeshed, carer's personal pain); (4) personal responses (patient eats to please family); (5) ceasing to be–starved to death; (6) being bereaved – the meaning now (meaning of cooking changed, patient remembered by using the old, shared cooking ware); (7) paradox (wavering pattern). This work did not specifically assess caregiver eating-distress, but provided insights regarding issues contributing to nutritional assessment in terminal care.

Pool and Froggatt conducted a literature review (no formal systematic methodology) that focused on anorexia and cachexia in patients with advanced cancer [16]. Anorexia seems to be a greater concern to carers than to patients. The preparation and serving food of is an expression of love and caring. Carers keep the belief that intake is necessary for survival, and retrospectively (bereaved) perceive anorexia as very distressing for the patient. Food plays a minimal role in comforting terminally ill patients, since they mainly do not suffer from hunger. This chapter discusses the importance of caregivers' eating-related distress in their coping with terminal illness.

Hughes and Neal focused their literature review (no formal systematic methodology) on the needs and wishes for food of patients with terminal illness and described nine food-related behaviours [17]. These included: (1) food-practice determinants: cultural, personal, social, situation, cash; (2) nourishment; (3) expression of friendship; (4) maintenance of interpersonal relationships; (5) to promote and maintain social status; (6) as a way to cope with stress and tension; (7) to influence the behaviour of others; (8) religious and creative expression; (9) 'channel theory': each household has a gatekeeper. The above-reported findings highlight the vast possible meanings of food and may guide sensible counselling.

An ongoing study by Strasser, Cerny and Kesselring explores elements of eating-related distress in patients with advanced cancer and cachexia, and in their relatives (those present > 50% during all meal times). It applies an inductive analytic approach with constant comparisons to analyse items appearing in ad verbatim transcripts of in-depth interviews (focus groups with couples, single patients, and widows). The preliminary findings reveal the wide-ranging distress patterns related to loss of appetite (disgust, taste changes, fluctuating, unpredictable), inability to eat (predictable but fear of starving), loss of weight (diffi-

cult to control, eating and weight not linked), insecurity about what is healthy (adaptation, learning), partnership (pressure, show caring by providing food), social contacts (practical limitations, changed normality), professionals (advice comes from other sources), and fighting a losing battle close to death. This (ongoing) study suggests: 1) observing the living space of patients and relatives; (2) provide team counselling for patients and relatives; (3) understand that eating-related distress is multidimensional, with relevant existential and social factors; (4) acknowledge that patients and relatives are innovative, with a limited role for professionals.

## Assessment Instruments for Eating-Related Distress

Assessment instruments for eating-related distress have not been established, but are under development, as discussed above [18].

Traditional instruments, such as the FAACT (Functional Assessment of Anorexia/Cachexia Therapy) for anorexia/cachexia, or widely used quality-of-life instruments, such as the EORTC-QlQ-c30, carry some items related to distress, but they were not specifically developed for the purpose of assessing distress. The FAACT [19], as an example, asks at least three distress-related questions: 'I am worried about my weight' (item 3), 'I am concerned how thin I look' (item 5), and 'my family or friends are pressuring me to eat' (item 8). In the general section of the FACT, there is a question regarding the impact of physical function on social contacts (item 3). In the EORTC-QlQ-c30, questions assessing interference with (physical) function (items 6, 7) or social contacts (items 26, 27) may depict issues related to cachexia and weakness, but not directly to eating. As a solitary symptom, only the impact of pain on daily life (item 19) is included in the EORTC-QLQ-C30, but there are no items related to the impact of eating. Only the presence and severity of eating-related symptoms (item 5, help in eating; item 13, loss of appetite; items 14, 15, nausea and vomiting; item 16, constipation) are assessed.

## Implications of Eating-Related Distress on Nutritional Counselling

The eating-related distress of patients with advanced, incurable cancer and of their partners seems to encompass multidimensional and individual issues potentially associated with different mechanism of anorexia/cachexia.

An improved definition of eating-related distress may increase the quality of palliative cancer care interventions focused on nutrition. In termi-

nal care, the cessation of oral intake needs to be respected, also as a sign of the autonomy and dignity of the patient. Likewise, the withdrawal of a pre-existing artificial nutrition requires careful communication, taking into account aspects of the meanings of food, understanding of the dying process, and issues of eating-related distress.

The importance of counselling and caring for relatives of the dying patients needs to be emphasised, fostering alternative ways to express love and compassion.

## References

1. Strasser F (2003) Pathophysiology of anorexia/cachexia syndrome. In: Doyle D, Hanks G, Cherny N et al (ed) Oxford textbook of palliative medicine, 3rd edn. Oxford University Press, Oxford, pp 520–533
2. Fearon KC, Barber MD, Moses AG (2001) The cancer cachexia syndrome. Surg Oncol Clin N Am 10:109–126
3. Robinson K, Bruera E (1995) The management of pain in patients with advanced cancer: the importance of multidimensional assessments. J Palliat Care 11:51–53
4. Strasser F, Bruera ED (2002) Update on anorexia / cachexia. Hematol Oncol Clin North Am 16:589–617
5. Holland JC (2001) Improving the human side of cancer care: psycho-oncology's contribution. Cancer J 7:458–471
6. Anonymous (2002) National cancer control programmes: policies and managerial guidelines, 2nd ed. World Health Organization, Geneva
7. Clark D (1999) 'Total pain,' disciplinary power and the body in the work of Cicely Saunders, 1958–1967. Soc Sci Med 49:727–736
8. Bruera E, Watanabe S (1994) New developments in the assessment of pain in cancer patients. Support Care Cancer 2:312–318
9. Cohen MZ, Williams L, Knight P et al (2004) Symptom masquerade: understanding the meaning of symptoms. Support Care Cancer 12:184–190
10. Bruera E, Schoeller T, Wenk R et al (1995) A prospective multi-center assessment of the Edmonton Staging System for cancer pain. J Pain Symptom Manage 10:348–355
11. Fainsinger RL, Nekolaichuk C, Lawlor P et al (2004) The Revised Edmonton Staging System for Cancer Pain, 3rd ed. EAPC Research Forum, Stresa (abs 27)
12. Okuyama T, Tanaka K, Akechi T et al (2001) Fatigue in ambulatory patients with advanced lung cancer: prevalence, correlated factors, and screening. J Pain Symptom Manage 22:554–564
13. Ellershaw J, Ward C (2003) Care of the dying patient: the last hours of life. Br Med J 326:30–34
14. McClement SE, Degner LF, Harlos MS (2003) Family beliefs regarding the nutritional care of a terminally ill relative: a qualitative study. J Palliat Med 6:737–748
15. Meares CJ (1997) Meaning of gradual cessation of oral intake in adult in-home hospice patients with terminal cancer as described by women primary caregivers. Oncol Nurs Forum 24:1751–1757
16. Poole K, Froggatt K (2002) Loss of weight and loss of appetite in advanced cancer: a problem for the patient, the carer, or the health professional? Palliat Med 16:499–506
17. Hughes N, Neal RD (2000) Adults terminal illness: their needs and wishes for food. J Adv Nurs 32:1101–1107
18. Strasser F, Dietrich L, Gisselbrecht D, Studerus E (2004) Development of an assessment instrument for eating-related distress of patients with cancer cachexia and their partners, 3rd ed. EAPC Research Forum, Stresa (abs 295)
19. Ribaudo JM, Cella D, Hahn EA et al (2000) Re-validation and shortening of the Functional Assessment of Anorexia/Cachexia Therapy (FAACT) questionnaire. Qual Life Res 9:1137–1146

# Challenges of Geriatric Oncology

Lodovico Balducci

## Introduction

The management of cancer in the older person is an increasingly common problem, as 60% of all neoplasms occur in individuals age 65 and older [1]. Aging is associated with a progressive decline in life-expectancy, functional reserve, and social resources, and an increased prevalence of comorbidity [2]. This process is highly individualised and poorly reflected in chronologic age. The diversity of the older population affects both clinical practice and clinical research, and underlies the main challenges of geriatric oncology. These include the formulation of individual treatment plans and of research protocols.

A classification of older individuals into groups of similar life-expectancy and functional reserve is key to the interpretation of the diversity of aging. The first section of this chapter illustrates current advances in geriatric assessment that may allow such classification. Thereafter, common precautions for the treatment of cancer in the elderly, and the most urgent questions to be tested in clinical trials are discussed.

## Clinical Assessment of the Older Cancer Patients

### Questions Related to the Clinical Assessment of the Older Person

Both in clinical practice and in clinical research, the answer to three basic questions determines whether an older person is a candidate for antineoplastic treatment:

- Is the patient going to die with cancer or of cancer?
- Is the patient going to live long enough to suffer the consequences of cancer?
- Is the patient able to tolerate the treatment?

Relevant questions also concern reversible barriers to treatment, including inadequate transportation, limited economic resources, and absence of a home caregiver able to react in the presence of emergencies, and additional risk factors, such as malnutrition, polypharmacy, memory disorders, depression, and poorly controlled comorbidity.

## The Comprehensive Geriatric Assessment

Originally, the answers to these questions were provided by a comprehensive geriatric assessment (CGA), including function, comorbidity, cognition, emotional, social and nutritional status, and medication review [2–3]. Prior to its adoption in geriatric oncology, in general geriatrics, the CGA reduced the risk of hospitalisation and of admission to adult living facilities [4] and may have improved the survival of older individuals [5–6]. In geriatric oncology, the CGA has unearthed a number of unsuspected conditions that might have interfered with the treatment of cancer in the majority of patients age 70 and older [7–9], has provided an estimate of life-expectancy and of treatment tolerance, and has allowed the institution of a common language in the description of older individuals [2, 10]. Ongoing clinical studies try to derive from the various elements of the CGA an individualised index predicting life-expectancy and risk of toxicity. Table 1 describes the basic elements of the geriatric assessment.

## New Forms of Geriatric Assessment

New forms of geriatric assessment that have emerged during the last 10 years include physical function and laboratory tests. A common example of the tests of physical function includes the 'timed

**Table 1.** Comprehensive Geriatric Assessment (CGA) and its implications

| | |
|---|---|
| *Functional status*<br>Activities of daily (ADL) and instrumental<br>activities of daily living (IADL) | Relation to life-expectancy, functional dependence<br>and tolerance of stress |
| *Comorbidity*<br>Number of comorbid conditions and comorbidity indices | Relation to life-expectancy and tolerance of stress |
| *Mental status*<br>Folstein mini-mental status | Relation to life-expectancy and dependence |
| *Emotional conditions*<br>Geriatric Depression Scale (GDS) | Relation to survival; may indicate motivation to<br>receive treatment |
| *Nutritional status*<br>Mini-nutritional assessment (MNA) | Reversible condition; possible relationship to survival |
| *Polypharmacy* | Risk of drug interactions |
| *Geriatric syndromes*<br>Delirium, dementia, depression, falls, incontinence,<br>spontaneous bone fractures<br>neglect and abuse, failure to thrive | Relationship to survival<br>Functional dependence |

get up and go test' [3]. A person is asked to get up from an armchair, walk 10 feet, return, and sit down again. A score of 1 is assigned to each one of these three findings; use of the arms for getting up, uncertain gait, and requiring more than 10 s to complete the full activity. The higher the sum of the scores, the higher is the risk of mortality and functional dependence. Other tests with prognostic value include handgrip and strength of the lower extremities.

Laboratory tests that measured increased circulating levels of interleukin (IL)-6 and D-dimer were found to predict an increased risk of functional dependence and mortality during the following 2 years in a population of home-dwelling persons age 70 and older [11]. While controversy lingers related to which cytokine best reflects aging, current studies involving older individuals should include at least an assessment of circulating levels of IL-6.

### The Cardiovascular Health Study and the First Clinical Classification of Older Individuals

The first classification of older individuals into groups of different risks of mortality, hospitalisa-

tion, functional dependence, and disability was validated in the Cardiovascular Health Study (CHS) [12] on the basis of five simple assessments (Table 2). More than 5000 individuals age 65 and older were followed for several years to study the risk factors of cardiovascular diseases in the elderly. At the time of enrollment, all subjects underwent a complex geriatric assessment that included the tests described in Table 2. After 3 and 7 years, it was clear that three groups of patients of different mortality and risk of functional dependence, hospitalisation, and disability could be recognised: those without abnormal tests (fit); those who had one or two abnormal parameters (pre-frail), and those with three or more abnormal parameters (frail). At a recent consensus conference on frailty, it was agreed to embrace this classification as a frame of reference for future studies in older individuals. It appears reasonable that this user-friendly cost-effective assessment be adopted both in clinical practice and clinical research involving older individuals with cancer.

While the CHS classification represents a major step toward a common language, several of its limitations should be addressed:

**Table 2.** Assessment of older individuals in the Cardiovascular Health Study (CHS)

| Assessment | Tests |
| --- | --- |
| Involuntary weight loss | ≥ 10 lbs during the previous year |
| Grip strength | By hand dynamometer: decreased grip strength is considered a value within the lowest quintile for persons of the same body mass index (BMI), age and gender |
| Slow walk | Time necessary to walk 15 feet; slow walk is considered a time within the highest quintile for persons of the same gender and height |
| Self-reported exhaustion | Score of the answer to the following questions:<br>- I feel without energy<br>- I cannot get going<br>How often have you felt this way in the last 2 weeks:<br>0 = 1 day or less<br>1 = 2–3 days<br>2 = 3–4 days<br>3 = most of the times<br>A score of 2 or 3 denotes self-reported exhaustion |
| Low energy levels | Present if a person has not performed any of the following activities during the past 2 weeks: walking, mowing the lawn, raking, gardening, hiking, jogging, biking, exercise cycling, dancing, aerobics, bowling, golf, single and double tennis, racquetball, callisthenics, swimming |

- The definition of frailty involves a wide array of functional status, from fully independent to fully dependent. This wide scope limits use of the CHS in clinical practice. Previous studies have demonstrated that dependence in activities of daily living (ADLs) and instrumental activities of daily living (IADLs), as well as comorbidity scores and geriatric syndromes are predictive of mortality and of chemotherapy-related toxicity [13–14]. In clinical decisions, these parameters should be maintained to identify patients for whom symptom management only is preferred. A subclassification of frailty into subgroups of different life-expectancy and functional reserve is an urgent research project (Fig. 1).

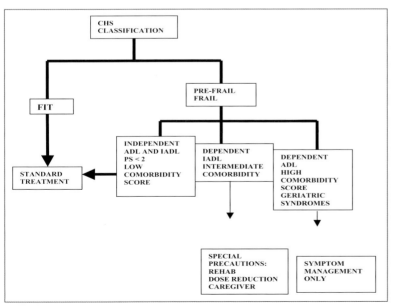

**Fig. 1.** Algorithm for the evaluation of the elderly person prior to chemotherapy

- The CHS did not address the reversibility of frailty and pre-frailty, an extremely important issue that should be examined in future studies.
- The CHS classification does not address the influence of comorbidity, malnutrition, and socio-economic situations on the management of older cancer patients.

In conclusion, the CHS assessment represents a minimal common denominator that should be integrated with other measures, according to clinical circumstances; in particular, the diagnosis of frailty and pre-frailty should be seen as a red flag for a more in-depth assessment.

## Clinical Parameters of Special Interest in the Older Cancer Patients

Among the comorbid conditions, anaemia and depression occupy a special place, as they are often reversible, easy to detect, and are associated with increased morbidity and mortality [15–17]. In light of recent studies demonstrating that haemoglobin levels < 13 gm/dl are an independent risk factor for death in women age 65 and older [15–16], it appears reasonable to consider haemoglobin levels < 13 gm/dl as indicative of anaemia in men and in women. In addition to reticulocyte count, a basic work-up should include iron, iron-binding capacity, ferritin, soluble transferrin, B12, folate levels, and creatinine clearance [15, 16]. In addition to being a risk factor for death, anaemia is a risk factor for functional dependence, cardio-vascular diseases, complications of cytotoxic chemotherapy, and possibly dementia [15].

Of the socio-economic conditions, the availability of a home caregiver is paramount [2]. A home caregiver able to respond to an emergency by providing transportation and care is recommended for all older individuals and definitely for those who are not 'fit.'

With the advent of effective cancer treatment, capable to produce prolonged remissions and even cure, it has become very important to assess the quality of long-term cancer survivorship. Antineoplastic treatment, especially cytotoxic chemotherapy, may cause long-term disability and chronic morbidity, more often in older than in younger individuals. In addition to health-related quality of life, quality of survivorship may be reflected in function, comorbidity, cognitive integrity, emotional health, and general feeling of well-being. Fatigue, the most common long-term complication of cancer chemotherapy, may represent the main threat to the well-being of older cancer survivors [18–19].

## The Estimate of Life-Expectancy

Short-term life-expectancy determines the institution of life-prolonging treatment, long-term life-expectancy that of curative treatment. Simple and reliable ways to calculate mortality risk, from which life-expectancy may be derived, were described by Walter et al. [20–21]. One-year mortality risk may be estimated from a number of parameters (Table 3), such as gender, function, comorbidity, renal function, and nutrition. A score is assigned to each parameter, and the risk of mortality is calculated from the sum of the scores. For long-term mortality, life-tables may be used. The risk of mortality for each age cohort is divided into quartiles, and the geriatric assessment allows the assignment of patients to the appropriate quartile.

**Table 3.** Estimate of 1 year mortality

A. Scoring system

| Risk factor | Odd ratio | p value | Score |
|---|---|---|---|
| Male | 1.4 (1.1–1.8) | 0.01 | 1 |
| ADL: 1–4 | 2.1 (1.6–2.8) | < 0.0001 | 2 |
| All | 5.7 (4.2–7.7) | < 0.0001 | 5 |
| Comorbidity: | | | |
| CHF | 2.0 (1.5–2.5) | < 0.001 | 2 |
| Solitary cancer | 2.6 (0.17–3.9) | < 0.001 | 3 |
| Metastatic cancer | 13.4 (6.2–39) | < 0.001 | 8 |
| Creatinine > 3.0 | 1.7 (1.2–2.5) | 0.01 | 2 |
| Albumin 3.0–3.4 | 1.7 (1.2–2.3) | 0.001 | 1 |
| < 3 | 2.1 (1.4–3.0) | < 0.001 | 1 |

B. Mortality risk according to the sum of scores

| Score | Mortality risk (%) |
|---|---|
| 0–1 | < 5 |
| 2–3 | 15 |
| 4–5 | 30–40 |
| 6+ | 60–70 |

## The Future of Geriatric Assessment

New insights in the biology of aging may suggest more reliable evaluation instruments. So far, the assessment of aging has been fragmented and limited to individual domains. The time may have come for a more global vision of aging. According to the most recent construct, aging involves a loss of entropy and of fractality, in addition to and as a consequence of the decline in functional reserve of multiple organ systems [22]. Loss of entropy means loss of ability to produce energy in excess, loss of fractality means loss of rapid coordination between different activities. Gait disturbance, in the presence of normal muscular strength as well as normal cerebellar and posterior column function, is perhaps the most typical manifestation of the loss of fractality. These losses act in concert to produce a progressive loss in the capacity of adaptation that eventually becomes incompatible with independent life and ultimately with life itself. Some simple measures of entropy have been proposed. If validated in the clinical arena, this measurements may provide a global estimate of aging and of its reversibility.

## Age and Tumour Biology

Aging may be associated with changes in tumour biology [2]. In at least five conditions (Table 4), the behaviour of the tumour and the prognosis of cancer change with the age of the patient [2]. Two observations related to Table 4 are in order. First, contrary to a common assumption that cancer in older patients is generally more benign, cancer may become more aggressive and more difficult to control with age. Second, at least two mechanisms may be involved in the pathogenesis of these changes. If cancer is considered to be a plant, the growth of the plant depends on the seed (the tumour cell) and the soil (the tumour host). Information related to the seed, such as the expression of the multidrug resistance gene (MDR-1) in leukaemic myeloblasts, or the concentration of hormone receptors and Her2/neu on breast cancer cells are useful prognostic indicators that may determine the management of cancer in individual cases. Further insight into the biology of the seed may be gained by studying the genome of the neoplastic cell by microarray techniques. Unfortunately, there are currently no useful clini-

**Table 4.** Neoplasms whose biology changes with age

| Neoplasm | Biology change | Mechanism |
|---|---|---|
| Acute myelogenous leukaemia (AML) | Increased prevalence of disease resistant to chemotherapy | Seed: increased prevalence of multi-drug resistance expression in myeloblasts |
| Non-Hodgkin's lymphoma | Decreased duration of remission following chemotherapy | Soil: increased concentration of IL-6 in the blood of older individuals Seed: possibly |
| Breast cancer | More indolent disease | Seed: increased prevalence of hormone-receptor-rich well-differentiated tumours Soil: endocrine senescence and immune senescence |
| Ovarian cancer | Decreased response rate to chemotherapy, duration of remission and survival | Unknown |
| Lung cancer | Presentation at earlier stages in older individuals | Possible seed: as lunge cancer develops preferentially in older ex-smokers, it is reasonable to expect a more indolent disease |

cal parameters to assess the influence of the host on tumour growth. Tumour–host interactions thus appear to be an area of important future investigations in geriatric oncology.

## Treatment-Related Considerations

Anti-neoplastic treatment may be local or systemic: local treatment involves surgery and radiation therapy, while systemic treatment consists of hormonal therapy, cytotoxic chemotherapy, biological therapy, and targeted therapy.

### Cancer Surgery and Aging

Although the risk of surgical complications seems to increase with the age of the patient, elective surgery appears reasonably safe at least up to age 80. The only possible exception to this statement involves total pneumonectomy, which is poorly tolerated by patients age 70 and older [23–24]. Not surprisingly, the main risk of age-related surgical complications is seen with emergency surgery, especially of the gastrointestinal tract for obstruction of the large bowel. The risk of septic death may be two- to three-fold higher for patients age 70 and older than for the younger ones. This finding emphasises the need for regular screening for colorectal cancer, as early detection may avoid emergency surgery in the majority of cases [2].

New developments in anaesthesia and in surgical techniques have rendered surgery safer for all individuals, including the oldest old [2].

### Radiation Therapy

Several large studies have demonstrated that the majority of patients age 70 and older, and even those over 80 may complete a full course of external beam irradiation without undue toxicity [25–27]. Special caution appears necessary in irradiating the chest and the pelvis, as the risk of mucositis may increase with the age of the patient; likewise, malnutrition should be prevented by identifying patients at increased nutritional risk and by assuring adequate gastrointestinal access when oesophageal obstruction or severe dysphagia

are predictable. Brachytherapy, which spares normal tissues to a large extent, may be even safer than external beam irradiation for older individuals, although three-dimensional simulation has minimised the complications even of this form of treatment.

It is not yet clear whether new radiation techniques, such as hyper-fractionation or combined chemo-radiation treatment, are as safe in individuals 70 and over as in younger ones.

### Cytotoxic Chemotherapy

Aging is associated with changes in the pharmacokinetics and pharmacodynamics of drugs, and with increased vulnerability of normal tissues to the complications of this form of treatment [28] (Table 5).

While intestinal absorption declines with age, this change does not seem to affect the bioavailability of oral drugs, at least in individuals up to age 80. This finding is important in view of the recent development of a number of oral cytotoxic agents, which may be particularly convenient for older individuals due to home administration and flexible and titratable doses. The volume of distribution of water-soluble drugs declines with age, due to a reduction in total body water and in serum albumin. The AUC of drugs may not

**Table 5.** Effects of age on the pharmacology of cytotoxic chemotherapy

A.  Pharmacokinetics
     Reduced absorption
     Reduced volume of distribution ($V_d$)
     Reduced renal excretion
     Reduced hepatic metabolism

B.  Pharmacodynamics
     Reduced rate of DNA repair
     Reduced rate of intracellular drug metabolism

C.  Increased vulnerability of normal tissues
     Myelotoxicity
     Mucositis
     Cardiotoxicity
     Peripheral and central neutoroxicity

change, but the peak concentration of these agents is increased and the risk of toxicity enhanced as a results of volume of distribution ($V_d$) alterations. The effects of $V_d$ changes may be ameliorated by correction of anaemia, when this is present. Several studies have shown that anaemia is an independent risk factor for chemotherapy-induced myelodepression [28], as many agents bind to red blood cells; consequently, anaemia is associated with increased concentration of circulating free drug. A decline in the glomerular filtration rate (GFR) is almost universal with aging, and may lead to an increased half-life of cytotoxic compounds, such as carboplatin, methotrexate, and bleomycin, whose parent compounds are excreted through the kidneys, and drugs that give origin to active or toxic metabolites excreted from the kidneys. For example, 80% of the activities of idarubicin and daunorubicin are metabolised in the liver and excreted from the biliary tract, but is due to renally excreted alcohols. Likewise, cytarabine in high doses gives origin to Ara-uridine, a metabolite that is toxic to the cerebellum and is eliminated by the kidney. Not surprisingly, the risk of cerebellar complications increases in the presence of renal insufficiency. It should be highlighted that in individuals age 60 and older the GFR may be reduced despite normal concentrations of serum creatinine, because lean body mass may decline with age. Marx recently compared different ways to calculate GFR on the basis of gender, age, and serum creatinine [29]. Compared with the gold standard of radioactive EDTA excretion, the Cockroft-Gault formula, which is commonly used, underestimated the GFR when it was below 50 ml/min [29]. It appears prudent to adjust the first dose of chemotherapy to renal function as determined according to this formula, with the provision that in the absence of toxicity subsequent doses should be increased to prevent the risk of under-treatment. Hepatic mass, hepatic circulation, and the activity of P450 reactions decline with age, and it is not clear how these parameters change the pharmacology of antineoplastic agents in older individuals. A number of studies failed to show age-related prolongation of the half life of drugs eliminated with the bile.

The repair of cisplatin-induced DNA adducts in circulating monocytes is delayed in people age 70 and older, indicating that the capacity of DNA repair declines with age, which may increase the toxicity of cytotoxic agents in older individuals [28]. Although the concentration and activity of drug metabolising enzymes may decline with aging, this possibility was never conclusively demonstrated.

The risk and severity of myelotoxicity, especially of neutropaenia, increases with age [28–30]. In three major cooperative groups, the ECOG, the SWOG, and the International Breast Cancer Study Group, age 65 and older was a risk factor for neutropaenia. Likewise, a review of the management in private practices in the USA of large-cell lymphoma with CHOP or CHOP-like combinations of chemotherapy indicated that the incidence of neutropaenia and neutropaenic infections almost doubled in individuals age 65 and older. Of serious concern is also the fact that hospitalisation for neutropaenic infections was longer for older individuals, suggesting that neutropaenia is more severe, more costly, more debilitating, and possibly more lethal in elderly patients. Fortunately, at least five randomised and controlled studies demonstrated that filgrastim reduced by 30–50% the risk of neutropaenia and neutropaenic infection, even in patients age 65 and older (Table 6). An alternative strategy to prevent chemotherapy-related toxicity, a reduction of the doses of cytotoxic agents, is not advisable, at least in the case of potentially curable neoplasms, such as large-cell lymphoma, breast cancer, and colorectal cancer, in the adjuvant setting. In these conditions, dose reduction has uniformly resulted in poorer survival and higher recurrence rates.

The risk of dysphagia and diarrhoea, especially from fluorinated pyrimidines, increases with age, and in a few cases it has been lethal. At present, there are no antidotes to this complication, but a number of provisions may reduce the risk and the severity of it. These include substitution of capecitabine for intravenous fluorouracil or fluorouridine, and early hospitalisation and fluid replacement prior to the development of dehydration. Capecitabine is a pro-drug of fluorouracil and is activated preferentially in neoplastic tissues, thus minimising the exposure of normal tissues to

**Table 6.** Effectiveness of filgrastim in the elderly

| Author | Number of patients | Patients with neutropaenia (%) | Patients with neutropaenic infection (%) |
|---|---|---|---|
| Zinzani et al. [31] | 350 | | |
| G-CSF | | 23 | 5 |
| No GCSF | | 56 | 21 |
| Zagonel et al. [32] | 126 | | |
| G-CSF | | 4.8 | 4.8 |
| No G-CSF | | 27.7 | 15.6 |
| Bertini [33] | 90 | | |
| G-CSF | | 22 | 2 |
| No G-CSF | | 44 | 9.5 |
| Osby  et al. [34] | 455 | | |
| G-CSF | | 62 | 31 |
| No G-CSF | | 92 | 47 |
| Doorduijn et al. [35] | 411 | | |
| G-CSF | | 20 | 20 |
| No G-CSF | | 32 | 32 |

*G-CSF*, granulocyte colony-stimulating factor

the active compounds. A number of antidotes to mucositis are currently undergoing investigation, including keratinocyte growth factor and an oral preparation of lysine.

While the risk of anthracycline-related cardiotoxicity increases with age, this complication is rare and no special provisions are recommended for its prevention. Administration of doxorubicin by continuous infusion has lessened the risk of cardiomyopathy, but is cumbersome and expensive, while prophylactic administration of dexrazoxane is associated with increased risk of mucositis and myelotoxicity, and might even protect the tumour. Liposomal anthracyclines appear promising for minimising the toxicity of these compounds, including cardiotoxicity, but experience with these drugs is limited so far.

No antidotes are available for peripheral neurotoxicity, beside substitution of neurotoxic agents with less toxic compounds of equivalent activity, such as carboplatin in lieu of cisplatin or taxotere in lieu of taxol. In older individuals, peripheral neurotoxicity may be disabling.

Cognitive disorders are among the most devastating geriatric syndromes. The concern that cognition may be affected by cytotoxic chemotherapy has emerged from a number of studies showing cognitive

compromise in peri-menopausal women with breast cancer who received adjuvant treatment. At least in part, this finding might have been a consequence of chemotherapy-precipitated menopause. In any case, the study of the cognitive effects of chemotherapy, and their potential reversal is a major priority in the management of older cancer patients.

Of special interest to the management of older cancer patients has been the development of new drugs with low toxicity risk. These include capecitabine, vinorelbine, taxanes in low doses, gemcitabine, and liposomal anthracyclines. These agents may provide effective palliation of symptoms even in patients who are frail, functionally dependent, and with significant comorbidity.

## Hormonal Therapy

Hormonal treatment is used for the management of breast, prostatic, and endometrial cancer. In the case of breast cancer, the main advances include the introduction of aromatase inhibitors and of the estrogen antagonist faslodex. All aromatase inhibitors appear to be superior to tamoxifen, both in the treatment of metastatic disease and in the adjuvant setting. When compared to tamoxifen, these agents are not associated with endometrial cancer, and have reduced risk of deep-vein and arterial thrombosis, hot flashes, and vaginal secretion. Of concern is the observation that the nonsteroidal aromatase inhibitors letrozole and anastrazol seem to enhance the risk of osteoporosis and bone fractures. The long-term effects of these compounds on cognition and serum lipids are unknown and cause some concerns, especially for women with long life-expectancy. Also, in the case of faslodex, the risk of endometrial cancer and thrombosis is significantly reduced compared to tamoxifen; while its effects on bones, lipids, and cognition are unknown. Faslodex is active in approximately 20% of patients whose cancer progressed whilst receiving tamoxifen. The role of this agent in the adjuvant setting has not been clarified.

In the case of prostate cancer, the only recent advance has been the approval of abarelix, an LH-RH antagonist for the management of life-threatening metastatic disease, including impending urinary obstruction or spinal cord compression. The main advantage of this compound over LH-RH analogs is the prevention of the initial testosterone spate and the risk of tumour progression.

### Biological Treatment

In addition to interferon (IFN)-α and IL-2 at high doses, whose use in older individuals is limited, angiogenesis inhibitors have emerged as forms of cancer treatment. Thalidomide, in combination with decadron appears to be a safer and more effective combination than melphalan and prednisone in the initial management of multiple myeloma. A major advantage of thalidomide in this setting has been the sparing of haematopoietic stem cells, which are destroyed by melphalan, thus allowing the possibility of high-dose chemotherapy and stem-cell rescue.

### Targeted Therapy

New insights in tumour biology have allowed target-specific metabolic processes that are essential to tumour survival. Targeted therapy includes naked and tagged monoclonal antibodies, and small molecules inhibiting key enzymes, such as tyrosine phosphokinase (TPK), farnesyl transferase, and histone deacetylase. Targeted therapy spares normal tissues, and is very promising for older individuals. Currently, rituximab and trastuzumab, alone or in combination with cytotoxic chemotherapy, have been proven effective and safe in the therapy of B-cell lymphoma and breast cancer, respectively. Likewise, the TPK inhibitor imanitib has improved the prognosis of patients with chronic myelogenous leukaemia while ameliorating at the same time the toxicity of standard treatment. Other promising compounds include radiotagged monoclonal antibodies in the management of refractory low-grade lymphoma.

### Conclusions

The main challenges of geriatric oncology include:

- Assessment of the older person able to predict life-expectancy, short- and long-term tolerance of treatment. A comprehensive geriatric assessment, including function, comorbidity, cognition, nutrition, pharmacy, and social support, is still the standard approach. Novel approaches, including the use of CHS classification, and of laboratory markers of aging promise to be more time- and cost-effective and should be included in future studies. Investigators should realise that this is an evolving field, influenced both by new insight into the biology of aging and by the medical and cultural environment.
- The study of long-term survivors represents a priority, as this outcome is no longer unusual, even for older individuals. Assessments of special interest include functional independence, cognition, emotional health, and overall quality of life.
- The influence of aging in the biology of cancer is almost uncharted ground. More insight into this field is essential for deciding which cancers represent a threat to a person's survival and function.
- The development of antidotes to myelotoxicity and of safer drugs has allowed more effective treatment of cancer in older individuals. The prevention of mucositis remains an important priority.
- The integration of new forms of treatment with more standard cytotoxic chemotherapy is one of the major new challenges of oncology, including geriatric oncology.

# References

1. Yancik R, Ries LA (2000) Aging and cancer in America. Demographic and epidemiologic perspectives. Hematol Oncol Clin N America 14:17–23
2. Balducci L, Extermann M (2004) A practical approach to the older cancer patient. Curr Probl Cancer 25:6–76
3. Balducci L, Extermann M (2003) The assessment of the older cancer patient. In: Overcash J, Balducci L (eds) The older cancer Patient. Springer medical Publisher, New York
4. Cohen HJ, Feussner JR, Weinberger M et al (2002) A controlled trial of inpatient and outpatient geriatric evaluation and management. N Engl J Med 346:905–912
5. Bernabei R, Gambassi G, Carbonin P (2002) A controlled trial of geriatric evaluation. N Engl J Med 347:371–373
6. Extermann M (2003) Comprehensive geriatric Assessment basics for the cancer professional. J Oncol Manag 12:13–17
7. Repetto L, Fratino L, Audisio RA et al (2002) Comprehensive geriatric assessment adds information to the Eastern Cooperative group performance status in elderly cancer patients. An Italian group for geriatric oncology study. J Clin Oncol 20:494–502
8. Ingram SS, Seo PH, Martell RE et al (2002) Comprehensive assessment of the elderly cancer patient: the feasibility of self-report methodology. J Clin Oncol 20:770–775
9. Extermann M, Overcash J, Lyman GH et al (1998) Comorbidity and functional status are independent in older cancer patients. J Clin Oncol 16:1582–1587
10. Balducci L, Yates J (2006) Guidelines for the management of older patients with cancer. Oncology, NCCN Proceedings, November, pp 221–227
11. Cohen HJ, Harris T, Pieper CF (2003) Coagulation and activation of inflammatory pathways in the development of functional decline and mortality in the elderly. Am J Med 114:180–187
12. Fried LP, Tangen CM, Walston J et al (2001) Frailty in older adults: evidence for a phenotype. J gerontol med Sci 56A:M146–M156
13. Extermann M, Chan H, Cantor AB et al (2002) Predictors of tolerance to chemotherapy in older cancer patients: a prospective pilot study. Eur J canceer 38:1466–1473
14. Chen H, Cantor A, Meyer J et al (2003) Can older cancer patients tolerate chemotherapy? A prospective pilot study. Cancer 97:1107–1114
15. Balducci L (2003) Anemia, cancer and aging. Cancer Control JHLMCC 10:478–486
16. Knight K, Wade S, Balducci L (2004) Prevalence and outcomes of anemia in cancer: a systematic review of the literature. Am J Med 116 Suppl 7A:11s–26s
17. Blazer DG, Hybels CF, Pieper CF (2001) The association of depression and mortality in elderly persons: a case for multiple independent pathways. J gerontol Med Sci 56A:M505–M509
18. Garman KS, Pieper Cf, Seo P et al (2003) Function in elderly cancer survivors depends on comorbidity. J gerontol Med Sci 58:M1119–M1124
19. Hewitt M, Rowland JH, Yancik R (2003) Cancer survivors in the United States: age health and disability. J Gerontol Med Sci 58:82–91
20. Walter LC, Brand RJ, Counsell SR et al (2001) Development and validation of a prognostic index for 1-year mortality in older adults after hospitalization. JAMA 285:2750–2756
21. Walter LC, Covinsky KE (2001) Cancer Screening in elderly patients, JAMA 285:2750–2756
22. Lipsitz LA (2004) Physiolocical complexity, aging and the path to frailty. Sci Aging Knowledge Environ (16) PE16
23. Wingo PA, Guest JL, McGinnis L et al (2000) Patterns of inpatient surgeries for the top four cancers in the United States. Cancer Causes Control 11:497–512
24. Fabri P (2005) Cancer surgery in the elderly. In: Balducci L, Lyman GH, Ershler WB (eds) Comprehensive geriatric oncology, 2nd ed. Taylor & Francis, New York, pp 399–405
25. Olmi P, Ausili Cefaro GP, Balzi M et al (1997) Radiotherapy in the aged. Clin Ger Med 13:143–168
26. Scalliet P, Pignon T (1998) Radiotherapy in the elderly. In: Balducci L, Lyman GH, Ershler WB (ed) Comprehensive geriatric oncology, Harwood Academic Publishers, Amsterdam, pp 421–428
27. Zachariah B, Balducci L (2000) Radiation therapy of the older patient. Hematol Oncol Clin N America 14:131–167
28. Cova D, Balducci L (2005) Cancer chemotherapy in the older patient. In: Balducci L, Lyman GH, Ershler WB (eds), Comprehensive geriatric oncology, 2nd ed. Taylor & Francis, New York, pp 463–488
29. Marx GM, Blake GM, Galani E et al (2004) Evaluation of the Cockroft-Gault Jelliffe and Wright formulae in estimating renal function in elderly cancer patients. Ann Oncol 15:291–295
30. Balducci L, Repetto L (2004) Increased risk of myelotoxicity in elderly patients with non-Hodgkin's Lymphoma. Cancer 100:6–11
31. Zinzani PL, Storti S, Zaccaria A et al (1999) Elderly aggressive-histology non-Hodgkin's lymphoma: first-line VNCOP-B regimen experience on 350 patients. Blood 94:33–38
32. Zagonel V, Babare R, Merola MC et al (1994) Cost-benefit of granulocyte colony-stimulating factor administration in older patients with non-Hodgkin's lymphoma treated with combination chemotherapy. Ann Oncol 5(Suppl 2):127–132
33. Bertini M (1993) Therapeutic strategies in intermediate grade lymphomas in elderly patients. The Italian Multiregional non Hodgkin's Lymphoma Study Group (IMRNHLSG). Hematol Oncol 11(Suppl 1):52–58
34. Osby E, Hagberg H, Kvaloy S et al; Nordic Lymphoma Group (2003) CHOP is superior to CNOP in elderly patients with aggressive lymphoma while outcome is unaffected by filgrastim treatment: results of a Nordic Lymphoma Group randomized trial. Blood 101:3840–3848
35. Doorduijn JK, van der Holt B, van Imhoff GW et al (2003) CHOP compared with CHOP plus granulocyte colony-stimulating factor in elderly patients with aggressive non-Hodgkin's lymphoma. J Clin Oncol 21:3041–3050

# SECTION 10
# TREATMENT OF CANCER CACHEXIA

# The Current Management of Cancer Cachexia

Giovanni Mantovani

## Mechanisms of Cancer-Related Anorexia/Cachexia

The anorexia/cachexia syndrome is one of the most common causes of death among patients with cancer and is present in 80% at death [1]. The term 'cachexia' derives from the Greek *kakòs*, which means 'bad', and *hexis*, meaning 'condition'. The characteristic clinical picture of anorexia, tissue wasting, loss of body weight accompanied by a decrease in muscle mass and adipose tissue, and poor performance status that often precedes death has been named cancer-related anorexia/cachexia (CAC) [2–5]. Since the 1980s, the previous concepts explaining CAC were replaced by a more complex insight, which stresses the interaction between metabolically active molecules produced by the tumour itself and the host immune response. One of the main features of the cachectic syndrome is anorexia, which may be so significant that spontaneous nutrition is totally inhibited. The pathogenesis of anorexia is most certainly multifactorial but not yet well understood. It seems to be attributable, in part, to intermediary metabolites (e.g. lactate, ketones, oligonucleotides) that accumulate along an abnormal metabolic pathway, or other substances released by the tumour itself or by normal cells in response to the tumour [3]. However, anorexia cannot by itself account for the complex organic alterations seen in CAC. Indeed, nutritional supplementation alone cannot effectively reverse the process of cachexia. An increased resting energy expenditure may contribute to body weight loss in patients with cancer and may explain the increased oxidation of fat tissue. Futile energy-consuming cycles, such as the Cori cycle, may contribute to this increased energy demand. Unlike starvation, body weight loss in patients with cancer arises equally from loss of muscle and fat, characterised by increased catabolism of skeletal muscle and decreased protein synthesis [6]. Catabolic factors capable of direct breakdown of muscle and adipose tissue appear to be secreted by cachexia-inducing tumours and may play an active role in the process of tissue degeneration [6].

## Metabolic Abnormalities

In addition to reduced food intake, important abnormalities in carbohydrate, protein and lipid biochemistry and metabolism and changes in energy metabolism have been observed, which may account for CAC.

The most important carbohydrate abnormalities are insulin resistance, increased glucose synthesis, gluconeogenesis and Cori cycle activity, and decreased glucose tolerance and turnover. The main pathological changes of protein metabolism include increased protein turnover, muscle catabolism, and liver and tumour protein synthesis, while muscle protein synthesis is decreased. The main abnormalities found in lipid metabolism are enhanced lipid mobilisation, decreased lipogenesis, decreased lipoprotein lipase activity, elevated triglycerides and decreased high-density lipoproteins, increased venous glycerol, and decreased glycerol clearance from the plasma [5, 7, 8].

## Proinflammatory Cytokines

Cancer-related anorexia/cachexia may result from circulating factors produced by the tumour, or by the host immune system in response to the tumour, such as cytokines released by lymphocytes and/or monocyte/macrophages.

A number of proinflammatory cytokines, including interleukin (IL)-1, IL-6, tumour necrosis factor-$\alpha$ (TNF-$\alpha$), interferon (IFN)-$\alpha$ and IFN$\gamma$, have been implicated in the pathogenesis of cachexia associated with human cancer. TNF-$\alpha$ was first identified by Rouzer and Cerami [9] as a specific circulating mediator of the wasting resulting from a chronic experimental infectious disease and named cachectin, which was subsequently found to be identical to TNF-$\alpha$. However, data from numerous clinical and laboratory studies suggest that the action of cytokines, although important, may not alone explain the complex mechanism of CAC [10–13].

IL-1 and TNF-$\alpha$ have been proposed as mediators of the host's response to inflammation [14]. Human IL-1 and TNF-$\alpha$ administered to healthy animals produced significant reduction in their food intake [15]. High serum levels of TNF-$\alpha$, IL-2 and IFN$\gamma$ have been found in patients or experimental animals with cancer [16], and although IL-6 levels appear to correlate with tumour progression in animal models [16], evidence has been provided to support a role for IL-6 as a cachectic factor in the development of cancer cachexia in an animal model system [17]. Chronically elevated levels of these factors, either alone or in combination, are capable of reproducing the different features of CAC [17–20].

More direct evidence of a cytokine involvement in CAC is provided by the observations that cachexia in experimental animal models [12, 21, 22] can be relieved by administration of specific cytokine antagonists. These studies revealed that cachexia can rarely be attributed to any one cytokine but rather is associated with a set of cytokines that work in concert. These cytokines seem to play central roles in both cachexia-related inflammation and the acute-phase response [23].

Additional factors and mechanisms thought to play a central role in CAC are the presence of a chronic systemic inflammatory state, circulating tumour-derived lipolytic and proteolytic factors, increased futile energy-consuming cycles, such as the Cori cycle, and a decreased food intake.

## Circulating Tumour-Derived Catabolic Factors

In addition to chronic proinflammatory factors, circulating factors, such as lipid-mobilising factors (LMF), and proteolysis-inducing factor (PIF) may play a role in the development of CAC. These are tumour-derived catabolic factors acting directly on adipose tissue and skeletal muscle, without affecting food intake [24–28].

## Systemic Inflammation

There is evidence that a chronic, low-grade, tumour-induced activation of the host immune system that shares numerous characteristics with the 'acute-phase response' found after major traumatic events and septic shock is involved in CAC. Septic shock is a situation characterised by an increased production of cytokines [29, 30], high levels of catecholamines, cortisol and glucagon [29, 31–33], increased peripheral amino acid mobilisation and hepatic amino acid uptake [29, 34], increased hepatic gluconeogenesis and acute-phase protein production [29, 35, 36], enhanced mobilisation of free fatty acids [37] and increased metabolism [38]. The acute-phase response is a systemic reaction to tissue injury, typically observed during inflammation, infection or trauma, characterised by the release of a series of hepatocyte-derived plasma proteins known as acute-phase reactants, including C-reactive protein, fibrinogen, complement factors B and C3, and by reduced synthesis of albumin and transferrin. An acute-phase response is observed in patients with cancer. In fact, the cytokines IL-1, IL-6 and TNF-$\alpha$ are regarded as the major mediators of acute-phase protein induction in the liver. Unfortunately, the role played by acute-phase proteins during cancer growth is still poorly understood.

## Decreased Food Intake

Malnutrition may be considered one hallmark of cancer cachexia and it is associated with anorexia, that is, loss of appetite and/or decreased food intake. Appetite is a complex function resulting from the contribution of peripheral and central nervous afferents in the ventral hypothalamus. Stimulation of the medial hypothalamic nucleus inhibits feeding, while stimulation of the lateral nucleus promotes food intake. Among peripheral afferents, oral stimulation by pleasant tastes elicits eating, whereas gastric distention inhibits it.

There is evidence that proinflammatory cytokines such as IL-1, IL-6 and TNF-α are involved in cancer-related anorexia and decreased food intake, but these cytokines do not seem to be the only mediators of CAC.

Since multiple factors are involved in the control of food intake, it is possible that there are also many factors contributing to the tumour-associated anorexia. Indeed, anorexigenic compounds are either released by the tumour into the circulation or the tumour itself may induce metabolic changes resulting in the release of such substances by host tissues. Changes in tryptophan levels in patients with cancer result in increased brain serotonin synthesis and, thus, serotonergic activity, which leads to reduced food intake. Other factors could be involved in promoting the inhibitory afferents to the hypothalamus by stimulating serotonergic and catecholaminergic fibres, such as increased lactate and fatty acid blood levels, both of which are associated with tumour burden. Few controlled clinical trials have investigated the incidence of cancer-related reduction of food intake: this fact may be because of the methodological difficulties associated with human diet analysis and the need for large patient and control groups.

### Role of Leptin and Neuropeptides

Loss of body weight is a strong stimulus to food intake in humans. Therefore, the presence of CAC in patients with cancer suggests a failure of the adaptive feeding response. A large amount of evidence has been provided in the last few years on the regulation of feeding and body weight. Leptin, a recently found hormone produced by the adipocyte ob gene, has been shown to be an essential component of the homeostatic regulation of body weight. Leptin acts to control food intake and energy expenditure via a neuropeptidergic effect or molecules within the hypothalamus. Complex interactions take place among the nervous, endocrine and immune systems inducing behavioural and metabolic responses [38–44].

Proinflammatory cytokines, proposed as mediators of CAC, may have a central role in long-term inhibition of feeding by mimicking the hypothalamic effect of excessive negative feedback signalling from leptin. This could be via continuous stimulation of anorexigenic neuropeptides such as serotonin- and corticotropin-releasing factor, as well as by inhibition of the neuropeptide Y orexigenic network consisting of opioid peptides and galanin, and the recently identified melanin-concentrating hormone, orexin and agouti-related peptide. Such abnormalities in the hypothalamic neuropeptide loop in tumour-bearing animals lead to the development of CAC.

Although the present therapeutic use of neuropeptide agonists/antagonists is obesity treatment, this area could also be an effective target for the treatment of CAC, particularly in combination with other agents with different mechanisms of action [45, 46].

A study by our group [47] demonstrated very low leptin levels associated with high levels of inflammatory cytokines in patients with advanced-stage cancer, several of whom had a significant body weight loss.

## Treatment of CAC

It is outside the scope of this chapter to review the current standard clinical management of patients with CAC. However, clinicians should consider the need to address the patient as a whole before planning a comprehensive treatment plan for CAC, including enteral and/or parenteral nutrition and pharmacological treatment, that is the use of orexigenic (appetite stimulants), anticatabolic (and anticytokine) and anabolic agents [48]. The management of CAC is challenging. This section examines therapies and drugs used in patients with CAC, distinguishing between those that are unproven, which are briefly mentioned, and those that have been proven to be effective or that are currently under investigation, which are discussed in greater detail.

### Unproven or Ineffective Treatments

It was hoped that enteral or parenteral nutritional support would circumvent cancer anorexia cachexia and alleviate malnutrition. However, the inability of hypercaloric feeding to increase lean mass, especially skeletal muscle mass, has been repeatedly demonstrated [49].

Dietary counselling, positioning of a fine-bore nasogastric tube and percutaneous gastrostomy (i.e. enteral nutrition), and total parenteral nutrition (TPN) are the possible options to counteract CAC by increasing food intake. However, none of these has proven to be effective.

Dietary counselling was reported to have no effect [6]. Nasogastric tube feeding showed a body weight increase in some studies [50] and a decrease in whole body protein breakdown in other studies [51]; however, the drawback to enteral tube feeding is the distress to the patients, especially in cases of long-term treatment [52].

Various systematic prospective studies that have evaluated the potential benefit of TPN have generally been disappointing [52–55]. Therefore, its use is not recommended in unselected patients, especially in view of the fact that TPN may itself have significant complications. However, it may be worthwhile further evaluating TPN in carefully defined settings, possibly in conjunction with other modalities such as synthetic progestagens or anabolic steroids [56]. Indeed, parenteral nutrition may facilitate administration of complete chemoradiation doses for oesophageal cancer [53] and may have beneficial effects in certain patients with decreased food intake because of mechanical obstruction of the gastrointestinal tract [57, 58]. Home parenteral nutrition can also be rewarding for such patients. Enteral nutrition has the advantages of maintaining the gut-mucosal barrier and immunological function, as well as having low adverse side-effects and low cost [57–59].

The effects of caloric intake on tumour development and growth are still being debated [60]. A clear benefit from nutritional support may thus be limited to a specific, small subset of patients with severe malnutrition who may require surgery or may have an obstructing, but potentially therapy-responsive tumour [1, 57, 61].

## Cyproheptadine

Based on the evidence that CAC is associated with increased serotonergic activity in the brain [62],

serotonergic blockade may be beneficial in reducing symptoms. One potentially interesting drug is cyproheptadine, a histamine antagonist with antiserotonergic properties and an appetite-stimulating effect. However, in a placebo-controlled clinical trial, cyproheptadine only induced a slight improvement of appetite without significant effect on body weight [63]. Its clinical use is not recommended, especially in view of its sedating effects. No other serotonin antagonists have been investigated in this patient population to date.

## Hydrazine

Hydrazine inhibits hepatic gluconeogenesis in rats by inhibiting the enzyme phosphoenolpyruvatecarboxykinase [64]. However, three large, randomised, placebo-controlled trials have failed to observe any beneficial effect on appetite or body weight in patients with cancer [65–67].

## Metoclopramide

Metoclopramide has been the most extensively used drug in patients with cancer for the prevention and treatment of chemotherapy-induced emesis and has yielded significant results [68]. As many patients with cancer have symptoms of delayed gastric emptying and gastroparesis that might increase the incidence of early satiety and negatively influence food intake [69–71], this prokinetic agent has been extensively studied in these patients. A recent randomised controlled trial reported that controlled-release metoclopramide every 12 hours was significantly more effective than immediate-release metoclopramide every 6 hours [72]. At present, the effectiveness of other prokinetic agents such as cisapride and domperidone needs to be demonstrated in randomised, controlled clinical trials.

## Cannabinoids (Dronabinol)

The active ingredient of marihuana, dronabinol ($\Delta$-9-tetrahydrocannabinol, THC) is known to have a positive effect on appetite, body weight and chemotherapy-induced nausea [73].

Dronabinol was first used as an antiemetic in patients with cancer; however, it was reported to have significant neurological and adverse effects including dizziness, euphoria and impairment of cognitive functions. Currently there is only one controlled trial comparing dronabinol vs megestrol acetate vs combination therapy in patients with CAC. This trial showed that oral megestrol acetate 800 mg/day provided superior anorexia palliation compared with oral dronabinol 2.5 mg twice daily, while combination therapy did not appear to confer additional benefit [74].

In the past, two open studies [75, 76] demonstrated some improvement in mood and appetite with no significant change in body weight. In the first study by Wadleigh et al. [75], with dronabinol in patients with advanced cancer, a subjective improvement in mood and appetite was observed at the higher dose studied, but all patients had a progressive body weight loss. In the second study, Nelson et al. [76] observed improved appetite and increased food intake using dronabinol 7.5 mg/day but the effect on body weight was not reported. A randomised controlled trial in patients with AIDS showed similar results [77]. Moreover, the significant adverse effects of this drug need to be taken into account. These include somnolence, mental confusion and cognitive status disturbances [77], which may worsen the mental status of patients with CAC, who are often receiving opioids and other psychoactive drugs.

## Drugs Commonly Used

### Progestagens

Progestagens were the first agents used and are the current first-line agents used in patients with CAC for which there is a track record of clinical research. An extensive amount of literature is available in patients with cancer, with the use of both megestrol and medroxyprogesterone.

Both drugs are synthetic progestagens that were first used to treat hormone-sensitive tumours [78, 79]. As a result of the observed body weight gain and appetite stimulation, independent of tumour response, in a number of patients receiving such therapy, several trials in the last two decades have addressed the use of progestagens for the management of CAC. The proposed mechanism of action of progestagens in CAC has not been completely elucidated. It may be related to glucocorticoid activity making these drugs similar to corticosteroids. Moreover, there is evidence that progestagens may stimulate appetite via neuropeptide Y in the central nervous system (ventromedial hypothalamus) [80]. Furthermore, they act, at least in part, by down-regulating the synthesis and release of proinflammatory cytokines, as shown by several experimental and clinical studies, including two of our studies [81, 82]. We have also previously published an overview of this topic [83].

In the first study [81], the effect of megestrol in patients with CAC was evaluated to determine its ability to increase appetite and body weight in patients with head and neck cancer with advanced-stage (III–IV) disease, treated with cisplatin-based neoadjuvant chemotherapy. Eleven male patients (mean age 57.8 years; range 43–69 years; Karnofsky performance status 90–100; body weight decrease > 10% of the ideal or customary body weight) were enrolled in the study. Ten patients were treated with megestrol during neoadjuvant chemotherapy and one was treated with megestrol during definitive locoregional radiation therapy administered at the end of primary chemotherapy. Clinical parameters evaluated before and after megestrol treatment included clinical response to chemotherapy after three cycles, body weight, appetite (using a visual analogue scale calibrated from 0 to 10), Karnofsky performance status, and quality of life (Spitzer's Quality-of-Life Index [QLI]). Serum levels as well as in vitro production of IL-1–$\alpha$ and $\beta$, IL-2, IL-6, TNF-$\alpha$ and sIL-2R were determined in patients before and after megestrol treatment and were compared with those of healthy individuals. Megestrol (160 mg tablets) was administered at a dosage of 320 mg/day during the interval between chemotherapy cycles, starting from the third day after the end of the cycle until the day before the next cycle (days 8–21) for a total of three consecutive cycles. During the cycles the dosage of megestrol ranged from 160 to 320 mg/day, based on clinical response. Of the 11 enrolled patients, nine (81.8%) were evaluable; two patients were not evaluable because of major protocol violations (drug intake was < 90% of that scheduled). Except for performance status, all parameters showed an improvement following treatment with megestrol. In particular, increases were observed in average body weight (6.3 kg or 13.2%), appetite (by a score of 2.4 or 38.6%), and Spitzer's QLI (by a score of 2.4 or 36.2%). The serum levels of cytokines studied were significantly higher in patients before megestrol treatment than in healthy individuals. Serum levels of all cytokines, as well as IL-6 production in vitro, decreased in patients after megestrol treatment. Our results strongly supported the hypothesis that the beneficial therapeutic effects of megestrol in patients with CAC may be due in part to its ability to down-regulate the synthesis and release of key cytokines involved in CAC.

The second study [82] addressed the question of whether the other synthetic progestagen more commonly used, medroxyprogesterone, at doses that are pharmacologically active in vitro (0.1, 0.2 and 0.4 mg/l), was able to influence the in vitro production and/or release of cytokines and serotonin (5-hydroxytryptamine) in patients with advanced-stage cancer. Ten patients with advanced-stage cancer at different sites were included in the study, which showed that the in vitro production of IL-1, IL-6, TNF-$\alpha$ and serotonin in these patients was significantly reduced in the presence of medroxyprogesterone. The concentration of medroxyprogesterone used in this study was within the range of plasma values seen in patients receiving oral medroxyprogesterone 1500/2000 mg/day. As shown in Table 1, megestrol has been the drug most widely studied for its effect on CAC, with eight randomised, double-blind, placebo-controlled trials [83–94], compared with medroxyprogesterone (two placebo-controlled studies) [95, 96].

Megestrol has shown a dose-related effect on appetite, body weight gain and subjective sensation of well-being with oral dosages ranging from 160 to 1,600 mg/day, with an optimal dosage of 480–800 mg/day. However, because a dosage of 160 mg/day has demonstrated a significant effect, the possible dose-related adverse effects of megestrol and the increased costs of higher dosages, we recommend, in agreement with Gagnon and Bruera

[48] and on the basis of our experience, starting treatment at a low dosage (160 mg/day) and regulating the dose upwards according to clinical response.

Some patients may require up to 320 mg/day and a very few will respond only to 480 mg/day.

Medroxyprogesterone was used at dosages ranging from 300 mg/day to 4000 mg/day. The placebo-controlled study of Simons et al. [96] used oral medroxyprogesterone 1000 mg/day and reported a significant improvement of appetite and body weight. We currently recommend a medroxyprogesterone dosage of 1000 mg/day orally (equivalent to megestrol 160 mg/day). Most published studies using megestrol or medroxyprogesterone in patients with CAC have used tablets rather than the oral suspension formulation. However, oncologists are increasingly using megestrol or medroxyprogesterone oral suspensions in their patients with malignancies because of improved compliance and decreased cost [97].

Both megestrol and medroxyprogesterone may induce adverse effects. These are an increased risk of thromboembolic events, peripheral oedema, breakthrough bleeding, hyperglycaemia, hypertension and Cushing's syndrome [98–100]. However, it is very rare that patients taking megestrol or medroxyprogesterone have to stop the drug because of adverse effects [84, 85, 87, 101].

As the bioavailability of megestrol acetate directly affects its efficacy and safety, the formulation was refined to enhance its pharmacokinetics. Such efforts yielded megestrol acetate in a tablet form, followed by a concentrated oral suspension form, and, very recently, an oral suspension form developed using nanocrystal technology. Nanocrystal technology was designed specifically to optimise drug delivery and enhance the bioavailability of drugs with poor water solubility. Megestrol acetate nanocrystal oral suspension has been approved by the US FDA for the treatment of cachexia in patients with AIDS; clinical trials in patients with cancer cachexia will be carried out very soon. Preclinical pharmacokinetic data suggest that the new megestrol acetate formulation has the potential to shorten significantly the time to clinical response and thus may improve outcomes in patients with anorexia-cachexia [102].

**Table 1.** Summary of randomised, prospective, placebo-controlled trials of progestagens in patients with cancer-related anorexia/cachexia

| Dosage | Duration of treatment | Study Design | No. of patients | Results | Adverse Effects | Reference Author |
|---|---|---|---|---|---|---|
| **Megestrol** | | | | | | |
| 480 mg/day | 1 wk | pc, co | 40 | Improved appetite, caloric intake, energy level, bodyweight, tricep skinfold and calf circumference. | Mild oedema, nausea (similar to placebo) | Bruera E, et al. 1990 |
| 800 mg/day | 1.6 mo | pc | 133 | Improved appetite, food intake, bodyweight; less nausea, less emesis compared with placebo | Oedema and thrombo-embolic events | Loprinzi CL, et al. 1990 |
| 1600 mg/day | 1 mo | pc | 89 | Increased appetite, food intake, greater change in prealbumin; no change in athropometrics except bodyweight; nutrition impact symptoms improved *vs* no change or worsening in placebo; no differences in QoL, positive response with crossover design | Oedema, DVT | Tchekmedyian NS, et al. 1992 |
| 240 mg/dy | 2 mo | pc | 150 | Bodyweight gain, increased appetite score, fewer patients with decreased performance status compared with lacebo | Oedema, DVT (no different from Placebo) | Feliu J, et al. 1992 |
| 160, 480 mg/day | 12 wk | pc | 240 | Improved appetite, mood and overall QoL at both doses; possibly less nausea, emesis compared with placebo; sustained improved QoL; increase in prealbumin | None reported | Beller E, et al. 1997 |
| 480 mg/day | 8 wk | pc | 55 | Sample too small for significant results | None reported | Schmoll E, et al. 1991 |
| 160 mg/day | 6 wk | pc | 64 | Maintained bodyweight and nutritional parameters during chemo/radiotherapy compared with parameters deterioration in placebo; QoL maintained with megestrol | None reported | Fietkau R, et al. 1997 |
| 160, 480, 800, 1280 mg/day | 66 days | rc | 342 | Improved appetite, food intake and bodyweight, decreased nausea | None reported | Loprinzi CL, et al. 1993 |
| 480 mg/day | 10 days | pc, co | 83 | Improved activity, appetite and well-being. No increase of bodyweight | None reported | Bruera E, et al. 1996 |
| 480 mg/day | 12 wk | pc | 38 | No Increase of bodyweight | None reported | McMillan DC, et al. 1994 |
| 160, 320 mg/day | 1 mo | rc | 122 | Increased appetite | None reported | Gebbia V, et al. 1996 |
| **Medrossiprogesterone** | | | | | | |
| 300 mg/day | 6 wk | pc | 60 | Increased appetite, serum retinol binding protein and serum thyroid binding prealbumin | None reported | Downer S, et al. 1993 |
| 500 mg/day | 12 wk | pc | 206 | Beneficial effect on appetite at 6 and 12 wk; bodyweight gain with medroxyprogesterone vs loss on placebo; no other measurable changes in QoL | None reported | Simons JPFHA, et al. 1996 |

*co*, crossover; *DVT*, deep vein thrombosis; *pc*, placebo-controlled; *QoL*, Quality of Life; *rc*, randomise, controlled (no placebo)

## Corticosteroids

Although several randomised, placebo-controlled studies (shown in Table 2) demonstrated that corticosteroids, including dexamethasone, prednisolone and methylprednisolone, induce a usually temporary (limited to a few weeks) effect on symptoms such as appetite, food intake, sensation of well-being and performance status, none of these studies showed a beneficial effect on body weight. [103–107].

In addition, corticosteroids have an antiemetic activity [108] and are able to reduce asthenia [103] and to control pain [109]. Their mechanism of action in CAC is not well understood, although the inhibition of prostaglandin (PG) activity [110] and the suppression of IL-1 [111, 112] and TNF [113] production are the most well-recognised targets. In view of the wide range of well-known adverse effects and cautions to be advised with these agents, they should be used in patients in the end-stage phase of cancer with short expected survival, with the attempt to improve quality of life without affecting body weight.

The type, dosage and route of administration of corticosteroids are not established, although low dosages, less than 1 mg/kg of prednisone equivalent, are recommended in clinical practice.

## Anticytokine Approaches to CAC Treatment

Proinflammatory cytokines such as IL-1, IL-6, and particularly, TNF-α have a prominent role in the pathogenesis of CAC. The specific neutralisation of these factors with antibodies in animal models of cachexia suggests that an anticytokine approach is worth pursuing, while taking into account that no single cytokine is responsible for all abnormalities found in CAC. However, in chronic human diseases such as cancer, the long-term administration of anticytokine antibodies could be of no practical use. Pentoxifylline and thalidomide are two agents with anticytokine activity currently being investigated as therapy for CAC.

## Anti-IL-6 Monoclonal Antibody

Currently, although the therapeutic impact on CAC of anti-IL-6 monoclonal antibody (mAb) therapy could be of clinical benefit in cancer patients, no published clinical trial using this approach is yet available [114].

## Anti-TNF-α mAb

On the basis of experimental data on the ability of anti-TNF-α mAb to neutralise the in vitro and in vivo biological effect on TNF-α [115] and animal studies carried out by Torelli et al. [116], a phase II multicentre, randomised, double-blind, placebo-controlled study evaluating the efficacy and safety of anti-TNF-α mAb to treat CAC in 90 patients with pancreatic cancer was carried out and completed in February 2006: the results are not yet known.

**Table 2.** Placebo-controlled trials of corticosteroids in cancer-related anorexia/cachexia [38]

| Drug | Dosage (mg) | Route | No. of patients | Significant symptoms outcomes | Effects on bodyweight | Reference |
|------|-------------|-------|-----------------|-------------------------------|-----------------------|-----------|
| Dexamethasone | 0.75 or 1.5 qid | PO | 116 | ↑ Appetite | Ni | [95] |
| Prednisolone[a] | 5 tid | PO | 61 | ↑ Appetite | Ni | [96] |
| Methylprednisolone[a] | 16 bid | PO | 40 | ↑ Pain Control ↑ Appetite, food intake and performance status | Nil Not measured | [97] |
| Methylprednisolone | 125 od | IV | 403 | ↑ Quality of life | Ni | [98] |
| Methylprednisolone | 125 od | IV | 173 | ↑ Quality of life | Ni | [99] |

[a] Crossover design
*bid*, twice daily; *IV*, intravenous; *od*, once daily; *PO*, oral; *qid*, 4 times daily; *tid*, 3 times daily; ↑, increase.

## Pentoxifylline

Pentoxifylline is a methylxantine derivative approved for the treatment of intermittent claudication, which was subsequently found to have anti-inflammatory and immune-modulating effects mediated by the inhibition of phosphodiesterase. It has been shown to inhibit TNF-α production in humans in response to experimentally administered endotoxin [117]. Recent preliminary investigations in patients with cancer have suggested a potential role for pentoxifylline. Intravenous administration of pentoxifylline in 14 patients with cancer who had high serum TNF-α levels significantly reduced the serum levels of this cytokine [118]. However, a recent double-blind, placebo-controlled trial of pentoxifylline therapy in patients with CAC did not show a beneficial effect on appetite or body weight [119].

## Thalidomide

Thalidomide was first clinically introduced as a sedative drug and in the 1960s it was withdrawn from use because of its established teratogenic effect. Thalidomide has complex immunomodulatory and anti-inflammatory properties. It has been shown to down-regulate the production of TNF-α and other proinflammatory cytokines, inhibit the transcription factor nuclear factor kB, down-regulate cyclo-oxygenase-2 and inhibit angiogenesis. In a recent randomised, placebo-controlled trial, thalidomide was found to be well tolerated and effective at attenuating loss of weight and lean body mass in 33 patients with cachexia due to advanced pancreatic cancer [120]. Randomised clinical trials with thalidomide in patients with CAC are awaited. That the mild sedative effect of thalidomide may make it difficult to mask the drug in placebo-controlled trials needs to be taken into account [48].

## Emerging Drugs

### Non-steroidal Anti-Inflammatory Drugs

Non-steroidal anti-inflammatory drugs (NSAIDs) are very widely used in patients with cancer for the treatment of fever and pain. They act by inhibiting PG production by the rate-limiting enzymes known as cyclo-oxygenases (COX). Because traditional NSAIDs inhibit both COX-1 and COX-2, these drugs induce adverse effects such as gastrointestinal injury up to ulceration, reduced appetite and consequent reduced body weight: indeed, these drugs may be considered a potential cause of anorexia in patients with cancer.

On the other hand, ibuprofen, an inhibitor of the enzyme COX-1, was found to decrease C-reactive protein [121], produce body weight gain [122] and improve survival in patients with cancer [123].

The administration of indomethacin (50 mg twice daily) to a heterogeneous group of advanced cancer patients in a randomised controlled study has been shown to be associated with a long improvement in survival [123].

To date, no other studies on the beneficial effects of NSAIDs in human CAC are available, although placebo-controlled trials with these drugs may be justified.

### COX-2 Selective Inhibitors (Celecoxib, Rofecoxib and Valdecoxib)

COX-2 is a bifunctional enzyme possessing both cyclo-oxygenase and peroxidase activities. Selective COX-2 inhibitors inhibit PG biosynthesis (anti-COX-2 activity) but do not, or only partially, affect the peroxidase activity of COX, which can generate proximate carcinogens. In experimental animals, selective inhibitors of COX-2 such as celecoxib reduce the formation of head and neck, colorectal, stomach, lung, breast and prostate tumours. In addition to preventing tumorigenesis, selective COX-2 inhibitors suppress the growth of established tumours. A selective COX-2 inhibitor was also observed to decrease the number and size of metastases. In most studies, selective COX-2 inhibitors decrease the rate of tumour growth rather than cause a reduction in tumour size [124–126]. Therefore, significant preclinical evidence strongly supports the potential role for these inhibitors for the treatment of cancer.

Currently, the COX-2 inhibitors are being studied in clinical trials to confirm their role in the prevention of cancer, particularly colon cancer [127], and in combination with chemotherapy and radia-

---

tion therapy to prove their effectiveness in cervical cancer, lung cancer and brain tumours [128].

Notwithstanding their potential interest also in the treatment of cancer cachexia, some questions have arisen on the clinical use of these agents because of their toxicity and particularly cardiovascular risks. For this reason, rofecoxib has been withdrawn by the manufacturer. Another drug in this class, valdecoxib, has shown an increased risk for cardiovascular events in patients after heart surgery. As regards celecoxib, in December 2004 the National Cancer Institute stopped celecoxib (Celebrex) administration in an ongoing clinical trial investigating a new use of the drug to prevent colon polyps because of an increased risk of cardiovascular events in patients taking Celebrex versus those taking a placebo. Patients in the clinical trial taking 400 mg of Celebrex twice daily had a 3.4 times greater risk of cardiovascular events compared to placebo. For patients in the trial taking 200 mg of Celebrex twice daily, the risk was 2.5 times greater. The average duration of treatment in the trial was 33 months. A similar ongoing study comparing Celebrex 400 mg once a day versus placebo, in patients followed for a similar period of time, has not shown increased risk. Based on the currently available data, the FDA has concluded in April 2005 that an increased risk of serious adverse cardiovascular events appears to be a class effect of non-steroidal anti-inflammatory drugs (NSAIDs; excluding aspirin). The FDA has requested that the package insert for all NSAIDs, including Celebrex, be revised to include a boxed warning to highlight the potential increased risk of cardiovascular events and the well-described risk of serious, and potentially life-threatening, gastrointestinal bleeding. The FDA has also requested that the package insert for all NSAIDs be revised to include a contraindication for use in patients immediately after coronary artery bypass (CABG) surgery. Consequently, the inclusion of celecoxib in clinical trials should be discouraged.

### Melatonin

In a recent controlled trial in 100 patients with metastatic cancer, melatonin was shown to reduce significantly body weight loss [129]. Melatonin may act by decreasing circulating levels of TNF [130].

### n-3 Fatty Acids

The supplementation of n-3 polyunsaturated fatty acids has been shown to inhibit IL-1 and TNF-α production through a blockade of the COX and lipo-oxygenase pathways.

Eicosapentaenoic acid (EPA) is the main component of this family and is found in large quantities in fish oil: at doses of 2–6 g daily it has been shown to lower the production of proinflammatory cytokines in healthy volunteers [131]. EPA is also able to down-regulate the acute-phase protein response [132, 133]. Its activity appears to be mediated by a blockade of the effects of proteolysis-inducing factor and lipid-mobilising factor [134]. In a study in patients with colorectal cancer, long-term treatment with EPA, docosahexaenoic acid (DHA) and α-linolenic acid induced a significant decrease in serum IL-1, IL-6, TNF-α and IFNα levels [135]. Two recent studies by Wigmore et al. [136, 137] reported the effects of n-3 fatty acid treatment in patients with pancreatic cancer who were losing weight. In the first study [136], oral supplementation with fish oil capsules (12 tablets per day, 18% EPA, 12% DHA) for 3 months led to a significant median body weight gain of 0.3 kg/month compared to a previous body weight loss of 2.9 kg/month. A significant reduction in acute-phase protein production was also observed. In the second study [137], 4 weeks of treatment with EPA reduced the C-reactive protein through the suppression of IL-6 production.

EPA has been shown to impair the growth of tumour cell lines in vitro and slow down the growth of experimental tumours in animal models [138, 139]. EPA has been found to stabilise weight in cachectic tumour-bearing mice independently of any anti-tumour effect [144]. In uncontrolled clinical trials with EPA or fish oil, a weight stabilisation was observed in weight-losing pancreatic cancer patients [136, 141].

Fearon et al. compared a protein- and energy-dense supplement enriched with n-3 fatty acids and antioxidants with an isocaloric isonitrogenous control supplement for their effects on weight, lean body mass (LBM), dietary intake, and quality of life in 200 cachectic patients with advanced pancreatic cancer. Intention-to-treat group comparisons indicated that, at the mean dose taken (1.4 cans/day), enrichment with n-3 fatty acids did not provide a therapeutic advantage and that both supplements were equally effective in arresting weight loss. Post hoc dose-response analysis suggests that, if taken in sufficient quantity (> 1.5 cans/day), only the n-3 fatty acid-enriched energy- and protein-dense supplement results in net gain of weight, lean tissue, and improved quality of life [142].

A clinical trial using an EPA supplement vs megestrol acetate vs both in 421 patients with cancer-associated wasting was carried out by the North Central Cancer Treatment Group and the National Cancer Institute in Canada and failed to demonstrate an improvement of weight or appetite with EPA supplement [143].

Recently, a phase III, double-blind, randomised comparator study was carried out as a multicentre multinational study to assess the benefit of a protein- and energy-dense supplement enriched with n-3 fatty acids and antioxidants versus standard nutritional product in 240 patients with stage IV non-small-cell lung cancer. The primary end-point was preservation of LBM. The patient accrual ended at the beginning of 2005 and the results are not yet known.

Further trials are required to examine the potential role of n-3-enriched supplements in the treatment of CAC.

## β2 Agonists

Clenbuterol is the most studied of the β2-adrenergic agonists. Treatment of tumour-bearing animals with salbutamol, salmeterol and clenbuterol had a positive effect on skeletal muscle mass, without influencing tumour growth or food intake [144].

One controlled trial reported that clenbuterol was able to improve muscle strength after orthopaedic surgery. These drugs, which are able to prevent or reverse muscle loss in sedentary people, such as patients with cancer, are potentially interesting and should be studied in clinical controlled trials. Clenbuterol could be used clinically in the treatment of patients with CAC.

In summary, the anabolic properties of β2-agonists are well established with the therapeutically relevant effects observed in animal models of cachexia. In addition, enhanced sensitivity to β2-agonists

in cachectic subjects may suggest that β2-agonists can be of importance in the treatment of CAC.

## Anabolic Agents

Anabolic agents have the potential to improve body composition by maintaining or improving lean body mass. These agents include growth hormone (GH), insulin-like growth factor (IGF)-1, testosterone, dihydrotestosterone and testosterone analogues.

## Growth Hormone and Insulin-Like Growth Factor

Strong positive effects on nitrogen balance and protein mass have been demonstrated with GH in different clinical situations [145]. Most of its anabolic effects on protein synthesis are mediated by IGF-1, produced by the liver [146]. In a study in 10 patients with cancer, GH administered for 3 days increased plasma IGF-1 levels and decreased urinary nitrogen losses; however, an improvement of nitrogen balance was observed only in patients not overtly cachectic [147]. The effects of IGF-1 in patients with CAC have not been studied to date.

## Anabolic Androgens

Anabolic androgens are synthetic derivatives of testosterone with more anabolic effect and less androgenic activity than testosterone itself. Although in other wasting diseases the anabolic steroids have shown a beneficial effect on body weight muscle mass and performance status, very few studies have been carried out to date in patients with cancer. In a randomised, prospective study in weight-losing patients with lung cancer, chemotherapy with or without nandrolone decanoate 200 mg weekly for 1 month was compared and no significant difference was observed in body weight loss between the study arms [148].

## Branched-Chain Amino Acids

The anabolic properties of branched-chain amino acids (BCAAs), and in particular of leucine, have been known for many years, but only recently have their molecular mechanisms been elucidated.

Consistent experimental and clinical data indicate that BCAAs, and particularly leucine and its metabolite b-hydroxy-b-methylbutyrate, are highly effective in preventing CAC by enhancing protein metabolism and promoting appetite and food intake [149].

## Specific Anticancer Treatments

Specific anticancer treatments may be employed in patients with advanced disease for palliation. Indeed, for instance, oral fluoropyrimidine tegafur/uracil prolonged survival and improved cancer cachexia in a colon-26-bearing murine cachexia model by decreasing the plasma levels of both IL-6 and tumour PGE2. These findings suggest that tegafur/uracil, at a low-toxic dose, could be useful in patients with CAC and poor performance status [150].

## Assessment of the Quality of Life

It is important that all the interventions used in patients with CAC, i.e. nutritional, pharmacological, supportive care, are not evaluated merely in terms of objective medical (i.e. physical) parameters, such as body weight gain, increased food intake, etc., and that the assessment of any therapy also takes into account the self-assessed patient evaluation of treatment outcome, that is quality of life (QoL). There are no published QoL questionnaires devoted to evaluating specific symptoms present in patients with CAC. Different QoL questionnaires have been used in the different studies addressing this issue. Simons et al. [96] utilised the European Organisation for Research and Treatment of Cancer Quality of Life Questionnaire C-30 (EORTC-QLQ-C30) [151], a widely used instrument developed for use in patients with cancer; Rowland et al. [152] used a patient-completed visual analogue QoL unit scale; Bruera et al. [153] used the Piper Fatigue Scale and the Functional Living Index-Cancer. Recently we have introduced the EQ-5D questionnaire in the QoL evaluation of cachectic patients. It is a standardised instrument applicable to a wide range of health conditions and treatments, which provides a simple descriptive profile and a single index value for health status. The EQ-

5D self-report questionnaire essentially consists of two pages comprising the EQ-5D descriptive system and the EQ-5D VAS. The EQ-5D descriptive system assesses five dimensions of health: mobility, self-care, usual activities, pain/discomfort, anxiety/depression; each dimension comprises three levels (no problems, some/moderate problems, extreme problems) and a unique health state score is defined by combining the level from each dimension. EQ-5D VAS records the respondent's self-rated health status on a vertical graduated (0–100) visual analogue scale (http.www.euroqol.org/eq5d). It is hoped that QoL questionnaires that specifically address the most significant symptoms present in patients with CAC will be designed and validated.

## Conclusions

Cancer-related anorexia/cachexia is a complex phenomenon, which involves a series of pathophysiological mechanisms such as major metabolic abnormalities, abnormal production and release of tumour byproducts and host cytokines, chronic activation and defective functioning of the host immune system, leading to a final outcome of 'cachexia'. Consequently, the management of CAC is a complex challenge, which may address the different causes underlying this clinical event, requiring clinicians to select for each individual patient the most appropriate treatment on the basis of known (e.g. serum cytokine level) or reasonably hypothesised causative factors. In this review, we have examined all the potential modalities of intervention from nutritional to pharmacological approaches, clearly distinguishing between unproven, investigational and well-established treatments. Among these latter there are progestagens, presently to be considered the most effective and well-tolerated drugs for CAC. Among the investigational agents, there are drugs such as anti-IL-6 mAb, anti-TNF-$\alpha$ mAb, thalidomide and formoterol, which acts on muscle mass and antagonises protein wasting. Finally, the aim of treatment in CAC should focus on symptomatic, subjective and QoL endpoints rather than just on objective (nutritional) ones, since patient survival is far beyond the scope of this treatment setting [48].

# References

1. Nelson KA (2000) The cancer anorexia-cachexia syndrome. Semin Oncol 27:64–68
2. Heber D, Byerley LO, Chi J (1986) Pathophysiology of malnutrition in the adult cancer patient. Cancer Res 58:1867–1873
3. Bruera E (1992) Clinical management of anorexia and cachexia in patients with advanced cancer. Oncology 49(Suppl 2):35–42
4. Brennan MR (1997) Uncomplicated starvation vs cancer cachexia. Cancer Res 37:2359–2364
5. Nelson K, Walsh D (1991) Management of the anorexia/ cachexia syndrome. Cancer Bull 43:403–406
6. Tisdale MJ (1997) Cancer cachexia: metabolic alterations and clinical manifestations. Nutrition 13:1–7
7. Devereaux DF, Redgrave TG, Tilton M et al (1984) Intolerance to administered lipids in tumor bearing animals. Surgery 100:292–297
8. Vlassara H, Spiegel RJ, Daval DS et al (1986) Reduced plasma lipoprotein lipase activity in patients with malignancy-associated weight loss. Horm Metab Res 18:698–703
9. Rouzer CA, Cerami A (1980) Hypertriglyceridemia associated with Trypanosoma brucei brucei infection in rabbits: role of defective triglyceride removal. Mol Biochem Parasitol 2:31–38
10. McNamara MJ, Alexander HR, Norton JA (1992) Cytokines and their role in the pathophysiology of cancer cachexia. JPEN J Parenter Enteral Nutr 16(Suppl 6):50S–55S
11. Tisdale MJ (1997) Biology of cachexia. J Natl Cancer Inst 89:1763–1773
12. Noguchi Y, Yoshikawa T, Matsumoto A et al (1996) Are cytokines possible mediators of cancer cachexia? Surg Today 26:467–475
13. Espat NJ, Copeland EM, Moldawer LL (1994) Tumor necrosis factor and cachexia: a current perspective. Surg Oncol 3:255–262
14. Moldawer LL, Gelin J, Schersten T et al (1987) Circulating interleukin 1 and tumor necrosis factor during inflammation. Am J Physiol 253:R922–R928
15. Moldawer LL, Andersson C, Gelin J (1988) Regulation of food intake and hepatic protein synthesis by recombinant-derived cytokines. Am J Physiol 254:6450–6456
16. Moldawer LL, Rogy MA, Lowry SF (1992) The role of cytokines in cancer cachexia. JPEN J Parenter Enteral Nutr 16:43S–49S
17. Strassmann G, Fong M, Kenney JS et al (1992) Evidence for the involvement of interleukin-6 in experimental cancer cachexia. J Clin Invest 89:1681–1684
18. Busbridge J, Dascombe MJ, Hoopkins S (1989) Acute central effects of interleukin-6 on body temperature, thermogenesis and food intake in the rat. Proc Nutr Soc 38:48A
19. Gelin J, Moldawer LL, Lonnroth C (1991) Role of endogenous tumor necrosis factor alfa and interleukin 1 for experimental tumor growth and the development of cancer cachexia. Cancer Res 51:415–421
20. McLaughlin CL, Rogan GJ, Ton J (1992) Food intake and body temperature responses of rat to recombinant interleukin 1 beta and a tripeptide interleukin 1 beta antagonist. Physiol Behav 52:1155–1160
21. Sherry BA, Gelin J, Fong Y (1991) Anticachectin/tumor necrosis factor alpha antibodies attenuate development of cancer cachexia. Cancer Res 51:415-421
22. Matthys P, Billiau A (1997) Cytokines and cachexia. Nutr 13:763–770
23. Moldawer LL, Copeland EM (1997) Proinflammatory cytokines, nutritional support, and the cachexia syndrome: interactions and therapeutic options. Cancer 79:1828–1839
24. Simons JP (1997) Cancer cachexia. Simons JP, Maastricht
25. Beck SA, Mulligan HD, Tisdale MJ (1990) Lipolytic factors associated with murine and human cancer cachexia. J Natl Cancer Inst 82:1922–1926
26. Beck SA, Groundwater P, Barton C et al (1990) Alterations in serum lipolytic activity of cancer patients with response to therapy. Br J Cancer 62:822–825
27. Taylor DD, Gercel-Taylor C, Jenis LG et al (1992) Identification of a human tumor-derived lipolysis-promoting factor. Cancer Res 52:829–834
28. Todorov PT, Cariuk P, McDevitt TM et al (1996) Characterization of a cancer cachectic factor. Nature 379:739–742
29. Byerley LO, Alcock NW, Starnes HF (1992) Sepsis induced cascade of cytokine mRNA expression: correlation with metabolic changes. Am J Physiol 261:E728–E735
30. Waage A, Brandtzaeg P, Halstensen A et al (1989) The complex pattern of cytokines in serum from patients with meningococcal septic shock. J Exp Med 169:333–338
31. Wilmore DW, Long JM, Mason AD et al (1974) Catecholamines: mediator of the hypermetabolic response to thermal injury. Ann Surg 180:653–668
32. Stoner HB, Barton RN, Little RA et al (1977) Measuring the severity of injury. BMJ 2:1247–1249
33. Wilmore DW, Moylan JA, Pruitt Bam Lindsey CA et al (1974) Hyperglucagonaemia after burns. Lancet 1:73–75
34. Rosenblatt S, Jr Clowes GH, George BC et al (1983) Exchange of amino acids by muscle and liver in sepsis. Arch Surg 118:167–175
35. Long CL (1997) Energy balance and carbohydrate metabolism in infection and sepsis. Am J Clin Nutr 30:1301–1310
36. Baumann H, Gauldie J (1994) The acute phase response. Immunol Today 15:74–80

37. Nordenstrom J, Carpentier YA, Askanazi J et al (1983) Free fatty acid mobilization and oxidation during total parenteral nutrition in trauma and infection. Ann Surg 198:725–735

38. Oliff A, Defeo-Jones D, Boyer M et al (1987) Tumor secreting human TNF/cachectin induce cachexia in mice. Cell 50:555–563

39. Campfield LA, Smith FJ,Guisez Y et al (1995) Recombinant mouse OB protein: evidence for a peripheral signal linking adiposity and central neural networks. Science 269:546–549

40. Stephens TW, Basinski M, Bristow PK et al (1995) The role of neuropeptide Y in the antiobesity action of the obese gene product. Nature 377:530–532

41. Halaas JL, Gajiwala KS, Maffei M et al (1995) Weight reducing effects of the plasma protein encoded by the obese gene. Science 269:543–546

42. Schwartz MW, Baskin DG, Bukowski TR et al (1996) Specificity of leptin action on elevated blood glucose levels and hypothalamic neuropeptide Y gene expression in ob/ob mice. Diabetes 45:531–535

43. Billington CJ, Briggs JE, Grace M, Levine AS (1991) Effects of intracerebroventricular injection of neuropeptide Y on energy metabolism. Am J Physiol 260(2Pt 2):R321–R327

44. Dryden S, Frankish H, Wang Q, Williams G (1994) Neuropeptide Y and energy balance: one way ahead for the treatment of obesity? Eur J Clin Invest 24:293–308

45. Inui A (1999) Cancer anorexia-cachexia syndrome: are neuropeptides the key? Cancer Res 15:4493–4501

46. Inui A (1999) Neuropeptide Y: a key molecule in anorexia and cachexia in wasting disorders? Mol Med Today 5:79–85

47. Mantovani G, Macciò A, Mura L et al (2000) Serum levels of leptin and proinflammatory cytokines in patients with advanced-stage cancer at different sites. J Mol Med 78:554–556

48. Gagnon B, Bruera E (1998) A review of the drug treatment of cachexia associated with cancer. Drugs 55:675–688

49. Kotler DP (2000) Cachexia. Ann Intern Med 133:622–634

50. Bennegard K, Eden E, Ekman L et al (1983) Metabolic response of whole body and peripheral tissues to enteral nutrition in weight-losing cancer and non cancer patients. Gastroenterology 85:92–99

51. Dresler CM, Jeevanandam M, Brennan MF (1987) Metabolic efficacy of enteral feeding in malnourished cancer and non cancer patients. Metabolism 36:82–88

52. Laviano A, Meguid MM (1996) Nutritional issues in cancer management. Nutrition 12:358–371

53. Klein S, Kinney J, Jeejeebhoy K et al (1997) Nutrition support in clinical practice: review of published data and recommendations for future research directions. Clin Nutr 16:193–218

54. Sikora SS, Ribeiro U, Kane JM 3rd et al (1998) Role of nutrition support during induction chemoradiation therapy in esophageal cancer. JPEN J Parenter Enteral Nutr 22:18–21

55. Lipman TO (1991) Clinical trials of nutritional support in cancer: parenteral and enteral therapy. Hematol Oncol Clin North Am 5:91–102

56. Nelson KA,Walsh D, Sheehan FA (1994) The cancer anorexia-cachexia syndrome. J Clin Oncol 12:213–225

57. Body JJ (1999) Metabolic sequelae of cancers (excluding bone marrow transplantation). Curr Opin Clin Nutr Metab Care 2:339–344

58. Body JJ (1999) The syndrome of anorexia-cachexia. Curr Opin Oncol 11:255–260

59. Nelson KA,Walsh D, Sheehan FA (1994) The cancer anorexia-cachexia syndrome. J Clin Oncol 12:213–225

60. Miller M (1998) Can reducing caloric intake also help reduce cancer? J Natl Cancer Inst 90:1766–1767

61. Nitenberg G, Raynard B (2000) Nutritional support of the cancer patient: issues and dilemmas. Crit Rev Oncol Hematol 34:137–168

62. Laviano A, Meguid MM,Yang ZJ et al (1996) Cracking the riddle of cancer anorexia. Nutrition 12:706–710

63. Kardinal CG, Loprinzi CL, Schaid DJ et al (1990) A controlled trial of cyproheptadine in cancer patients with anorexia and/or cachexia. Cancer 65:2657–2662

64. Ray PD, Hanson RL, Lardy HA (1970) Inhibition by hydrazine of gluconeogenesis in the rat. J Biol Chem 245:690–696

65. Kosty MP, Fleishman SB, Herndon JE et al (1994) Cisplatin, vinblastine and hydrazine sulfate in advanced, non-small-cell lung cancer: a randomized placebo controlled, double-blind phase III study of the cancer and leukemia group B. J Clin Oncol 12:1113–1120

66. Loprinzi CL, Kuross AS, O'Fallon JR et al (1994) Randomized placebo-controlled evaluation of hydrazine sulfate in patients with advanced colorectal cancer. J Clin Oncol 12:1121–1125

67. Loprinzi CL, Goldberg RM, Su JQ et al (1994) Placebo controlled trial of hydrazine sulfate in patients with newly diagnosed non-small-cell lung cancer. J Clin Oncol 12:1126–1129

68. Gralla RJ, Itri LM, Prisko SE et al (1981) Antiemetic efficacy of high-dose metoclopramide: randomized trials with placebo and prochlorperazine in patients with chemotherapy-induced nausea and vomiting. N Engl J Med 305:905–909

69. Grosvenor M, Bulcavage L, Chlebowski RT (1989) Symptoms potentially influencing weight loss in a cancer population. Cancer 63:330–334

70. Shivshanker K, Bennett RW, Hayne TP (1983) Tumor associated gastroparesis: correction with metoclopramide. Am J Surg 145:221–225

71. Nelson KA, Walsh TD, Sheehan FG et al (1993) Assessment of upper gastrointestinal motility in the cancer associated dyspepsia syndrome. J Palliat Care 9:27–31

72. Bruera E, MacBachern T, Spachynski K et al (1994)

Comparison of the efficacy, safety and pharmacokinetics of controlled release and immediate release metoclopramide for the management of chronic nausea in patients with advanced cancer. Cancer 74:3204–3211

73. Foltin RW, Fishman MW, Byrne MF (1988) Effects of smoked marijuana on food intake and body weight of humans living in a residential laboratory. Appetite 11:1–14

74. Jatoi A, Windschitl HE, Loprinzi CL, et al (2002) Dronabinol versus megestrol acetate versus combination therapy for cancer-associated anorexia: a North Central Cancer Treatment Group study. Support Care Cancer 10:71–75

75. Wadleigh R, Spaulding M, Lembersky B et al (1990) Dronabinol enhancement of appetite and cancer patients. Proc Am Soc Clin Oncol 9:331 (abs)

76. Nelson K, Walsh D, Deeter P et al (1994) A phase II study of deltanine-tetrahydrocannabinol for appetite stimulation in cancer-associated anorexia. J Palliat Care 10:14–18

77. Beal JE, Olson R, Laubenstein L et al (1995) Dronabinol as a treatment for anorexia associated with weight loss in patients with AIDS. J Pain Symptom Manage 10:89–97

78. Cavalli G, Goldhirsch A, Jungi F et al (1984) Randomized trial of low-versus-high-dose medroxyprogesterone acetate in the treatment of postmenopausal patients with advanced breast cancer. In: Pellegrini A, Robustelli Della Cuna G (eds) Role of medroxyprogesterone in endocrine-related tumors, vol 3. Raven Press, New York, pp 79–89

79. Tchekmedyian NS, Tait N, Moody M et al (1987) Highdose megestrol acetate: a possible treatment for cachexia. JAMA 257:1195–1198

80. McCarthy HD, Crowder RE, Dryden S et al (1994) Megestrol acetate stimulates food and water intake in the rat: effects on regional hypothalamic neuropeptide Y concentrations. Eur J Pharmacol 265:99–102

81. Mantovani G, Macciò A, Bianchi A et al (1995) Megestrol acetate in neoplastic anorexia/cachexia: clinical evaluation and comparison with cytokine levels in patients with head and neck carcinoma treated with neoadjuvant chemotherapy. Int J Clin Lab Res 25:135–141

82. Mantovani G, Macciò A, Esu S et al (1997) Medroxyprogesterone acetate reduces the in vitro production of cytokines and serotonin involved in anorexia/cachexia and emesis by peripheral blood mononuclear cells of cancer patients. Eur J Cancer 33:602–607

83. Mantovani G, Macciò A, Lai P et al (1988) Cytokine activity in cancer-related anorexia/cachexia: role of megestrol acetate and medroxyprogesterone acetate. Semin Oncol 25(2 Suppl 6):45–52

84. Bruera E, MacMillan K, Hanson J et al (1990) A controlled trial of megestrol acetate on appetite, caloric intake, nutritional status and other symptoms in patients with advanced cancer. Cancer 66:1279–1282

85. Loprinzi CL, Ellison NM, Shaid DJ et al (1990) Controlled trial of megestrol acetate for the treatment of cancer, anorexia and cachexia. J Natl Cancer Inst 82:1127–1132

86. Tchekmedyian NS, Hakman M, Siau J et al (1992) Megestrol acetate in cancer anorexia and weight loss. Cancer 69:1268–1274

87. Feliu J, Gonzalez-Baron M, Berrocal A (1992) Usefulness of megestrol acetate in cancer cachexia and anorexia. Am J Clin Oncol 15:436–460

88. Beller E, Tattersall M, Kumley T et al (1997) Improved quality of life with megestrol acetate in patients with endocrine-insensitive advanced cancer: a randomised placebo-controlled trial. Ann Oncol 8:277–283

89. Schmoll E, Wilke H, Thole R (1991) Megestrol acetate in cancer cachexia. Semin Oncol 1(Suppl 2):32–34

90. Fietkau R, Riepi M, Kettner H (1997) Supportive use of megestrol acetate in patients with head and neck cancer during radio(chemo)therapy. Eur J Cancer 33:75–79

91. Loprinzi CL, Michalak JC, Shaid DJ (1993) Phase three evaluation of four doses of megestrol acetate as therapy for patients with cancer anorexia and/or cachexia. J Clin Oncol 11:762–767

92. Bruera E, Ernst S, Hagen N et al (1996) Symptomatic effects of megestrol acetate (MA): a double-blind, crossover study. Proc Am Soc Clin Oncol 15:531 (abs)

93. McMillan DC, Simpson JM, Preston T et al (1994) Effect of megestrol acetate on weight loss, body composition and blood screen of gastrointestinal cancer patients. Clin Nutr 85–89

94. Gebbia V, Testa A, Gebbia N (1996) Prospective randomised trial of two levels of megestrol acetate in the management of anorexia-cachexia syndrome in patients with metastatic cancer. Br J Cancer 73:1576–1580

95. Downer S, Joel S, Allbright A et al (1993) A double blind placebo controlled trial of medroxyprogesterone acetate (MPA) in cancer cachexia. Br J Cancer 67:1102–1105

96. Simons JP, Aaronson NK, Vansteenkiste JF et al (1996) Effect of medroxyprogesterone acetate on appetite, weight, and quality of life in advanced-stage non-hormone-sensitive cancer: a placebo-controlled multicenter study. J Clin Oncol 14:1077–1084

97. Ottery FD, Walsh D, Strawford A (1998) Pharmacologic management of anorexia/cachexia. Semin Oncol 25(Suppl 6):35–44

98. De Vita Jr VT, Hellman S, Rosenberg SA (1997) Cancer principles and practice of oncology. Vol 1, 5th ed. Lippincott-Raven, Philadelphia

99. Bruera E, Fainsinger RL (1993) Clinical management of cachexia and anorexia. In: Doyle D, Hanks G, MacDonald N (eds) Oxford textbook of palliative medicine. Oxford Medical Publications, London, pp 330–337

100. Steer KA, Kurtz AB, Honour JW (1995) Megestrol-induced Cushing's syndrome. Clin Endocrinol 42:91–93

101. Heckmayr M, Gatzeneier U (1992) Treatment of cancer weight loss in patients with advanced lung cancer. Oncology 49(Suppl 2):32–34

102. Femia RA, Goyette RE (2005) The science of megestrol acetate delivery: potential to improve outcomes in cachexia. Bio Drugs 19:179–87

103. Moertel CG, Schutt AJ, Reitemeier RJ, Hahn RG (1974) Corticosteroid therapy of preterminal gastrointestinal cancer. Cancer 33:1607–1609

104. Willox JC, Corr J, Shaw J et al (1984) Prednisolone as an appetite stimulant in patients with cancer. Br Med J (Clin Res Ed) 288:27

105. Bruera E, Roca E, Cedaro L et al (1985) Action of oral methylprednisolone in terminal cancer patients: a prospective randomized double-blind study. Cancer Treat Rep 69:751–754

106. Della Cuna GR, Pellegrini A, Piazzi M (1989) Effect of methylprednisolone sodium succinate on quality of life in preterminal cancer patients: a placebo-controlled, multicenter study. The Methylprednisolone Preterminal Cancer Study Group. Eur J Cancer Clin Oncol 25:1817–1821

107. Popiela T, Lucchi R, Giongo F (1989) Methylprednisolone as palliative therapy for female terminal cancer patients. The Methylprednisolone Female Preterminal Cancer Study Group. Eur J Cancer Clin Oncol 25:1823–1829

108. Bruera ED, Roca E, Cedaro L et al (1983) Improved control of chemotherapy-induced emesis by the addition of dexamethasone to metoclopramide in patients resistant to metoclopramide. Cancer Treat Rep 67:381–383

109. Watanabe S, Bruera E (1994) Corticosteroids as adjuvant analgesics. J Pain Symptom Manage 9:442–445

110. Fuinsinger R (1996) Pharmacological approach to cancer cachexia and cachexia. In: Bruera E, Higginson I (eds) Cachexia-anorexia in cancer patients. Oxford University Press, Oxford, pp 128–140

111. Plata-Salaman CR (1991) Dexamethasone inhibits food intake suppression induced by low doses of interleukin-1 beta administered intracerebroventricularly. Brain Res Bull 27:737–738

112. Uehara A, Sekiya C, Takasugi Y et al (1989) Anorexia induced by interleukin 1: involvement of corticotropinreleasing factor. Am J Physiol 257(3 Pt 2):R613–R617

113. Han J, Thompson P, Beutler B (1990) Dexamethasone and pentoxifylline inhibit endotoxin-induced cachectin/tumor necrosis factor synthesis at separate points in the signaling pathway. J Exp Med 172:391–394

114. Trikha M, Corringham R, Klein B, Rossi JF. (2003) Targeted anti-interleukin-6 monoclonal antibody therapy for cancer: a review of the rationale and clinical evidence. Clin Cancer Res 9:4653–4665

115. Siegel SA, Shealy DJ, Nakada MT et al (1995) The mouse/human chimeric monoclonal antibody cA2 neutralizes TNF in vitro and protects transgenic mice from cachexia and TNF lethality in vivo. Cytokine 7:15–25

116. Torelli GF, Meguid MM, Moldawer LL et al (1999) Use of recombinant human soluble TNF receptor in anorectic tumor-bearing rats. Am J Physiol 277:R850–R855

117. Zabel P, Wolter DT, Schonharting MM, Schade UF (1989) Oxpentifylline in endotoxaemia. Lancet 2:1474–1477

118. Lissoni P, Ardizzoia A, Perego MS et al (1993) Inhibition of tumor necrosis factor-alpha secretion by pentoxifylline in advanced cancer patients with abnormally high blood levels of tumor necrosis factor-alpha. J Biol Regul Homeost Agents 7:73–75

119. Goldberg RM, Loprinzi CL, Mailliard JA et al (1995) Pentoxifylline for treatment of cancer anorexia and cachexia? A randomized, double-blind, placebo-controlled trial. J Clin Oncol 13:2856–2859

120. Gordon JN, Trebble TM, Ellis RD et al (2005) Thalidomide in the treatment of cancer cachexia: a randomised placebo controlled trial. Gut 54:540–545

121. Wigmore SJ, Falconer JS, Plester CE et al (1995) Ibuprofen reduces energy expenditure and acute-phase protein production compared with placebo in pancreatic cancer patients. Br J Cancer 72:185–188

122. McMillan DC, O'Gorman P, Fearon KC, McArdle CS (1997) A pilot study of megestrol acetate and ibuprofen in the treatment of cachexia in gastrointestinal cancer patients. Br J Cancer 76:788–790

123. Lundholm K, Gelin J, Hyltander A et al (1994) Anti-inflammatory treatment may prolong survival in undernourished patients with metastatic solid tumors. Cancer Res 54:5602–5606

124. Masferrer JL, Leahy KM, Koki AT et al (2000) Antiangiogenic and antitumor activities of cyclooxygenase-2 inhibitors. Cancer Res 60:1306–1311

125. Moore RJ, Zweifel B, Heuvelman DM et al (2000) Enhanced antitumor activity by co-administration of celecoxib and chemotherapeutic agents cyclophosphamide and 5-FU. Proc Am Assoc Cancer Res 41:409

126. Kishi K, Petersen S, Petersen C et al (2000) Preferential enhancement of tumor radioresponse by a cyclooxygenase-2 inhibitor. Cancer Res 60:1326–1331

127. Reddy BS, Hirose Y, Lubet R et al (2000) Chemoprevention of colon cancer by specific cyclooxygenase-2 inhibitor, celecoxib, administered during different stages of carcinogenesis. Cancer Res 60:293–297

128. Dicker AP (2003) COX-2 inhibitors and cancer therapeutics: potential roles for inhibitors of COX-2 in combination with cytotoxic therapy: reports from a symposium held in conjunction with the Radiation Therapy Oncology Group, June 2001 Meeting. Am J

Clin Oncol 26:S46–S47

129. Lissoni P, Paolorossi F, Tancini G et al (1996) Is there a role for melatonin in the treatment of neoplastic cachexia? Eur J Cancer 32A:1340–1343

130. Lissoni P, Barni S, Tancini G et al (1994) Role of the pineal gland in the control of macrophage functions and its possible implication in cancer: a study of interactions between tumor necrosis factor-alpha and the pineal hormone melatonin. J Biol Regul Homeost Agents 8:126–129

131. Meydani SN, Lichtenstein AH, Cornwall S et al (1993) Immunologic effects of national cholesterol education panel step-2 diets with and without fish-derived N-3 fatty acid enrichment. J Clin Invest 92:105–113

132. Wigmore SJ, Fearon KC, Ross JA (1997) Modulation of human hepatocyte acute phase protein production in vitro by n-3 and n-6 polyunsaturated fatty acids. Ann Surg 225:103–111

133. Barber MD, Ross JA, Preston T et al (1999) Fish oil-enriched nutritional supplement attenuates progression of the acute-phase response in weight-losing patients with advanced pancreatic cancer. J Nutr 129:1120–1125

134. Tisdale MJ (1996) Inhibition of lipolysis and muscle protein degradation by EPA in cancer cachexia. Nutrition 12:S31–S33

135. Purasiri P, Murray A, Richardson S et al (1994) Modulation of cytokine production in vivo by dietary essential fatty acids in patients with colorectal cancer. Clin Sci (Lond) 87:711–717

136. Wigmore SJ, Ross JA, Falconer JS et al (1996) The effect of polyunsaturated fatty acids on the progress of cachexia in patients with pancreatic cancer. Nutrition 12:S27–S30

137. Wigmore SJ, Fearon KC, Maingay JP, Ross JA (1997) Down-regulation of the acute-phase response in patients with pancreatic cancer cachexia receiving oral eicosapentaenoic acid is mediated via suppression of interleukin-6. Clin Sci (Lond) 92:215–221

138. Falconer JS, Ross JA, Fearon KC et al (1994) Effect of eicosapentaenoic acid and other fatty acids on the growth in vitro of human pancreatic cancer cell lines. Br J Cancer 69:826–832

139. de Bravo MG, de Antueno RJ, Toledo J et al (1991) Effects of an eicosapentaenoic and docosahexaenoic acid concentrate on a human lung carcinoma grown in nude mice. Lipids 26:866–870

140. Beck SA, Smith KL, Tisdale MJ (1991) Anticachectic and antitumor effect of eicosapentaenoic acid and its effect on protein turnover. Cancer Res 51:6089–6093

141. Barber MD, Wigmore SJ, Ross JA et al (1997) Eicosapentaenoic acid attenuates cachexia associated with advanced pancreatic cancer. Prostaglandin Leukot Essent Fatty Acids 57:204

142. Fearon KC, Von Meyenfeldt MF, Moses AG et al (2003) Effect of a protein and energy dense N-3 fatty acid enriched oral supplement on loss of weight and lean tissue in cancer cachexia: a randomised double blind trial. Gut 52:1479–1486

143. Jatoi A, Rowland K, Loprinzi CL et al; North Central Cancer Treatment Group (2004) An eicosapentaenoic acid supplement versus megestrol acetate versus both for patients with cancer-associated wasting: a North Central Cancer Treatment Group and National Cancer Institute of Canada collaborative effort. J Clin Oncol 22:2469–2476

144. Carbo N, Lopez-Soriano J, Tarrago T et al (1997) Comparative effects of beta2-adrenergic agonists on muscle waste associated with tumor growth. Cancer Lett 115:113–118

145. Ziegler TR, Wilmore DW (1993) Anabolic effects of growth hormone administration in adults. In: Muller EE, Cocchi D, Locatelli V (eds) Growth hormone and somatomedins during lifespan. Springer Verlag, Berlin, pp 312–328

146. Froesch ER, Schmid C, Schwander J et al (1985) Actions of insulin-like growth factors. Ann Rev Physiol 47:443–467

147. Tayek JA, Brasel JA (1995) Failure of anabolism in malnourished cancer patients receiving growth hormone: a clinical research center study. J Clin Endocrinol Metab 80:2082–2087

148. Ottery FD (1996) Supportive nutritional management of the patient with pancreatic cancer. Oncology 10:26–32

149. Laviano A, Muscaritoli M, Cascino A et al (2005) Branched-chain amino acids: the best compromise to achieve anabolism? Curr Opin Clin Nutr Metab Care 8:408–414

150. Nukatsuka M, Fujioka A, Saito H et al (1996) Prolongation of survival period and improvement of cancer cachexia by long-term administration of UFT. Cancer Lett 104:197–203

151. Aaronson NK, Ahmedzai S, Bergman B et al (1993) The European Organization for Research and Treatment of Cancer QLQC30: a quality-of-life instrument for use in international clinical trials in oncology. J Natl Cancer Inst 85:365–376

152. Rowland Jr KM, Loprinzi CL, Shaw EG et al (1996) Randomized double-blind placebo-controlled trial of cisplatin and etoposide plus megestrol acetate/placebo in extensive-stage small cell lung cancer: a north central cancer treatment group study. J Clin Oncol 14:135–141

153. Bruera E, Ernst S, Hagen N et al (1998) Effectiveness of megestrol acetate in patients with advanced cancer: a randomized, double-blind, crossover study. Cancer Prev Control 2:74–78

# The Role of Artificial Nutrition Support in the Cancer Patient

Federico Bozzetti

## Background

Patients with cancer often suffer from progressive involuntary weight loss, which is called cancer wasting. Clinical features of this syndrome include anorexia, early satiety, depletion of lean and fat body mass, muscle weakness, fatigue and impaired immune function. It occurs in 30–90% of cancer patients depending on location, stage, type, grade, spread and anticancer treatment [1]. Patients with cancer of lung, pancreas, head-and-neck area and upper gastrointestinal tract often suffer from wasting [2–5].

Wasting among cancer patients is shown to be associated with shorter survival time, increased length of hospital stay, increased postoperative complications, impaired immune function and reduced quality of life [5–11]. In a recent study by Andreyev et al., 1555 patients with gastrointestinal cancer receiving chemotherapy were studied retrospectively [6]. Their results showed that patients with weight loss had significantly increased chemotherapy-induced toxicity and decreased response to therapy, duration of therapy, performance status, survival and quality of life. In other studies it is furthermore suggested that wasting is the cause of death in up to 23% of cancer patients [7, 9, 12, 13].

The progressive, involuntary weight loss seen is cancer wasting is a complex, multifactorial syndrome, occurring through a variety of mechanisms associated with the tumour, the host response to the tumour, and its treatment [1, 14–17]. Although the mechanisms are still not fully understood, both reduced food intake and metabolic disturbances are thought to contribute to the development of wasting [1, 14]. Metabolic disturbances associated with cancer affect both energy expenditure and the metabolism of protein, fat and carbohydrate [1, 15].

A number of studies have assessed food intake of cancer patients. Results show that both protein and energy intake are reduced in these patients, and can depend on tumour site and treatment [22].

Reduced food intake may be caused by systemic effects of disease (anorexia, altered taste and smell, early satiety, nausea or vomiting, pain), local effects of the tumour (dysphagia, gastrointestinal obstruction) or psychological factors (fear, anxiety, depression) [14, 23]. Furthermore, anticancer treatment (both chemotherapy and radiation therapy) induces several side-effects such as anorexia, alteration in taste and smell, fatigue or mucositis, which can decrease food intake [1]. A variety of medications may interfere with nutrition, by decreasing appetite and impairing digestion and absorption of nutrients. Taste alterations are reported in 15–100% of all cancer patients, receiving different cancer treatments [24–31]. Decreased taste or taste loss is reported in 13–50% of cancer patients receiving different treatments [25, 26, 28, 30] and seems to involve all four taste modalities (sweet, salty, sour, bitter) [23, 30–33]. Due to taste alterations or taste loss, preference for foods or nutritional supplements may also change.

Although it has been known since the beginning of the history of medicine that wasting is often associated with malignant disease, it was only at the start of the century that the first investigations on nitrogen balance in cancer patients began to be published [34–36].

The first systematic attempts at feeding cancer patients parenterally or enterally date back to the period 1949–1956, by Waddell and Grillo [37], Bolker [38], Pareira et al. [39, 40], Terepka and Waterhouse [41] and subsequently Watkin and Steinfield [42].

## Effects of Nutritional Support on the Nutritional Status

The rationale for using artificial nutrition (total parenteral nutrition, TPN, or enteral nutrition, EN) in cancer patients is primarily based on the assumption that, although the final outcome of cancer patients mainly reflects the prognosis of the primary tumour, concomitant malnutrition can affect survival by increasing the complications of the oncological therapy, reducing tolerance to these treatments and, in some cases, decreasing both the length and the quality of survival.

This approach tends to parallel cancer wasting with undernutrition, a concept that is partially true, since reduced intake only partially accounts for the onset and progression of wasting. Nevertheless, the modern use of drugs or nutriceuticals as agents capable of modulating the production of cytokines involved in the mechanisms of wasting would be ineffective if patients were not metabolically supported by adequate provision of macronutrients.

The effects of TPN and EN on nutritional status have been reviewed in previous publications [43, 44] and are summarised in Tables 1 and 2. The beneficial effects of TPN are more evident when compared in controlled studies to a standard oral diet (Table 3). It is noteworthy that there is a nutritional benefit even when a vigorous nutritional support is being administered to patients undergoing an oncological therapy (Table 4).

A number of studies have examined specific protein kinetics response to TPN in malnourished cancer patients. Whole-body protein turnover has been shown to increase with TPN [45–48], but whole-body protein synthesis has been reported both to increase [49–51] and to decrease [48]. Whole-body protein catabolism has been reported to decrease in cancer patients on TPN [48, 49]. Few studies have investigated the two components of protein kinetics, namely the muscle compartment and the extra-muscle compartment. Shaw et al. [50] have reported an increase in whole-body protein synthesis and in the fractional synthetic rate of protein in muscle, with no change in whole-body protein catabolism.

In our experience in severely malnourished patients with gastric cancer [52], whole-body protein synthesis and catabolism did not significantly change from 'before' to 'during' TPN, even when the net balance moved from negative to positive. In contrast, the skeletal muscle protein synthesis as well as the protein synthesis rate increased significantly, converting the net balance to a positive value.

Generally it has been shown that TPN does not increase the serum level of proteins, albumin [53, 54], transferrin, cholinesterase or ceruloplasmin.

As regards TPN and immunological response, Monson et al. [55] have reported an increase of lymphocyte blastogenesis and production of the helper T lymphocyte lymphokine interleukin-2 after 7 days of a TPN regimen, but also a significant impairment of basal natural killer and interleukin-2-activated natural killer activity. In contrast, we published a study showing that a 10-day course of TPN was able to restore to normal a depressed basal or interleukin- or interferon-stimulated natural killer activity in wasting cancer patients [56].

Jeevanandam et al. [48] have shown that a 10-day course of TPN containing 29 non-protein kcal/kg/day + 1.6 g amino acid/kg/day significantly decreased protein breakdown (by 50 and 59%) and increased protein synthesis (by 21 and 33%) in cancer and non-cancer patients, respectively, while it increased protein turnover (by 15%) in cancer patients only. The utilisation efficiency of infused amino acids for synthesis of body proteins was 39% in both cancer and non-cancer patients.

Taken as a whole, the data indicate that TPN and EN are usually able to prevent a further deterioration of the nutritional state and may sometimes improve some metabolic indices. These outcomes are probably dependent on the length of the nutritional support, the biological aggressiveness of the tumour and the effectiveness of the available oncological therapy.

It must be emphasised that even when the nutritional benefit often seems to be limited to maintaining a 'status quo', it does so in patients who would otherwise be condemned to a progressive chronic 'auto-cannibalism' without nutritional support. However, the nutritional response of cancer patients is always more sluggish and limited

**Table 1.** Effects of TPN on the nutritional status of cancer patients

| Variable | Response |
|---|---|
| Body weight | Always increase |
| Body fat | Usually increase |
| Muscle mass | |
|    Anthropometry | No change or increase |
|    Urinary creatinine or 3-CH$_3$-histidine | No change or decrease |
| Lean body mass | |
|    Nitrogen balance | Always positive |
|    Total body nitrogen | No change or increase |
| Whole-body K | Increase or no change |
| Serum protein | |
|    Total protein | No change |
|    Albumin | Usually no change |
|    Transferrin | Usually no change |
|    Prealbumin | No change or increase |
|    Retinol-binding protein | Usually increase or no change |
|    Cholinesterase and ceruloplasmin | No change |
| Immune humoral response | |
|    IgA, C$_3$, C$_4$ | No change |
|    IgG, IgM, IgA | No change or sometimes increase |
| Non-specific cellular response | |
|    Neutrophils, total lymphocytes | |
|    B, T lymphocytes | |
|    Helper T, suppressor T, chemotaxis | No change |
|    Phagocytosis killing index | |
|    Natural killer | No change or increase |

than that of undernourished non-cancer patients (Table 5).

Only a few studies, which were randomised [48, 57, 58], prospective and controlled [59], have compared TPN and EN (Table 6). It appeared that TPN was more effective than EN in promoting weight gain [57], even though this gain may be simply due to accrual of fat or water. Nevertheless, TPN was able to maintain a better nitrogen balance and plasma amino acid level [48, 57] and a positive balance of K, Na, Cl, P and Mg [59].

Burt's 1983 study [46] did not find any difference between EN and TPN as far as protein whole-body flux, protein synthesis and catabolism were concerned. However, during the control (basal) period, whole-body protein catabolism was uniformly and significantly higher than synthesis and during the period of nutritional repletion through EN or TPN the rate of whole-body synthesis tended to be greater than that of catabolism. In addition, during the period of nutritional support, the percentage of nitrogen entering the metabolic pool

**Table 2.** Effects of EN on the nutritional status of cancer patients

| Variable | Response |
|---|---|
| Body weight | Usually increase, sometimes no change |
| Body fat | Increase or no change |
| Muscle mass | |
| Anthropometry | No change, sometimes increase |
| Urinary creatinine or 3-CH$_3$-histidine | No change |
| 3-CH$_3$-histidine efflux from the leg | Decrease |
| Tyrosine, AA and BCAA efflux from the leg | No change |
| Lean body mass | |
| Nitrogen balance | Usually positive or equilibrium |
| Total body nitrogen | No change |
| Whole-body K | Increase or no change |
| Serum protein | |
| Total protein | No change or increase |
| Albumin | Usually no change, sometimes increase or decrease |
| TIBC, CHE, TBPA | No change or increase |
| Ceruloplasmin | No change |
| Immune humoral response | |
| IgG, IgA, IgM, CH$_{50}$ | No change |
| C$_3$-C$_4$, C$_3$PA | Increase |
| Non-specific cellular response | Increase or no change |

*TIBC*, total iron-binding capacity; *CHE*, cholinesterase; *TBPA*, thyroxine-binding prealbumin

that was derived from catabolism of protein was significantly decreased in both EN and TPN groups.

The study by Dresler et al. [60] showed that before nutritional repletion, the flux of nitrogen entering the metabolic pool originated solely from the breakdown of body protein and about 75% of this flux was utilised in protein synthesis. However, when an exogenous supply of amino acids was introduced in cancer patients, utilisation efficiency decreased to 58% during EN, and to 39–43% in cancer patients during TPN. Therefore it appeared to be an advantage for the enteral route in terms of utilisation for synthesis of body proteins.

Overall, both EN and TPN tend to stabilise the nutritional status and whole-body protein economics and, depending on the type of metabolic parameter that is adopted, TPN or EN appears to be slightly more effective.

## Effects of Nutritional Support on Clinical Outcome

### Effects of Nutritional Support in Cancer Patients Submitted to Surgery

The rationale for perioperatively treating malnourished cancer patients with artificial nutrition

**Table 3.** Nutritional effects of TPN versus a standard oral diet (SOD)

| Variable | TPN | SOD |
|---|---|---|
| Weight | ↑ or = | = or ↓ |
| N balance | Positive | Negative |
| Total body K | = | = |
| Urinary 3-methylhistidine | ↓ | = |
| Total protein | = or ↑ | = or ↓ |
| Albumin | = or ↓ | = or ↓ |
| Transferrin | ↑ or = | = or ↓ ↑ |
| CHE, RBP | ↑ | ↓ |
| TBPA | = | = |
| Ceruloplasmin, Fibrinogen, IgA | = | = |
| IgG, IgM, C₃a | ↑ | = |

*CHE*, cholinesterase; *RBP*, retinol-binding protein; *TBPA*, thyroxine-binding prealbumin; ↑, increase; ↓, decrease; = no change

**Table 4.** Effects of TPN and EN in cancer patients receiving chemotherapy or radiotherapy

| Variable | Type of nutrition | Response |
|---|---|---|
| Body weight | TPN | Increase or no change |
|  | EN | Increase or no change |
| Body fat | TPN | Increase |
| Muscular mass | TPN | Increase |
| Lean body mass | | |
|   Nitrogen balance | TPN | Positive |
|   Total body nitrogen | TPN | No change |
| Serum protein | | |
|   Total protein | | |
|   Albumin | | |
|   Transferrin | TPN | No change |
|   Retinol-binding protein | | |
| Immune humoral response | | |
|   IgA, IgM | TPN | Increase |

mainly relies on the following assumptions: (1) malnourished cancer patients are at higher risk of postoperative complications (especially infections); (2) cancer malnutrition can be reversed through the use of a nutritional support and consequently the surgical risk can be reduced.

However, the value of the above statements is limited, since malnutrition is not the only (and

**Table 5.** Response to TPN and EN in cancer versus non-cancer patients

| Variable | TPN | | EN | |
|---|---|---|---|---|
| | Cancer | Non-cancer | Cancer | Non-cancer |
| Weight | ↑ | ↑↑ | ↑ | ↑ or ↑↑ |
| Arm circumference | | | | |
| Triceps skinfold | ↑ | ↑ | = or ↑ | ↑ |
| Arm muscle area | ↑ | ↑↑ | ↑ | ↑ |
| Creatinine-height index | ↑ | ↑↑ | ↑ | ↑ |
| N balance | + | + | + | + |
| Total body K | - | - | ↑ | ↑ |
| Tyrosine balance | - | - | = | + |
| Albumin | ↑ | ↑↑ | ↑ | ↑ |
| Prealbumin | = | = | = | = |
| Retinol-binding protein | = | = | - | - |
| Balance of: | | | | |
| Na | + | + | - | + |
| K | + | + | - | + |
| Cl | + | + | - | + |
| Mg | + | ++ | - | + |
| P | + | + | + | + |
| Ca | = | = | + | + |

↑↑, strong increase; ↑, increase; ↓, decrease; = no change; +, positive; –, negative

also perhaps not the most important, except in extreme cases) cause of surgical complications. Cancer malnutrition can probably be reversed by artificial nutrition but this is less easy and it takes more time than in non-cancer patients. Moreover, the length of the preoperative hospital stay has been correlated with increased surgical infection rates. Finally, we do not know whether the parameters of nutritional assessment we use to define a malnourished patient (weight loss, low serum albumin, lymphocyte number, etc.) are the same ones that are pathogenetically involved in the defective defence of the host against the microorganisms, and consequently whether we should aim at normalising them with artificial nutrition before carrying out a surgical intervention on the patient. Furthermore, it is a common experience that the more severe the malnutrition, the more advanced the stage of the tumour [62], so that the chance of performing an explorative surgery that makes useless the benefit of artificial nutrition is magnified in severely malnourished patients.

Because of all these intrinsic difficulties, the results of randomised clinical trials have been disparate; only by pooling all these trials together, as has been done in meta-analyses [63, 64], is it possible to find a statistically significant advantage in terms of reduction of the complication rate in patients receiving TPN, while reduction in mortality is dubious.

A review of 21 studies on preoperative artificial nutrition in cancer patients revealed that 16 were randomised clinical trials, but only six focused on malnourished patients with gastrointestinal tract cancers [65–70]. Two of these were non-randomised studies involving patients with oesophageal carcinoma who had metabolic [65] and clinical benefits [68]. The other four studies included a randomised clinical trial in patients with gastrointestinal carcinoma, which showed a reduction in septic complications only in those patients who had weight loss > 10% [70], and three [66, 67, 71] that showed no reduction in complications.

**Table 6.** Prospective studies on the metabolic effects of EN vs TPN [1–4]

| Nutritional parameter | EN | TPN | p |
|---|---|---|---|
| Balance of: | | | |
| N | + | + | |
| P | + | More + | 0.05 |
| K | - | + | 0.05 |
| Na | - | + | 0.05 |
| Cl | - | + | 0.05 |
| Ca | + | - | |
| Mg | - | + | 0.05 |
| Δ H$_2$O | + | + | |
| Δ Albumin | No change | + | |
| Δ CHI | + | + | |
| Δ TSF | + | + | |
| Δ MMA | + | | |
| N balance | + after 7 days | + after 1 day | |
| Weight | ↑ 1% after 30 days | ↑ 6% after 30 days | |
| Albumin | ↑ 7.4% | ↑ 6.3% | |
| Glucose turnover rate | ↑ × 4 | ↑ × 4 | |
| Gluconeogenesis from alanine | Suppressed | Suppressed | |
| Weight | No change | ↑ | 0.05 |
| N balance | No change | ↑ | 0.03 |
| Albumin | ↓ | No change | |
| Transferrin | No change | No change | |
| Ceruloplasmin | No change | No change | |
| TBK | No change | No change | |
| 3 Met-His | No change | No change | |

EN vs TPN (kg/day): 38 kcal and 0.9–1.2 vs 1.2–1.8 g AA [59]
EN vs TPN (kg/day): 63 vs 62 kcal and 2.1 vs 1.5 g AA [57]
EN vs TPN (kg/day): 49 vs 49 and 1.5–2 vs 2.5 g AA [46]

*CHI*, creatinine/height index; *TSF*, triceps skinfold; *MMA*, muscle mass area; *TBK*, total body potassium; *3 Met-His* 3, methylhistidine; ↑, increase; ↓, decrease; +, positive; -, negative

The discrepancy in the results obtained by these randomised studies involving TPN in the pre- and postoperative periods [66, 67, 70] may be related to the different lengths of preoperative feeding (11 days, 3 days and > 5 days). For example, the lowest rate of septic complications occurred in the group that received preoperative parenteral nutrition for the longest period of time.

Recently, a prospective randomised study involving cirrhotic patients who were submitted to wide hepatic resections for hepatocarcinoma reported that preoperative nutritional support can reduce postoperative complications [72], but the control group was probably disadvantaged by the administration of an excess protein-energy-free saline infusion.

We studied 90 patients with gastrointestinal cancer and weight loss ≥ 10% and showed that pre-operative TPN (10 days, calorie regimen at 1.5 × resting metabolic expenditure, kcal/N = 150/1, glucose/fat ratio 70:30) was able to reduce both overall complication rate and mortality at a statistically significant level [79].

### Artificial Nutrition as an Adjunctive Therapy in Patients Receiving Chemotherapy or Radiation Therapy

A recent meta-analysis was performed by the American Gastrointestinal Association [74] on the impact of TPN in patients receiving oncological therapy.

Twenty-seven randomised controlled trials (RCT) assessing the impact of TPN on a total of 1050 patients were reviewed: 19 studied TPN in patients receiving chemotherapy, three investigated cancer patients being treated with radiation therapy, and four were on patients undergoing bone marrow transplantation.

Results showed that there was no apparent effect of TPN on mortality in the overall series, even if a single RCT in patients undergoing bone marrow transplantation [75] showed an increase of survival in the fed patients. There was, however, a poorer response to chemotherapy in particular (absolute risk difference -7%; confidence intervals -12%, -1%) in TPN patients.

### TPN in Incurable, Aphagic, Cancer Patients

The use of TPN in such patients is controversial. Common experience shows that while patients with benign intestinal failure survive thanks to long-term home TPN, cancer patients die despite TPN.

However, there are circumstances in some lethal diseases, where survival is more dependent on the provision of nutrients and prevention of a progressive nutritional deprivation than on progression of the primary disease.

This can be the case in some cancer patients who are aphagic because of chronic intestinal obstruction due to peritoneal carcinomatosis, without involvement of vital organs such liver, lung or brain, and who have an acceptable performance status.

It is not clear whether TPN should be considered a therapy or basic humane care in these circumstances. In both cases a randomised comparison between TPN and no TPN is not possible: in fact, can a RCT be performed if some nutritionists deem TPN to be a life-saving procedure, some oncologists a futile treatment and some palliativists simple basic humane care [76]?

To my knowledge, only one RCT [77, 78] assessed the value of TPN provided to patients with end-stage malignancies receiving no specific cancer therapy. The treated patients lived significantly longer (46 days) than the control patients (7 days).

Although cancer patients account for the highest percentage of subjects receiving home TPN in many European countries [79] and in the USA, very few studies have investigated the effect of nutritional support on survival [80–84], and only two on the quality of life [81, 85].

Data showed that median survival ranged from 2.5 months [83] to over 5 months [81], with 30% of patients surviving longer than 6–7 months [81–83], a period that hardly would be expected in aphagic wasted patients without nutritional support.

Quality of life was maintained at acceptable levels and obviously declined in the last weeks of life [82].

## References

1. Nitenberg G, Raynard B (2000) Nutritional support of the cancer patients: issues and dilemmas. Crit Rev Oncol Hematol 34:137–168
2. Barber MD, Ross JA, Fearon KC (1999) Cancer cachexia. Surg Oncol 8:133–141
3. DeWys WD (1980) Nutritional care of the cancer patient. JAMA 244:374–376
4. Brookes GB (1985) Nutritional status – a prognostic indicator in head and neck cancer. Otolaryngol Head Neck Surg 93:69–74
5. Van Bokhorst-de van der Schueren MA, van Leeuwen PA, Sauerwein HP et al (1997) Assessment of malnutrition parameters in head and neck cancer and their relation to postoperative complications. Head Neck 19:419–425
6. Andreyev HJ, Norman AR, Oates J, Cunningham D

(1998) Why do patients with weight loss have a worse outcome when undergoing chemotherapy for gastrointestinal malignancies? Eur J Cancer 34:503–509

7. Dewys WD, Begg C, Lavin PT et al (1980) Prognostic effect of weight loss prior to chemotherapy in cancer patients. Eastern Cooperative Oncology Group. Am J Med 69:491–497

8. Jagoe RT, Goodship TH, Gibson GJ (2001) The influence of nutritional status on complications after operations for lung cancer. Ann Thoracic Surg 71:936–943

9. Ovesen L, Hannibal J, Mortesen RL (1993) The interrelationship of weight loss, dietary intake, and quality of life in ambulatory patients with cancer of the lung, breast and ovary. Nutr Cancer 10:159–167

10. Robinson G, Goldstein M, Levine GM (1987) Impact of nutritional status on DRG length of stay. JPEN J Parenter Enteral Nutr 1:49–51

11. Shaw-Stiffel TA, Zarny LA, Pleban WE et al (1993) Effect of nutrition status and other factors on length of hospital stay after major gastrointestinal surgery. Nutrition 9:140–145

12. O'Gorman P, McMillan DC, McArdle CS (1998) Impact of weight loss, appetite, and the inflammatory response on quality of life in gastrointestinal cancer patients. Nutr Cancer 32:76–80

13. Iganaki J, Rodrguez V, Bodey GP (1974) Proceedings: Causes of death in cancer patients. Cancer 33:568–573

14. Tisdale MJ (2001) Cancer anorexia and cachexia. Nutrition 17:438–442

15. Mutlu EA, Mobarhan S (2000) Nutrition in the care of the cancer patient. Nutr Clin Care 3:3–23

16. Fearon KCH (2001) Nutritional support in cancer. Clin Nutr 20:187–190

17. Rivadeneira DE, Evoy D, Fahey TJ 3rd et al (1998) Nutritional support of the cancer patient. CA Cancer J Clin 48:69–80

18. Bosaeus I, Daneryd P, Svanberg E, Lundholm K (2001) Dietary intake and resting energy expenditure in relation to weight loss in unselected cancer patients. Int J Cancer 93:380–383

19. Giacosa A, Frascio F, Sukkar SG, Roncella S (1996) Food intake and body composition in cancer cachexia. Nutrition 12:S20–S23

20. Ripamonti C, Fulfaro F (1998) Taste alterations in cancer patients. J Pain Symptom Manage 16:349–351

21. Ripamonti C, Zecca E, Brunelli C et al (1998) Randomized, controlled clinical trial to evaluate the effects of zinc sulphate on cancer patients with taste alterations caused by head and neck irradiation. Cancer 82:1938–1945

22. Sitzia J, North C, Stanley J, Winterberg N (1997) Side effects of CHOP in the treatment of non-Hodgkin's lymphoma. Cancer Nurs 20:430–439

23. Mattsson T, Arvidson K, Heimdahl A et al (1992) Alteration in taste acuity associated with allogeneic bone marrow transplantation. J Oral Pathol Med 21:33–37

24. Lockhart PB, Clark JR (1990) Oral complications following neoadjuvant chemotherapy in patients with head and neck cancer. NCI Monogr 9:99–101

25. Lees J (1999) Incidence of weight loss in head and neck cancer patients on commencing radiotherapy treatment at a regional oncology centre. Eur J Cancer Care (Engl) 8:133–136

26. Fanning J, Hilgers RD (1993) High-dose cisplatin carboplatin chemotherapy in primary advanced epithelial ovarian cancer. Gynecol Oncol 51:182–186

27. Epstein JB, Robertson M, Emerton S et al (2001) Quality of life and oral function in patients treated with radiation therapy for head and neck cancer. Head Neck 23:389–398

28. DeWys WD, Walters K (1975) Abnormalities of taste sensation in cancer patients. Cancer 36:1888–1896

29. Trant AS, Serin J, Douglass HO (1982) Is taste related to anorexia in cancer patients? Am J Clin Nutr 36:45–58

30. Gallagher P, Tweedle DE (1983) Taste threshold and acceptability of commercial diets in cancer patients. JPEN J Parenter Enteral Nutr 7:361–363

31. Tomita Y, Osaki T (1990) Gustatory impairment and salivary gland pathophysiology in relation to cancer treatment. Int J Oral Maxillofac Surg 19:299–304

32. Ovesen L, Hannibal H, Sorensen M (1991) Taste thresholds in patients with small-cell lung cancer. J Cancer Res Clin Oncol 117:70–72

33. Ovesen L, Sorensen M, Hannibal J, Allingstrup L (1991) Electrical taste detection thresholds and chemical smell detection thresholds in patients with cancer. Cancer 68:2260–2265

34. Edsall DL (1905) Case of acute leukaemia. Am J Med Sci 130:589–600

35. Musser JH, Edsall DL (1905) Study of metabolism of leukaemia under influence of X-ray. Tr Ass Am Phys 20:294–321

36. Murphy JB, Means JH, Aub JC (1917) Effect of roentgen ray and radium therapy on metabolism of patient with lymphatic leukaemia. Arch Intern Med 19:890–900

37. Waddell WR, Grillo HC (1959) Metabolic effect of fat emulsion. Am J Clin Nutr 7:43–49

38. Bolker N (1953) Nitrogen balance in malignant disease. Am J Roentgen 69:839–848

39. Pareira MD, Conrad EJ, Hicks W, Elman R (1954) Therapeutic nutrition and tube feeding. J Am Med Assoc 156:810–816

40. Pareira MD, Conrad EJ, Hicks W, Elman R (1955) Clinical response and changes in nitrogen balance, body weight, plasma protein and haemoglobin following tube feeding in cancer cachexia. Cancer 8:803–808

41. Terepka AR, Waterhouse C (1956) Metabolic observations during the forced feeding of patients with cancer. Am J Med 20:225–238

42. Watkin D, Steinfield JL (1965) Nutrient and energy metabolism in patients with and without cancer

during hyperalimentation with fat administered intravenously. Am J Clin Nutr 16:182–212

43. Bozzetti F (1989) Effects of artificial nutrition on the nutritional status of cancer patients. JPEN J Parent Ent Nutr 13:406–420

44. Bozzetti F (1992) Nutritional support in adult cancer patients. Clin Nutr 11:167–179

45. Burt ME, Gorschboth CM, Brennan MF (1982) A controlled, prospective, randomized trial comparing the metabolic effects of enteral and parenteral nutrition in the cancer patient. Cancer 49:1092–1105

46. Burt ME, Stein TP, Brennan MF (1983) A controlled, randomized trial evaluating the effects of enteral and parenteral nutrition on protein metabolism in cancer-bearing man. J Surg Res 34:303–314

47. Burt ME, Brennan MF (1984) Nutritional support of the patient with esophageal cancer. Semin Oncol 11:127–135

48. Jeevanandam M, Legaspi A, Lowry SF (1988) Effect of total parenteral nutrition on whole body protein kinetics in cachetic patients with benign or malignant disease. JPEN J Parenter Enteral Nutr 12:229–236

49. Shaw JHF, Wolfe RR (1988) Whole-body protein kinetics in patients with early and advanced gastrointestinal cancer: the response to glucose infusion and total parenteral nutrition. Surgery 103:148–155

50. Shaw JHF, Humberstone DA, Douglas RG, Koea J (1991) Leucine kinetics in patients with benign disease, non-weight-losing cancer, and cancer cachexia: studies at the whole-body and tissue level and the response to nutritional support. Surgery 109:37–50

51. Hyltander A, Warnold I, Eden E, Lundholm K (1991) Effect on whole-body protein synthesis after institution of intravenous nutrition in cancer and non-cancer patients who lose weight. Eur J Cancer 27:16–21

52. Bozzetti F, Gavazzi C, Ferrari P, Dworzak F (2000) Effect of total parenteral nutrition on the protein kinetics of patients with cancer cachexia. Tumori 86:408–411

53. Fan ST, Law WY, Wong KK, Chan WP (1989) Preoperative parenteral nutrition in patients with oesophageal cancer: a prospective, clinical trial. Clin Nutr 8:23–27

54. Gray G, Meguid M (1990) Can total parenteral nutrition reverse hypalbuminemia in oncology patients? Nutr 6:225–228

55. Monson JRT, Ramsden CW, MacFie J et al (1986) Immunorestorative effect of lipid emulsions during total parenteral nutrition. Br J Surg 73:843–846

56. Bozzetti F, Cozzaglio L, Villa ML et al (1995) Restorative effect of total parenteral nutrition on natural killer cell activity in malnourished cancer patients. Eur J Cancer 12:2023–2027

57. Lim STK, Choa RG, Lan KH, Ong GB (1981) Total parenteral nutrition versus gastrostomy in the preoperative preparation of patients with carcinoma of the oesophagus. Br J Surg 68:69–72

58. Pearlstone DB, Lee J, Alexander RH et al (1995) Effect of enteral and parenteral nutrition on amino acid levels in cancer patients. JPEN J Parenter Enteral Nutr 19:204–208

59. Nixon DW, Lawson DH, Kutner M et al (1981) Hyperalimentation of the cancer patient with protein-calorie undernutrition. Cancer Res 41:2038–2045

60. Dresler CM, Jeevanandam M, Brennan MF (1987) Metabolic efficacy or enteral feeding in malnourished cancer and non-cancer patients. Metabolism 36:82–88

61. Jeevanandam M, Horowitz GD, Lowry SF et al (1985) Cancer cachexia: effect of total parenteral nutrition on whole body protein kinetics in man. JPEN J Parenter Enteral Nutr 9:108

62. Bozzetti F, Migliavacca S, Scotti A et al (1982) Impact of cancer, type, site, stage and treatment on the nutritional status of patients. Ann Surg 196:170–179

63. Klein S, Simes J, Blackburn GL (1986) Total parenteral nutrition and cancer clinical trials. Cancer 58:1378–1386

64. McGeer AJ, Detsky AS, O'Rourke K (1990) Parenteral nutrition in cancer patients undergoing chemotherapy: a meta-analysis. Nutrition 6:233–240

65. Haffejee AA, Angorn IB (1977) Oral alimentation following intubation for esophageal cancer. Ann Surg 186:165–170

66. Holter AR, Fisher JE (1977) The effects of perioperative hyperalimentation on complications in patients with carcinoma and weight loss. J Surg Res 23:31–34

67. Thompson BR, Julian TB, Stremple JF (1981) Perioperative parenteral nutrition in patients with gastrointestinal cancer. J Surg Res 30:497–500

68. Daly JM, Massar E, Giacco G et al (1982) Parenteral nutrition in esophageal cancer patients. Ann Surg 196:206–208

69. Meijerink WJHJ, Von Meyenfeldt MF, Rouflart MMJ, Soeters PB (1992) Efficacy of perioperative nutritional support. Lancet 340:187–188

70. Von Meyenfeldt MF, Meijerink WJHJ, Rouflart MMJ et al (1992) Perioperative nutritional support: a randomized clinical trial. Clin Nutr 11:180–186

71. Fan ST, Law WY, Wong KK, Chan WP (1989) Preoperative parenteral nutrition in patients with oesophageal cancer: a prospective, clinical trial. Clin Nutr 8:23–27

72. Fan ST, Lo CM, Lai EC et al (1994) Perioperative nutritional support in patients undergoing hepatectomy for hepatocellular carcinoma. N Eng J Med 331:1547–1552

73. Bozzetti F, Gavazzi C, Miceli R et al (2000) Perioperative total parenteral nutrition in malnourished, gastrointestinal cancer patients: a randomized, clinical trial. JPEN J Parenter Enteral Nutr 24:7–14

74. Koretz RL, Lipam TO, Klein S (2001) AGA technical review on parenteral nutrition. Gastroenterology

121:970–1001

75. Weisdorf SA, Lysne J, Wind D et al (1987) Positive effect of prophylactic total parenteral nutrition on long-term outcome of bone marrow transplantation. Transplantation 43:833–838

76. Bozzetti F (2003) Home total parenteral nutrition in incurable cancer patients: a therapy, a basic humane care or something in between? Clin Nutr 22:109–111

77. Solassol C, Joyeux H, Dubois JB (1979) Total parenteral nutrition (TPN) with complete nutritive mixtures: an artificial gut in cancer patients. Nutr Cancer 1:13–18

78. Solassol C, Joyeux H (1979) Artificial gut with complete nutritive mixtures as a major adjuvant therapy in cancer patients. Acta Chir Scand 494:186–188

79. Van Gossum A, Vahedi KK, Abdel-Malik et al (2001) ESPEN-HAN Working Group. Clinical, social and rehabilitation status of long-term home parenteral nutrition patients: results of a European multicentre survey. Clin Nutr 20:205–210

80. Cozzaglio L, Balzola F, Cosentino F et al (1997) Outcome of cancer patients receiving home par-

enteral nutrition. Italian Society of Parenteral and Enteral Nutrition (SINPE). JPEN J Parenter Enteral Nutr 21:339–342

81. Scolapio JS, Fleming CR, Kelly DG et al (1999) Survival of home parenteral nutrition-treated patients: 20 years of experience at the Mayo Clinic. Mayo Clin Proc 74:217–222

82. Bozzetti F, Cozzaglio L, Biganzoli E et al (2002) Quality of life and length of survival in advanced cancer patients on home parenteral nutrition. Clin Nutr 21:269–271

83. Pasanisi F, Orban A, Scalfi L et al (2001) Predictors of survival in terminal-cancer patients with irreversible bowel obstruction receiving home parenteral nutrition. Nutrition 17:581–584

84. Torelli GF, Campos AC, Meguid MM (1999) Use of TPN in terminally ill cancer patients. Nutrition 15:665–667

85. Gervasio S, Finocchiaro C, Galletti R et al (2002) Home parenteral nutrition (HPN) in advanced cancer patients: effects on nutritional status, quality of life and predictors of survival. Clin Nutr 21(Suppl 1):78

# The Role of Appetite Stimulants for Cancer-Related Weight Loss

Jamie H. Von Roenn

## Introduction

Involuntary weight loss and its end-stage manifestation, the anorexia and cachexia syndrome, is a frequent complication of cancer. The incidence of weight loss varies both with the primary site of the malignancy and its stage. At presentation, 15–48% of cancer patients report weight loss, while more than 80% of those with advanced disease note involuntary weight loss [1]. A weight loss of as little as 5% from premorbid weight predicts a poor prognosis, particularly among patients with lymphoma, lung, breast or gastrointestinal malignancies. Weight loss of less than 5% adversely impacts survival, with the greatest effect seen in those patients with good performance status [1]. Involuntary weight loss adversely affects quality of life as well [2–4].

Curative therapy for the underlying malignancy reverses cancer-related weight loss. Unfortunately, for the majority of patients with advanced disease, cure is not yet a possibility, highlighting the need for effective interventions for involuntary weight loss. The pathophysiology of cancer-related weight loss is multifactorial. The mechanism of weight loss varies with the primary site, resulting from complex interactions between decreased energy intake, lipolytic and proteolytic factors produced by the tumour, hormonal abnormalities, and cytokine alterations in the context of metabolic abnormalities that result in progressive loss of skeletal muscle.

The challenge is to understand the pathophysiology of cancer-related weight loss and the anorexia and cachexia syndrome to the extent that targeted therapies can be developed and utilised to reverse this devastating complex. From a pathophysiological point of view, pharmacological treatments for cancer-related weight loss can be cate-gorised as: (1) medications to treat symptoms that interfere with caloric intake; (2) appetite stimulants; (3) drugs that affect intermediary metabolism or specific humoral inflammatory responses; and (4) anabolic agents.

This chapter will focus on pharmacological stimulants of appetite for the management of cancer-related weight loss.

Anorexia occurs in up to 85% of patients with advanced cancer, making it among the most common symptoms [5]. Identifying and treating reversible symptoms that contribute to anorexia, such as nausea, bloating or depression, to name a few, is the first step in the treatment of patients with involuntary weight loss. The impact of aggressive symptom control on energy intake has not been prospectively evaluated, but symptom control clearly improves caloric intake and quality of life for some patients. Treatment of symptoms alone, however, is often inadequate to maintain or replenish weight and/or total body protein mass.

Caloric supplementation may seem a reasonable approach to treat cancer-associated weight loss. However, the striking differences between starvation, an absolute lack of energy intake and cachexia highlight the inadequacy of caloric supplementation as a treatment for cancer-related cachexia. In starvation, the body adapts by decreasing energy expenditure and preserving muscle mass relative to fat mass. In the setting of involuntary weight loss and cancer, energy expenditure may remain elevated in spite of inadequate energy intake, and skeletal muscle loss and fat mass are progressively lost with relative maintenance of visceral mass. Furthermore, clinical trials of aggressive caloric supplementation, whether parenterally or enterally, do not demonstrate significant reversal of cancer-associated weight loss for the majority of patients.

## Orexigenic Agents

Recognising the frequent link between decreased appetite and weight loss, early clinical trials of pharmacological interventions for cancer-associated weight loss focused on orexigenic agents. The best-studied agents include cyproheptadine, corticosteroids, dronabinol and megestrol acetate, alone and/or in combination.

### Cyproheptadine

Cyproheptadine is an antihistaminic, antiserotonergic agent approved in the USA for the treatment of allergic disorders and in Europe, in geriatric patients, for essential anorexia and in adolescents for anorexia nervosa. Theoretically, cyproheptadine decreases the cerebral production of tryptophan and serotonin, potential mediators of anorexia. A randomised, double-blind, placebo-controlled trial performed by the North Central Oncology Group tested this hypothesis. Two hundred and ninety-five patients with advanced cancer were randomised to receive either placebo or oral cyproheptadine 8 mg three times daily. Though well tolerated, cyproheptadine led to minimal improvements in appetite without a corresponding increase in body weight [6].

### Corticosteroids

Corticosteroids, an important palliative intervention for patients with advanced cancer, stimulate appetite. Multiple randomised, placebo-controlled trials of corticosteroids, at a variety of doses and schedules, have tested their appetite-stimulating properties (Table 1) [7–11]. Corticosteroids consis-

tently improve appetite, though short-lived (4–8 weeks), without measurable increase in weight gain. In general, treatment with corticosteroids is associated with an improvement in overall sense of well-being. They may be of particular benefit for patients who have other steroid-responsive symptoms, such as nausea, asthenia or pain, particularly bone or visceral pain.

Corticosteroids, however, have significant potential for toxicity, which increases with the total dose and duration of therapy. Prolonged use of steroids produces progressive muscle wasting, electrolyte imbalances and fluid retention. The neuropsychiatric complications of steroids are varied, and occasionally severe. Mild neuropsychiatric symptoms are frequent, occurring in up to 50% of patients [12]. Organic mood disorders and delirium are the most severe neuropsychiatric toxicities of steroids. These events generally occur within the first two weeks of treatment and resolve with dose reduction.

The most effective dose or formulation of steroids for treatment of anorexia is unclear. As noted above, multiple steroid formulations and doses effectively stimulate appetite. Dexamethasone is generally considered the steroid of choice because of its limited mineral corticoid activity and relatively low cost. Dexamethasone is best administered as a single morning dose with breakfast to avoid the insomnia associated with evening steroid administration. Steroids are not indicated to treat anorexia in patients with a survival anticipated to be greater than 8 weeks. For patients with very advanced cancer and limited survival, less than 2 months, corticosteroids may be an excellent therapy choice for the palliation of anorexia. For bedridden patients in particular, corticosteroids may be the

**Table 1.** Corticosteroid trials

| Author | Steroid/dose | Appetite | Weight |
|---|---|---|---|
| Moertel [7] | Dexamethasone 0.75–1.5 mg PO QID | ≠ | No change |
| Wilcox [8] | Prednisolone 5 mg PO TID | ≠ | No change |
| Bruera [9] | Methylprednisolone | ≠ | No change |
| Robustelli Della Cuna [10] | Methylprednisolone | ≠ | No change |
| Popiela [11] | Methylprednisolone 125 mg IV/day | ≠ | No change |

best therapeutic option, as exacerbation of muscle wasting is not of particular concern. Corticosteroids are also a particularly useful therapy consideration for patients who require co-analgesia with an anti-inflammatory agent (e.g., the patient with painful bone metastases).

## Cannabinoids

Dronabinol (delta-9-tetrahydrocannabinol), a synthetic cannabinoid, has been used both as an antiemetic (with potency similar to that of prochlorperazine) and as an appetite stimulant in patients with both HIV- and cancer-related weight loss [13–17]. Appetite stimulation with dronabinol treatment was suggested by data from phase II studies in patients with cancer-related anorexia [15]. In a 6-week, dose-ranging study, 30 patients with advanced cancer received 2.5 mg of dronabinol daily, 2.5 mg twice daily, or 5 mg once a day. Weight loss continued in all treatment groups, although the rate of weight loss was decreased compared to baseline weight changes. Mood and appetite were improved in patients who were treated with 5 mg daily.

The only randomised, placebo-controlled study of dronabinol as an appetite stimulant was carried out in patients with AIDS-related wasting [17]. One hundred and thirty-nine patients were enrolled, 88 of whom (63%) were evaluable for efficacy. Dronabinol 2.5 mg twice daily, as compared with placebo, led to greater improvement in patient-reported appetite ($p = 0.01$), a trend towards weight gain after 6 weeks of treatment (+0.1 kg and -0.4 kg, respectively; $p = 0.21$), improvement in mood ($p = 0.005$), and decreased nausea ($p = 0.05$). Forty-three per cent of the dronabinol-treated patients, as compared with 13% of the placebo-treated patients ($p < 0.001$), experienced treatment-related toxicities. Neurological toxicity, occurring in 35% of the dronabinol-treated patients versus 9% of those receiving placebo ($p < 0.001$), was the primary basis for the difference in toxicity rates across the study arms. Dose reductions were required by 18% of the dronabinol-treated group for neurological toxicity. Euphoria, dizziness, thinking abnormalities and somnolence were the most frequent dose-limiting toxicities.

After completion of the 6-week, randomised study, patients were eligible to receive up to 1 year of open-label dronabinol. Of the 90 patients for whom data are available from the study extension, patient-reported appetite stimulation was maintained for at least 6 months and was associated with an increase in body weight of at least 2 kg in 39% of the patients. However, the lack of objective measures of increased appetite (e.g., increases in caloric intake) or evidence of weight gain in the majority of dronabinol-treated patients suggests limited usefulness of this agent.

Appetite stimulation by cannabinoids is highly variable and does not generally translate into weight gain. Toxicities are significant, particularly in elderly patients, who appear more sensitive to dronabinol's neurological toxicity.

If a decision is made to prescribe dronabinol, it has reasonably good tolerance at a dose of dronabinol 2.5 mg three times daily. Elderly patients, however, should probably be started at a lower dose, 2.5 mg once daily, with escalation as tolerated.

## Megestrol Acetate

Megestrol acetate is a synthetic, orally available progestational agent used widely for the treatment of hormone-responsive malignancies. With conventional dose, 160 mg daily, megestrol acetate results in stimulation of appetite and weight gain in about 30% of patients with advanced breast cancer [18]. In patients with cancer-related weight loss and hormone-insensitive tumours, a similar proportion, 25–30% of patients, report appetite stimulation and weight gain with standard doses [18].

A phase I/II study of megestrol acetate 480–1600 mg daily in patients with advanced cancer observed a marked increase in appetite and weight with treatment [19]. In fact, 81% of patients enrolled on this trial gained 2 kg or more. Multiple, randomised, placebo-controlled trials have demonstrated significant appetite improvement and weight gain with megestrol acetate therapy in patients with advanced cancer (Table 2). A randomised, double-blind, placebo-controlled trial of megestrol acetate 800 mg daily in patients with cancer-associated anorexia and cachexia was conducted by the North Central Oncology Group [20].

**Table 2.** Cancer cachexia placebo-controlled trials of megestrol acetate (*MA*)

| Author | N | MA Dose | Appetite | Weight |
|---|---|---|---|---|
| Loprinzi [20] | 133 | 800 mg vs placebo | ↑ | ↑ Mean = 1.4 kg (MA group) |
| Bruera [21] | 40 | 480 mg (crossover trial) | ↑ | ↑ |
| Tchekmedyian [22] | 89 | 1600 mg | ↑ | ↑ |

*N*, number of patients

One hundred and thirty-three patients with advanced cancer were randomly assigned to megestrol acetate 800 mg or placebo for 3 months. Megestrol acetate-treated patients reported greater appetite ($p = 0.003$) and caloric intake ($p = 0.009$) as compared to patients treated with placebo. A weight gain of 15 pounds or greater over enrollment weight was observed in 16% of patients treated with megestrol acetate, as compared to 2% of placebo-treated patients. Megestrol acetate-treated patients experienced decreased nausea and vomiting. No clinically significant toxicities were observed and ascribed to treatment, with the exception of mild oedema.

Bruera et al. reported a double-blind, placebo-controlled, crossover trial of megestrol acetate 480 mg daily or placebo for 7 days [21]. Forty patients with advanced, non-hormone-responsive tumours and cancer-associated cachexia were enrolled. Appetite, pain, nausea, depression, energy level, and sense of well-being were assessed by patient reports using a visual analogue scale, and nutritional status, caloric intake and side-effects were recorded. Megestrol acetate resulted in significant improvement in appetite, caloric intake, nutritional status and energy as compared to placebo. As in previous trials, toxicity was minimal, consisting of mild oedema in three patients and nausea in two.

High-dose megestrol acetate, 1600 mg daily, for anorexia treatment was evaluated in 89 patients with hormone-insensitive malignancies [22]. After 1 month of therapy, patients reported improvement in appetite and food intake, as compared to those receiving placebo. A three-item questionnaire assessing appetite, food intake, and concern about weight revealed a greater level of improvement in all of these parameters with megestrol acetate treatment as compared to placebo.

The improvement in appetite and weight gain observed with megestrol acetate has been reported across a range of dose levels. A randomised study of megestrol acetate at doses of 160, 480, 800 and 1280 mg per day demonstrated a positive dose-response effect between megestrol acetate dose and patient-determined appetite and food intake [23]. However, the highest dose tested, 1280 mg per day, did not provide benefit over and above that seen with the 800 mg per day dose. No statistically significant differences in toxicity were observed across treatment groups. Specifically, no dose-related increase in either thromboembolic events or oedema was reported.

Numerous studies of megestrol acetate for the treatment of cachexia have consistently demonstrated improvement in appetite and weight gain [19–23]. However, the composition of this weight gain, as evaluated by dual X-ray absorptiometry and tritiated body water methodologies, is primarily fat mass [24]. There is no significant increase in total body water. The megestrol acetate trials in patients with advanced cancer and cachexia have by and large failed to show significant toxicity. However, important endocrinological effects have been reported.

Megestrol acetate has glucocorticoid effects, which may result in depression of the pituitary adrenal axis and exacerbation of glucose intolerance [25–27]. When megestrol acetate is discontinued, the patient should be closely observed because of the potential for a steroid withdrawal syndrome.

A study of megestrol acetate in patients with AIDS-related wasting demonstrated a drop in cortisol levels to nearly undetectable levels in patients in whom plasma megestrol acetate levels were >150 ng/ml [28]. The frequency of endocrinological toxicity appears related to total drug exposure: higher doses over a more prolonged treatment period lead to greater risk. In addition, in men, a decrease in testosterone is routinely identified after 1 week of therapy, even with doses as low as megestrol acetate 160 mg daily. While no significant differences in the incidence of thromboembolic phenomena in the high-dose, placebo-controlled studies of megestrol acetate have been reported, concerns remain about this risk, particularly in patients with metastatic adenocarcinoma and its increased risk for thrombosis [19, 21, 23].

The 'optimal' dose of megestrol acetate for cancer-related weight loss is unclear. Megestrol acetate, oral suspension, milligram for milligram is approximately 10% more bioavailable than the tablet formulation [29]. An intermediate dose of megestrol acetate 400 mg daily, titrated up or down based on response, is a reasonable starting point. It is important to note, however, that 25% of patients reach their maximum weight change after 6 weeks of treatment [30].

### Combination Therapy

Combination therapy with megestrol acetate and dronabinol offers no advantage over treatment with megestrol acetate alone [31]. A randomised, placebo-controlled study of megestrol acetate 800 mg and placebo, versus oral dronabinol 2.5 mg twice daily and placebo, or both active agents, enrolled 469 patients with advanced cancer and weight loss. Megestrol acetate proved superior to dronabinol as an orexigenic agent, and combination treatment offered no advantage over treatment with megestrol acetate alone. Megestrol acetate-treated patients reported greater appetite improvement and weight gain, compared with dronabinol-treated patients: 75% versus 49% ($p = 0.001$) for appetite and 11% versus 3% ($p = 0.02$) for number with greater than 10% increase in weight over baseline, respectively. An unblinded, randomised study in patients with AIDS-related weight loss, again comparing combination megestrol acetate and dronabinol to either agent alone, demonstrated weight gain only in those patients receiving megestrol acetate 750 mg daily, whether alone or in combination with dronabinol [32].

## Conclusions

In summary, megestrol acetate is the most potent available orexigenic agent and leads to improvement in quality of life for patients with advanced cancer and weight loss. Unfortunately, in spite of the significant weight gain observed with megestrol acetate treatment, the weight gain is predominantly due to an increase in fat mass and, therefore, unlikely to produce improvement in strength or survival. A clear role for dronabinol is difficult to define. Glucocorticoids are of greatest benefit for patients with the most advanced cancer, particularly for those who are bed bound.

When considering treatment for patients with anorexia and weight loss, the intervention for a particular patient should be chosen based on the patient's treatment goals and prognosis. For the patient with very limited survival (weeks), whose primary goal is to increase the enjoyment of eating, either megestrol acetate or corticosteroids may be useful. For the majority of patients, however, treatment is intended to improve oral intake, weight, and ideally function. To achieve this, an approach that combines an orexigenic agent with an anabolic agent may be of greater benefit. Further studies will be necessary to define new agents as well as potential beneficial combinations.

# References

1. Dewys WD, Begg C, Lavin PT et al (1980) Prognostic effect of weight loss prior to chemotherapy in cancer patients. Am J Med 69:491–497

2. MacDonald N, Baracos VE, Plata-Salaman CR, Tisdale MJ (2000) Cachexia-anorexia workshop. Vancouver, British Columbia, Canada. November 7-9-1997. Nutrition 16:1006–1020

3. Kotler DP (2000) Cachexia. Ann Int Med 133:622–634

4. Nixon DW, Lawson DH, Kutner M et al (1981) Hyperalimentation of the cancer patient with protein-calorie under-nutrition. Cancer Res 41:2038–2045

5. Bruera E, Fainsinger RL (1993) Clinical management of cachexia and anorexia. In: Doyle D, Hanks G, MacDonald N (eds) Oxford textbook of palliative medicine. Oxford Medical Publications, London, pp 330–337

6. Kardinal C, Loprinzi C, Shaid DS et al (1980) A controlled trial of cyproheptadine in cancer patients with anorexia. Cancer 65:2657–2662

7. Moertel C, Schulte A, Reitemeier R (1974) Corticosteroid therapy of preterminal gastrointestinal cancer. Cancer 33:1607–1609

8. Wilcox JC, Corr J, Shaw J (1984) Prednisone as an appetite stimulant in patients with cancer. BMJ 288:27

9. Bruera E, Roca E, Cedaro L et al (1985) Action of oral methylprednisolone in terminal cancer patients: a prospective randomized double-blind study. Cancer Treat Rep 69:751–754

10. Robustelli Della Cuna GR, Pellegrini A, Piazzi M (1989) Effect of methylprednisolone sodium succinate on quality of life in pre-terminal cancer patients: a placebo controlled, multi-center study. Eur J Cancer Clin Oncol 25:1817–1821

11. Popiela T, Lucchi R, Giongo F (1989) Methylprednisolone as palliative therapy for female terminal cancer patients. Eur J Cancer Clin Oncol 25:1923–1929

12. Stiefel FC, Breitbart WS, Holland JC (1989) Corticosteroids in cancer: neuropsychiatric complications. Cancer Invest 7:479–491

13. Sallan SE, Cronin C, Zelan M, Zinberg NE (1976) Antiemetics in patients receiving chemotherapy for cancer: a randomized comparison of delta-9 tetrahydrocannabinol and prochlorperazine. N Engl J Med 302:135–138

14. Wadleigh R, Spaulding M, Lembersky B et al (1990) Dronabinol enhancement of appetite in cancer patients. Proc Am Soc Clin Oncol 9:331 (Abs 1280)

15. Nelson K, Walsh D, Deeter P, Sheehan F (1994) A phase II study of delta-9-tetrahydrocannabinol for appetite stimulation in cancer-associated anorexia. J Palliat Care 10:14–18

16. Gorter R, Seefrid M, Volberding P (1992) Dronabinol effects on weight in patients with HIV infection. AIDS 6:127–128

17. Beal JE, Olson R, Laubernstein L et al (1995) Dronabinol as a treatment for anorexia associated with weight loss in patients with AIDS. J Pain Symptom Manage 10:89–97

18. Gregory EJ, Cohen SC, Oives DW (1985) Megestrol acetate therapy for advanced breast cancer. J Clin Oncol 3:155–160

19. Tchekmedyian NS, Tait A, Mandy M, Aisner J (1987) High dose megestrol acetate: a possible treatment for cachexia. JAMA 9:1195–1998

20. Loprinzi CL, Ellison NM, Schaid DJ et al (1990) Controlled trial of megestrol acetate for the treatment of cancer anorexia and cachexia. J Natl Cancer Inst 82:1127–1132

21. Bruera E, MacMillan K, Kuehn N et al (1990) A controlled trial of megestrol acetate on appetite, calorie intake, nutritional status and other symptoms in patients with advanced cancer. Cancer 66:1279–1282

22. Tchekmedyian NS, Tait N, Moody M et al (1986) Appetite stimulation with megestrol acetate in cachectic cancer patients. Semin Oncol 13:37–43

23. Loprinzi CL, Michalak JC, Schaid DJ et al (1993) Phase III evaluation of four doses of megestrol acetate as therapy for patients with cancer anorexia and/or cachexia. J Clin Oncol 11:762–767

24. Loprinzi CL, Schaid DJ, Dose AM et al (1993) Body-composition changes in patients who gain weight while receiving megestrol acetate. J Clin Oncol 11:152–154

25. Mann M, Koller E, Murgo A et al (1997) Glucocorticoid-like activity of megestrol. Arch Intern Med 157:1651–1656

26. Loprinzi CL, Jensen MD, Jiang NS, Schaid DJ (1992) Effect of megestrol acetate on the human pituitary-adrenal axis. Mayo Clin Proc 67:1160–1162

27. Lang I, Zielinski CC, Templ H et al (1990) Medroxyprogesterone acetate lowers plasma corticotropin and cortisol but does not suppress anterior pituitary responsiveness to human corticotropin releasing factor. Cancer 66:1949–1953

28. Engelson ES, Pi-Sunyer FX, Kotler DP (1995) Effects of megestrol acetate therapy on body composition and circulating testosterone concentration in patients with AIDS. AIDS 9:1107–1108

29. Graham KK, Mikolich DJ, Fisher AE et al (1994) Pharmacologic evaluation of megestrol acetate oral suspension in cachectic AIDS patients. J Acquir Immune Defic Syndr 7:580–586

30. Von Roenn JH, Armstrong D, Kotler DP et al (1994) Megestrol acetate in patients with AIDS-related cachexia. Ann Int Med 121:393–399

31. Jatoi A, Windschitl HE, Loprinzi CL et al (2002) Dronabinol versus megestrol acetate versus combination therapy for cancer-associated anorexia: a North Central Cancer Treatment Group study. J Clin Oncol 20:567–573

32. Timpone JG, Wright DJ, Li N et al (1997) The safety and pharmacokinetics of single-agent and combination therapy with megestrol acetate and dronabinol for the treatment of HIV wasting syndrome. AIDS Res Hum Retroviruses 13:305–315

# Palliative Management of Anorexia/Cachexia and Associated Symptoms

Florian Strasser

## Introduction

The focus of palliative care is illness-oriented, with the main aim being to relieve suffering. In contrast, the disease-oriented approach aims to improve the natural course of a disease and the length of life. Caring for nutritional issues of patients with advancing, progressive and terminal illness improves when the nutritional interventions focus on the effects of the illness on patients and relatives, and do not target curative or disease-oriented endpoints (such as weight, oral intake). This brief chapter highlights the concept of palliative care, issues of palliative nutritional endpoints and decision making, the potential importance of treatment of symptoms and syndromes such as constipation as causes for secondary anorexia/cachexia, issues of palliative symptom and syndrome management, and terminal care.

## Palliative Care Concept

The World Health Organization (WHO) recently published an updated definition of palliative care, which highlights the multidimensional approach, multidisciplinarity, and its applicability earlier in the course of the disease rather than in the terminal phase only (Table 1) [1].

Palliation can also be understood as prevention of unnecessary suffering. Proactive screening for distressing symptoms and complications can begin at the diagnosis of an advanced, progressive and incurable disease, not just in the very terminal phase. Specialist palliative care services, in association with disease specialists [2], can provide assessment and management of psycho-physical symptoms and socio-spiritual needs of patients during the course of the illness and at the end of life [3].

**Table 1.** WHO definition of palliative care

Provides relief from pain and other distressing symptoms

Affirms life and regards dying as a normal process

Intends neither to hasten nor to postpone death

Integrates the psychological and spiritual aspects of patient care

Support system: help patients live as actively as possible until death

Support system: help the family cope during the patient's illness and in their own bereavement

Uses a team approach to address the needs of patients and their families, including bereavement counselling, if indicated

Will enhance quality of life, may positively influence the course of illness

Is applicable early in the course of illness, in conjunction with other therapies that are intended to prolong life, such as chemotherapy or radiation therapy, and includes those investigations needed better to understand and manage distressing clinical complications

## Palliative Nutritional Endpoints and Decision Making

A careful multidimensional evaluation is the basis for treatment decisions for patients with advanced illness, such as cancer, suffering from anorexia, cachexia and related symptoms (see also Chp. 9.11 'Eating-related Distress of Patients with Advanced, Incurable Cancer and Their Partners').

In order to prioritise anorexia/cachexia in the present (and often rapidly fluctuating) context, the patient should be assessed considering concurring physical (anorexia, fatigue, asthenia, body image, chronic nausea), psychological–emotional (anxiety, worthlessness, anhedonia), social (meal-ritual, express love through cooking) and spiritual–existential (bread of life) symptoms and distress.

The natural history of the disease and its complications need to be taken into account including the actual and future disease-specific treatment options and plans. Adequate communication skills need to be applied in order to guide the patient and the family within their coping style, cultural background, and preferences of decision making [4]. Further influencing factors include co-morbidities and general conditions such as the living situation of the patient and available social and financial resources.

The subsequently developed comprehensive management approach involves team interactions and agreement with the patient and family about treatment goals and meaningful outcomes. The goals of the intervention may concentrate predominantly on changes in body image, focus on improvement of function, consist in the control of a specific symptom (sensation of anorexia, decreased food intake, chronic nausea), or aim to improve overall quality of life.

These aspects of palliative care, the multidimensional assessment, caring and treatment of patients with advanced, progressive disease and weight loss, may be insufficiently recognised by focusing mainly on the influence of catabolic–metabolic processes and pharmacological and nutritional treatments. Relevant endpoints of palliative nutritional interventions are individual priorities and may include primarily eating-related symptoms such as loss of appetite, chronic nausea, fullness or taste alterations, but also social function (social withdrawal from meals, tensions in the partnership), joy of eating (feelings of guilt, powerlessness and helplessness to fulfil calorie requirements, 'terror' of the weight scale (the distress caused by monitoring weight too closely), uncertainty about healthy food), emotional issues (eating-related distress), body image, physical and role function (fatigue, weakness), or existential issues (perceived starving to death). A helpful intervention is the normalisation of the experience and counselling patients and their relatives about the causes of these endpoints.

Since palliative care concepts apply early in the course of a disease, both palliative and curative interventions are possible in a generally palliative, or illness-oriented situation. The clear definition about the goals of an intervention is important to avoid both extremes: neglect and overactivity. The focus on amount of intake, optimisation of nutrients or weight is curative in nature, since it does not aim to relieve primarily suffering. Treatment of the sensation of loss of appetite, decreasing the distress related to social interactions associated with meals, is palliative in nature. However, the optimal management of constipation leading to (almost) complete reversal of anorexia, or stenting the colon to improve bowel obstruction, aim to relieve suffering but are curative in nature. In both cases a pure palliative approach to relieve anorexia, visceral pain, and nausea in constipation and bowel obstruction would probably be of minor quality in many patients.

With regards to the decision whether to provide artificial nutritional interventions in the palliative care context, guidelines are not standardised. This issue has recently been put on the agenda of the European Association of Palliative Care (www.eapcnet.org).

As an example, a practical approach towards providing nutritional interventions in patients with advanced cancer may include the following elements: (1) relative importance of a starvational component (bowel obstruction [5, 6], radiotherapy for head and neck cancers, intake, surgery [7, 8], high-dose chemotherapy [9]); (2) probability of a reversible inflammation (infection, treatment-responsive cancer disease); (3) expected life expectancy [10]; (4) integrity of the upper and lower gastrointestinal tract; (5) goals of the nutritional intervention and meaningful outcomes; (6) dietary counselling (assessment of nutritional status, dietary and educational needs, provision of educational and nutritional supplements, alleviate anxiety and conflict around patient's inability to consume what would normally be considered as normal diet) [11]; (7) discussion of the option of enteral nutrition in patients with a starvational component and functioning bowel; (8) consideration of parenteral nutrition for a selected patient group (predominantly starvational component, accurate estimation of life expectancy, a good understanding of the individual indication, effects and side-effects, the impossibility of using enteral nutrition, after appropriate discussion with the patient and his or her family, psychological impact of withdrawal of parenteral nutrition); (9) ethical principles (autonomy [right to medically futile treatment?], beneficience [does the intervention really do more good than harm?], non-maleficence [side-effects and complications of the intervention] and justice [are the potentially high treatment costs justified considering economical limitations of the society?]).

## Treatment of Symptoms and Constipation as Causes for Secondary Anorexia/Cachexia

In patients with advanced, progressive, incurable disease, the causes of anorexia, decreased oral intake and loss of weight are complex. Besides the primary (paraneoplastic) catabolic processes, a number of important causes for loss of appetite or weight may occur, such as severe symptoms (i.e. pain, shortness of breath, depression), syndromes (i.e. constipation, mucositis, bowel obstruction) or prolonged bed rest [12]. Poor assessment of interfering symptoms (see Chp. 9.11) by not acknowledging risk factors for symptom expression and insufficient symptom management (i.e. pain, depression, social distress), or negligence of the syndromes constipation [13] or sedation [14] can lead to sub-standard management.

## Palliative Symptom and Syndrome Management

Eating-related symptoms encompass a wealth of possible symptoms, which can be individually very different in severity and predominance. Their management follows multidimensional principles.

For palliative treatment of anorexia, the progestins are still the most effective drugs, but with limited effects on other nutritional endpoints. It remains to be discussed with the patient, whether the pure improvement of the sensation of appetite is a meaningful endpoint considering the side-effects and price. Corticosteroids are effective, but only for a few weeks, then side-effects gain importance. Prokinetics are helpful for chronic nausea in a subgroup of patients. Newer treatments have the

potential to change this map of limited evidence-based treatment options.

Constipation often causes symptoms such as anorexia, early satiety or nausea before it is perceived as a symptom (feeling of incomplete evacuation, fullness of the bowel, etc.). It needs to be diagnosed as a syndrome (history, X-ray abdomen, rectal examination), not as a symptom.

## Terminal Care

Decrease of oral (nutritional) intake in terminal patients can cause considerable psychosocial distress to patients and relatives, also with philosophical and religious connotations. Adequate education and counselling addressing the anxiety of family members that a relative is 'starving to death' is often important. Reframing families from the concept that terminal cachexia from 'starving to death' towards an understanding of the complex catabolic abnormalities in cachexia is a useful strategy ('The administration of more food will not result in additional fat or muscle synthesis because of the generally irreversible underlying abnormalities'). This reframing can decrease emotional and social distress of patients and relatives and can maintain the social benefits of meal times.

Adequate mouth care and small amounts of ice chips or sips of cold beverages gain importance in the terminal phase. Hypodermoclysis can be very useful in maintaining adequate hydration at home at little cost and with minimal invasiveness [15].

## Conclusions

Palliative, multidimensional concepts of anorexia and cachexia carry the potential to optimise quality of life of patients with advanced cancer until death through: (1) establishing more targeted multidimensional interventions, (2) improved decision making, and (3) research projects tailored to this patient population testing several hypotheses, i.e. eating-related distress, diagnosis and impact of secondary anorexia/cachexia, multidimensional individually targeted treatments, and specific drugs.

# References

1. Anonymous (2002) National cancer control programmes: policies and managerial guidelines, 2nd ed. World Health Organization, Geneva
2. Maltoni M, Amadori D (2001) Palliative medicine and medical oncology. Ann Oncol 12:443–450
3. Marwick C (2001) IOM calls for improvements in palliative care. J Natl Cancer Inst 93:1128
4. Bruera E, Sweeney C, Calder K et al (2001) Patient preferences versus physician perceptions of treatment decisions in cancer care. J Clin Oncol 19:2883–2885
5. Pasanisi F, Orban A, Scalfi L et al (2001) Predictors of survival in terminal-cancer patients with irreversible bowel obstruction receiving home parenteral nutrition. Nutrition 17:581–584
6. King LA, Carson LF, Konstantinides N et al (1993) Outcome assessment of home parenteral nutrition in patients with gynecologic malignancies: what have we learned in a decade of experience? Gynecol Oncol 51:377–382
7. Heyland DK, Montalvo M, MacDonald S et al (2001) Total parenteral nutrition in the surgical patient: a meta-analysis. Can J Surg 44:102–111
8. Daly JM, Weintraub FN, Shou J et al (1995) Enteral nutrition during multimodality therapy in upper gastrointestinal cancer patients. Ann Surg 221:327–338
9. Charuhas PM, Fosberg KL, Bruemmer B et al (1997) A double-blind randomized trial comparing outpatient parenteral nutrition with intravenous hydration: effect on resumption of oral intake after marrow transplantation. JPEN J Parenter Enteral Nutr 21:157–161
10. Glare P, Virik K, Jones M et al (2003) A systematic review of physicians' survival predictions in terminally ill cancer patients. BMJ 327:195
11. Ovesen L, Allingstrup L, Hannibal J et al (1993) Effect of dietary counseling on food intake, body weight, response rate, survival, and quality of life in cancer patients undergoing chemotherapy: a prospective, randomized study. J Clin Oncol 11:2043–2049
12. Strasser F (2003) Pathophysiology of anorexia/cachexia syndrome. In: Doyle D, Hanks G, Cherny N et al (eds) Oxford textbook of palliative Medicine, 3rd edn. Oxford University Press, Oxford, pp 520–533
13. Strasser F (2003) Management of specific symptoms and syndromes: constipation. In: Bruera E, Fisch M (eds) Cambridge handbook of advanced cancer care. Cambridge University Press, Cambridge, pp 397–497
14. Lawlor PG, Gagnon B, Mancini IL et al (2000) Occurrence, causes, and outcome of delirium in patients with advanced cancer: a prospective study. Arch Intern Med 160:786–794
15. Bruera E, Legris MA, Kuehn N, Miller MJ (1990) Hypodermoclysis for the administration of fluids and narcotic analgesics in patients with advanced cancer. J Pain Symptom Manage 5:218–220

# Pharmaco-Nutritional Supports for the Treatment of Cancer Cachexia

Max Dahele, Kenneth C.H. Fearon

## Introduction

### Background

Cancer cachexia is a major symptom burden for patients with cancer. Cachexia occurs in up to one half of all patients diagnosed with cancer [1] and is more frequent in patients with lung and upper-gastrointestinal cancer. Cancer cachexia results from the interaction of the host and the tumour. However, the nature of this interaction is incompletely understood [2–5], including the dynamics of the host response (activation of the systemic inflammatory response, metabolic, immune and neuroendocrine changes) and those tumour characteristics or tumour-derived products that influence expression of the syndrome (e.g. proteolysis-inducing factor [PIF]). The relative importance of individual mediators and pathways in different patients or tumour types is unclear, as is the reason why individuals with apparently similar tumours should show considerable variation in their tendency to develop cachexia. As ability to discriminate the relative importance in vivo of different mediators improves, so too should the ability to develop appropriately targeted therapy.

The aim of this chapter is to discuss the support of the cachectic cancer patient using the pharmacological effect of a variety of nutrients in addition to conventional pharmacological agents. However, cachectic patients must first be identified, appropriate treatment selected and agreed with patients, compliance maximised and adequate follow-up put in place.

## The Diagnosis of Cancer Cachexia and its Implications

The hallmarks of cachexia are involuntary weight loss, disproportionate skeletal muscle wasting and anorexia/early satiety. However, not all patients will conform to the stereotypical image of 'cachexia'; for example, they may still be technically overweight despite having lost a substantial mass of lean tissue or they may be relatively weight-stable despite significant physiological change.

Pre-treatment weight loss has long been identified as an important prognostic factor in oncology [6] and the objective clinical consequences of cachexia are profound – reduced survival, impaired response to anti-cancer therapy, impaired immunity, lower performance status, increased symptomatology, reduced physical activity, impaired quality of life. It is important to identify potentially reversible conditions that can exacerbate cachexia (e.g. mechanical causes of inadequate nutritional intake, malabsorption, metabolic disorders such as hypercalcaemia, and depression) and to manage adequately other problems that may confront cancer patients (e.g. pain, nausea, constipation and infection). Common treatment-related side-effects (e.g. gastrointestinal sequelae of chemotherapy or radiotherapy such as nausea, mucositis, diarrhoea, food aversion) should also be anticipated. In addition, there is a suggestion that some cytotoxic drugs may themselves generate cachexia-like side-effects [7].

## Hurdles to the Nutritional Management of Cancer Cachexia

The therapy of cancer cachexia poses a real challenge to all who confront it. A holistic approach to patient care that includes an assessment of social and functional parameters in addition to the medical and nutritional status of the patient is important to maximise patient function and independence. This is likely to require structured, multidisciplinary patient care, and attention to service organisation and economic analyses may be needed to support the introduction of cachexia therapies into patient care. The routine formal assessment of functional nutritional status is uncommon in medicine but objective tools that can also guide therapy are available [8]. Practical approaches to cancer nutrition should be highlighted and encouraged [9].

Cancer patients will see many different health professionals and this is a challenge when it comes to providing education about cachexia. In medicine, nutrition has not always received the recognition it deserves and this has been acknowledged for some time now [10]. Patients frequently access biologically active complementary/alternative medicines but there may not always be robust information on their safety or efficacy and their interaction with conventional therapy is often incompletely understood [11, 12].

## Physiological Disturbance in Cancer Cachexia – Targets for Specialised Nutritional Therapy and Pharmacological Intervention

Weight loss in cancer patients suggests an imbalance in energy supply and demand. Energy expenditure (demand) in patients is largely governed by their resting energy expenditure (REE) and the energy expended on physical activity. Cancer patients may be hypo- or hyper-metabolic and it is possible that this may be influenced by tumour type or the stage of illness. Cachectic cancer patients may exhibit relative glucose intolerance and insulin resistance and demonstrate increased glucose and protein turnover. These metabolic abnormalities may become more pronounced as the disease progresses and are associated with an energy cost.

An increase in the REE may not be reflected in the patient's total energy expenditure (TEE). Physical activity is a variable quantity and may be curtailed in ill patients (although the dynamics of this relationship are not completely understood). Such a reduction in physical activity is highly likely to impact on patients' function, independence and quality of life. Furthermore, it may also exacerbate functional decline as inactivity is linked to muscle atrophy. The other side of the energy balance equation is supply and, for a variety of reasons (see below), many patients with cachexia may have an inadequate nutritional intake.

Physiologically, the breakdown of body tissue in cachexia reflects excessive catabolism and/or inadequate anabolic activity. Persistence of these changes may eventually be detrimental to the patient's function and overall well-being. Possible mediators of catabolism are endogenous corticosteroids, PIF, lipid-mobilising factor (LMF) and proinflammatory cytokines. Inadequate anabolic activity might reflect an impaired response to anabolic mediators such as anabolic-androgenic steroids, growth hormone or insulin or an inadequate supply of energy and macro/micronutrients. For many patients with advanced cancer, alleviating cachexia by tumour cure is unfortunately not possible at this time. Therefore as the tumour persists so will the physiological disturbance and it seems likely that attempts to modulate cachexia with conventional nutritional supplementation alone will be unsuccessful.

## Challenges in Treating Cancer Cachexia

Many single cachexia therapies have been tested in isolation and have met with limited or no success. It seems likely that a combination of therapies, perhaps individualised according to pathophysiological abnormalities, will ultimately be required to modulate the cachectic process.

Whilst the focus on weight loss in cancer cachexia is understandable (it is tangible, easy to measure and related to 'clinical outcomes'), it is nevertheless possible that weight loss is an insensitive marker for the physiological dysfunction driving cachexia and that by the time a patient manifests significant weight loss, the cachectic process is firmly established and is likely to be more difficult to slow or reverse. Furthermore, the functional implications of focusing on weight gain are unclear. Abnormalities in REE have now been identified early in the disease process [13]. There is a requirement for practical early markers of the cachectic process in cancer patients as this group of patients may in fact have the most to gain from cachexia therapy.

Strategically, there is a need for consensus on the research definition of cancer cachexia and for the identification of prognostic criteria that will allow for meaningful stratification of the syndrome. While greater understanding of the molecular pathophysiology of the syndrome will suggest new therapeutic targets, there is also a clear need to define appropriate criteria of therapeutic success. The relevance of end-points currently applied to cancer cachexia to both patients and researchers also needs to be established. For example, does weight gain mean longer survival, increased response to anti-cancer therapy, better functional status or improved quality of life? Which body compartments should be targeted? Do these compartments retain 'normal' functional potential, for example, is cachectic muscle performance or efficiency impaired? How should various interventions (e.g. pharmacological and exercise therapy [14–17]) be integrated? It will be important to establish how cachexia therapy combines and interacts with conventional anti-cancer treatment. The intent of anti-cancer treatment is frequently palliative. Therefore, patient-centred end-points (e.g. function and 'quality of life') are important.

## Nutritional Therapy

### Background

Patients with advanced cancer may have an inadequate nutritional intake and fail to increase appropriately their intake in response to increased resting energy demands [18]. Intake may be reduced by 'primary' mechanisms induced by the cachexia syndrome (and manifesting as anorexia or early satiety) or may be 'secondary' to problems such as mechanical gut obstruction or impaired swallowing, nausea, constipation, depression, gastrointestinal fungal infection and treatment side-effects (e.g. opiates, antibiotics, chemotherapy, radiotherapy). Such secondary problems should be proactively sought and appropriately managed. In addition, the medical team should also be alert to the risk of deteriorating nutritional status when patients are hospitalised [19, 20].

The pathogenesis of 'primary' anorexia/early satiety and the control of human appetite are incompletely understood. At the present time,

cytokines (including interleukins 1β and 6 [IL-1β, IL-6] and tumour necrosis factor-alpha [TNF-α]), the balance of central neurotransmitters (e.g. serotonin) and neuropeptides (e.g. neuropeptide Y) and hormones (e.g. leptin and ghrelin) have all been implicated [21].

As with any other intervention, the guiding concept for nutritional intervention must be 'first do no harm'. There has been some concern that nutritional support might promote tumour growth [22–24]. In studying pharmaco-nutritional support it should be ascertained that the experimental therapy itself or the means by which it is delivered does not worsen patient outcome.

In supporting cachectic cancer patients, the optimal intake of macro- and micronutrients remains to be established and many patients receive 'conventional' nutritional products. There are several theoretical reasons why this may not be optimal. These include the observations that systemic inflammation increases the requirement for certain amino acids [25] and that high-energy phosphate compounds may be reduced in tumour-bearing rats [26].

## Conventional Nutritional Support

The broad aims of nutritional support for cachectic cancer patients are to improve function and well-being, to reduce morbidity and mortality and to strengthen patients for further challenges that may be imposed upon them. A number of trials have studied conventional nutritional support in cancer patients, several in patients receiving anti-tumour therapy. These therapies may themselves be regarded as 'stressors' that can continue for weeks or months. Furthermore, many cancer interventions may exacerbate reductions in energy and nutrient intake. Surgical patients may be fasted for prolonged periods perioperatively and both chemotherapy and radiotherapy may induce side-effects such as anorexia, nausea, vomiting, mucositis, taste change or lethargy (depending of course on the drugs being used and the location, treatment volume and dose of radiotherapy) [27]. Current understanding as to how nutrition and chemotherapy interact is incomplete [28–30]. Intuitively a nutritionally replete patient should do better but this has not been easy to demonstrate.

Early nutritional intervention studies focused on using parenteral nutrition (PN) to increase nutritional intake. Initial promising results were not supported by later prospective studies [31]. There is some theoretical evidence that nutritional therapy can modulate chemotherapy [32, 33] but in trials of patients undergoing chemotherapy PN does not appear to increase survival, or to improve response rates or toxicity. It may actually be associated with a detrimental outcome and an increased risk of sepsis [34, 35]. In studies where PN has been associated with decreased survival, the spectre of nutrition-induced tumour progression has been raised [36]. It is generally agreed that PN should be reserved for specific indications [31].

It is now appreciated that the gut plays an important role in systemic immunity. In common with other tissues, if the gut is not used it will atrophy and so this is the case with PN. Impaired gut integrity and subsequent bacterial translocation may be one important negative consequence of PN and this may be exacerbated by cancer therapy (e.g. radiotherapy or chemotherapy) or cancer-related complications (e.g. bowel obstruction) [31]. The oral/enteral route has advantages over PN as the gut is used. It is also cheaper and (relatively) user-friendly. Studies of oral nutrition in chemotherapy patients have identified challenges in overcoming systemic and gastrointestinal symptoms. Nonetheless, increases in energy and protein intake can be achieved but these have not been shown to improve outcome [37, 38]. The energy and protein density of an oral supplement may be important in determining net benefit. In a recent study of nutritional supplementation in treatment-naïve patients with advanced pancreatic cancer (not receiving cytotoxic therapy), the control arm received a high protein and caloric-dense oral nutritional supplement and patients' weight loss was halted [39].

On current evidence it seems that, at best, conventional oral nutritional supplementation may stabilise weight in malnourished wasting patients but that this may not be reflected by an improvement in conventional outcomes. Assuming that the outcomes are appropriate, why should this be? Cancer can clearly induce profound physiological dysregulation in susceptible individuals and patients who develop cachexia may be unable to use effectively the energy and nutrients provided in conventional supplements. There are mixed data concerning this matter. In a heterogenous group of cancer patients it was suggested that PN was able to increase both fat and lean body mass [40]. However, other investigators have suggested that, while PN can promote net protein synthesis in depleted non-cancer patients, it is unable to achieve nitrogen equilibrium [41] in weight-losing cancer patients. In addition cachectic patients may synthesise protein less well from PN [42], and standard PN may be insufficient to increase protein synthesis in weight-losing cancer and non-cancer patients [43]. Some investigations have suggested there is little difference between the response of cancer and non-cancer patients to artificial feeding [44, 45] while others have shown a partial block to the accretion of lean tissue [46].

Despite being inconclusive, the data suggest that at least a proportion of cachectic cancer patients are unable to utilise effectively the nutrition they ingest and research is now yielding suggestions as to why this may be the case. For example, one explanation for the difficulty in generating increased lean body mass (muscle) is that inflammatory cytokines are reprioritising nitrogen metabolism to increase hepatic acute-phase protein synthesis at the expense of peripheral lean tissues [47]. These metabolic challenges are compounded by tumour-specific products (e.g. PIF), which increase lean tissue catabolism at a time when nutritional intake is reduced. However, even if additional energy and nutrients alone can stabilise weight, ongoing physiological abnormalities and the overall symptom burden may preclude substantial improvements in function, quality of life or even prognosis.

## Refining Oral Nutritional Support

For any oral nutritional supplement to be effective it must be consumed and unfortunately patients with advanced cancer frequently demonstrate anorexia, early satiety and alteration in taste and food preference. These obstacles to increasing oral nutritional intake suggest that appetite and desire for food will often need to be improved if an oral nutritional supplement is to have any chance of benefit. This could be particularly important in patients also receiving anti-cancer therapies, which may further limit nutritional intake. Gastrointestinal tract function may also be abnormal and patients should be asked about their medication (e.g. opiates) and symptoms of early satiety/fullness. Of course, nutrition does not just come as a supplement. Recognising eating as a social activity and paying due attention to practical food issues such as the selection, storage, preparation and timing of eating is an important part of optimising nutritional intake.

Refining oral nutritional support has generally involved adding specific nutrients at supra-physiological levels in order to modulate metabolic or immune function [48]. Thus the aim is to use nutrients as drugs, hence the term pharmaconutrition or 'nutraceuticals' [49]. However, the composition of the complete nutritional matrix including the macronutrients is also likely to be important and requires to be optimised [50, 51].

## Omega-3 Fatty Acids and Oral Nutritional Support

The eicosanoids are biologically active substances that, in addition to other roles in malignancy, are important mediators of the systemic inflammatory response [52]. Their production can be modulated by dietary polyunsaturated fatty acids (lipids), particularly the omega n-6 and n-3 fatty acids. Omega-6 fatty acids tend to produce highly 'inflammatory' eicosanoids, whereas those derived from n-3 fatty acids are considerably less so [53]. Altering the balance of eicosanoids in vivo through the manipulation of dietary lipids may therefore affect systemic inflammation. Although there may be variation between individuals [54], n-3 fatty acids appear to be able to reduce levels of proinflammatory cytokines and C-reactive protein [55]. They also modulate PIF-mediated ubiquitin-proteasome proteolysis, possibly via the transcription factor NF-κB [56–58] and influence hepatic protein synthesis [47]. There is also some evidence to suggest they may have anti-tumour activity themselves [59, 60] and down-regulate the toxicity of chemotherapy [61, 62].

Studies in cachectic pancreatic cancer patients

have suggested that, when given at doses 20–40 times the normal Western dietary intake, n-3 fatty acids are well tolerated [63] and can stabilise patients' weight [64]. On the basis that successful cachexia therapy has to address both metabolic changes and reduced food intake, the combination of a conventional oral nutritional supplement with n-3 fatty acids and antioxidants was developed. The recommended daily intake of two cans provides 620 kcal, 32 g protein and 2.2 g eicosapentaenoic acid (EPA).

This combination supplement has now been tested in two large-scale randomised studies. Intention-to-treat analysis of an 8-week treatment period of cachectic patients with advanced pancreatic cancer ($n = 200$) showed no advantage from a mean intake of 1.4 cans/day of the n-3-enriched supplement when compared with an isocaloric, isonitrogenous control. Both supplements arrested weight loss to the same extent. Mean n-3 intake was suboptimal, however, and post-hoc analysis suggested that, in those patients who did achieve the desirable supplement intake (providing 2 g EPA/day), weight and lean tissue increased and quality of life improved. In addition, it seems that there may have been deviation in reported EPA and supplement intake in the control population, further complicating interpretation [39]. A subgroup of patients underwent further physiological study and, in those receiving the n-3-enriched supplement, physical activity was significantly increased [65]. Increased activity may be particularly beneficial in cachectic patients as inactivity is a risk factor for muscle atrophy [66].

A second large randomised study (reported in abstract) compared the same supplement with megestrol acetate or a combination of the two in a heterogenous population [67]. The combination of an appetite stimulant with the specialised nutritional supplement seems logical and intuitively beneficial. However, it was no better than megestrol acetate alone. Finally, a study using fish oil capsules alone showed no benefit from 2 weeks of n-3 fatty acid supplementation in advanced cancer in comparison with placebo [68]. However, it is possible that the brevity and lack of conventional nutritional support in this study may have affected the outcome.

Thus, while there is much in vitro and animal

experimental evidence to support the use of n-3 fatty acids on an intention-to-treat basis, the case for benefit from n-3 fatty acid supplementation has not yet been proven. The major obstacle is oral delivery of an adequate dose. Other remaining questions include when in the disease course is the best time to study the effect of n-3 fatty acids? How can patients who may benefit from n-3 fatty acids be identified? What is the optimum duration of supplementation? How best can n-3 fatty acids be delivered to the patient? What is the interaction between n-3 fatty acids and anti-cancer therapies? Should n-3 fatty acids be combined with other agents (e.g. anabolic agents) and, if so, how? What is the optimum clinical model with which to assess their effects? In addition, the optimum macro-micronutrient supplement mix to accompany n-3 fatty acids remains to be established.

### Hydroxy-Beta-Methylbutyrate, Arginine and Glutamine

Hydroxy-beta-methylbutyrate (HMB) is a leucine derivative, which, in common with arginine and glutamine, may favourably modulate protein turnover. The combination had already shown activity in weight-losing patients with acquired immunodeficiency syndrome [69] and has recently been tested against an isonitrogenous non-essential amino acid control supplement in weight-losing cancer patients ($n = 32$). After 4 weeks of administration, patients receiving the experimental supplement had increased their fat-free mass (FFM) and weight and this net gain was maintained to the end of the 24-week study. Control patients lost weight and FFM. This combination awaits further study and characterisation [70] in cancer cachexia, including its effects on tumour growth [71, 72]. Its safety has recently been assessed [73].

### Additional Approaches

Glutamine is an amino acid with various physiological effects (e.g. metabolic, immune and gut integrity) and supplementation in cancer patients has recently been reviewed extensively [74]. The specific role of immune-modifying nutritional supplementation in surgery has recently been

reviewed [75, 76]. There have been suggestions that patients with upper gastrointestinal cancer undergoing surgery may benefit from this approach: however, further studies are needed to characterise this intervention. Any role for using 'probiotics' as a therapy in cancer cachexia remains to be established.

## Pharmacological Therapy for Cancer Cachexia

### Background

A plethora of disparate agents have been or are being studied and some of the more common are described. It is not possible to be exhaustive and the reader is directed to recent literature [77–79]. The division of drugs into separate areas of activity may be somewhat artificial as many of them are likely to act via several different pathways and have multiple effects on the host. Key aims of integrated pharmaco-nutritional support for cancer cachexia are to optimise patient function and general well-being, and to influence morbidity and possibly survival with acceptable side-effects. In order to achieve these aims, end-points need to be clearly defined and understood: for example, what do improvements in appetite or weight mean? Are function or quality or life improved as a result? If not, what is the meaning to patients of improvements in these parameters? It is important to realise that many studies in cancer cachexia therapy have been conducted in patients with far advanced cancer. If there were to be a shift to the earlier diagnosis of cachexia and initiation of 'physiology-modifying therapy', then the therapeutic ratio of agents may change. The optimum combinations of pharmacological agents, 'conventional nutrition' and nutraceuticals remain to be established.

### Appetite Stimulants

#### Progestational Agents

Megestrol acetate and medroxyprogesterone acetate are synthetic progestagens that also have some mineralocorticoid activity. Megestrol acetate has been favoured and is one of the most studied therapies in cancer cachexia [80]. Originally used as a therapy in hormone-sensitive tumours, the observation that in a substantial number of patients appetite and weight increased led to it being studied in cancer cachexia [81]. It has been widely promoted as a therapy for cachexia and anorexia, although whether patient function or quality of life is improved is less clear. Appetite can be increased after only a short period of treatment [82]. Improvements in well-being may also occur in some patients without obvious changes in nutritional status [83]. Although it has not been assessed in all studies, there appears to be little impact on lean body mass, which is currently thought to be the most important body compartment in modulating function. In fact, a detrimental effect on muscle has been demonstrated in elderly males [84] and the weight gain seems largely secondary to increased fat and some fluid [85]. This is consistent with observations in AIDS patients [86, 87]. Megestrol acetate has also been shown to induce male hypogonadism [88] and there are theoretical reasons as to why this may not be beneficial to cachectic cancer patients.

Although megestrol acetate may improve general well-being [83], there is conflicting evidence of its impact on quality of life [89–91]. Whilst the progestagens seem to be quite well tolerated (it is possible that in some cases this may reflect brief study duration), there have been concerns over increased risks of thromboembolic disease (TED). There is also a possibility of adrenal suppression in some patients [92, 93]. The interaction of progestational agents with chemotherapy requires further study [94] and the benefits of combining them with other agents or resistance exercise remain to be established. It is unclear how these drugs exert their effects but they may modulate cytokines [95], insulin-like growth factor [96], or neuropeptides [97]. While it is not possible to advocate the generalised use of these agents on the available data, certain carefully selected patients, particularly those with significant anorexia, may benefit from them. The possible increase in TED should inform patient selection and counselling. The potential for tumour progression in some patients should also be borne in mind [98]. Whether progestagens should be combined with testosterone or specialised nutrition, for example, remains to be determined, as does optimum dosing and duration of therapy [99].

### Corticosteroids

Several corticosteroids have been used in cancer cachexia [100–102] with documented improvements in mood and appetite. However, their impact may not last beyond a few weeks and they can cause substantial morbidity. While undesirable effects such as increased protein catabolism, myopathy and immune suppression will render these agents unsuitable for many with cancer cachexia, the risk/benefit ratio may be acceptable in certain situations, in which case dexamethasone is a reasonable choice.

### Other Appetite Stimulants

Other appetite stimulants that have been investigated include dronabinol [103, 104] and cyproheptadine [105]. There is currently little evidence to recommend the general use of these drugs. Recommendations on the use of appetite stimulants in oncology have been published recently [106].

### Anabolic Drugs

#### Anabolic-Androgenic Steroids and Other Anabolic Steroids

Anabolic steroids are analogues of testosterone that can increase lean body mass [107, 108] and increase weight and activity in hypogonadal males [109, 110]. Although a proportion of cancer patients may be hypogonadal [111], the role of these drugs and how they should be combined with other modalities (e.g. physical therapy, nutrition and anti-inflammatory/anti-catabolic therapies) in cancer cachexia is currently unclear. As with other anabolic agents there has been some concern that tumour growth may be promoted. There has also been wariness of potential toxicity. Once again, present data can lend support to opposing points of view. In two contemporary studies, oxandrolone was reported to improve weight, lean body mass, performance status and quality of life [112, 113] but fluoxymesterone (an anabolic corticosteroid) seemed unimpressive in a trial comparing it with dexamethasone and megestrol acetate [114]. At the moment, these drugs need further study to identify their place in treating cancer cachexia. In particular, it is unclear which drugs are optimal and how they should be administered (e.g. alone or in combination), which route of administration is to be preferred, what doses are optimal, what nutrients should be combined with anabolic steroids and, if appropriate, whether they should be integrated with physical therapy.

### Recombinant Human Growth Hormone

This is an anabolic agent that has been little studied in oncology [115], possibly in part due to concerns over tumour growth promotion, although these effects are still uncertain [116–119]. Its physiological effects include increased fat metabolism and enhanced protein synthesis and it has been studied in HIV/AIDS wasting, where it has increased lean body mass and improved laboratory exercise parameters [120]. Its role in cancer patients is currently unclear.

### Other Anabolic Drugs

This category of unproven drugs includes insulin alone or in combination [121–123] and clenbuterol [124, 125]. Myostatin is a powerful inhibitor of skeletal muscle growth that may be a potential therapeutic target [126].

### Anti-cytokine and Anti-inflammatory Agents

Pentoxifylline and hydrazine sulphate both appear to modulate TNF but contemporary evidence does not support their use in weight-losing cancer patients [127–130].

Thalidomide and melatonin [131–134] are two agents for which there is some early evidence of clinical benefit. Melatonin has been studied in combination with chemotherapy and may modulate efficacy and toxicity [135]. Along with thalidomide it is a candidate for further study. Neither agent can currently be recommended for routine

use in cancer cachexia. Although much of the available evidence suggests that multiple pathways are likely to be important, TNF has been afforded a key role in cachexia. Antibodies to TNF are now available and signal a further approach to cachexia therapy. At this time their potential is unknown [136–138].

Both progestagens and the polyunsaturated fatty acid EPA [139] have anti-cytokine properties and have been discussed above. EPA is also an anti-inflammatory agent. Non-steroidal anti-inflammatory drugs (NSAIDs) have been studied alone and in combination with other drugs and there are data to support a role for them in the management of cachexia [140–143]. An NSAID and progestagen combination has activity in patients with advanced gastrointestinal cancer with effects on weight and quality of life and the combination deserves further study [144]. Selective cyclo-oxygenase-2 (COX-2) inhibitors may also modulate cachexia with an improved side-effect profile over traditional NSAIDs but they require further investigation [145–147]. While there is experimental evidence in tumour-bearing animals that NSAIDs may beneficially affect skeletal muscle mass [148], it is also important to note that the interaction between inflammation and muscle repair is incompletely understood [149] and there are suggestions that the COX-2 pathway is important in skeletal muscle regeneration [150].

Macrolide antibiotics can reduce inflammation; they may also have anti-tumour effects and modulate anti-cancer therapy [151–154] and they stimulate gastric emptying. Whether or not a possible anti-cachexia effect is independent of antibacterial activity is uncertain. This class of drugs has already been used in small clinical trials of advanced cancer and appears worthy of further study [155, 156]. The cholesterol-lowering statins also have anti-inflammatory activity, but did not prevent muscle wasting in a rat model [157].

### Additional Agents

Angiotensin-converting enzyme inhibitors are currently under investigation in cancer cachexia. They have a number of possible physiological effects including anti-inflammatory activity, suppression of tumour growth, angiogenesis inhibition and beneficial effects on muscle function [158, 159].

Adenosine 5'-triphosphate has been studied with some evidence of benefit in patients with advanced lung cancer [160, 161]. Another way of increasing high-energy phosphate compounds may be by supplementing with oral creatine. This is recognised as having beneficial effects in certain types of athletic performance (although there are conflicting reports [162, 163]), and in a clinical study of older men it improved their muscular performance [164]. There have been some concerns over safety, which has been reviewed recently [165].

Recombinant human erythropoietin (and darbopoietin) may be used to overcome anaemia and promote exercise capacity as part of an overall strategy to improve performance [166–168]. However, it also has growth factor properties and there have been recent concerns over possible deleterious effects on tumours [169, 170].

Any therapeutic role for nitric oxide modulation remains to be determined [171, 172].

Beta-blockers have been suggested as agents that might modulate REE in hypermetabolic cachectic patients. It is possible that this may in part be mediated by the autonomic nervous system [173–175]. These agents require further study [176].

## Conclusions

Optimising nutritional therapy (including the nutraceutical component), pharmacological therapy and other modalities (such as physical therapy) and identifying effective combinations of these remain a challenge in cancer cachexia. Similarly, the means by which these diverse approaches should be integrated into patient care and combined with anti-tumour therapies remains to be resolved. The efficient assessment of potential therapies may benefit from regular horizon scanning, prioritisation of therapeutic targets and strategies for the rational selection of combinations [147, 177, 178], the strengthening of ties with other disciplines and cooperative studies. Experience to date suggests that attempts at obtaining consensus on the duration of clinical trials, defining optimum end-points, standardising assessment methods and trying to stratify patients by predominant metabolic abnormalities may all be worthwhile endeavours.

## References

1. Palesty JA, Dudrick SJ (2003) What we have learned about cachexia in gastrointestinal cancer. Dig Dis 21:198–213
2. Inui A (2002) Cancer anorexia-cachexia syndrome: current issues in research and management. CA Cancer J Clin 52:72–91
3. Crown AL, Cottle K, Lightman SL et al (2002) What is the role of the insulin-like growth factor system in the pathophysiology of cancer cachexia, and how is it regulated? Clin Endocrinol (Oxf) 56:723–733
4. Brink M, Anwar A, Delafontaine P (2002) Neurohormonal factors in the development of catabolic/anabolic imbalance and cachexia. Int J Cardiol 85:111–121; discussion 121–124
5. Heber D, Byerley LO, Tchekmedyian NS (1992) Hormonal and metabolic abnormalities in the malnourished cancer patient: effects on host-tumor interaction. JPEN J Parenter Enteral Nutr 16:60S–64S
6. Dewys WD, Begg C, Lavin PT et al (1980) Prognostic effect of weight loss prior to chemotherapy in cancer patients. Eastern Cooperative Oncology Group.

Am J Med 69:491
7. Tohgo A, Kumazawa E, Akahane K et al (2002) Anticancer drugs that induce cancer-associated cachectic syndromes. Expert Rev Anticancer Ther 2:121–129
8. Bauer J, Capra S (2003) Comparison of a malnutrition screening tool with subjective global assessment in hospitalised patients with cancer – sensitivity and specificity. Asia Pac J Clin Nutr 12:257–260
9. Ottery FD (1996) Definition of standardized nutritional assessment and interventional pathways in oncology. Nutrition 12:S15–S19
10. Davis CH (1994) The report to Congress on the appropriate federal role in assuring access by medical students, residents, and practicing physicians to adequate training in nutrition. Public Health Rep 109:824–826
11. Werneke U, Earl J, Seydel C et al (2004) Potential health risks of complementary alternative medicines in cancer patients. Br J Cancer 90:408–413
12. Cassidy A (2003) Are herbal remedies and dietary supplements safe and effective for breast cancer

patients? Breast Cancer Res 5:300–302

13. Jatoi A, Daly BD, Hughes VA et al (2001) Do patients with nonmetastatic non-small cell lung cancer demonstrate altered resting energy expenditure? Ann Thorac Surg 72:348–351

14. Ardies CM (2002) Exercise, cachexia, and cancer therapy: a molecular rationale. Nutr Cancer 42:143–157

15. Al-Majid S, McCarthy DO (2001) Cancer-induced fatigue and skeletal muscle wasting: the role of exercise. Biol Res Nurs 2:186–197

16. Al-Majid S, McCarthy DO (2001) Resistance exercise training attenuates wasting of the extensor digitorum longus muscle in mice bearing the colon-26 adenocarcinoma. Biol Res Nurs 2:155–166

17. Daneryd P (2002) Epoetin alfa for protection of metabolic and exercise capacity in cancer patients. Semin Oncol 29:69–74

18. Bosaeus I, Daneryd P, Svanberg E, Lundholm K (2001) Dietary intake and resting energy expenditure in relation to weight loss in unselected cancer patients. Int J Cancer 93:380–383

19. Braunschweig C, Gomez S, Sheean PM (2000) Impact of declines in nutritional status on outcomes in adult patients hospitalized for more than 7 days. J Am Diet Assoc 100:1316–1322

20. Ravera E, Bozzetti F, Ammatuna M, Radaelli G (1987) Impact of hospitalization on the nutritional status of cancer patients. Tumori 73:375–380

21. Laviano A, Meguid MM, Rossi-Fanelli F (2003) Cancer anorexia: clinical implications, pathogenesis, and therapeutic strategies. Lancet Oncol 4:686–694

22. McNurlan MA, Heys SD, Park KG et al (1994) Tumour and host tissue responses to branched-chain amino acid supplementation of patients with cancer. Clin Sci (Lond) 86:339–345

23. Heys SD, Park KG, McNurlan MA et al (1991) Stimulation of protein synthesis in human tumours by parenteral nutrition: evidence for modulation of tumour growth. Br J Surg 78:483–487

24. Park KG, Heys SD, Blessing K et al (1992) Stimulation of human breast cancers by dietary L-arginine. Clin Sci (Lond) 82:413–417

25. Preston T, Slater C, McMillan DC et al (1998) Fibrinogen synthesis is elevated in fasting cancer patients with an acute phase response. J Nutr 128:1355–1360

26. Hochwald SN, Harrison LE, Port JL et al (1996) Depletion of high energy phosphate compounds in the tumor-bearing state and reversal after tumor resection. Surgery 120:534–541

27. Donaldson SS, Lenon RA (1979) Alterations of nutritional status: impact of chemotherapy and radiation therapy. Cancer 43:2036–2052

28. Samuels SE, Knowles AL, Tilignac T et al (2000) Protein metabolism in the small intestine during cancer cachexia and chemotherapy in mice. Cancer Res 60:4968–4974

29. Nelson K, Walsh D, Sheehan F (2002) Cancer and chemotherapy-related upper gastrointestinal symptoms: the role of abnormal gastric motor function and its evaluation in cancer patients. Support Care Cancer 10:455–461

30. Lawson DH, Nixon DW, Kutner MH et al (1981) Enteral versus parenteral nutritional support in cancer patients. Cancer Treat Rep 65:101–106

31. Mercadante S (1998) Parenteral versus enteral nutrition in cancer patients: indications and practice. Support Care Cancer 6:85–93

32. Torosian MH, Jalali S, Nguyen HQ (1990) Protein intake and 5-fluorouracil toxicity in tumor-bearing animals. J Surg Res 49:298–301

33. Torosian MH, Mullen JL, Miller EE et al (1988) Reduction of methotrexate toxicity with improved nutritional status in tumor-bearing animals. Cancer 61:1731–1735

34. De Cicco M, Panarello G, Fantin D et al (1993) Parenteral nutrition in cancer patients receiving chemotherapy: effects on toxicity and nutritional status. JPEN J Parenter Enteral Nutr 17:513–518

35. McGeer AJ, Detsky AS, O'Rourke K (1990) Parenteral nutrition in cancer patients undergoing chemotherapy: a meta-analysis. Nutrition 6:233–240

36. Chlebowski RT (1985) Critical evaluation of the role of nutritional support with chemotherapy. Cancer 55:268–272

37. Evans WK, Nixon DW, Daly JM et al (1987) A randomized study of oral nutritional support versus ad lib nutritional intake during chemotherapy for advanced colorectal and non-small-cell lung cancer. J Clin Oncol 5:113–124

38. Ovesen L, Allingstrup L, Hannibal J et al (1993) Effect of dietary counseling on food intake, body weight, response rate, survival, and quality of life in cancer patients undergoing chemotherapy: a prospective, randomized study. J Clin Oncol 11:2043–2049

39. Fearon KC, Von Meyenfeldt MF, Moses AG et al (2003) Effect of a protein and energy dense N-3 fatty acid enriched oral supplement on loss of weight and lean tissue in cancer cachexia: a randomised double blind trial. Gut 52:1479–1486

40. Cohn SH, Gartenhaus W, Vartsky D et al (1981) Body composition and dietary intake in neoplastic disease. Am J Clin Nutr 34:1997–2004

41. Shaw JH (1988) Influence of stress, depletion, and/or malignant disease on the responsiveness of surgical patients to total parenteral nutrition. Am J Clin Nutr 48:144–147

42. Jeevanandam M, Legaspi A, Lowry SF et al (1988) Effect of total parenteral nutrition on whole body protein kinetics in cachectic patients with benign or malignant disease. JPEN J Parenter Enteral Nutr 12:229–236

43. Hyltander A, Warnold I, Eden E, Lundholm K (1991) Effect on whole-body protein synthesis after institution of intravenous nutrition in cancer and non-cancer patients who lose weight. Eur J Cancer

27:16–21

44. Bennegard K, Eden E, Ekman L et al (1983) Metabolic response of whole body and peripheral tissues to enteral nutrition in weight-losing cancer and noncancer patients. Gastroenterology 85:92–99

45. Edstrom S, Bennegard K, Eden E, Lundholm K (1982) Energy and tissue metabolism in patients with cancer during nutritional support. Arch Otolaryngol 108:697–699

46. Nixon DW, Lawson DH, Kutner M et al (1981) Hyperalimentation of the cancer patient with protein-calorie undernutrition. Cancer Res 41:2038–2045

47. Barber MD, Preston T, McMillan DC et al (2004) Modulation of the liver export protein synthetic response to feeding by an n-3 fatty-acid-enriched nutritional supplement is associated with anabolism in cachectic cancer patients. Clin Sci (Lond) 106:359–364

48. Heys SD, Walker LG, Smith I, Eremin O (1999) Enteral nutritional supplementation with key nutrients in patients with critical illness and cancer: a meta-analysis of randomized controlled clinical trials. Ann Surg 229:467–477

49. McCarthy DO (2003) Rethinking nutritional support for persons with cancer cachexia. Biol Res Nurs 5:3–17

50. Tisdale MJ, Brennan RA (1988) A comparison of long-chain triglycerides and medium-chain triglycerides on weight loss and tumour size in a cachexia model. Br J Cancer 58:580–583

51. Smith HJ, Greenberg NA, Tisdale MJ (2004) Effect of eicosapentaenoic acid, protein and amino acids on protein synthesis and degradation in skeletal muscle of cachectic mice. Br J Cancer 91:408–412

52. Ross JA, Fearon KC (2002) Eicosanoid-dependent cancer cachexia and wasting. Curr Opin Clin Nutr Metab Care 5:241–248

53. Calder PC (2002) Dietary modification of inflammation with lipids. Proc Nutr Soc 61:345–358

54. Grimble RF, Howell WM, O'Reilly G et al (2002) The ability of fish oil to suppress tumor necrosis factor alpha production by peripheral blood mononuclear cells in healthy men is associated with polymorphisms in genes that influence tumor necrosis factor alpha production. Am J Clin Nutr 76:454–459

55. Wigmore SJ, Fearon KC, Maingay JP, Ross JA (1999) Down-regulation of the acute-phase response in patients with pancreatic cancer cachexia receiving oral eicosapentaenoic acid is mediated via suppression of interleukin-6. Clin Sci (Lond) 92:215–221

56. Tisdale MJ (2004) Cancer cachexia. Langenbecks Arch Surg 389:299–305

57. Lazarus DD, Destree AT, Mazzola LM et al (1999) A new model of cancer cachexia: contribution of the ubiquitin-proteasome pathway. Am J Physiol 277:E332–E341

58. Whitehouse AS, Tisdale MJ (2003) Increased expression of the ubiquitin-proteasome pathway in murine myotubes by proteolysis-inducing factor (PIF) is associated with activation of the transcription factor NF-kappaB. Br J Cancer 89:1116–1122

59. Togni V, Ota CC, Folador A et al (2003) Cancer cachexia and tumor growth reduction in Walker 256 tumor-bearing rats supplemented with N-3 polyunsaturated fatty acids for one generation. Nutr Cancer 46:52–58

60. Jho DH, Babcock TA, Tevar R et al (2002) Eicosapentaenoic acid supplementation reduces tumor volume and attenuates cachexia in a rat model of progressive non-metastasizing malignancy. JPEN J Parenter Enteral Nutr 26:291–297

61. Hardman WE, Moyer MP, Cameron IL (2002) Consumption of an omega-3 fatty acids product, INCELL AAFA, reduced side-effects of CPT-11 (irinotecan) in mice. Br J Cancer 86:983–988

62. Hardman WE (2002) Omega-3 fatty acids to augment cancer therapy. J Nutr 132:3508S–3512S

63. Barber MD, Fearon KC (2001) Tolerance and incorporation of a high-dose eicosapentaenoic acid diester emulsion by patients with pancreatic cancer cachexia. Lipids 36:347–351

64. Wigmore SJ, Barber MD, Ross JA et al (2000) Effect of oral eicosapentaenoic acid on weight loss in patients with pancreatic cancer. Nutr Cancer 36:177–184

65. Moses AW, Slater C, Preston T et al (2004) Reduced total energy expenditure and physical activity in cachectic patients with pancreatic cancer can be modulated by an energy and protein dense oral supplement enriched with n-3 fatty acids. Br J Cancer 90:996–1002

66. Ferrando AA, Stuart CA, Sheffield-Moore M, Wolfe RR (1999) Inactivity amplifies the catabolic response of skeletal muscle to cortisol. J Clin Endocrinol Metab 84:3515–3521

67. Jatoi A, Rowland KM, Loprinzi CL et al (2003) An eicosapentaenoic acid (EPA)-enriched supplement versus megestrol acetate (MA) versus both for patients with cancer-associated wasting. A collaborative effort from the North Central Cancer Treatment Group (NCCTG) and the National Cancer Institute of Canada. Proc Am Soc Clin Oncol 22:743 (abs 2987)

68. Bruera E, Strasser F, Palmer JL et al (2003) Effect of fish oil on appetite and other symptoms in patients with advanced cancer and anorexia/cachexia: a double-blind, placebo-controlled study. J Clin Oncol 21:129–134

69. Clark RH, Feleke G, Din M et al (2000) Nutritional treatment for acquired immunodeficiency virus-associated wasting using beta-hydroxy beta-methylbutyrate, glutamine, and arginine: a randomized, double-blind, placebo-controlled study. JPEN J Parenter Enteral Nutr 24:133–139

70. May PE, Barber A, D'Olimpio JT et al (2002) Reversal of cancer-related wasting using oral supplementation with a combination of beta-hydroxy-

beta-methylbutyrate, arginine, and glutamine. Am J Surg 183:471–479

71. Gomes-Marcondes MC, Ventrucci G, Toledo MT et al (2003) A leucine-supplemented diet improved protein content of skeletal muscle in young tumor-bearing rats. Braz J Med Biol Res 36:1589–1594

72. Bartlett DL, Charland S, Torosian MH (1995) Effect of glutamine on tumor and host growth. Ann Surg Oncol 2:71–76

73. Rathmacher JA, Nissen S, Panton L et al (2004) Supplementation with a combination of beta-hydroxy-beta-methylbutyrate (HMB), arginine, and glutamine is safe and could improve hematological parameters. JPEN J Parenter Enteral Nutr 28:65–75

74. Yoshida S, Kaibara A, Ishibashi N, Shirouzu K (2001) Glutamine supplementation in cancer patients. Nutrition 17:766–768

75. Calder PC (2003) Immunonutrition. BMJ 327:117–118

76. McCowen KC, Bistrian BR (2003) Immunonutrition: problematic or problem solving? Am J Clin Nutr 77:764–770

77. Argiles JM, Almendro V, Busquets S, Lopez-Soriano FJ (2004) The pharmacological treatment of cachexia. Curr Drug Targets 5:265–277

78. MacDonald N, Easson AM, Mazurak VC et al (2003) Understanding and managing cancer cachexia. J Am Coll Surg 197:143–161

79. Strasser F, Bruera ED (2002) Update on anorexia and cachexia. Hematol Oncol Clin North Am 16:589–617

80. Pascual Lopez A, Roque i Figuls M, Urrutia Cuchi G et al (2004) Systematic review of megestrol acetate in the treatment of anorexia-cachexia syndrome. J Pain Symptom Manage 27:360–369

81. Aisner J, Parnes H, Tait N et al (1990) Appetite stimulation and weight gain with megestrol acetate. Semin Oncol 17:2–7

82. De Conno F, Martini C, Zecca E et al (1998) Megestrol acetate for anorexia in patients with far-advanced cancer: a double-blind controlled clinical trial. Eur J Cancer 34:1705–1709

83. Bruera E, Ernst S, Hagen N et al (1998) Effectiveness of megestrol acetate in patients with advanced cancer: a randomized, double-blind, crossover study. Cancer Prev Control 2:74–78

84. Lambert CP, Sullivan DH, Freeling SA et al (2002) Effects of testosterone replacement and/or resistance exercise on the composition of megestrol acetate stimulated weight gain in elderly men: a randomized controlled trial. J Clin Endocrinol Metab 87:2100–2106

85. Loprinzi CL, Schaid DJ, Dose AM et al (1993) Body-composition changes in patients who gain weight while receiving megestrol acetate. J Clin Oncol 11:152–154

86. Oster MH, Enders SR, Samuels SJ et al (1994) Megestrol acetate in patients with AIDS and cachexia. Ann Intern Med 121:400–408

87. Von Roenn JH, Knopf K (1996) Anorexia/cachexia in patients with HIV: lessons for the oncologist. Oncology (Huntingt) 10:1049–1056; discussion 1062–1064, 1067–1068

88. Engelson ES, Pi-Sunyer FX, Kotler DP (1995) Effects of megestrol acetate therapy on body composition and circulating testosterone concentrations in patients with AIDS. AIDS 9:1107–1108

89. Beller E, Tattersall M, Lumley T et al (1997) Improved quality of life with megestrol acetate in patients with endocrine-insensitive advanced cancer: a randomised placebo-controlled trial. Australasian Megestrol Acetate Cooperative Study Group. Ann Oncol 8:277–283

90. Tomiska M, Tomiskova M, Salajka F et al (2003) Palliative treatment of cancer anorexia with oral suspension of megestrol acetate. Neoplasma 50:227–233

91. Vadell C, Segui MA, Gimenez-Arnau JM et al (1998) Anticachectic efficacy of megestrol acetate at different doses and versus placebo in patients with neoplastic cachexia. Am J Clin Oncol 21:347–351

92. Meacham LR, Mazewski C, Krawiecki N (2003) Mechanism of transient adrenal insufficiency with megestrol acetate treatment of cachexia in children with cancer. J Pediatr Hematol Oncol 25:414–417

93. Orme LM, Bond JD, Humphrey MS et al (2003) Megestrol acetate in pediatric oncology patients may lead to severe, symptomatic adrenal suppression. Cancer 98:397–405

94. Rowland KM Jr, Loprinzi CL, Shaw EG et al (1996) Randomized double-blind placebo-controlled trial of cisplatin and etoposide plus megestrol acetate/placebo in extensive-stage small-cell lung cancer: a North Central Cancer Treatment Group study. J Clin Oncol 14:135–141

95. Mantovani G, Macciò A, Lai P et al (1998) Cytokine involvement in cancer anorexia/cachexia: role of megestrol acetate and medroxyprogesterone acetate on cytokine downregulation and improvement of clinical symptoms. Crit Rev Oncog 9:99–106

96. Helle SI, Lundgren S, Geisler S et al (1999) Effects of treatment with megestrol acetate on the insulin-like growth factor system: time and dose dependency. Eur J Cancer 35:1070–1075

97. McCarthy HD, Crowder RE, Dryden S, Williams G (1994) Megestrol acetate stimulates food and water intake in the rat: effects on regional hypothalamic neuropeptide Y concentrations. Eur J Pharmacol 265:99–102

98. Tassinari D, Fochessati F, Panzini I et al (2003) Rapid progression of advanced 'hormone-resistant' prostate cancer during palliative treatment with progestins for cancer cachexia. J Pain Symptom Manage 25:481–484

99. Maltoni M, Nanni O, Scarpi E et al (2001) High-dose progestins for the treatment of cancer anorexia-cachexia syndrome: a systematic review of randomised clinical trials. Ann Oncol 12:289–300

100. Willox JC, Corr J, Shaw J et al (1984) Prednisolone as an appetite stimulant in patients with cancer. Br Med J (Clin Res Ed) 288:27

101. Della Cuna GR, Pellegrini A, Piazzi M (1989) Effect of methylprednisolone sodium succinate on quality of life in preterminal cancer patients: a placebo-controlled, multicenter study. The Methylprednisolone Preterminal Cancer Study Group. Eur J Cancer Clin Oncol 25:1817–1821

102. Moertel CG, Schutt AJ, Reitemeier RJ, Hahn RG (1974) Corticosteroid therapy of preterminal gastrointestinal cancer. Cancer 33:1607–1609

103. Jatoi A, Windschitl HE, Loprinzi CL et al (2002) Dronabinol versus megestrol acetate versus combination therapy for cancer-associated anorexia: a North Central Cancer Treatment Group study. J Clin Oncol 20:567–573

104. Walsh D, Nelson KA, Mahmoud FA (2003) Established and potential therapeutic applications of cannabinoids in oncology. Support Care Cancer 11:137–143

105. Kardinal CG, Loprinzi CL, Schaid DJ et al (1990) A controlled trial of cyproheptadine in cancer patients with anorexia and/or cachexia. Cancer 65:2657–2662

106. Desport JC, Gory-Delabaere G, Blanc-Vincent MP et al (2003) Standards, options and recommendations for the use of appetite stimulants in oncology (2000). Br J Cancer 89(Suppl 1):S98–S100

107. Basaria S, Wahlstrom JT, Dobs AS (2001) Clinical review 138: anabolic-androgenic steroid therapy in the treatment of chronic diseases. J Clin Endocrinol Metab 86:5108–5117

108. Langer CJ, Hoffman JP, Ottery FD (2001) Clinical significance of weight loss in cancer patients: rationale for the use of anabolic agents in the treatment of cancer-related cachexia. Nutrition 17:S1–S20

109. Mudali S, Dobs AS (2004) Effects of testosterone on body composition of the aging male. Mech Ageing Dev 125:297–304

110. Franchimont P, Kicovic PM, Mattei A, Roulier R (1978) Effects of oral testosterone undecanoate in hypogonadal male patients. Clin Endocrinol (Oxf) 9:313–320

111. Simons JP, Schols AM, Buurman WA, Wouters EF (1999) Weight loss and low body cell mass in males with lung cancer: relationship with systemic inflammation, acute-phase response, resting energy expenditure, and catabolic and anabolic hormones. Clin Sci (Lond) 97:215–223

112. Tchekmedyian S, Fesen M, Price LM, Ottery FD (2003) Ongoing placebo-controlled study of oxandrolone in cancer-related weight loss. Int J Radiat Oncol Biol Phys 57:S283-S284

113. Muurahainen N, Mulligan K (1998) Clinical trials update in human immunodeficiency virus wasting. Semin Oncol 25:104–111

114. Loprinzi CL, Kugler JW, Sloan JA et al (1999) Randomized comparison of megestrol acetate versus dexamethasone versus fluoxymesterone for the treatment of cancer anorexia/cachexia. J Clin Oncol 17:3299–3306

115. Binnerts A, Uitterlinden P, Hofland LJ et al (1990) The in vitro and in vivo effects of human growth hormone administration on tumor growth of rats bearing a transplantable rat pituitary tumor (7315b). Eur J Cancer 26:269–276

116. Bartlett DL, Stein TP, Torosian MH (1995) Effect of growth hormone and protein intake on tumor growth and host cachexia. Surgery 117:260–267

117. Fiebig HH, Dengler W, Hendriks HR (2000) No evidence of tumor growth stimulation in human tumors in vitro following treatment with recombinant human growth hormone. Anticancer Drugs 11:659–664

118. Ng B, Wolf RF, Weksler B et al (1993) Growth hormone administration preserves lean body mass in sarcoma-bearing rats treated with doxorubicin. Cancer Res 53:5483–5486

119. Torosian MH (1993) Growth hormone and prostate cancer growth and metastasis in tumor-bearing animals. J Pediatr Endocrinol 6:93–97

120. Mulligan K, Tai VW, Schambelan M (1999) Use of growth hormone and other anabolic agents in AIDS wasting. JPEN J Parenter Enteral Nutr 23:S202–S209

121. Bartlett DL, Charland S, Torosian MH (1994) Growth hormone, insulin, and somatostatin therapy of cancer cachexia. Cancer 73:1499–1504

122. Piffar PM, Fernandez R, Tchaikovski O et al (2003) Naproxen, clenbuterol and insulin administration ameliorates cancer cachexia and reduces tumor growth in Walker 256 tumor-bearing rats. Cancer Lett 201:139–148

123. Moley JF, Morrison SD, Norton JA (1985) Insulin reversal of cancer cachexia in rats. Cancer Res 45:4925–4931

124. Carbo N, Lopez-Soriano J, Tarrago T et al (1997) Comparative effects of beta2-adrenergic agonists on muscle waste associated with tumour growth. Cancer Lett 115:113–118

125. Hyltander A, Svaninger G, Lundholm K (1993) The effect of clenbuterol on body composition in spontaneously eating tumour-bearing mice. Biosci Rep 13:325–331

126. Zimmers TA, Davies MV, Koniaris LG et al (2002) Induction of cachexia in mice by systemically administered myostatin. Science 296:1486–1488

127. Goldberg RM, Loprinzi CL, Mailliard JA et al (1995) Pentoxifylline for treatment of cancer anorexia and cachexia? A randomized, double-blind, placebo-controlled trial. J Clin Oncol 13:2856–2859

128. Kosty MP, Fleishman SB, Herndon JE 2nd et al (1994) Cisplatin, vinblastine, and hydrazine sulfate in advanced, non-small-cell lung cancer: a randomized placebo-controlled, double-blind phase III study of the Cancer and Leukemia Group B. J Clin Oncol 12:1113–1120

129. Loprinzi CL, Kuross SA, O'Fallon JR et al (1994) Randomized placebo-controlled evaluation of

hydrazine sulfate in patients with advanced colorectal cancer. J Clin Oncol 12:1121–1125

130. Loprinzi CL, Goldberg RM, Su JQ et al (1994) Placebo-controlled trial of hydrazine sulfate in patients with newly diagnosed non-small-cell lung cancer. J Clin Oncol 12:1126–1129

131. Khan ZH, Simpson EJ, Cole AT et al (2003) Oesophageal cancer and cachexia: the effect of short-term treatment with thalidomide on weight loss and lean body mass. Aliment Pharmacol Ther 17:677–682

132. Zhou S, Kestell P, Tingle MD, Paxton JW (2002) Thalidomide in cancer treatment: a potential role in the elderly? Drugs Aging 19:85–100

133. Fanelli M, Sarmiento R, Gattuso D et al (2003) Thalidomide: a new anticancer drug? Expert Opin Investig Drugs 12:1211–1225

134. Lissoni P (2002) Is there a role for melatonin in supportive care? Support Care Cancer 10:110–116

135. Lissoni P, Barni S, Mandala M et al (1999) Decreased toxicity and increased efficacy of cancer chemotherapy using the pineal hormone melatonin in metastatic solid tumour patients with poor clinical status. Eur J Cancer 35:1688–1692

136. Siegel SA, Shealy DJ, Nakada MT et al (1995) The mouse/human chimeric monoclonal antibody cA2 neutralizes TNF in vitro and protects transgenic mice from cachexia and TNF lethality in vivo. Cytokine 7:15–25

137. Anker SD, Coats AJ (2002) How to RECOVER from RENAISSANCE? The significance of the results of RECOVER, RENAISSANCE, RENEWAL and ATTACH. Int J Cardiol 86:123–130

138. Mann DL, McMurray JJ, Packer M et al (2004) Targeted anticytokine therapy in patients with chronic heart failure: results of the Randomized Etanercept Worldwide Evaluation (RENEWAL). Circulation 109:1594–1602

139. Jho DH, Cole SM, Lee EM, Espat NJ (2004) Role of omega-3 fatty acid supplementation in inflammation and malignancy. Integr Cancer Ther 3:98–111

140. Preston T, Fearon KC, McMillan DC et al (1995) Effect of ibuprofen on the acute-phase response and protein metabolism in patients with cancer and weight loss. Br J Surg 82:229–234

141. Eli Y, Przedecki F, Levin G et al (2001) Comparative effects of indomethacin on cell proliferation and cell cycle progression in tumor cells grown in vitro and in vivo. Biochem Pharmacol 61:565–571

142. Lundholm K, Daneryd P, Korner U et al (2004) Evidence that long-term COX-treatment improves energy homeostasis and body composition in cancer patients with progressive cachexia. Int J Oncol 24:505–512

143. Lundholm K, Gelin J, Hyltander A et al (1994) Anti-inflammatory treatment may prolong survival in undernourished patients with metastatic solid tumors. Cancer Res 54:5602–5606

144. McMillan DC, Wigmore SJ, Fearon KC et al (1999) A prospective randomized study of megestrol acetate and ibuprofen in gastrointestinal cancer patients with weight loss. Br J Cancer 79:495–500

145. Davis TW, Zweifel BS, O'Neal JM et al (2004) Inhibition of cyclooxygenase-2 by celecoxib reverses tumor-induced wasting. J Pharmacol Exp Ther 308:929–934

146. Hussey HJ, Tisdale MJ (2000) Effect of the specific cyclooxygenase-2 inhibitor meloxicam on tumour growth and cachexia in a murine model. Int J Cancer 87:95–100

147. Lundholm K, Daneryd P, Bosaeus I et al (2004) Palliative nutritional intervention in addition to cyclooxygenase and erythropoietin treatment for patients with malignant disease: effects on survival, metabolism, and function. Cancer 100:1967–1977

148. McCarthy DO, Whitney P, Hitt A, Al-Majid S (2004) Indomethacin and ibuprofen preserve gastrocnemius muscle mass in mice bearing the colon-26 adenocarcinoma. Res Nurs Health 27:174–184

149. Prisk V, Huard J (2003) Muscle injuries and repair: the role of prostaglandins and inflammation. Histol Histopathol 18:1243–1256

150. Bondesen BA, Mills ST, Kegley KM, Pavlath GK (2004) The COX-2 pathway is essential during early stages of skeletal muscle regeneration. Am J Physiol Cell Physiol 287:C475–C483

151. Hamada K, Mikasa K, Yunou Y et al (2000) Adjuvant effect of clarithromycin on chemotherapy for murine lung cancer. Chemotherapy 46:49–61

152. Ianaro A, Ialenti A, Maffia P et al (2000) Anti-inflammatory activity of macrolide antibiotics. J Pharmacol Exp Ther 292:156–163

153. Suzaki H, Asano K, Ohki S et al (1999) Suppressive activity of a macrolide antibiotic, roxithromycin, on pro-inflammatory cytokine production in vitro and in vivo. Mediators Inflamm 8:199–204

154. Boffa DJ, Luan F, Thomas D et al (2004) Rapamycin inhibits the growth and metastatic progression of non-small cell lung cancer. Clin Cancer Res 10:293–300

155. Sakamoto M, Mikasa K, Majima T et al (2001) Anti-cachectic effect of clarithromycin for patients with unresectable non-small cell lung cancer. Chemotherapy 47:444–451

156. Mikasa K, Sawaki M, Kita E et al (1997) Significant survival benefit to patients with advanced non-small-cell lung cancer from treatment with clarithromycin. Chemotherapy 43:288–296

157. Muscaritoli M, Costelli P, Bossola M et al (2003) Effects of simvastatin administration in an experimental model of cancer cachexia. Nutrition 19:936–939

158. Onder G, Penninx BW, Balkrishnan R et al (2002) Relation between use of angiotensin-converting enzyme inhibitors and muscle strength and physical function in older women: an observational study. Lancet 359:926–930

159. Yoshiji H, Kuriyama S, Fukui H (2002) Perindopril: possible use in cancer therapy. Anticancer Drugs

13:221–228

160. Agteresch HJ, Burgers SA, van der Gaast A et al (2003) Randomized clinical trial of adenosine 5'-triphosphate on tumor growth and survival in advanced lung cancer patients. Anticancer Drugs 14:639–644

161. Walsh TD, Rivera NI (2002) Adenosine triphosphate for cancer cachexia. Curr Oncol Rep 4:231–232

162. Izquierdo M, Ibanez J, Gonzalez-Badillo JJ, Gorostiaga EM (2002) Effects of creatine supplementation on muscle power, endurance, and sprint performance. Med Sci Sports Exerc 34:332–343

163. Lemon PW (2002) Dietary creatine supplementation and exercise performance: why inconsistent results? Can J Appl Physiol 27:663–681

164. Gotshalk LA, Volek JS, Staron RS et al (2002) Creatine supplementation improves muscular performance in older men. Med Sci Sports Exerc 34:537–543

165. Terjung RL, Clarkson P, Eichner ER et al (2000) American College of Sports Medicine roundtable. The physiological and health effects of oral creatine supplementation. Med Sci Sports Exerc 32:706–717

166. Evans WJ (2002) Physical function in men and women with cancer. Effects of anemia and conditioning. Oncology (Huntingt) 16:109–115

167. Kotasek D, Steger G, Faught W et al (2003) Aranesp 980291 Study Group. Darbepoetin alfa administered every 3 weeks alleviates anaemia in patients with solid tumours receiving chemotherapy; results of a double-blind, placebo-controlled, randomised study. Eur J Cancer 39:2026–2034

168. Daneryd P, Svanberg E, Korner U et al (1998) Protection of metabolic and exercise capacity in unselected weight-losing cancer patients following treatment with recombinant erythropoietin: a randomized prospective study. Cancer Res Dec 58:5374–5379

169. Yasuda Y, Fujita Y, Matsuo T et al (2003) Erythropoietin regulates tumour growth of human malignancies. Carcinogenesis 24:1021–1029. Erratum in: Carcinogenesis 24:1567

170. Brower V (2003) Erythropoietin may impair, not improve, cancer survival. Nat Med 9:1439

171. Cahlin C, Gelin J, Delbro D et al (2000) Effect of cyclooxygenase and nitric oxide synthase inhibitors on tumor growth in mouse tumor models with and without cancer cachexia related to prostanoids. Cancer Res 60:1742–1749

172. Terao H, Asano K, Kanai K et al (2003) Suppressive activity of macrolide antibiotics on nitric oxide production by lipopolysaccharide stimulation in mice. Mediators Inflamm 12:195–202

173. Gambardella A, Tortoriello R, Pesce L et al (1999) Intralipid infusion combined with propranolol administration has favorable metabolic effects in elderly malnourished cancer patients. Metabolism 48:291–297

174. Brooks SL, Neville AM, Rothwell NJ et al (1981) Sympathetic activation of brown-adipose-tissue thermogenesis in cachexia. Biosci Rep 1:509–517

175. Hyltander A, Korner U, Lundholm KG (1993) Evaluation of mechanisms behind elevated energy expenditure in cancer patients with solid tumours. Eur J Clin Invest 23:46–52

176. Hyltander A, Daneryd P, Sandstrom R et al (2000) Beta-adrenoceptor activity and resting energy metabolism in weight losing cancer patients. Eur J Cancer 36:330–334

177. Pinto JA Jr, Folador A, Bonato SJ et al (2004) Fish oil supplementation in F1 generation associated with naproxen, clenbuterol, and insulin administration reduce tumor growth and cachexia in Walker 256 tumor-bearing rats. J Nutr Biochem 15:358–365

178. Cerchietti LC, Navigante AH, Peluffo GD et al (2004) Effects of celecoxib, medroxyprogesterone, and dietary intervention on systemic syndromes in patients with advanced lung adenocarcinoma: a pilot study. J Pain Symptom Manage 27:85–95

# A Critical Assessment of the Outcome Measures and Goals of Intervention in Cancer Cachexia

Kenneth C.H. Fearon, Richard J.E. Skipworth

## Introduction

Cancer cachexia is a multifactorial, multifaceted problem for which there is no uniform pathophysiological or clinical definition [1]. It is generally accepted as a complex syndrome with several cardinal features, including anorexia, early satiety, severe weight loss, muscle wasting, ischaemia, anaemia and oedema [2]. The essential characteristic that distinguishes cachexia from simple starvation is that the features of cachexia cannot be readily reversed by nutritional support alone [3].

Cachexia appears even more complex when we attempt to judge the success or failure of any proposed therapy for its amelioration. The Food and Drug Administration has recently indicated that, in order for a treatment to be licensed for the management of cachexia, there must be a documented improvement in both the nutritional and functional status of a patient so treated [4]. But what outcome variables should we measure to assess this improvement?

## Measures of Nutritional and Functional Status

Classically, nutritional status has been assessed by simple measurements of body weight, body mass index (BMI), anthropometry or body composition (e.g. lean body mass [LBM], body cell mass [BCM]). More advanced methods of assessing physiological/metabolic aspects of nutritional status have also been advocated, including resting energy expenditure (REE), muscle fatigue, immune function and protein kinetics. Nutritional outcomes that have been assessed in cachexia intervention trials have included a variety of these anthropometric/biochemical [5–8] and physiological variables [8–10] (Fig. 1).

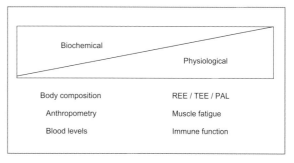

**Fig. 1.** Nutritional outcomes. *REE*, resting energy expenditure; *TEE*, total energy expenditure; *PAL*, physical activity level

Clinically useful end-points to assay changes in functional status have proved more controversial. One basic method that simply relies on subjective questioning of patients about current activities is physician-assessed performance score (PS) (e.g. the Karnofsky PS score or the World Health Organization [WHO] PS score).

Objective techniques used to assess functional status in cachexia intervention trials have included treadmill tests [11, 12] and handgrip dynamometry [13]. Recently, spontaneous physical activity has been proposed as a more useful index of patient-orientated quality of life (QoL) [1]. This proposition will be discussed later in this chapter.

## The Challenge of Nutritional Intervention Trials in Cancer Cachexia

In general, trials of clinical nutrition begin with the observation that a particular disease and/or its treatment are associated with adverse clinical outcomes. It is also observed that, during the course of this disease, patients demonstrate deteriorating nutritional status. The hypothesis is then derived that disease-related deterioration in nutritional status may contribute to the overall adverse clinical outcomes. The challenge in clinical trials is to develop a nutritional intervention of sufficient efficacy that not only does the measured nutritional status of patients improve significantly, but the effect of this improved nutritional status on adverse clinical outcomes can also be demonstrated (Fig. 2).

## Reaching a Consensus on Primary Outcomes for Cachexia Studies

Outcome measures are 'the results of health care processes' [14]. They are a measure of change and represent the difference from one point in time (usually before an intervention) to another point in time (usually following an intervention) [15]. Outcome measures should be standardised, with explicit instructions for administration and scoring [16].

When developing a *primary outcome* for studies in cachexia, it is crucial to remember that it represents the outcome of prime importance. As such, it should be a significant and relevant endpoint, which is clearly stated and defined. It should

also have a reasonable chance of being proven (c.f. power analysis) by the proposed intervention trial. In contrast, a *surrogate outcome* is an observation marker that is believed to relate to the primary end-point. It can be clinical, physiological, chemical or biological. Surrogate outcomes should be easy to identify and should be a good proxy or true predictor of the primary outcome.

The primary clinical outcome measures that have been used in clinical nutrition trials include variables that are either patient-, doctor- or service-focused (Fig. 3). Patient-focused outcomes may include QoL variables [17] or measures of patient independence [18]. Doctor-focused outcomes include measures of patient survival [19], the incidence of complications [20] and the length of hospital stay [21]. Service-focused outcomes include assessments of the cost effectiveness of any new treatment and the financial viability of the introduction of such a treatment to medical practice [22]. Unfortunately, the direct measurement of any of these variables is often a difficult and costly exercise. This problem, compounded by the multiple potential confounding influences on such outcomes, renders a trial of appropriate statistical power dauntingly large, complex and expensive.

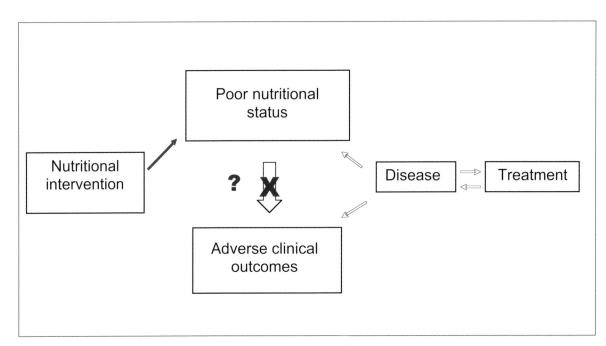

**Fig. 2.** Challenges in clinical nutrition trials. Challenges denoted in red colour

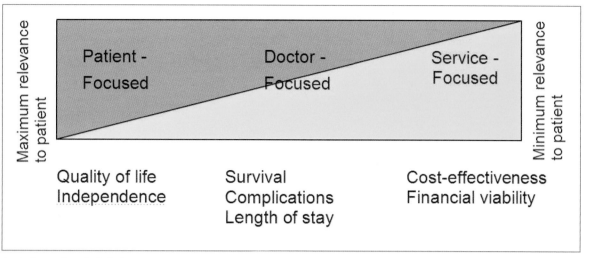

**Fig. 3.** Examples of clinical outcomes

This has often led investigators and pharmaceutical companies to abandon the direct measurement of adverse clinical outcomes in favour of simpler, cheaper studies. For example, if assessing the efficacy of a new nutritional intervention, the temptation has been to focus on changing adverse nutritional status and then to assume a direct relationship between nutritional status and adverse clinical outcomes, independent of the disease process. This model, although less complex and therefore less costly, is flawed as it leans towards the examination of surrogate end-points rather than important primary outcomes. It also relies on an assumption that is highly debatable! The failure to address clinical end-points as primary outcomes in cachexia trials has led to the current *status quo* in which intervention studies have little impact on clinical practice.

## The Use of Outcome Measures: The Current Status Quo

Recently, there has been considerable interest in the potential therapeutic value of eicosapentaenoic acid (EPA), an omega n-3 polyunsaturated fatty acid with anti-inflammatory/anti-catabolic properties, for the treatment of cancer cachexia. A series of clinical studies has been conducted to assess the efficacy of EPA, and this body of litera-

ture provides a useful resource from which we can review the current outcome measures reported in cachexia trials. Table 1 documents the main outcome variables measured in four of these studies [5–8]. Immediately we can see that there is no consensus as to which outcomes should actually be included in a trial of anti-cachexia therapy. Neither is there a standard methodology for assessing these outcomes. For example, nutritional status was assessed by two different methods: change in either body weight or LBM. As can be seen in Table 1, although change in body weight was documented in all four studies, LBM was measured in only two. Food intake was assessed using either a 3-day diet diary or a linear analogue scale to document self-reported appetite. It was variably addressed in the different trials by different methods. Patient function was assessed using either self-reported physical function as part of a QoL questionnaire, or physician-reported PS, using the Karnofsky or WHO scales. It was variably documented by three of the trials, and it was not addressed at all by one major study. Global QoL and survival duration from the initiation of treatment were documented by most of the studies, but not all. The obvious conclusions are that uncertainty surrounds both the methodology of assessing seemingly simple outcomes and the question of which variables should be examined in the first instance.

**Table 1.** Outcome measures reported in recent eicosapentaenoic acid studies

|                          | Nutrition |     | Intake |     | Function |     | Global | Survival |
|                          | Weight | LBM | Appetite | FI | PA | PS | QoL |          |
|--------------------------|:------:|:---:|:--------:|:--:|:--:|:--:|:---:|:--------:|
| Burns 2004 [5] (n=43)    | √      | -   | -        | -  | √  | -  | -   | √        |
| Jatoi 2004 [6] (n=429)   | √      | -   | √        | -  | -  | -  | √   | √        |
| Bruera 2003 [7] (n=60)   | √      | √   | √        | √  | -  | √  | √   | -        |
| Fearon 2003 [8] (n=200)  | √      | √   | √        | √  | √  | √  | √   |          |

LBM, lean body mass; FI, diet diary food intake; PA, self-reported physical function; PS, performance score; QoL, quality of life

The situation is equally confusing when we consider the use of *primary* outcomes in these four studies. Weight was used as the primary outcome in two of the trials, LBM in another, and no primary outcome variable was stated in the fourth study. Clearly there is no agreement concerning the identity of the primary outcome variable in cachexia intervention trials.

## The Pros and Cons of Current Outcome Measures

In the development of primary outcome variables for future cachexia intervention studies, it is useful to consider the relative advantages and disadvantages of outcomes currently being used. If we consider change in weight in the assessment of nutritional status, it becomes obvious that the current situation is inadequate to address the subtleties of cachexia. Despite being the most intuitive of all the outcomes currently employed, and perhaps the simplest to measure in a sensitive, objective manner, it remains difficult to determine exactly how much weight gain is required in the individual patient to be *clinically* significant, rather than *statistically* significant. Equally, total body weight represents the sum of a variety of different body compartments, and therefore documentation of a change in weight does not identify the specific

nature of tissue lost or gained. This is particularly relevant to the study of cachexia, a syndrome in which patients may demonstrate a relative, if not absolute, expansion of extracellular water space [23]. The use of LBM as a primary end-point is perhaps superior to body weight alone as it reflects, at least to some degree, the functional protein mass in the body. It can be estimated either directly or indirectly by a variety of techniques, including anthropometry, bioelectrical impedance analysis, isotope dilution or dual-energy X-ray absorptiometry (DEXA) [24, 25]. However, as LBM is not a measure of a specific tissue mass, and also includes the mass of the extracellular water space, it is subject to some of the same criticisms as total body weight. As a patient becomes more oedematous, a change in LBM may be independent of the protein content of that mass. Furthermore, the functional significance of a change in lean tissue mass is still not clearly established.

If we consider PS as an example of outcomes used to assess functional status, the overall picture is no clearer. PS tools have shown some value as prognostic indicators [26], and attempts have been made to validate such tools as global markers of functional status [27]. However, despite growing interest in the functional assessment of cancer patients [28], it remains unclear exactly what PS scores measure and how they relate to true levels of patient activity. It has been suggested that PS suffers from being too narrow a tool [29], and that conventional PS scores are less informative in older patients. There is therefore an overwhelming need to develop new primary outcomes to assess accurately the impact of cachexia therapies.

## The Importance of Patient-Centred Outcomes

The real value of any cachexia intervention can only be truly measured by assessing the day-to-day impact on the individual patient, whether that be an impact on QoL or patient independence. Over the past 20 years, the importance of such patient-centred outcomes has become evident. Studies have shown that cancer patients receiving palliative care are interested not only in the quantity of their remaining life, but also the quality. For example, in a recent survey of patients with advanced lung cancer, only 22% of patients chose palliative chemotherapy, in preference to supportive care alone, to benefit from the associated 3-month survival advantage [30]. In contrast, 68% of patients chose chemotherapy if it substantially reduced adverse symptoms without prolonging life.

QoL is a very complex issue to address. It is a multidimensional construct that includes clinical, psychological, physical, cognitive, emotional, spiritual and social domains. It is therefore best measured using tools that assess multiple domains of patient well-being [31–33], as well as common symptoms of cancer and its treatment (e.g. pain, nausea, fatigue). It is generally accepted that QoL is a subjective phenomenon, which is best assessed by the individual patient. Indeed, studies have shown that considerable disparities exist between concurrent ratings of QoL made by patients and their physicians [34, 35]. Various attempts have been made to develop a crude assessment of overall QoL, and these are generally known as global QoL measurements [36]. However, when determining the impact of a nutritional intervention on QoL, rather than measuring global QoL (which is likely to be influenced by many other factors independent of nutritional status [37]), it might be more relevant to assay the intensity of a specific symptom that is readily influenced by nutritional status. The physical function of a patient is one

such proximal index of QoL that might be useful in application to cachexia intervention trials [1] (see later).

## When Should the Primary Outcome Be Assessed?

In general, cachexia intervention trials study patients over a period of weeks, looking for a change in either body composition, functional status or a combination of the two. However, there is no agreement regarding how long any interventional study should be. To detect a measurable change in body composition usually requires a trial lasting 6–8 weeks. In the four EPA trials examined above, the duration of the intervention ranged from 2 to 12 weeks [5–8]. Assessment of functional status may have an advantage, as it tends to improve ahead of changes in body composition and therefore may be demonstrable over a shorter timescale (e.g. days). However, no matter which variable is selected as primary outcome, cachectic cancer patients are generally so unwell when entered into intervention trials that less than 50% are still assessable at 8 weeks from treatment initiation [8]. This fact suggests that there is a probable selective attrition of the patient population, a problem that has not been adequately addressed by refinement of trial methodology.

## The Standard of Care in Cachexia Trials

When designing an intervention trial it is important to bear in mind the hypothesis that the trial is attempting to prove. Most commonly, an intervention is compared with a placebo; the two cohorts of patient subjects should otherwise receive the same standard of care. However, the standard of care pertaining to the general management of cachexia remains currently undefined. The issue of standardisation of care in cancer cachexia is a complex field that can be divided into general medical issues and specific issues. General medical issues include patients' pain, constipation, depression, fatigue, malabsorption and diabetes, to name but a few. All must be adequately controlled if any effect of an anti-cachectic intervention is going to be demonstrated in a consistent and controlled manner. Equally, the concomitant use of oral supplements, dietary advice, anti-inflammatory drugs, exercise, appetite stimulants, anabolic agents or treatments of anaemia must also be strictly regulated and recorded, as these inputs may alter the eventual outcome. If these elements are not carefully controlled, they may form a source of bias and possibly contribute to the negative (or positive) outcome of any intervention trial.

## Development of a Novel Profile of Cancer Cachexia for Use in Trial Design

The likelihood of detecting a clinically significant change in any outcome variable will be influenced by the characteristics of the patients entered into the trial. To reflect the complex nature of cancer cachexia, a multifactorial profile of cachexia might be a more sensitive method of characterising patients who might then be entered into intervention trials. We propose the inclusion of three profile components: weight loss, reduced food intake and the presence of systemic inflammation.

### Weight Loss

Most clinical intervention trials in cancer cachexia utilise the presence of 5% weight loss as the principal entry criterion. However, it remains unclear which aspects of the cachexia syndrome relate best to function or prognosis. Evidently it would be useful to develop a profile of cachexia that allows one to target patients who, as a result of their cachexia syndrome, are at most risk from adverse function or prognosis. We have previously characterised extensively the incidence of, and the mechanisms behind, the development of weight loss in patients with unresectable pancreatic cancer [38, 39]. This patient population forms a useful paradigm of cachexia due to the extremely high incidence of weight loss and the almost uniform pattern of wasting between patients [39]. In our studies, 85% of patients had lost a median of 14% of their pre-illness stable weight at diagnosis. However, it is of interest to note that weight loss

alone is not an independent prognostic indicator in this group of patients [40]. We have therefore hypothesised that a more detailed and complete profile of the cachexia syndrome might yield study results that reflect the dominance of cachexia as a causative agent in the adverse clinical outcome of these patients. The markers of cachexia that we believe to be important in these patients include not only weight loss, but also reduced food intake and the presence of systemic inflammation (serum C-reactive protein [CRP] > 10 mg/l).

### Reduced Food Intake

Anorexia and reduced food intake have long been recognised as essential components of the cachexia syndrome [41]. Indeed, anorexia is present in 15–40% of cancer patients at diagnosis [42]. However, difficulties in the accurate determination of food intake by free-living human subjects have hampered study of the contribution of reduced food intake to overall wasting [43–45]. The issue is complicated further by substantial inter-individual variation in patient total energy expenditure (TEE) [46, 47], and therefore food intake. One interesting study examined the features of cachexia that correlated with survival following a 4-month follow-up of cancer patients undergoing outpatient palliative care ($n = 297$) [48]. In this patient group, weight loss and persistent hypermetabolism were found to be significantly associated with a shorter duration of survival. The baseline nutritional intake of the patients at the start of the study was 26 kcal/kg per day or approximately 1560 kcal/day. Dietary intake did not differ between normo- and hypermetabolic patients and it was not related to tumour type or gender. Patients able to increase their energy intake demonstrated a significant prolongation of survival. This study therefore identified a daily food intake of greater than approximately 1500 kcal as a significantly favourable prognostic variable.

The reason why 1500 kcal/day is an important variable in determining patient well-being in cachexia is apparent from recent studies of TEE and its component parts. Using a combination of doubly-labelled water (to measure TEE), and indirect calorimetry (to estimate REE) in free-living human subjects, it is possible to measure the energy expended on physical activity. When REE is expressed as a ratio in relation to TEE, this is known as the physical activity level (PAL) (Fig. 4). Recently, we demonstrated that, in patients with advanced pancreatic cancer and weight loss, average TEE was 1700 kcal/day, average REE was 1400 kcal/day, and average food intake was 1500 kcal/day [49]. Thus, the net result was a persistent negative energy balance of approximately 200 kcal/day per patient. Measured PAL (mean 1.24 [SD 0.04]) was much lower than that recorded in healthy adults of similar age (mean 1.62 [SD 0.28]) [50]. These levels are comparable with those observed in patients with spinal cord injury living at home [51] or in patients with cerebral palsy [52]. In this scenario, it seems that any increase in physical activity towards normal levels would simply worsen the established negative energy balance. In contrast, any increase in food intake from approximately 1500 kcal/day towards at least 1700 kcal/day would result in the restoration of positive energy balance, which for self-evident, physiologi-

cal reasons, might well prolong the patient's ultimate duration of survival.

## Systemic Inflammation

Over the past two decades, it has become apparent that the presence of systemic inflammation is a significant adverse prognostic factor in a variety of major disease processes, including both atherosclerosis [53] and cancer [54], the two major causes of mortality in western society. It has been shown in a variety of tumour types (e.g. pancreatic [54], gastric [55], oesophageal [56], colorectal [57], non-small cell lung cancer [58], breast [59], renal [60]) that the presence of systemic inflammation is associated with a shortened overall duration of survival. Moreover, the severity of such inflammation also correlates with survival duration [61]. It has been shown in an animal model of cancer cachexia [62], and to some extent in humans [63–65], that proinflammatory mediators play a dominant pathophysiological role. Patients with systemic inflammation exhibit an elevated REE

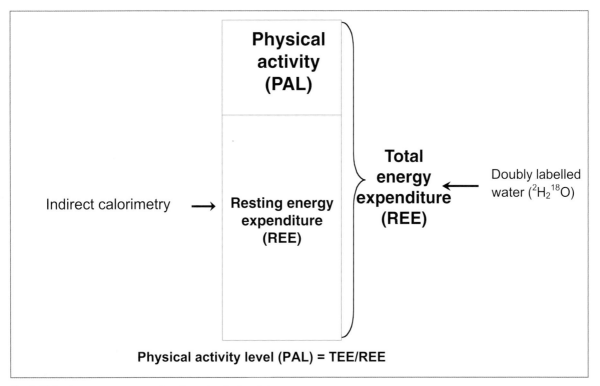

**Fig. 4.** Objective measurement of patient physical activity

and a reduced food intake [38, 66]. Thus, both sides of the energy balance equation are affected by systemic inflammation in such a way as to maximise the negative net result. From both a mechanistic and observational standpoint, it seems that systemic inflammation is highly likely to be important in the profile of a patient with cancer cachexia.

## Using the New Composite Cachexia Profile

Against this background we have recently examined whether the presence of weight loss, reduced food intake and systemic inflammation describes a patient population with both reduced nutritional and functional status. As can be seen in Table 2, indices of nutritional and functional status were all significantly reduced if patients demonstrated the composite profile of cachexia (i.e. weight loss, reduced food intake and systemic inflammation). Within this same patient cohort, the presence of the composite cachexia profile was the single most powerful predictor of adverse survival duration (unpublished results). Thus, a patient demonstrating weight loss, reduced food intake and systemic inflammation (Fig. 5) demands active therapy on the basis that these features characterise a group with particularly adverse function and prognosis. The development of a clear mathematical model demonstrating the importance of such features in the cachexia syndrome marks a new level in our ability to characterise the syndrome and may help in the design of cachexia intervention trials.

## Physical Activity as a Primary, Patient-Centred Outcome in Cachexia Intervention Trials

Many cachexia intervention trials have focused solely on changes in nutritional status as the primary end-point. However, regulatory authorities are also interested in improving patients' QoL [4]. An important domain of QoL that may be strongly influenced by nutritional status is physical function. To improve physical activity in cancer cachexia, a number of areas may be targeted (Fig. 6). LBM (the patient's 'engine') may be maximised either by size and/or by the efficiency of its func-

tion. Food intake (the patient's 'fuel') may be maximised by increasing the total supply of macronutrients (more calories) and/or improving the energy quality/density of the food. Finally, medical, nursing or physiotherapy staff may attempt to

**Table 2.** Nutritional and functional patient characteristics ($n = 170$), according to a multifactor definition of cancer cachexia

| Cachexia definition (all three criteria met) | ≥ 10% weight loss ≤ 1500 kcal/day ≥ 10 mg/l CRP | | |
|---|---|---|---|
| | No ($n = 133$) | Yes ($n = 37$) | $p$ value |
| Body composition Lean body mass (kg) | 44.3 | 39.6 | 0.003 |
| Objective function | | | |
| Grip strength (kg$^2$) | 27.9 | 22 | < 0.001 |
| KPS | 76.3 | 67 | < 0.001 |
| Health status | | | |
| EQ-5D$_{VAS}$ | 58.9 | 43 | < 0.001 |
| Subjective function | | | |
| EORTC: Physical function | 69.1 | 53.3 | < 0.001 |
| EORTC: Dyspnoea | 17.2 | 35.1 | 0.001 |
| EORTC: Fatigue | 47.7 | 69.1 | < 0.001 |

Patients were required to fulfil all three criteria (weight loss, dietary intake, elevated C-reactive protein [CRP]) of the multifactor cachexia definition, and were studied for differences in body composition and objective and subjective indices of functional status.
*KPS*, Karnofsky performance score; *EQ-5D$_{VAS}$*, visual analogue scale rating of EQ-5D health-related quality-of-life questionnaire; *EORTC*, the European Organization for Research and Treatment of Cancer questionnaire

- Weight loss (10 or 15%)
- Food intake (< 1500 kcal/day)
- Systemic inflammation (CRP>10 mg/l)

**Fig. 5.** Key markers of cachexia. *CRP*, C-reactive protein

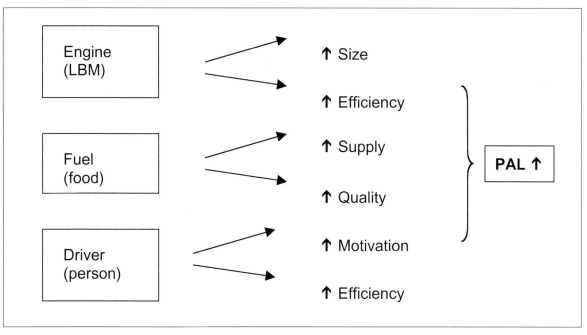

**Fig. 6.** Improving physical activity in cancer cachexia. *LBM*, lean body mass; *PAL*, physical activity level

motivate the cachectic patient to mobilise, or instruct the patient on how to utilise their limited energy reserves more efficiently.

In a recent intervention trial, Moses and co-workers demonstrated that the baseline PAL of cachectic pancreatic cancer patients was very low (with patients spending prolonged periods at rest or in bed) [49]. Patients were randomised to receive either an energy- and protein-dense oral nutritional supplement, or the same supplement enriched with a pharmacological dose of EPA. The combined regimen was designed not only to improve patients' food intake but also to address some of the underlying metabolic abnormalities that contribute to the syndrome of cachexia (e.g. systemic inflammation). Patients receiving the conventional supplement did not demonstrate increased PAL. However, PAL did increase significantly in those patients receiving the combined regimen, to values commensurate for sedentary office workers [67]. This is one of the few randomised studies that has used objective methodology and shown that a nutritional intervention can

improve physical function in advanced cancer patients.

## Conclusions

Cachexia is a multidimensional problem, and therefore the characterisation of cachectic patients must be performed in a fashion that reflects this (i.e. includes weight loss, food intake and systemic inflammation). In any intervention trial of anti-cachexia therapy, the primary outcome should be patient-focused. Physical activity level is an example of one such health-related quality-of-life variable that can be altered by therapeutic interventions to cachexia. The testing of novel therapeutic agents must be executed within the context of a defined background of best supportive care. Finally, future intervention trials in cachexia must address the current lack of standardised and defined inclusion criteria and outcome variables.

# References

1. Dahele M, Fearon KCH (2004) Research methodology: cancer cachexia syndrome. Palliat Med 18:409–417
2. Tisdale MJ (2002) Cachexia in cancer patients. Nat Rev Cancer 2:862–871
3. Nixon DW, Lawson DH (1983) Nutritional support of the cancer patient. Hosp Formul 8:616–619
4. Anonymous (1997) Workshop: clinical trials for the treatment of secondary wasting and cachexia: selection of appropriate endpoints. May 22-23, Bethesda
5. Burns CP, Halabi S, Clamon G et al (2004) Phase II study of high-dose fish oil capsules for patients with cancer-related cachexia. Cancer 101:370–378
6. Jatoi A, Rowland K, Loprinzi CL et al (2004) North Central Cancer Treatment Group. An eicosapentaenoic acid supplement versus megestrol acetate versus both for patients with cancer-associated wasting: a North Central Cancer Treatment Group and National Cancer Institute of Canada collaborative effort. J Clin Oncol 22:2469–2476
7. Bruera E, Strasser F, Palmer JL et al (2003) Effect of fish oil on appetite and other symptoms in patients with advanced cancer and anorexia/cachexia: a double-blind, placebo-controlled study. J Clin Oncol 21:129–134
8. Fearon KC, Von Meyenfeldt MF, Moses AG et al (2003) Effect of a protein and energy dense N-3 fatty acid enriched oral supplement on loss of weight and lean tissue in cancer cachexia: a randomised double blind trial. Gut 52:1479–1486
9. Tayek JA, Bistrian BR, Hehir DJ et al (1986) Improved protein kinetics and albumin synthesis by branched chain amino acid-enriched total parenteral nutrition in cancer cachexia. A prospective randomized crossover trial. Cancer 58:147–157
10. Daneryd P (2002) Epoetin alfa for protection of metabolic and exercise capacity in cancer patients. Semin Oncol 29:69–74
11. Lundholm K, Daneryd P, Bosaeus I et al (2004) Palliative nutritional intervention in addition to cyclooxygenase and erythropoietin treatment for patients with malignant disease: Effects on survival, metabolism and function. Cancer 100:1967–1977
12. Daneryd P, Svanberg E, Korner U et al (1998) Protection of metabolic and exercise capacity in unselected weight-losing cancer patients following treatment with recombinant erythropoietin: a randomised prospective study. Cancer Res 58:5374–5379
13. Edelman MJ, Gandara DR, Meyers FJ et al (1999) Serotonergic blockade in the treatment of the cancer anorexia-cachexia syndrome. Cancer 86:684–688
14. Baumberg L, Long A, Jefferson J (1995) International workshop: culture and outcomes. Barcelona, 9-10 June 1995; Leeds: European Clearing House on Health Outcomes
15. Kendall N (1997) Developing outcome assessments: a step-by-step approach. NZ J Physiol 25:11–17
16. McDowell I, Newell C (1997) Measuring Health - a guide to rating scales and questionnaires, 2nd edn. Oxford University Press, New York
17. Vadell C, Segui MA, Gimenez-Arnau JM et al (1998) Anticachectic efficacy of megestrol acetate at different doses and versus placebo in patients with neoplastic cachexia. Am J Clin Oncol 21:347–351
18. De Conno F, Martini Z, Zecca E et al (1998) Megestrol acetate for anorexia in patients with far-advanced cancer: a double-blind controlled clinical trial. Eur J Cancer 34:1705–1709
19. Gebbia V, Testa A, Gebbia N (1996) Prospective randomised trial of two dose levels of megestrol acetate in the management of anorexia-cachexia syndrome in patients with metastatic cancer. Br J Cancer 73:1576–1580
20. Loprinzi CL, Kugler JW, Sloan JA et al (1999) Randomized comparison of megestrol acetate versus dexamethasone versus fluoxymesterone for the treatment of cancer anorexia/cachexia. J Clin Oncol 17:3299–3306
21. Moskovitz DN, Kim YI (2004) Does perioperative immunonutrition reduce postoperative complications in patients with gastrointestinal cancer undergoing operations? Nutr Rev 62:443–447
22. Laviano A, Muscaritoli M, Rossi-Fanelli F (2005) Phase II study of high-dose fish oil capsules for patients with cancer-related cachexia: a Cancer and Leukaemia Group B study (comment). Cancer 103:651–652
23. Fearon KC, Preston T (1990) Body composition in cancer cachexia. Infusionstherapie 17:63–66
24. Koch J (1998) The role of body composition measurements in wasting syndromes. Semin Oncol 25:12–19
25. Pichard C, Kyle UG (1998) Body composition measurements during wasting diseases. Curr Opin Nutr Metab Care 1:357–361
26. Buccheri G, Ferrigno D, Tamburini M (1996) Karnofsky and ECOG performance status scoring in lung cancer: a prospective, longitudinal study of 536 patients from a single institution. Eur J Cancer 32A:1135–1141
27. Yates JW, Chalmer B, McKegney FP (1980) Evaluation of patients with advanced cancer using the Karnofsky performance status. Cancer 45:2220–2224
28. Batel-Copel LM, Kornblith AB, Batel PC, Holland JC (1997) Do oncologists have an increasing interest in the quality of life of their patients? A literature review of the last 15 years. Eur J Cancer 33:29–32
29. Schaafsma J, Osoba D (1994) The Karnofsky Performance Status Scale re-examined: a cross validation with the EORTC-C30. Qual Life Res 3:413–424
30. Silvestri G, Pritchard R, Welch HG (1998)

Preferences for chemotherapy in patients with advanced non-small cell lung cancer: descriptive study based on scripted interviews. BMJ 317:771–775

31. Cella DF, Bonomi AE (1995) Measuring quality of life: 1995 update. Oncology 9:47–60

32. Osoba D (1994) Lessons learned from measuring health-related quality of life in oncology. J Clin Oncol 12:608–616

33. Moinpour CM (1994) Measuring quality of life: an emerging science. Semin Oncol 21:48–63

34. Kahn SB, Houts PS, Harding SP (1992) Quality of life and patients with cancer: a comparative study of patient versus physician perceptions and its implications for cancer education. J Cancer Educ 7:241–249

35. Stephens RJ, Hopwood P, Girling DJ, Machin D (1997) Randomized clinical trials with quality of life endpoints: are doctors' ratings of patient's physical symptoms interchangeable with patients' self-ratings? Qual Life Res 6:225–236

36. Hyland ME, Sodergren SC (1996) Development of a new type of global quality of life scale, and comparison of performance and preference for 12 global scales. Qual Life Res 5:469–480

37. Somerfield M, Jatoi A, Nguyen PL et al (2003) Hazards of quality-of-life data for clinical decision making. J Clin Oncol 21:82–83

38. Wigmore SJ, Plester CE, Ross JA, Fearon KC (1997) Contribution of anorexia and hypermetabolism to weight loss in anicteric patients with pancreatic cancer. Br J Surg 84:196–197

39. Wigmore SJ, Plester CE, Richardson RA, Fearon KC (1997) Changes in nutritional status associated with unresectable pancreatic cancer. Br J Cancer 75:106–109

40. Brennan MF, Kattan MW, Klimstra D, Conlon K (2004) Prognostic nomogram for patients undergoing resection for adenocarcinoma of the pancreas. Ann Surg 240:293–298

41. Laviano A, Meguid MM, Rossi-Fanelli F (2003) Cancer anorexia: clinical implications, pathogenesis, and therapeutic strategies. Lancet Oncol 4:686–694

42. DeWys WD (1977) Anorexia in cancer patients. Cancer Res 37:2354–2358

43. Westerterp KR, Goris AH (2002) Validity of the assessment of dietary intake: problems of misreporting. Curr Opin Clin Nutr Metab Care 5:489–493

44. Kaskoun MC, Johnson RK, Goran MI (1994) Comparison of energy intake by semiquantitative food-frequency questionnaire with total energy expenditure by the doubly labelled water method in young children. Am J Clin Nutr 60:43–47

45. McCrory MA, Hajduk CL, Roberts SB (2002) Procedures for screening out inaccurate reports of dietary energy intake. Public Health Nutr 5:873–882

46. Goran MI, Beer WH, Wolfe RR et al (1993) Variation in total energy expenditure in young healthy free-living men. Metabolism 42:487–496

47. Goran MI (1995) Variation in total energy expenditure in humans. Obes Res 3:59–66

48. Bosaeus I, Daneryd P, Lundholm K (2002) Dietary intake, resting energy expenditure, weight loss and survival in cancer patients. J Nutr 132:3465S–3466S

49. Moses AW, Slater C, Preston T et al (2004) Reduced total energy expenditure and physical activity in cachectic patients with pancreatic cancer can be modulated by an energy and protein dense oral supplement enriched with n-3 fatty acids. Br J Cancer 90:996–1002

50. Gibney ER (2000) Energy expenditure in disease: time to revisit? Proc Nutr Soc 59:199–207

51. Mollinger LA, Spurr GB, el Ghatit AZ et al (1985) Daily energy expenditure and basal metabolic rates of patients with spinal cord injury. Arch Phys Med Rehabil 66:420–426

52. Stallings VA, Zemel BS, Davies JC et al (1996) Energy expenditure of children and adolescents with severe disabilities: a cerebral palsy model. Am J Clin Nutr 64:627–634

53. Libby P (2002) Inflammation in atherosclerosis. Nature 420:868–874

54. Falconer JS, Fearon KC, Ross JA et al (1995) Acute-phase protein response and survival duration of patients with pancreatic cancer. Cancer 75:2077–2082

55. Rashid SA, O'Quigley J, Axon AT, Cooper EH (1982) Plasma protein profiles and prognosis in gastric cancer. Br J Cancer 45:390–394

56. Ikeda M, Natsugoe S, Ueno S et al (2003) Significant host- and tumor-related factors for predicting prognosis in patients with esophageal carcinoma. Ann Surg 238:197–202

57. McMillan DC, Canna K, McArdle CS (2003) Systemic inflammatory response predicts survival following curative resection of colorectal cancer. Br J Surg 90:215–219

58. Forrest LM, McMillan DC, McArdle CS et al (2004) Comparison of an inflammation-based prognostic score (GPS) with performance status (ECOG) in patients receiving platinum-based chemotherapy for inoperable non-small cell lung cancer. Br J Cancer 90:1704–1706

59. Heys SD, Ogston KN, Simpson WG et al (1998) Acute phase proteins in patients with large and locally advanced breast cancer treated with neo-adjuvant chemotherapy: response and survival. Int J Oncol 13:589–594

60. Bromwich E, McMillan DC, Lamb GW et al (2004) The systemic inflammatory response, performance status and survival in patients undergoing alpha-interferon treatment for advanced renal cancer. Br J Cancer 91:1236–1238

61. McMillan DC, Elahi MM, Sattar N et al (2001) Measurement of the systemic inflammatory response predicts cancer-specific and non-cancer survival in patients with cancer. Nutr Cancer 41:64–69

62. Todorov P, Cariuk P, McDermott T et al (1996) Characterization of a cancer cachectic factor. Nature 379:739–742

63. Wigmore SJ, Todorov PT, Barber MD et al (2000) Characteristics of patients with pancreatic cancer expressing a novel cancer cachectic factor. Br J Surg 87:53–58

64. O'Riordain MG, Falconer JS, Maingay J et al (1999) Peripheral blood cells from weight-losing cancer patients control the hepatic acute phase response by a primarily interleukin-6 dependent mechanism. Int J Oncol 15:823–827

65. Barber MD, Fearon KCH, Ross JA (1999) Relationship of serum levels of interleukin-6, soluble interleukin-6 receptor and tumour necrosis factor receptors to the acute-phase protein response in advanced pancreatic cancer. Clin Sci 96:83–87

66. Falconer JS, Fearon KC, Plester CE et al (1994) Cytokines, the acute-phase response, and resting energy expenditure in cachectic patients with pancreatic cancer. Ann Surg 219:325–331

67. Black AE, Coward WA, Cole TJ, Prentice AM (1996) Human energy expenditure in affluent societies: an analysis of 574 doubly-labelled water measurements. Eur J Clin Nutr 50:72–92

# Meeting the Amino Acid Requirements for Protein Anabolism in Cancer Cachexia

Vickie E. Baracos

## Cachexia, Cachexia Therapy and Protein Nutrition

A large fraction of patients with advanced cancer develop cachexia [1], a wasting syndrome characterised by anorexia, asthenia, and profound losses of adipose tissue and skeletal muscle mass. The association of cachexia syndrome with poor prognosis, loss of functional status and poor quality of life has motivated researchers to develop therapeutic strategies for this problem [2].

One principle of cachexia therapy is based upon the concept that cancer cachexia is, at least in part, a form of malnutrition. Thus, total parenteral nutrition may be provided in cases of complete gastrointestinal failure and enteral nutritional support (delivered by nasogastric tube or percutaneous gastrostomy) is used to circumvent upper gastrointestinal tract deficit, obstruction or injury. When oral intake is ongoing, agents that promote spontaneous food intake form the first line of support, such as glucocorticoids [3], progestational agents [4–10] and dronabinol [5, 6]. Dietary supplementation approaches include the application of specific foods or nutrients that may be deficient in patients capable of oral intake. The polyunsaturated n-3 fatty acids derived from fish oils (either alone or incorporated in enteral formulae) have been the subject of several recent clinical trials [11–14].

The current thinking on cachexia syndromes places great emphasis on losses of body nitrogen especially from skeletal muscle. Reduced nitrogen balance in cancer cachexia results from a fundamental metabolic shift, which results in decreased anabolism and increased catabolism; the simultaneous presence of both of these defects results in the most rapid muscle atrophy. A multi-modal strategy that stimulates protein synthesis, provides energy and building blocks for net protein anabolism, and normalises proteolysis, would be required for effective therapy. However, while the major focus of clinical anti-cachexia therapy is the retention or gain of lean body mass, the consideration of dietary protein level and amino acid composition necessary to these ends is surprisingly absent from the literature. Although 20 or so anti-cachexia agents are currently used in clinical practice or are under investigation [2], proteins and/or amino acids have barely been considered. Only one study to date has used amino acid therapy as a primary anti-cachexia agent in cancer patients [15], and neither appetite stimulants nor anabolic agents have been delivered concurrently with a protein/amino acid supply designed to fully realise their potential efficacy. Considering the importance of lean body mass in the minds of cachexia researchers, the lack of attention to protein nutrition seems inexplicable.

## Dietary Intake of Proteins in Patients with Cancer

The typical nutrient intakes of individuals with advanced cancer have not been widely studied. This would appear to be an important deficit, as it is obvious that no anti-cachexia strategy is likely to be entirely effective unless coupled with adequate intake of essential nutrients, including proteins, and any need for supplementation must necessarily be considered in the context of the level of intake. A couple of relevant citations on dietary intakes of cancer patients may be found in the recent literature. Fearon (2003) reported the typical protein and energy intake of patients with unresectable pancreatic cancer who completed 3-day dietary records [16]. On average, total energy intakes were 1500–1600 kcal/day and protein intakes were 60–63 g protein/day, to provide an overall protein:energy

(P:E) ratio of 0.040. These data are highly consistent with our results (Hutton et al., unpublished observations) in a population of 96 patients with solid tumours (mostly lung and gastrointestinal) with advanced disease, who had average intakes of 1578 kcal and 63 g protein/day and a P:E of 0.040. Most recently, Lundholm et al. presented selected intake data on 309 patients with solid tumours mostly of gastrointestinal origin, and the energy intake of this group was 1600–1700 kcal/day: the protein intakes were not reported [17].

## What are the Dietary Protein Requirements of Cancer Patients?

Dietary protein and amino acid requirements of cancer patients have never been formally determined, and we have argued elsewhere that this is an important deficit in the literature that would hopefully draw the attention of nutritional scientists with appropriate expertise [18]. Methods for the determination of human protein requirements continue to advance conceptually and technically, and the subset of these that are minimally invasive merit particular scrutiny for use, since patients with advanced malignancy may not tolerate extensive or invasive investigations. The indicator amino acid oxidation approach has been extensively developed for clinical use by Ball and co-workers [19, 20]. This method is based on the principle that the oxidation of an indicator amino acid is high when a test amino acid is limiting for protein synthesis, and that indicator oxidation decreases to reach a low and constant value once amino acid requirements are met [19, 21]. Using this technique, breath and urine are the only samples required following the consumption of diet with a varying amount of the study amino acid and administration of the indicator amino acid tracer [19, 21]. The indicator amino acid oxidation technique has been used to determine amino acid requirements in healthy adults and in individuals with metabolic disorders and has found particular application in highly vulnerable populations such as premature neonates and children [19, 21].

The plasma amino acid response to an infusion of an amino acid mixture is an indirect approach that has also been used to identify the amino acids that limit protein synthesis [22, 23]. This method is based on the differential behaviour of infused amino acids depending on whether the infusion oversupplies or undersupplies amino acids relative to requirements. If an amino acid is undersupplied, its plasma concentration will not rise during an amino acid infusion, because of its use for protein synthesis. By contrast, infusion of an amino acid that is already present at or above required amounts, will result in a steep rise in its plasma concentration. This approach has been used in HIV/AIDS patients [22] and was also used to manipulate parenteral amino acid formulation to meet the specific needs of hospitalised patients in an intensive care unit [23]. The linear regression of plasma plateau concentrations of amino acids in response to an amino acid infusion was used to determine which amino acids were oversupplied or undersupplied in each individual patient. A parenteral amino acid formulation that corrected these imbalances was then given for 5 days and resulted in improved nitrogen balance [23]. The identification of limiting amino acids in cancer is an important step in determining appropriate dietary supplements that will promote lean tissue gain: however, to date this has not been accomplished in cancer patients.

Until such time as the amino acid requirements of cancer patients are empirically determined, a suitable starting point might be the recommended protein requirements of healthy persons in the range of ages of the average age of cancer diagnosis (65 years in Canada) and average age of cancer death (69 years), and thereafter to consider any factors that would tend to alter protein requirements relative to that value. Conventional dietary recommendations include protein intake for weight maintenance plus a factor for disease. For example, the *Clinical Guide to Oncology Nutrition* of the American Dietetic Association suggests a protein intake of 1.0–1.5 g protein/kg body weight per day [24], depending on patient, disease and treatment factors. It has been a long-standing convention to express protein intake as a constant function of body weight (i.e. per kg of body weight): however, Millward [25, 26] suggests that a nutrient density (i.e. P:E ratio) may be more useful to provide a basis for suggesting protein intakes. Based on the assumption that the energy requirement is the major determinant of total intake, then if the protein requirement is expressed as a P:E ratio, the recommended intakes can be adjusted taking into account the factors that impact on energy requirements such as age, gender, body weight and activity level. The reader is referred to the work of Millward and Jackson [26] for the full details underlying this concept.

If one were to accept the arguments presented by Millward and Jackson, then a healthy 60- to 70-year-old man or woman weighing 70 kg with a low physical activity level of 1.5 times the basal metabolism value would require a dietary P:E ratio of at least 0.12 to maintain N balance. This might be considered to be a minimum amount, for the following reasons. The calculations by Millward are based on the assumption of energy balance, and do not take into account that at low energy intakes amino acids are diverted to energy-yielding reactions. The average energy intakes of advanced pancreatic cancer patients are in the vicinity of determined basal metabolic rate (22–25 kcal/kg body weight per day) and thus a significant fraction of individuals are not taking in enough energy even to match basal metabolism requirements [16, 27]. Also, the definition used by Millward and Jackson for calculation of the P:E ratio of sedentary persons is a physical activity level of 1.5 times basal metabolism value and there is evidence that the physical activity level of advanced cancer patients is of the order of 1.25 [27]. Finally, no factor is added to these suggested protein intakes for the presence of disease.

## A Role for Aggressive Protein Supplementation?

Based on the foregoing, it might be concluded that dietary protein intakes in patients with advanced cancer are largely insufficient. The protein intakes in the population appear to be in the 60 g/day range and the P:E ratio approximately 0.04. The approach of the American Dietetic Association recommended protein intakes would be up to 90–100 g/day. Taking the approach of Millward and Jackson and the energy intakes of advanced cancer patients indicated above (1600 kcal/day), then a P:E ratio of just 0.1 would correspond to about 150 g protein/day, and this value is about 2.5-fold higher and 1.5 standard deviations higher than the average protein intake of typical cancer patient populations.

Aggressive protein supplementation remains to be systematically tested in advanced cancer patients. Eubanks-May et al. [15] produced the first report of targeted amino acid supplementation in patients with cancer cachexia. A population of patients with solid tumours of mixed types were randomised to daily treatment with 31 g of a mixture of arginine, glutamine and a metabolite of leucine or an isonitrogenous control containing alanine, serine, glutamate and glycine. There is some evidence to suggest that arginine, glutamine and leucine (as well as some other amino acids) may be limiting amino acids in the tumour-bearing state [18]. Whether this mixture is ideal remains to be established: however, the test group gained an average of 2.5 kg of lean body mass after 12 weeks of supplementation, while patients on the control treatment lost lean body mass. The reported gain of lean body mass by amino acids alone in the absence of any orexigenic or anabolic therapy also suggests that protein intake per se may be limiting. These results must be substantiated by larger and more systematic studies of protein nutrition in cancer patient populations and further supported by studies of requirements that will define the ideal amino acid mixture needed to underpin successful cachexia therapy.

## References

1.  Dunlop R (1996) Clinical epidemiology of cancer cachexia. In: Bruera E, Higginson I (eds) Cachexia-Anorexia in Cancer Patients. Oxford University Press, Oxford, pp 76–82
2.  MacDonald N, Easson NM, Mazurak VC et al (2003) Understanding and managing cancer cachexia. J Am Coll Surg 197:143–161
3.  Loprinzi CL, Kugler JW, Sloan JA et al (1999) Randomized comparison of megestrol acetate versus dexamethasone versus fluoxymesterone for the treatment of cancer anorexia/cachexia. J Clin Oncol 17:3299–3306
4.  Tchekmedyian NS, Hickman M, Siau J et al (1990) Treatment of cancer anorexia with megestrol aceta-

te: impact on quality of life. Oncology 4:185–192

5. Jatoi A, Windschitl HE, Loprinzi CL et al (2002) Donabinol versus megestrol acetate versus combination therapy for cancer-associated anorexia: a North Central Cancer Treatment Group study. J Clin Oncol 20:567–573

6. Timpone JG, Weight DJ, Li N et al (1997) The safety and pharmacokinetics of single-agent and combination therapy with megestrol acetate and dronabinol for the treatment of HIV wasting syndrome. The DATRI 004 study group: division of AIDS treatment research initiative. AIDS Res Hum Retroviruses 13:305–315

7. Loprinzi CL, Michalak JC, Schaid DK et al (1993) Phase III evaluation of four doses of megestrol acetate as therapy for patients with cancer anorexia and/or cachexia. J Clin Oncol 11:762–767

8. Bruera E, Ernst S, Hagen N et al (1998) Effectiveness of megestrol acetate in patients with advanced cancer: a randomized, double-blind, crossover study. Cancer Prev Control 2:74–78

9. Bruera E, Macmillan K, Kuehn N et al (1990) A controlled trial of megestrol acetate on appetite, caloric intake, nutritional status, and other symptoms in patients with advanced cancer. Cancer 15:1279–1282

10. Azcona C, Castro L, Crespo E et al (1996) Megestrol acetate therapy for anorexia and weight loss in children with malignant solid tumors. Aliment Pharmacol Ther 4:577–586

11. Wigmore SJ, Barber MD, Ross JA et al (2000) Effect of oral eicosapentanoic acid on weight loss in patients with pancreatic cancer. Nutr Cancer 36:177–184

12. Barber MD, Ross JA, Voss AC et al (1999) The effect of an oral nutritional supplement enriched with fish oil on weight-loss in patients with pancreatic cancer. Br J Cancer 81:80–86

13. Burns CP, Halabi S, Clamon GH et al (1999) Phase I clinical study of fish oil fatty acid capsules for patients with cancer cachexia: Cancer and Leukemia Group B Study 9473. Clin Cancer Res 5:3942–3947

14. Bruera E, Strasser F, Palmer JL et al (2003) Effect of fish oil on appetite and other symptoms in patients with advanced cancer and anorexia/cachexia: a double-blind, placebo-controlled study. J Clin Oncol 21:129–134

15. Eubanks-May P, Barber A, D'Olimpio J et al (2002) Reversal of cancer-related wasting using oral supplementation with a combination of b-hydroxy-b-methylbutyrate, arginine, and glutamine. Am J Surg 183:471–479

16. Fearon KC, Von Meyenfeldt MF, Moses AG et al (2003) Effect of a protein and energy dense N-3 fatty acid enriched oral supplement on loss of weight and lean tissue in cancer cachexia: a randomised double blind trial. Gut 52:1479–1486

17. Lundholm K, Daneryd P, Bosaeus I et al (2004) Palliative nutritional intervention in addition to cyclooxygenase and erythropoietin treatment for patients with malignant disease: effects on survival, metabolism and function. Cancer 100:1967–1977

18. Mackenzie M, Baracos VE (2003) Cancer-associated cachexia: altered metabolism of protein and amino acids. In: Cynober L (ed) Amino acid metabolism and therapy in health and diseases, 2nd edn. CRC Press, Boca Raton, pp 339–354

19. Brunton JA, Ball RO, Pencharz PB (1998) Determination of amino acid requirements by indicator amino acid oxidation: applications in health and disease. Curr Opin Clin Nutr Metab Care 1:449–453

20. Zello GA, Wykes LJ, Ball RO, Pencharz PB (1995) Recent advances in methods of assessing dietary amino acid requirements for adult humans. J Nutr 125:2907–2915

21. Bross R, Ball RO, Pencharz PB (1998) Development of a minimally invasive protocol for the determination of phenylalanine and lysine kinetics in humans during the fed state. J Nutr 128:1913–1919

22. Laurichesse H, Tauveron I, Gourdon F et al (1998) Threonine and methionine are limiting amino acids for protein synthesis in patients with AIDS. J Nutr 128:1342–1348

23. Berard MP, Pelletier A, Ollivier JM et al (2002) Qualitative manipulation of amino acid supply during total parenteral nutrition in surgical patients. JPEN J Parenter Enteral Nutr 26:136–143

24. Martin C (1999) Calorie, protein, fluid and micronutrient requirements. In: McCallum PD, Polisena CG (eds) The clinical guide to oncology nutrition. The American Dietetic Association, Chicago, pp 45–47

25. Millward DJ (2004) Macronutrient intakes as determinants of dietary protein and amino acid adequacy. J Nutr 134(6S):1588S–1596S

26. Millward DJ, Jackson AA (2004) Protein and energy ratios of current diets in developed and developing countries compared with a safe protein:energy ratio: implications for recommended protein and amino acid intakes. Public Health Nutr 7:387–405

27. Moses AW, Slater C, Preston T et al (2004) Reduced total energy expenditure and physical activity in cachectic patients with pancreatic cancer can be modulated by an energy and protein dense oral supplement enriched with n-3 fatty acids. Br J Cancer 90:996–1002

# The Role of Branched-Chain Amino Acids and Serotonin Antagonists in the Prevention and Treatment of Cancer Cachexia

Alessandro Laviano, Antonia Cascino, Michael M. Meguid, Isabella Preziosa, Filippo Rossi Fanelli

## Introduction

Cachexia is pervasive among patients suffering from chronic diseases, including cancer, liver cirrhosis and chronic renal failure. The development of cachexia dramatically impacts on the clinical course of the underlying disease, by increasing morbidity and mortality, and impinging on patients' quality of life. Also, weight loss influences outcome by increasing drug-induced toxicity and impeding completion of the therapeutic schedule. Particularly in cancer patients, weight loss is a reliable predictor for toxicity from treatment and shorter survival [1].

Effective anti-cachexia therapies are needed. Intuitively, the best possible approach is any that may prevent or antagonise the molecular mechanisms triggering the occurrence of wasting. Many weapons of lean body mass destruction have been discovered and characterised (e.g. cytokines, ubiquitin-proteasome pathway, NF-kB, myostatins), but many more may still be undiscovered. Their identification and the characterisation of their mutual interactions are the goals of anti-cachexia research for the next years, ultimately allowing our patients to '*brawny* go where no one has gone before'.

A novel approach to the treatment of cachexia is based on ameliorating one of its determinants, anorexia. Anorexia, together with profound changes in protein, lipid and glucose metabolisms, contributes to the development of malnutrition and eventually cachexia by significantly reducing energy intake. Although restoring energy intake to normal via appetite stimulants or artificial nutrition is not associated with stabilisation or improvement of lean body mass wasting, at least in cancer patients, recent data seem to suggest that enhancing appetite via modulation of brain neurochemistry, and particularly brain serotonin, may lead to preservation of muscle mass [2].

## Role of Brain Serotonin in Energy Intake Control

A simplistic view of energy intake regulation is that ingested nutrients are sensed at different levels of the gastrointestinal tract, including the liver. This information, together with that arising from adipose tissue, is transmitted to the brain via a series of routes (neuronal input, hormones, peptides), and is integrated in the hypothalamus, where the appropriate behavioural response is triggered. Actually, the picture is far more complex, since the hypothalamus consists of different areas and nuclei, and within each of them a set of effectors (neurotransmitters, neuromodulatory peptides and transmembrane proteins) interact [3].

For several decades, hypothalamic serotonin systems have been implicated in the suppression of feeding [4]. Serotonin is a monoamine acting as neurotransmitter and involved in different biological responses. Although the exact role of serotonin in the central regulation of food intake and body weight still awaits further clarification, its involvement in this process has been repeatedly confirmed. Now it is clear that serotonin acts in conjunction with neuropeptides and peripheral hormones to bring about physiological states such as hunger, satiation and satiety [5]. Supporting this view, it has been shown recently that fenfluramine, a serotonergic drug, acts in the arcuate nucleus of hypothalamus (the integrating centre receiving information from the periphery) by stimulating a specific neuronal population, the pro-opiomelanocortin (POMC) neurons, which is a critical circuit involved in mediating satiety under physiological conditions [6].

Beside its role in influencing food intake, hypothalamic serotonin appears also to impact energy expenditure. In a recent report, Ohliger-Frerking et al. studied dorsal raphe nucleus serotonergic neurons projecting to the hypothalamus to influence feeding [7]. They showed that the neurons from obese Zucker rats exhibited both a larger depolarisation and increased firing rate in response to phenylephrine than did cells from lean rats, thus suggesting that dorsal raphe nucleus serotonergic neurons of obese rats have an enhanced adrenergic drive. Furthermore, serotonin reduces food intake and augments sympathetic activity, thus promoting weight loss [8].

## Role of Brain Serotonin in Disease-Associated Anorexia

Considering disease-associated anorexia as a pathological and persistent form of satiety, it is intuitive to speculate that the pathogenesis of anorexia could be related to a derangement of the physiological mechanism mediating satiety. As a consequence, much scientific effort has been devoted to clarify the involvement of hypothalamic appetite-suppressing circuits in the onset of anorexia. Many studies have been conducted in animal models of cancer anorexia, but it is reasonable to translate the results obtained to other diseases. Therefore, it appears that disease-associated anorexia is related to the inability of the hypothalamus to respond appropriately to consistent peripheral signals, primarily due to the hyperactivation of the melanocortin system. This derangement could be triggered by cytokines.

The mechanisms by which cytokines negatively influence energy intake are currently under investigation. As proposed by Inui, cytokines may play a pivotal role in long-term inhibition of feeding by mimicking the hypothalamic effect of excessive negative feedback signalling [9]. This could be done by persistent stimulation of the POMC anorexigenic pathway. Recent data suggest that hypothalamic serotonergic neurotransmission may be critical in linking cytokines and the melanocortin system [6]. Thus, it could be speculated that during disease, cytokines increase hypothalamic serotonergic activity, which in turn contributes to persistent activation of POMC neurons, leading to the onset of anorexia and reduced food

intake. In humans, the demonstration of the involvement of brain serotonin in anorexia is more difficult since serotonergic activity cannot be easily measured in vivo. Thus, the activity of the hypothalamic serotonergic system is inferred by cerebrospinal fluid (CSF) levels of tryptophan.

Tryptophan is the precursor of serotonin, whose synthesis is strictly dependent on the availability of tryptophan [10]. In anorectic cancer patients, plasma and particularly CSF concentrations of tryptophan are increased when compared to controls and non-anorectic cancer patients [11, 12]. After tumour removal, plasma tryptophan normalises and food intake improves [13]. Similar data have been obtained in patients with liver cirrhosis. In this clinical setting, the presence of anorexia was associated with higher plasma levels of tryptophan than in non-anorectic patients with liver cirrhosis [14]. Also, brain tryptophan availability, which predicts brain tryptophan levels, was higher in anorectic than in non-anorectic patients. In uremic patients, persistently high brain serotonin levels appear to be related to the onset of anorexia and reduced food intake [15]. When considered together, these data suggest that brain serotonin could represent a key factor involved in the pathogenesis of cancer anorexia and thus provide an interesting therapeutic target.

## Antiserotonergic Therapies Targeting Anorexia and Cachexia

Disease-associated anorexia might be therapeutically approached by interfering with the neurochemical events downstream of cytokine activation. Serotonergic hypothalamic neurotransmission represents a suitable example, and it is therefore tempting to speculate that by interfering with hypothalamic serotonin release, food intake might be improved. Hypothalamic serotonin synthesis strictly depends on the brain availability of its precursor, the amino acid tryptophan [10]. An increase of plasma and brain tryptophan levels, leading to increased brain serotonergic activity, has been demonstrated in different diseases and linked to the presence of anorexia and reduced food intake. Tryptophan crosses the blood–brain barrier via a specific transport mechanism shared with the other neutral amino acids, including the branched-chain amino acids (BCAA). Thus, by artificially increasing the plasma levels of the competing amino acids, a reduction of tryptophan brain entry could be achieved, leading to a reduction of hypothalamic serotonin synthesis and release, which in turn would result in amelioration of cancer anorexia. To test this hypothesis, tumour-bearing rats were fed with a BCAA-enriched diet, and their feeding behaviour was compared with that of tumour-bearing rats receiving an isocaloric, isonitrogenous standard diet. The results obtained showed that BCAA-enriched diet delayed the development of anorexia by 2 days when compared to standard diet (unpublished observations). To test further the clinical relevance of BCAA, anorectic cancer patients were orally supplemented with BCAA or placebo for 7 days, while simultaneously recording their energy intake [16]. Anorexia significantly improved after 3 days of treatment only in cancer patients receiving BCAA, leading to a significant improvement of energy intake. These encouraging results must be considered as preliminary, since they were obtained in a small population during a short study period, and need to be validated in larger trials. However, they confirm the feasibility of interfering with hypothalamic neurotransmission to influence energy intake. Indeed, more fascinating results were later obtained in uremia and in liver cirrhosis.

During chronic renal failure, derangements of plasma amino acid profile occur and a reduction of circulating levels of BCAA is frequently observed. Interestingly, the reduction of plasma BCAA is associated with the presence of anorexia [17]. It is therefore tempting to speculate that by supplementing uremic patients with BCAA, energy intake and nutritional status can be improved. Hiroshige et al. studied 44 elderly patients on chronic haemodialysis [17]. Among them, 28 patients with low plasma albumin levels (< 3.5 g/dl) were classified as the malnourished group; they also suffered from anorexia. The other 16 patients did not complain of anorexia and were classified as the well-nourished group. Hiroshige et al. then performed a 12-month, double-blind,

placebo-controlled study on the malnourished group. Fourteen patients received daily oral BCAA supplementation (12 g/day) or a placebo in random order in a cross-over trial for 6 months. Lower plasma levels of BCAA and lower protein and caloric intakes were found in the malnourished group as compared to the well-nourished group. In BCAA-treated malnourished patients, anorexia and poor oral protein and calorie intakes improved within a month, concomitant with the improvement of plasma BCAA levels over the values in well-nourished patients. After 6 months of BCAA supplementation, anthropometric indices (body fat percentage, lean body mass) showed a statistically significant increase and mean plasma albumin concentration increased from 3.3 g/dl to 3.9 g/dl. After changing BCAA for a placebo, spontaneous oral food intake decreased, but the favourable nutritional status persisted for the next 6 months. In 14 patients initially treated with placebo, no significant changes in nutritional parameters were observed during the first 6 months. However, positive results were obtained by BCAA supplementation during the subsequent 6 months, and mean plasma albumin concentration increased from 3.2 g/dl to 3.8 g/dl. These data are particularly important because they demonstrate that BCAA supplementation results not only in improved food intake but also in improved nutritional status. Such encouraging results were replicated also in cirrhotic patients.

A multicentre, randomised study comparing 1-year nutritional supplementation with BCAA against lactoalbumin or maltodextrins was recently performed in 174 patients [18]. Primary outcomes were the prevention of a combined endpoint (death and deterioration to exclusion criteria), the need for hospital admission, and the duration of hospital stay. Secondary outcomes were nutritional parameters, laboratory data and Child-Pugh score, anorexia, health-related quality of life, and need for therapy. Interestingly, treatment with BCAA significantly reduced the combined event rates compared with lactoalbumin. The average hospital admission rate was lower in the BCAA arm compared with control treatments. In patients who remained in the study, nutritional parameters and liver function tests were, on average, stable or improved during treatment with BCAA and the Child-Pugh score decreased. Also, anorexia and health-related quality of life (SF-36 questionnaire) improved. In particular, anorexia was reported in more than 50% of all cases and was not different between groups. Its prevalence decreased with BCAA from 52 to 25% and remained unchanged with lactoalbumin and maltodextrins. Treatment groups did not score differently on SF-36 questionnaire at baseline. Treatment with BCAA had a significant effect on role limitation/physical, and other scales improved significantly when compared with baseline. Physical functioning and role limitation/emotional also improved. No significant changes were observed in subjects treated with lactoalbumin or maltodextrins. Finally, there was a shift toward better scoring of health only in subjects actively treated with BCAA, with the percentage of patients scoring health as poor decreasing from 19 to 3%. Similarly, after 1 year of continuous treatment with BCAA, the percentage of patients believing that their health had improved during the preceding 12 months had increased from 29 to 52%, and the percentage believing that their health had worsened had decreased from 43 to 18%.

When considered together, these data suggest that the antiserotonergic approach to the treatment of disease-associated anorexia is effective and results in significant clinical outcomes, far beyond mere increase of energy intake. The observed improvement of nutritional status and particularly of lean body mass could be explained at least in part by the excitatory effects of serotonin on hypothalamic melanocortin receptors [6], whose function has been linked to cachexia [19]. By reducing brain serotonergic activity via BCAA, it is conceivable that melanocortin receptors are less activated, leading to reduced peripheral muscle wasting. However, recent data suggest that BCAA, and particularly leucine, may influence muscle wasting by directly inhibiting intracellular proteolytic factors.

Considering the role of brain serotonin in the pathogenesis of disease-associated anorexia and cachexia, antiserotonergic drugs might be as effective as BCAA in improving food intake and nutritional status. However, this approach bears some

limitations. Firstly, antiserotonergic drugs must target the specific serotonin receptor involved in the pathogenesis of anorexia, the best candidate for this role being the 5-HT(2C) receptor. The need for selectivity may explain the failure of cyproheptadine in the treatment of anorexia in cancer patients (for review see [20]). Secondly, provided that the given antiserotonergic drug selectively targets 5-HT(2C) receptors, then it must reach the hypothalamus in adequate concentrations to block the receptors. This may be difficult to achieve, particularly if adequate brain concentrations are reached only when using suprapharmacological peripheral doses, which may lead to the development of side-effects.

Promising and in early clinical trials is blockade of type 3 serotonergic receptors, which appear more involved in mediating nausea and emesis rather than in controlling energy balance [4]. Ondansetron is a type 3 serotonergic receptor antagonist widely used in cancer patients in the prevention and treatment of chemotherapy-induced nausea and vomiting. Edelman et al. [21] studied 27 patients with advanced cancer and weight loss. Patients were not receiving antineoplastic treatment, but received oral ondansetron. Unfortunately, weight loss continued, but after 1 month of treatment patients scored better on an hedonic scale, suggesting that they were enjoying food more. However, large and placebo-controlled trials are needed to establish whether these positive results reflected a true orexigenic effect attributable exclusively to ondansetron, thus prompting more interest in this class of drugs.

## Role of Brain Monoamines in Disease-Associated Anorexia-Cachexia

More data support a role for hypothalamic neurotransmission as an effective therapeutic target in the treatment of anorexia. Using in vivo microdialysis, Blaha et al. showed that intrahypothalamic serotonin concentrations are increased in anorectic tumour-bearing rats [22]. In the same study, they also showed a more complex derangement of hypothalamic monoaminergic neurotransmission, since dopamine levels were also found to be depressed [22]. This evidence may give the neurochemical explanation for the results obtained in anorectic cancer patients, whose food intake has been restored and quality of life improved by the administration of dopamine (L-DOPA) at a dosage ranging from 375 750 mg/day [23, 24]. Although not obtained in prospective randomised clinical trials, these data are very intriguing and further support the 'monoaminergic' approach to the treatment of anorexia.

The nitric oxide system and the production of eicosanoids might be of importance for the pathogenesis of disease-associated anorexia. Supporting this view, animal and clinical studies show that nitric oxide synthase and cyclo-oxygenase inhibitors, including indomethacin, decrease tumour growth and improve anorexia [25, 26]. However, evidence that nitric oxide and eicosanoids act directly on cells in the central nervous system is lacking. Also, the nitric oxide mechanism may involve tumour growth and thereby secondarily influence appetite. Finally, nitric oxide and eicosanoid influences on appetite appear related to serotonin metabolism [27, 28], and the prostaglandin $E_2$ receptor EP3 has been identified on serotonergic neuronal cell bodies in the raphe nucleus [29]. Thus, nitric oxide and eicosanoid pathways could not be completely alien from the cytokine-monoamine system.

## Supplementation of BCAA as Anti-cachectic Therapy

Beyond their prophagic effects, BCAA appear to exert anti-catabolic effects by inhibiting intracellular proteolytic pathways. The anti-catabolic properties of BCAA, and in particular of leucine, have been known for many years, but only recently have their molecular mechanisms been elucidated. Animal studies showed that a leucine-enriched diet ameliorates protein content and body composition in an experimental tumour model [30]. These results appear to be mediated not only by the increased stimulation of protein synthesis, but also by the concomitant attenuation of protein degradation [31]. Indeed, BCAA and leucine in particular significantly influence the expression and activity of the main intracellular proteolytic pathway, i.e. the ubiquitin-proteasome system [31]. Further supporting the potentials of BCAA as anti-cachectic agents, it has been demonstrated recently in vitro that β-hydroxy-β-methylbutyrate (HMB), a leucine metabolite, is highly effective in inhibiting proteolysis, its activity being similar to that of a well-established anti-cachectic agent, eicosapentaenoic acid [32].

These intriguing experimental results have been successfully repeated in humans under different catabolic conditions. Paddon-Jones et al. investigated the role of essential amino acid supplementation in reducing bedrest-induced muscle catabolism [33]. It is important to note that the suggested supplementation of essential amino acids included a large daily dose of BCAA (approximately 18 g/day). After 28 days of bedrest, the fractional synthetic rate of supplemented patients was higher than that of the control group [33]. Also, lean leg mass was maintained throughout the study period only in the supplemented group [33]. Finally, strength loss was more pronounced in the control group than in the supplemented group [33].

To investigate, in a randomised controlled trial, any benefit of the long-term administration of BCAA in patients undergoing chemoembolisation for hepatocellular carcinoma, Poon et al. decided to supplement cancer patients with a low dose of BCAA (11 g/day) for 1 year [34]. Data obtained were then compared and showed a difference from those obtained in the control group. Although the interpretation of the results is limited by the design of the study, which is not blind and placebo-controlled, hepatocellular carcinoma patients receiving BCAA showed lower morbidity, higher serum albumin and better quality of life than the control group [34].

When considered together, these data suggest that BCAA have significant anti-anorectic and anti-cachectic effects, and their supplementation may represent a viable intervention not only for cancer patients, but also for those individuals at risk of sarcopenia due to immobility or prolonged bedrest consequent to trauma, orthopaedic or neurological diseases.

## References

1. Ross PJ, Ashley S, Norton A et al (2004) Do patients with weight loss have a worse outcome when undergoing chemotherapy for lung cancers? Br J Cancer 90:1905–1911

2. Laviano A, Meguid MM, Rossi Fanelli F (2003) Cancer anorexia: clinical implications, pathogenesis, and therapeutic strategies. Lancet Oncol 4:686–694

3. Schwartz MW, Woods SC, Porte DJr et al (2000) Central nervous system control of food intake. Nature 404:661–671

4. Giorgetti M, Tecott LH (2004) Contributions of 5-HT2C receptors to multiple actions of central serotonin systems. Eur J Pharmacol 488:1–9

5. Havel PJ, Larsen PJ, Cameron JL (2000) Neuroendocrinology. In: Conn PM, Freeman ME (eds) Physiology and medicine. Humana Press, Totowa, pp 335–352

6. Heisler LK, Cowley MA, Tecott LH et al (2002) Activation of central melanocortin pathways by fenfluramine. Science 297:609–611

7. Ohliger-Frerking P, Horowitz JM, Horwitz BA (2002) Enhanced adrenergic excitation of serotonergic dorsal raphe neurons in genetically obese rats. Neurosci Lett 332:107–110

8. Bray GA (2000) Reciprocal relation of food intake and sympathetic activity: experimental observations and clinical implications. Int J Obes Relat Metab Disord 24(Suppl 2):S8–S17

9. Inui A (1999) Cancer anorexia-cachexia syndrome: are neuropeptides the key? Cancer Res 59:4493–4501

10. Diksic M, Young SN (2001) Study of the brain serotonergic system with labelled alpha-methyl-L-tryptophan. J Neurochem 78:1185–1200

11. Rossi Fanelli F, Cangiano C, Ceci F et al (1986) Plasma tryptophan and anorexia in human cancer. Eur J Cancer Clin Oncol 22:89–95

12. Cangiano C, Cascino A, Ceci F et al (1990) Plasma and CSF tryptophan in cancer anorexia. J Neural Transm (Gen Sect) 81:225–233

13. Cangiano C, Testa U, Muscaritoli M et al (1994) Cytokines, tryptophan and anorexia in cancer patients before and after surgical tumor ablation. Anticancer Res 14:1451–1456

14. Laviano A, Cangiano C, Preziosa I et al (1997) Plasma tryptophan levels and anorexia in liver cirrhosis. Int J Eating Disord 21:181–186

15. Aguilera A, Selgas R, Codoceo R et al (2000) Uremic anorexia: a consequence of persistently high brain serotonin levels? The tryptophan/serotonin disorder hypothesis. Perit Dial Int 20:810–816

16. Cangiano C, Laviano A, Meguid MM et al (1996) Effects of administration of oral branched-chain amino acids on anorexia and caloric intake in cancer patients. J Natl Cancer Inst 88:550–552

17. Hiroshige K, Sonta T, Suda T et al (2001) Oral supplementation of branched-chain amino acids improves nutritional status in elderly patients on chronic haemodialysis. Neprhol Dial Transplant 16:1856–1862

18. Marchesini G, Bianchi G, Merli M et al (2003) Nutritional supplementation with branched-chain amino acids in advanced cirrhosis: a double-blind, randomized trial. Gastroenterology 124:1792–1801

19. Marks DL, Butler AA, Turner R et al (2003) Differential role of melanocortin receptor subtypes in cachexia. Endocrinology 144:1513–1523

20. Laviano A, Meguid MM (1996) Nutritional issues in cancer management. Nutrition 12:358–371

21. Edelman MJ, Gandara DR, Meyers FJ et al (1999) Serotonergic blockade in the treatment of the cancer anorexia-cachexia syndrome. Cancer 86:684–688

22. Blaha V, Yang ZJ, Meguid MM et al (1998) Ventromedial nucleus of hypothalamus is related to the development of cancer-induced anorexia: in vivo microdialysis study. Acta Medica (Hradec Kralove) 41:3–11

23. Herreros R, Serrat I, Boronat A (1999) L-DOPA and cancer anorexia. Palliat Med 13:83–84

24. Lozano RH, Jofre IS (2002) Novel use of L-DOPA in the treatment of anorexia and asthenia associated with cancer. Palliat Med 16:548

25. Cahlin C, Gelin J, Delbro D et al (2000) Effect of cyclooxigenase and nitric oxide synthase inhibitors on tumor growth in mouse tumor models with and without cachexia related to prostanoids. Cancer Res 60:1742–1749

26. Lundholm K, Gelin J, Hyltander A et al (1994) Anti-inflammatory treatment may prolong survival in undernourished patients with metastatic solid tumors. Cancer Res 54:5602–5606

27. Squadrito F, Calapai G, Altavilla D et al (1994) Central serotoninergic system involvement in the anorexia induced by NG-nitro-L-arginine, an inhibitor of nitric oxide synthase. Eur J Pharmacol 255:51–55

28. Lugarini F, Hrupka BJ, Schwartz GJ et al (2002) A role for cyclooxygenase-2 in lipopolysaccharide-induced anorexia in rats. Am J Physiol Regul Integr Comp Physiol 283:R862–R868

29. Nakamura K, Li YQ, Kaneko T et al (2001) Prostaglandin E3 receptor protein in serotonin and catecholamine cell groups: a double immunofluorescence study in the rat brain. Neuroscience 103:763–775

30. Gomes-Marcondes MCC, Ventrucci G, Toledo MT et al (2003) A leucine-supplemented diet improved protein content of skeletal muscle in young tumor-bearing rats. Braz J Med Biol Res 36:1589–1594

31. Ventrucci G, Mello MAR, Gomes-Marcondes MCC (2004) Proteasome activity is altered in muscle tissue of tumour-bearing rats fed a leucine-rich diet. Endocr Relat Cancer 11:887–895

32. Smith HJ, Wyke SM, Tisdale MJ (2003) Mechanism of the attenuation of Proteolysis-Inducing Factor stimu-

lated protein degradation in muscle by b-hydroxy-b-methylbutyrate. Cancer Res 64:8731–8735

33.  Paddon-Jones D, Sheffield-Moore M, Urban RJ et al (2004) Essential amino acid and carbohydrate supplementation ameliorates muscle protein loss in humans during 28 days bedrest. J Clin Endocrinol Metab 89:4351–4358

34.  Poon RT-P, Yu W-C, Fan S-T, Wong J (2004) Long-term oral branched chain amino acids in patients undergoing chemoembolization for hepatocellular carcinoma: a randomized trial. Aliment Pharmacol Ther 19:779–788

# An Update on Therapeutics: The Cancer Anorexia/Weight Loss Syndrome in Advanced Cancer Patients

Aminah Jatoi, Karin F. Giordano, Phuong L. Nguyen

## The Impetus Behind Studying and Treating the Cancer Anorexia/Weight Loss Syndrome

Experienced oncologists acknowledge that the cancer anorexia/weight loss syndrome predicts a shorter survival for patients with advanced, incurable disease. Several powerful, well-conducted studies have borne out this clinical impression. DeWys et al. focused on weight loss in a multi-institutional, retrospective review of 3047 cancer patients and observed that loss of more than 5% of premorbid weight predicted an early demise [1]. This prognostic effect occurred independently of tumour stage, tumour histology and patient performance status. Weight loss was also associated with a trend towards lower chemotherapy response rates.

Anorexia carries this same prognostic effect. Chang recently reviewed the predictive capability of various cancer symptoms and found that, similar to weight loss, anorexia, or loss of appetite, also predicts an early demise for the cancer patient [2]. Thus, the impetus for studying the cancer anorexia/weight loss syndrome rests in part in the hope that effective treatment will improve survival.

In addition to improving survival, there is another rationale for investigating this syndrome. Walsh et al. found that for patients with advanced and incurable cancer, anorexia is one of the most pervasive and bothersome symptoms at the very end of life [3]. In their review of 1000 cancer patients at the end of life, Walsh et al. found that anorexia occurred in 60% of patients and ranked third as the most troubling symptom, out-ranked only by pain and fatigue. In addition, several studies have shown that weight loss is associated with a decline in functional status. Finkelstein et al. observed that recent weight loss of > 5% among cancer patients was associated with a significant decline in functional status, as assessed by patient questionnaire data ($p = 0.004$) [4]. In lung cancer patients, Sarna et al. found that weight loss was associated with decreased functional status over a 30-week period [5]. Hence, the primary goals of treating the anorexia/weight loss syndrome are to improve both survival and quality of life in patients with advanced, incurable cancer.

## A Brief Overview of Current Treatment Options

To date, treatment attempts have yielded only modest success. Trials that have evaluated caloric supplementation have not shown this approach to be meritorious. For example, in a randomised study, Ovesen et al. found that cancer patients who received nutritional counselling consumed more calories, but that this additional consumption did not yield improvements in tumour response rates, survival or quality of life [6]. Similarly, several clinical trials have investigated total parenteral nutrition in chemotherapy-treated patients with advanced cancer and have found that this intervention, too, is ineffective. In fact, an analysis of these studies with total parenteral nutrition prompted the American College of Physicians to issue a consensus recommendation that total parenteral nutrition not be given to advanced cancer patients who are receiving chemotherapy [7].

Pharmacological agents have become the next resort from a therapeutic and clinical trials perspective. Progesterones and corticosteroids have been the most extensively studied but are limited in their benefits at best (Table 1). For example, megestrol acetate improves appetite in only 20–30% of cancer patients after subtracting a placebo effect [8]. Placebo-controlled trials with this agent demonstrate no improvement in sur-

**Table 1.** Agents with proven but limited efficacy

---

Corticosteroids

Progesterones

---

vival and no improvement in global quality of life. To date, randomised, placebo-controlled trials with corticosteroids, as well as other progestational agents, have been equally disappointing. Thus, there is a clear need to investigate other innovative strategies.

## A Brief Overview of Mechanisms To Explain the Cancer Anorexia/Weight Loss Syndrome

Recent strategies for treating the cancer anorexia/weight loss syndrome have relied heavily on an improved understanding of mechanisms of disease. How does cancer cause weight loss, debility and anorexia? A variety of different mediators have been described. Todorov et al. have discovered a 24-kilodalton proteoglycan derived from the MAC16 tumour line [9] and have labelled this mediator proteolysis-inducing factor (PIF). Although only a few studies have focused on PIF, antibodies to this substance appear to prevent weight loss in tumour-bearing animal models. Clinical data suggest that PIF is specific to cancer-associated wasting, as it is not found in cancer patients without weight loss nor in patients who are losing weight as a result of other diseases. To our knowledge, no clinical studies that have specifically focused on PIF inhibition have been reported thus far.

In addition to this mediator, other mediators that appear to play an active role in cancer-associated anorexia/weight loss include tumour necrosis factor-alpha (TNF-$\alpha$), interleukin (IL)-1$\beta$, IL-6 and ciliary neurotrophic factor [10–13]. The former has received notable attention of late because of animal studies that suggest inhibition of TNF-$\alpha$ is associated with an improvement in both appetite and weight. For example, Torelli et al. observed that an agent that targets the p55 soluble receptor improves appetite and attenuates

weight loss in tumour-bearing animals. TNF-$\alpha$ spawns a variety of other events, such as activation of the ubiquitin-proteasome system, and thereby leads to lean tissue wasting [14].

From the standpoint of appetite, it appears that the cancer patient's hormonal milieu is altered in the setting of the anorexia/weight loss syndrome. For example, in a North Central Cancer Treatment Group study in 73 advanced cancer patients with the anorexia/weight loss syndrome, it appeared preliminarily that neuropeptide Y, a potent orexigenic agent, was depressed [15]. Mean circulating neuropeptide Y concentrations (± standard deviations) were 466 pg/ml ± 161 pg/ml in cancer patients compared to concentrations of 560 pg/ml ± 151 pg/ml in historical controls ($p = 0.004$). Other hormone concentrations such as leptin and cholecystokinin were no different between cancer patients and controls. Nonetheless, this exploratory study suggests that hormonal mechanisms may be at work in causing anorexia in patients with this syndrome.

Over the past few years, the medical literature has drawn upon the above mechanisms in an effort to yield potentially promising treatment strategies. Some of these efforts, as well as the mechanisms that have supported their further study, are summarised below.

## What's New in the Clinical Management of the Cancer Anorexia/Weight Loss Syndrome?

### Hormonal Therapy

Although the benefits of progestational agents and corticosteroids have been modest, preliminary investigations suggest that other hormonal interventions merit further testing (Table 2). First, melatonin is secreted by the pineal gland and plays an important role in neuroendocrine regulation. Lissoni et al. examined the effects of melatonin in 100 patients with metastatic cancer. When administered at an oral dose of 20 mg/day, melatonin appeared to stabilise weight [16]. Patients who were receiving supportive care exclusively had much higher rates of notable weight loss (10% or more of baseline weight loss) ($p < 0.01$). The

**Table 2.** Promising agents that require further testing

Melatonin

Oxandrolone

Thalidomide

Tumour necrosis factor inhibitors

Non-steroidal anti-inflammatory drugs

Adenosine triphosphate

Creatine

inflammatory cytokine TNF-α appeared to drop in melatonin-treated patients, a finding that suggests a potential mechanism of action to explain the preliminary favourable weight effects seen with the administration of this hormone [17]. In another study performed by this same group, 70 patients with advanced non-small cell lung cancer were randomly assigned to receive cisplatin and etoposide versus this same chemotherapy combination along with melatonin 20 mg/day [18]. A larger percentage of melatonin-treated patients manifested weight stability. Taken together, these two studies strongly suggest that melatonin qualifies for further study in advanced cancer patients with weight loss.

Another hormonal agent that has received increasing attention in the treatment of this syndrome is oxandrolone. Von Roenn recently studied this anabolic androgenic steroid in 37 cancer patients. In a phase II study design, all patients received oxandrolone 10 mg orally twice a day [19]. This agent appeared to be well tolerated, and this preliminary investigation suggested that weight gain occurred in 84% of patients. An increase in lean tissue occurred in half of these patients who gained weight. Whether these promising results occur from general effects of this hormone on altering the cancer patient's hormonal milieu with consequential repercussions on appetite stimulation or from an entirely different mechanism of action is unclear. Nonetheless, these promising data led to a phase III trial that is nearing completion. Earlier studies had suggested that other androgens, such as fluoxymesterone, were not effective in treating the cancer anorexia/weight loss syndrome [20]. However, von Roenn et al. have

presented animal data to show that oxandrolone is far more specific in its androgen receptor binding capability and therefore potentially more capable of treating this syndrome. This more specific hormone-receptor binding might explain the favourable effects of oxandrolone and heightens the anticipation of maturing phase III data.

### Tumour Necrosis Factor-Alpha Inhibition

Thalidomide also deserves further investigation. Promising trials in AIDS patients have led to further investigation of this agent among cancer patients. Thalidomide treatment has resulted in weight gain and possibly maintenance of functional status in AIDS patients. Laboratory studies suggest that this agent shortens the half-life of TNF-a mRNA [21], although this drug has also demonstrated dose-dependent, bi-directional regulation of TNF-α.

Four studies in cancer patients are especially noteworthy. First, Bruera et al. evaluated a cohort of 72 cancer patients who received thalidomide 100 mg/night over 10 days [22]. Thirty-five patients dropped out of the study as a result of cancer-related morbidity. However, among the remaining patients, the majority reported improvement in insomnia (69%), nausea (44%) and loss of appetite (63%). As many as 53% reported an improvement in their overall sense of well-being. A comparison of symptom improvement between thalidomide-treated and historical megestrol acetate-treated patients suggests a trend in favour of thalidomide: mean difference ± standard deviation: -1.09 ± 2.67 versus 0.04 ± 1.71 for nausea ($p = 0.05$); -2.21 ± 2.83 versus -1.03 ± 2.49 for appetite ($p = 0.073$); and -1.65 ± 3.19 versus -0.61 ± 1.42 for sense of well-being ($p = 0.033$), respectively. This study was neither randomised nor double-blinded, but its specific focus on quality of life and symptom control strategies suggests that thalidomide may be of benefit to cancer patients independently of any potential antineoplastic effects.

In a second study, Mahmoud et al. observed an improvement in appetite with thalidomide 50–100 mg per day in 15 cancer patients [23]. Additionally, in a third study, Boasberg et al. observed weight stability in15 cancer patients who were treated with thalidomide 100–200 mg per day [24].

Finally, Khan et al. studied 11 patients with unresectable oesophageal cancer [25]. All patients were treated sequentially with an isocaloric diet for 2 weeks followed by thalidomide 200 mg orally daily. Among the ten evaluable patients, nine lost weight. However, during the subsequent 2 weeks, eight of these ten patients began to gain weight. Body composition assessed with dual X-ray absorptiometry indicated an augmentation of lean tissue.

Despite such promising data, the routine use of thalidomide for the cancer anorexia/weight loss syndrome does not yet comprise the standard of care. Thalidomide carries with it side-effects including somnolence, rash, sensorimotor-peripheral neuropathy and constipation, as well as less frequent side-effects including mood changes, dry mouth, headache, nausea, oedema, dry skin, pruritus, bradycardia, thyroid dysfunction and alterations in serum glucose levels. Teratogenicity is also a concern, although markedly less so in patients with advanced cancer. Since part of the goal of treating the cancer anorexia/weight loss syndrome is improvement in quality of life, the toxicity profile of any potential agent should be well established and minimal before it is routinely prescribed in this setting. Additionally, a large phase III trial that demonstrates definite improvements in quality of life and survival has not yet been reported.

But the above promising data have spurred further investigation into TNF-$\alpha$ blockade. The agents etanercept and infliximab have been used extensively for other medical indications, and the underlying hypothesis behind recent clinical trials is that these agents can be used to treat the cancer anorexia/weight loss syndrome. Both are specific inhibitors of TNF-$\alpha$. The animal data from Torelli et al., as alluded to above [14], specifically evaluated blockade of the TNF-$\alpha$ p55 soluble receptor and demonstrated improvement in appetite and weight in tumour-bearing animals. Currently, the North Central Cancer Treatment Group is conducting two large placebo-controlled trials with each of these agents [26]. Preliminary results are anticipated by the year 2006.

## Other Anti-inflammatory Agents

One of the most promising studies to look at anti-inflammatory agents was a landmark trial from Lundholm et al. [27]. In a placebo-controlled trial, these investigators found that indomethacin resulted in an improvement in survival in advanced cancer patients with the anorexia/weight loss syndrome. Since then, other studies have suggested that non-steroidal anti-inflammatory agents may play a role in treating this syndrome [28]. Although direct antineoplastic effects may be at work in achieving these benefits, the implication that the cancer anorexia/weight loss syndrome is mediated by inflammation suggests that these agents might also be directly treating this syndrome. Further confirmatory clinical studies and further mechanistic studies with these agents in this setting are indicated.

## Other Agents

Adenosine 5'-triphosphate (ATP), administered as a continuous infusion over many hours appears to show promise in patients with advanced non-small cell lung cancer. The rationale for this approach is two-fold. First, non-small cell lung cancer patients manifest an increase in metabolic rate that leads to wasted energy and subsequent weight loss. ATP is a key energy source, and perhaps its administration may compensate for the depletion of energy sources, although it remains unclear if intravenous ATP enters the cell. Second, empiric data from earlier trials with ATP suggested that this agent may be enhancing weight stability in non-small cell lung cancer patients. In an effort to test this agent further for the cancer anorexia/weight loss syndrome, Agteresch et al. randomly assigned 58 patients to receive either ATP or no ATP [29]. The study was not double-blinded, but a 0.2-kg increase in weight was noted over a 4-week period in the ATP-treated group. In contrast, a 1-kg drop in weight occurred in the group that did not receive ATP. In addition, strength and quality of life were more favourable in the ATP-treated patients. A promising agent, ATP deserves further investigation in this setting.

Another agent that merits further investigation, despite the fact that it has not yet been studied in cancer patients, is creatine. Commonly used by 'body builders', creatine is about to undergo active clinical investigation for the cancer anorexia/weight loss syndrome. In a collaborative trial, the North Central Cancer Treatment Group and the National Cancer Institute of Canada are about to open a phase III, placebo-controlled trial to study this amino acid derivative. Although potential mechanisms of action have not been well characterised, over 50 clinical trials have investigated creatine supplementation in other disease settings. Empiric observations suggest that creatine merits testing in the clinical setting in cancer patients and in aggregate can be summarised with the five following observations [30, 31]. First, creatine supplementation is associated with weight gain, including augmentation of lean tissue, in healthy individuals. Second, creatine promotes athletic performance in healthy individuals. Third, individuals with bulky musculature benefit less from creatine, an observation that suggests why not all studies have been totally consistent in finding improvements in athletic performance and suggests that there is perhaps merit in studying this agent in wasting cancer patients. Fourth, the agent has been shown to be relatively safe in healthy populations, with the most commonly reported adverse event being a mild, transient elevation of creatine after a loading dose. Fifth, in other disease states, such as McArdle's disease and congestive heart failure, as well as other muscle disorders, preliminary data suggest that creatine may be beneficial for patients with muscle wasting. Taken together, these preliminary data imply that further study of creatine is indicated in cancer patients.

## References

1. DeWys WD, Begg C, Lavin PT et al (1980) Prognostic effect of weight loss prior to chemotherapy in cancer patients. Eastern Cooperative Oncology Group. Am J Med 69:491–497
2. Chang VT (2000) The value of symptoms in prognosis of cancer patients. Topics in palliative care, Volume 4. Oxford University Press, Oxford
3. Walsh D, Donnelly S, Rybicki L (2000) The symptoms of advanced cancer: relation to age, gender, and performance status in 1000 patients. Support Care Cancer 8:175–179
4. Finkelstein DM, Cassileth BR, Bonomi PD et al (1988) A pilot study of the functional living index-cancer (FLIC) scale for the assessment of quality of life for metastatic lung cancer patients. Am J Clin Oncol 11:630–633
5. Sarna L, Lindsey AM, Dean H et al (1994) Weight change and lung cancer: relationships with symptom distress, functional status, and smoking. Res Nurs Health 17:371–379
6. Ovesen L, Allingstrup L, Hannibal J et al (1993) Effect of dietary counseling on food intake, body weight, response rate, survival, and quality of life in cancer patients undergoing chemotherapy: a prospective, randomized study. J Clin Oncol 11:2043–2049
7. Anonymous (1989) Parenteral nutrition in patients receiving cancer chemotherapy. Ann Intern Med 110:734–736
8. Loprinzi CL, Ellison NM, Schaid DJ et al (1990) Controlled trial of megestrol acetate for the treatment of cancer anorexia and cachexia. J Natl Cancer Inst 82:1127–1132
9. Todorov P, Cariuk P, McDevitt T et al (1996) Characterization of a cancer cachectic factor. Nature 379:739–742
10. Falconer JS, Fearon KC, Plester CE (1994) Cytokines, the acute-phase response, and resting energy expenditure in cachectic patients with pancreatic cancer. Ann Surg 219:325–331
11. Hellerstein MK, Meydani SN et al (1989) Interleukin1-induced anorexia in the rat. Influence of prostaglandins. J Clin Invest 84:228–235
12. Fong Y, Moldawer LL, Marano M et al (1989) Cachectin/TNF or IL-1 alpha induces cachexia with redistribution of body proteins. Am J Physiol 256:R659–R665
13. Greenberg AS, Nordan RP, McIntosh J et al (1992) Interleukin 6 reduces lipoprotein lipase activity in adipose tissue of mice in vivo and in 3T3-L1 adipocytes: a possible role for interleukin 6 in cancer cachexia. Cancer Res 52:4113–4116
14. Torelli GF, Meguid MM, Moldawer LL et al (1999) Use of recombinant human soluble TNF receptor in anorectic tumor-bearing rats. Am J Physiol 277:R850–R855
15. Jatoi A, Loprinzi CL, Sloan JA et al (2001) Neuropeptide Y, leptin, and cholecystokinin 8 in patients with advanced cancer and anorexia: a North Central Cancer Treatment Group exploratory investigation. Cancer 92:629–633
16. Lissoni P, Chilelli M, Villa S et al (2003) Five years survival in metastatic non-small cell lung cancer patients treated with chemotherapy alone or che-

motherapy and melatonin: a randomized trial. J Pineal Res 35:12–15

17. Braczkowski R, Zubelewicz B, Romanowski W et al (1995) Modulation of tumor necrosis factor-alpha toxicity by the pineal hormone melatonin in metastatic solid tumor patients. Ann NY Acad Sci 768:334–336

18. Lissoni P, Paolorossi F, Ardizzoia A et al (1997) A randomized study of chemotherapy with cisplatin plus etoposide versus chemoendocrine therapy with cisplatin, etoposide and the pineal hormone melatonin as a first-line treatment of advanced non-small cell lung cancer in patients with a poor clinical state. J Pineal Res 23:15–19

19. Von Roenn JH, Tchekmedyian S, Ke-Ning S et al (2002) Oxandralone in cancer-related weight loss: improvement in weight, body cell mass, performance status, and quality of life. Proc Soc Clin Oncol #1450

20. Loprinzi CL, Kugler JW, Sloan JA et al (1999) Randomized comparison of megestrol acetate versus dexamethasone versus fluoxymesterone for the treatment of cancer anorexia/cachexia. J Clin Oncol 17:3299–3306

21. Moreira AL, Sampaio EP, Zmuidzinas A et al (1993) Thalidomide exerts its inhibitory effects on tumor necrosis factor by enhancing mRNA degradation. J Exp Med 177:1675–1680

22. Bruera E, Neumann CM, Pituskin E et al (1999) Thalidomide in patients with cachexia due to terminal cancer: preliminary report. Ann Oncol 10:857–859

23. Mahmoud FA, Walsh D, Davis S et al (2003) A dose titration study of thalidomide in cancer anorexia. Proc Am Soc Clin Oncol #3170

24. Boasberg P, O'Day S, Weisberg M et al (2000) Thalidomide induced cessation of weight loss and improved sleep in advanced cancer patients with cachexia. Proceedings of the American Society of Clinical Oncology, 2396

25. Khan ZH, Simpson EJ, Cole AT et al (2003) Oesophageal cancer and cachexia: the effect of short-term treatment with thalidomide on weight loss and lean body mass. Aliment Pharmacol Ther 17:677–682

26. Jatoi A, Sideras K, Nguyen PL (2006) Tumor necrosis factor alpha as a treatment target for the cancer anorexia/weight loss syndrome. Supportive Cancer Therapy (in press)

27. Lundholm K, Gelin J, Hyltander A et al (1994) Anti-inflammatory treatment may prolong survival in undernourished patients with metastatic solid tumors. Cancer Res 54:5602–5606

28. Lundholm K, Daneryd P, Korner U et al (2004) Evidence that long-term COX-treatment improves energy homeostasis and body composition in cancer patients with progressive cachexia. Int J Oncol 24:505–512

29. Agteresch HJ, Rietveld T, Kerkhofs LG et al (2002) Beneficial effects of adenosine triphosphate on nutritional status in advanced lung cancer patients: a randomized clinical trial. J Clin Oncol 20:371–378

30. Juhn MS, Tarnopolsky M (1998) Potential side effects of oral creatine supplementation: a critical review. Clin J Sport Med 8:298–304

31. Juhn MS, Tarnopolsky M (1998) Oral creatine supplementation and athletic performance: a critical review. Clin J Sport Med 8:286–297

# Medroxyprogesterone Acetate in Cancer Cachexia

Giorgio Lelli, Benedetta Urbini, Daniela Scapoli, Germana Gilli

## Introduction

For a long time the use of testosterone-derivative drugs (nandrolone decanoate and others) has been indicated for patients with cancer anorexia-cachexia syndrome (CACS) on the basis of a truly protein anabolic effect [1], but the above drugs have a limited use because of some severe side-effects (liver damage, endocrine effects).

More recently, the use of corticosteroids has been proposed: nevertheless, none of the studies on the effects of corticosteroids in CACS has demonstrated a body weight gain, but only short-lasting benefits in terms of appetite and sensation of well-being, compared to a wide range of adverse effects [2].

## Mechanism of Action of High-Dose Progestins in CACS

Our early experience (first half of the 1980s) has clearly demonstrated that the use of 'high' doses (i.e. more than 500 mg daily intramuscularly, IM or orally, PO) of medroxyprogesterone acetate (MPA) in the treatment of advanced breast cancer patients can increase body weight in about 50% of treated patients [3]. It was associated with a better appetite and performance status and seemed to be unrelated to a direct antineoplastic effect (Fig. 1, *top*). Therefore, we assumed that high-dose MPA had an anabolic effect, similar to that observed with testosterone derivatives [1, 2]. Nevertheless, some questions concerning the body weight

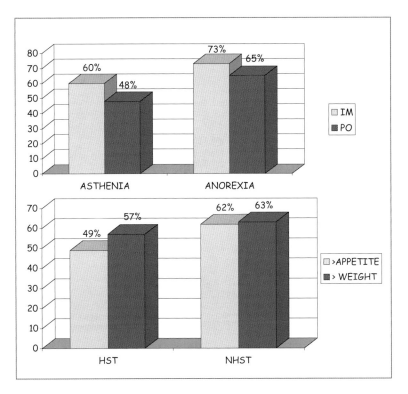

**Fig. 1.** High-dose (≥ 500 mg/day) medroxyprogesterone acetate in cancer patients. *Top* Subjective remission in breast cancer patients. *Bottom* Improvement in appetite/body weight in hormone-sensitive tumours (*HST*) or non-hormone-sensitive tumours (*NHST*). (Modified from [3, 4])

increase arose from these observations:

1. Is it related to or independent from the anti-tumour effect of MPA?
2. Is it based on a 'true' anabolic effect or a steroidal effect?
3. To what extent is it due to fluid and electrolyte retention?

The first question has been answered in a trial on a group of 65 patients with non-hormone-sensitive tumours, undergoing treatment with 2000 mg/day of MPA (Fig. 1, *bottom*): appetite (anorexia) improved in 62% of patients, while body weight increased significantly (more than 0.5 kg) in 63% [4].

In order to try to demonstrate a 'true' anabolic effect, a group of 10 patients with advanced non-hormone-sensitive cancer was submitted to treatment with high-dose MPA (> 500 mg/day, PO or IM) for 30 days. Before and after treatment, anthropometric parameters (body weight, skinfold plicometry, muscular strength) and metabolic parameters (protein, calories and nitrogen intake, measured by dietary survey; urinary nitrogen excretion measured by Kieldahl's method, and nitrogen balance) were registered. While anthropometric parameters showed no significant increase, except for muscular strength (24.4 kg before, 29.1 kg after, $p < 0.02$), we clearly demonstrated [5] a significant improvement in the nitrogen balance, protein and caloric intake (Fig. 2). Finally, in another group of 10 advanced cancer patients, no detectable effect on water and salt metabolism was demonstrated [6] by the evaluation of the exchangeable sodium pool with the $^{22}$Na method.

A possible explanation of the 'true' anti-cachectic effect of this drug was found by some authors [7, 8] who studied the influence of MPA administration on the various pro-cachectic cytokines, showing a down-regulatory effect on the synthesis and release of interleukin (IL)-1, IL-2, IL-6, tumour necrosis factor-$\alpha$ (TNF-$\alpha$) and serotonin.

## Side-Effects and Preferred Schedule of High-Dose MPA

High-dose progestins are well tolerated (Table 1); very rarely, the treatment must be interrupted because of the appearance of severe side-effects. Thromboembolic phenomena have been observed employing the intramuscular route only. MPA

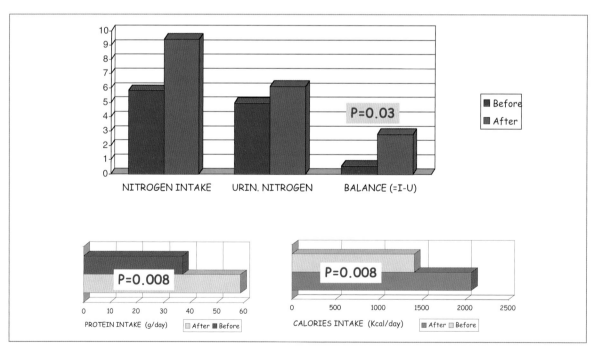

**Fig. 2.** High-dose ($\geq$ 500 mg/day) medroxyprogesterone acetate as an anabolic agent: nitrogen balance (*top*), protein and caloric intake (*bottom*). (Modified from [5]). *I – U*, intake – urinary

**Table 1.** Side-effects of high-dose MPA (296 patients). (Modified from [3])

| Side-effect | Percentage |
|---|---|
| Sweating | 16% |
| Fine tremors | 12.5% |
| Vaginal spotting | 10% |
| Cushing face | 8% |
| Cramps | 7% |
| Gluteal abscess | 7%[a] |
| Gastric intolerance | 4%[b] |
| Insomnia | 2% |
| Constipation | 2% |
| Itching | 1% |
| Thrombophlebitis | 0.5%[a] |

[a]By IM route, [b]PO

should generally be avoided only in cases of severe liver damage, previous ipercoagulability status or severe hypertension [3, 6]. One possible advantage of MPA over megestrol acetate (MA) is that it can be given in an intramuscular depot formulation in order to simplify the administration

for non-compliant patients and to maintain good drug plasma levels [3]. Nevertheless, in patients with a life expectancy of at least 4 weeks, the dose level of 1000 mg daily orally should be considered a 'golden standard', considering that following oral administration MPA is rapidly, even if not completely, absorbed, depending on the particle size of the oral formulation, according to our experience [3].

## Controlled Trials on MPA

Placebo-controlled trials [9–13] on the effect of MPA treatment on anorexia and body weight generally confirmed an improvement in both parameters (Table 2). It is important to remark that in three studies [9–11] MPA was administered during chemotherapy, and that in the same studies an improvement in quality of life was reported. Nevertheless, in contrast with our previous experience, those authors [13] who analysed body composition demonstrated that the bulk of the weight gain was due to increased body fat, while fat-free mass was not significantly influenced by the treatment.

**Table 2.** Random studies on MPA

| Author (ref.) | No. of patients | Dose of MPA | Results | | |
|---|---|---|---|---|---|
| | | | Anorexia | Body weight | Other parameters |
| Downer [9] | 60[a] | 300 mg/day PO[b] | $p = 0.015$ (6 weeks) | $p < 0.05$ (6 weeks) | NC in: PS, EN, mood |
| Kornek [10] | 31[a] | 500 mg/day PO[b] | 60% vs 43% | +3 kg/12 weeks ($p = 0.06$) | Improved QoL (40% vs 14%, NS) |
| Neri [11] | 279[a] | 1000 mg/day PO | NR | $p = 0.001$ | Improved PS |
| Simons [12, 13] | 206 | 1000 mg/day PO[b] | $p = 0.01$ (12 weeks) | + 0.6 kg/12 weeks ($p = 0.04$) | EN: $p = 0.01$ FAT: $p = 0.009$ FFM: NC REE: $p = 0.009$ |

[a]Concurrent chemotherapy, [b]tablets
*NC*, no change; *NR*, not reported; *NS*, not significant; *PS*, performance status; *EN*, energy; *FAT*, fat mass; *FFM*, fat-free mass; *REE*, resting energy expenditure; *QoL*, quality of life

## Conclusions and Future Perspectives

The role of MPA in the treatment of CACS has been the subject of many critical reviews [14, 15]. Nevertheless, the evaluation criteria of the above-cited drugs are mainly based on the weight increase and appetite stimulation. Therefore, a new insight into the mechanism of action of MPA, MA and other agents is urgently needed, because no definitive answer yet exists to the question of the true 'anabolic' effect of these drugs. Moreover, there are no trials available comparing MPA and MA, even if the efficacy of both drugs has been demonstrated in several studies. Very recently [16], the combination of MPA with other new agents, in particular with the cyclo-oxygenase-2 (COX-2) inhibitors, has been suggested as a way of ameliorating the efficacy of the treatment in cancer cachexia.

In conclusion, we consider it mandatory that studies on MPA, like on the other anabolic agents, should continue with a better consideration of the outcome results, possibly with a better understanding of body composition and cytokine levels before and after treatment.

### Acknowledgements

We thank Professor F. Pannuti for his continuous commitment in focusing and transmitting attention to palliative care, symptom evaluation and management, and for having stimulated our interest in medroxyprogesterone acetate.

## References

1. Kochakian CD (1976) II Metabolic effects. In: Kochakian CD (ed) Anabolic Steroids. Springer Verlag, Berlin, pp 5–72
2. Mantovani G, Macciò A, Massa E, Madeddu C (2001) Managing cancer-related anorexia/cachexia. Drugs 61:499–514
3. Pannuti F, Martoni A, Camaggi CM et al (1982) High dose medroxyprogesterone acetate in oncology. History, clinical use and pharmacokinetics In: Cavalli F, McGuire WL, Pannuti F (eds) Proceedings of the International Symposium on Medroxyprogesterone Acetate. Excerpta Medica, Amsterdam, pp 5–43
4. Pannuti F, Burroni P, Fruet F et al (1980) Anabolizing and antipain effect of the short-term treatment with medroxyprogesterone acetate (MAP) at high oral doses in oncology. Panminerva Med 22:149
5. Lelli G, Angelelli B, Giambiasi ME et al (1983) The anabolic effect of high dose medroxyprogesterone acetate in oncology. Pharmacol Res Commun 15:561–568
6. Lelli G, Angelelli B, Zanichelli L et al (1984) The effect of high dose medroxyprogesterone acetate on water and salt metabolism in advanced cancer patients. Chemioterapia 3:327–329
7. Mantovani G, Macciò A, Lai P et al (1998) Cytokine activity in cancer-related anorexia/cachexia: role of megestrol acetate and medroxyprogesterone acetate. Semin Oncol 25(Suppl 6):45–52
8. Kurebayashi J, Yamamoto S, Otsuki T et al (1999) Medroxyprogesterone acetate inhibits interleukin 6 secretion from KPL-4 human breast cancer cells both in vitro and in vivo: a possible mechanism of the anticachectic effect. Br J Cancer 79:631–636
9. Downer S, Joel S, Albright A et al (1993) A double blind placebo controlled trial of medroxyprogesterone acetate (MPA) in cancer cachexia. Br J Cancer 67:1102–1105
10. Kornek GV, Schenk T, Ludwig H et al (1996) Placebo-controlled trial of medroxyprogesterone acetate in gastrointestinal malignancies and cachexia. Onkologie 19:164–168
11. Neri B, Garosi VL, Intini C (1997) Effect of medroxyprogesterone acetate on the quality of life of the oncologic patient: a multicentric cooperative study. Anticancer Drugs 8:459–465
12. Simons J, Aaronson NK, Vansteenkiste JF et al (1996) Effects of medroxyprogesterone acetate on appetite, weight and quality of life in advanced stage non hormone sensitive cancer: a placebo controlled multicenter study. J Clin Oncol 14:1077–1084
13. Simons JP, Schols AM, Hoefnagels JM et al (1988) Effects of medroxyprogesterone acetate on food intake, body composition, and resting energy expenditure in patients with advanced, nonhormone-sensitive cancer. Cancer 82:553–560
14. Gagnon B, Bruera E (1998) A review of the drug treatment of cachexia associated with cancer. Drugs 55:675–688
15. Maltoni M, Nanni O, Scarpi E et al (2001) High-dose progestins for the treatment of cancer anorexia-cachexia syndrome. A systematic review of randomized clinical trials. Ann Oncol 12:289–300
16. Cerchietti LC, Navigante AH, Peluffo GD et al (2004) Effects of celecoxib, medroxyprogesterone, and dietary intervention on systemic syndromes in patients with advanced lung adenocarcinoma: a pilot study. J Pain Symptom Manage 27:85–95

# Progestagens and Corticosteroids in the Management of Cancer Cachexia

Davide Tassinari, Marco Maltoni

## Introduction

Over the past few years, many authors have approached the problem of the treatment of cancer cachexia focusing on either the knowledge of the main pathogenetic events, or the outcomes of the treatment in terms of symptoms or improvement in quality of life [1–8]. The relevance of clinical investigations of cancer anorexia-cachexia has epidemiological and clinical roots, considering that it is very frequent in advanced and terminal disease (up to 40% of patients with advanced disease, and more than 80% of terminal patients), and that its clinical manifestations often represent a source of great concern for both patients and relatives [1–5]. The clinical approach to cancer anorexia-cachexia has been directed towards different targets, and it can be aetiological, pathogenetic or symptomatic according to the attention paid to tumour growth, the main pathogenetic events, or the clinical behaviour of the syndrome. However, it is mandatory to define both the biological and clinical rationale of the different therapeutic options, and the outcomes of every therapeutic approach, using an evidence-based model. There are two main questions concerning clinical research in cancer anorexia-cachexia:

- Does a treatment exist that could act against the main pathogenetic events and influence the clinical outcome behaviour of cancer cachexia?
- What are the main outcomes of a treatment against cancer cachexia, and are these outcomes actually based on evidence-based tools?

The need for an evidence-based palliative medicine represents one of the main topics of palliative care, as it would be incorrect to avoid an evidence-based model when making decisions in clinical practice. On the other hand, methodologically correct clinical research can be hard in palliative care, because of the peculiar characteristics of patients with advanced or terminal disease. The treatment of cancer cachexia with corticosteroids or progestagens is based on a quite solid evidence of activity. However, despite the large number of trials supporting their use in clinical practice, some aspects still remain undefined and deserve to be looked at in more depth.

## Biological Rationale of Medical Treatment of Cancer Cachexia

Recently, many authors have investigated the different pathogenetic events responsible for the clinical behaviour of cancer cachexia, and suggested a role for both tumour cells and immuno-mediated responses to tumour growth, as important events in the pathogenesis of the syndrome [1, 7, 9–41]. Although the main pathogenetic events are not fully understood and the relationship between tumour factors and host inflammatory cytokines still remains undefined, a role of different tumour products and an immuno-mediated action of the monocyte-macrophage system seem to be involved in the pathogenesis of cancer cachexia (Fig. 1). Besides the speculative value of the biological knowledge about the role of host and tumour cytokines, the efforts of clinical researchers have been addressing the possibility of down-regulating the pro-cachectic action of cytokines, favouring a control of the clinical manifestations of the syndrome. To this end, progestagens and corticosteroids (and also non-steroidal anti-inflammatory drugs, eicosapentaenoic acid, melatonin and thalidomide) have been evaluated and proposed as active options in the treatment of cachexia-related

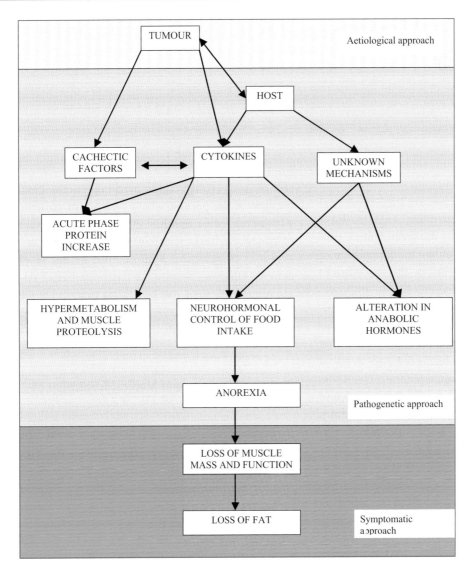

**Fig. 1.** Main pathogenetic events and sites of action of therapeutic options

symptoms [24–26, 42–57]. Two considerations can be made, coupling the biological dimension and the clinical approach:

– Besides representing a pathogenetic treatment, a treatment addressed towards one or more steps in the pathogenesis of the clinical syndrome might also be considered a kind of 'target treatment' in palliative care [42–44, 46, 47]
– The different sites of action of the different molecules might represent the starting point for a poly-pharmacotherapy against different steps in the same cascade [55–57].

The concept of a treatment designed on the basis of the biological characterisation of the dis-

ease represents one of the main topics of modern oncology, and some different models of clinical research and clinical practice support the activity and effectiveness of such an approach in the treatment of solid and haematological cancers [58–66]. There are two fields that might represent an interesting dimension in the pathogenetic approach to the palliative treatment of cancer cachexia:

– The use of biological markers to select the patients with the highest probability of response to the treatment (predictive value of the marker)
– The use of biological markers as surrogate endpoints of response.

This kind of approach has recently been evaluated in clinical research, and some preliminary results seem promising, but it would be hasty to state that the treatment of cancer cachexia as a 'target approach' is possible [57, 67]. Indeed, the reasons limiting a 'target approach' are various, and not well known. Besides the role of cytokines (interleukin 1, interleukin 6, interferon gamma and tumour necrosis factor alpha) in the pathogenesis of cachexia, some other mechanisms might play a pathogenetic role together with or instead of the cytokine cascade, favouring a low activity of an 'anti-cytokines' approach, or a mechanism of 'escape' in some patients [1, 68]. However, the possible variables occurring in the 'cytokine-mediated' anorexia-cachexia syndrome probably represent one of the main reasons supporting a target approach. An improvement in clinical results might be achievable by selecting patients using biological predictive factors of response, when we are able to detect biological markers in daily clinical practice [31–39, 42–44].

## Outcomes of a Palliative Treatment of Cancer Cachexia

Although a 'target approach' to cancer cachexia is still too far off to be validated definitively, the assessment of the outcome of a treatment represents an interesting field of investigation in clinical practice. The definition of an outcome in palliative medicine may be considered a general problem, but cancer cachexia represents one of the most paradigmatic examples in this field of clinical research. Some years ago, the consensus data of the Outcomes Working Group of the American Society of Clinical Oncology (ASCO) distinguished the outcomes of a treatment into patient outcomes (survival and quality of life) and cancer outcomes (response rate), and gave higher priority to patient outcomes [69]. Although the guidelines of the working group did not strictly concern palliative care, they can be translated into the palliative care dimension, as similar documents have never been produced for palliative care. It follows that quality of life should be identified as the main patient outcome, and quality-of-life assessment should represent the primary end-point of a trial in palliative care. However, although quality of life can surely represent the main end-point whenever an improvement in survival is not reasonably expected, the way by which quality of life should be assessed in clinical research and in daily clinical practice is not yet well defined [70, 71]. Some preliminary differences are worthy of being defined:

- The activity of a treatment defines if the treatment could act
- The efficacy of a treatment defines how much a treatment should act
- The effectiveness of a treatment defines if the treatment actually acts in clinical practice [72, 73].

On the one hand, activity, efficacy and effectiveness are strictly related to each other; on the other hand, they are very different from a methodological point of view:

- The activity of a treatment is defined by phase II trials
- The efficacy of a treatment is defined by phase III trials
- The effectiveness of a treatment is defined by phase IV trials.

Moreover, the main outcomes and the surrogate outcomes of a medical approach should be defined in clinical research, and the relationship between main and surrogate outcomes represents an open question not yet fully answered [74–79]. Indeed, there are no definitive data distinguishing main and surrogate end-points in quality-of-life assessment, and the relationship between symptom control and quality of life in an outcome analysis is still unclear. Symptom assessment surely represents the core of the validated instruments for quality-of-life assessment, but it cannot represent by itself a validated instrument for quality-of-life assessment. It follows that symptom assessment can be an index of activity of a treatment, or a surrogate end-point of quality of life, but quality of life must be considered either the main outcome of a treatment in palliative care, or the main index of efficacy of the treatment [74]. If we assume that symptom assessment represents an index of activity, and quality of life an index of efficacy of a treatment, we can re-analyse the clinical trials investigating corticosteroids or progestagens in cancer anorexia-cachexia, revisiting the results from an outcome point of view.

## Clinical Evidence of Activity, Efficacy and Safety of a Palliative Treatment with Corticosteroids or Progestagens in Cancer Anorexia-Cachexia Syndrome

Much biological evidence supports the activity of corticosteroids and progestagens in the treatment of cancer anorexia-cachexia through the inhibition of the cytokine cascade, which concurs with the clinical manifestations of the syndrome [42–44]. However, although the role of progestagens and corticosteroids as pathogenetic treatments of cancer cachexia is well defined, it may be interesting to review the clinical role of the two categories of drugs using an 'evidence-based' approach, and focusing on the outcomes of the two treatments. The first step is the definition of the levels of evidence and the grading of the recommendations, as identified by the main groups of research in clinical oncology [80, 81]. Table 1 shows the levels of evidence and the grading of the recommendations used by the Italian Association of Medical Oncology (AIOM), the European Society of Medical Oncology (ESMO) and ASCO. Although an evidence-based approach can be applied only in part to the particular dimension of palliative care, there are few

doubts about the need for an evidence-based palliative medicine. Consequently, we shall review the outcomes of the palliative treatment with corticosteroids or progestagens against cancer cachexia from an evidence-based point of view [82, 83].

### Activity, Efficacy and Safety of Corticosteroids in Palliative Treatment of Cancer Cachexia

Although many data support the use of corticosteroids in palliative care, their use is only supported in part by evidence-based rules [84]. The two main reasons for this limit are:
– The use of corticosteroids goes back to a 'pre-evidence-based' era in medicine, and, like some other old approaches, it could be assigned to a kind of 'traditional knowledge' in medicine
– The 'experience-based' evidence of their use in clinical practice (methodologically the opposite of the 'evidence-based' approach) is so high that it would be hard for their use not to be considered as the 'standard procedure' in 'evidence-based' confirmatory randomised trials.

Many interesting randomised clinical trials support the use of corticosteroids in the treatment of cancer cachexia [85–89]. Although the pivotal

**Table 1.** Levels of evidence and grading of recommendations

| Grading of recommendations | Level of evidence | Type of evidence |
|---|---|---|
| A | I | Evidence is obtained from meta-analysis of multiple, well-designed, controlled studies. Randomised trials with low false-positive and low false-negative errors (high power) |
| B | II | Evidence is obtained from at least one well-designed experimental study. Randomised trials with high false-positive and/or negative errors (low power) |
| | III | Evidence is obtained from well-designed, quasi experimental studies such as non-randomised, controlled single-group, pre-post, cohort, time or matched case-control series |
| C | IV | Evidence is from well-designed, non-experimental studies such as comparative and correlational descriptive and case studies |
| D | V | Evidence is from case reports and clinical examples |

trial of Moertel et al. dates back to 1974 [85], and other important trials were published in the 1980s [86–89], some considerations can be made approaching the results from an outcome point of view. All trials showed that corticosteroids (dexamethasone or prednisolone, or methylprednisolone) induce a temporary benefit against different cachexia-related symptoms, improving the appetite, food intake, sensation of well-being, and performance status. Conversely, no trial demonstrated an improvement in body weight. Moreover, the trials of Robustelli della Cuna and Popiela [88, 89] approached the dimension of quality-of-life assessment during the treatment, and tried to go beyond symptom assessment in the outcome assessment in palliative care. Besides these interesting results detailed in Table 2, there is much evidence that corticosteroids can act against some other symptoms, that are related to, but not constitutive of, cancer cachexia, such as asthenia, or nausea and vomiting [90–93]. It follows that corticosteroids are very useful in some different conditions of clinical practice, when cachexia coexists with other syndromes such as asthenia, nausea and vomiting, or dyspnoea. Such a versatility of corticosteroids is only partially known from a pathophysiological point of view. As concerns cancer cachexia, corticosteroids may be supposed to act by inhibiting the immune response and cytokine cascade, and acting on the central nervous system. However, other characteristics can partially counterbalance the data of activity. The above-mentioned trials and some others reported that the activity against cachexia-related symptoms is limited to a few weeks, and the relevant side-effects (peptic ulcer, cataract, opportunistic infections, glucose intolerance, myopathy) can often make it difficult to use corticosteroids in clinical practice. It follows that corticosteroids can surely be considered an active and probably efficacious approach against cancer cachexia, but shortness of action and side-effects suggest their use is limited to patients with advanced disease and expected short duration of survival [8, 94]. Finally, type, dosage and route of administration remain ill defined, and low dosages (less than 1 mg/kg of prednisone equivalent) seem recommendable in daily clinical practice [8].

**Table 2.** Randomised clinical trials of corticosteroids in cancer cachexia

| References | Molecule | Trial design | Number of patients | Main outcomes | Level of evidence (Table 1) |
|---|---|---|---|---|---|
| Moertel et al. [85] | Oral dexamethasone[a] | PCCT | 116 | Improve appetite | II |
| Willox et al. [86] | Oral prednisolone[b] | PCCT COD | 61 | Improve appetite | II |
| Bruera et al. [87] | Oral methylprednisolone[c] | PCCT COD | 40 | Improve appetite Improve food intake Improve pain control Improve performance status | II |
| Robustelli della Cuna et al. [88] | Parenteral methylprednisolone[d] | PCCT | 403 | Improve quality of life | I |
| Popiela et al. [89] | Parenteral methylprednisolone[d] | PCCT | 173 | Improve quality of life | I |

*PCCT*, placebo-controlled clinical trial; *COD*, cross-over design
Dosages: [a]0.75–1.5 mg four times daily; [b]5 mg three times daily; [c]16 mg twice daily; [d]125 mg four times daily

## Activity, Efficacy and Safety of Progestagens in Palliative Treatment of Cancer Cachexia

The use of progestagens in the palliative treatment of cancer cachexia has been largely investigated in the past few years, and to date they represent the treatment of choice [1–6, 8, 9, 94]. However, despite the large amount of data about activity, efficacy and safety of medroxyprogesterone acetate or megestrol acetate [95–111], and the supposed down-regulation of the cytokine cascade as their main mechanism of action [42–44], some considerations can be made. Unlike what has been observed about the clinical evidence of efficacy of corticosteroids in cancer cachexia, many randomised trials support the efficacy of progestagens, and two meta-analyses have been published in recent years, demonstrating their palliative role [95, 96]. Nevertheless, two issues are to be highlighted in the evaluation of the evidence of efficacy of progestagens in cancer cachexia:

- Evidence suggests that progestagens can down-regulate the cytokine cascade, but there are no data supporting the role of cytokine dosage as a predictive factor of response
- There is much evidence that progestagens can improve appetite and weight gain in patients with cancer cachexia, but the evidence is not enough to relate such an improvement to an improvement of quality of life.

In our systematic review of the literature, we selected 15 randomised clinical trials published before June 1999. All trials assessed the effect of progestagens on body weight, and all trials but two evaluated appetite improvement as an end-point of the treatment. Although weight gain or appetite improvement were evaluated differently in the different trials (the differences consisted in the time or the method of assessment), a significant role of progestagens was observed in both (Table 3). Quality of life was assessed in nine trials [97–105], but a positive role of high doses of progestagens was observed in just two [101, 102] (Table 4). We tried to understand the reasons for the lack of correlation between weight gain or appetite improvement and quality of life, and identified three possible factors:

- Insufficient sensitivity of the instruments used for quality-of-life assessment (the instruments used in the trials were not validated for the terminal phase of neoplastic disease)
- Duration of the treatment and follow-up too short to evaluate the impact of the treatment on overall quality of life
- Secondary relevance of cancer cachexia in the status of terminal or pre-terminal patients.

Another issue can help in understanding the reasons for such a discrepancy in the outcomes of the palliative approach with progestagens to cancer cachexia. Quality of life is probably the main end-point of a therapeutic approach in palliative care. Moreover, it represents a multidimensional aspect of the patient's life, and health-related quality of life is what we usually try to assess in clinical research [114]. Symptom improvement is one of the main domains in the health-related improvement in quality of life, but it does not represent the quality of life by itself. Likewise, symptom assessment plays an important role in quality-of-life assessment, but it cannot be considered the quality-of-life assessment by itself. It follows that symptom assessment can be considered an index of activity of a treatment against a clinical syndrome, while health-related quality of life is the main index of efficacy. Likewise, symptom assessment can be assumed as a surrogate outcome of quality of life, that should be assessed *within*, but not *instead of*, quality-of-life assessment [74]. In any case, to date progestagens represent the treatment of choice of cancer cachexia, and they can be considered one of the most active options, but the dosage of the treatment still remains undefined. In an interesting (even though questionable) trial, Loprinzi et al. tried to investigate the problem of the most active dosage of megestrol acetate in cancer cachexia, comparing four doses in 342 patients [106]. The patients were randomised to receive oral megestrol acetate at doses of 160, 480, 800 and 1280 mg/day and were evaluated monthly for response. The trial demonstrated a positive dose–response effect on appetite stimulation, but no significant effect on weight gain (only a trend in favour of high doses was shown), without any difference in the occurrence of side-effects. In particular, an improvement was observed up to 800 mg/day, while no further improvement was observed for higher doses. Despite these interest-

**Table 3.** Randomised clinical trials of progestagens in cancer cachexia

| Author | Number of patients | Arms | Outcomes | Level of evidence (Table 1) |
|---|---|---|---|---|
| Bruera et al. [97] | 84 | MA 480 mg vs placebo | Weight gain Improve appetite | II |
| De Conno et al. [98] | 42 | MA 160 mg vs placebo | Weight gain Improve appetite | II |
| Simons et al. [99] | 206 | MPA 1000 mg vs placebo | Weight gain Improve appetite | I |
| Vedell et al. [100] | 150 | MA 160 mg vs MA 480 mg vs placebo | Weight gain Improve appetite | I |
| Beller et al. [101] | 240 | MA 160 mg vs MA 480mg vs placebo | Weight gain Improve appetite Improve quality of life | I |
| Kornek et al. [102] | 31 | MPA 500 mg vs placebo | Weight gain Improve appetite Improve quality of life | II |
| Rowland et al. [103] | 243 | MA 800 mg vs placebo | Weight gain | I |
| Tchekmedyian et al. [104] | 89 | MA 1600 mg vs placebo | Weight gain Improve appetite | II |
| Westman et al. [105] | 255 | MA 320 mg vs placebo | Weight gain Improve appetite | I |
| Feliu et al. [107] | 150 | MA 240 mg vs placebo | Weight gain Improve appetite | I |
| Schmoll et al. [108] | 91 | MA 480 mg vs MA 960 mg vs placebo | Weight gain Improve appetite | II |
| Downer et al. [109] | 60 | MPA 300 mg vs placebo | Weight gain Improve appetite | II |
| Loprinzi et al. [110] | 133 | MA 800 mg vs placebo | Weight gain Improve appetite | I |
| Neri et al. [111] | 279 | MPA 1000 mg vs placebo | Weight gain | I |
| Bruera et al. [112] | 40 | MA 480 mg vs placebo | Weight gain Improve appetite | II |
| Jatoi et al. [113] | 469 | MA 800 mg vs DBN 5 mg vs MA 800 mg + DBN 5 mg | Weight gain Improve appetite Improve quality of life | I |

*MA*, megestrol acetate; *MPA*, medroxyprogesterone acetate; *DBN*, dronabinol

**Table 4.** Randomised clinical trials with quality of life as end-point

| Author | Number of patients | Arms | Quality-of-life assessment | Results |
|---|---|---|---|---|
| Bruera et al. [97] | 84 | MA 480 mg vs placebo | Functional living index – cancer | No differences in quality-of-life assessment |
| De Conno et al. [98] | 42 | MA 160 mg vs placebo | Therapy impact questionnaire | No differences in quality-of-life assessment |
| Simons et al. [99] | 206 | MPA 1000 mg vs placebo | EORTC-QLQ-C30 questionnaire | No differences in quality-of-life assessment |
| Vedell et al. [100] | 150 | MA 160 mg vs MA 480 mg vs placebo | Seven linear analogue self-assessment scales | No differences in quality-of-life assessment |
| Beller et al. [101] | 240 | MA 160 mg vs MA 480 mg vs placebo | Six linear analogue self-assessment scales | Improvement in overall quality of life of patients treated with MA |
| Kornek et al. [102] | 31 | MPA 500 mg vs placebo | Functional living index – cancer | Improvement in overall quality of life of patients treated with MPA |
| Rowland et al. [103] | 243 | MA 800 mg vs placebo | Visual analogue quality-of-life scale | No differences in quality-of-life assessment |
| Tchekmedyian et al. [104] | 89 | MA 1600 mg vs placebo | 29-item, patient-rated linear analogue scale | No differences in quality-of-life assessment |
| Westman et al. [105] | 255 | MA 320 mg vs placebo | EORTC-QLQ-C30 | No differences in quality-of-life assessment |
| Jatoi et al. [113] | 469 | MA 800 mg vs DBN 5 mg vs MA 800 mg + DBN 5 mg | FACT-cachexia | Improvement in quality-of-life assessment for MA or MA + DBN |

*MA*, megestrol acetate; *MPA*, medroxyprogesterone acetate; *DBN*, dronabinol

ing and methodologically correct results, on the basis of pharmacoeconomic considerations the authors suggested starting with lower doses of megestrol acetate, reserving higher doses to resistant patients. Some consideration can be made in this regard:

– There is a positive correlation between outcome and dosage (at least up to 800 mg/day), and this methodologically correct result could be applied to clinical practice. Moreover, the lack of a dose-related incidence of side-effects reinforces the conclusions of the trial for a clinical application

– The considerations of the authors regarding a clinically non-significant (although statistically

significant) difference in the outcomes in the four arms, though questionable, is reasonable. It follows that it might be acceptable from a clinical point of view to start with lower doses of megestrol acetate (160 mg/day), reserving higher doses for resistant patients

– The use of a cost-minimisation analysis (that needs comparable outcomes to be applied among the different hypotheses) is quite incorrect and unfit for this kind of application.

The trial of Loprinzi et al. correctly approaches the problem of the proper dose of megestrol acetate, and suggests a correct instrument to guide clinicians in daily clinical practice. Conversely, the final considerations may be considered correct from a clinical and biological point of view, but incorrect from a pharmacoeconomic point of view, because of the improper use of a pharmacoeconomic analysis in a setting that does not require such considerations.

Finally, all data in the literature indicate that high doses of progestagens are usually safe, and serious side-effects are not frequent in clinical practice [8, 9, 95–112]. Both medroxyprogesterone acetate and megestrol acetate increase the risk of thromboembolic events, peripheral oedema, breakthrough bleeding, hyperglycaemia, hypertension and Cushing's syndrome, but patients taking high doses of progestagens have to stop the treatment sporadically because of the occurrence of serious side-effects [8].

### Corticosteroids or High Doses of Progestagens: The Best Choice in Clinical Practice?

In the previous paragraphs we have reviewed the evidence supporting the use of corticosteroids or progestagens in the treatment of cancer anorexia-cachexia, supplying either the evidence of activity and efficacy (if any), or the limits of their use in clinical practice. The next step is the evidence-based analysis of the reasons for selecting one approach rather than another in clinical practice. Most reviews suggest some assumptions that are worthy of critical analysis:

- The effect of corticosteroids against cachexia-related symptoms is generally fast but short, usually limited to a few weeks. Moreover, the serious side-effects frequently occurring in chronic treatments limit their indication to patients with advanced disease and short expected survival [8, 9]
- The relative latency of action and the higher activity and safety of progestagens in comparison with corticosteroids make them the treatment of choice for patients with an expected survival greater than 3–4 weeks. This assumption is supported by either clinical or pharmacoeconomic considerations, as corticosteroids cost less than progestagens [8, 9, 94].

Loprinzi et al. analysed the different profile of corticosteroids (dexamethasone), progestagens (megestrol acetate) and anabolic corticosteroids (fluoxymesterone) in a trial involving 496 patients with cancer cachexia, randomly assigned to these three treatment options [115]. The results are interesting:

- Fluoxymesterone induced a significantly lower appetite enhancement and did not have a favourable toxic profile
- Megestrol acetate and dexamethasone induced similar appetite enhancement and similar changes in non-fluid weight status, with a non-significant trend favouring megestrol acetate for both parameters
- Dexamethasone had more corticosteroid-type toxicity and a higher rate of drug discontinuation than megestrol acetate, because of toxicity and/or patient refusal
- Megestrol acetate had a higher rate of deep venous thrombosis than dexamethasone.

To understand better when and why to choose corticosteroids or progestagens in clinical practice, the data of Loprinzi merit integration with those reported by De Conno et al. in a randomised, placebo-controlled trial comparing the clinical response of megestrol acetate and placebo in 42 patients evaluated at 7 and 14 days after beginning the treatment [98]. Appetite improvement started significantly earlier in patients treated with megestrol acetate than in those receiving placebo. It follows that both these trials may modify, at least in part, the current clinical habit reported by qualitative review literature:

- Both progestagens and corticosteroids can act against cachexia-related symptoms in the early and late phases of the disease
- The actual clinical advantage of progestagens is the lower occurrence of serious side-effects and the lower rate of discontinuation of the treatment
- Although the cost of corticosteroids is lower than that of progestagens, a correct analysis of cost minimisation (assuming an equal effect between dexamethasone and megestrol acetate, as reported by Loprinzi et al. [115]), which includes either the pharmaceutical costs or those for the treatment of side-effects, seems to favour progestagens as the treatment of choice in cancer cachexia.

On the basis of these observations, progestagens

should be considered as first-choice treatment in cancer cachexia, whereas the use of corticosteroids should be limited to patients with short life expectancy, because of their worse safety profile.

## Conclusions

Cancer anorexia-cachexia syndrome represents a relevant problem in the treatment of patients with advanced neoplastic disease. In the past few years, many authors have investigated the mechanisms underlying the clinical manifestations of the syndrome and its relevance in terms of quality of life. Much evidence supports the role of corticosteroids and progestagens in the treatment of the syndrome, and there are guidelines that address the choice in daily clinical practice. Nevertheless, some dimensions remain undefined and merit further investigations. A crucial, open question is the definition of the treatment in clinical practice. Although the identification of primary and surrogate outcomes in palliative care is not limited to cancer cachexia, it is important to observe that a palliative treatment against cachexia, even though able to improve cachexia-related symptoms, probably does not improve patient quality of life. Likewise, our 'evidence-based' knowledge is often based on surrogate end-points of clinical efficacy. These limits do not allow us to state that corticosteroids or progestagens are effective therapeutic options in the palliative approach to cancer cachexia, although a lot of evidence supports a high activity of both of them (and particularly of progestagens). Many efforts must be made to define better the outcomes of the palliative treatments, and the recovery of quality of life as the main outcome in palliative care, as well as the inclusion of symptom improvement in a comprehensive quality-of-life assessment, will be the challenge of the next years. To date, corticosteroids, and mostly progestagens, are the most active options in the treatment of cancer cachexia, and they have to be considered the standard options for the next clinical trials. Two possible scenarios may be suggested for the dimension of future clinical trials:

– A 'biological' characterisation of the patients based on the identification of predictive markers of response. The outcomes might be improved by selecting the patients to be treated on the basis of the predictive value of response to a particular treatment

– A review of clinical outcomes in palliative care, focusing on 'health-related' quality of life as well as on symptom improvement, as a better approach to patients and their relatives in the latter stages of the patient's life.

At present, clinical evidence of activity supports the use of progestagens as the standard option in the treatment of cancer cachexia, and starting from such an evidence base we should continue to improve our knowledge on the outcome research in cancer cachexia.

## References

1. Laviano A, Meguid MM, Rossi-Fanelli F (2003) Cancer anorexia: clinical implications, pathogenesis and therapeutic strategies. Lancet Oncol 4:686–694
2. Inui A (2002) Cancer anorexia-cachexia syndrome: current issues in research and management. CA Cancer J Clin 52:72–91
3. Nelson KA (2000) The cancer anorexia-cachexia syndrome. Semin Oncol 27:64–68
4. Davis MP, Dickerson D (2000) Cachexia and anorexia: cancer's covert killer. Support Care Cancer 8:180–187
5. Puccio M, Nathanson L (1997) The cancer cachexia syndrome. Semin Oncol 24:277–287
6. Kotler DP (2000) Cachexia. Ann Intern Med 133:622–634
7. Dunlop RJ, Campllell CW (2000) Cytokines and advanced cancer. J Pain Symptom Manage 20:214–232
8. Mantovani G, Macciò A, Massa E, Madeddu C (2001) Managing cancer-related anorexia/cachexia. Drug 61:499–514
9. Jatoi A, Loprinzi CL (2002) Anorexia/weight loss. In: Berger AM, Portenoy RK, Weissman DE (eds) Principles and practice of palliative care and supportive oncology, 2nd edn. Lippincott Williams and Wilkins, Philadelphia, pp 169–177
10. Strasser F (2004) Pathophysiology of the anorexia/cachexia syndrome. In: Doyle D, Hanks G, Cherny N, Calman K (eds) Oxford textbook of palliative medicine, 3rd edn. Oxford University Press, New York, pp 520–533
11. Rink TJ (1994) In search of a satietary factor. Nature

372:406–407

12. Spina M, Merlo-Pick E, Chan RKW et al (1996) Appetite suppressing effect of urocortin, a CRF-related neuropeptide. Science 273:1561–1564

13. Beck SA, Mulligan HD, Tisdale MJ (1990) Lipolytic factors associated with murine and human cancer cachexia. J Natl Cancer Inst 82:1922–1926

14. Todorov P, Cariuk P, McDevitt T et al (1996) Characterisation of a cancer cachectic factor. Nature 379:739–742

15. Khan S, Tisdale MJ (1999) Catabolism of adipose tissue by a tumor produced lipid mobilising factor. Int J Cancer 80:444–447

16. Hussey HJ, Tisdale MJ (1999) Effect of a cachectic factor on carbohydrate metabolism and attenuation by eicosapentaenoic acid. Br J Cancer 80:1231–1235

17. Belisario JE, Katz M, Chenker E et al (1991) Bioactivity of skeletal muscle proteolysis inducing factor in the plasma proteins from cancer patients with weight loss. Br J Cancer 63:705–710

18. Todorov PT, Deacon M, Tisdale MJ (1997) Structural analysis of a tumor produced sulfated glycoprotein capable of initiating muscle protein degradation. J Biol Chem 272:12279–12288

19. Cariuk P, Lorite MJ, Todorov PT et al (1997) Induction of cachexia in mice by a product isolated from the urine of cachectic cancer patients. Br J Cancer 6:606–613

20. Lorite MJ, Thomson MG, Drake JL et al (1998) Mechanism of muscle protein degradation induced by a cancer cachectic factor. Br J Cancer 78:850–856

21. Lorite MJ, Cariuk P, Tisdale MJ (1997) Induction of muscle protein degradation by a tumor factor. Br J Cancer 76:1035–1040

22. Wigmore SJ, Todorov PT, Barber MD et al (2000) Characteristics of patients with pancreatic cancer expressing a novel cancer cachectic factor. Br J Surg 87:53–58

23. Groundwater P, Beck SA, Barton C et al (1990) Alteration of serum and urinary lipolytic activity with weight loss in cachectic cancer patients. Br J Cancer 62:816–821

24. Cahlin C, Korner A, Axelsson H et al (2000) Experimental cancer cachexia: the role of host-derived cytokines interleukin-6, interleukin-12, interferon-gamma and tumor necrosis factor alpha evaluated in gene knockout bearing mice on C57B1 background and eicosapentaenoic-dependent cachexia. Cancer Res 60:5488–5493

25. Smith HJ, Lorite MJ, Tisdale MJ (1997) Effect of a cancer cachectic factor on protein synthesis/degradation in murine C2C12 myoblast: modulation by eicosapentaenoic acid. Cancer Res 59:5507–5513

26. Beck SA, Smith KL, Tisdale MJ (1991) Anticachectic and antitumor effect of eicosapentaenoic acid and its effect on protein turnover. Cancer Res 51:6089–6093

27. Nakashima J, Tachibana M, Ueno M et al (1998) Association between tumor necrosis factor in serum and cachexia in patients with prostatic cancer. Clin Cancer Res 4:1743–1748

28. Soda K, Kawakami M, Kashii A et al (1995) Manifestations of cancer cachexia induced by colon adenocarcinoma are not fully ascribable to interleukin 6. Int J Cancer 28:332–336

29. Tisdale MJ (1998) New cachectic factor. Curr Opin Clin Nutr Metab Care 1:253–256

30. Albrect JT, Canada TW (1996) Cachexia and anorexia in malignancy. Hematol Oncol Clin North Am 10:791–800

31. Naguchi Y, Yoshikawa T, Matsumoto A et al (1996) Are cytokines possible mediators of cancer cachexia? Surg Today 26:467–475

32. Nomura K, Noguchi Y, Yoshikawa T et al (1997) Plasma interleukin-6 is not a mediator of changes in lipoprotein lipase activity in cancer patients. Hepatogastroenterology 44:1519–1526

33. Argiles GM, Lopez-Soriano FJ (1999) The role of cytokines in cancer cachexia. Med Res Rev 19:223–248

34. Shibata M, Takekawa M (1999) Increased serum concentrations of circulating soluble receptor for interleukin-2 and its effect as a prognostic indicator in cachectic patients with gastric and colorectal cancer. Oncology 56:54–58

35. Bossola M, Muscaritoli M, Bellantone R et al (2000) Serum tumor necrosis factor-alpha levels in cancer patients are discontinuous and correlate with weight loss. Eur J Clin Invest 30:1107–1112

36. Maltoni M, Fabbri L, Nanni O et al (1997) Serum levels of tumor necrosis factor alpha and other cytokines do not correlate with weight loss and anorexia in cancer patients. Support Care Cancer 5:130–135

37. Mantovani G (2000) Cachexia and anorexia. Support Care Cancer 8:506–507

38. Espat NJ, Copeland EM, Moldawer LL et al (1994) Tumor necrosis factor and cachexia: a current perspective. Surg Oncol 3:255–262

39. McNamara MJ, Alexander HR, Norton JA (1992) Cytokines and their role in the pathophysiology of cancer cachexia. JPEN J Parenter Enteral Nutr 16(Suppl 6):50–53

40. Moldawer LL, Rogy MA, Lowry SF et al (1992) The role of cytokines in cancer cachexia. JPEN J Parenter Enteral Nutr 16:43–49

41. Plata-Salaman CR (1992) Central nervous system mechanism contributing to the cachexia-anorexia syndrome. Nutrition 16:43–49

42. Mantovani G, Macciò A, Lai P et al (1998) Cytokines involvement in cancer anorexia/cachexia: role of megestrol acetate and medroxy-progesterone acetate on cytokine down-regulation and improvement of clinical symptoms. Crit Rev Oncog 9:99–106

43. Mantovani G, Macciò A, Esu S et al (1997) Medroxyprogesterone acetate reduces the in vitro production of cytokines and serotonin involved in anorexia/cachexia and emesis by peripheral blood

mononuclear cells of cancer patients. Eur J Cancer 33:602–607

44. Mantovani G, Macciò A, Lai P et al (1998) Cytokine activity in cancer related anorexia/cachexia: role of megestrol acetate and medroxyprogesterone acetate. Semin Oncol 25(Suppl 6):45–52

45. Peuckmann V, Fisch M, Bruera E (2000) Potential novel uses of thalidomide: focus on palliative care. Drugs 60:273–292

46. Schimdt H, Rush B, Simonian G (1996) Thalidomide inhibits TNF response and increases survival following endotoxins in rats. J Surg Res 63:143–146

47. Bruera E, Neumann C, Pitukskin E et al (1999) Thalidomide in patients with cachexia due to terminal cancer: preliminary report. Ann Oncol 10:857–859

48. Lissoni P, Paolorossi F, Tancini G et al (1996) Is there a role for melatonin in the treatment of neoplastic cachexia? Eur J Cancer 32A:1340–1343

49. Neri B, DeLeonardis V, Gemelli MT et al (1998) Melatonin as biological response modifier in cancer patients. Anticancer Res 18:1329–1332

50. Tisdale M (1996) Inhibition of lypolysis and muscle protein degradation by EPA in cancer cachexia. Nutrition 12(Suppl 1):531–533

51. DeDeckerre E (1999) Possible beneficial effect of fish and fish N-3 polyunsaturated fatty acids in breast and colorectal cancer. Eur J Cancer Prev 80:1231–1235

52. Barber M, Ross J, Vossa C et al (1999) The effect of an oral nutritional supplement enriched with fish oil on weight-loss in patients with pancreatic cancer. Br J Cancer 81:80–86

53. Moertel CG, Schutt AJ, Reitemeir RJ et al (1974) Corticosteroid therapy of preterminal gastrointestinal cancer. Cancer 33:1607–1609

54. Ettingen AB, Portenoy RK (1988) The use of corticosteroids in the treatment of symptoms associated with cancer. J Pain Symptom Manage 3:99–103

55. Lissoni P, Brivio F, Ardizzoia A et al (1993) Subcutaneous therapy with low-dose interleukin-2 plus the neurohormone melatonin in metastatic gastric cancer patients with low performance status. Tumori 79:401–404

56. McMillian DC, O'Gorman P, Fearon KCF et al (1997) A pilot study of megestrol acetate and ibuprofen in the treatment of cachexia in gastrointestinal cancer patients. Br J Cancer 76:788–790

57. Cerchietti LCA, Navigante AH, Peluffo GD et al (2004) Effects of celecoxib, medroxyprogesterone and dietary intervention on systemic syndromes in patients with advanced lung adenocarcinoma: a pilot study. J Pain Symptom Manage 27:85–95

58. Arteaga CL, Moulder SL, Yakes M (2002) HER (erbB) tyrosine kinase inhibitors in the treatment of breast cancer. Semin Oncol 29(Suppl 11):4–10

59. Pegram MD, Reese DM (2002) Combined biological therapy of breast cancer using monoclonal antibodies directed against HER2/neu protein and vascular endothelial growth factor. Semin Oncol 29(Suppl 11):29–37

60. Ligibel JA, Winer EP (2002) Trastuzumab/chemotherapy combination in metastatic breast cancer. Semin Oncol 29(Suppl 11):38–43

61. Ritter CA, Arteaga CL (2003) The epidermal growth factor receptor-tyrosine kinase: a promising therapeutic target in solid tumors. Semin Oncol 30(Suppl 1):3–11

62. Cella D (2003) Impact of ZD1839 on non small cell lung cancer related symptoms as measured by the functional assessment of cancer therapy lung scale. Semin Oncol 30(Suppl 1):39–48

63. Douglass EC (2003) Development of ZD1839 in colorectal cancer. Semin Oncol 30(Suppl 6):17–22

64. Grunwald V, Hidalgo M (2003) Development of the epidermal growth factor receptor inhibitor OSI-774. Semin Oncol 30(Suppl 6):23–31

65. Swaton C (2004) Cell-cycle targeted therapies. Lancet Oncol 5:27–36

66. Johnson P, Glennie M (2003) The mechanism of action of rituximab in the elimination of tumor cells. Semin Oncol 30(Suppl 2):3–8

67. Tassinari D, Sartori S, Maltoni M et al (2004) Target therapies in palliative care: from a clinical to a biological approach. J Pain Symptom Manage 28:195–197

68. Rubin H (2003) Cancer cachexia: its correlations and causes. Proc Natl Acad Sci USA 100:5384–5389

69. Anonymous (1996) Outcomes of cancer treatment for technology assessment and cancer treatment guidelines. Amercian Society of Clinical Oncology. J Clin Oncol 14:671–679

70. Kaasa S, Loge JH (2003) Quality of life in palliative care: principles and practice. Palliat Med 17:11–20

71. Kaasa S, Loge JH (2002) Quality of life assessment in palliative care. Lancet Oncol 3:175–182

72. Cochrane AL (1972) Effectiveness and efficiency: random reflection on health services. Royal Society of Medicine, London

73. Haynes B (1999) Can it work? Does it work? Is it worth it? BMJ 319:652–653

74. Tassinari D (2003) Surrogate end point of quality of life assessment: have we really found what we are looking for? Health Qual Life Outcomes 1:71

75. Tassinari D, Poggi B, Fantini M et al (2003) Can we really consider quality of life as an outcome of palliative care? J Pain Symptom Manage 26:886–887

76. Tassinari D, Panzini I, Sartori S, Ravaioli A (2003) Surrogate outcomes in quality of life research: where we will end up? J Clin Oncol 21:1894–1895

77. Tassinari D, Panzini I, Ravaioli A et al (2002) Quality of life at the end of life: how is the solution far away? J Clin Oncol 20:1704–1705

78. Hwang SS, Chang VT, Fairclough DL et al (2003) Longitudinal quality of life in advanced cancer patients: pilot study results from a VA medical center. J Pain Symptom Manage 25:225–235

79. Goodwin DM, Higginson IJ, Myers K et al (2003)

Effectiveness of palliative day care in improving pain, symptom control and quality of life. J Pain Symptom Manage 25:202–212

80. Cook DJ, Guyatt GH, Laupacis A, Sackett DL (1992) Rules of evidence and clinical recommendations on the use of antithrombotic agents. Chest 102(Suppl 4):305S–311S

81. Harbour R, Miller J (2001) A new system for grading recommendations in evidence based guidelines. BMJ 323:334–336

82. Tassinari D, Maltoni M, Amadori D (2002) Prediction of survival in terminally ill cancer patients: why we cannot avoid an evidence-based palliative medicine. Ann Oncol 13:1322–1323

83. Kaasa S, De Conno F (2001) Palliative care research. Eur J Cancer 37(Suppl 8):153S–159S

84. Henriksen H, Gamborg H, Leikersfeldt G (2003) Corticosteroids in palliation of preterminal and terminal cancer patients. Evidence or empiricism? Ugeskr Laeger 165:3913–3917

85. Moertel C, Schutt AG, Reiteneier RJ et al (1974) Corticosteroid therapy of pre-terminal gastrointestinal cancer. Cancer 33:1607–1609

86. Willox J, Corr J, Shaw J et al (1984) Prednisolone as an appetite stimulant in patients with cancer. BMJ 288:27

87. Bruera E, Roca E, Cedaro L et al (1985) Action of oral methylprednisolone in terminal cancer patients: a prospective randomized double blind study. Cancer Treat Rep 69:751–754

88. Robustelli della Cuna G, Pellegrini A, Piazzi M (1989) Effect of methylprednisolone sodium succinate on quality of life in pre-terminal cancer patients: a placebo controlled multicenter study. Eur J Cancer Clin Oncol 25:1823–1829

89. Popiela T, Lucchi R, Giongo F (1989) Methylprednisolone as palliative therapy for female terminal cancer patients. Eur J Cancer Clin Oncol 25:1823–1829

90. Barnes EA, Bruera E (2002) Fatigue in patients with advanced cancer: a review. Int J Gynecol Cancer 12(5):424–428

91. Bruera E, Neumann CM (1998) Management of specific symptom complexes in patients receiving palliative care. CMAJ 158:1717–1726

92. Bruera ED, MacEachern TJ, Spachynski KA et al (1994) Comparison of the efficacy, safety, and pharmacokinetics of controlled release and immediate release metoclopramide for the management of chronic nausea in patients with advanced cancer. Cancer 74:3204–3211

93. Watanabe S, Bruera E (1994) Corticosteroids as adjuvant analgesics. J Pain Symptom Manage 9:442–445

94. Bruera E, Sweeney C (2004) Pharmacological interventions in cachexia and anorexia. In: Doyle D, Hanks G, Cherny N, Calman K (eds) Oxford textbook of palliative medicine, 3rd edn. Oxford University Press, New York, pp 552–560

95. Maltoni M, Nanni O, Scarpi E et al (2001) High-dose progestins for the treatment of cancer anorexia-cachexia syndrome: a systematic review of randomized clinical trials. Ann Oncol 12:289–300

96. Lopez AP, Roquè-i-Figuls M, Urrutia Cuchi G et al (2004) Systematic review of megestrol acetate in the treatment of anorexia-cachexia syndrome. J Pain Symptom Manage 27:360–369

97. Bruera E, Ernst S, Hagen N et al (1998) Effectiveness of megestrol acetate in patients with advanced cancer: a randomized double blind, crossover study. Cancer Prev Control 2:74–78

98. De Conno F, Martini C, Zecca E et al (1998) Megestrol acetate for anorexia in patients with far-advanced cancer: a double-blind controlled clinical trial. Eur J Cancer 34:1705–1709

99. Simons JPFHA, Aaronson NK, Vansteenkiste JF et al (1996) Effects of medroxyprogesterone acetate on appetite, weight and quality of life in advanced-stage non-hormone-sensitive cancer: a placebo-controlled multicentric study. J Clin Oncol 14:1077–1084

100. Vedell C, Segui MA, Gimenez-Arnau JM et al (1998) Anticachectic efficacy of megestrol acetate at different doses and versus placebo in patients with neoplastic cachexia. Am J Clin Oncol 21:347–351

101. Beller E, Tattersall M, Lumley T et al (1997) Improved quality of life with megestrol acetate in patients with endocrine-insensitive advanced cancer: a randomised placebo-controlled trial. Australasian megestrol acetate cooperative study group. Ann Oncol 8:277–283

102. Kornek GV, Schenk T, Ludwig H et al (1996) Placebo-controlled trial of medroxyprogesterone acetate in gastrointestinal malignancies and cachexia. Onkologie 19:164–168

103. Rowland KM, Loprinzi CL, Shaw EG et al (1996) Randomized double-blind placebo-controlled trial of cisplatin and etoposide plus megestrol acetate/placebo in extensive-stage small-cell lung cancer: a North Central Cancer Treatment Group study. J Clin Oncol 14:135–141

104. Tchekmedyian NS, Hickman M, Siau J et al (1992) Megestrol acetate in cancer anorexia and weight loss. Cancer 69:1268–1274

105. Westman G, Bergman B, Albertsson M et al (1999) Megestrol acetate in advanced progressive hormone-insensitive cancer. Effects on the quality of life: a placebo-controlled randomised multicentre trial. Eur J Cancer 35:586–595

106. Loprinzi CL, Michalak D, Schaid DJ et al (1993) Phase III evaluation of four doses of megestrol acetate as therapy for patients with cancer anorexia and/or cachexia. J Clin Oncol 11:762–767

107. Feliu J, Gonzalez-Baron M, Berrocal A et al (1992) Usefulness of megestrol acetate in cancer cachexia and anorexia. Am J Clin Oncol 15:436–440

108. Schmoll E (1992) Risks and benefit of various therapies for cancer anorexia. Oncology 49:43–45

109. Downer S, Joel S, Allbright A et al (1993) A double

blind placebo controlled trial of medroxyprogesterone acetate (MPA) in cancer cachexia. Br J Cancer 67:1102–1105

110. Loprinzi CL, Ellison NM, Schaid DJ et al (1990) Controlled trial of megestrol acetate for the treatment of cancer anorexia and cachexia. J Natl Cancer Inst 82:1127–1132

111. Neri B, Garosi VL, Intini C (1997) Effect of medroxyprogesterone acetate on the quality of life of the oncologic patient: a multicentric cooperative study. Anticancer Drugs 8:459–465

112. Bruera E, MacMillan K, Kuehn N et al (1990) A controlled trial of megestrol acetate on appetite, caloric intake, nutritional status and other symptoms in patients with advanced cancer. Cancer 66:1279–1282

113. Jatoi A, Windschitl HE, Loprinzi CL et al (2002) Dronabinol versus megestrol acetate versus combination therapy for cancer-associated anorexia: a North Central Cancer Treatment Group Study. J Clin Oncol 20:567–573

114. Cella D, Chang CH, Lai JS et al (2002) Advances in quality of life measurements in oncology patients. Semin Oncol 29(Suppl 8):60–68

115. Loprinzi CL, Kugler JW, Sloan JA et al (1999) A randomized comparison of megestrol acetate versus dexamethasone, versus fluoxymesterone for the treatment of cancer anorexia/cachexia. J Clin Oncol 17:3299–3306

# COX-2 Inhibitors in Cancer Cachexia

Giovanni Mantovani

## Introduction

Cyclo-oxygenase-2 (COX-2) is an enzyme catalysing the synthesis of prostaglandins (PGs) from arachidonic acid. Cells contain genes coding for two isoforms of COX (COX-1 and COX-2). COX-1 is expressed constitutively in most tissues and appears to be responsible for the production of PGs that mediate normal physiological functions, such as maintenance of the integrity of the gastric mucosa and regulation of renal blood flow. In contrast, COX-2 is undetectable in most normal tissues: it is induced by cytokines, growth factors, oncogenes and tumour promoters, and it contributes to the synthesis of PGs in inflamed and neoplastic tissues [1]. COX-2 is induced in many human tumours and is associated with aberrant angiogenesis in a number of pathological settings, especially those involving inflammation. It has been well demonstrated that dysregulation of COX-2 expression correlates with development of gastrointestinal cancers. Several studies reported that COX-2 expression is increased in human colorectal adenocarcinomas: it has been detected in 80–90% of colorectal adenocarcinomas and in 40–50% of premalignant adenomas [2]. Several studies suggest that COX-2, by inducing $PGE_2$ synthesis, contributes to the development of certain types of tumour [3, 4]. PGs appear to be important in the pathogenesis of cancer because they affect mitogenesis, cell adhesion, immune surveillance and apoptosis [5–8]. Cancers such as cancer of the head and neck, breast, lung and colon form more PGs than the normal tissues from which they arise [9–11].

## COX-2 Selective Inhibitors (Celecoxib, Rofecoxib and Valdecoxib)

Cyclo-oxygenase-2 is a bifunctional enzyme possessing both cyclo-oxygenase and peroxidase activities. Selective COX-2 inhibitors inhibit PG biosynthesis (anti-COX-2 activity) but do not, or only partially, affect the peroxidase activity of COX, which can generate proximate carcinogens. In experimental animals, selective inhibitors of COX-2 such as celecoxib reduce the formation of head and neck, colorectal, stomach, lung, breast and prostate tumours. In addition to preventing tumorigenesis, selective COX-2 inhibitors suppress the growth of established tumours. A selective COX-2 inhibitor was also observed to decrease the number and size of metastases. In most studies, selective COX-2 inhibitors decrease the rate of tumour growth rather than cause a reduction in tumour size [12–14].

Therefore, significant preclinical evidence strongly supports the potential role for these inhibitors in the treatment of cancer. Currently, the COX-2 inhibitors are being studied in clinical trials to confirm their role in the prevention of cancer, particularly colon cancer, and in combination with chemotherapy and radiation therapy to prove their effectiveness in cervical cancer, lung cancer and brain tumours [15].

Notwithstanding their potential interest also in the treatment of cancer cachexia, some questions have arisen on the clinical use of these agents because of their toxicity and particularly cardiovascular risks. For this reason, rofecoxib has been withdrawn by the manufacturer. Another drug in this class, valdecoxib, has shown an increased risk for cardiovascular events in patients after heart surgery. As regards celecoxib, in December 2004 the National Cancer Institute stopped celecoxib (Celebrex) administration in an ongoing clinical trial investigating a new use of the drug to prevent colon polyps because of an increased risk of cardiovascular events in patients taking Celebrex versus those taking a placebo. Patients in the clinical trial taking 400 mg of Celebrex twice daily had a 3.4 times greater risk of cardiovascualr events compared to placebo. For patients in the trial taking 200 mg of Celebrex twice daily, the risk was 2.5 times greater. The average duration of treatment in the trial was 33 months. A similar ongoing study comparing Celebrex 400 mg once a day versus placebo, in patients followed for a similar period of time, has not shown increased risk. Consequently, the Food and Drug Administration (FDA) issued an alert on December 17, 2004 (http://www.fda.gov/bbs/topics/news/2004/NEW01 144.html). Based on the currently available data, FDA has concluded in April 2005 that an increased risk of serious adverse CV events appears to be a class effect of non-steroidal anti-inflammatory drugs (NSAIDs) (excluding aspirin). FDA has requested that the package insert for all NSAIDs, including Celebrex, be revised to include a boxed warning to highlight the potential increased risk of CV events and the well described risk of serious, and potentially life-threatening, gastrointestinal bleeding. FDA has also requested that the package insert for all NSAIDs be revised to include a contraindication for use in patients immediately postoperative from coronary artery bypass (CABG) surgery. Consequently the inclusion of celecoxib in clinical trials should be discouraged.

## COX-2 Inhibitors in Cancer Cachexia

### Experimental Evidence

Additionally, it has been suggested that the COX-2 inhibitors could have a potential role in counteracting cancer cachexia [16].

Indeed, there is increasing evidence that eicosanoids such as PGs have a role in the development of cachexia. Review of the literature showed a study from as early as 1975 demonstrating that indomethacin (a non-steroidal anti-inflammatory,

NSAID) was able to inhibit levels of urinary $PGE_2$ metabolites and this reduction correlated with reduced serum hypercalcaemia [17], a condition often associated with cachexia. Prostaglandin release is a component of the signalling cascade in skeletal muscle protein turnover in vitro, which suggests these agents may play a role in pathologies of muscle catabolism, and therefore wasting (for review see [18]). Aside from direct effects on muscle biology, PGs can also regulate the expression of proinflammatory cytokines, such as interleukin-6 (IL-6) and tumour necrosis factor-$\alpha$ (TNF$\alpha$) [19]. NSAIDs have been shown to block the protein catabolic effects of serum from cachectic mice [20] and have been reported to prevent muscle protein breakdown in some tumour-bearing rats, with no observed increase in food intake [21], although this observation does not seem to be universally confirmed [22].

Selective COX-2 inhibitors such as celecoxib have been demonstrated to have potent anti-tumour (prevention) and growth inhibitory effects in preclinical tumour models [23–28]. Davies et al. [16] observed in numerous models that tumour-bearing animals treated with COX-2 inhibitors retained body weight and overall health compared with vehicle-treated animals. This held true even when treated tumours eventually exceeded the size in which vehicle-treated animals had to be sacrificed. The same authors have conducted specific studies in two tumour models where cachexia is apparent to explore the possible effects of COX-2 inhibition on tumour-induced wasting. It was observed that acute treatment of severely cachectic tumour-bearing animals with the COX-2 inhibitor celecoxib maintained or reduced serum calcium levels and produced a rapid and significant weight gain (reversal of weight loss) compared with tumour-matched vehicle-treated animals. In one model, this also correlated with reduced circulating IL-6 observable as early as 24 h after initiation of treatment. These data suggest that COX-2-derived PGs can mediate cachexia and further suggest a possible benefit for the use of celecoxib in the treatment of tumour-induced wasting.

In an experimental model in mice, COX-2 inhibitors have been found to result in preserved food intake and maintenance of body weight during inflammation [29]. The COX-2 inhibitor meloxicam was capable of directly antagonising the process of muscle catabolism in cancer cachexia of mice induced by proteolysis-inducing factor [30].

Okamoto studied the effects of the COX-2 inhibitor Zaltoprofen on the cachectic symptoms of the rodent 'sickness behaviour' model, which is superimposable on cancer cachexia, and obtained an improvement in the loss of body weight [31].

## Clinical Evidence

As for human studies, short-term administration of the NSAID ibuprofen reduced hypermetabolism and acute-phase response in patients with colon cancer and pancreatic cancer, suggesting an anti-cachectic benefit via lowering energy expenditure [32–34]. Another study by Lundholm et al. found a survival advantage from indomethacin treatment among late-stage cancer patients, although cachexia was not specifically addressed [35]. A prospective study comparing megestrol acetate versus megestrol acetate/ibuprofen was recently done in gastrointestinal cancer patients [36]. Of those evaluable at 12 weeks (38%), there was a decrease in weight (median 2.8 kg) in the megestrol acetate/placebo group compared with an increase (median 2.3 kg) in the megestrol acetate/ibuprofen group. There was also an improvement in the EuroQol-EQ-5D quality-of-life scores of the latter group.

However, chronic use of traditional NSAIDs is not widespread in cancer patients due to concerns about inhibition of COX-1 activity and possible adverse effects on mucosal (especially gastrointestinal) and haematological tissues, particularly in the context of chemotherapy. The discovery of the inducible form of COX-2 and subsequent development of selective COX-2 inhibitors raises the possibility of safely reducing tumour-mediated PG levels, which may lead to control of some aspects of cachexia.

In a retrospective case-control analysis performed on a database of material collected consecutively, Lundholm et al. found that weight-losing untreated cancer patients had elevated resting energy expenditure compared to undernourished non-cancer patients. This difference became significantly reduced by long-term indomethacin treatment. Heart rate was correspondingly decreased, while systolic blood pressure increased

following indomethacin treatment of cancer patients. Total body fat was more preserved, while lean body mass was uninfluenced by long-term indomethacin administration to cancer patients. All these beneficial effects were parallel to a decrease in systemic inflammation (C-reactive protein, erythrocyte sedimentation rate) in cancer patients on indomethacin. Systemic inflammation and resting energy metabolism predicted weight loss in progressive cancer. These data support the concept that COX treatment may offer beneficial metabolic effects to weight-losing cancer patients by attenuation of resting metabolism and improved appetite due to decreased systemic inflammation [37].

A very recent study was reported by Cerchietti et al. [38]. The aim of this study was to ameliorate some of the cachectic symptoms in a homogeneous group of lung adenocarcinoma patients using a multitargeted therapy. Fifteen patients with evidence of cancer anorexia-cachexia syndrome (CACS) were studied. CACS was defined as the presence of weight loss, anorexia, fatigue, performance status $\geq 2$ and acute-phase protein response. Patients received medroxyprogesterone acetate (MPA, 500 mg twice daily), celecoxib (200 mg twice daily), plus oral food supplementation for 6 weeks. After treatment, 13 patients either had stable weight ($\pm$ 1%) or had gained weight. There were significant differences in improvement of body weight-change rate, nausea, early satiety, fatigue, appetite and performance status. Patients who had any kind of lung infection showed higher levels of IL-10 compared to non-infected patients ($p = 0.039$). The results suggest that patients with advanced lung adenocarcinoma, treated with MPA, celecoxib and dietary intervention, might have considerable improvement in certain CACS symptoms.

Moreover, the results of animal studies have demonstrated that, as well as decreasing the production of cytokines, the consumption of n-3 fatty acids can also reduce cancer-induced cachexia via a mechanism suppressing arachidonic acid production. The mechanism by which n-3 fatty acids act is to suppress the production of arachidonic acid from linoleic acid by competing more successfully than linoleic acid for the activity of the $\Delta 5$ and $\Delta 6$ desaturases [39].

# References

1. Herschman HR (1996) Prostaglandin synthase 2. Biochim Biophys Acta 1299:125–140
2. Sano H, Kawahito Y, Wilder RL et al (1995) Expression of cyclooxygenase-1 and -2 in human colorectal cancer. Cancer Res 55:3785–3789
3. Lupulescu A (1996) Prostaglandins, their inhibitors and cancer. Prostaglandins Leukot Essent Fatty Acids 54:83–94
4. Bennett A (1986) The production of prostanoids in human cancers, and their implications for tumor progression. Prog Lipid Res 25:539–542
5. Eling TE, Thompson DC, Foureman GL et al (1990) Prostaglandin H synthase and xenobiotic oxidation. Annu Rev Pharmacol Toxicol 30:1–45
6. Tsujii M, DuBois RN (1995) Alterations in cellular adhesion and apoptosis in epithelial cells overexpressing prostaglandin endoperoxide synthase 2. Cell 83:493–501
7. Weitzman SA, Gordon LI (1990) Inflammation and cancer: role of phagocyte-generated oxidants in carcinogenesis. Blood 76:655–663
8. Kambayashi T, Alexander HR, Fong M, Strassmann G (1995) Potential involvement of IL-10 in suppressing tumor-associated macrophages. Colon-26-derived prostaglandin E2 inhibits TNF-alpha release via a mechanism involving IL-10. J Immunol 154:3383–3390
9. Tsujii M, Kawano S, Tsuji S et al (1998) Cyclooxygenase regulates angiogenesis induced by colon cancer cells. Cell 93:705–716
10. Gallo O, Franchi A, Magnelli L et al (2001) Cyclooxygenase-2 pathway correlates with VEGF expression in head and neck cancer. Implications for tumor angiogenesis and metastasis. Neoplasia 3:53–61
11. Eling TE, Curtis JF (1992) Xenobiotic metabolism by prostaglandin H synthase. Pharmacol Ther 53:261–273
12. Masferrer JL, Leahy KM, Koki AT et al (2000) Antiangiogenic and antitumor activities of cyclooxygenase-2 inhibitors. Cancer Res 60:1306–1311
13. Moore RJ, Zweifel B, Heuvelman DM et al (2000) Enhanced antitumor activity by co-administration of celecoxib and chemotherapeutic agents cyclophosphamide and 5-FU. Proc Am Assoc Cancer Res 41:409
14. Kishi K, Petersen S, Petersen C et al (2000) Preferential enhancement of tumor radioresponse by a cyclooxygenase-2 inhibitor. Cancer Res 60:1326–1331
15. Dicker AP (2003) COX-2 inhibitors and cancer therapeutics: potential roles for inhibitors of COX-2 in combination with cytotoxic therapy: reports from a symposium held in conjunction with the Radiation Therapy Oncology Group June 2001 Meeting. Am J Clin Oncol 26:S46–S47
16. Davis TW, Zweifel BS, O'Neal JM et al (2004) Inhibition of COX-2 by celecoxib reverses tumor induced wasting. J Pharmacol Exp Ther 308:929–934
17. Seyberth HW, Segre GV, Sweetmen BJ et al (1975) Prostaglandins as mediators of hypercalcemia associated with certain types of cancer. N Engl J Med 293:1278–1285
18. Thompson MG , Palmer RM (1998) Signalling pathways regulating protein turnover in skeletal muscle. Cell Signal 10:1–11
19. Rothwell NJ (1992) Eicosanoids, thermogenesis and thermoregulation. Prostaglandins Leukot Essent Fatty Acids 46:1–7
20. Smith KL, Tisdale MJ (1993) Mechanism of muscle protein degradation in cancer cachexia. Br J Cancer 68:314–318
21. Homem-de-Bittencourt Jr PI, Pontieri V, Curi R, Lopes OU (1989) Effects of aspirin-like drugs on Walker 256 tumor growth and cachexia in rats. Braz J Med Biol Res 22:1039–1042
22. McCarthy DO (1999) Inhibitors of prostaglandin synthesis do not improve food intake or body weight of tumor-bearing rats. Res Nurs Health 22:380–387
23. McEntee MF, Chiu CH, Whelan J (1999) Relationship of b-catenin and Bcl-2 expression to sulindac-induced regression of intestinal tumors in Min mice. Carcinogenesis 20:635–640
24. Williams CS, Mann M, DuBois RN (1999) The role of cyclooxygenases in inflammation, cancer and development. Oncogene 18:7908–7916
25. Jacoby RF, Seibert K, Cole CE et al (2000) The cyclooxygenase-2 inhibitor celecoxib is a potent preventive and therapeutic agent in the min mouse model of adenomatous polyposis. Cancer Res 60:5040–5044
26. Masferrer J (2001) Approach to angiogenesis inhibition based on cyclooxygenase–2. Cancer J 7(Suppl 3):S144–S150
27. Leahy KM, Ornberg RL, Wang Y et al (2002) Cyclooxygenase-2 inhibition by celecoxib reduces proliferation and induces apoptosis in angiogenic endothelial cells in vivo. Cancer Res 62:625–631
28. Zweifel BS, Davis TW, Ornberg RL, Masferrer JL (2002) Direct evidence for a role of cyclooxygenase 2-derived prostaglandin E2 in human head and neck xenograft tumors. Cancer Res 62:6706–6711
29. Johnson PM, Vogt SK, Burney MW, Muglia LJ (2002) COX-2 inhibition attenuates anorexia during systemic inflammation without impairing cytokine production. Am J Physiol Endocrinol Metab 282:E650–E656
30. Hussey HJ, Tisdale MJ (2000) Effect of the specific cyclooxygenase-2 inhibitor meloxicam on tumour growth and cachexia in a murine model. Int J Cancer 87:95–100
31. Okamoto T (2002) NSAID zaltoprofen improves the

decrease in body weight in rodent sickness behavior models: proposed new applications of NSAIDs (Review). Int J Mol Med 9:369–372

32. McMillan DC, Leen E, Smith J et al (1995) Effect of extended ibuprofen administration on the acute phase protein response in colorectal cancer patients. Eur J Surg Oncol 21:531–534

33. Preston T, Fearon KC, McMillan DC et al (1995) Effect of ibuprofen on the acute-phase response and protein metabolism in patients with cancer and weight loss. Br J Surg 82:229–234

34. Wigmore SJ, Falconer JS, Plester CE et al (1995) Ibuprofen reduces energy expenditure and acute-phase protein production compared with placebo in pancreatic cancer patients. Br J Cancer 72:185–188

35. Lundholm K, Gelin J, Hyltander A et al (1994) Anti-inflammatory treatment may prolong survival in undernourished patients with metastatic solid tumors. Cancer Res 54:5602–5606

36. McMillan DC, Wigmore SJ, Fearon KC et al (1999) A prospective randomized study of megestrol acetate and ibuprofen in gastrointestinal cancer patients with weight loss. Br J Cancer 79:495–500

37. Lundholm K, Daneryd P, Korner U et al (2004) Evidence that long-term COX-treatment improves energy homeostasis and body composition in cancer patients with progressive cachexia. Int J Oncol 24:505–512

38. Cerchietti LC, Navigante AH, Peluffo GD et al (2004) Effects of celecoxib, medroxyprogesterone, and dietary intervention on systemic syndromes in patients with advanced lung adenocarcinoma: a pilot study. J Pain Symptom Manage 27:85–95

39. Hague TA, Christoffersen BO (1984) Effect of dietary fats in arachidonic acid and eicosapentaenoic acid biosynthesis and conversion of C22 fatty acids in isolated liver cells. Biochim Biophys Acta 796:205–217

# Anti-TNF-α Antibody and Cancer Cachexia

Mark de Witte, Mark Anderson, Don Robinson

## Cancer Cachexia

Cachexia is characterised by accelerated loss of adipose tissue and skeletal muscle in the context of a chronic inflammatory response [1–3]. It is a common complication of advanced cancer [4]. About half of all cancer patients suffer from this syndrome, which is among the most debilitating and life-threatening complications [5]. The key feature of this syndrome is weight loss, but other symptoms, such as anorexia, fatigue, vomiting and anaemia, and accelerated malnutrition with depletion of whole-body lipid and protein stores are frequently observed. Cancer cachexia contributes to immobility, a propensity to infection, shortened duration of survival, and overall decreased quality of life [6].

Cachexia may be responsible for one third of cancer deaths, independent of tumour burden or metastases, and therefore is a critical factor to consider when initiating treatment modalities for this population [7]. Patients with cancer cachexia often have specific problems that lead to a reduction in nutritional intake. However, nutritional supplements alone cannot correct cachexia. In a meta-analysis of published trials, patients undergoing total parenteral nutrition while receiving chemotherapy showed decreased survival, a poorer tumour response, and significant increases in infectious complications [8].

Earlier chapters in this book have presented strong evidence in support of the hypothesis that there is a causal relationship between the proinflammatory cytokine tumour necrosis factor-α (TNF-α) and cancer cachexia. Proinflammatory cytokines can become pathogenic when dysregulated in malignant disease [9, 10].

In vitro tests, animal experiments and epidemiological studies have important roles in identifying associations between biological factors, but they may not provide credible mechanistic explanations; because of unknown effects of confounding factors, they may not establish causation. How should association data be interpreted and reported, and how might they direct progress in the management of cancer cachexia? The value of association data derives from their roles in helping to design prospective, controlled investigations to test the strength of the associations and the hypotheses underlying biological causation [11]. The factors that confound the interpretation of association studies can be elucidated via carefully designed, stringently conducted clinical trials. We will improve our understanding of clinical trial results as we increase knowledge of the cellular and molecular biology of cancer, cancer cachexia, and the inter-related signalling pathways that may be modulated by biological agents such as monoclonal antibodies.

The definitive treatment of cancer cachexia is removal of the causative tumour. When curative resection is not possible, systemic medical interventions are indicated but none has been successful. An optimal therapeutic agent would target the agonistic pathways of both the causative tumour and the consequent dysregulated metabolism of the wasting syndrome. Orexigenic agents, corticosteroids, progestational and anabolic agents have been investigated clinically, but, unfortunately, they provide only slight benefit, and upon completion of the studies, nutritional parameters return to baseline.

There are four approved drug products for the treatment of cachexia: oxandrolone, dronabinol, megestrol acetate and growth hormone. Oxandrolone, an anabolic steroid, is used to promote weight gain and offset protein catabolism. Dronabinol and megestrol acetate were approved initially for the anorexia associated with human immunodeficiency virus (HIV)/acquired immunodeficiency syndrome (AIDS) and since have been used to treat anorexia associated with cachexia. Growth hormone has been shown to produce a positive change in lean body mass in clinical trials. However, these drug products have not been studied intensively in cancer patients, and none has been approved for cancer cachexia [12, 13].

Patients with pancreatic cancer have among the highest incidence of weight loss of any group of patients with cancer, with approximately 80–90% losing weight during the course of their illness [14, 15]. In pancreatic cancer patients the onset of cachexia usually is long before the tumour is diagnosed. Erosion of skeletal muscle is a major contributory factor in the poor prognosis of these patients, often leading to hypostatic pneumonia and respiratory failure. The depletion of lean body mass limits their ability to tolerate cytotoxic regimens, both in dose and duration [16]. Arresting the syndrome of cachexia should have great clinical impact in pancreas cancer [17].

# TNF-α and Cancer Cachexia

The pathogenesis of cancer cachexia has not been fully elucidated. However, numerous cytokines produced by activated lymphocytes, monocytes, macrophages and/or tumour cells, including TNF-α, interleukin (IL)-1, IL-6 and interferon (IFN)-α, have been implicated as mediators of the syndrome [18–21].

TNF-α was originally named 'cachectin' when identified as a circulating mediator of wasting in an animal model of chronic parasitic infection [22, 23]. In subsequent studies it was found that continuous infusions of TNF-α in rats resulted in the development of anorexia, loss of body weight, protein, lipid and cell mass, leading to death [24–26]. Oliff et al. established an animal model using a tumour cell line that continually produced low concentrations of TNF-α. When this cell line was transplanted into nude mice, 80% of the animals developed severe, progressive weight loss and ultimately died with the pathological and histological characteristics of cancer-induced

cachexia [19].

Llovera et al. found that implantation of the Lewis lung carcinoma in gene knockout mice deficient in TNF-α demonstrated a different pattern of wasting compared to tumour-implanted wild-type mice [27]. In the knockout mice, protein degradation occurred at a lower rate and the ubiquitin-proteasome system was activated to a lesser degree. These observations suggest that TNF-α mediates the excessive wasting of lean tissue in cancer. In another study, Llovera et al. found that TNF-α led to a doubling of expression of ubiquitin genes in skeletal muscle [26]. This finding supports the critical role of the ubiquitin-proteasome system in the destruction of most skeletal muscle proteins in a variety of wasting conditions [1].

Through a series of in vitro and in vivo experiments in mice, Guttridge et al. found that TNF-α interferes with the muscle repair process by suppressing MyoD expression. This suppression is mediated by the activation of the transcription factor NF-κB [28]. MyoD is essential for skeletal muscle differentiation and for repair of damaged tissue, and it may be particularly important for the replenishing of wasted muscle [29].

Serum TNF-α levels are not always detectable in cancer patients with cachexia and their correlation with weight loss has not been demonstrated consistently. The inability to detect circulating cytokines is attributed to their low rate of production, their short half-life and rapid clearance from plasma, or their localised paracrine production [30]. However, it has been reported that TNF-α is intermittently or discontinuously detectable in patients with gastrointestinal cancer and that its levels correlate with the severity of weight loss [31]. The serum level of TNF-α was significantly higher in patients with advanced-stage cancer than in healthy individuals [32]. A significant inverse correlation was shown between the detectability of serum TNF-α levels and serum albumin levels, haemoglobin levels, body mass index, and performance status in 110 patients with prostate cancer [33]. In this study, patients with elevated serum TNF-α levels had a significantly shorter median time of survival than did patients in whom serum TNF-α was undetectable.

Falconer et al. demonstrated that the spontaneous production of TNF-α by isolated peripheral blood mononuclear cells (PBMCs) was significantly greater in pancreatic cancer patients even though circulating TNF could not be detected in the same patients [34]. A study in patients with pancreatic cancer showed that more patients with metastatic disease had detectable serum levels of TNF-α compared to those with non-metastatic disease. Patients with detectable serum TNF-α levels had significantly lower body weight and body mass index, lower haematocrit and haemoglobin values, and lower serum total protein and albumin levels compared to those with undetectable TNF-α levels [35].

Over the past 20 years, following its initial discovery, a growing body of evidence has identified TNF-α as a key mediator in the pathogenesis of cachexia syndrome. Thus, it is a rational hypothesis that blocking the effects of TNF-α may delay or stop the progression of cancer cachexia.

## Anti-TNF-α Treatment of Cancer Cachexia

Several studies have demonstrated the role of anti-TNF-α treatment in animal models of cachexia. Sherry et al. studied the effect of anti-TNF-α immunoglobulin treatment in C57B1/6 mice bearing a methylcholanthrene-induced sarcoma that produced TNF-α. The anti-TNF-α treatment resulted in a significant reduction of weight loss, protein loss and fat loss. It was concluded that neutralising endogenous TNF-α production with antibodies offers the potential to reduce tissue wasting associated with neoplastic disease [36].

An animal study testing the ability of TNF-α antibody blockade to ameliorate cachexia in nude mice bearing xenografted human melanoma A375S2 tumours was performed by Centocor Inc. [37]. The murine antibody A2 (mA2), an anti-human TNF-α antibody (murine version of infliximab) and chimeric V1q (cV1q), an anti-mouse TNF-α antibody, were used to treat tumour-bearing animals. The combination of anti-human TNF-α (mA2) and anti-mouse TNF-α (cV1q) significantly inhibited weight loss in human melanoma tumour-bearing animals compared to

control antibody-treated animals. These findings indicate that TNF-α participates in weight loss in human melanoma tumour-bearing animals and that antibody blockade of TNF-α activity attenuates tumour-induced cachexia in this model.

Siegel et al. (1995) evaluated the ability of the anti-TNF-α monoclonal antibody infliximab to neutralise the in vitro and in vivo biological effects of TNF-α. It was found that repeated administration of infliximab to transgenic mice that constitutively express human TNF-α achieved significant weight gain and prevented subsequent mortality compared with the control group [38].

Torelli et al. (1999) examined food intake and body weight among tumour-bearing rodents treated with a dimeric, pegylated 55-kDa TNF-α inhibitor. Tumour-bearing rodents received either active agent or vehicle alone. Mice that received the TNF-α inhibitor consumed more calories ad libitum over a 1-week period than those receiving only vehicle. The mice that received the TNF-α inhibitor had an increase in body weight [39].

Anti-TNF-α treatment has shown therapeutic effect in the treatment of cachexia associated with *Trypanosoma cruzi* infection [40], AIDS and/or tuberculosis [2, 41].

A pilot study of anti-TNF-α therapy in patients with myelofibrosis with myeloid metaplasia reported that etanercept, a soluble TNF-α receptor fusion protein that blocks TNF activity, can palliate constitutional symptoms such as drenching night sweats, profound fatigue, and unintentional weight loss. Improvements were seen in seven of seven patients with unintentional weight loss, and 10 of 20 patients with fatigue [42].

A prospective clinical study in rheumatoid arthritis (RA) showed evidence that anti-TNF-α therapy was associated with weight gain in 40 of 46 patients (87.5%). Thirty of these patients received intravenous infliximab (3 mg/kg) at weeks 0, 2, 6, and then every 8 weeks, and 16 patients received subcutaneous etanercept 25 mg twice weekly. Mean follow-up time was 10.7 months. The mean initial weight was 70.1 kg and the mean final weight was 73.3 kg, corresponding to a mean weight gain of 3.2 kg [43].

## Anti-TNF-α Therapy and Malignancy

There are many fascinating paradoxes in biology; one is that the cytokine protein TNF-α can promote cancer progression when produced endogenously and chronically at physiological levels within the tumour microenviroment, but can be cytotoxic to cancer cells when delivered in pharmacological doses in controlled settings, such as isolated limb perfusion [44, 45]. Thus, there can be concern that anti-TNF-α therapy could promote growth of existing cancer by blockade of a protein that possibly could be inducing tumour necrosis. There is evidence to counter this concern. Progressing tumours have evaded immune control for years and the inflammatory response to tumour-induced tissue injury, ineffectual in eliminating the neoplasia, may have become converted, as it were, to serve as a source of paracrine growth factors for malignant cells. The role of TNF-α as a tumour promoter has been reported [9, 46–48]. TNF-α was implicated in tumour growth in a murine model by the observation that TNF-α knockout mice are highly resistant to the induced generation of skin tumours. The presence of functional TNF-α has no effect on DNA mutation rates or tumour initiation, but instead profoundly influences tumour promotion. TPA was shown to induce TNF-α in skin keratinocytes of wild-type mice. The production of activating protein-1 (AP-1) transcription pathway-induced gene products such as granulocyte-macrophage colony-stimulating factor (GM-CSF), matrix metalloproteinase (MMP)-3 and MMP-9 is important for the tumour-promoting effect. Anti-tumour effects were observed following pharmacological intervention with a neutralising anti-mouse TNF-α antibody.

A number of studies have indicated that cytokines such as TNF-α may contribute to the pathogenesis of both solid and haematological malignancies and paraneoplastic complications [9, 49–51]. TNF-α can function as a growth factor for hairy cell leukaemia cells and multiple myeloma cells, or as a progression factor for B cell leukaemia [52–55]. Anti-TNF-α antibody treatment has been shown to lower tumour burden in hairy cell leukaemia [56]. Preclinical studies of pancreatic carcinogenesis indicated that supra-physiological levels of TNF-α have cytotoxic effects on tumour cells, but at physiological levels, TNF-α can stimulate pancreatic cancer cell growth via growth factor and growth factor receptor upregulation [57].

Anti-TNF-α therapy with infliximab in humans does not alter the number or function of cells potentially involved in tumour surveillance, including T cells, NK cells, B cells, monocytes and macrophages [58–60]. The action of infliximab is specific to TNF-α; infliximab does not cross-react with lymphotoxin-α (TNF-β), thus avoiding any potential tumorigenic complications from inhibiting lymphotoxin-α [61].

## Potential Risks of Anti-TNF-α Therapy

Infliximab is a chimeric (human–murine) IgG1κ monoclonal antibody with an approximate molecular weight of 149100 daltons, in the pharmacological class of selective immunosuppressive agents. It is composed of human-constant and murine-variable regions and binds specifically to human TNF-α with an association constant of $10^{-10}$ M (Fig. 1). Infliximab has a well-documented safety profile throughout clinical development and in post-marketing safety surveillance for the approved indications of Crohn's disease and RA [62–65].

However, the potential impact of immunosuppressive, anti-TNF-α treatment on the development of infections, autoimmunity, underlying cancer, and any new malignancy must be monitored closely in any proposed study. The biological basis of concern pertaining to immunosuppression warrants heightened vigilance and consideration of the benefit-to-risk ratio when prescribing anti-TNF therapies.

Because of the adaptive, protective purpose of inflammation, pharmacological inhibition of this proinflammatory cytokine could have adverse effects in the host, unrelated to the target disease of the anti-TNF-α therapy. The risk of reactivation of latent tuberculosis is addressed in the prescribing information for infliximab [66]. Pre-emptive systemic antifungal therapy is recommended for patients receiving infliximab for treatment of graft-versus-host disease [67]. Smith and Skelton

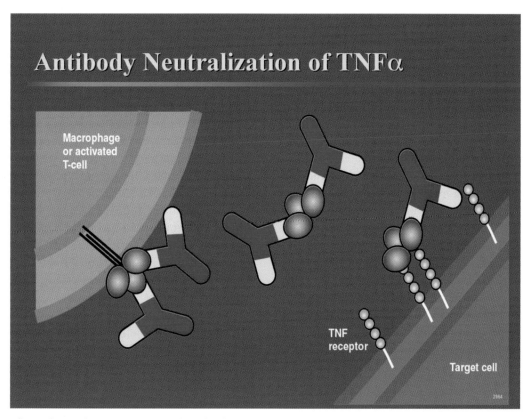

**Fig. 1.** Infliximab is a chimeric monoclonal antibody, which binds to tumour necrosis factor-alpha. Infliximab has been shown to bind to all three forms of TNF-α: transmembrane, soluble and receptor-bound

reported cases of squamous cell carcinoma (SCC) that became evident and grew rapidly during an initial period of etanercept therapy for RA [68]. The tumours may have been present, but occult and controlled, prior to disruption of immunological control. Etanercept could disable innate antitumour surveillance by blockade of both lymphotoxin α, and the direct cytotoxic effects of TNF-α and/or by inhibition of the TH1 cytokine pattern and impairment of cytotoxic T cells. All cases of SCC were in chronically UV-damaged, actinic skin predisposed to tumorigenesis by long-term, low-level production of TNF-α. No new SCCs developed in patients who continued treatment for more than 1 year, suggesting prolonged anti-TNF-α therapy could be preventive of cutaneous malignancies.

Pharmacovigilance data on etanercept, infliximab and adalimumab were reviewed by the FDA in 2003, with a focus on lymphoproliferative disease in patients treated with these anti-TNF-α

agents, relative to the rate expected in populations with immune-mediated diseases [69]. The potential role of TNF-α-blocking therapy in the long-term development of malignancies is not known. A prospective study of 18 572 RA patients treated with anti-TNF-α therapy plus methotrexate reported an increased standard incidence ratio (SIR) compared to patients not receiving methotrexate or biologics, but confidence intervals overlapped for all treatments [70]. Patients with highly active disease and/or chronic exposure to immunosuppressant therapies may have severalfold higher risk for development of lymphoma, thus caution should be exercised when considering use of anti-TNF-α agents in patients with a history of malignancy or who develop malignancy during treatment.

The FDA reported on the risks of histoplasmosis [71], lymphoma [72], and/or listeriosis [73]. The Mayo clinic reviewed the safety of infliximab in 500 Crohn's patients treated with infliximab

[74]. The biological basis of concern warrants heightened vigilance and consideration of the benefit-to-risk ratio when prescribing anti-TNF therapies.

The role of TNF-α in cisplatin-mediated renal injury was demonstrated in a mouse model. Treatment of animals with TNF-α synthesis inhibitors or anti-TNF-α antibodies prevented kidney damage in the model [75].

TNF-α appears to play a complex role in side-effects of radiotherapy as well and anti-TNF-α treatments may be useful in their management [76, 77]. TNF-α is also a known activator of osteoclasts [78] and mediator of neuropathic pain [79]. An intriguing pair of clinical cases in which etanercept was used to treat refractory metastatic bone pain suggest that anti-TNF-α agents may be useful to control cancer pain [80]. The potential value of anti-TNF-α agents in these debilitating conditions presents broad opportunities to improve cancer care.

## Objectives for a Clinical Trial

There is concordance of opinion amongst physicians, clinical scientists and regulatory health authorities on the value of multicentre, randomised, controlled clinical trials, with adequate statistical power and preferably double-blinded, to determine the true effects of an intervention with therapeutic intent. To evaluate treatment of a complex syndrome such as cachexia, rather than a distinct or singular abnormality, those design features may be considered requisite. Restrictive protocol eligibility criteria and stratification on prognostic factors must be used to limit the impact of various co-morbidities, concomitant medications, patient histories and physicians' treatment patterns and skills. Patients with eating disorders, infections, maldigestion, malabsorption or diarrhoea, adrenal or thyroid diseases should be excluded. Efforts to limit disparities among the patients may reduce confounding variables but also will limit the validity of generalisations about the results from the 'sample' studied to the wider population with cancer cachexia. End-points should be assessed frequently so that time-to-event estimates may be as precise as possible.

In some situations, prospective, controlled trials could be unethical because some patients would need to be allocated to study groups hypothesised to be less beneficial than other groups. Early-phase clinical studies that precede evidence of clinical efficacy must be based upon strong evidence from animal and laboratory studies that demonstrate the predicted effects with acceptable toxicity. By adding the experimental treatment or placebo to the standard treatment for the disease, all randomised patients can receive ethical and appropriate medical care while the potential added benefit of the investigational treatment can be evaluated objectively. The potential adverse effects and/or interactions of the combined therapies must be assessed.

Treatment of cancer cachexia with the anti-TNF-α monoclonal antibody infliximab is being investigated in a multicenter, randomised, double-blind, and placebo-controlled study. The therapeutic goals of anti-TNF-α treatment in patients with cancer cachexia are to inhibit the systemic inflammatory response and catabolic processes, with intent to improve patients' physical functioning, nutritional health and overall quality of life. Thereby, ultimately and most importantly, survival may be prolonged, and with such quality as to be worth prolonging.

Cancer cachexia involves systemic manifestations and multiorgan, multisystem pathological consequences of TNF-α produced by the tumour and by activated immune cells throughout the patient. This implies widely distributed and/or high levels of TNF-α in metabolically (catabolically) active tissues, and intra/peri-tumoral. The doses and schedule of infliximab will define the pharmacokinetic profile in a metabolically dysregulated population of patients with cancer cachexia. The pharmacokinetic, pharmacodynamic and clinical results may suggest an effective dose and schedule of anti-TNF therapy.

Adult patients with previously untreated, surgically unresectable, locally advanced or metastatic adenocarcinoma of the pancreas, who have experienced involuntary weight loss of ≥ 10% compared to their stable weight before illness, or loss of 5% body weight within 90 days, are being treated.

Weight loss should be documented, if possible, not only self-reported. The overall goals are to evaluate the safety and efficacy for treating cachexia when infliximab is administered concomitantly with standard gemcitabine chemotherapy, and to provide a basis for the selection of a functional (or performance) end-point, representative of clinical benefit in the context of a debilitating syndrome of wasting.

The primary objective of the study is to evaluate the effects of treatment on a critical hallmark of cachexia, the patients' loss of lean body mass. Lean body mass is a biologically rational end-point and logical target measure for the efficacy assessment of anti-TNF-α therapy. Loss of metabolically active lean tissue, including skeletal/respiratory muscle, is associated with worsened performance status, a higher incidence of infections and toxicities due to chemotherapy, progressive impairment of function, dependence on caregivers, and markedly decreased survival time. Clinical evidence of preservation of lean body mass in these cancer patients would provide proof of the concept that blocking the actions of TNF-α systemically with infliximab can inhibit the proteolytic pathways of cachexia.

Major secondary objectives of the study are to evaluate the safety of infliximab in a concomitant regimen with gemcitabine, time to tumour progression, survival, quality of life and tumour response. Additionally, this study will evaluate the feasibility and value of a basic physical performance end-point, the 6-minute walk test (American Thoracic Society guideline) [81], as a measure of clinical benefit.

The potential impact on the underlying cancer of combining anti-TNF-α antibody with chemotherapy is not known. Could the anti-tumour activity of the chemotherapy be impaired by interference with its mechanism of action or by alteration of its metabolism and pharmacokinetics? If possible, reliable and appropriate animal models should be used in experiments to test for interactions. Researchers must understand the biochemical pathways of the anti-tumour chemotherapy and any plausible biological rationale for interference by the anti-cytokine immunotherapy. Thus, in this study the time to tumour progression

is monitored closely as both a measure of efficacy and of safety. An independent, unblinded, safety monitoring committee oversees the study and regularly reviews safety data. The committee consists of two medical oncologists, a bioethicist and a statistician. Should there be unexpected evidence of accelerated progression of cancer, or exacerbation of complications in patients treated with gemcitabine plus infliximab, compared to patients treated with gemcitabine plus placebo, the active combination regimen could be considered unsafe. Conversely, evidence of longer median time to tumour progression in the patients treated with the active combination would support the hypothesis that blocking the effector functions of endogenous TNF-α with antibody may inhibit the tumour growth.

Until completion of the study and analyses of all the results, the primary and major secondary end-points are considered of equal importance. Evaluated together, they should provide decisive knowledge of the biological effects and clinical benefit of infliximab added to standard chemotherapy in pancreas cancer patients (Fig. 2, 3).

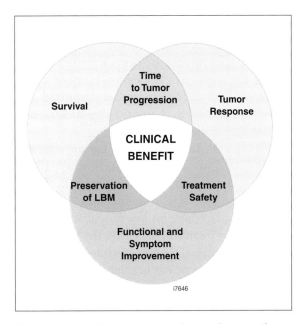

**Fig. 2.** Inter-related outcomes or endpoints that contribute to overall assessment of benefit to a cancer patient

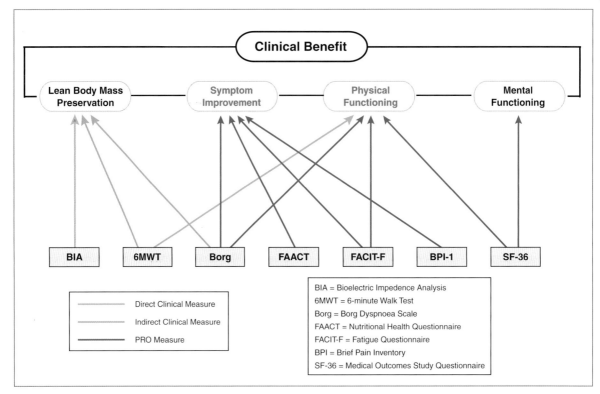

**Fig. 3.** Multiple methods and instruments used to assess clinical benefit. *PRO*, patients reported outcomes

## Assessing the Overall Benefit to the Patient

The impact of a monoclonal antibody blocking and neutralising TNF-α on the symptoms and physical functioning of cancer patients with cachexia is not known. An approach exploring the convergence of clinical and patient-reported outcomes can be used to clarify the clinical benefit of an anti-TNF-α therapy [82–84].

Biological cancer therapies are particularly appropriate for the triangulation approach because their side-effect profiles are markedly less adverse than cytotoxic chemotherapies. Therefore, assessments of symptoms and functioning are less influenced by treatment toxicities. The lower toxicity profile of biologics offers advantages to regulatory authorities as well as healthcare providers [83, 85]. The association of upregulated cytokines, particularly TNF-α, with cancer symptom development is reliable [86–88]. The results of studies of anti-TNF-α, as monotherapy or in combination with other anti-cancer agents, should be integrated tightly to clarify the biological mechanism of action, assess overall treatment effects by both objective and subjective measures, explore end-points important to regulatory agencies and providers of care [85, 89–91] and define clinically meaningful differences in measures of patient-reported outcomes.

Genomic and proteomic signatures someday soon may allow individualisation of anti-cancer therapy with accurate, pre-treatment identification of patients who will respond to targeted therapies. Until that time, the success of a clinical trial will continue to depend on the following factors: careful selection of the scientific question to be answered, a restricted focus on that question, the validity of the trial end-points, the clinical relevance and practicality of the trial design and the rigour with which the investigators adhere to the protocol.

# References

1. Tisdale MJ (2000) Biomedicine. Protein loss in cancer cachexia. Science 289:2293–2294

2. Kotler DP (2000) Cachexia. Ann Intern Med 133:622–634

3. Ross JA, Fearon KC (2002) Eicosanoid-dependent cancer cachexia and wasting. Curr Opin Clin Nutr Metab Care 5:241–248

4. Fearon KC, Moses AG (2002) Cancer cachexia. Int J Cardiol 85:73–81

5. Inui A (2002) Cancer anorexia–cachexia syndrome: current issues in research and management. CA Cancer J Clin 52:72–91

6. Wigmore SJ, Ross JA, Falconer JS et al (1996) The effect of polyunsaturated fatty acids on the progress of cachexia in patients with pancreatic cancer. Nutrition 12:S27–S30

7. Pirisi A (2000) US researchers find key link in muscle-wasting syndrome. Lancet 356:1249

8. McGeer AJ, Detsky AS, O'Rourke K (1990) Parenteral nutrition in cancer patients undergoing chemotherapy: a meta–analysis. Nutrition 6:233–240

9. Balkwill F (2002) Tumor necrosis factor or tumor promoting factor? Cytokine Growth Factor Rev 13:135–141

10. Szlosarek PW, Balkwill FR (2003) Tumour necrosis factor alpha: a potential target for the therapy of solid tumours. Lancet Oncol 4:565–573

11. Anonymous (2004) Fact or fiction: biochemistry to the rescue. Lancet Oncol 5:197

12. Mann M (1999) Approved pharmacologic interventions for wasting: an overview and lessons learned. J Nutr 129:303S–305S

13. MacDonald N, Easson AM, Mazurak VC et al (2003) Understanding and managing cancer cachexia. J Am Coll Surg 197:143–161

14. Falconer JS, Fearon KC, Ross JA et al (1995) Acute-phase protein response and survival duration of patients with pancreatic cancer. Cancer 75:2077–2082

15. Wigmore SJ, Plester CE, Richardson RA et al (1997) Changes in nutritional status associated with unresectable pancreatic cancer. Br J Cancer 75:106–109

16. Andreyev HJ, Norman AR, Oates J et al (1998) Why do patients with weight loss have a worse outcome when undergoing chemotherapy for gastrointestinal malignancies? Eur J Cancer 34:503–509

17. Kern S, Hruban R, Hollingsworth MA et al (2001) A white paper: the product of a pancreas cancer think tank. Cancer Res 61:4923–4932

18. Tamura S, Ouchi KF, Mori K et al (1995) Involvement of human interleukin 6 in experimental cachexia induced by a human uterine cervical carcinoma xenograft. Clin Cancer Res 1:1353–1358

19. Oliff A, Defeo-Jones D, Boyer M et al (1987) Tumors secreting human TNF/cachectin induce cachexia in mice. Cell 50:555–563

20. Sharma R, Anker SD (2002) Cytokines, apoptosis and cachexia:the potential for TNF antagonism. Int J Cardiol 85:161–171

21. Argiles JM, Moore-Carrasco R, Busquets S et al (2003) Catabolic mediators as targets for cancer cachexia. Drug Discov Today 8:838–844

22. Rouzer CA, Cerami A (1980) Hypertriglyceridemia associated with Trypanosoma brucei brucei infection in rabbits: role of defective triglyceride removal. Mol Biochem Parasitol 2:31–38

23. Beutler B, Greenwald D, Hulmes JD et al (1985) Identity of tumour necrosis factor and the macrophage-secreted factor cachectin. Nature 316:552–554

24. Tracey KJ, Wei H, Manogue KR et al (1988) Cachectin/tumor necrosis factor induces cachexia, anemia, and inflammation. J Exp Med 167:1211–1227

25. Darling G, Fraker DL, Jensen JC et al (1990) Cachectic effects of recombinant human tumor necrosis factor in rats. Cancer Res 50:4008–4013

26. Llovera M, Lopez–Soriano FJ, Argiles JM (1993) Effects of tumor necrosis factor-alpha on muscle-protein turnover in female Wistar rats. J Natl Cancer Inst 85:1334–1339

27. Llovera M, Garcia-Martinez C, Lopez–Soriano J et al (1998) Protein turnover in skeletal muscle of tumour–bearing transgenic mice overexpressing the soluble TNF receptor-1. Cancer Lett 130:19–27

28. Guttridge DC, Mayo MW, Madrid LV et al (2000) NF-kappaB-induced loss of MyoD messenger RNA: possible role in muscle decay and cachexia. Science 289:2363–2366

29. Megeney LA, Kablar B, Garrett K et al (1996) MyoD is required for myogenic stem cell function in adult skeletal muscle. Genes Dev 10:1173–1183

30. Argiles JM, Lopez–Soriano J, Busquets S et al (1997) Journey from cachexia to obesity by TNF. FASEB J 11:743–751

31. Bossola M, Muscaritoli M, Bellantone R et al (2000) Serum tumour necrosis factor-alpha levels in cancer patients are discontinuous and correlate with weight loss. Eur J Clin Invest 30:1107–1112

32. Mantovani G, Macciò A, Mura L et al (2000) Serum levels of leptin and proinflammatory cytokines in patients with advanced-stage cancer at different sites. J Mol Med 78:554–561

33. Nakashima J, Tachibana M, Ueno M et al (1998) Association between tumor necrosis factor in serum and cachexia in patients with prostate cancer. Clin Cancer Res 4:1743–1748

34. Falconer JS, Fearon KC, Plester CE et al (1994) Cytokines, the acute–phase response, and resting energy expenditure in cachectic patients with pancreatic cancer. Ann Surg 219:325–331

35. Karayiannakis AJ, Syrigos KN, Polychronidis A et al (2001) Serum levels of tumor necrosis factor–alpha and nutritional status in pancreatic cancer patients.

Anticancer Res 21:1355–1358

36. Sherry BA, Gelin J, Fong Y et al (1989) Anticachectin/tumor necrosis factor-alpha antibodies attenuate development of cachexia in tumor models. FASEB J 3:1956–1962

37. Trikha M (2002) Combined blockade of human and mouse TNF inhibits cancer cachexia in nude mice. Centocor Technical Report Biorestr 315 (Internal Centocor Report), Centocor Inc, Malvern

38. Siegel SA, Shealy DJ, Nakada MT et al (1995) The mouse/human chimeric monoclonal antibody cA2 neutralizes TNF in vitro and protects transgenic mice from cachexia and TNF lethality in vivo. Cytokine 7:15–25

39. Torelli GF, Meguid MM, Moldawer LL et al (1999) Use of recombinant human soluble TNF receptor in anorectic tumor-bearing rats. Am J Physiol 277:R850–R855

40. Truyens C, Torrico F, Angelo–Barrios A et al (1995) The cachexia associated with Trypanosoma cruzi acute infection in mice is attenuated by anti-TNF-alpha, but not by anti-IL-6 or anti-IFN-gamma antibodies. Parasite Immunol 17:561–568

41. Haslett PA (1998) Anticytokine approaches to the treatment of anorexia and cachexia. Semin Oncol 25:53–57

42. Steensma DP, Mesa RA, Li CY et al (2002) Etanercept, a soluble tumor necrosis factor receptor, palliates constitutional symptoms in patients with myelofibrosis with myeloid metaplasia: results of a pilot study. Blood 99:2252–2254

43. Fonseca J, Canhao H, Resende C et al (2002) Weight gain associated with the administration of tumor necrosis factor alpha antagonists in patients with rheumatoid arthritis. EULAR (Annual European Congress of Rheumatology). Arthritis Reum 46:S170 (abs)

44. Eggermont AM, de Wilt JH, ten Hagen TL (2003) Current uses of isolated limb perfusion in the clinic and a model system for new strategies. Lancet Oncol 4:429–437

45. Eggermont AM, ten Hagen TL (2003) Tumor necrosis factor-based isolated limb perfusion for soft tissue sarcoma and melanoma: ten years of successful anti-vascular therapy. Curr Oncol Rep 5:79–80

46. Arnott CH, Scott KA, Moore RJ et al (2004) Expression of both TNF-alpha receptor subtypes is essential for optimal skin tumour development. Oncogene 23:1902–1910

47. Malik ST, Griffin DB, Fiers W et al (1989) Paradoxical effects of tumour necrosis factor in experimental ovarian cancer. Int J Cancer 44:918–925

48. Scott KA, Moore RJ, Arnott CH et al (2003) An anti-tumor necrosis factor-alpha antibody inhibits the development of experimental skin tumors. Mol Cancer Ther 2:445–451

49. Montserrat E (1997) Chronic lymphoproliferative disorders. Curr Opin Oncol 9:34–41

50. Holden RJ, Pakula IS, Mooney PA (1998) An immuno-logical model connecting the pathogenesis of stress, depression and carcinoma. Med Hypotheses 51:309–314

51. Tselepis C, Perry I, Dawson C et al (2002) Tumour necrosis factor-alpha in Barrett's oesophagus: a potential novel mechanism of action. Oncogene 21:6071–6081

52. Barak V, Nisman B, Polliack A (1999) The tumor necrosis factor family and correlation with disease activity and response to treatment in hairy cell leukemia. Eur J Haematol 62:71–75

53. Schiller JH, Bittner G, Spriggs DR (1992) Tumor necrosis factor, but not other hematopoietic growth factors, prolongs the survival of hairy cell leukemia cells. Leuk Res 16:337–346

54. Hideshima T, Chauhan D, Schlossman R et al (2001) The role of tumor necrosis factor alpha in the pathophysiology of human multiple myeloma: therapeutic applications. Oncogene 20:4519–4527

55. Foa R, Massaia M, Cardona S et al (1990) Production of tumor necrosis factor-alpha by B-cell chronic lymphocytic leukemia cells: a possible regulatory role of TNF in the progression of the disease. Blood 76:393–400

56. Huang D, Reittie JE, Stephens S et al (1992) Effects of anti-TNF monoclonal antibody infusion in patients with hairy cell leukaemia. Br J Haematol 81:231–234

57. Friess H, Guo XZ, Nan BC et al (1999) Growth factors and cytokines in pancreatic carcinogenesis. Ann NY Acad Sci 880:110–121

58. Cope AP, Londei M, Chu NR et al (1994) Chronic exposure to tumor necrosis factor (TNF) in vitro impairs the activation of T cells through the T cell receptor/CD3 complex; reversal in vivo by anti-TNF antibodies in patients with rheumatoid arthritis. J Clin Invest 94:749–760

59. D'Haens G, Ceuppens J, Colpaert S et al (1997) Restoration of decreased in vitro lymphocyte proliferative response to mycobacteria and mitogens after single infusion of chimeric anti–TNF alpha antibodies in Crohn's disease. Gastroenterology 112:A595 (abs)

60. Meenan J, Hommes D, van Dullemen H (1997) The influence of TNF alpha mAb, cA2, on circulating lymphocyte populations. Gastroenterology 112:A1039 (abs)

61. Knight DM, Trinh H, Le J et al (1993) Construction and initial characterization of a mouse-human chimeric anti-TNF antibody. Mol Immunol 30:1443–1453

62. Nahar IK, Shojania K, Marra CA et al (2003) Infliximab treatment of rheumatoid arthritis and Crohn's disease. Ann Pharmacother 37:1256–1265

63. Hommes DW, van Deventer SJ (2003) Infliximab therapy in Crohn's disease:safety issues. Neth J Med 61:100–104

64 Mikuls TR, Moreland LW (2003) Benefit–risk assessment of infliximab in the treatment of rheumatoid arthritis. Drug Saf 26:23–32

65. Khanna D, McMahon M, Furst DE (2004) Safety of tumour necrosis factor-alpha antagonists. Drug Saf

27:307–324

66. Anonymous (2003) REMICADE® (infliximab) package insert. Centocor Inc, Malvern

67. Marty FM, Lee SJ, Fahey MM et al (2003) Infliximab use in patients with severe graft-versus-host disease and other emerging risk factors of non-Candida invasive fungal infections in allogeneic hematopoietic stem cell transplant recipients: a cohort study. Blood 102:2768–2776

68. Smith KJ, Skelton HG (2001) Rapid onset of cutaneous squamous cell carcinoma in patients with rheumatoid arthritis after starting tumor necrosis factor alpha receptor IgG1-Fc fusion complex therapy. J Am Acad Dermatol 45:953–956

69. Kavanaugh A, Keystone EC (2003) The safety of biologic agents in early rheumatoid arthritis. Clin Exp Rheumatol 21:S203–S208 (abs)

70. Wolfe F, Michaud K (2003) Lymphoma in rheumatoid arthritis: the effect of methotrexate and anti-TNF therapy in 18,572 patients. Arthritis Rheum 48:S242 (abs)

71. Lee JH, Slifman NR, Gershon SK et al (2002) Life-threatening histoplasmosis complicating immunotherapy with tumor necrosis factor alpha antagonists infliximab and etanercept. Arthritis Rheum 46:2565–2570

72. Brown SL, Greene MH, Gershon SK et al (2002) Tumor necrosis factor antagonist therapy and lymphoma development: twenty-six cases reported to the Food and Drug Administration. Arthritis Rheum 46:3151–3158

73. Slifman NR, Gershon SK, Lee JH et al (2003) Listeria monocytogenes infection as a complication of treatment with tumor necrosis factor alpha-neutralizing agents. Arthritis Rheum 48:319–324

74. Colombel JF, Loftus EV Jr, Tremaine WJ et al (2004) The safety profile of infliximab in patients with Crohn's disease: the Mayo clinic experience in 500 patients. Gastroenterology 126:19–31

75. Ramesh G, Reeves WB (2002) TNF-alpha mediates chemokine and cytokine expression and renal injury in cisplatin nephrotoxicity. J Clin Invest 110:835–842

76. Delanian S, Porcher R, Balla-Mekias S et al (2003) Randomized, placebo-controlled trial of combined pentoxifylline and tocopherol for regression of superficial radiation-induced fibrosis. J Clin Oncol 21:2545–2550

77. Rube CE, van Valen F, Wilfert F et al (2003) Ewing's sarcoma and peripheral primitive neuroectodermal tumor cells produce large quantities of bioactive tumor necrosis factor-alpha (TNF-alpha) after radiation exposure. Int J Radiat Oncol Biol Phys 56:1414–1425

78. Azuma Y, Kaji K, Katogi R et al (2000) Tumor necrosis factor-alpha induces differentiation of and bone resorption by osteoclasts. J Biol Chem 275:4858–4864

79. Schafers M, Lee DH, Brors D et al (2003) Increased sensitivity of injured and adjacent uninjured rat primary sensory neurons to exogenous tumor necrosis factor-alpha after spinal nerve ligation. J Neurosci 23:3028–3038

80. Tobinick EL (2003) Targeted etanercept for treatment–refractory pain due to bone metastasis: two case reports. Clin Ther 25:2279–2288

81. Anonymous (2002) American Thoracic Society statement: guidelines for the six-minute walk test. Am J Respir Crit Care Med 166:111–117

82. Cella D, Eton DT, Lai JS et al (2002) Combining anchor and distribution-based methods to derive minimal clinically important differences on the Functional Assessment of Cancer Therapy (FACT) anemia and fatigue scales. J Pain Symptom Manage 24:547–561

83. Johnson JR, Williams G, Pazdur R (2003) End points and United States Food and Drug Administration approval of oncology drugs. J Clin Oncol 21:1404–1411

84. Steer CB, Marx GM, Harper PG (2001) Is there quality in clinical benefit? Ann Oncol 12:1191–1193

85. Patrick-Miller LJ (2003) Is there a role for the assessment of health-related quality of life in the clinical evaluation of novel cytostatic agents? Clin Cancer Res 9:2040–2048 Commentary re: LoRusso PM (2003) Improvements in quality of life and disease-related symptoms in phase I trials of the selective oral epidermal growth factor receptor tyrosine kinase inhibitor ZD1839 in non-small cell lung cancer and other solid tumors. Clin Cancer Res 9:1990–1994

86. Cleeland CS, Bennett GJ, Dantzer R et al (2003) Are the symptoms of cancer and cancer treatment due to a shared biologic mechanism? A cytokine-immunologic model of cancer symptoms. Cancer 97:2919–2925

87. Pfitzenmaier J, Vessella R, Higano CS et al (2003) Elevation of cytokine levels in cachectic patients with prostate carcinoma. Cancer 97:1211–1216

88. Raison CL, Miller AH (2003) Depression in cancer: new developments regarding diagnosis and treatment. Biol Psychiatry 54:283–294

89. Chassany O, Sagnier P, Marquis P et al (2002) Patient reported outcomes: the example of health-related quality of life. A European guidance document for the improved integration of health-related quality of life assessments in the drug regulatory process. Drug Inf J 36:209–238

90. Hirschfeld S, Pazdur R (2002) Oncology drug development: United States Food and Drug Administration perspective. Crit Rev Oncol Hematol 42:137–143

91. Revicki DA, Osoba D, Fairclough D et al (2000) Recommendations on health-related quality of life research to support labeling and promotional claims in the United States. Qual Life Res 9:887–900

# A Phase II Study with Antioxidants, both in the Diet and Supplemented, Pharmaco-nutritional Support, Progestagen and Anti-COX-2 Showing Efficacy and Safety in Patients with Cancer-Related Anorexia-Cachexia and Oxidative Stress

Giovanni Mantovani, Clelia Madeddu, Antonio Macciò, Giulia Gramignano, Maria Rita Lusso, Elena Massa, Giorgio Astara, Roberto Serpe

## Introduction

Cancer-related anorexia-cachexia syndrome (CACS) is a complex syndrome characterised by progressive weight loss with depletion of host reserves of skeletal muscle and, to a lesser extent, adipose tissue, anorexia, reduced food intake, poor performance status and quality of life that often precedes death [1]. At the time of diagnosis, 80% of patients with upper gastrointestinal cancers and 60% with lung cancer have already experienced substantial weight loss [2]. The prevalence of cachexia increases from 50 to > 80% before death and in > 20% cachexia is the main cause of death [2]. CACS results from the interaction of the host and the tumour. However, its nature is incompletely understood [3–6], including the dynamics of host response (activation of systemic inflammatory response, metabolic, immune and neuroendocrine changes) and those tumour characteristics or tumour-derived products that influence expression of the syndrome (e.g. proteolysis-inducing factor, PIF). The relative importance of individual mediators and pathways in different patients or tumour types is unclear, as is the reason why individuals with apparently similar tumours should show considerable variation in their tendency to develop cachexia.

CACS is the net result of profound metabolic changes characterised by breakdown of skeletal muscle and abnormalities in protein, fat and carbohydrate metabolism, alongside changes in energy metabolism. Circulating factors produced by the tumour, or by the host immune system in response to the tumour, such as cytokines released by lymphocytes and/or monocytes/macrophages, tumour-derived PIF and lipid-mobilising factor (LMF) play a crucial role among the causal factors. Moreover, a chronic systemic inflammatory state induced by a low-grade tumour-sustained activation of the host immune system with the production of eicosanoids and acute-phase reactants takes place during CACS and in turn contributes to its progression and worsening.

Among proinflammatory cytokines, those mainly involved include interleukin (IL)-1, IL-6, tumour necrosis factor (TNF)-$\alpha$, interferon (IFN)-$\alpha$ and IFN-$\gamma$ [7–11]. They may act with a central role in long-term inhibition of feeding by mimicking the hypothalamic effect of excessive negative feedback signalling from leptin.

Several mechanisms may lead to oxidative stress (OS) in cancer patients. The first, altered energy metabolism, may account for symptoms such as anorexia/cachexia, nausea and vomiting that prevent a normal nutrition and thereby a normal supply of nutrients such as glucose, proteins and vitamins, leading eventually to accumulation of free radicals that are known as reactive oxygen species (ROS), such as hydroxyl radicals, superoxide radicals, and others.

The second mechanism is a non-specific chronic activation of the immune system with an excessive production of proinflammatory cytokines, which in turn may increase the ROS production [12]. Indeed, a chronic inflammatory condition associated with increased OS has been suggested as one of the triggering mechanisms behind the tumour-induced immune suppression [13]. Recently, several studies have reported that the chronic inflammation that occurs in patients with advanced cancer may be attributable to OS, which can adversely affect the immune functions. Indeed, free oxygen radicals produced by macrophages were able to inhibit non-specific and tumour-specific cytotoxicity and down-regulate signal molecules [14–17]. Therapeutic interventions aimed at protecting the immune system in cancer patients from OS-induced cell damage may enhance their immune competence.

A third mechanism may be the result of the use of antineoplastic drugs: many of them, particularly alkylating agents and cisplatin, are able to produce an excess of ROS and therefore lead to OS [18]. Several studies have shown that chemotherapy and radiation therapy are associated with increased formation of ROS and depletion of critical plasma and tissue antioxidants [19].

Thus, the hypothesis may arise that the body redox systems, which include antioxidant enzymes and low molecular weight antioxidants, may be dysregulated in cancer patients and that this imbalance might enhance disease progression. Regarding the mechanisms linking OS and cachexia in cancer, the following evidence has been provided: (a) in a murine model of muscle wasting and cachexia, TNF-$\alpha$ has been shown to induce OS and nitric oxide synthase; moreover, TNF-$\alpha$-induced cachexia could be prevented with the antioxidants D-$\alpha$-tocopherol or the nitric oxide synthase inhibitor nitro-L-arginine [20]; (b) an enhanced protein degradation is seen in skeletal muscle of cachectic mice given TNF-$\alpha$, which seems to be mediated by OS: there is some evidence that this may be a direct effect and is associated with an increase in total cellular ubiquitin-conjugated muscle proteins [21]; (c) a high rate of glycolytic activity and lactate production is commonly seen in the skeletal muscle tissue in practically all catabolic conditions, including cancer [22–25].

CACS/OS has been dealt with comprehensively in a number of our previous papers and the following evidence has been provided: (1) a clinically significant OS takes place in advanced cancer patients, as shown by increased levels of ROS and decreased levels of glutathione peroxidase (GPx) [26, 27]; (2) CACS is very frequent in advanced disease and it is associated with high levels of proinflammatory cytokines [12, 28, 29]; (3) both CACS and OS alone and in combination are highly predictive of clinical outcome and survival [29]; (4) the antioxidant agents $\alpha$-lipoic acid (ALA), carbo-

cysteine lisine salt and vitamins A, C and E administered to cancer patients alone or in combination were able to reduce ROS levels and increase GPx activity, while reducing serum levels of proinflammatory cytokines, i.e. they were effective on OS [27]; (5) ALA and N-acetyl cysteine (NAC) were able to correct in vitro the most significant functional defects of peripheral blood mononuclear cells isolated from advanced-stage cancer patients, i.e. the defective response to anti-CD3 mAb and the defective membrane expression of CD25 and CD95 [30].

Many single therapies against CACS and OS have been tested in isolation and have met with limited or no success. It seems likely that a combination of therapies, addressed to the different pathophysiological targets, will be required to fight the cachectic process.

## Aim of the Study

The aim of the present study was to test the efficacy and safety of an integrated treatment based on a pharmaco-nutritional support, antioxidants and drugs, all administered orally, in a population of advanced cancer patients with CACS/OS. The efficacy was assessed in terms of clinical response, improvement of nutritional/functional variables, changes in laboratory variables (indicators of CACS/OS) and improvement of quality of life (QL). The interim results of the study have already been published [31] and the final results will be published in May 2006 [32].

## Patients and Methods

### Study Design

An open non-randomised phase II study was designed according to the Simon two-stage design for $P_1 - P_0 = 0.20$: considering $P_0$ (i.e. non-effective treatment) as a total response of ≤ 40% of patients and $P_1$ (i.e. effective treatment) as a total response of at least 60% of patients, the treatment should be considered effective if at least 21 out of 39 patients are 'responders'. The study was approved by the Ethical Committee of the Policlinico Universitario, University of Cagliari, and written informed consent was obtained by all patients prior to inclusion in the study.

## Patient Eligibility

Inclusion criteria were as follows: 18–80 years; histologically confirmed tumour of any site at advanced stage, especially cancers inducing early cachexia (head and neck and gastrointestinal cancers); loss of at least 5% of their ideal (or pre-illness) body weight in the last 3 months (early 'clinical' or overt cachexia); and/or with abnormal values of proinflammatory cytokines, ROS, and antioxidant enzymes predictive of the onset of clinical cachexia; any antineoplastic therapy with curative or palliative intent (chemotherapy or hormone therapy) or supportive care; life expectancy of > 4 months.

Exclusion criteria were: pregnancy; significant comorbidities; mechanical obstruction to feeding; medical treatments inducing significant changes of patient metabolism or body weight.

## Treatment Plan

The integrated treatment consisted of the following:
- Diet with high polyphenol content (300 mg/day) obtained by alimentary sources or supplemented per os by tablets (one tablet Quercetix, Elbea Pharma, Milan, Italy)
- Antioxidant treatment: ALA (Tiobec, Laborest, Nerviano, Milan, Italy) 300 mg/day per os plus carbocysteine lysine salt (Fluifort, Dompè, Milan, Italy) 2.7 g/day per os plus vitamin E (Sursum 400, Abiogen Pharma, Pisa, Italy) 400 mg/day per os plus vitamin A 30 000 IU/day per os plus vitamin C 500 mg/day per os
- Pharmaco-nutritional support per os (ProSure, Abbott Laboratories, North Chicago, IL, USA) enriched with n-3 fatty acids (eicosapentaenoic acid [EPA] 1.1 g and docosahexaenoic acid 0.46 g, 310 kcal per can): two cans/day
- Progestagen: medroxyprogesterone acetate (MPA; Provera, Pfizer, Milan, Italy) 500 mg/day per os
- Selective cyclo-oxygenase (COX)-2 inhibitor Celecoxib (Celebrex, Pfizer) 200 mg/day per os.

The polyphenols have been included for their high activity as antioxidants [33]: among them, the quercetin is the most effective. The objective of the oral pharmaco-nutritional supplement is to integrate the energetic/proteic intake with the supplementation of n-3 fatty acids, which are able to inhibit cytokine production (TNF-α). Treatment with MPA has been proven to inhibit the cytokine production and to act positively on patient cenestesis [34]. The selected antioxidant treatment has been shown to be effective in reducing blood levels of ROS and increasing blood levels of physiological antioxidant enzymes in a series of our previous articles [26, 27, 30]. The COX-2 selective inhibitor Celecoxib has been chosen for its ability, shown both in experimental and clinical studies, to inhibit cancer-related inflammatory mediators (prostaglandin E$_2$), angiogenesis, and therefore cancer progression: clinical data in the treatment of CACS have been published recently [35].

The treatment duration was 4 months: this was considered adequate both to exploit its effects and to meet patient compliance.

## Study End-Points

The end-points of the study were efficacy and safety. The following were efficacy variables: (a) clinical, (b) nutritional/functional, (c) laboratory and (d) QL.

The following changes of variables after treatment compared to before were considered significant for response to treatment:
(a) *Clinical variables.* Objective clinical response (RECIST): an improvement or at least disease stability starting at minimum from stable disease [36]. Performance status (PS) according to ECOG scale [37]: an improvement of 1 unit.
(b) *Nutritional/functional variables.* Body weight: an increase of at least 5%. Lean body mass (LBM) by bioimpedentiometry: an increase of at least 10%. Appetite evaluated by visual analogue scale ranging from 0 to 10: an increase of at least 2 units. Resting energy expenditure (REE: kcal/day) by indirect calorimetry (calculated only in a subset of patients): a decrease of at least 10%. Grip strength by dynamometer: an increase of at least 30%.

(c) *Laboratory variables.* Serum levels of proinflammatory cytokines (IL-6 and TNF-α): a decrease of at least 25%. Serum levels of leptin: an increase of at least 100%. Blood levels of ROS by FORT test: a decrease of at least 80–100 FORT units. Evaluation by photometer of the erythrocyte levels of the antioxidant enzyme GPx: an increase of at least 2000 units (or 50%).

(d) *Evaluation of QL* by the following questionnaires: European Organization for Research and Treatment of Cancer (EORTC) QLQ-C30 version 3: an increase of at least 25% of the score. Euro QL EQ-5D: an increase of at least 25% of the scores of both EQ-5D$_{index}$ and EQ-5D$_{VAS}$. Multidimensional Fatigue Symptom Inventory-Short Form (MFSI-SF) [38]: a decrease of at least 25% of the score.

*Timing of evaluation of above variables.* The clinical, nutritional/functional, laboratory and QL variables were evaluated before treatment and at 1, 2 and 4 months.

## Criteria for Considering Patients as 'Responders', 'High Responders' or 'Non-responders'

The patients were considered as 'high responders' if the following changes occurred after treatment:
- Improvement of clinical response plus improvement of PS, or improvement of clinical response plus stability of PS, or stability of clinical response plus improvement of PS
- Improvement of at least three nutritional/functional variables with stability of the other variables
- Improvement of three or more laboratory variables (including at least proinflammatory cytokines and ROS) independently from the changes of the other variables
- Improvement of the scores of (at least) two or more QL questionnaires and no worsening of the others.

The patients were considered as 'responders' if the following changes occurred after treatment:
- No change or even slight worsening of the clinical response, which, however, does not reach progressing disease (PD) plus no change of PS < 2 or improvement of PS ≥ 2
- Improvement of at least three nutritional/func-

tional variables plus stability of one and worsening of one, or improvement of at least three plus stability of the other two, or improvement of at least two plus stability of the other three
- Improvement of at least two laboratory variables (including at least proinflammatory cytokines and ROS) independently from the changes of the other variables
- Improvement of the scores of at least one QL questionnaire with no change of the others or worsening of no more than one.

All patients who did not meet the above criteria were considered 'non-responders'.

## Methods

### Evaluation of LBM by Bioimpedentiometry

The impedance measurements were conducted with a bioelectric impedance analyser series 101 (using the standard four-electrode arrangement at 800 mA and 50 kHz). Body composition data analysed by the bioelectric impedance analyser are derived from correlations of resistance (R) and reactance (Xc). During the bioelectric impedance analyser measurement, the subjects lay supine with arms and legs angled outward so that the medial surface of the limbs did not touch the rest of the body. For conventional whole-body measurement, the electrodes are placed between the hand and the foot of the dominant side.

### REE by Indirect Calorimetry

The REE includes the basal energy expenditure plus the energy required for eating, minimal physical activity, and thermogenic effect of food. We used a Deltatrac metabolic monitor (Datex Ohmeda, Helsinki, Finland) that evaluates oxygen consumption and carbon dioxide production by applying the Harris-Benedict formulas.

### Assessment of Serum Levels of Proinflammatory Cytokines and Leptin

Proinflammatory cytokines (IL-6 and TNF-α) were evaluated by ELISA assay using monoclonal antibodies for two different epitopes of the cytokine molecules. The absorbance of the sample was analysed by a spectrophotometer at 450 nm. Serum leptin levels were determined with an ELISA assay using a monoclonal antibody specific for human leptin. The absorbance was measured by a spectrophotometer at $450 \pm 10$ nm. More details about the techniques are reported in our previous studies [28, 29].

Blood levels of ROS were determined using the FORT test: the radical species produced by the reaction, which are directly proportional to the quantity of lipid peroxides present in the sample, interact with an additive (phenylenediamine derivative), which forms a radical molecule evaluable by spectrophotometer at 505 nm (Form CR 2000, Callegari, Parma, Italy). Results are expressed as FORT units, where 1 FORT unit corresponds to 0.26 mg/l of $H_2O_2$ [39]. Erythrocyte levels of GPx were measured by photometer using a commercially available kit (Ransod, Randox Lab, Crumlin, UK).

## Statistical Analysis

The benefit obtained by treated patients was evaluated using the paired Student's t test or Wilcoxon ranks test when appropriate (baseline vs posttreatment values).

Correlations between changes of LBM and clinical (PS), nutritional/functional (appetite, grip stength), laboratory variables (IL-6, TNF-α, leptin, ROS and GPx) and QL questionnaires were tested using two-sided Spearman's ranks correlation analysis, using Bonferroni's correction for multiple tests. Moreover, the same correlations were made between changes of fatigue and changes of the above-cited variables. Significant relationships would have been examined by multivariate linear regression analysis. Significance was determined at 5%, 1% and 0.1% levels, two-sided.

## Results

### Patients

From July 2002 to January 2005, 39 patients completed the treatment and all were evaluable. Patient clinical characteristics are listed in Table 1.

**Table 1.** Patient clinical characteristics

|  | No. | % |
|---|---|---|
| Patients enrolled | 39 | |
| Male/female | 23/16 | |
| Age | | |
|   Mean ± SD:  58.9 ± 9.1 | | |
|   Range:  42–78 | | |
| Weight | | |
|   Mean ± SD:  55.8 ± 10.5 | | |
|   Range:  36–76 | | |
| BMI | | |
|   Mean ± SD:  21.8 ± 4.4 | | |
|   Range:  14.4–32.1 | | |
|   BMI < 18.5 | 9 | 23.1 |
|   BMI 18.5–25 | 25 | 64.1 |
|   BMI 25–30 | 5 | 12.8 |
| Weight loss before study entry | | |
|   > 10% | 5 | 12.8 |
|   5–10% | 9 | 23.1 |
|   < 5% | 3 | 7.7 |
| Tumour site | | |
|   Head and neck | 17 | 43.6 |
|   Lung | 8 | 20.5 |
|   Ovary | 3 | 7.7 |
|   Breast | 3 | 7.7 |
|   Stomach | 2 | 5.1 |
|   Pancreas | 2 | 5.1 |
|   Liver | 2 | 5.1 |
|   Kidney | 1 | 2.6 |
|   Uterine sarcoma | 1 | 2.6 |
| Stage | | |
|   IIIA | 1 | 2.6 |
|   IV | 38 | 97.4 |
| ECOG PS | | |
|   0 | 2 | 5.1 |
|   1 | 27 | 69.2 |
|   2 | 10 | 25.7 |

*BMI*, body mass index; *ECOG PS*, Eastern Cooperative Oncology Group Performance Status

### Study End-Points

#### Efficacy

*Clinical variables.* Objective response was evaluated in all 39 patients: after treatment 16 patients improved (six patients changed from PD to stable disease [SD] and ten patients changed from PD to partial response [PR] or complete response [CR]), seven patients remained unchanged (SD) and 16 patients worsened to PD. PS remained unchanged (0 or 1) in 22 patients, PS remained 2 in four patients, whereas it improved (from 2 to 1) in seven patients and worsened in six patients. PS was assessed by the same clinician for all patients at all times to minimise reporters' inherent bias.

*Nutritional/functional variables.* The results are reported in Table 2 and Fig. 1. The body weight increased significantly from baseline as well as the LBM and appetite, while the grip strength did not show significant changes. A decrease of REE at the end of treatment was found in two of five patients studied.

*Laboratory variables.* The results are reported in Table 2 and Figs 2 and 3. Proinflammatory cytokines IL-6 and TNF-α decreased significantly, while leptin increased significantly. ROS and GPx showed a trend toward a decrease and increase, respectively, but the changes were not significant.

*Quality of life variables.* The QL variables are reported in Table 3. Overall QL, and in particular EORTC-QLQ-C30 as well as EQ-5D$_{VAS}$ and fatigue, improved after treatment.

*Correlations between changes of LBM and clinical (PS), nutritional/functional (appetite, grip strength), laboratory (IL-6, TNF-α, leptin, ROS and GPx) and QL variables.* A significant negative relationship was found only between LBM and IL-6 changes (Table 4). Therefore, multivariate regression analysis was not performed.

*Correlations between changes of fatigue and clinical (PS), nutritional/functional (appetite, grip strength) and laboratory (IL-6, TNF-α, leptin, ROS and GPx) variables.* No significant relationship was found (Table 5).

## Safety

Overall, the treatment was quite well tolerated by patients. No patient complained of serious adverse events nor was withdrawn from the study due to toxicity. One patient interrupted MPA after 2

**Table 2.** Nutritional/functional and laboratory variables evaluated after 1, 2, and 4 months of treatment on 39 patients

| Variable | Baseline | After 1 month | p value | After 2 months | p value | After 4 months | p value |
|---|---|---|---|---|---|---|---|
| Body weight (kg) | 55.1 ± 10 | 56.5 ± 10.5 | 0.001 | 56.4 ± 9.7 | 0.036 | 57 ± 9.8 | 0.031 |
| LBM (kg) | 38 ± 9 | 38.9 ± 9 | 0.059 | 39.4 ± 8.9 | 0.045 | 39.7 ± 8.7 | 0.024 |
| Grip strength (kg) | 28.0 ± 10.4 | 27.8 ± 9.5 | 0.879 | 27.9 ± 9.3 | 0.673 | 28.1 ± 9.5 | 0.827 |
| Appetite | 5.5 ± 2.5 | 6.6 ± 2.2 | 0.005 | 6.8 ± 1.9 | 0.001 | 7.0 ± 1.6 | 0.004 |
| IL-6 (pg/ml) | 12.5 ± 9.9 | 8.8 ± 8.7 | 0.002 | 7.5 ± 8.6 | 0.003 | 7.4 ± 8.5 | 0.007 |
| TNFa (pg/ml) | 22.2 ± 16.6 | 19.5 ± 16 | 0.204 | 15.8 ± 13 | 0.020 | 14 ± 11.7 | 0.015 |
| Leptin (ng/ml) | 5.9 ± 6.1 | 8.9 ± 10.6 | 0.008 | 10.2 ± 13.3 | 0.031 | 13.6 ± 13.3 | < 0.001 |
| ROS (FORT U) | 468.5 ± 97.2 | 436.6 ± 92.5 | 0.033 | 437.7 ± 89.6 | 0.087 | 444.1 ± 93.6 | 0.162 |
| GPx (U/l) | 8206.6 ± 2322.3 | 8339.3 ± 2411.8 | 0.726 | 8295.9 ± 2314.1 | 0.848 | 8849.2 ± 2629 | 0.211 |

Data are reported as mean ± standard deviation. Significance was considered for $p < 0.05$, as calculated with Student's t test for paired data (post-treatment values vs baseline values). Significance for IL-6, TNF-α and leptin was calculated using Wilcoxon ranks test. *LBM,* lean body mass; *IL-6,* interleukin-6; *TNF-α,* tumour necrosis factor-α; *ROS,* reactive oxygen species; *GPx,* glutathione peroxidase

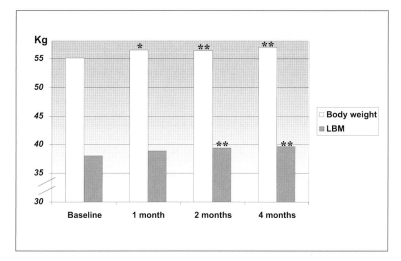

**Fig. 1.** Body weight and LBM values after 1, 2 and 4 months of treatment compared to baseline. The body weight and LBM are shown in kilograms (kg). * $p \leq$ 0.01; ** $p < 0.05$, as calculated by Student's t-test for paired data (post-treatment data versus baseline)

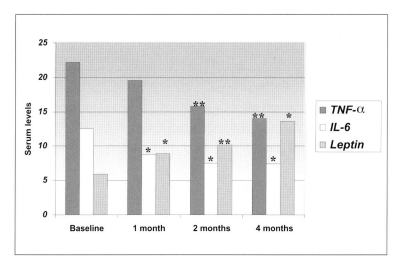

**Fig. 2.** Serum levels of TNF-$\alpha$ (pg/ml), IL-6 (pg/ml) and leptin (ng/ml) after 1, 2 and 4 months of treatment compared to baseline. * $p \leq 0.01$; ** $p < 0.05$, as calculated by Wilcoxon ranks test (post-treatment data versus baseline)

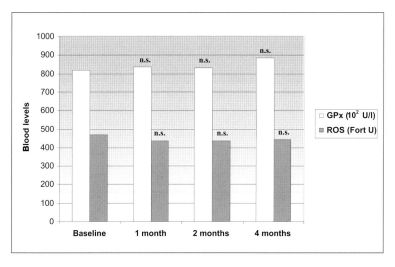

**Fig. 3.** Blood levels of GPx and ROS after 1, 2 and 4 months of treatment compared to baseline. *n.s.*, non-significant, as calculated by Student's t-test for paired data (post-treatment data versus baseline)

**Table 3.** Quality of life variables assessed after 1, 2 and 4 months of treatment in 39 patients

| Questionnaire | Baseline | After 1 month | *p* value | After 2 month | *p* value | After 4 month | *p* value |
|---|---|---|---|---|---|---|---|
| EORTC QLQ-C30 | $65.9 \pm 16.3$ | $72.4 \pm 15.6$ | 0.008 | $71.8 \pm 14.6$ | 0.020 | $70.9 \pm 14.6$ | 0.044 |
| EQ-5Dindex | $0.50 \pm 0.4$ | $0.58 \pm 0.4$ | 0.175 | $0.56 \pm 0.4$ | 0.340 | $0.59 \pm 0.4$ | 0.114 |
| EQ-5Dvas | $49.4 \pm 21.4$ | $58.9 \pm 22.7$ | 0.016 | $58.6 \pm 20.6$ | 0.015 | $58.7 \pm 19.4$ | 0.009 |
| MFSI-SF | $20.1 \pm 22.1$ | $14.4 \pm 20.3$ | 0.125 | $11.8 \pm 17.2$ | 0.022 | $10.8 \pm 14.4$ | 0.004 |

The global QL score for each questionnaire is reported as mean $\pm$ SD. For EORTC QLQ-C30, EQ5Dindex and EQ-5Dvas the increasing score corresponds to improvement of quality of life, while for MSFI-SF the decrease of QL score corresponds to amelioration of fatigue. Significance was considered at $p < 0.05$, as calculated with Student's t test for paired data (post-treatment values vs baseline). *EORTC QLQ-C30*, European Organization for Research and Treatment of Cancer QLQ-C30; *EQ-5D*, Euro QL-5D, *MFSI-SF* Multidimensional Fatigue Symptom Inventory-Short Form

**Table 4.** Correlation between LBM changes and changes of clinical (ECOG PS), nutritional/functional (appetite, grip strength), laboratory (IL-6, TNF-$\alpha$, leptin, ROS, GPx) and quality of life variables

| | Spearman's r | *p* value |
|---|---|---|
| Clinical variables | | |
| ECOG PS | -0.09 | 0.568 |
| Nutritional/functional variables | | |
| Appetite | 0.08 | 0.664 |
| Grip strength | 0.01 | 0.949 |
| Laboratory variables | | |
| IL-6 | -0.40 | 0.013 |
| TNF-$\alpha$ | -0.17 | 0.321 |
| Leptin | 0.26 | 0.121 |
| ROS | 0.11 | 0.529 |
| *GPx* | 0.05 | 0.747 |
| QL questionnaires | | |
| EORTC QLQ-C30 | 0.17 | 0.303 |
| EQ-5D$_{index}$ | 0.02 | 0.913 |
| EQ-5D$_{vas}$ | 0.28 | 0.097 |
| MFSI-SF | 0.21 | 0.271 |

The results show a significant correlation between LBM changes and IL-6 levels. In contrast, the changes of other variables did not show a significant correlation with LBM changes. Correlation analysis was performed by Spearman rank correlation test. Results were considered significant at $p < 0.05$. *ECOG PS*, Eastern Cooperative Oncology Group Performance Status; *IL-6*, interleukin-6; *TNF-$\alpha$*, tumour necrosis factor-$\alpha$; *ROS*, reactive oxygen species; *GPx*, glutathione peroxidase; *EORTC QLQ-C30*, European Organization for Research and Treatment of Cancer QLQ-C30; *EQ-5D*, Euro QL-5D; *MFSI-SF*, Multidimensional Fatigue Symptom Inventory-Short Form

**Table 5.** Correlation between MFSI-SF score changes and changes of clinical (ECOG PS), nutritional/functional (LBM, appetite, grip strength) and laboratory (IL-6, TNF-$\alpha$, leptin, ROS, GPx) variables

| | Spearman's r | *p* value |
|---|---|---|
| Clinical variables | | |
| ECOG PS | 0.10 | 0.582 |
| Nutritional/functional variables | | |
| LBM | 0.21 | 0.271 |
| Appetite | -0.16 | 0.410 |
| Grip strength | -0.22 | 0.276 |
| Laboratory variables | | |
| IL-6 | -0.21 | 0.275 |
| TNF-$\alpha$ | 0.23 | 0.221 |
| Leptin | -0.10 | 0.622 |
| ROS | 0.31 | 0.103 |
| GPx | -0.07 | 0.728 |

Correlation analysis was performed by Spearman rank correlation test. Results were considered significant at $p < 0.05$. *ECOG PS*, Eastern Cooperative Oncology Group Performance Status; *LBM*, lean body mass; *IL-6*, interleukin-6; *TNF-$\alpha$*, tumour necrosis factor-$\alpha$; *ROS*, reactive oxygen species; *GPx*, glutathione peroxidase

months because of deep-vein thrombosis in the leg. So far, the treatment has been demonstrated to be safe without significant side-effects and achieved an optimal compliance by patients as assessed by count of both tablets/cans returned.

## Assessment of 'Responders' and 'Non-responders'

At the end of the study, 22 out of 39 patients were responders (17 'responders' and five 'high responders'), while the minimum required was 21 out of 39: therefore the treatment was effective. It should be taken into account that, as already reported in Sect. 'Patients and Methods', the response criteria were arbitrary, although they were carefully built up by us.

In our study we have used two different types of statistical evaluation: the first assessed the treatment efficacy comparing the mean ± standard deviation values of the different variables before and after treatment and the second in terms of patient 'responders' and 'non-responders'.

The second evaluation was used for the final assessment of the treatment efficacy in accordance with the Simon two-stage phase II design selected for this study.

## Discussion

Cancer-related anorexia-cachexia and oxidative stress are two of the most important features of advanced cancer and are both predictive of a poor patient clinical outcome, i.e. survival. Moreover, the resulting malnutrition and the loss of LBM worsen the quality of life mainly by negatively affecting the patient's physical activity and also impair recovery by decreasing tolerance to therapy and increasing complications. Thus far, attempts at correcting CACS with enteral nutrition with nasogastric tube or percutaneous gastrostomy, or total parenteral nutrition, have generally been disappointing [40–44]. Likewise, attempts at drug therapy for CACS with a variety of agents have had limited success: consequently, we have tried to select an innovative approach that was at the same time based on a solid background and feasible in an outpatient setting. In the present phase II study, we used multiple feasible and potentially effective tools available against CACS/OS to test their efficacy: if positive results are obtained, we will proceed with a randomised phase III study.

The present study demonstrates that the treatment administered was effective in inducing a significant increase not only of total body weight but rather LBM: indeed, the body weight increase (1.9 kg) was almost completely sustained by a parallel increase of LBM (1.7 kg). This should translate into a parallel improvement in functioning, as suggested by our preliminary unpublished results obtained by physical activity assessment with appropriate equipment, and therefore QL.

The decrease of IL-6 after treatment was the only variable significantly correlated with LBM. This finding further strengthens the role of proinflammatory cytokines in the pathophysiology of CACS/OS. The increase of leptin after treatment confirms its inverse association with proinflammatory cytokines, which has been already reported in several of our previous papers [28, 29].

The QL improved significantly after treatment: this was particularly relevant for fatigue. However, it it worth noting that there was no correlation between changes of fatigue and changes of any of the other variables studied.

Two points are to be considered on the sample patients included: (1) the tumour site was relatively heterogeneous, so preventing the likelihood of numerous dropouts inherent to rapidly progressive tumours with very poor prognosis, such as pancreatic cancer; (2) more than half of the patients were in the range of normal body weight (BMI < 25), i.e. were not overtly cachectic, though almost half of them had a significant loss of body weight as compared to pre-illness body weight.

We shall now try to explain how the different components of our treatment may have acted on the different targets involved. The first components were several antioxidant agents selected on the basis of our and others' previous experimental and clinical evidence of activity, administered both through alimentary sources and/or supplementation. The second component was a pharmaco-nutritional support or 'nutraceutical' enriched with n-3 fatty acids, which appear to be able to reduce levels of proinflammatory cytokines [45], modulate PIF-mediated ubiquitin-proteasome proteolysis, possibly via the transcription factor NF-kappaB [46–48] and influence hepatic 'acute-phase' protein synthesis [49]. There is also some evidence to suggest they may have anti-tumour activity themselves [50, 51] and down-regulate the toxicity of chemotherapy [52, 53]. Studies on cachectic pancreatic cancer patients have suggested that, when given at doses 20–40 times the normal western dietary intake, n-3 fatty acids are well tolerated [54] and can stabilise patients' body weight [55]. On the basis that a successful cachexia therapy has to address both metabolic changes and reduced food intake, the combination of a conventional oral nutritional supplement with n-3 fatty acids and antioxidants was developed. The recommended daily intake of two cans provides 620 kcal, 32 g protein and 2.2 g EPA. This combination supplement has recently been tested in two large-scale randomised studies. In the first overall randomised trial, LBM did not change significantly [56] in a patient population in which compliance with the experimental supplement averaged 1.4 cans/day, while in a substudy the administration of the supplement enriched with EPA was associated with an increase in physical activity, which may reflect improved quality of life [57]. Increased activity is particularly beneficial in cachectic patients, as inactivity is a risk factor for muscle atrophy [58]. The second study compared the same supplement with megestrol acetate or a combination of the two: however, the combination was not better than megestrol acetate alone [59]. Thus, while there is much in vitro and animal experimental evidence to support the use of n-3 fatty acids, the case for benefit from their supplementation has not yet been proven definitively. The major obstacle is oral delivery of an adequate dose: in addition, the optimum macro-micronutrient supplement mix to accompany n-3 fatty acids remains to be established.

It is worth noting that in our study, 66.6% of patients consumed two cans/day and the mean consumption was 1.5 cans/day: the probable reasons why LBM increased significantly in our study compared with results obtained by Fearon [56] where it did not, were the better compliance of our patients to pharmaco-nutritional supplement and

the longer duration of treatment (4 months vs 8 weeks).

The third component of our treatment was the synthetic progestagen MPA, which is currently the only approved agent in Europe as well as the most widely used against CACS: it has been shown to be successful to a certain extent in reversing body weight loss, although this occurs as a result of an increase in fat mass and water retention rather than the preservation of LBM [60, 61]. The reason to have included MPA in our treatment approach was, apart from the above-cited indications, its ability, which was demonstrated for the first time in one of our experimental studies, to down-regulate the production and/or release of proinflammatory cytokines as well as serotonin, both heavily involved with CACS [34]. However, in administering MPA, the increased risk of thromboembolic events, peripheral oedema, breakthrough bleeding, hyperglycaemia and hypertension must be taken into account, which therefore entails a careful patient selection. The dosage of MPA we have used (500 mg/day) is in the mean range of the currently recommended dosages and in our hands it has been shown to be safe: indeed, only one patient had to discontinue MPA due to leg deep-vein thrombosis.

The rationale for including COX-2 inhibitors is reported in Sect. 'Patients and Methods'. Notwithstanding their potential interest also in the treatment of cancer cachexia, some questions have arisen recently on the clinical use of these agents because of their toxicity and particularly cardiovascular risks. It is to be noted that at the dosage (200 mg/day) and for the time duration (4 months) used in our study, the treatment is to be considered completely safe (http://www.fda.gov/bbs/topics/news/2004/NEW01144.html). In a recent study by Cerchietti et al. [35], 15 patients with evidence of CACS received MPA 500 mg twice daily, celecoxib 200 mg twice daily plus oral food supplementation for 6 weeks: an increase of body weight was observed as well as an improvement in fatigue, appetite and performance status.

Among the potentially useful agents not used in this study, anti-TNF-α monoclonal antibody is now under approval in the USA for the treatment of CACS: a multicentre randomised clinical trial to test its effectiveness in cachectic pancreatic cancer patients has recently completed patient accrual.

The methodological issues to be considered aside from the combined approach used in the present study include the best way to assess the degree of CACS, its appropriate characterisation by measuring all possible contributing factors (a 'CACS staging system') and the best ways to assess caloric intake, nutrition status, patient functioning and well-being. Considering that both CACS and OS are clinically relevant in terms of their impact on both patient QL and survival, the search for a potentially effective treatment on both these endpoints must be considered critical among the not yet available oncological treatments with a high impact.

It is also to be taken into account that the treatment tested is simple, easy to administer, based mainly on alimentary sources, relatively low-cost pharmaco-nutritional support and low-cost drugs: therefore, it may be considered as having a favourable cost-benefit profile while achieving an optimal patient compliance.

The results of the present study are very encouraging, although they should be considered with some caution taking into account that this is an uncontrolled study.

Based on the results reported above, a phase III randomised study was started in February 2005 as a multicentre trial involving 10–12 Italian oncology departments, with the aim of testing the safety and efficacy of an integrated approach of CACS/OS to improve both objective clinical symptoms such as LBM and subjective symptoms such as functioning and QL. The study has been approved by the Ethical Committee of the Policlinico Universitario, University of Cagliari, Italy and each patient has to sign an informed consent before study entry.

The patient eligibility criteria are the same as those of the phase II study: patients 18–80 years old, with histologically confirmed advanced-stage tumour of any site, especially cancers inducing early cachexia (head and neck and gastrointestinal cancers) who have lost at least 5% of their ideal (or pre-illness) body weight in the last 3 months (early 'clinical' or overt cachexia), and/or with abnormal values of proinflammatory cytokines, ROS and antioxidant enzymes, predictive of the onset of clinical cachexia, treated either with antineoplastic therapy (chemotherapy or hormone therapy) or supportive care or off-treatment, with a life expectancy of more than 4 months.

Exclusion criteria are the following: severe uncontrolled comorbidities, mechanical obstruction to feeding, concomitant medical treatments that induce a significant change of body weight and metabolism (such as corticosteroid treatment), diabetes, female patients of childbearing age, positive history of thromboembolic events.

Eligible patients are to be randomised to the following five arms of treatment. Polyphenols (300 mg/day) + antioxidant agents, including ALA 400 mg/day per os + carboxycysteine 2.7 g/day per os (or mesna 1800 mg/day per os) + vitamin E 400 mg/day per os + vitamin A 30 000 IU and vitamin C 500 mg/day per os, are administered to all patients. The following are added to each arm:

Arm 1: Medroxyprogesterone acetate 500 mg/day per os;

Arm 2: Pharmaco-nutritional support containing EPA and docosahexaenoic acid (DHA), high-calorie, high-protein content, two cans/day;

Arm 3: L-Carnitine 4 g/day;

Arm 4: Thalidomide 200 mg/day;

Arm 5: Medroxyprogesterone acetate + pharmaco-nutritional support + L-Carnitine + thalidomide.

The treatment duration is 16 weeks.

The aim of the phase III study is to evaluate the efficacy of each arm of treatment for the following key variables:
- Clinical: Objective clinical response, PS by ECOG/Karnofsky, progression-free survival
- Nutritional/functional: LBM, grip strength by dinamometer, a detailed evaluation of daily activity and the corresponding energy expenditure assessed by a physical activity meter
- Laboratory: Proinflammatory cytokines IL-6, TNF-$\alpha$ and leptin
- Quality of life: EORTC QLQ-C30, EQ5D$_{index}$ and EQ5D$_{vas}$; fatigue by MFSI-SF.

The key variables have to be evaluated before treatment and at 4, 8, 16 and 24 weeks.

Hypothesising a difference between arms of

20%, considering an alpha-type error of 0.05 and a beta-type error of 0.20, 95 patients will be enrolled for each arm. The comparison between arms for the key end-point parameters will be made using the ANOVA test or the Kruskall-Wallis test for non-parametric variables. Survival (overall survival and progression-free survival) will be evaluated starting from the date of enrollment in the study using the Kaplan-Meier method. Moreover, the benefit obtained by the patients enrolled in each arm following the treatment will be evaluated using the paired Student's t test or Wilcoxon signed rank test when appropriate (pre-treatment vs post-treatment values). Significance will be

determined at 5%, 1% and 0.1% levels (e.g. chi-square test, two-sided).

The study is ongoing and up to May 2006 82 patients have been enrolled. The end of accrual is scheduled for the beginning of 2007.

We are confident that this study will be successful in improving both objective clinical symptoms such as LBM and subjective symptoms such as functioning and QL.

The ultimate goal should be that of translating the results obtained in advanced cancer patients into a prevention trial in a population of individuals at risk of developing CACS/OS.

# References

1. Dewys WD, Begg C, Lavin PT et al (1980) Prognostic effect of weight loss prior to chemotherapy in cancer patients. Eastern Cooperative Oncology Group. Am J Med 69:491–497
2. Bruera E (1997) ABC of palliative care. Anorexia, cachexia, and nutrition. BMJ 315:1219–1222
3. Inui A (2002) Cancer anorexia-cachexia syndrome: current issues in research and management. CA Cancer J Clin 52:72–91
4. Crown AL, Cottle K, Lightman SL et al (2002) What is the role of the insulin-like growth factor system in the pathophysiology of cancer cachexia, and how is it regulated? Clin Endocrinol (Oxf) 56:723–733
5. Brink M, Anwar A, Delafontaine P (2002) Neurohormonal factors in the development of catabolic/anabolic imbalance and cachexia. Int J Cardiol 85:111–121; discussion 121–124
6. Heber D, Byerley LO, Tchekmedyian NS (1992) Hormonal and metabolic abnormalities in the malnourished cancer patient: effects on host-tumor interaction. JPEN J Parenter Enteral Nutr 16:60S–64S
7. Moldawer LL, Gelin J, Schersten T, Lundholm KG (1987) Circulating interleukin 1 and tumor necrosis factor during inflammation. Am J Physiol 253:R922–R928
8. Strassmann G, Fong M, Kenney JS, Jacob CO (1992) Evidence for the involvement of interleukin 6 in experimental cancer cachexia. J Clin Invest 89:1681–1684
9. Busbridge J, Dascombe MJ, Hoopkins S (1989) Acute central effects of interleukin-6 on body temperature, thermogenesis and food intake in the rat. Proc Nutr Soc 38:48A
10. Gelin J, Moldawer LL, Lonnroth C et al (1991) Role of endogenous tumor necrosis factor alpha and interleukin 1 for experimental tumor growth and the development of cancer cachexia. Cancer Res 51:415–421
11. McLaughlin CL, Rogan GJ, Tou J et al (1992) Food intake and body temperature responses of rats to recombinant human interleukin-1 beta and a tripeptide interleukin-1 beta antagonist. Physiol Behav 52:1155–1160
12. Mantovani G, Macciò A, Lai P et al (1998) Cytokine activity in cancer-related anorexia/cachexia: role of megestrol acetate and medroxyprogesterone acetate. Semin Oncol 25:45–52
13. Malmberg KJ, Lenkei R, Petersson M et al (2002) A short-term dietary supplementation of high doses of vitamin E increases T helper 1 cytokine production in patients with advanced colorectal cancer. Clin Cancer Res 8:1772–1778
14. Kono K, Salazar-Onfray F, Petersson M et al (1996) Hydrogen peroxide secreted by tumor-derived macrophages down-modulates signal-transducing zeta molecules and inhibits tumor-specific T cell- and natural killer cell-mediated cytotoxicity. Eur J Immunol 26:1308–1313
15. Aoe T, Okamoto Y, Saito T (1995) Activated macrophages induce structural abnormalities of the T cell receptor-CD3 complex. J Exp Med 181:1881–1886
16. Otjuji M, Kimura Y, Aoe T et al (1996) Oxidative stress by tumor-derived macrophages suppresses the expression of CD3 e chain of T-cell receptor complex and antigen-specific T-cell responses. Proc Natl Acad Sci USA 93:13119–13124
17. Bingisser RM, Tilbrook PA, Holt PG, Kees UR (1998) Macrophage-derived nitric oxide regulates T cell activation via reversible disruption of the Jak3/STAT5 signaling pathway. J Immunol 160:5729–5734
18. Weijl NI, Cleton FJ, Osanto S (1997) Free radicals and antioxidants in chemotherapy-induced toxicity. Cancer Treat Rev 23:209–240
19. Sabitha KE, Shyamaladevi CS (1999) Oxidant and antioxidant activity changes in patients with oral cancer and treated with radiotherapy. Oral Oncol

35:273–277

20. Buck M, Chojkier M (1996) Muscle wasting and dedifferentiation induced by oxidative stress in a murine model of cachexia is prevented by inhibitors of nitric oxide synthesis and antioxidants. EMBO J 15:1753–1765

21. Tisdale MJ (2001) Loss of skeletal muscle in cancer: biochemical mechanisms. Front Biosci 6:D164–D174

22. Shaw JH, Wolfe RR (1987) Glucose and urea kinetics in patients with early and advanced gastrointestinal cancer: the response to glucose infusion, parenteral feeding, and surgical resection. Surgery 101:181–191

23. Tayek JA (1992) A review of cancer cachexia and abnormal glucose metabolism in humans with cancer. J Am Coll Nutr 11:445–456

24. Wilmore DW, Aulick LH (1978) Metabolic changes in burned patients. Surg Clin North Am 58:1173–1187

25. Roth E, Mühlbacher F, Rauhs R et al (1982) Metabolic disorders in severe abdominal sepsis: glutamine deficiency in skeletal muscle. Clin Nutr 1:25–41

26. Mantovani G, Macciò A, Madeddu C et al (2002) Quantitative evaluation of oxidative stress, chronic inflammatory indices and leptin in cancer patients: correlation with stage and performance status. Int J Cancer 98:84–91

27. Mantovani G, Macciò A, Madeddu C et al (2003) The impact of different antioxidant agents alone or in combination on reactive oxygen species, antioxidant enzymes and cytokines in a series of advanced cancer patients at different sites: correlation with disease progression. Free Radic Res 37:213–223

28. Mantovani G, Macciò A, Mura L et al (2000) Serum levels of leptin and proinflammatory cytokines in patients with advanced-stage cancer at different sites. J Mol Med 78:554–561

29. Mantovani G, Macciò A, Madeddu C et al (2001) Serum values of proinflammatory cytokines are inversely correlated with serum leptin levels in patients with advanced stage cancer at different sites. J Mol Med 79:406–414

30. Mantovani G, Macciò A, Melis G et al (2000) Restoration of functional defects in peripheral blood mononuclear cells isolated from cancer patients by thiol antioxidants alpha-lipoic acid and N-acetyl cysteine. Int J Cancer 86:842–847

31. Mantovani G, Madeddu C, Macciò A et al (2004) Cancer-related anorexia/cachexia syndrome and oxidative stress: an innovative approach beyond current treatment. Cancer Epidemiol Biomarkers Prev 13:1651–1659

32. Mantovani G, Maccio A, Madeddu C et al (2006) A Phase II study with antioxidants, both in the diet and supplemented, pharmaco-nutritional support, progestagen and anti-COX-2 showing efficacy and safety in patients with cancer-related anorexia/cachexia (CACS) and oxidative stress (OS). Cancer Epidemiol Biomarkers Prev 15:1030-1034

33. Higdon JV, Frei B (2003) Tea catechins and polyphe-nols: health effects, metabolism, and antioxidant functions. Crit Rev Food Sci Nutr 43:89–143

34. Mantovani G, Macciò A, Esu S et al (1997) Medroxyprogesterone acetate reduces the in vitro production of cytokines and serotonin involved in anorexia/cachexia and emesis by peripheral blood mononuclear cells of cancer patients. Eur J Cancer 33:602–607

35. Cerchietti LC, Navigante AH, Peluffo GD et al (2004) Effects of celecoxib, medroxyprogesterone, and dietary intervention on systemic syndromes in patients with advanced lung adenocarcinoma: a pilot study. J Pain Symptom Manage 27:85–95

36. Therasse P, Arbuck SG, Eisenhauer EA et al (2000) New guidelines to evaluate the response to treatment in solid tumors. European Organization for Research and Treatment of Cancer, National Cancer Institute of the United States, National Cancer Institute of Canada. J Natl Cancer Inst 92:205–216

37. Oken MM, Creech RH, Tormey DC et al (1982) Toxicity and response criteria of the Eastern Cooperative Oncology Group. Am J Clin Oncol 5:649–655

38. Stein KD, Martin SC, Hann DM, Jacobsen PB (1998) A multidimensional measure of fatigue for use with cancer patients. Cancer Pract 6:143–152

39. Alberti A, Bolognini L, Macciantelli D, Caratelli M (2000) The radical cation of N,N-diethyl-para-phenylendiamine: a possible indicator of oxidative stress in biological samples. Res Chem Intermed 26:253–267

40. Mantovani G, Macciò A, Massa E, Madeddu C (2001) Managing cancer-related anorexia/cachexia. Drugs 61:499–514

41. Laviano A, Meguid MM (1996) Nutritional issues in cancer management. Nutrition 12:358–371

42. Klein S, Kinney J, Jeejeebhoy K et al (1997) Nutrition support in clinical practice: review of published data and recommendations for future research directions. Summary of a conference sponsored by the National Institutes of Health, American Society for Parenteral and Enteral Nutrition, and American Society for Clinical Nutrition. Am J Clin Nutr 66:683–706

43. Sikora SS, Ribeiro U, Kane JM 3rd et al (1998) Role of nutrition support during induction chemoradiation therapy in esophageal cancer. JPEN J Parenter Enteral Nutr 22:18–21

44. Lipman TO (1991) Clinical trials of nutritional support in cancer. Parenteral and enteral therapy. Hematol Oncol Clin North Am 5:91–102

45. Wigmore S, Fearon, KC, Maingay JP, Ross JA (1999) Down-regulation of the acute-phase response in patients with pancreatic cancer cachexia receiving oral eicosapentaenoic acid is mediated via suppression of interleukin-6. Clin Sci (Lond) 92:215–221

46. Tisdale MJ (2004) Cancer cachexia. Langenbecks Arch Surg 389:299–305

47. Lazarus D, Destree AT, Mazzola LM et al (1999) A

new model of cancer cachexia: contribution of the ubiquitin-proteasome pathway. Am J Physiol 277(2 Pt 1):E332–E341

48. Whitehouse AS, Tisdale MJ (2003) Increased expression of the ubiquitin-proteasome pathway in murine myotubes by proteolysis-inducing factor (PIF) is associated with activation of the transcription factor NF-kappaB. Br J Cancer 89:1116–1122

49. Barber MD, Preston T, McMillan DC et al (2004) Modulation of the liver export protein synthetic response to feeding by an n-3 fatty-acid-enriched nutritional supplement is associated with anabolism in cachectic cancer patients. Clin Sci (Lond) 106:359–364

50. Togni V, Ota CC, Folador A et al (2003) Cancer cachexia and tumor growth reduction in Walker 256 tumor-bearing rats supplemented with N-3 polyunsaturated fatty acids for one generation. Nutr Cancer 46:52–58

51. Jho DH, Babcock TA, Tevar R et al (2002) Eicosapentaenoic acid supplementation reduces tumor volume and attenuates cachexia in a rat model of progressive non-metastasizing malignancy. JPEN J Parenter Enteral Nutr 26:291–297

52. Hardman WE, Moyer MP, Cameron IL (2002) Consumption of an omega-3 fatty acids product, INCELL AAFA, reduced side-effects of CPT-11 (irinotecan) in mice. Br J Cancer 86:983–988

53. Hardman WE (2002) Omega-3 fatty acids to augment cancer therapy. J Nutr 132:3508S–3512S

54. Barber MD, Fearon KC (2001) Tolerance and incorporation of a high-dose eicosapentaenoic acid diester emulsion by patients with pancreatic cancer cachexia. Lipids 36:347–351

55. Wigmore SJ, Barber MD, Ross JA et al (2000) Effect of oral eicosapentaenoic acid on weight loss in patients with pancreatic cancer. Nutr Cancer 36:177–184

56. Fearon KC, Von Meyenfeldt MF, Moses AG et al (2003) Effect of a protein and energy dense N-3 fatty acid enriched oral supplement on loss of weight and lean tissue in cancer cachexia: a randomised double blind trial. Gut 52:1479–1486

57. Moses AW, Slater C, Preston T et al (2004) Reduced total energy expenditure and physical activity in cachectic patients with pancreatic cancer can be modulated by an energy and protein dense oral supplement enriched with n-3 fatty acids. Br J Cancer 90:996–1002

58. Ferrando AA, Stuart CA, Sheffield-Moore M, Wolfe RR (1999) Inactivity amplifies the catabolic response of skeletal muscle to cortisol. J Clin Endocrinol Metab 84:3515–3521

59. Jatoi ARK, Rowland K, Loprinzi CL et al (2003) An eicosapentaenoic acid (EPA)-enriched supplement versus megestrol acetate (MA) versus both for patients with cancer-associated wasting. A collaborative effort from the North Central Cancer Treatment Group (NCCTG) and the National Cancer Institute of Canada. Proc Am Soc Clin Oncol 22:743 (abs 2987)

60. Downer S, Joel S, Allbright A et al (1993) A double blind placebo controlled trial of medroxyprogesterone acetate (MPA) in cancer cachexia. Br J Cancer 67:1102–1105

61. Simons JP, Aaronson NK, Vansteenkiste JF et al (1996) Effects of medroxyprogesterone acetate on appetite, weight, and quality of life in advanced-stage non-hormone-sensitive cancer: a placebo-controlled multicenter study. J Clin Oncol 14:1077–1084

# SECTION 11
# TREATMENT OF CACHEXIA IN THE ELDERLY

# Treatment of Cachexia in the Elderly

Shing-Shing Yeh, Michael W. Schuster

## Treatment of Weight Loss and Cachexia in the Elderly

Numerous studies have shown that weight loss is associated with an increase in mortality [1–4]. Treating weight loss in the elderly can ameliorate many medical conditions. For example, rehabilitation time following post-hip fractures has been shown to decrease with nutritional supplementation [5]. In hospitalised geriatric patients, nutritional supplementation resulted in improvement in serum protein, nutritional status, and decreased mortality [6]. In a subset of geriatric inpatients, low serum albumin with weight loss predicts those patients at highest risk for dying during the subsequent 2 years [7]. Riquelme and Torres et al. [8] carried out a multivariate analysis of risk and prognostic factors in community-acquired pneumonia in the elderly and found that age by itself was not a significant factor related to prognosis. Among the significant risk factors, only nutritional status is amenable to medical intervention. In the cachectic elderly, medical, cognitive, and psychiatric disorders may diminish self-sufficiency in activities of daily living (ADL), thus reducing the quality of life and increasing the frequency of secondary procedures, hospitalisations, and need for skilled care [2, 9]. The understanding of the pathophysiology of geriatric cachexia has increased and has resulted in effective and safe nutritional measures.

## Physiological Causes of Weight Loss in the Elderly

The regulation of food intake changes with age and involve mechanisms that are complex and multifactorial, making the treatment of weight loss more challenging. Weight loss and poor food intake in the elderly may be due to the following [10, 11] (Tables 1, 2):

1. Changes associated with normal aging (reduced basal hunger, decreased gastric emptying time, failure to adjust food intake after periods of overfeeding or underfeeding)
2. Endocrine disturbances (hyperthyroidism, hyperparathyroidism, hypoadrenalism)
3. Medications (theophylline, lithium, digoxin, chemotherapy agents for cancer treatment, antibiotics, and many other medications that distort normal smell and taste perception)
4. Dementia and related behavioural disturbances
5. Psychiatric problems (depression, anorexia nervosa, alcoholism, late-life paranoia)
6. Gastric, intestinal, and related problems (swallowing disorders, missing dentures, pain, malabsorption, diarrhoea, constipation)
7. Systemic-disease-related dysphagia (strokes, Parkinson's disease, achalasia, scleroderma)
8. Dysgeusia (age-related decline in taste and smell)
9. Chronic diseases (chronic obstructive pulmonary disease, congestive heart failure, rheumatoid arthritis, HIV, cancers)
10. Dysfunction (inability to feed oneself, limited income, poor eyesight, poor diet)
11. Infections (acute and chronic diseases, HIV, gastritis, cholecystitis).

The Council for Nutritional Strategies in Long-Term Care has developed an algorithm for the assessment of undernutrition in long-term care settings. This algorithm was published in a supplement to the Annals of Long-Term Care, 2004, and addresses the diagnosis of weight loss. The first step in the management of weight loss in the elderly is to attempt to identify and treat any specific underlying treatable or contributing conditions (e.g. endocrine diseases, medication, polypharma-

**Table 1.** Causes of involuntary weight loss in the elderly; the 9 'D's'. (Adapted from [11])

| |
| --- |
| Dysgeusia |
| Dentition |
| Dysphagia |
| Depression |
| Drugs |
| Dementia |
| Diseases |
| Diarrhoea (malabsorption) |
| Dysfunction |

**Table 2.** Treatable causes of malnutrition ('meals on wheels'). (Adapted from [10])

| | |
| --- | --- |
| M | Medication effect |
| E | Emotional problems (depression) |
| A | Anorexia tardive (nervosa, alcoholism) |
| L | Late-life paranoia |
| S | Swallowing disorders |
| O | Oral factors (e.g., poorly fitting dentures, caries) |
| N | No money |
| W | Wandering and other dementia related behaviours |
| H | Hyperthyroidism, hypothyroidism, hyperparathyroidism, hypoadrenalism |
| E | Enteric problems (malabsorption) |
| E | Eating problems (inability to feed oneself) |
| L | Low-salt, low-cholesterol diets |
| S | Stones, social problems (e.g., isolation, inability to obtain preferred foods) |

cy, depression, dentition, constipation, dehydration diarrhoea, systemic diseases, infections, and social support for providing food and feeding). However, Kayser-Jones et al. found that a lack of attention to individual food preferences, inadequate staffing, and a lack of feeding assistance were major factors accounting for weight loss in the elderly [12].

These are some of the important issues that need to be addressed first.

## Nutritional Supplementation

Rolls and Dimeo found that even healthy elderly men consumed significant less baseline energy compared to young men [13–16]. Roberts et al. found that healthy elderly men had both a short-term (7 weeks) and a long-term (6 months) impairment in adjusting their food intake after an episode of either overfeeding or underfeeding. Encouraging the elderly to take in extra food (with verbal prompts, physical assistance, or appetite stimulants) at mealtime over a period of 4–6 weeks, then allowing them to eat at their own volition could promote weight gain. Since the elderly are not able to adjust their food intake after a period of overfeeding for at least 6 months, they will continue exceeding their eating needs and thus, increase weight [14–16]. The elderly men in the study did not decrease food intake even after they were given supplements before meals. As a result, they obtained 10–30% extra energy from the 'preload' (supplements) and still were able to take in their usual amount of food at mealtime. Providing an energy-dense nutritional supplement 30–90 min before a meal can thus increase energy intake in elderly people.

McCrory et al. found that a wide variety of sweets, snacks, condiments, and high-carbohydrate entrees coupled with a smaller variety of vegetables promoted long-term increase in energy intake and body fat [17]. Providing nutritional supplements consisting of a wide variety of sweets and carbohydrates may be helpful as the second step for the treatment of weight loss. In addition, loss of taste and smell are common in the elderly, and medications and medical conditions play a major role in taste losses and distortions [18]. Thus, the use of flavour-enhanced food has a correspondingly positive effect on food intake.

Resistance at meal times in demented patients is widely reported [19], and behavioural disturbances play a role in low body weight and weight loss in demented patients [19]. Providing feeding assistance and using feeding assistants may promote intake in the demented population [20].

## Tube Feeding

Tube feeding has been indicated in persons with neuromuscular diseases (with impaired swallowing or gag reflex), postoperative patients, individuals who are unable to eat, and patients using ventilators. Feeding-tube-associated side effects include aspiration, diarrhoea, and vomiting [21]. Numerous studies have been aimed at determining the benefits of tube feeding [22]. Mitchell et al. found no evidence that tube feeding prolonged survival, especially if dysphagia is the main indication [23]. Only a small subset of nursing-home residents benefit from tube feeding [23].

## Parenteral Nutrition

Parenteral nutrition can be given to the elderly immediately after acute disease if they are incapable of taking in adequate calories or fluid for a short period of time [24]. This must be only a temporary measure and cannot be sustained for more than a few weeks. Peripheral parenteral nutrition only provides a limited amount of calories and the infusion site has to be changed frequently; thus, its benefit is restricted [25, 26].

## Pharmacological Interventions

The effects of nutritional support on the prevention and treatment of cancer and AIDS cachexia have been extensively investigated [27–33]. However, nonselective nutritional support with total parenteral nutrition (TPN) or percutaneous endoscopic gastrostomy (PEG)-tube insertion, with their associated complications, has failed to provide benefit [34].

Understanding the role of cytokines in mediating cachexia in cancer and AIDS may also provide new insights into nutritional therapy and pharmacotherapy for the treatment of geriatric cachexia [35–38].

Pharmacological treatment agents for cachexia can be divided into five categories: (1) appetite stimulants, (2) direct cytokine inhibitors, (3) anabolic amino acids, (4) indirect cytokine inhibitors, and (5) miscellaneous agents as metabolic stimulants or supplements (Table 3).

## Treatment with Appetite Stimulants

### Megestrol Acetate

Megestrol acetate (MA) is a synthetic derivative of a naturally occurring progestational agent and is similar to progesterone. MA treatment of patients with cancer increases appetite and non-fluid weight gain in a dose-dependent manner, and is well-tolerated in patients with advanced malignant diseases [39–44].

Von Roenn et al. found that treating patients with MA for AIDS-related anorexia/ cachexia not only increased weight, but also improved body image, sense of well-being, and pleasure from eating [45–47]. The Food and Drug Administration (FDA) has approved the use of MA for the treatment of anorexia, cachexia, and/or an unexplained significant weight loss in patients with a diagnosis of AIDS. A few studies have shown that treating cachexia in the elderly with MA improved quality of life and weight gain [48–51]. Lambert et al. found that MA appears to have an anti-anabolic effect on muscle size, even when combined with testosterone replacement. Resistance exercise attenuated this reduction in muscle mass [52].

Although the mechanism(s) by which MA promotes weight gain is unknown, Hamburger et al. suggested that it either blocks tumour necrosis factor (TNF) or reverses the effects of TNF by inducing adipocyte differentiation [53]. Reitmeier and Hartenstein found that MA increases body weight by increasing fat and body cell mass rather than by fluid retention [54]. Beck and Tisdale [55] reported that the weight gain associated with MA can be blocked by co-treatment with TNF-α in NMRI mice.

It is not surprising that progesterone plays an important role in nutritional status. Lapp and Thomas found, for example, that higher progesterone concentrations are common in late pregnancy and result in decreased interleukin (IL)-6 levels to 40–50% of controls [56].

Mantovani et al. [57–60] reported that the appetite, weight, and sense of well-being of cancer

**Table 3.** Possible pharmacological treatment agents for geriatric cachexia

| Appetite stimulant | Direct cytokine inhibitors | Indirect cytokine-inhibitors (metabolic stimulants) |
| --- | --- | --- |
| Dronabinol | Pentoxifylline | Testosterone |
| Megestrol acetate | Thalidomide<br>N-3 fatty acids<br>Fish oil<br>Monoclonal antibodies against specific cytokines<br>*N*-acetylcysteine<br>Specific cytokine-receptor antagonists | Anabolic steroids<br>Growth hormone<br>Insulin-like growth factor-1 |

| Anabolic amino acids | Miscellaneous |
| --- | --- |
| Ornithine oxoglutarate | Cyproheptadine |
| Branched-chain amino acids | Hydralazine sulfate |
| Glutamine and arginine | Creatine<br>Melatonin<br>β-Blockers<br>NSAID/COX inhibitors<br>ACE inhibitors<br>Ghrelin<br>Anandamide<br>Ponalrestat |
| | ATP |
| | Cyclic plasma perfusion |
| | Other cytokine-related substances |

*ACE*, angiotensin-converting enzyme; *ATP*, adenosine 5'-triphosphate; *COX*, cyclooxigenase; *NSAID*, non-steroidal anti-inflammatory drug

patients improved with MA. In addition, cytokine levels in these patients decreased with MA treatment, but not with chemotherapy alone. They [57–60] also found that medroxyprogesterone acetate reduces the in vitro production of pro-inflammatory cytokines (IL-1, IL-6, TNF-α, and serotonin) from peripheral mononuclear cells of cancer patients. Yeh et al. observed a correlation between cytokine levels, nutritional status, and appetite in patients treated with MA [38, 61]. By contrast, in a 6-week trial of MA, Loprinzi et al. did not find evidence that MA down-regulates IL-6 in patients with cancer-associated anorexia and weight loss [62]. McCarthy et al. [63] showed that MA stimulates food and water intake, and this effect may involve neuropeptide Y (a potent feeding-stimulating substance). In another animal study, Costa et al. [64] demonstrated that MA stimulation of appetite may involve calcium channels in the ventromedial hypothalamus.

Although prolonged use of MA appears to be safe, therapy with this drug can result in clinical manifestations of glucocorticoid-like activity [65]. Studies of the effects of long-term administration of MA have shown that it may cause venous thromboembolism, hyperglycaemia, secondary adrenal suppression, and adrenal insufficiency [66–75]. Short-term administration (12 weeks) of MA in a preliminary pilot study of geriatric nursing-home residents with cachexia (69 patients) revealed the drug to be safe and without apparent evidence of adrenal suppression [48, 51].

## Dronabinol

The use of dronabinol (a cannabinoid derivative) has been reported anecdotally to lead to weight gain and appetite stimulation [76, 77]. Volicer et al. [78] found that dronabinol treatment increased the body weight of Alzheimer's patients. Morley et al. [50] suggested that dronabinol has a particularly good profile for persons with anorexia who are at the end of life. The drug should initially be given at a low dose (2.5 mg) in the evening. The dose should be increased to 5 mg per day if no improvement in appetite is seen after 2–4 weeks. Jatoi et al. found that MA provided superior anorexia palliation among advanced cancer patients compared with dronabinol alone and combination therapy did not appear to confer additional benefit [79]. Dronabinol has been used by HIV patients and approved by the FDA as an appetite stimulant and anti-emetic in these patients [76, 80, 81]. The main side effects are euphoria, somnolence, sedation, fatigue, and hallucinations [78]. Effects such as sedation, dizziness, and hallucinations make the drug less ideally suited for the geriatric population.

## Indirect Cytokine Inhibitors (Metabolic Stimulants)

### Anabolic Agents and Testosterone

The use of anabolic drugs, such as methyltestosterone, oxandrolone, and stanozolol, has been explored in clinical trials with cachectic AIDS patients. Studies showed that nandrolone decanoate decreases the weight loss associated with cancer and HIV [82–84]. The main side effects were masculinisation, fluid retention, and hepatic toxicity [83, 85–87]. The efficacy of nandrolone decanoate unknown in geriatric patients. However, Batterham and Garsia studied the effects of nandrolone decanoate and MA in HIV patients with weight loss and concluded that both drugs resulted in an increase in fat-free mass greater than that obtained with dietary counselling alone [82]. Oxandrolone has been studied for treating weight loss in patients with HIV infection, cachectic chronic obstructive pulmonary disease (COPD) patients, and cancer patients with weight loss [35, 88–96]. Earthman et al. found that oxandrolone therapy in HIV infection improves weight, quality of life, and lean body mass, with minimal adverse effects [97].

Testosterone has been used as a treatment for cachexia and weight loss in HIV patients with positive results concerning weight and gain of lean muscle mass, but with unknown clinically meaningful changes in muscle function and disease outcome in HIV-infected men [98–102]. Morley et al. safely administered testosterone to older men with hypogonadism and noted an increase in the upper-arm strength of this population [52, 103]. Dolan et al. found that testosterone administration increased muscle strength in low-weight HIV-infected women and suggested that it may be a useful adjunctive therapy to maintain muscle function in this group of patients [104, 105].

In elderly men, an additional problem associated with the use of testosterone-like drugs might be an exacerbation of prostate cancer, which would therefore limit its use.

### Growth Hormone and Insulin-Like Growth Factor-1

Growth hormone (GH) and insulin-like growth factor (IGF)-1 stimulate amino-acid uptake and protein synthesis in muscle and improve myocyte proliferation and differentiation in animal studies [106, 107]. The FDA recently granted accelerated approval for a form of recombinant human GH (rhGH) to treat AIDS wasting. Preliminary reports from Schambelan and co-workers in AIDS patients have all been positive [108–112]. The combined GH and IGF-1 doses used in studies in adult males with HIV-associated weight loss had mixed results in producing a sustained anabolic response [113–120]. In fact, after trauma, the anti-catabolic action of rhGH is associated with a potentially harmful decrease in muscle glutamine production and increased mortality [116]. Use of the rhGH for elderly patients with a low somatomedin C or IGF improved lean muscle mass, but not functional ability. Moreover, frequent side effects were seen [121]. Morley and co-workers [122] demonstrated that rhGH, which is a very expensive therapy, led to nitrogen retention and weight gain in malnourished older patients. The effects of GH may be mediated through IGF-1. However, the combination of GH and IGF-1 did not result in consistent appetite stimulation [123]. Peripheral oedema, hyperglycaemia, carpal tunnel syndrome, and gynecomastia were the major adverse effects.

## Anabolic Amino Acids

### Ornithine Oxoglutarine

Brocker et al. randomised 194 elderly patients at two centres to ornithine oxoglutarine (OrnOx) or placebo and noted improved appetite and weight gain in the group of convalescing, ambulatory patients who received the drug [124]. OrnOx works by increasing amino acid and insulin levels; therefore, a major side effect may be hypoglycaemia.

### Glutamine and Arginine

Glutamine is one of the most abundant amino acids in the body. It is important for maintaining a healthy immune status, protein metabolism, and gastrointestinal mucosal integrity [125–128]. Arginine has been shown to stimulate the immune system, enhance wound healing, and decrease the rate of tumour growth. Several prospective, randomised, double-blind studies in cancer and HIV patients found positive weight gain after supplementing patients' diets with glutamine and arginine [129–134]. Since glutamine is an essential nutrient for cell growth, its exogenous supplementation might be used by rapidly growing tumour cells in patients with cancer. This, in turn, may lead to increased levels of pro-inflammatory cytokines that, in turn, may exacerbate cachexia [135]. The efficacy of glutamine in treating geriatric cachexia is unknown.

### Branched-Chain Amino Acids

Other attempts at improving anorexia with nutritional substrates such as branched-chain amino acids (BCAA), which have been used in TPN, are still under investigation. BCAA can compete with tryptophan (the precursor of serotonin in the central nervous system, thus reducing serotonin production and increasing food intake [136]. Tayek et al. found that BCAA-enriched formulas improved albumin synthesis and may favourably influence protein metabolism in cancer cachexia [137]. Once again, the efficacy of BCAA in the geriatric setting is unknown.

## Direct Cytokine Inhibitors

Patients with advanced HIV infection or those with opportunistic infections have elevated TNF-$\alpha$ levels, and there is a correlation with the development of wasting [138, 139]. Pharmacological manipulation of TNF-$\alpha$ regulation has been proposed as a means of stabilising or reversing the wasting process.

### Pentoxifylline

Pentoxifylline decreases TNF-$\alpha$ production by suppressing TNF-$\alpha$ mRNA transcription [140]. Studies using pentoxifylline to treat cancer- and HIV-associated cachexia demonstrated that it did not improve appetite, weight, or sense of well-being [141–143]. It may have even have an adverse effect on the course of opportunistic infections. Sathe and Sarai [144, 145] found that pentoxifylline treatment led to impairment in TNF-$\alpha$ secretion and, thereby, increased the mycobacterial load in macrophages of AIDS patients with disseminated Mycobacterium avium-intracellulare complex infection. Gastrointestinal disturbances were among the major adverse effects. The failure of pentoxifylline in the HIV-induced cachexia trial does not rule it out as a possible agent for cachexia treatment in the elderly, but its potential effectiveness is less likely.

### Thalidomide

Thalidomide also decreases TNF-$\alpha$ production by increasing degradation of TNF-$\alpha$ mRNA [146]. It reduces serum C-reactive protein and IL-6 [147]. Reyes-Teran et al. [148] carried out a double-blind, placebo-controlled study with 23 HIV-infected wasting patients and found a significant weight gain and improved Karnofsky scores in the thalidomide-treated group. There was no significant change in viral load and absolute CD4+ cells count. However, 29% of the treatment group developed a rash. Other well-known side effects are peripheral neuropathy, somnolence, and constipation. Vivid memories of thalidomide-induced teratogenicity several decades ago make it very difficult to revive this medication for general use. The exact role of thalidomide in the treatment of cancer and cancer cachexia in the elderly remains to be elucidated [149, 150].

## N-3 Fatty Acids and Fish Oil

N-3 fatty acids, mainly from fish oils, interfere with the cyclooxygenase ($PGE_2$ production) and lipooxygenase metabolic pathways. They also inhibit cytokine synthesis and activity [151, 152]. Dinarello [153] and Endres [154] found that N-3 fatty acids improved food intake in rats with IL-1-induced anorexia. Tisdale and Dhesi also reported that using omega-3 fatty acids stopped the weight loss in an experimental cachexia model [155]. While the role of N-3 fatty acids in the treatment of cancer cachexia remains unclear [156], their potential role in the treatment of cancer cachexia is promising [157, 158].

## N-Acetylcysteine

This compound is effective in replenishing depleted glutathione levels and regulates levels of pro-inflammatory cytokines, such as TNF, IL-1, and IL-6 [159]. N-Acetylcysteine may therefore be of clinical benefit in the treatment of cachexia [159].

## Miscellaneous Agents

### Cyproheptadine

Cyproheptadine is both an antihistamine and an antiserotonergic reagent. It is effective in treating selected groups of children with anorexia and, reportedly, affects central appetite centres. Yet, the results of clinical trials in cancer patients have been disappointing [160]. The side effects of sedation and dizziness make this drug less likely to be used in the geriatric population. Moreover, its efficacy is unproven despite its widespread usage in this group of patients.

### Hydrazine Sulfate

Hydrazine sulfate is an inhibitor of gluconeogenesis. Clinical trials in cancer patients, however, failed to show benefit in cancer cachexia [161, 162]. The efficacy of hydrazine sulfate in the geriatric population has not been studied.

## Melatonin

Melatonin down-regulates TNF levels. In a randomised trial of 100 patients with metastatic cancer [163], Lissoni et al. showed that melatonin, given at a dose of 20 mg orally every evening, resulted in a statistically significant decrease in TNF levels in patients treated with study drug compared to the placebo group. Of even more interest was the fact that the melatonin-treated patients had significantly less weight loss. Its use in geriatric cachexia remains unknown.

## Creatine

Creatine is a physiologically active substance required for muscle contraction. The proper amount of creatine phosphate in the muscle allows high rates of adenosine resynthesis; therefore, it plays a vital role in the performance of high-intensity exercise. Creatine supplementation has not consistently been shown to enhance performance in exercise tasks, but it may increase performance in situations in which the availability of creatine phosphate is important [164, 165–168]. Short-term creatine supplementation appears to increase body mass in young males, although the initial increase is most likely water weight. Long-term creatine supplementation, in conjunction with physical training involving resistance exercise, may increase lean body mass [169–171]. Its use in geriatric cachexia is not yet known.

## β-Blockers

Wasting in cancer patients is multifactorial, but is caused, at least in part, by increased β(1)- and β(2)-adrenoceptor activity, as well as elevated basal metabolic rate and altered host metabolism [172–174]. Weight gain in response to β-blocker therapy in the hypertensive population may be attributable to decreased resting energy expenditure, inhibition of lipolysis, and decreased insulin sensitivity [175, 176]. β-Blocker therapy has also been shown to reverse excess protein catabolism after severe burns and may increase skeletal muscle mass [176–178]. Hryniewicz et al. were able to partially reverse cachexia by β-adrenergic-receptor blocker therapy in patients with chronic heart failure [179]. β-Blocker treatment potentially prevents further weight loss in cachectic geriatric patients [180]; however, there may be an exacerbation of sick sinus syndrome in some of these patients.

### NSAIDs/COX Inhibitors

Cachexia has also effectively been attenuated by cyclooxygenase-2 (COX-2) inhibitor treatment in established animal cancer models [181–184], and this class of drugs may play an important role in cachexia treatment [185, 186]. A study of cachectic cancer patients in Sweden who were given indomethacin found a significant prolongation in their survival compared to placebo-treated patients [187].

### Angiotensin-Converting-Enzyme (ACE) Inhibitors

Body wasting is a clinical feature of a variety of chronic illnesses like congestive heart failure. Treatment of cardiac cachexia with ACE inhibitors has been found to be somewhat successful [188, 189]. The potential role of these inhibitors in the treatment of cachexia is promising but is still under investigation in cancer and HIV-infected patients.

### Ghrelin

Ghrelin, an endogenous ligand for the GH secretagogue receptor, was recently identified in the rat stomach. Ghrelin exhibits gastroprokinetic activity with structural resemblance to motilin in addition to potent orexigenic activity through its action on hypothalamic neuropeptide Y (NPY) and Y(1) receptor; this effect was lost after vagotomy [190]. Peripherally administered ghrelin blocked IL-1β-induced anorexia and produced positive energy balance by promoting food intake and decreasing energy expenditure [190]. Ghrelin, which is negatively regulated by leptin and IL-1β, is secreted by the stomach and increases arcuate NPY expression, which in turn acts through Y(1) receptors to increase food intake and decrease energy expenditure. Gastric peptide ghrelin may, thus, functions as part of the orexigenic pathway downstream from leptin and is a potential therapeutic target not only for obesity, but also for anorexia and cachexia [190].

### Anandamide

Hao et al. reported a possible role of the endocannabinoid anandamide on modulating the behavioural and neurochemical consequences of semi-starvation in an animal study. They found that low-dose anandamide (0.001 mg/kg) could improve food intake and cognitive function. Anandamide-treated mice consumed 44% more food each day. The hypothalami of these animals contained significantly increased concentrations of norepinephrine, dopamine, and 5-hydroxytryptamine (5-HT). In the hippocampus, anandamide significantly increased norepinephrine and dopamine, but decreased 5-HT. The fact that low-dose anandamide improved food intake, cognitive function, and reversed some of the neurotransmitter changes caused by diet restriction suggests its possible use in the treatment of cachexia [191]. Phase II studies in humans have yet to be done.

### Ponalrestat

Lipoprotein lipase (LPL) is a key regulatory enzyme responsible for the hydrolysis of triglyceride (TG)-rich lipoproteins. The reduction in LPL activity is observed in tumour-bearing animals and cancer patients with cachexia, suggesting an involvement of LPL in inducing cancer cachexia [192]. Kawamura et al. demonstrated that tumour-induced cachexia in mice is inhibited by ponalrestat [193–195]. This suggests that ponalrestat, a LPL-activating agent, has a therapeutic potential for the treatment of cachexia, although no human trials have been conducted.

## Adenosine 5′-triphosphate (ATP)

Cancer cachexia is associated with elevated lipolysis, proteolysis, and gluconeogenesis. ATP infusion has been found to significantly inhibit loss of body weight, fat mass, and fat-free mass in patients with advanced lung cancer [196]. Agteresch et al. found that regular infusions of ATP inhibited loss of body weight and improved quality of life in patients with non-small-cell lung cancer (NSCLC) [196]. ATP treatment was associated with a significant increase in survival in the subgroup of weight-losing patients with stage IIIB NSCLC [197].

## Cyclic Plasma Perfusion

Anaemia-inducing substance (AIS) is a protein of approximately 50000 molecular weight that is secreted by malignant tumour tissue and depresses erythrocyte and immunocompetent cell functions. Ishiko and et al. reported enhanced AIS activity and lipolytic activity as the tumours grew and suggested that AIS is one of the substances involved in the enhanced lipolytic activity seen in advanced-tumour-bearing rabbits [198]. AIS can be removed by cyclic plasma perfusion adsorption in animal studies [198, 199]. This mode of treatment resulted in reduced muscle wasting and increased lean body mass, and induced angiogenesis in the adipose tissue in tumour-bearing rabbits [200, 201]. No human trials have been reported.

## Other Cytokine-Related Substances

Interleukin-1 receptor agonist A, IL-15, and Decoy nuclear factor κB [202, 203] have been employed to reverse cancer cachexia in animal models with some success. IL-15, which is known to favour muscle-fibre hypertrophy, antagonised enhanced muscle-protein breakdown in a cancer cachexia model [203]. The alterations in protein-breakdown rates induced by IL-15 were associated with an inhibition of the ATP-ubiquitin-dependent proteolytic pathway and resulted in a preventive effect on muscle-protein wasting [203, 204]. The nuclear factor-κB (NF-κB) family of transcription factors is involved in multiple cellular processes, including cytokine gene expression, cellular adhesion, cell-cycle activation, apoptosis and oncogenesis. Suppression of NF-κB results in attenuation of cancer cachexia in a mouse tumour model [205–207]. All studies involving cytokine-related substances showed improved food intake, but no single agent alone was able to reverse all the changes seen in the tumour-bearing state. Combinations of drugs, such as a PGE$_2$ inhibitor with an anti-cytokine antibody, or IL-15 gene transfer and anti-IL-6 antibody, or substances that act upon more than one pro-inflammatory cytokine, may be needed to augment the anti-cachectic effect.

## Conclusions

Weight loss is associated with increased mortality and is a major problem in the geriatric population. Feelings of well-being and the pleasure derived from eating positively affect the quality of life of older individuals. The connection between eating and good health has been understood for hundreds of years and transcends all cultures. Furthermore, it is understood that when the elderly stop eating, their death is imminent. The first step in management of elderly weight loss is to attempt to identify and treat any specific underlying treatable or contributing conditions. Providing an energy-dense nutritional supplement 30–90 min before a meal can increase energy intake in elderly people. Use of flavour-enhanced food also has a positive effect on food intake. Providing feeding assistance and using feeding assistants may promote food intake in demented patients.

A better understanding of the role of pro-inflammatory cytokines in mediating cancer- and HIV-induced cachexia may provide an explanation for geriatric cachexia and the increased levels of negative regulatory cytokines, as well as possible pharmacological treatment for this condition. Overlapping physiological activities make it unlikely that a single substance is the sole cause of cachexia. Several different cytokines produce the same response. The potential involvement of IL-6, TNF-α, IL-1, serotonin, PGE$_2$, and other cytokines (IL-10, IL-4, IL-15) in the pathophysiology of ageing, chronic diseases, and wasting calls for research on ways to suppress the secretion, dysregulation, or downstream effects of these compounds.

Anti-cytokine antibodies have been used to reverse cancer cachexia in animal models with some success. Studies showed improvement in food intake, but no single antibody alone was able to reverse all the changes seen in the tumour-bearing state. Combination studies, such as those that combined a PGE$_2$ inhibitor with an anti-cytokine antibody or IL-10 gene transfer and an anti-IL-6 antibody, have demonstrated augmentation of the anti-cachexia effect. Further investigation with specific nutritional manipulations, and the administration of specific steroids, neuropeptides, and peptide hormones are promising. Further research will be needed to fully evaluate the safety and efficacy of these interventions and to determine what their effect is in the treatment of geriatric cachexia.

**Acknowledgements**
The authors thank Sherri Lovitts for her help in preparing the manuscript.

# References

1. Sullivan DH, Walls RC (1994) Impact of nutritional status on morbidity in a population of geriatric rehabilitation patients. J Am Geriatr Soc 42:471–477
2. Sullivan DH (1995) Impact of nutritional status on health outcomes of nursing home residents. J Am Geriatr Soc 43:195–196
3. Sullivan DH, Walls RC, Bopp MM (1995) Protein-energy undernutrition and the risk of mortality within one year of hospital discharge: a follow-up study. J Am Geriatr Soc 43:507–512
4. Sullivan DH (1995) The role of nutrition in increased morbidity and mortality. Clin Geriatr Med 11:661–674
5. Bastow MD, Rawlings J, Allison SP (1983) Benefits of supplementary tube feeding after fractured neck of femur: a randomized controlled trial. Br Med J 287:1589–1592
6. Woo J, Ho SC, Mak YT et al (1994) Nutritional status of elderly patients during recovery from chest infection and the role of nutritional supplementation assessed by a prospective randomized single-blind trial. Age Ageing 23:40–48
7. McMurtry C, Rosenthal A (1995) Predictors of 2-year mortality among older male veterans on a geriatric rehabilitation unit. J Am Geriatr Soc 43:1123–1126
8. Riquelme R, Torres A, El-Ebiary M et al (1996) Community-acquired pneumonia in the elderly. Am J Respir Crit Care Med 154:1450–1455
9. Sullivan D, Walls R (1994) Impact of nutritional status on morbidity in a population of geriatric rehabilitation patients. J Am Geriatr Soc 42:471–477
10. Morley J, Kraenzle D (1994) Causes of weight loss in a community nursing home. J Am Geriatr Soc 42:583–585
11. Robbins LJ (1989) Evaluation of weight loss in the elderly. Geriatrics 44:31–34, 37
12. Kayser-Jones J (2001) Starved for attention. Reflect Nurs Leadersh 27:10–14, 45
13. Rolls BJ, Dimeo KA, Shide DJ (1995) Age-related impairments in the regulation of food intake. Am J Clin Nutr 62:923–931
14. Moriguti JC, Das SK, Saltzman E et al (2000) Effects of a 6-week hypocaloric diet on changes in body composition, hunger, and subsequent weight regain in healthy young and older adults. J Gerontol A Biol Sci Med Sci 55:B580–B587
15. Roberts SB, Fuss P, Heyman MB et al (1994) Control of food intake in older men. JAMA 272:1601–1606
16. Roberts SB (2000) Regulation of energy intake in relation to metabolic state and nutritional status. Eur J Clin Nutr 54(Suppl 3):S64–S69
17. McCrory MA, Fuss PJ, McCallum JE et al (1999) Dietary variety within food groups: association with energy intake and body fatness in men and women. Am J Clin Nutr 69:440–447
18. Schiffman SS (1997) Taste and smell losses in normal aging and disease. JAMA 278:1357–1362
19. White HK, McConnell ES, Bales CW, Kuchibhatla M (2004) A 6-month observational study of the relationship between weight loss and behavioral symptoms in institutionalized Alzheimer's disease subjects. J Am Med Dir Assoc 5:89–97
20. Simmons, SF, Osterweil D, Schnelle JF (2001) Improving food intake in nursing home residents with feeding assistance: a staffing analysis. J Gerontol A Biol Sci Med Sci 56:M790–M794
21. Murphy DJ, Santilli S (1998) Elderly patients' preferences for long-term life support. Arch Fam Med 7:484–488
22. Abitbol V, Selinger-Leneman H, Gallais Y et al (2002) Percutaneous endoscopic gastrostomy in elderly patients. A prospective study in a geriatric hospital. Gastroenterol Clin Biol 26:448–453
23. Mitchell, SL, Tetroe JM (2000) Survival after percutaneous endoscopic gastrostomy placement in older persons. J Gerontol A Biol Sci Med Sci 55:M735–M739
24. Gomez Ramos, MJ, Saturno Hernandez PJ (2002) Parenteral nutrition in a general hospital: quality criteria and factors associated with compliance. Med Clin (Barc) 119:686–689
25. Shintani S, Fumimura Y, Shiigai T et al (2001) Feeding methods for long-term bedridden patients

with dysphagia under home health care - percutaneous endoscopic gastrostomy (PEG) and intravenous hyperalimentation (IVH). Gan To Kagaku
Ryoho 28(Suppl 1):61–64

26. Ling PR, Khaodhiar L, Bistrian BR et al (2001)
    Inflammatory mediators in patients receiving long-
    term home parenteral nutrition. Dig Dis Sci
    46:2484–2489

27. McNamara M, Alexander H, Norton J (1992)
    Cytokines and their role in the pathophysiology of
    cancer cachexia. JPEN J Parenter Enteral Nutr
    16(Suppl 6):S50–S55

28. Tisdale M (1997) Biology of cachexia. J Natl Cancer
    Inst 89:1763–1773

29. Tisdale M, McDevitt TM, Todorov PT et al (1996)
    Catabolic factors in cancer cachexia. In vivo
    10:131–136

30. Tisdale MJ (2003) The 'cancer cachectic factor.'
    Support Care Cancer 11:73–78

31. Tisdale MJ (2002) Cachexia in cancer patients. Nat
    Rev Cancer 2:862–871

32. Tisdale MJ (2001) Cancer anorexia and cachexia.
    Nutrition 17:438–442

33. Kotler DP, Grunfeld C (1995) Pathophysiology and
    treatment of the AIDS wasting syndrome. AIDS Clin
    Rev 96:229–275

34. Tokuda Y, Koketsu H (2002) High mortality in
    hospitalized elderly patients with feeding tube pla-
    cement. Intern Med 41:613–616

35. Yeh SS, Hafner A, Schuster MW et al (2003)
    Relationship between body composition and cytoki-
    nes in cachectic patients with chronic obstructive
    pulmonary disease. J Am Geriatr Soc 51:890–891

36. Yeh SS, Schuster MW (1999) Geriatric cachexia: the
    role of cytokines. Am J Clin Nutr 70:183–197

37. Yeh SS, Schuster MW (2000) Reply to JL Caddell. Am
    J Clin Nutr 71:852–853

38. Yeh SS, Wu SY, Levine DM et al (2001) The correla-
    tion of cytokine levels with body weight after mege-
    strol acetate treatment in geriatric patients. J
    Gerontol A Biol Sci Med Sci 56:M48–M54

39. Morgan L (1985) Megestrol acetate versus tamoxifen
    in advanced breast cancer in postmenopausal
    patients. Semin Oncol 12:43–47

40. Muss HB, Case LD, Capizzi RL et al (1990) High-ver-
    sus standard dose megestrol acetate in woman with
    advanced breast cancer: a phase III trial of the
    Piedmont Oncology Association. J Clin Oncol
    8:1797–1805

41. Tchekmedyian NS, Zahyna D, Halpert C, Heber D
    (1992) Clinical aspects of nutrition in advanced can-
    cer. Oncology 49(Suppl 2):3–7

42. Tchekmedyian NS, Hickman M, Siau J et al (1992)
    Megestrol acetate in cancer anorexia and weight
    loss. Cancer 69:1268–1274

43. Tchekmedyian NS, Tait N, Moody M, Aisner J (1987)
    High-dose megestrol acetate. A possible treatment
    for cachexia. JAMA 257:1195–1198

44. Pascual Lopez A, Roque i Figuls M, Urrutia Cuchi G

et al (2004) Systematic review of megestrol acetate
in the treatment of anorexia-cachexia syndrome. J
Pain Symptom Manage 27:360–369

45. Von Roenn JH, Armstrong D, Kotler DP et al (1994)
    Megestrol acetate in patients with AIDS-related
    cachexia. Ann Intern Med 121:393–399

46. Von Roenn JH (1994) Randomized trials of mege-
    strol acetate for AIDS-associated anorexia and
    cachexia. Oncology 51:19–24

47. Von Roenn JH, Murphy RL, Weber KM et al (1988)
    Megestrol acetate for treatment of cachexia associa-
    ted with human immunodeficiency virus (HIV)
    infection. Ann Intern Med 10:840–841

48. Yeh SS, Wu SY, Lee TP et al (2000) Improvement in
    quality-of-life measures and stimulation of weight
    gain after treatment with megestrol acetate oral
    suspension in geriatric cachexia: results of a double-
    blind, placebo-controlled study. J Am Geriatr Soc
    48:485–492

49. Simmons SF, Walker KA, Osterweil D (2004) The
    effect of megestrol acetate on oral food and fluid
    intake in nursing home residents: a pilot study. J Am
    Med Dir Assoc 5:24–30

50. Morley JE (2002) Orexigenic and anabolic agents.
    Clin Geriatr Med 18:853–866

51. Karcic E, Philpot C, Morley JE (2002) Treating mal-
    nutrition with megestrol acetate: literature review
    and review of our experience. J Nutr Health Aging
    6:191–200

52. Lambert CP, Sullivan DH, Freeling SA et al (2002)
    Effects of testosterone replacement and/or resistan-
    ce exercise on the composition of megestrol acetate
    stimulated weight gain in elderly men: a randomi-
    zed controlled trial. J Clin Endocrinol Metab
    87:2100–2106

53. Hamburger AW, Parnes H, Gordon GB et al (1988)
    Megestrol acetate induced differentiation of 3T3-L1
    adipocytes in vitro. Semin Oncol 15:76–78

54. Reitmeier M, Hartenstein R (1990) Megestrol acetate
    and determination of body composition by bioelec-
    trical impedance analysis in cancer cachexia. Proc
    Am Soc Clin Oncol 9:325 (abs)

55. Beck S, Tisdale M (1990) Effect of megestrol acetate
    on weight loss induced by tumor necrosis factor
    alpha and a cachexia-inducing tumor (MAC16) in
    NMRI mice. Br J Cancer 62:420–424

56. Lapp CA, Thomas ME, Lewis JB (1995) Modulation
    by progesterone of interleukin-6 production by gin-
    gival fibroblasts. J Periodontol 66:279–284

57. Mantovani G, Macciò A, Lai P et al (1998) Cytokine
    involvement in cancer anorexia/cachexia: role of
    megestrol acetate and medroxyprogesterone acetate
    on cytokine downregulation and improvement of
    clinical symptoms. Crit Rev Oncog 9:99–106

58. Mantovani G, Macciò A, Lai P et al (1998) Cytokine
    activity in cancer-related anorexia/cachexia: role of
    megestrol acetate and medroxyprogesterone acetate.
    Semin Oncol 25(Suppl 6):45–52

59. Mantovani G, Macciò A, Esu S et al (1997)

Medroxyprogesterone acetate reduces the in vitro production of cytokines and serotonin involved in anorexia/cachexia and emesis by peripheral blood mononuclear cells of cancer patients. Eur J Cancer 33:602–607

60. Mantovani G (1997) Serum levels of cytokines and weightloss/anorexia in cancer patients. Support Care Cancer 5:422–423

61. Yeh SS, Wu SS, Levine DM et al (2000) Quality of life and stimulation of weight gain after treatment with megestrol acetate: correlation between cytokine levels and nutritional status, appetite, and in geriatric patients. J Nutr Health Aging 4:246–251

62. Jatoi A, Yamashita J, Sloan JA et al (2002) Does megestrol acetate down-regulate interleukin-6 in patients with cancer-associated anorexia and weight loss? A North Central Cancer Treatment Group investigation. Support Care Cancer 10:71–75

63. McCarthy HD, Crowder RE, Dryden S, Williams G (1994) Megestrol acetate stimulates food and water intake in the rat: effects on regional hypothalamic neuropeptide Y concentrations. Eur J Pharmacol 265:99–102

64. Costa AM, Spence KT, Plata-Salaman CR, Ffrench-Mullen JM (1995) Residual Ca2+ channel current modulation by megestrol acetate via a G-protein alpha s-subunit in rat hypothalamic neurones. J Physiol 487:291–303

65. Meacham LR, Mazewski C, Krawiecki N (2003) Mechanism of transient adrenal insufficiency with megestrol acetate treatment of cachexia in children with cancer. J Pediatr Hematol Oncol 25:414–417

66. McKone EF, Tonelli MR, Aitken ML (2002) Adrenal insufficiency and testicular failure secondary to megestrol acetate therapy in a patient with cystic fibrosis. Pediatr Pulmonol 34:381–383

67. Pimentel G, Santos E, Arastu M, Cowan JA (1996) Hyperglycemia in an AIDS patient taking megestrol. Hosp Pract (Off Ed) 31:27–28

68. Hervas R, Cepeda C, Pulido F (2004) Cushing syndrome secondary to megestrol acetate in a patient with AIDS. Med Clin (Barc) 122:638–639

69. Kropsky B, Shi Y, Cherniack EP (2003) Incidence of deep-venous thrombosis in nursing home residents using megestrol acetate. J Am Med Dir Assoc 4:255–256

70. Thomas DR (2004) Incidence of venous thromboembolism in megestrol acetate users. J Am Med Dir Assoc 5:65–66; author reply 66–67

71. Bennett RG (2003) Megestrol complications. Chest 123:309–310; author reply 310

72. Naing KK, Dewar JA, Leese GP (1999) Megestrol acetate therapy and secondary adrenal suppression. Cancer 86:1044–1049

73. Mann M, Koller E, Murgo A et al (1997) Glucocorticoid-like activity of megestrol. A summary of Food and Drug Administration experience and a review of the literature. Arch Intern Med 157:1651–1656

74. Gonzalez Del Valle L, Herrero Ambrosio A, Martinez

75. Hernandez P et al (1996) Hyperglycemia induced by megestrol acetate in a patient with AIDS. Ann Pharmacother 30:1113–1114

75. Loprinzi CL, Fonseca R, Jensen MD (1996) Megestrol acetate-induced adrenal suppression. J Clin Oncol 14:689

76. Gorter RW (1999) Cancer cachexia and cannabinoids. Forsch Komplementarmed 6(Suppl 3):21–22

77. Gorter R (1998) Cannabis and cannabidiol: interview with Robert Gorter, MD. Interview by Fred Gardner. AIDS Treat News 305:4–6

78. Volicer L, Stelly M, Morris J et al (1997) Effects of dronabinol on anorexia and disturbed behavior in patients with Alzheimer's disease. Int J Geriatr Psychiatry 12:913–919

79. Jatoi A, Windschitl HE, Loprinzi CL et al (2002) Dronabinol versus megestrol acetate versus combination therapy for cancer-associated anorexia: a North Central Cancer Treatment Group study. J Clin Oncol 20:567–573

80. Beal JE, Olson R, Laubenstein L et al (1995) Dronabinol as a treatment for anorexia associated with weight loss in patients with AIDS. J Pain Symptom Manage 10:89–97

81. Struwe M, Kaempfer SH, Geiger CJ et al (1993) Effect of dronabinol on nutritional status in HIV infection. Ann Pharmacother 27:827–831

82. Batterham MJ, Garsia R (2001) A comparison of megestrol acetate, nandrolone decanoate and dietary counselling for HIV associated weight loss. Int J Androl 24:232–240

83. Lyden E, Cvetkovska E, Westin T et al (1995) Effects of nandrolone propionate on experimental tumor growth and cancer cachexia. Metabolism 44:445–451

84. Gruzdev BM, Ivannikov EV, Gorbacheva ES (1999) Anabolic therapy in patients with HIV infections. Ter Arkh 71:35–37

85. Gold J, High HA, Li Y et al (1996) Safety and efficacy of nandrolone decanoate for treatment of wasting in patients with HIV infection. AIDS 10:745–752

86. Johansen KL, Mulligan K, Schambelan M (1999) Anabolic effect of nandrolone decanoate in patients receiving dialysis. JAMA 281:1275–1281

87. Strawford A, Barbieri T, Neese R et al (1999) Effects of nandrolone decanoate therapy in borderline hypogonadal men with HIV-associated weight loss. J Acquir Immune Defic Syndr Hum Retrovirol 20:137–146

88. Berger JR, Pall L, Hall CD et al (1996) Oxandrolone in AIDS-wasting myopathy. AIDS 10:1657–1662

89. Bonkovsky HL, Fiellin DA, Smith GS et al (1991) A randomized, controlled trial of treatment of alcoholic hepatitis with parenteral nutrition and oxandrolone. I. Short-terms effect on liver function. Am J Gastroenterol 86:1200–1208

90. Demling RH, Orgill DP (2000) The anticatabolic and wound healing effects of the testosterone analog oxandrolone after severe burn injury. J Crit Care 15:12–17

91. Romeyn M, Gunn N 3rd (2000) Resistance exercise and oxandrolone for men with HIV-related weight loss. JAMA 284:176

92. Yeh SS, DeGuzman B, Kramer T (2002) Reversal of COPD-associated weight loss using the anabolic agent oxandrolone. Chest 122:421–428

93. Krasner DL, Belcher AE (2000) Oxandrolone restores appetite. An increase in weight helps heal wounds. Am J Nurs 100:53

94. Demling R, De Santi L (1998) Closure of the 'non-healing wound' corresponds with correction of weight loss using the anabolic agent oxandrolone. Ostomy Wound Manage 44:58–62, 64, 66 passim

95. Langer CJ, Hoffman JP, Ottery FD (2001) Clinical significance of weight loss in cancer patients: rationale for the use of anabolic agents in the treatment of cancer-related cachexia. Nutrition 17(1 Suppl):S1–S20

96. Mwamburi DM, Gerrior J, Wilson IB et al (2004) Comparing megestrol acetate therapy with oxandrolone therapy for HIV-related weight loss: similar results in 2 months. Clin Infect Dis 38:895–902

97. Earthman CP, Reid PM, Harper IT et al (2002) Body cell mass repletion and improved quality of life in HIV-infected individuals receiving oxandrolone. JPEN J Parenter Enteral Nutr 26:357–365

98. Grinspoon S, Corcoran C, Parlman K et al (2000) Effects of testosterone and progressive resistance training in eugonadal men with AIDS wasting. A randomized, controlled trial. Ann Intern Med 133:348–355

99. Bhasin S, Storer TW, Javanbakht M et al (2000) Testosterone replacement and resistance exercise in HIV-infected men with weight loss and low testosterone levels. JAMA 283:763–770

100. Bhasin S, Storer TW, Asbel-Sethi N et al (1998) Effects of testosterone replacement with a nongenital, transdermal system, Androderm, in human immunodeficiency virus-infected men with low testosterone levels. J Clin Endocrinol Metab 83:3155–3162

101. Coodley GO, Coodley MK (1997) A trial of testosterone therapy for HIV-associated weight loss. AIDS 11:1347–1352

102. Bennell KL, Brukner PD, Malcolm SA (1996) Effect of altered reproductive function and lowered testosterone levels on bone density in male endurance athletes. Br J Sports Med 30:205–208

103. Morley JE, Perry HM 3rd, Kaiser FE et al (1993) Effects of testosterone replacement therapy in old hypogonadal males: a preliminary study. J Am Geriatr Soc 41:149–152

104. Dolan S, Wilkie S, Aliabadi N et al (2004) Effects of testosterone administration in human immunodeficiency virus-infected women with low weight: a randomized placebo-controlled study. Arch Intern Med 164:897–904

105. Schurgin S, Dolan S, Perlstein A et al (2004) Effects of testosterone administration on growth hormone pulse dynamics in human immunodeficiency virus-infected women. J Clin Endocrinol Metab 89:3290–3297

106. Svanberg E, Ohlsson C, Kimball SR, Lundholm K (2000) rhIGF-1/IGFBP-3 complex, but not free rhIGF-1, supports muscle protein biosynthesis in rats during semistarvation. Eur J Clin Invest 30:438–446

107. Wang W, Iresjo BM, Karlsson L, Svanberg E (2000) Provision of rhIGF-1/IGFBP-3 complex attenuated development of cancer cachexia in an experimental tumor model. Clin Nutr 19:127–132

108. Tai VW, Schambelan M, Algren H et al (2002) Effects of recombinant human growth hormone on fat distribution in patients with human immunodeficiency virus-associated wasting. Clin Infect Dis 35:1258–1262

109. Lo JC, Mulligan K, Noor MA et al (2001) The effects of recombinant human growth hormone on body composition and glucose metabolism in HIV-infected patients with fat accumulation. J Clin Endocrinol Metab 86:3480–3487

110. Mulligan K, Tai VW, Schambelan M (1999) Use of growth hormone and other anabolic agents in AIDS wasting. JPEN J Parenter Enteral Nutr 23:S202–S209

111. Mulligan K, Tai VW, Schambelan M (1998) Effects of chronic growth hormone treatment on energy intake and resting energy metabolism in patients with human immunodeficiency virus-associated wasting - a clinical research center study. J Clin Endocrinol Metab 83:1542–1547

112. Schambelan M, Mulligan K, Grunfeld C et al (1996) Recombinant human growth hormone in patients with HIV-associated wasting. A randomized, placebo-controlled trial. Serostim Study Group. Ann Intern Med 125:873–882

113. Cominelli S, Raguso CA, Karsegard L et al (2002) Weight-losing HIV-infected patients on recombinant human growth hormone for 12 wk: a national study. Nutrition 18:583–586

114. Crown AL, Cottle K, Lightman SL et al (2002) What is the role of the insulin-like growth factor system in the pathophysiology of cancer cachexia, and how is it regulated? Clin Endocrinol (Oxf) 56:723–733

115. Roubenoff R (2000) Acquired immunodeficiency syndrome wasting, functional performance, and quality of life. Am J Manag Care 6:1003–1016

116. Biolo G, Iscra F, Bosutti A et al (2000) Growth hormone decreases muscle glutamine production and stimulates protein synthesis in hypercatabolic patients. Am J Physiol Endocrinol Metab 279:E323–E332

117. Mynarcik DC, Frost RA, Lang CH et al (1999) Insulin-like growth factor system in patients with HIV infection: effect of exogenous growth hormone administration. J Acquir Immune Defic Syndr 22:49–55

118. Windisch PA, Papatheofanis FJ, Matuszewski KA (1998) Recombinant human growth hormone for

AIDS-associated wasting. Ann Pharmacother 32:437–445

119. Ellis KJ, Lee PD, Pivarnik JM et al (1996) Changes in body composition of human immunodeficiency virus-infected males receiving insulin-like growth factor I and growth hormone. J Clin Endocrinol Metab 81:3033–3038

120. Von Roenn JH, Knopf K (1996) Anorexia/cachexia in patients with HIV: lessons for the oncologist. Oncology (Huntingt) 10:1049–1056; discussion 1062–1064, 1067–1068

121. Papadakis MA, Grady D, Black D et al (1996) Growth hormone replacement in healthy older men improves body composition but not functional ability. Ann Intern Med 124:708–716

122. Kaiser FE, Silver AJ, Morley JE (1991) The effect of recombinant human growth hormone on malnourished older individuals. J Am Geriatr Soc 39:235–240

123. Waters D, Danska J, Hardy K et al (1996) Recombinant human growth hormone, insulin-like growth factor 1, and combination therapy in AIDS-associated wasting. Ann Intern Med 125:865–872

124. Brocker P, Vellas B, Albarede JL, Poynard T (1994) A two-centre, randomized, double-blind trial of ornithine oxoglutarate in 194 elderly, ambulatory, convalescent subjects. Age Ageing 23:303–306

125. Boelens PG, Fonk JC, Houdijk AP et al (2004) Primary immune response to keyhole limpet haemocyanin following trauma in relation to low plasma glutamine. Clin Exp Immunol 136:356–364

126. Sahni M, Guenther HL, Fleisch H et al (1993) Bisphosphonates act on rat bone resorption through the mediation of osteoblasts. J Clin Invest 91:2004–2011

127. Lai YN, Yeh SL, Lin MT et al (2004) Glutamine supplementation enhances mucosal immunity in rats with Gut-Derived sepsis. Nutrition 20:286–291

128. Akisu M, Baka M, Huseyinov A, Kultursay N (2003) The role of dietary supplementation with L-glutamine in inflammatory mediator release and intestinal injury in hypoxia/reoxygenation-induced experimental necrotizing enterocolitis. Ann Nutr Metab 47:262–266

129. Rathmacher JA, Nissen S, Panton L et al (2004) Supplementation with a combination of beta-hydroxy-beta-methylbutyrate (HMB), arginine, and glutamine is safe and could improve hematological parameters. JPEN J Parenter Enteral Nutr 28:65–75

130. May PE, Barber A, D'Olimpio JT et al (2002) Reversal of cancer-related wasting using oral supplementation with a combination of beta-hydroxy-beta-methylbutyrate, arginine, and glutamine. Am J Surg 183:471–479

131. Clark RH, Feleke G, Din M et al (2000) Nutritional treatment for acquired immunodeficiency virus-associated wasting using beta-hydroxy beta-methylbutyrate, glutamine, and arginine: a randomized, double-blind, placebo-controlled study. JPEN J Parenter Enteral Nutr 24:133–139

132. von Meyenfeldt MF (1999) Nutritional support during treatment of biliopancreatic malignancy. Ann Oncol 10(Suppl 4):273–277

133. Vazquez P, Gomez de Segura IA, Cos A et al (1996) Response of the intestinal mucosa to different enteral diets in situations of surgical stress and malnutrition. Nutr Hosp 11:321–327

134. Kinscherf R, Hack V, Fischbach T et al (1996) Low plasma glutamine in combination with high glutamate levels indicate risk for loss of body cell mass in healthy individuals: the effect of N-acetyl-cysteine. J Mol Med 74:393–400

135. Austgen TR, Chen MK, Dudrick PS et al (1992) Cytokine regulation of intestinal glutamine utilization. Am J Surg 163:174–179, discussion 179–180

136. Smith QR (1991) The blood-brain barrier and the regulation of amino acid uptake and availability to brain. Adv Exp Med Biol 291:55–71

137. Tayek JA, Bistrian BR, Hehir DJ et al (1986) Improved protein kinetics and albumin synthesis by branched chain amino acid-enriched total parenteral nutrition in cancer cachexia. A prospective randomized crossover trial. Cancer 58:147–157

138. Grunfeld C, Feingold KR (1991) The metabolic effects of tumor necrosis factor and other cytokines. Biotherapy 3:143–158

139. Grunfeld C, Kotler DP (1992) Wasting in the acquired immunodeficiency syndrome. Semin Liver Dis 12:175–187

140. Doherty GM, Jensen JC, Alexander HR et al (1991) Pentoxifylline suppression of tumor necrosis factor gene transcription. Surgery 110:192–198

141. Landman D, Sarai A, Sathe SS (1994) Use of pentoxifylline therapy for patients with AIDS-related wasting: pilot study. Clin Infect Dis 18:97–99

142. Goldberg RM, Loprinzi CL, Mailliard JA et al (1995) Pentoxifylline for treatment of cancer anorexia and cachexia? A randomized, double-blind, placebo-controlled trial. J Clin Oncol 13:2856–2859

143. Kruse A, Rieneck K, Kappel M et al (1995) Pentoxifylline therapy in HIV seropositive subjects with elevated TNF. Immunopharmacology 31:85–91

144. Sathe SS, Tsigler D, Sarai A, Kumar P (1995) Pentoxifylline impairs macrophage defense against Mycobacterium avium complex. J Infect Dis 172:863–866

145. Sathe SS, Sarai A, Tsigler D, Nedunchezian D (1994) Pentoxifylline aggravates impairment in tumor necrosis factor-alpha secretion and increases mycobacterial load in macrophages from AIDS patients with disseminated Mycobacterium avium-intracellulare complex infection. J Infect Dis 170:484–487

146. Greig NH, Giordano T, Zhu X et al (2004) Thalidomide-based TNF-alpha inhibitors for neurodegenerative diseases. Acta Neurobiol Exp (Wars) 64:1–9

147. Kedar I, Mermershtain W, Ivgi H (2004) Thalidomide reduces serum C-reactive protein and

interleukin-6 and induces response to IL-2 in a fraction of metastatic renal cell cancer patients who failed IL-2-based therapy. Int J Cancer 110:260–265

148. Reyes-Teran G, Sierra-Madero JG, Martinez del Cerro V et al (1996) Effects of thalidomide on HIV-associated wasting syndrome: a randomized, double, blind, placebo-controlled clinical trial. AIDS 10:1501–1507

149. Zhou S, Kestell P, Tingle MD, Paxton JW (2002) Thalidomide in cancer treatment: a potential role in the elderly? Drugs Aging 19:85–100

150. Khan ZH, Simpson EJ, Cole AT et al (2003) Oesophageal cancer and cachexia: the effect of short-term treatment with thalidomide on weight loss and lean body mass. Aliment Pharmacol Ther 17:677–682

151. Sauer LA, Dauchy RT, Blask DE (2000) Mechanism for the antitumor and anticachectic effects of n-3 fatty acids. Cancer Res 60:5289–5295

152. Meydani SN, Endres S, Woods MM et al (1991) Oral (n-3) fatty acid supplementation suppresses cytokine production and lymphocyte proliferation: comparison between young and older women. J Nutr 121:547–555

153. Dinarello CA, Endres S, Meydani SN et al (1990) Interleukin-1, anorexia, and dietary fatty acids. Ann N Y Acad Sci 587:332–338

154. Endres S, Ghorbani R, Kelley VE et al (1989) The effect of dietary supplementation with n-3 polyunsaturated fatty acids on the synthesis of interleukin-1 and tumor necrosis factor by mononuclear cells. N Engl J Med 320:265–271

155. Tisdale MJ, Dhesi JK (1990) Inhibition of weight loss by omega-3 fatty acids in an experimental cachexia model. Cancer Res 50:5022–5026

156. Costelli P, Llovera M, Lopez-Soriano J et al (1995) Lack of effect of eicosapentaenoic acid in preventing cancer cachexia and inhibiting tumor growth. Cancer Lett 97:25–32

157. Fearon KC, Von Meyenfeldt MF, Moses AG et al (2003) Effect of a protein and energy dense N-3 fatty acid enriched oral supplement on loss of weight and lean tissue in cancer cachexia: a randomised double blind trial. Gut 52:1479–1486

158. Jatoi A, Rowland K, Loprinzi CL et al (2004) An eicosapentaenoic acid supplement versus megestrol acetate versus both for patients with cancer-associated wasting: a North Central Cancer Treatment Group and National Cancer Institute of Canada collaborative effort. J Clin Oncol 22:2469–2476

159. Roederer M, Staal FJ, Raju PA et al (1990) Cytokine-stimulated human immunodeficiency virus replication is inhibited by N-acetyl-L-cysteine. Proc Natl Acad Sci U S A 87:4884–4888

160. Kardinal CG, Loprinzi CL, Schaid DJ et al (1990) A controlled trial of cyproheptadine in cancer patients with anorexia and/or cachexia. Cancer 65:2657–2662

161. Loprinzi CL, Kuross SA, O'Fallon JR et al (1994) Randomized placebo-controlled evaluation of hydrazine sulfate in patients with advanced colorectal cancer. J Clin Oncol 12:1121–1125

162. Loprinzi CL, Goldberg RM, Su JQ et al (1994) Placebo-controlled trial of hydrazine sulfate in patients with newly diagnosed non-small-cell lung cancer. J Clin Oncol 12:1126–1129

163. Lissoni P, Paolorossi F, Tancini G et al (1996) Is there a role for melatonin in the treatment of neoplastic cachexia? Eur J Cancer 32A:1340–1343

164. Maughan R (1995) Creatine supplementation and exercise performance. International journal of sport nutrition 5:94–101

165. Engelhardt M, Neumann G, Berbalk A, Reuter I (1998) Creatine supplementation in endurance sports. Med Sci Sports Exerc 30:1123–1129

166. Greenhaff PL, Casey A, Short AH et al (1993) Influence of oral creatine supplementation of muscle torque during repeated bouts of maximal voluntary exercise in man. Clin Sci (Lond) 84:565–571

167. Birch R, Noble D, Greenhaff PL (1994) The influence of dietary creatine supplementation on performance during repeated bouts of maximal isokinetic cycling in man. Eur J Appl Physiol Occup Physiol 69:268–276

168. Greenhaff PL (1995) Creatine and its application as an ergogenic aid. Int J Sport Nutr 5:S100–S110

169. Terjung RL, Clarkson P, Eichner ER et al (2000) American College of Sports Medicine roundtable. The physiological and health effects of oral creatine supplementation. Med Sci Sports Exerc 32:706–717

170. Williams MH, Branch JD (1998) Creatine supplementation and exercise performance: an update. J Am Coll Nutr 17:216–234

171. Redondo DR, Dowling EA, Graham BL et al (1996) The effect of oral creatine monohydrate supplementation on running velocity. Int J Sport Nutr 6:213–221

172. Hyltander A, Daneryd P, Sandstrom R et al (2000) Beta-adrenoceptor activity and resting energy metabolism in weight losing cancer patients. Eur J Cancer 36:330–334

173. Roe S, Cooper AL, Morris ID, Rothwell NJ (1996) Mechanisms of cachexia induced by T-cell leukemia in the rat. Metabolism 45:645–651

174. Szabo K (1979) Clinical experiences with beta adrenergic blocking therapy on burned patients. Scand J Plast Reconstr Surg 13:211–215

175. Lamont LS, Brown T, Riebe D, Caldwell M (2000) The major components of human energy balance during chronic beta-adrenergic blockade. J Cardiopulm Rehabil 20:247–250

176. Reichel K, Rehfeldt C, Weikard R et al (1993) Effect of a beta-agonist and a beta-agonist/beta-antagonist combination on muscle growth, body composition and protein metabolism in rats. Arch Tierernahr 45:211–225

177. Arbabi S, Ahrns KS, Wahl WL et al (2004) Beta-blocker use is associated with improved outcomes in

adult burn patients. J Trauma 56:265–269; discussion 269–271

178. Kawakami M, He J, Sakamoto T, Okada Y (2001) Catecholamines play a role in the production of interleukin-6 and interleukin-1alpha in unburned skin after burn injury in mice. Crit Care Med 29:796–801

179. Hryniewicz K, Androne AS, Hudaihed A, Katz SD (2003) Partial reversal of cachexia by beta-adrenergic receptor blocker therapy in patients with chronic heart failure. J Card Fail 9:464–468

180. Gambardella A, Tortoriello R, Pesce L et al (1999) Intralipid infusion combined with propranolol administration has favorable metabolic effects in elderly malnourished cancer patients. Metabolism 48:291–297

181. Hussey HJ, Tisdale MJ (2000) Effect of the specific cyclooxygenase-2 inhibitor meloxicam on tumour growth and cachexia in a murine model. Int J Cancer 87:95–100

182. Cahlin C, Gelin J, Delbro D et al (2000) Effect of cyclooxygenase and nitric oxide synthase inhibitors on tumor growth in mouse tumor models with and without cancer cachexia related to prostanoids. Cancer Res 60:1742–1719

183. Gelin J, Moldawer LL, Lonnroth C et al (1991) Role of endogenous tumor necrosis factor alpha and interleukin 1 for experimental tumor growth and the development of cancer cachexia. Cancer Res 51:415–421

184. Gelin J, Andersson C, Lundholm K (1991) Effects of indomethacin, cytokines, and cyclosporin A on tumor growth and the subsequent development of cancer cachexia. Cancer Res 51:880–885

185. Wang W, Lonnroth C, Svanberg E, Lundholm K (2001) Cytokine and cyclooxygenase-2 protein in brain areas of tumor-bearing mice with prostanoid-related anorexia. Cancer Res 61:4707–4715

186. Cahlin C, Korner A, Axelsson H et al (2000) Experimental cancer cachexia: the role of host-derived cytokines interleukin (IL)-6, IL-12, interferon-gamma, and tumor necrosis factor alpha evaluated in gene knockout, tumor-bearing mice on C57 Bl background and eicosanoid-dependent cachexia. Cancer Res 60:5488–5493

187. Lundholm K, Gelin J, Hyltander A et al (1994) Anti-inflammatory treatment may prolong survival in undernourished patients with metastatic solid tumors. Cancer Res 54:5602–5606

188. Adigun AQ, Ajayi AA (2001) The effects of enalapril-digoxin-diuretic combination therapy on nutritional and anthropometric indices in chronic congestive heart failure: preliminary findings in cardiac cachexia. Eur J Heart Fail 3:359–363

189. Anker SD, Negassa A, Coats AJ et al (2003) Prognostic importance of weight loss in chronic heart failure and the effect of treatment with angiotensin-converting-enzyme inhibitors: an observational study. Lancet 361:1077–1083

190. Asakawa A, Inui A, Kaga T et al (2001) Ghrelin is an appetite-stimulatory signal from stomach with structural resemblance to motilin. Gastroenterology 120:337–345

191. Hao S, Avraham Y, Mechoulam R, Berry EM (2000) Low dose anandamide affects food intake, cognitive function, neurotransmitter and corticosterone levels in diet-restricted mice. Eur J Pharmacol 392:147–156

192. Kawamura I, Yamamoto N, Sakai F et al (1999) Activation of lipoprotein lipase and inhibition of B16 melanoma-induced cachexia in mice by ponalrestat, an aldose reductase inhibitor. Anticancer Res 19:341–348

193. Kawamura I, Lacey E, Yamamoto N et al (1999) Ponalrestat, an aldose reductase inhibitor, inhibits cachexia syndrome induced by colon26 adenocarcinoma in mice. Anticancer Res 19:4105–4111

194. Kawamura I, Yamamoto N, Sakai F et al (1999) Effect of lipoprotein lipase activators bezafibrate and NO-1886, on B16 melanoma-induced cachexia in mice. Anticancer Res 19:4099–4103

195. Kawamura I, Lacey E, Inami M et al (1999) Ponalrestat, an aldose reductase inhibitor, inhibits cachexia syndrome in nude mice bearing human melanomas G361 and SEKI. Anticancer Res 19:4091–4097

196. Agteresch HJ, Dagnelie PC, van der Gaast A et al (2000) Randomized clinical trial of adenosine 5'-triphosphate in patients with advanced non-small-cell lung cancer. J Natl Cancer Inst 92:321–328

197. Agteresch HJ, Burgers SA, van der Gaast A et al (2003) Randomized clinical trial of adenosine 5'-triphosphate on tumor growth and survival in advanced lung cancer patients. Anticancer Drugs 14:639–644

198. Ishiko O, Yasui T, Hirai K et al (1999) Lipolytic activity of anemia-inducing substance from tumor-bearing rabbits. Nutr Cancer 33:201–205

199. Ishiko O, Hirai K, Nishimura S et al (1999) Elimination of anemia-inducing substance by cyclic plasma perfusion of tumor-bearing rabbits. Clin Cancer Res 5:2660–2665

200. Ishiko O, Sumi T, Yoshida H et al (2001) Angiogenesis in the adipose tissue of tumor-bearing rabbits treated by cyclic plasma perfusion. Int J Oncol 19:785–790

201. Ishiko O, Yoshida H, Sumi T et al (2001) Expression of skeletal muscle cells apoptosis regulatory proteins in plasma-perfused VX2 carcinoma-bearing rabbits. Anticancer Res 21:2363–2368

202. Josephs MD, Solorzano CC, Taylor M et al (2000) Modulation of the acute phase response by altered expression of the IL-1 type 1 receptor or IL-1ra. Am J Physiol Regul Integr Comp Physiol 278:R824–R830

203. Carbo N, Lopez-Soriano J, Costelli P et al (2000) Interleukin-15 antagonizes muscle protein waste in tumour-bearing rats. Br J Cancer 83:526–531

204. Figueras M, Busquets S, Carbo N et al (2004)

Interleukin-15 is able to suppress the increased DNA fragmentation associated with muscle wasting in tumour-bearing rats. FEBS Lett 569:201–206

205. Schwartz SA, Hernandez A, Mark Evers B (1999) The role of NF-kappaB/IkappaB proteins in cancer: implications for novel treatment strategies. Surg Oncol 8:143–153

206. Kawamura I, Morishita R, Tsujimoto S et al (2001) Intravenous injection of oligodeoxynucleotides to the NF-kappaB binding site inhibits hepatic metastasis of M5076 reticulosarcoma in mice. Gene Ther 8:905–912

207. Kawamura I, Morishita R, Tomita N et al (1999) Intratumoral injection of oligonucleotides to the NF kappa B binding site inhibits cachexia in a mouse tumor model. Gene Ther 6:91–97

# Treatment of Sarcopenia and Cachexia in the Elderly

Charles P. Lambert, William J. Evans, Dennis H. Sullivan

## Introduction

Cachexia is defined as physical wasting with loss of muscle mass and weight that is caused by disease [1]. It is common for elderly individuals who have disease to exhibit cachexia. Additionally, muscle mass loss is characteristic of the conditions of frailty and sarcopenia. Sarcopenia is the age-related loss of muscle mass [2]. Physical frailty has been characterised by Fried et al. [3] as a condition that results from reduced strength, reduced gait velocity, reduced physical activity, weight loss, and exhaustion. Clearly, sarcopenia and frailty could be classified as cachectic conditions because they are associated with muscle mass loss. This chapter will describe the causes of sarcopenia, treatment of sarcopenia, causes of cachexia in elderly individuals, and treatment of cachexia in elderly individuals.

## Causes of Sarcopenia

### Aging, Protein Synthesis, and Protein Breakdown

There is a reduction in muscle mass as one ages, with detectable changes occurring after the age of 50 [4]. This loss of muscle mass is related to reduced protein synthesis with age, increased protein breakdown, or a combination of the two. Based on recent results [5], it appears that basal protein synthesis is similar between young and old. Earlier research [6–10], however, suggested that protein synthesis is reduced in the elderly compared to the young. Recent results using the microdialysis approach to examine the release of 3- methylhistidine into the interstitial fluid suggest that skeletal muscle protein breakdown is substantially elevated in old relative to young [11]. The causes of these changes in protein metabolism with age have not been completely elucidated but potential causative factors are discussed below.

## Denervation

Aging is associated with a reduction in α-motor neurons or denervation and concomitant reduction in muscle strength [12]. The effect of denervation on skeletal muscle is to reduce protein synthesis and, to a greater extent, increase muscle protein degradation [13]. This increase in muscle protein degradation as a result of denervation occurs primarily through the ATP-dependent ubiquitin-proteasome pathway [14].

## Reduction in Testosterone, Growth Hormone, and IGF-1

It is clear that a reduction in the testosterone concentration in healthy young individuals will result in a loss of fat-free mass and muscle strength [15]. It is also well-known that there is a reduction in testosterone of at least 1% per year after the age of 50 in normal healthy men [4]. Furthermore, it has been reported that reduced testosterone concentrations are related to reduced fat-free mass, appendicular skeletal muscle mass, and muscle strength in elderly individuals [16–19]. Additionally, growth hormone decreases with age. This results in a reduction in fat-free mass and an increase in visceral fat mass in the abdominal region [20–22]. An additional manifestation of the reduction in growth hormone is a reduction in circulating insulin-like growth factor (IGF)-1. Statistically significant inverse correlations have been observed between increasing age and IGF-1 concentrations [23]. It is believed that the effects of growth hormone on fat-free mass and fat mass are mediated through IGF-1. Thus, a decline in the circulating concentration of this growth factor would be expected to reduce muscle mass.

## Elevation in Proinflammatory Cytokines

Normal aging is associated with an increase in the proinflammatory cytokines interleukin (IL)-6 and tumour necrosis factor (TNF)-α [24] and a reduction in muscle mass. Therefore, it is possible that the elevation in proinflammatory cytokines, which can induce proteolysis in skeletal muscle, may contribute to the decline in muscle mass with age. Visser et al. [25] reported that IL-6 and TNF-α concentration were inversely related to muscle mass and muscle strength in 3075 elderly individuals. Furthermore, Greiwe et al. [26] reported that TNF-α in muscle is elevated in frail elders and that resistance training decreased the resting TNF-α concentration. It has also been demonstrated that IL-6 and IGF-1 and their interaction were significant predictors of handgrip strength and muscle power [27]. IGF-1 was an independent predictor of muscle function only in subjects in the lowest IL-6 tertile, suggesting that the effect of IGF-1 on muscle function depends on the IL-6 level [27]. Payette et al. [28] reported that the IL-6 concentration was a significant predictor of sarcopenia in women age 72–92. Thus, these findings, taken collectively, suggest that elevations in proinflammatory cytokines, namely IL-6 and TNF-α, are related to sarcopenia.

## Inadequate Protein Intake

There are relatively recent data to suggest that the intake of protein at the RDA (0.8g/kg/day) is insufficient to maintain muscle mass in the elderly [29]. Additionally, in young people it was found that the myosin content, represented by type IIX fibres, was 51% lower in individuals who ingested protein at a rate of ~0.6 g/kg/day than in individuals who consumed protein at a rate of ~1.5 g/kg/day [30]. The diets were isoenergetic and 4 weeks in length. Thus, it appears that inadequate protein intake can result in muscle mass losses in the elderly and in the young. Moreover, it appears that elderly individuals do not ingest adequate amounts of protein, as ~33% of men and women over the age of 60 eat

less than 0.8 g/kg/day and ~15% eat less than 0.6 g/kg/day [31].

## Inadequate Energy Intake

It is clear that in many elderly individuals there is a reduction in appetite. According to data from the US Department of Agriculture, a large proportion of the elderly do not meet the recommended level of dietary energy intake [32]. Hughes et al. [33] reported that over 9.4 years elderly individuals who lost weight also lost fat-free mass. Specifically, a loss of 1 kg of body weight was associated with a loss of 0.32 kg of fat-free mass in men and of 0.22 kg in women. Thus, from these studies it appears that inadequate voluntary energy intake is a contributing factor to the process of sarcopenia.

## Apoptosis

There is some evidence that at least some of the loss of muscle fibres in aging that contributes to sarcopenia is due to apoptosis [34–36]. However, the time course and magnitude of the effect of apoptosis in aging human muscle, in vivo, is unknown.

## Interventions to Reverse Sarcopenia

### Resistance Exercise Training

Resistance exercise training, which involves exercises with high loads (~80% of maximal force generating capacity) and low repetitions (≤ 8–10 repetitions), is a potent stimulator of muscle mass accrual [37, 38] and muscle strength gains [39–42] in the elderly. One way in which muscle mass is increased is by an increase in muscle protein synthesis. Yarasheski et al. [10] reported that 2 weeks of resistance training in the elderly increased muscle protein synthesis by 153%. From 16 studies in which men and women performed resistance training (8–12 weeks), the range for the increase in strength was 15.6–134%, with the mean being 58% improvement and the median for the increase in strength being 52.6% [43]. Improvements in strength occur via an increase in the ability to activate the muscles maximally (increased motor-unit recruitment and increased motor-unit firing rates) and to an increase in muscle size. During the first 8–12 weeks of resistance exercise training, the increase in the ability to activate the muscles plays a much greater role in increasing strength than the increase in muscle size. After ~12 weeks of resistance training, the increase in muscle size is the predominant mechanism for the increase in muscle strength [44].

Besides increasing muscle strength, it is clear that resistance exercise training can improve physical function in the elderly, such as improving gait speed, stair climbing speed, and the ability to rise from a chair. This is important as these are the functional activities that are impaired by sarcopenia.

The duration of resistance training studies is relatively short, typically ~12 weeks. One question that arises is how long do the strength improvements persist after cessation of a resistance exercise training program? Trappe et al. [45] found an increase in strength of 53% and an increase in muscle mass of 7% as a result of 12 weeks of resistance training (3 days per week) in elderly men. During 6 months of detraining (absence of training), there was a reduction in strength of 11% and muscle mass decreased by 5%. However, resistance training just 1 day per week for 6 months after the training phase, using the regimen employed during the training phase, resulted in maintenance of muscle strength and mass. Thus, the gains made during resistance training studies are relatively short-lived but can be maintained by infrequent training sessions.

## Testosterone Replacement

Data from the Baltimore Longitudinal Study on Aging (890 men), suggested that 20% of the men over 60 years of age, 30% over 70 years, and 50% over 80 years were hypogonadal, as defined by a total testosterone level < 325 ng/dl (11.3 nmol/l), [46]. It is widely believed that total testosterone declines 1% per year after the age of 50 years [4]. Thus, the decline in testosterone follows a time course similar to the decline in muscle strength and muscle mass. Many individuals believe that it is the decline in testosterone over time that results

in a reduction in muscle mass and muscle strength, and that by administering replacement doses of testosterone these parameters can be restored.

Morley et al. [47] studied 37 men aged 69–89 years old. Twenty-six of the men had a mean total testosterone level of < 272 ng/dl. They were administered 200 mg of testosterone enanthate every 2 weeks for 3 months. Alternating cases was the method used to assign subjects to treatment or placebo groups. The authors reported a nine-fold increase in bioavailable testosterone and a significant increase in right-hand muscle strength. Sih et al. [48] reported that 12 months of testosterone replacement (biweekly injections of 200 mg) in hypogonadal elderly men resulted in a significant increase in bilateral grip strength. Bhasin et al. [49] examined the effects of 10 weeks of testosterone replacement (100 mg/week) on body composition and strength in seven hypogonadal men aged 19–47 in an open-labelled non-randomised study. By day 15, serum testosterone had increased from 71.9 to 509 ng/ml. After 10 weeks, there was an 8.8 % increase in fat-free mass, an 11% increase in triceps cross-sectional area, and a 7% increase in thigh cross-sectional area. Strength on the bench press increased by 22% and that on the squat exercise by 45%. The caveat from the study of Bhasin et al. [49] is that these men had extremely low testosterone concentrations (mean = 71.9 ng/ml). As described above, the investigators from the Baltimore Longitudinal Study on Aging used a testosterone concentration of < 325 ng/l as the cut off for hypogonadism [46]. Thus, because the testosterone concentration was so low in the study of Bhasin et al. [49], and presumably muscle mass and muscle strength were extremely low, the response of these parameters to the administration of 100 mg testosterone/week may have been greater than that seen in other investigations. Brodsky et al. [50] studied testosterone replacement (3 mg/kg every 2 weeks) in hypogonadal men (total testosterone < 200 ng/ml). They reported a 15% increase in fat-free mass and a 13% increase in appendicular muscle mass. Tenover [51] used a double-blind randomised controlled trial to study the effects of testosterone replacement (100 mg/week; 3 months) in men age 57–76 who had low or borderline low serum testosterone (≤ 13.9 nmol/l; 400 ng/dl). A small (3%) increase in lean body mass and no change in grip strength were reported. In an open-labelled trial without a control group, Urban et al. [52] administered 100 mg of testosterone per week over 4 weeks to elderly men with a serum testosterone concentration of ≤ 480 ng/dl. Significant increases in strength in the hamstrings and quadriceps of both legs were observed. In contrast to the positive benefits observed in most studies, Snyder et al. [53] reported that, despite a 70% increase in testosterone concentration over 36 months in men over the age of 65 (using a testosterone patch), there was no significant improvement in muscle strength despite a significant increase in lean body mass. Thus, from these data it appears that testosterone replacement is likely an effective intervention for reversing sarcopenia. However, whether it is a better and/or safer alternative than resistance training remains to be determined.

## Other Potential Anabolic Interventions to Reverse Sarcopenia

### Other Androgens

#### Dehydroepiandrosterone

Welle et al. [54] reported that the administration of 5.5 mmol dehydroepiandrosterone (DHEA)/day for 4 weeks had no significant effect on body weight or lean body mass, as measured via two methods. Furthermore, there was no effect of DHEA on resting metabolic rate, total energy expenditure, or the rate of incorporation of leucine into muscle protein. Morales et al. [55] gave 50 mg DHEA/day of over 6 months to men and women age 40–70 and found an increase in the bioavailability of IGF-1. In a subsequent study [56], the same authors examined the effects of 6 months of treatment of 100 mg of DHEA to men and women age 50–65 years. In men, there was a 15% increase in knee muscle strength and a 13.9% increase in lumbar back strength but no improvement in women. Flynn et al. [57] administered 100 mg DHEA/day to men age 60–84 for 9 months, but found no significant change in lean body mass or

fat mass. The reason for the discrepancy in results is unknown. However, it appears that the administration of DHEA produces equivocal findings with regard to body composition and muscle strength; it is therefore not recommended as an efficacious treatment for sarcopenia.

### Growth Hormone and IGF-1

There are three studies that compared growth hormone (GH) administration with resistance training (RT) to RT alone. Yarasheski et al. [58] had men with low serum IGF-1 age 67 years complete 16 weeks of resistance training with GH administration or RT alone. They found no differences in the increase in the rate of vastus lateralis protein synthesis or isotonic and isokinetic strength between groups. Fat-free mass increased more in the RT + GH group than the RT group but this was attributed to an increase in non-contractile protein and fluid retention. Hennessey et al. [59] also reported no effect of GH administration with RT relative to RT alone with regard to strength improvements in elderly individuals (age 71.3 years). Strength improved by 55.6% in the GH + RT group and 47.8% in the RT alone group. Of possible importance, however, was the increase in the proportion of type II muscle fibres seen in the RT + GH group, as type II fibre atrophy and loss are observed in older individuals. Lange et al. [60] found no beneficial effect of RT + GH on muscle mass or strength relative to RT alone in individuals 74 years of age. They did find, however, similar to the findings of Hennessey et al. [59], a significant increase in the myosin heavy chain IIx isoform. Thompson et al. [61] reported improvements in indicators of anabolic changes in elderly women given IGF I and/or GH when these substances were administered for 4 weeks. However, there were side effects of these treatments such as joint swelling/pain, headaches, lethargy, and bloatedness. Sullivan et al. [62] studied the effects of combined GH and IGF-1 administration on undernourished frail elderly patients. Due to the many side effects, four out of the 13 subjects had to be withdrawn from the study. Brill et al. [63] examined the administration of testosterone, GH, or a combination of GH + testosterone on muscle strength and functional status (30 m walk time and stair-climbing ability). There were no improvements in isokinetic strength but improvements in the 30-m walk and stair-climbing ability as a result of the experimental treatments were observed. Blackman et al. [64] examined the effects of 26 weeks of testosterone, GH, or a combination of the two on strength and VO$_2$max (a measure of maximal aerobic exercise capacity). While there was a significant increase in muscle strength and VO$_2$max as a result of testosterone and GH administration, many side effects were reported. Svensson et al. [65] reported that 5 years of GH administration led to a persistent increase in isometric, concentric isokinetic knee flexor strength, and grip strength. They did not report any side effects.

These studies, taken together, suggest that GH or IGF-1 administration is of little benefit for increasing muscle mass or strength in elderly individuals. The combination of testosterone replacement and GH administration may be somewhat efficacious, but the side effects associated with GH administration suggest that the potential benefits are not worth the risks.

## Causes of Cachexia in Elderly Individuals

Compounding the effects of sarcopenia in many elderly individuals are disease states or acute illnesses that can lead to accelerated muscle mass loss and a state of cachexia. Acute illness appears to result in the loss of weight and muscle mass very rapidly whereas cachexia caused by chronic disease is a much slower process (unpublished observations). Among the chronic illnesses causing cachexia are chronic heart failure (CHF), chronic obstructive pulmonary disease (COPD), and cancer. The causes of cachexia in CHF appear to be elevations in TNF-α, IL-6, norepinephrine, epinephrine, and cortisol. Furthermore, anabolic stimuli, such as IGF-1 and DHEA, are reduced in CHF patients [66]. A potential causative factor in these humoral changes is tissue hypoxia [66]. In non-obese CHF patients, inadequate energy and protein intake are observed [67]. A common finding of COPD is an increase in resting energy

expenditure. It has been reported that increased levels of IL-6, IL-8, TNF-α, and C-reactive protein are associated with increased resting energy expenditure [68, 69]. However, nutritional interventions to offset the increased resting energy expenditure have been of scarce benefit. Additionally, low levels of circulating IGF and testosterone are also prevalent in COPD [70]. Evidence suggests that elevated proinflammatory cytokines exert their catabolic effects via the ATP-dependent ubiquitin-proteasome pathway for muscle proteolysis [71, 72]. It is also believed that proinflammatory cytokines also act by causing the production of reactive oxidative species in skeletal muscle [73]. It appears, as in CHF, that hypoxaemia is the trigger for the humoral changes observed in COPD, causing increased proinflammatory cytokines, decreased anabolic hormones, and increased reactive oxygen species leading to increased oxidative stress [74]. Also, apoptosis has been implicated in the muscle wasting of COPD [75]. With regard to cancer, it appears that the reduction in food intake is not able to explain all of the weight loss that occurs with cancer [76]. A reduction in protein synthesis due to amino acids being used for synthesis of acute-phase proteins has been suggested [76]. As in CHF and COPD, elevations of proinflammatory cytokines are thought to play a role in the cachexia of cancer [76]. Additionally, with cancer, there is release of lipid mobilising factor and proteolysis-inducing factor from the tumour [76]. Proinflammatory cytokines activate the ATP-dependent ubiquitin-proteasome pathway in COPD [74] and cancer [76] but probably not in CHF [77]. Also, apoptosis in muscle has been shown in CHF [77] and COPD [75]. Proteolysis-inducing factor has also been implicated in muscle apoptosis in cancer [78].

## Treatment of Cachexia Caused by Disease

### Chronic Heart Failure

#### Exercise Training

Gielen et al. [79] reported that 6 months of aerobic exercise training reduced skeletal-muscle TNF-α by 37%, IL-6 by 42%, and IL-1β by 48% in muscle;

inducible nitric oxide synthase was reduced by 52%. These adaptations clearly favour a reduced inflammatory response, which in turn should result in reduced cachexia. Pu et al. [80] examined the effect of 10 weeks of progressive resistance training on muscle-related changes in CHF. They found non-significant trends for increases in type I and type II muscle fibre areas and a 43.4% increase in muscle strength. Although these investigators did not measure intramuscular cytokine or growth factor concentrations, they did see improvements in functional tests, such as a 13% improvement in the 6-min walk test and significant improvements in treadmill exercise time to exhaustion. Thus, it appears that aerobic and resistance exercise are very effective interventions to reduce the effects of cachexia in CHF patients.

## Other Interventions To Reduce Cachexia in Chronic Heart Failure

Anker et al. [81] examined the effects of angiotensin-converting-enzyme (ACE) inhibitors on cachexia in CHF patients. These investigators reported that administration of these agents resulted in a reduction in weight loss in these individuals. The proposed mechanism is that ACE inhibitors increase catecholamine levels and improve endothelial function, such that blood flow to muscle is maintained and apoptosis, tissue damage, and oxidative stress are prevented by reducing ischaemia, and maintaining nutrient delivery to the muscle. Supporting this concept are data from Adigun and Ajayi [82], who found that the combination of enalpril (an ACE inhibitor)-digoxin-diuretic resulted in increased upper-arm and mid-thigh circumferences in individuals with CHF. To our knowledge, there are no studies evaluating nutritional supplementation in CHF.

## Chronic Obstructive Pulmonary Disease

### Testosterone and Anabolic Steroids

Yeh et al. [83] administered oxandrolone (10 mg, twice/day) for 16 weeks to individuals with COPD-induced weight loss. At week 16, they found that seven of 11 subjects had gained weight and the

mean gain in fat-free mass was 3.24 kg. Ferreira et al. [84] administered 250 mg of testosterone at baseline and gave 12 mg of stanozolol a day for 27 weeks. Nine out of 10 subjects that received testosterone/stanozolol gained weight (+ 1.8 kg) while the control group lost 0.4 kg. Lean body mass increased in the treated group as did arm- and thigh-muscle circumference. There was no change, however, in the 6 min walk distance or maximal exercise capacity. Creutzberg [85] administered nandrolone decanoate (ND) every 2 weeks for 8 weeks and found a greater increase in fat-free mass and cellular mass in the ND group, but muscle function, exercise capacity, and health status were similar in the ND and control groups. Thus, it appears from these data that the administration of androgens is efficacious in the treatment of the cachexia caused by COPD.

### Nutritional Support

Saudny-Unterberger [86] administered nutritional support (10 kcal/kg/day) over 2 weeks in COPD patients who were admitted for an exacerbation of their disease. Forced vital capacity increased in the treatment group by 8.7% whereas it decreased by 3.5% in the control group. There were no changes in handgrip strength or respiratory muscle but there was a trend towards an improvement in general well-being. No measures of body weight or fat-free mass were made. Creutzberg et al. [87] characterised the factors that appeared to be related to non-response to a nutritional intervention (extra 500–750 kcal/day) in individuals with COPD. They reported that the systemic inflammatory response (serum TNF-receptor 55, and intracellular adhesion molecule), aging and relative level of anorexia were associated with the non-responsiveness to nutritional intervention. In an 8-week pulmonary rehabilitation program, Creutzberg et al. [88] evaluated the administration of two or three liquid nutritional supplements a day, with a mean intake provided by the supplements of 2812 ± 523 kJ/24 h, on body composition and function in individuals with COPD. An increase in body weight of 2.1 kg and of fat-free mass of 1.1 kg was reported. Handgrip strength increased by 1.2 kg and peak power output on a cycle ergometer increased by 7 Watts. As a part of this study, it was also reported that glucocorticoid treatment reduced the anabolic response to nutritional supplementation. Steiner et al. [89] studied the effects of nutritional supplementation (570 kcal of a carbohydrate-rich supplement/day) and endurance walking on body composition in 85 COPD patients. They reported that individuals who performed endurance walking and received the supplement had no increase in lean body mass but there was an increase in lean body mass in those that received the supplement alone. Weisberg et al. [90] administered 800 mg of the progestational appetite stimulant megestrol acetate to COPD patients. They gained 3.2 kg of body weight but most of it was body fat. Additionally, the weight gain resulted in a reduction in the distance walked in the 6-min walk test. From these studies, it is unclear whether an increase in energy intake alone is adequate to attenuate or reverse cachexia associated with COPD.

### Nutritional Support and Anabolic Steroids

Schols et al. [91] studied 217 patients with COPD over 8 weeks in three groups: nutritional supplementation (420 kcal), nutritional supplementation and anabolic steroids (25 mg ND for women and 50 mg for men biweekly), and placebo. Low-intensity aerobic exercise was performed by all groups. There was a significant increase in arm-muscle circumference in the combined anabolic steroids and nutritional support. Maximal inspiratory mouth pressure increased in both treatment groups in the first 4 weeks but after 8 weeks only the combined treatment group was different from placebo. Thus, it appears that it is efficacious to combine anabolic steroids and nutritional supplementation for the treatment of cachexia related to COPD.

## Miscellaneous Treatments for Cachexia Caused by Aging, CHF, and COPD

### Omega-3 Fatty Acids

High doses of the omega-3 fatty acid eicosapentaenoic acid (EPA), in combination with energy supplementation, have been shown to be beneficial in attenuating the weight loss associated with pancreatic cancer [92, 93]. This appears to occur by an inhibition of the ATP-dependent ubiquitin pathway for muscle proteolysis [94] and by decreasing the increase in resting energy expenditure induced by the acute-phase response [95]. However, there have been no trials of EPA in treating the weight loss associated with aging, CHF, or COPD.

### Thalidomide

TNF-$\alpha$ plays a significant role in many chronic inflammatory diseases and thalidomide acts to reduce concentrations of TNF-$\alpha$ by degrading the TNF-$\alpha$ mRNA [96]. Thalidomide has been shown to be successful in the treatment of cachexia associated with HIV infection [97, 98]. There is one report of thalidomide use in CHF [99]. In that study, CHF patients were given 200 mg of thalidomide for 6 weeks. Plasma TNF-$\alpha$ concentrations were reduced by 43% and left ventricular ejection fraction increased by 31% in these patients. Thus, thalidomide would appear promising as an anti-cachectic agent. No trials have been reported to date using thalidomide to treat COPD or age-related cachexia.

### Etanercept

Etanercept (Enbrel) is fusion protein that reduces the bioactivity of TNF-$\alpha$. It has been used effectively and safely to reduce the disease progression of rheumatoid arthritis [100]. Two studies in CHF patients (RENAISSANCE and RECOVER [101]) examining the efficacy of etanercept have been conducted. Both found no beneficial effect of this drug. Studies have not been conducted with this drug in COPD or age-related cachexia.

### Pentoxifylline

This drug has been used routinely in treating peripheral vascular disease [102] and acts to reduce TNF gene transcription [103]. More recent data [104] suggest that pentoxifylline ultimately reduces whole-body proteolysis in chronically uraemic patients. It has also been shown to improve pulmonary gas exchange in COPD patients but its effect on cachexia in these patients is unknown. Furthermore, there have been no clinical trials evaluating this agent in CHF or aging.

## Creatine

Creatine is an amin oacid derivative found in relatively large quantities in meat. It has been used in the last ~10 years to improve exercise capacity in tasks that are brief but of high-intensity. Creatine acts to increase muscle phosphocreatine levels [105] and may increase the rate of phosphocreatine resynthesis [106]; both of these effects result in improved, brief, high-intensity, intermittent exercise capacity [105]. Additionally, a combination of creatine ingestion and resistance exercise training has been shown to result in greater muscle-mass gains than resistance training alone in young individuals [107]. Creatine administration has been combined with resistance training in the elderly, with one investigation finding no effect [108] and others finding improvements in lean body mass and strength [109, 110]. Thus, further investigation as to the potential anabolic actions of creatine and resistance training in older adults is warranted.

There is one report of creatine supplementation being used in patients with heart failure. Andrews et al. [111] reported that creatine ingestion by such patients significantly increased muscle endurance. Whether or not long-term creatine ingestion combined with resistance training attenuates cachexia in CHF requires further investigation. No studies have been carried out to examine the effects of creatine administration in COPD.

## N-Acetylcysteine

This non-specific antioxidant has been shown to delay fatigue in humans by reducing oxidative stress [112], but other studies have found no effect [113, 114]. A recent report, however, suggests that N-acetylcysteine can decrease the circulating TNF-α concentration and augment strength gains in elderly individuals [115]. There have been no reports of using this antioxidant in CHF or COPD but, because these conditions are considered to be inflammatory in nature and inflammatory conditions cause the production of reactive oxygen species, N-acetylcysteine may be a therapeutic option.

## Conclusions

Sarcopenia, or the age-related loss of muscle mass, is a consequence of normal aging. This process, however, may be attenuated and possibly reversed by resistance training and/or androgen replacement. Adequate protein intake and energy intake may also be useful in the attenuation of sarcopenia. Cachexia, the loss of weight and muscle mass as a result of disease, can be the result of acute illness or chronic diseases such as CHF, COPD, or cancer. Cachexia may be attenuated by aerobic or resistance exercise training, anabolic drugs, nutritional energy supplementation, various anti-cytokine drugs, or anti-catabolic/anabolic nutritional supplements. Clearly further research is warranted in the treatment of sarcopenia and cachexia.

## References

1. MedicineNet.com, vol 2004
2. Rosenberg IH (1989) Summary comments. Am J Clin Nutr 50:1231–1233
3. Fried LP, Tangen CM, Walston J et al (2001) Frailty in older adults: evidence for a phenotype. J Gerontol A Biol Sci Med Sci 56:M146–M156
4. Morales A, Heaton JP, Carson CC 3rd (2000) Andropause: a misnomer for a true clinical entity. J Urol 163:705–712
5. Volpi E, Sheffield-Moore M, Rasmussen BB, Wolfe RR (2001) Basal muscle amino acid kinetics and protein synthesis in healthy young and older men. JAMA 286:1206–1212
6. Welle S, Thornton C, Jozefowicz R, Statt M (1993) Myofibrillar protein synthesis in young and old men. Am J Physiol 264:E693–E698
7. Welle S, Thornton C, Statt M (1995) Myofibrillar protein synthesis in young and old human subjects after three months of resistance training. Am J Physiol 268:E422–E427
8. Balagopal P, Rooyackers OE, Adey DB et al (1997) Effects of aging on in vivo synthesis of skeletal muscle myosin heavy-chain and sarcoplasmic protein in humans. Am J Physiol 273:E790–E800

9. Hasten DL, Pak-Loduca J, Obert KA, Yarasheski KE (2000) Resistance exercise acutely increases MHC and mixed muscle protein synthesis rates in 78–84 and 23–32 yr olds. Am J Physiol Endocrinol Metab 278:E620–E626

10. Yarasheski KE, Zachwieja JJ, Bier DM (1993) Acute effects of resistance exercise on muscle protein synthesis rate in young and elderly men and women. Am J Physiol 265:E210–E214

11. Trappe T, Williams R, Carrithers J et al (2004) Influence of age and resistance exercise on human skeletal muscle proteolysis: a microdialysis approach. J Physiol 554:803–813

12. Doherty TJ, Vandervoort AA, Taylor AW, Brown WF (1993) Effects of motor unit losses on strength in older men and women. J Appl Physiol 74:868–874

13. Goldspink DF (1976) The effects of denervation on protein turnover of rat skeletal muscle. Biochem J 156:71–80

14. Medina R, Wing SS, Goldberg AL (1995) Increase in levels of polyubiquitin and proteasome mRNA in skeletal muscle during starvation and denervation atrophy. Biochem J 307:631–637

15. Mauras N, Hayes V, Welch S et al (1998) Testosterone deficiency in young men: marked alterations in whole body protein kinetics, strength, and adiposity. J Clin Endocrinol Metab 83:1886–1892

16. Melton LJ, 3rd, Khosla S, Riggs BL (2000) Epidemiology of sarcopenia. Mayo Clin Proc 75:S10–S12; discussion S12–S13

17. Perry HM 3rd, Miller DK, Patrick P, Morley JE (2000) Testosterone and leptin in older African-American men: relationship to age, strength, function, and season. Metabolism 49:1085–1091

18. Baumgartner RN, Waters DL, Gallagher D et al (1999) Predictors of skeletal muscle mass in elderly men and women. Mech Ageing Dev 107:123–136

19. Iannuzzi-Sucich M, Prestwood KM, Kenny AM (2002) Prevalence of sarcopenia and predictors of skeletal muscle mass in healthy, older men and women. J Gerontol A Biol Sci Med Sci 57:M772–M777

20. Iranmanesh A, Lizarralde G, Veldhuis JD (1991) Age and relative adiposity are specific negative determinants of the frequency and amplitude of growth hormone (GH) secretory bursts and the half-life of endogenous GH in healthy men. J Clin Endocrinol Metab 73:1081–1088

21. Veldhuis JD, Liem AY, South S et al (1995) Differential impact of age, sex steroid hormones, and obesity on basal versus pulsatile growth hormone secretion in men as assessed in an ultrasensitive chemiluminescence assay. J Clin Endocrinol Metab 80:3209–3222

22. Veldhuis JD, Iranmanesh A, Weltman A (1997) Elements in the pathophysiology of diminished growth hormone (GH) secretion in aging humans. Endocrine 7:41–48

23. Corpas E, Harman SM, Blackman MR (1993) Human growth hormone and human aging. Endocr Rev 14:20–39

24. Roubenoff R, Harris TB, Abad LW et al (1998) Monocyte cytokine production in an elderly population: effect of age and inflammation. J Gerontol A Biol Sci Med Sci 53:M20–M26

25. Visser M, Pahor M, Taaffe DR et al (2002) Relationship of interleukin-6 and tumor necrosis factor-alpha with muscle mass and muscle strength in elderly men and women: the Health ABC Study. J Gerontol A Biol Sci Med Sci 57:M326–M332

26. Greiwe JS, Cheng B, Rubin DC et al (2001) Resistance exercise decreases skeletal muscle tumor necrosis factor alpha in frail elderly humans. FASEB J 15:475–482

27. Barbieri M, Ferrucci L, Ragno E et al (2003) Chronic inflammation and the effect of IGF-1 on muscle strength and power in older persons. Am J Physiol Endocrinol Metab 284:E481–E487

28. Payette H, Roubenoff R, Jacques PF et al (2003) Insulin-like growth factor-1 and interleukin 6 predict sarcopenia in very old community-living men and women: the Framingham Heart Study. J Am Geriatr Soc 51:1237–1243

29. Campbell WW, Trappe TA, Wolfe RR, Evans WJ (2001) The recommended dietary allowance for protein may not be adequate for older people to maintain skeletal muscle. J Gerontol A Biol Sci Med Sci 56:M373–M380

30. Brodsky IG, Suzara D, Hornberger TA et al (2004) Isoenergetic dietary protein restriction decreases myosin heavy chain IIx fraction and myosin heavy chain production in humans. J Nutr 134:328–334

31. Roubenoff R, Hughes VA (2000) Sarcopenia: current concepts. J Gerontol A Biol Sci Med Sci 55:M716–M724

32. Weimer J (1998) Factors Affecting Nutrient Intake of the Elderly. Washington, D.C., US Department of Agriculture, Economic Research Service, Economic Research Service

33. Hughes VA, Frontera WR, Roubenoff R et al (2002) Longitudinal changes in body composition in older men and women: role of body weight change and physical activity. Am J Clin Nutr 76:473–481

34. Leeuwenburgh C (2003) Role of apoptosis in sarcopenia. J Gerontol A Biol Sci Med Sci 58:999–1001

35. Pollack M, Phaneuf S, Dirks A, Leeuwenburgh C (2002) The role of apoptosis in the normal aging brain, skeletal muscle, and heart. Ann N Y Acad Sci 959:93–107

36. Dirks A, Leeuwenburgh C (2002) Apoptosis in skeletal muscle with aging. Am J Physiol Regul Integr Comp Physiol 282:R519–R527

37. Moritani T, deVries HA (1980) Potential for gross muscle hypertrophy in older men. J Gerontol 35:672–682

38. Ivey FM, Roth SM, Ferrell RE et al (2000) Effects of age, gender, and myostatin genotype on the hypertrophic response to heavy resistance strength trai-

ning. J Gerontol A Biol Sci Med Sci 55:M641–M648

39. Flynn MG, Fahlman M, Braun WA et al (1999) Effects of resistance training on selected indexes of immune function in elderly women. J Appl Physiol 86:1905–1913

40. Frontera WR, Meredith CN, O'Reilly KP et al (1988) Strength conditioning in older men: skeletal muscle hypertrophy and improved function. J Appl Physiol 64:1038–1044

41. Harridge SD, Kryger A, Stensgaard A (1999) Knee extensor strength, activation, and size in very elderly people following strength training. Muscle Nerve 22:831–839

42. Trappe S, Williamson D, Godard M et al (2000) Effect of resistance training on single muscle fiber contractile function in older men. J Appl Physiol 89:143–152

43. Lambert CP, Evans WJ (2002) Effects of aging and resistance exercise on determinants of muscle strength. Journal of the American Aging Association 25:73–78

44. Sale DG (1988) Neural adaptation to resistance training. Med Sci Sports Exerc 20:S135–S145

45. Trappe S, Williamson D, Godard M (2002) Maintenance of whole muscle strength and size following resistance training in older men. J Gerontol A Biol Sci Med Sci 57:B138–B143

46. Harman SM, Metter EJ, Tobin JD et al (2001) Longitudinal effects of aging on serum total and free testosterone levels in healthy men. Baltimore Longitudinal Study of Aging. J Clin Endocrinol Metab 86:724–731

47. Morley JE, Perry HM, 3rd, Kaiser FE et al (1993) Effects of testosterone replacement therapy in old hypogonadal males: a preliminary study. J Am Geriatr Soc 41:149–152

48. Sih R, Morley JE, Kaiser FE et al (1997) Testosterone replacement in older hypogonadal men: a 12-month randomized controlled trial. J Clin Endocrinol Metab 82:1661–1667

49. Bhasin S, Storer TW, Berman N et al (1997) Testosterone replacement increases fat-free mass and muscle size in hypogonadal men. J Clin Endocrinol Metab 82:407–413

50. Brodsky IG, Balagopal P, Nair KS (1996) Effects of testosterone replacement on muscle mass and muscle protein synthesis in hypogonadal men - a clinical research center study. J Clin Endocrinol Metab 81:3469–3475

51. Tenover JS (1992) Effects of testosterone supplementation in the aging male. J Clin Endocrinol Metab 75:1092–1098

52. Urban RJ, Bodenburg YH, Gilkison C et al (1995) Testosterone administration to elderly men increases skeletal muscle strength and protein synthesis. Am J Physiol 269:E820–E826

53. Snyder PJ, Peachey H, Hannoush P et al (1999) Effect of testosterone treatment on body composition and muscle strength in men over 65 years of age. J Clin

Endocrinol Metab 84:2647–2653

54. Welle S, Jozefowicz R, Statt M (1990) Failure of dehydroepiandrosterone to influence energy and protein metabolism in humans. J Clin Endocrinol Metab 71:1259–1264

55. Morales AJ, Nolan JJ, Nelson JC, Yen SS (1994) Effects of replacement dose of dehydroepiandrosterone in men and women of advancing age. J Clin Endocrinol Metab 78:1360–1367

56. Morales AJ, Haubrich RH, Hwang JY et al (1998) The effect of six months treatment with a 100 mg daily dose of dehydroepiandrosterone (DHEA) on circulating sex steroids, body composition and muscle strength in age-advanced men and women. Clin Endocrinol (Oxf) 49:421–432

57. Flynn MA, Weaver-Osterholtz D, Sharpe-Timms KL et al (1999) Dehydroepiandrosterone replacement in aging humans. J Clin Endocrinol Metab 84:1527–1533

58. Yarasheski KE, Zachwieja JJ, Campbell JA, Bier DM (1995) Effect of growth hormone and resistance exercise on muscle growth and strength in older men. Am J Physiol 268:E268–E276

59. Hennessey JV, Chromiak JA, DellaVentura S et al (2001) Growth hormone administration and exercise effects on muscle fiber type and diameter in moderately frail older people. J Am Geriatr Soc 49:852–858

60. Lange KH, Andersen JL, Beyer N et al (2002) GH administration changes myosin heavy chain isoforms in skeletal muscle but does not augment muscle strength or hypertrophy, either alone or combined with resistance exercise training in healthy elderly men. J Clin Endocrinol Metab 87:513–523

61. Thompson JL, Butterfield GE, Marcus R et al (1995) The effects of recombinant human insulin-like growth factor-I and growth hormone on body composition in elderly women. J Clin Endocrinol Metab 80:1845–1852

62. Sullivan DH, Carter WJ, Warr WR, Williams LH (1998) Side effects resulting from the use of growth hormone and insulin-like growth factor-I as combined therapy to frail elderly patients. J Gerontol A Biol Sci Med Sci 53:M183–M187

63. Brill KT, Weltman AL, Gentili A et al (2002) Single and combined effects of growth hormone and testosterone administration on measures of body composition, physical performance, mood, sexual function, bone turnover, and muscle gene expression in healthy older men. J Clin Endocrinol Metab 87:5649–5657

64. Blackman MR, Sorkin JD, Munzer T et al (2002) Growth hormone and sex steroid administration in healthy aged women and men: a randomized controlled trial. JAMA 288:2282–2292

65. Svensson J, Stibrant Sunnerhagen K, Johannsson G (2003) Five years of growth hormone replacement therapy in adults: age- and gender-related changes

in isometric and isokinetic muscle strength. J Clin Endocrinol Metab 88:2061–2069

66. Anker SD, Sharma R (2002) The syndrome of cardiac cachexia. Int J Cardiol 85:51–66

67. Aquilani R, Opasich C, Verri M et al (2003) Is nutritional intake adequate in chronic heart failure patients? J Am Coll Cardiol 42:1218–1223

68. Di Francia M, Barbier D, Mege JL, Orehek J (1994) Tumor necrosis factor-alpha levels and weight loss in chronic obstructive pulmonary disease. Am J Respir Crit Care Med 150:1453–1455

69. Schols AM, Buurman WA, Staal van den Brekel AJ et al (1996) Evidence for a relation between metabolic derangements and increased levels of inflammatory mediators in a subgroup of patients with chronic obstructive pulmonary disease. Thorax 51:819–824

70. Creutzberg EC, Casaburi R (2003) Endocrinological disturbances in chronic obstructive pulmonary disease. Eur Respir J Suppl 46:76s–80s

71. Chai J, Wu Y, Sheng ZZ (2003) Role of ubiquitin-proteasome pathway in skeletal muscle wasting in rats with endotoxemia. Crit Care Med 31:1802–1807

72. Llovera M, Carbo N, Lopez-Soriano J et al (1998) Different cytokines modulate ubiquitin gene expression in rat skeletal muscle. Cancer Lett 133:83–87

73. Reid MB, Li YP (2001) Tumor necrosis factor-alpha and muscle wasting: a cellular perspective. Respir Res 2:269–272

74. Debigare R, Cote CH, Maltais F (2001) Peripheral muscle wasting in chronic obstructive pulmonary disease. Clinical relevance and mechanisms. Am J Respir Crit Care Med 164:1712–1717

75. Agusti AG, Sauleda J, Miralles C et al (2002) Skeletal muscle apoptosis and weight loss in chronic obstructive pulmonary disease. Am J Respir Crit Care Med 166:485–489

76. Tisdale MJ (2002) Cachexia in cancer patients. Nat Rev Cancer 2:862–871

77. Libera LD, Zennaro R, Sandri M et al (1999) Apoptosis and atrophy in rat slow skeletal muscles in chronic heart failure. Am J Physiol 277:C982–C986

78. Smith HJ, Tisdale MJ (2003) Induction of apoptosis by a cachectic-factor in murine myotubes and inhibition by eicosapentaenoic acid. Apoptosis 8:161–169

79. Gielen S, Adams V, Mobius-Winkler S et al (2003) Anti-inflammatory effects of exercise training in the skeletal muscle of patients with chronic heart failure. J Am Coll Cardiol 42:861–868

80. Pu CT, Johnson MT, Forman DE et al (2001) Randomized trial of progressive resistance training to counteract the myopathy of chronic heart failure. J Appl Physiol 90: 2341–2350

81. Anker SD, Negassa A, Coats AJ et al (2003) Prognostic importance of weight loss in chronic heart failure and the effect of treatment with angiotensin-converting-enzyme inhibitors: an observational study. Lancet 361:1077–1083

82. Adigun AQ, Ajayi AA (2001) The effects of enalapril-digoxin-diuretic combination therapy on nutritional and anthropometric indices in chronic congestive heart failure: preliminary findings in cardiac cachexia. Eur J Heart Fail 3:359–363

83. Yeh SS, Hafner A, Schuster MW et al (2003) Relationship between body composition and cytokines in cachectic patients with chronic obstructive pulmonary disease. J Am Geriatr Soc 51:890–891

84. Ferreira IM, Verreschi IT, Nery LE et al (1998) The influence of 6 months of oral anabolic steroids on body mass and respiratory muscles in undernourished COPD patients. Chest 114:19–28

85. Creutzberg EC, Wouters EF, Mostert R et al (2003) A role for anabolic steroids in the rehabilitation of patients with COPD? A double-blind, placebo-controlled, randomized trial. Chest 124:1733–1742

86. Saudny-Unterberger H, Martin JG, Gray-Donald K (1997) Impact of nutritional support on functional status during an acute exacerbation of chronic obstructive pulmonary disease. Am J Respir Crit Care Med 156:794–799

87. Creutzberg EC, Schols AM, Weling-Scheepers CA et al (2000) Characterization of nonresponse to high caloric oral nutritional therapy in depleted patients with chronic obstructive pulmonary disease. Am J Respir Crit Care Med 161:745–752

88. Creutzberg EC, Wouters EF, Mostert R et al (2003) Efficacy of nutritional supplementation therapy in depleted patients with chronic obstructive pulmonary disease. Nutrition 19:120–127

89. Steiner MC, Barton RL, Singh SJ, Morgan MD (2003) Nutritional enhancement of exercise performance in chronic obstructive pulmonary disease: a randomised controlled trial. Thorax 58:745–751

90. Weisberg J, Wanger J, Olson J et al (2002) Megestrol acetate stimulates weight gain and ventilation in underweight COPD patients. Chest 121:1070–1078

91. Schols AM, Soeters PB, Mostert R et al (1995) Physiologic effects of nutritional support and anabolic steroids in patients with chronic obstructive pulmonary disease. A placebo-controlled randomized trial. Am J Respir Crit Care Med 152:1268–1274

92. Barber MD, Ross JA, Voss AC et al (1999) The effect of an oral nutritional supplement enriched with fish oil on weight-loss in patients with pancreatic cancer. Br J Cancer 81:80–86

93. Fearon KC, Von Meyenfeldt MF, Moses AG et al (2003) Effect of a protein and energy dense N-3 fatty acid enriched oral supplement on loss of weight and lean tissue in cancer cachexia: a randomised double blind trial. 52:1479–1486

94. Whitehouse AS, Smith HJ, Drake JL, Tisdale MJ (2001) Mechanism of attenuation of skeletal muscle protein catabolism in cancer cachexia by eicosapentaenoic acid. Cancer Res 61:3604–3609

95. Wigmore SJ, Ross JA, Falconer JS et al (1996) The effect of polyunsaturated fatty acids on the progress of cachexia in patients with pancreatic cancer.

Nutrition 12:S27–S30

96. Calabrese L, Fleischer AB (2000) Thalidomide: current and potential clinical applications. Am J Med 108:487–495

97. Haslett P, Hempstead M, Seidman C et al (1997) The metabolic and immunologic effects of short-term thalidomide treatment of patients infected with the human immunodeficiency virus. AIDS Res Hum Retroviruses 13:1047–1054

98. Reyes-Teran G, Sierra-Madero JG, Martinez del Cerro V et al (1996) Effects of thalidomide on HIV-associated wasting syndrome: a randomized, double-blind, placebo-controlled clinical trial. AIDS 10:1501–1507

99. Gullestad L, Semb AG, Holt E et al (2002) Effect of thalidomide in patients with chronic heart failure. Am Heart J 144:847–850

100. Bathon JM, Genovese MC (2003) The Early Rheumatoid Arthritis (ERA) trial comparing the efficacy and safety of etanercept and methotrexate. Clin Exp Rheumatol 21:S195–S197

101. Anker SD, Coats AJ (2002) How to RECOVER from RENAISSANCE? The significance of the results of RECOVER, RENAISSANCE, RENEWAL and ATTACH. Int J Cardiol 86:123–130

102. Frampton JE, Brogden RN (1995) Pentoxifylline (oxpentifylline). A review of its therapeutic efficacy in the management of peripheral vascular and cerebrovascular disorders. Drugs Aging 7:480–503

103. Doherty GM, Jensen JC, Alexander HR et al (1991) Pentoxifylline suppression of tumor necrosis factor gene transcription. Surgery 110:192–198

104. Biolo G, Ciocchi B, Bosutti A et al (2002) Pentoxifylline acutely reduces protein catabolism in chronically uremic patients. Am J Kidney Dis 40:1162–1172

105. Casey A, Constantin-Teodosiu D, Howell S et al (1996) Creatine ingestion favorably affects performance and muscle metabolism during maximal exercise in humans. Am J Physiol 271:E31–E37

106. Greenhaff PL, Bodin K, Soderlund K, Hultman E (1994) Effect of oral creatine supplementation on skeletal muscle phosphocreatine resynthesis. Am J Physiol 266:E725–E730

107. Volek JS, Duncan ND, Mazzetti SA et al (1999) Performance and muscle fiber adaptations to creatine supplementation and heavy resistance training. Med Sci Sports Exerc 31:1147–1156

108. Bermon S, Venembre P, Sachet C et al (1998) Effects of creatine monohydrate ingestion in sedentary and weight-trained older adults. Acta Physiol Scand 164:147–155

109. Brose A, Parise G, Tarnopolsky MA (2003) Creatine supplementation enhances isometric strength and body composition improvements following strength exercise training in older adults. J Gerontol A Biol Sci Med Sci 58:11–19

110. Chrusch MJ, Chilibeck PD, Chad KE et al (2001) Creatine supplementation combined with resistance training in older men. Med Sci Sports Exerc 33:2111–2117

111. Andrews R, Greenhaff P, Curtis S et al (1998) The effect of dietary creatine supplementation on skeletal muscle metabolism in congestive heart failure. Eur Heart J 19:617–622

112. Reid MB, Stokic DS, Koch SM et al (1994) N-acetylcysteine inhibits muscle fatigue in humans. J Clin Invest 94:2468–2474

113. Medved I, Brown MJ, Bjorksten AR et al (2003) N-acetylcysteine infusion alters blood redox status but not time to fatigue during intense exercise in humans. J Appl Physiol 94:1572–1582

114. Medved I, Brown MJ, Bjorksten AR, McKenna MJ (2004) Effects of intravenous N-acetylcysteine infusion on time to fatigue and potassium regulation during prolonged cycling exercise. J Appl Physiol 96:211–217

115. Hauer K, Hildebrandt W, Sehl Y et al (2003) Improvement in muscular performance and decrease in tumor necrosis factor level in old age after antioxidant treatment. J Mol Med 81:118–125

# Management of Weight Loss in Older Persons

Osama QuBaiah, John E. Morley

## Introduction

The causes of significant weight loss in older persons are: (1) anorexia/starvation, (2) sarcopenia, (3) cachexia, and (4) dehydration. Thus, the first step in management of weight loss is to make the diagnosis. Depression, which is the most common cause of weight loss in older persons [1, 2], can be treated with antidepressants, which can also reverse weight loss, but monoamine oxidase inhibitors and mirtazapine (Remeron) appear to have specific orexigenic effects. The management of cachexia in older persons is extraordinarily complex, and involves both treatment of the underlying disease and specific nutritional therapy. Similarly, severe anorexia, often due to cytokine excess, must be treated.

When older persons lose weight, simple approaches like making sure that they can carry out activities of daily living, such as shopping, food preparation, and feeding, are the basic starting point for appropriate management. Other strategies to increase food intake by the elderly include the use of taste enhancers [3], eating with a companion [4], and, in nursing homes, enhancing the environment [5].

Specific treatments for conditions causing weight loss are given in Table 1. In persons with sarcopenia, resistance exercise is the treatment of choice. Testosterone increases muscle mass and strength in older men with sarcopenia [6, 7]. It should be recognised that in older persons a ratio of blood urea nitrogen (BUN) to creatinine greater than 10:1 commonly occurs due to bleeding from the gut, renal deterioration, and congestive heart failure. Therefore, the BUN:creatinine ratio is a poor measurement of dehydration in older persons.

Older persons with weight loss should receive a multivitamin supplement. In a meta-analysis by the Cochrane Collaboration [8], caloric supplementation was shown to produce a small increase in weight and to decrease mortality. When caloric supplements are given between meals, the total number of calories ingested is higher than in the absence of such supplements [9].

**Table 1.** Specific treatments for conditions causing weight loss in older persons

| Condition | Treatment |
| --- | --- |
| Depression | Antidepressants or electroconvulsive therapy |
| Late-life paranoia | Low-dose anti-psychotics |
| Dysphagia | Consider altered consistency of food, but remember that this may decrease quality of life; enteral feeding |
| Hypercalcaemia | Consider hyperparathyroidism |
| Hyperthyroidism | Radioactive iodine |
| Bacterial overgrowth | Antibiotics |
| *C. difficile* diarrhoea | Mitronidazole or antibiotics |
| *Helicobacter pylori* | Antibiotics plus protonics |
| Pancreatic insufficiency | Enzyme replacement |
| Pheochromocytoma | Surgery |

## Enteral Feeding

In general there are three indications for enteral feeding [10]: (1) patients with neuromuscular disease may have impaired swallowing or gag reflexes; (2) patients with hypermetabolic states, such as those induced by cancer or cachexia, may be unable to meet their nutritional needs by eating alone; (3) patients who are unable to eat, such as those who are ventilator-dependent, postoperative, or have tumours of the upper gastrointestinal tract.

In the elderly, the most common indication for enteral feeding is dysphagia with frequent aspiration. The only absolute contraindication to enteral feeding is mechanical obstruction of the gut. Enteral feeding is preferred over parenteral feeding because it maintains the functional and structural integrity of the gastrointestinal tract, is more physiological, easier to use, and costs less. There is controversy over whether enteral nutrition improves the outcome of older persons with dementia who are losing weight [11–15].

There are three approaches to use enteral feeding. The first and most common is to use enteral feeding as the sole source of nutrition. A second approach is to use it to supplement oral intake, and the third is to combine enteral and parenteral nutrition.

Access to the gut can be achieved by nasogastric, nasointestinal, percutaneous gastric, or percutaneous jejunal routes. Percutaneous gastrostomy is the preferred route when enteral feeding is expected to last longer than four weeks. Nasogastric tubes are not preferred over the long run because they are uncomfortable. Longer tubes that cross the pylorus into the duodenum or jejunum offer few advantages for reducing complications or improving nutrition. These tubes obviate the advantage of the stomach as a reservoir, require an infusion pump, and are frequently dislodged. Most oral medications cannot be used with percutaneous jejunal tubes, which are usually surgically inserted at the time of laparotomy. They are often used when upper gastrointestinal problems exist, or in patients in whom aspiration is a major problem.

Feedings can be administered intermittently or continuously. Intermittent feedings are more convenient for the nursing staff, do not require infusion pumps, permit more patient mobility, better simulate normal eating patterns with fasting periods, and may be more physiological [16]. Disadvantages include diarrhoea, vomiting, and possibly a higher risk of aspiration pneumonia. The average volume of intermittent feedings should be between 240 and 400 ml. The gastric residual should be checked before each feeding, and if greater than 200 ml for a nasogastric tube or 100 ml for a gastrostomy tube, the patient should be monitored closely. If a patient has not been fed in the last five days, feedings should begin as low-volume, continuous flow at a rate of 25–50 ml/h. Residual volume in the stomach should be monitored every 2–4 h, and feeding halted if the residual volume exceeds 1.5 times the hourly rate. When caloric needs have been met, feedings can be switched to intermittent.

## Complications of Enteral Feeding

In the largest study, the overall complication rate was 11.7% [17]. Of these, 6.2% were gastrointestinal, 3.5% were mechanical, and 2 % were metabolic.

## Mechanical Complications

Nasogastric tubes carry a higher risk of self-extubation and patient discomfort. Mechanical displacement of a gastrostomy tube may also occur. The tube can only be replaced 3 weeks or longer after the original placement, as the tract is still immature before that. An attempt at replacement can be made within 6–12 h after the event, but otherwise the patient should be referred to a specialist. Mechanical clogging has only been observed with the use of premixed formulas (e.g. Pulmocare, Ensure, Ensure Plus, Osmolite, and Enrich).

## Pulmonary Complications

A previous study found that 19% of nasogastric tube placements were not in the stomach or duodenum [18]. In elderly patients and in patients without an intact gag reflex, pneumothorax, pleural penetration, empyema, and bronchopleural fistula may occur. The placement of the tube should not be determined by insufflation over the stomach as this is frequently misleading; instead, placement should be confirmed radiologically.

Aspiration is the most serious pulmonary complication of tube feedings. As many as 40% of deaths associated with tube feedings result directly from aspiration pneumonia [19, 20]. Risk factors for aspiration include diabetes, pancreatitis, vagotomy, malnutrition, decreased gag reflex, a change in the level of consciousness, and gastric retention. Gastric retention can be treated with a low-fat formula or a prokinetic agent, such as metoclopramide. Formula-associated risks include high-nutrient-density formulas [21], hypo- and hyperosmolar solutions [22], and cold formulas. With long-term use, aspiration occurs in 44% of patients with nasogastric tubes and in 56% of patients with gastrostomy tubes. Duodenally placed tubes are not better than gastrostomy tubes. Jejunal tubes placed distal to the ligament of Treitz are not generally thought to prevent aspiration. One study that reviewed the literature regarding the use of enteral feeding to prevent aspiration concluded that there is no evidence to support that approach in a conscious patient with neurological dysphagia [23, 24]. The authors of the review suggested using tube feedings only in patients with recurrent pneumonia, with extremely uncomfortable cough during meals, or with an impaired level of consciousness.

## Gastrointestinal Complications

Diarrhoea was the most frequently reported gastrointestinal complication, but there are conflicting explanations as to its cause. Osmolarity, rate of delivery, $H_2$ blockers, antibiotics, and fibre content have all been suggested. The association between $H_2$ blockers and diarrhoea might be due to the development of bacterial overgrowth when the gastric pH exceeds 4. Sorbitol-containing drugs are often overlooked as a cause of diarrhoea. When significant diarrhoea occurs *Clostridium difficile* colitis should be ruled out first. Several studies

have shown that there is no effect when the osmolarity is varied between 145 and 430 mOsm [25] or when the formula composition is changed [26].

## Metabolic Complications

Hyperglycaemia, hypercapnia, electrolyte abnormalities, and re-feeding syndrome are metabolic complications that can occur with enteral feeding. Complications are seen more often in diabetics and in patients receiving formulas with high caloric density. In diabetics, the use of hyperosmolar formulas can lead to hyperosmolar nonketotic coma. High carbohydrate concentrations may increase respiratory quotients and increase carbon dioxide production. Re-feeding syndrome is characterised by dehydration, hypernatraemia, hyperchloraemia, and azotaemia. Its most common cause is the use of high-protein formulas with low water intake. This syndrome is seen among severely malnourished patients, such as alcoholics, when potassium and phosphorus requirements are high because of the intracellular shift that occurs when nutrients are replenished.

## Parenteral Feeding

Parenteral feeding may be helpful during acute hospital admissions in older persons. Often, only a small number of calories are ingested by the elderly during hospitalisation, either due to the underlying disease or to medical interventions. We have found peripheral parenteral nutrition to be a particularly useful method to supplement calories, and with minimal side effects. In malnourished older persons, parenteral vitamin supplements may decrease delirium. Nonetheless, in general, providing calories through the gut is preferable to using parenteral feeding, except for very short periods of time.

## Orexigenics

Numerous appetite stimulants have been used in older persons. There is no evidence that cyproheptadine can enhance appetite. Dronabinol (a synthetic tetrahydrocannabinol) produces an increase in hunger and possibly a mild increase in weight gain in older persons [27]. Because of its analgesic and anti-nausea properties and the general feeling of well being it produces, dronabinol is an excellent drug for palliative care.

**Table 2.** Orexigenics available for management of anorexia

---

Megestrol acetate or medroxyprogesterone

Dronabinol

Oxoglutarate

Cyproheptadine

Anabolic steroids, e.g., nandrolone, testosterone, oxandrolone

---

The use of anabolic steroids in older persons is controversial. Testosterone enhances muscle mass, but there are no controlled trials on the use of anabolic steroids, such as oxandrolone, by older persons. Moreover, anabolic steroids can cause liver dysfunction.

Megestrol acetate or medroxyprogesterone acetate are the orexigenic drugs of choice. Megestrol produces weight gain in older persons [28, 29], most likely by cytokine inhibition [29]. We recommend its use in all persons with elevated C-reactive protein. The major side effects of megestrol are a small increase in the incidence of deep-vein thrombosis, a decline in cortisol production, and male hypogonadism.

An overview of orexigenic treatment for the elderly is given in Table 2. Table 3 lists anticytokine agents that may be useful to treat cachexia.

**Table 3.** Anticytokine agents

---

Progestagens

Thalidomide

Pentoxiphylline

NSAIDs

Eicosapentaenoic acid

Cytokine antibodies

Soluble cytokine receptors

---

*NSAIDs*, non-steroidal anti-inflammatory drugs

## Conclusions

As weight loss is a marker for mortality in older persons, aggressive treatment is essential. Tables 4 and 5 review our guidelines for the treatment of weight loss in nursing home residents [30]. There is a need for controlled trials to more clearly delineate the appropriate management of weight loss in the elderly.

**Table 4.** Clinical guide to prevent and manage malnutrition in long-term care. The information in this table is aimed at nursing staff, dietary staff. and dietitians, and follows the strategy evaluate, document, and treat

# Clinical Guide to Prevent and Manage Malnutrition in Long-Term Care

## FOR NURSING STAFF AND DIETARY STAFF AND DIETITIANS (EVALUATE, DOCUMENT AND TREAT)

*The American Dietetic Association supports the Clinical Guide to Prevent and Manage Malnutrition in Long-Term Care.*
*Representatives from the American Dietetic Association were instrumental in its development.*

*These Guidelines were developed by the Council for Nutrition.*
*A special committee of The Gerontological Society of America (GSA) served as critical reviewers and provided input and modification of the final Guidelines.*
*While GSA does not endorse specific clinical measures, we support the principles underlying these Guidelines and their potential to improve nutrition in the nursing home.*

---

**Trigger Conditions**

Involuntary 5% weight loss in 30 days or 10% in 180 days or less
or
BMI ≤ 21
or
Resident leaves 25% or more of food uneaten at two thirds of meals
(Assess over 7 days, based on 2000 cal/day)

Put on weekly weight monitoring program/
Proceed with documentation utilizing Nursing Nutritional Checklist

**Suggestions for family:**
- Visit at meal time
- Help feed
- Discuss alternate food sources
- Review food preferences
- Recommend favorite foods or comfort foods
- Discuss quality of life issues and treatment goals

*This is a tool to assist in compliance. This is not an endorsement of the HCFA mandated criteria. It should be noted that because malnutrition in long-term care is multifactorial, any treatment that is initiated should be monitored for efficacy, and nursing interventions should proceed simultaneously with medical interventions.*

Quality indicator conditions:
- Fecal impactions, Infection (UTI, URI, pneumonia, GI)
- Tube feeding, decline in ADL's or pressure ulcer on low risk resident

Check hydration status
minimum 1500 cc fluid/day unless contraindicated
(For tube feeding patients, approximately 75%
of the total tube feeding volume should be considered free fluid)

Inform physician/dietitian

**Checklist for nurse to provide physician/dietitian:**

- Temperature
- Constipation
- Fecal impaction
- Drug list
- Mood/behavior
- Food/fluid intake
- Vomiting/nausea
- Indigestion
- Skin condition
- Swallowing problem

- Appetite assessment
- Infection – UTI, URI, GI
- Pain
- Albumin < 3.4 g/dL
- Cholesterol < 160 mg/dL
- Hgb < 12 g/dL
- Serum transferrin < 180*

\* Included in MDS

**Physician considerations:**
- Albumin
- Complete blood count
- Blood urea nitrogen
- Creatinine
- Hemoglobin
- Hematocrit
- Serum transferrin
- Cholesterol
- Consultation by dietitian
- Consult Clinical Guide for Physicians, Pharmacists, and Dietitians

Food/environmental considerations

**Food considerations:**
- Stop therapeutic diet
- Food preferences (e.g., ethnic)
- Consistency changes based on assessed needs
- Offer meal substitutes
- Snacks (between meals and HS)
- Medications not given at meal time
- Supplements not given at meal time
- Food served at proper temperature
- Food palatability (consider taste enhancers)
- Encourage family involvement in feeding

**Other:**
- Taste/sensory changes
- Ill-fitting dentures, missing teeth
- Motor agitation, tremors, wandering

**Environmental considerations:**
- Surroundings quiet and calm, comfortable
- Positive dining room atmosphere
- Well lighted
- Caregivers are friendly and polite
- Residents are happy with the meals and meal service
- Staff directs conversation to resident at meal time
- Dining room service not rushed
- Assistance encouraged
- Prompt service and assistance
- Compatible companions

Needs feeding assistance
Meal time assistance, restorative dining program

Dysphagia/aspiration
Swallowing evaluation/food consistency change,
thickened liquids, special feeding program,
enteral/parenteral feeding

Caloric-dense foods
Exercise program for appetite stimulation

*While presented for simplicity as a linear guide in two parts, many of the suggestions can be done simultaneously, and the order in which this approach is taken can be varied dependent on individual resident needs.*

Between-meal liquid calorically dense supplements

Consider other treatment options, e.g. hospitalize or palliative care
Document reason

**Table 4.** *continue*

# Nursing Nutritional Checklist (for use in Care Planning)

*The American Dietetic Association supports the Nursing Nutritional Checklist (for use in Care Planning).*
*Representatives from the American Dietetic Association were instrumental in its development.*

*This Nursing Nutritional Checklist (for use in Care Planning) was developed by the Council for Nutrition.*
*A special committee of The Gerontological Society of America (GSA) served as critical reviewers and provided input and modification of the final Checklist.*
*While GSA does not endorse specific clinical measures, we support the principles underlying this Checklist and its potential to improve nutrition in the nursing home.*

| Problem List (check all that apply) | Suggested Action Plan (check when completed) |
|---|---|
| ○ 1. Patient has ≥ 5% involuntary weight loss in 30 days? | ○ 1-4 . Monitor weight weekly. Continue to step #5 on problem list |
| ○ 2. Patient has ≥10% involuntary weight loss in 180 days or less. | |
| ○ 3. BMI is ≤ 21. (703 x weight in lbs/height in inches² **or** weight in kilograms/height in meters²) | |
| ○ 4. Resident leaves 25% or more food on tray? (in last 7 days) | |
| 5. Quality Indicators — Does patient have:<br>○ A. Fecal impaction in last 7 days<br>○ B. Infection (UTI, URI, Pneumonia, GI) in last 7 days<br>○ C. Tube feeding<br>○ D. Functional ADL decline<br>○ E. Development of pressure ulcer in low risk patient | 5.<br>○ A. Implement bowel program<br>○ B. Get physician order for U/A<br>○ C. Contact dietitian for assessment<br>○ D. Consider OT/PT assessment<br>○ E. Implement skin program |
| ○ 6. Patient takes in ≤1500cc fluid/day for the last 7 days? Is patient on fluid restriction? | ○ 6. Develop systematic plan to ensure adequate fluid intake (e.q., 300 mL with meals and 240 mL between meals) |
| ○ 7. Available labwork completed in the last 30 days:<br>Hgb _____     Albumin _____<br>Hct _____     Cholesterol _____<br>Serum WBC _____     U/A:<br>Sodium _____     Urine WBC _____<br>Potassium _____     Spec. Gravity _____<br>Glucose _____     Leuk. Esterase _____<br>BUN _____     Other _____<br>Creatinine _____ | ○ 7. Notify physician of values |
| 8. Nursing assessment of physical/psychological problems<br>○ A. Skin (pressure ulcers and skin tears)<br>○ B. Presence of fever (2° above baseline)<br>○ C. Presence of diarrhea<br>○ D. Presence of constipation<br>○ E. Takes drugs other than multivitamins/minerals<br>○ F. Symptoms of depression/anxiety<br>○ G. Loss of usual appetite<br>○ H. Presence of nausea/vomiting<br>○ I. Presence of dysphagia/choking<br>○ J. Ill-fitting dentures, missing teeth, periodontal disease | 8.<br>○ A. Implement skin program<br>○ B. Implement facility protocol<br>○ C. Implement facility protocol<br>○ D. Implement facility protocol<br>○ E. Contact pharmacy consultant for drug review<br>○ F. Evaluate for depression/anxiety (short geriatric mini depression scale)<br>○ G. Implement care plan to increase appetite<br>○ H. Implement facility protocol<br>○ I. Contact dietitian for evaluation<br>○ J. Contact dentist or dental technician |
| ○ 9. Not satisfied with food currently offered (for example, ethnic preferences) | ○ 9. Stop therapeutic diets and provide preferred foods/food substitutions |
| ○ 10. Patient needs meal time assistance | ○ 10. Provide timely, polite assistance during dining<br>○ Provide tray set up<br>○ Provide partial assistance/supervision (evaluate resident/staff ratio and supervision by licensed professional staff)<br>○ Provide total assistance (consider resident/staff ratio and supervision by licensed professional staff)<br>○ Consider training staff to provide meal time assistance |
| ○ 11. Patient has motor agitation, tremors, or wanders | ○ 11. Consider OT evaluation<br>○ Provide meal time assistance<br>○ Provide self-help feeding devices<br>○ Offer finger foods |
| ○ 12. Presence of environmental distractions or meal time environment concerns | ○ 12. Minimize environmental distractions<br>○ Provide compatible companions |
| ○ 13. Inadequate lighting in the dining room | ○ 13. Evaluate location in dining room |
| ○ 14. Patient needs 30–60 minutes to eat | ○ 14. Implement dining program, e.g. special area to eat for impaired residents or two meal time sessions |
| ○ 15. Patient is unable to tolerate current food consistency | ○ 15. Contact dietitian for texture screen |
| ○ 16. Supplements are given at meal time | ○ 16. Give liquid supplements in a pattern that optimizes nutrient intake |
| ○ 17. Medications are given at meal time | ○ 17. Contact pharmacist for appropriate administration time |
| ○ 18. Impaired visual acuity | ○ 18. Assure resident is wearing clean glasses at meal time<br>○ Provide meal time assistance (see #10) |
| ○ 19. Impaired hearing | ○ 19. Ensure that hearing aid is in place and working at meal time |
| ○ 20. Patient has a decline in taste and smell | ○ 20. Season foods<br>○ Serve food at proper temperature |

○ **When problem list is completed, contact physician, dietitian and pharmacist as appropriate with suggested action plan.**

Completed by: _____     Date: _____

**Table 5.** Clinical guide to prevent and manage malnutrition in long-term care. The information in this table is aimed at physicians, pharmacists, and dietitians, and follows the strategy evaluate, document, and treat

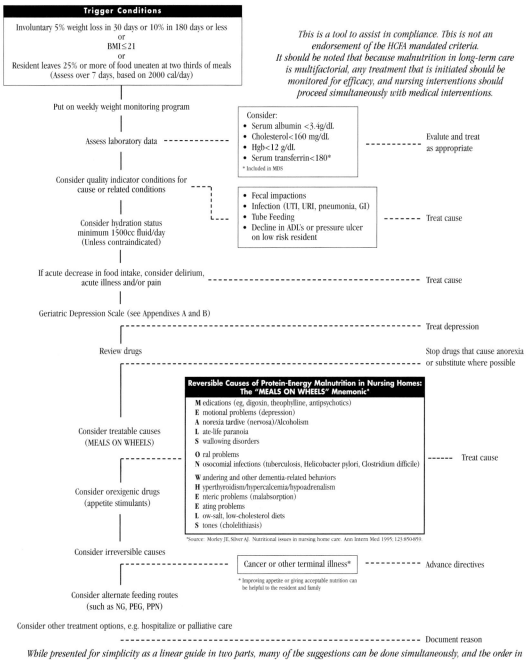

# Clinical Guide to Prevent and Manage Malnutrition in Long-Term Care
## FOR PHYSICIANS, PHARMACISTS, AND DIETITIANS (EVALUATE, DOCUMENT AND TREAT)

*The American Dietetic Association supports the Clinical Guide to Prevent and Manage Malnutrition in Long-Term Care. Representatives from the American Dietetic Association were instrumental in its development.*

*These Guidelines were developed by the Council for Nutrition.*
*A special committee of The Gerontological Society of America (GSA) served as critical reviewers and provided input and modification of the final Guidelines. While GSA does not endorse specific clinical measures, we support the principles underlying these Guidelines and their potential to improve nutrition in the nursing home.*

**Trigger Conditions**

Involuntary 5% weight loss in 30 days or 10% in 180 days or less
or
BMI≤21
or
Resident leaves 25% or more of food uneaten at two thirds of meals
(Assess over 7 days, based on 2000 cal/day)

*This is a tool to assist in compliance. This is not an endorsement of the HCFA mandated criteria. It should be noted that because malnutrition in long-term care is multifactorial, any treatment that is initiated should be monitored for efficacy, and nursing interventions should proceed simultaneously with medical interventions.*

Put on weekly weight monitoring program

Assess laboratory data - - - - - - - - - - - -

Consider:
• Serum albumin <3.4g/dL
• Cholesterol<160 mg/dL
• Hgb<12 g/dL
• Serum transferrin<180*
\* Included in MDS

- - - - - - - - - Evalute and treat as appropriate

Consider quality indicator conditions for cause or related conditions

• Fecal impactions
• Infection (UTI, URI, pneumonia, GI)
• Tube Feeding
• Decline in ADL's or pressure ulcer on low risk resident

- - - - - - - Treat cause

Consider hydration status
minimum 1500cc fluid/day
(Unless contraindicated)

If acute decrease in food intake, consider delirium, acute illness and/or pain - - - - - - - - - - - - - - - - - - - - - - - - - - - - - Treat cause

Geriatric Depression Scale (see Appendixes A and B)

- - - - - - - - - - - - - - - - - - - - - - - - - - - - - Treat depression

Review drugs

- - - - - - - - - - - - - - - - - - - - - - - - - - - - - Stop drugs that cause anorexia
or substitute where possible

**Reversible Causes of Protein-Energy Malnutrition in Nursing Homes: The "MEALS ON WHEELS" Mnemonic\***

**M** edications (eg, digoxin, theophylline, antipsychotics)
**E** motional problems (depression)
**A** norexia tardive (nervosa)/Alcoholism
**L** ate-life paranoia
**S** wallowing disorders

**O** ral problems
**N** osocomial infections (tuberculosis, Helicobacter pylori, Clostridium difficile)

**W** andering and other dementia-related behaviors
**H** yperthyroidism/hypercalcemia/hypoadrenalism
**E** nteric problems (malabsorption)
**E** ating problems
**L** ow-salt, low-cholesterol diets
**S** tones (cholelithiasis)

\*Source: Morley JE, Silver AJ. Nutritional issues in nursing home care. Ann Intern Med 1995;123:850-859.

Consider treatable causes
(MEALS ON WHEELS)

- - - - - - Treat cause

Consider orexigenic drugs
(appetite stimulants)

Consider irreversible causes

Cancer or other terminal illness\* - - - - - - - - - - Advance directives

\* Improving appetite or giving acceptable nutrition can be helpful to the resident and family

Consider alternate feeding routes
(such as NG, PEG, PPN)

Consider other treatment options, e.g. hospitalize or palliative care

- - - - - - - - - - - - - - - - - - - - - - - - - - - - - - - - - - - - - Document reason

*While presented for simplicity as a linear guide in two parts, many of the suggestions can be done simultaneously, and the order in which this approach is taken can be varied dependent on individual resident needs.*

# References

1. Morley JE, Kraenzle D (1994) Causes of weight loss in a community nursing home. J Am Geriatr Soc 42:583–585
2. Wilson MMG, Vaswani S, Liu D et al (1998) Prevalence and causes of undernutrition in medical outpatients. Am J Med 104:56–63
3. Mathey MFAM, Siebelink E, de Fraaf C, Van Staveren WA (2001) Flavor enhancement of food improves dietary intake and nutritional status of elderly nursing home residents. J Gerontol Med Sci 56A:M200–M205
4. Suda Y, Marske CE, Flaherty JH et al (2001) Examining the effect of intervention to nutritional problems of the elderly living in an inner city area: a pilot project. J Nutr Health Aging 5:118–123
5. Wilson MM, Purushothaman R, Morley JE (2002) Effect of liquid dietary supplements on energy intake in the elderly. Am J Clin Nutr 75:944–947
6. Morley JE, Perry HM (2003) Androgen treatment of male hypogonadism in older males. J Steroid Biochem Molecular Biol 85:367–373
7. Wittert GA, Chapman IM, Haren MT et al (2003) Oral testosterone supplementation increases muscle and decreases fat mass in healthy elderly males with low-normal gonadal status. J Gerontol Med Sci 58A:618–625
8. Milne AC, Potter J, Avenell A (2002) Protein and energy supplementation in elderly people at risk from malnutrition. Cochrane Database of Systematic Reviews (3):CD003288
9. Wilson MM, Purushothaman R, Morley JE (2002) Effect of liquid dietary supplements on energy intake in the elderly. Am J Clin Nutr 75:944–947
10. Haddad RY, Thomas DR (2002) Enteral nutrition and enteral tube feeding: review of the evidence. Clin Geriatr Med 18: 867–881
11. Hebuterne X (2002) Inserting a percutaneous endoscopic gastrotomy tube in an elderly patient may be a difficult decision. Gastroenterol Clin Biol 26:439–442
12. Skelly RH (2002) Are we using percutaneous endoscopic gastrostomy appropriately in the elderly? Curr Opin Clin Nutr Metab Care 5:35–42
13. Dwolatzky T, Berezovski S, Friedmann R et al (2001) A prospective comparison of the use of nasogastric and percutaneous endoscopic gastrostomy tubes for long-term enteral feeding in older people. Clin Nutr 20:535–540
14. Finucane TE, Christmas C, Travis K (1999) Tube feeding in patients with advanced dementia – a review of the evidence. J Am Med Assoc 282:1363–1370
15. Mitchell SL, Kiely DK, Lipsitz LA (1997) The risk factors and impact on survival of feeding tube placement in nursing home residents with severe cognitive impairment. Arch Int Med 157:327–332
16. Rombeau JL (1984) Nasoenteric tube feeding. WB Saunders, Philadelphia, p 261
17. Cataldi-Betcher EL, Seltzer MH, Slocum BA et al (1983) Complications occurring during enteral nutrition support: a prospective study. J Parenter Enter Nutr 7:546–552
18. Benya R, Langer S, Mobarhan S (1990) Flexible nasogastric feeding tube tip malposition immediately after placement. J Parenter Enter Nutr 14:108–109
19. Ciocon JO, Silverstone FA, Graver LM et al (1988) Tube feedings in elderly patients: indications, benefits, and complications. Arch Inern Med 148:429–433
20. Chowdhury Mosiuddin A, Batey R (1996) Complications and outcome of percutaneous endoscopic gastrostomy in different patient groups. J Gastroenterol Hepatol 11:835–839
21. Hunt JN, Stubbs DF (1975) The volume and energy content of meals as determinations of gastric emptying. J Physiol (London) 245:209–225
22. Davenport HW (1977) Physiology of the digestive tract, 4th ed. Year Book Medical Publishers, Chicago
23. Finucane TE, Bynum JP (1996) Use of tube feeding to prevent aspiration pneumonia. Lancet 348:1421–1424
24. Lipman TO (1983) The fate of enteral feeding tubes. Nutrition Supplement Service 3:71
25. Keohane PP, Attrill H, Love M et al (1984) Relationship between osmolality of diet and gastrointestinal side effects in enteral nutrition. BMJ 288:678–680
26. Zarling EJ, Parmar JR, Mobarhan S et al (1986) Effect of enteral formula rate, osmolality, and chemical composition upon clinical tolerance and carbohydrate absorption in normal subjects. JPEN J Parenter Enteral Nutr 10:588–590
27. Morley JE (2002) Orexigenic and anabolic agents. Clin Geriatr Med 18: 853–866
28. Karcic E, Philpot C, Morley JE (2002) Treating malnutrition with megestrol acetate: literature review and review of our experience. J Nutr Health Aging 6:191–200
29. Yeh SS, Wu SY, Levine DM et al (2001) The correlation of cytokine levels with body weight after megestrol acetate treatment in geriatric patients. J Gerontol Med Sci 56A:M48–M54
30. Thomas DR, Ashmen W, Morley JE, Evans WJ (2000) Nutritional management in long-term care: development of a clinical guideline. Council for Nutritional Clinical Strategies in Long-Term Care. J Gerontol A Med Sci 55A:M752–M734

# SECTION 12
# A GLOBAL PERSPECTIVE FOR THE TREATMENT OF CACHEXIA

# Cachexia: Therapeutic Immunomodulation Beyond Cytokine Antagonism

Stephan von Haehling, Stefan D. Anker

## Introduction

Cachexia is frequently observed in a number of different chronic illnesses. Although a final common pathway has not yet been established, a number of features have been recognised irrespective of underlying aetiology. These aspects of the disease include activation of the immune system, muscle wasting through the ubiquitin-proteasome pathway and endothelial dysfunction. Targeting these aspects of cachexia involves downstream signalling of proinflammatory cytokines, proteasome inhibition and possibly the use of 3-hydroxy-3-methylglutaryl coenzyme A (HMG-CoA) reductase inhibitors (statins). Apart from their cholesterol-lowering features, the latter class of drugs has recently been shown to improve endothelial dysfunction, to induce endothelial progenitor cells, and to have anti-inflammatory properties. These features have recently been termed pleiotropic effects of statins. It is therefore tempting to speculate that cachectic patients will benefit from treatment with statins, and possibly also from immunosuppression per se.

## Proteasome-Dependent Protein Degradation

Cachexia is frequently accompanied by elevated levels of proinflammatory cytokines [1–5]. Indeed, tumour necrosis factor-$\alpha$ (TNF-$\alpha$) appears to play a key role in the development of this perturbation [6]. TNF-$\alpha$ was first described in 1975 and termed cachectin for its ability to induce weight loss and anorexia in mice [7]. This syndrome, however, was reversed when the injection of TNF-$\alpha$ was discontinued. In chronic heart failure, for example, which often leads to cardiac cachexia, TNF-$\alpha$ leads to reduced peripheral blood flow [8], increased apop-

tosis [9] and lower skeletal muscle mass [10, 11]. Moreover, proinflammatory cytokine activation relates to prognosis in chronic heart failure independently of whether cachexia is present or not [12, 13]. Other proinflammatory mediators, such as interleukin (IL)-1$\beta$ and IL-6, also appear to contribute to both the development and the progression of cachexia [14]. Interestingly, the latter cytokine is the most potent mediator to induce the acute-phase response [15]. Maintaining the acute-phase response requires an excess of essential amino acids, which yields loss of body proteins [16]. Since skeletal muscle accounts for almost half of the body protein mass, this compartment is intensively affected.

The predominant pathway of protein turnover and degradation in eukaryotic cells is the ubiquitin-proteasome pathway (Fig. 1). The impact of protein degradation through this pathway has been demonstrated in vivo for cachexia in AIDS [17], sepsis [18], cancer [19] and renal failure [20]. Interestingly, cytokine signals, such as TNF-$\alpha$, IL-1 and IL-6 stimulate the ubiquitin-proteasome pathway in muscle [21–23]. It is still a matter of debate whether these signals act directly or whether they are secondary to the influence of cytokine-induced glucocorticoids [24]. The finding that protein degradation by the proteasome does not yield free amino acids but peptides suggests that a number of other factors may also be important in the regulation of muscle protein breakdown [25].

## Proteasome Inhibitors

Protein degradation by the proteasome complex represents a potential target for therapeutic interventions. Indeed, proteasome inhibitors have been available since 1994. The first clinical data from phase I studies became accessible in 2002. Four

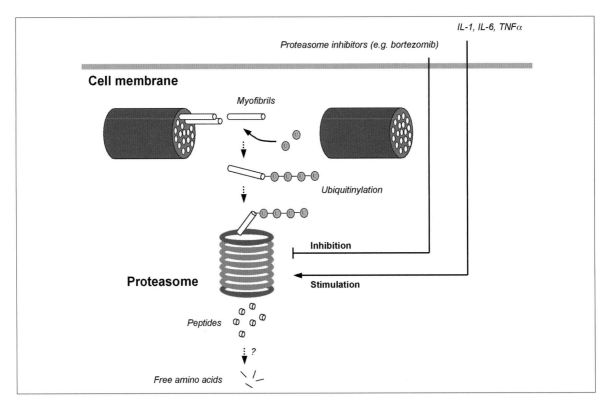

**Fig. 1.** Muscle wasting in man. An unknown stimulus, possibly TNF-α binding to its receptors, causes ubiquitin binding to myofibrils. These proteins are then directed to the proteasome complex. The proteasome releases peptides, which are further broken down to free amino acids by yet unidentified mechanisms. Several proinflammatory cytokines are known to induce proteasome activity while proteasome inhibitors block it

classes of proteasome inhibitors have been described so far [26, 27]:

1. Peptide aldehydes primarily inhibit the chymotrypsin-like activity of the proteasome, which is one of its specific proteolytic sites. Removing the peptide aldehyde restores the proteolytic activity.
2. Lactacystin and its active derivative β-lactone are more specific, but irreversible inhibitors of the proteasome. They act as pseudosubstrates that are covalently bound to one of the subunits of the proteasome [28].
3. Vinyl sulfone has been shown to inhibit the proteasome complex irreversibly in a similar manner to lactacystin [29]. In a human lymphoma cell line prolonged inhibition of the proteasome by vinyl sulfone led to the appearance of cell variants with a distinct proteolytic system [29].
4. Dipeptide boronic acid analogues have been shown to block proteasome activity via

reversible binding to its active sites. Indeed, bortezomib (also known as PS-341) from this class of proteasome inhibitors is the only such drug that has been used in clinical trials so far. A phase I study in 43 patients with different types of advanced solid tumour malignancies showed a safe and reasonable treatment regimen with this substance [30]. Side-effects were diarrhoea and sensory neurotoxicity, both of which are dose-limiting toxicities. Unfortunately, the authors did not report differences in body weight before and after treatment. Another study revealed that in vivo administration of bortezomib induced proteasome inhibition in a time-dependent manner and that the inhibition was also related to both the dose in milligrams per square meter of body surface area and the absolute dose of bortezomib [31]. This study also revealed that patients treated with bortezomib require careful monitoring of electrolyte abnormalities and late toxicities [31].

More recent work has illustrated the role of bortezomib in relapsed, refractory multiple myeloma [32]. In this multicentre, open-label, non-randomised phase II trial, 202 patients were enrolled and received 1.3 mg of bortezomib per square meter of body surface area twice weekly for up to eight cycles. The response rate was 35%. Myeloma protein became undetectable in seven patients, and in 12 patients myeloma protein was detectable only by immunofixation. Therefore, the authors of this study conclude that bortezomib is active in patients with relapsed multiple myeloma that is refractory to conventional chemotherapy [32].

Peptide aldehydes, lactacystin and β-lactone have been shown to block up to 90% of the degradation of abnormal proteins and short-lived proteins in the cell [29]. Unfortunately, it is not possible to block specifically myofibril degradation in skeletal muscle.

## Targeting Intracellular Signal Transduction

Nuclear factor-κB (NF-κB) is one of the principal transcription factors to transduce TNF-α signals into the cells. Moreover, it also activates gene transcription of cytokines, acute-phase response proteins, and cell adhesion molecules [33]. The complex interactions of NF-κB and other transcription factors are responsible for the inhibition and enhancement of certain genes. However, a coincident activation of several transcription factors is generally regarded necessary for maximal gene expression [34].

NF-κB was first described in 1986. It was so named because of being necessary for immunoglobulin kappa light chain transcription in B cells [35]. NF-κB is a heterodimer consisting of two subunits, which are, in unstimulated cells, bound to an inhibitory protein IκB. Therefore, it is kept in an inactivated form in the cytoplasm with its nuclear localisation signal being masked [36]. Once activated, IκB is phosphorylated and rapidly degraded in the ubiquitin-proteasome pathway. The free NF-κB complex can translocate into the nucleus, where NF-κB binds to κB DNA sequences (NF-κB responding elements).

Several approaches appear promising when targeting the intracellular signal transduction of TNF-α. Thus, IκB degradation, NF-κB translocation, or NF-κB DNA binding may be useful targets. In fact, genetic overexpression of IκB blocks NF-κB-dependent processes. Fumar acid, which blocks the nuclear translocation of NF-κB, has a high anti-inflammatory capacity [37]. Most recently, activation of NF-κB by overexpression of a IκB phosphorylating kinase has been shown sufficiently to block myogenesis, thus illustrating the link between NF-κB and cachexia development [38]. However, complete inhibition of NF-κB has proven detrimental; knockout studies targeting the major subunits of NF-κB show severe immunodeficiency in mice, which was lethal in some cases [39].

## Immunosuppressive Substances

### Immunomodulatory Cytokines

Some cytokines possess immunosuppressive properties. The most important such substance is IL-10, which was first described in 1989 as a cytokine synthesis inhibitory factor [39]. It has been suggested that IL-10 is a natural dampener of the immune response [40]. Binding of IL-10 to its receptor activates different tyrosine kinases. IL-10 potently suppresses the production of TNF-α, IL-1β and IL-6, which finally inhibits the onset of the acute-phase response [42]. In human cachexia a potential benefit of IL-10 treatment has not been investigated so far, although it has proven clinically beneficial in several immunological disorders [43, 44]. Over the past few years, five proteins have been discovered, which show 20–28% amino acid identity to IL-10 [45]. These proteins, like IL-10, belong to the family of class 2 cytokines. They have recently been termed IL-19, IL-20, IL-22, IL-24 and IL-26, respectively [45]. However, the physiological role of these substances has not yet been identified convincingly.

Transforming growth factor-β (TGF-β) is another cytokine with immunosuppressive features [46]. It has an essential role in the development, homeostasis and repair of nearly all tissues. The principal action of TGF-β is the inhibition of leukocyte activation. However, TGF-β is also capable of stimulating the synthesis and secretion of extracellular matrix proteins. Moreover, it blocks TNF-α and IL-6 production from lipopolysaccharide (LPS)-stimulated whole blood [47]. Interestingly, TGF-β injection into mice yields progressive suppression of erythropoiesis, which was associated with both increased plasma levels of TNF-α and progressive cachexia [48]. A similar study in nude mice found that the injection of more than 2 mg/day TGF-β led to generalised intestinal fibrosis and cachexia, although this was not accompanied by elevated TNF-α levels [49]. This is grounds to apprehend that TGF-β application is detrimental in cachectic patients.

IL-4 and IL-13 are closely related, and both affect the morphology, surface receptor expression and cytokine synthesis of monocytes and macrophages. Both cytokines inhibit the production of IL-1β, IL-6, IL-8 and other proinflammatory cytokines in models of ex vivo stimulated monocytes [68]. IL-4 has been found to protect from the development of cachexia in a model of IL-4 knockout mice following infection with *Schistosoma mansoni* [50]. Indeed, the magnitude of weight loss was significantly increased compared to uninfected IL-4 knockout mice and wild-type mice. Therefore, it is not surprising that the mortality of the IL-4 knockout mice was also increased [50].

## Glucocorticoids

Glucocorticoids freely penetrate cell membranes, and after entering the target cell they bind to a cytosolic glucocorticoid receptor. This receptor eventually serves as a transcription factor. However, the anti-inflammatory action of these substances is not strictly dependent on DNA binding of the hormone–receptor complex. Moreover, glucocorticoids also activate other transcription factors, such as NF-κB [51], and it appears that side-effects are mostly attributable to the transactivating characteristics of glucocorticoid receptors that require DNA binding.

Glucocorticoids are widely used in the treatment of inflammatory and immune diseases for their ability to suppress immune activation. Interestingly, they seem to relieve anorexia and asthenia [52]. Glucocorticoids have also been found to stimulate food intake in patients with cancer cachexia [52]. However, most studies have shown a limited effect of up to 4 weeks on symptoms such as appetite, food intake, well-being and performance [53, 54]. Unfortunately, these studies failed to show beneficial effects on body weight. One of the key mechanisms of glucocorticoid action might be the induction of IκB synthesis [55, 56]. Furthermore, IκB might be able to remove actively NF-κB from its DNA binding site. Another mode of glucocorticoid action involves direct protein–protein interaction [57]. Transcription factors such as NF-κB seem to bind to glucocorticoid receptors in the cytosol [45]. Proinflammatory genes may therefore be suppressed due to masking of transactivating domains. Dexamethasone, for example, is a potent synthetic glucocorticoid. Indeed, it blocks TNF-α/IL-1-dependent induction and translocation of NF-κB [58]. Not surprisingly, dexamethasone also inhibits the LPS-induced activation of NF-κB [47]. However, the application of glucocorticoids for the treatment of cachexia remains controversial. The most important issue is that prolonged use may lead to weakness and osteoporosis, diabetes and even delirium.

## Calcineurin Inhibitors

Calcineurin inhibitors are immunosuppressive substances largely used after transplantation and during the course of certain autoimmune disorders. The most important drugs from this class of agents are the nephrotoxic cyclosporin A and tacrolimus. They pass freely through cell membranes. Tacrolimus is more potent than cyclosporin A. Unfortunately, both cyclosporin A and tacrolimus share a narrow range between subtherapeutic and toxic plasma concentration, and therefore frequent drug monitoring is required [59].

Cyclosporin A is a small peptide of fungal origin. Its major targets are T cells [60], whose cyclophilins are strongly bound. Cyclophilins are involved in protein folding. Cyclosporin-cyclophilin complexes inhibit calcineurin. This, in turn, yields inhibition of both activation and nuclear translocation of NF-AT, which is involved in IL-2, IL-4 and TNF-α transcription [61]. The actions on other cell types are less well understood, although cyclosporin appears to be able to inhibit the proteasome in murine macrophage cell lines. In these cells, cyclosporin A has also been found to suppress LPS-induced IκB degradation. Therefore, inhibition of proteasome activity seems to be the mechanism by which cyclosporin A prevents NF-κB activation [62, 63]. These data are in keeping with other reports that showed a dose-dependent inhibition of IL-1β and TNF-α production in an animal model [64]. Other workers have confirmed these data using U937 monocyte cells, in which cyclosporin A reduced the secretion of IL-1β, IL-6, IL-8 and TNF-α [65]. In human alveolar macrophages, cyclosporin A was able to inhibit the production of IL-8 and TNF-α as well [66]. A further study demonstrated that cyclosporin A injected into rats with inflammation-induced cachexia prevented the sustained loss of body weight and adipose tissue [67].

Tacrolimus (FK506) shares some of the actions of cyclosporin A. It is a macrolide antibiotic, which mainly inhibits T-cell activation via association with calcineurin. Tacrolimus binds to FK506-binding protein (FKBP), and the FKBP–calcineurin complex inhibits NF-AT activation [68]. Similar to cyclosporin A, tacrolimus has been shown to reduce TNF-α production by certain cell types [69], although this does not appear to be its principal mode of action.

Sirolimus is not a calcineurin inhibitor per se. It is, like tacrolimus, a macrolide antibiotic [70], but it acts at a later stage at inhibiting T-cell proliferation [71]. Sirolimus also binds to FKBP, although the sirolimus–FKBP complex does not inhibit calcineurin. Sirolimus failed to affect the LPS-stimulated TNF-α production in a whole blood model [72].

## Statins

Statins are the drugs most often prescribed to treat hypercholesterolaemia. The mechanism by which this class of drugs blocks cholesterol biosynthesis is competitive inhibition of HMG-CoA reductase (Fig. 2). This enzyme catalyses the rate-limiting

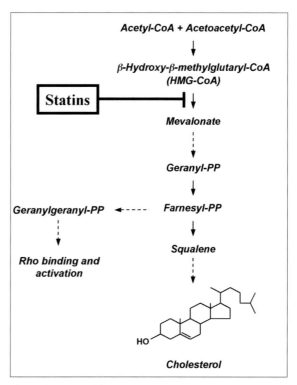

**Fig. 2.** Cholesterol biosynthesis. The rate-limiting step of this pathway is 3-hydroxy-3-methylglutaryl-CoA (HMG-CoA) reductase activity. Statins competitively inhibit this enzyme. Intermediates from cholesterol biosynthesis are used as attachments to different proteins and enzymes. *CoA*, coenzyme A; *PP*, pyrophosphate

step in cholesterol biosynthesis in the liver and other tissues. Indeed, statins bind to HMG-CoA reductase at nanomolecular concentrations. This leads to the displacement of the natural substrate (HMG-CoA), which itself binds at micromolar concentrations [73]. Blocking the enzyme leads to a significant reduction in plasma low-density lipoprotein (LDL) levels. In general, LDL levels are reduced by another 7% with each doubling of the dose [74]. However, it has become clear that lipid reduction alone cannot entirely account for the benefits of statin therapy.

### Statin Development and Classification

In search of a substance that lowers plasma cholesterol levels, Endo et al. tested more than 6000 fungi species, which finally, in 1973, led to the discovery of ML-236B [75]. ML-236B was subsequently termed mevastatin; however, due to its severe side-effects, it never reached the market. Nevertheless, mevastatin is still frequently used in in vitro studies. Lovastatin (mevinolin) was the first statin to be approved by the Food and Drug Administration (FDA) in 1987. Currently, lovastatin, simvastatin, pravastatin, fluvastatin and atorvastatin are available (Fig. 3). The new substance, rosuvastatin, was approved by the FDA in August 2003. Pitavastatin, as a very recent addition to the group, is currently available in Japan only. Statins are well tolerated and generally considered safe. Cerivastatin, however, was withdrawn from the market in August 2001, because it had the highest incidence of the overall rare side-effect rhabdomyolysis, and it is assumed to be involved in a total of 52 deaths worldwide [76]. Early data suggested that cholesterol reduction with statins may cause an increase in the incidence of cancer [77]. Furthermore, experimental data suggested that statins could increase the occurrence of several types of cancer in rodents [78]. However, data from a meta-analysis [79] and a recent analysis from the Scandinavian Simvastatin Survival Study (4S) have helped large-ly to dispel this concern. In fact, in the 4S data there was no difference in mortality from and incidence of cancer between the simvastatin and the placebo group 10 years after study termination [80].

Statins are currently subdivided according to different characteristics, such as their chemical structure (open ring vs closed ring structure), their origin (synthetic vs natural, the latter being derived from fungal fermentation), and their solubility (hydrophilic vs lipophilic, Fig. 3). Lipophilic statins would be expected to penetrate cell membranes more effectively, thus eliciting more pleiotropic effects [81]. However, the evidence suggests otherwise, because hydrophilic statins and lipophilic ones appear to share the same pleiotropic activity. Furthermore, only statins with an open ring structure inhibit HMG-CoA reductase and lead to a decrease in plasma cholesterol. Statins with a closed-ring structure must undergo metabolisation to an open ring structure before activity is initiated, although these substances may still confer pleiotropic effects before metabolisation occurs.

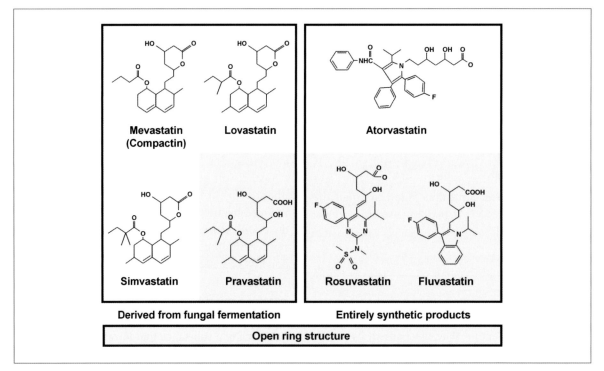

**Fig. 3.** Chemical structure and classification of statins. Statins are subgrouped according to their origin (natural vs synthetic), their chemical structure (open vs closed ring) and their solubility (lipophilic vs hydrophilic). See text for details

## Statin-Mediated Effects on Inflammatory Markers

Several clinical trials have shown that statins reduce plasma levels of the acute-phase reactant C-reactive protein (CRP). In a population of 5742 patients enrolled in a randomised, double-blind, placebo-controlled trial of lovastatin in the primary prevention of acute coronary events, Ridker et al. found that lovastatin reduced the median level of CRP by 14.8% (95% confidence interval: 12.5–17.4%, $p < 0.001$) as compared to the placebo group during the first year of treatment [82]. This effect was unrelated to any change in lipid levels. This finding was still significant in a group of 1702 men and women with no prior history of cardiovascular disease [83]. After 24 weeks of double-blind, placebo-controlled treatment, pravastatin reduced median CRP levels by 16.9% in this cohort ($p < 0.001$ vs placebo). In a similar study, atorvastatin and pravastatin were recently found to reduce CRP levels significantly among 3745 patients with acute coronary syndromes within 30 days of initiation [84]. Atorvastatin 80 mg once daily was more effective than pravastatin 40 mg once daily at 30 days (median CRP level: 1.6 vs 2.3 mg/l, $p < 0.001$) and 4 months (1.3 vs 2.1 mg/l, $p < 0.001$). Interestingly, the achieved CRP and LDL levels were independent of each other.

Early data from a study in six adults with hypercholesterolaemia indicated that pravastatin treatment over 7 weeks decreases LPS-stimulated production of TNF-$\alpha$ (from 25.3 ± 11.7 ng/ml at baseline to 17.6 ± 7.1 ng/ml, $p = 0.028$) and IL-6 (from 100.0 ± 56.2 ng/ml to 72.2 ± 51.0 ng/ml, $p = 0.046$) in vitro [85]. Several other workers have since confirmed the capability of statins to attenuate proinflammatory cytokine activation in patients with visceral obesity [86], coronary artery disease [87, 88], acute coronary syndromes [89], idiopathic dilated cardiomyopathy [90], and in heart transplant recipients [91]. Although the overall trend points toward a decrease in TNF-$\alpha$ and IL-6 production under statin therapy, some studies provided neutral results regarding these markers [86, 89].

## Effects on Re-endothelialisation

Statins have been shown to decrease neointimal thickening in models of carotid injury [92, 93] and also to reduce clinical events and angiographic restenosis after coronary stent implantation [94]. These effects were attributed to inhibition of smooth muscle cell proliferation [95]. However, recent research has provided insights into the profound effects of statins on endothelial cell function. Simvastatin and pravastatin have been demonstrated to activate phosphorylation of the protein kinase Akt in human umbilical vein endothelial cells [96]. Akt is involved in endothelial cell survival and blood vessel development [97]. It also protects cardiomyocytes from apoptosis [98] and activates endothelial nitric oxide production [99, 100]. Daily intraperitoneal simvastatin injection led to enhanced Akt signalling in the ischaemic rabbit limb after femoral artery resection. This led to a highly significant promotion of capillary formation after 40 days of treatment (simvastatin: 253 ± 23 capillaries/mm$^2$ vs control: 163 ± 9 capillaries/mm$^2$, $p < 0.01$) [96]. Another study confirmed the role of Akt [101]. In this study, serum starvation was used to induce apoptosis in cultured endothelial progenitor cells. Simvastatin reduced the percentage of apoptotic cells from 24 ± 5% to 6 ± 1% ($p < 0.02$), which was mediated by Akt signalling [101].

On the other hand, statins appear directly to mobilise bone marrow-derived endothelial progenitor cells. Atorvastatin, for example, has recently been shown to increase the number of circulating endothelial progenitor cells in vivo during 4 weeks of follow-up in 15 patients with coronary artery disease [102]. Indeed, statin treatment was associated with a 1.5-fold increase in the number of circulating cells after 1 week, and this was followed by sustained increased levels to threefold throughout the 4-week study period ($p<0.05$) [102]. In a study conducted in 34 male Sprague-Dawley rats, simvastatin treatment produced dose-dependent accelerated re-endothelialisation of balloon-injured arterial segments [103]. After 2 weeks, the re-endothelialised area of statin-treated rats was 12.3 ± 1.8 mm$^2$ (66.6 ± 9.9%) of the total denuded area. In contrast, the re-endothelialised area in the no-statin group measured 5.4 ± 1.1 mm$^2$ (31.6 ± 5.9%) of the denuded area ($p < 0.01$) [103].

## Statin-Mediated Effects on Proteasome-Dependent Protein Degradation

A recent report has demonstrated a role of statins in the inhibition of proteasome-dependent protein degradation [104]. Indeed, mevastatin induced degenerative changes and reduced the viability of terminally differentiated murine neuroblastoma cells by inhibiting proteasome activity. Pravastatin, however, having an open ring structure, affected neither the degeneration and viability of these cells nor their proteasome activity.

## Statin-Mediated Effects on Endothelial Function

The vascular endothelium is an important source of mediators, which maintain an antithrombotic surface, regulate vascular tone, modulate inflammatory responses, and inhibit proliferation of vascular smooth muscle cells [105]. Nitric oxide (NO) is the most important such mediator. It is constitutively produced by endothelial nitric oxide synthase (eNOS). Statins have recently been found to improve the availability of NO, which leads to an improved endothelial function [106]. Some effects appear to be attributable to the inhibition of cholesterol biosynthesis. Indeed, substrates downstream from mevalonate in the synthesis cascade supply a number of metabolic pathways [106, 107]. Geranylgeranyl-pyrophosphate is one such substrate, which serves as a lipid attachment to Rho, the latter being a GTP-binding protein. This protein coordinates a number of different cellular responses by interacting with downstream targets [108]. Rho is involved in stress fibre formation [109], monocyte adhesion and transmigration through the endothelium [110, 111]. Moreover, statins appear to have antioxidant properties, which also improve endothelial function.

Atorvastatin, for example, has been shown to upregulate the expression of catalase at both the mRNA and protein level in cultured rat aortic vascular smooth muscle cells [112]. These findings have to be seen in light of the fact that statins have been shown directly [113] (and indirectly [114–116]) to induce eNOS transcription and activity.

## Thalidomide

Thalidomide was first synthesised by Kunz in 1954 [117] and it took some years until its teratogenic effects became apparent. Therefore, thalidomide is now mostly known for its tragic associations. Indeed, malformation of the unborn can be induced by a single dose of the drug [83]. The substance was initially developed as a sedative. However, thalidomide has been used over the past years in the treatment of erythema nodosum leprosum, a serious complication of leprosy thought to be mainly mediated by TNF-α [118]. Indeed, thalidomide has been shown to inhibit selectively the production of TNF-α by LPS-stimulated human monocytes in vitro, leaving other proinflammatory cytokines such as IL-1β and IL-6 unaltered [119]. This effect seems to be mediated by selective TNF-α mRNA degradation [120]. Other modes of action have lately been described, which include upregulation of IL-2, IL-4 and IL-5 secretion, inhibition of mitogen-stimulated peripheral mononuclear cells and the enhancement of T-cell responses. Some amino-substituted thalidomide analogues seem to have fewer side-effects and a greater potential to suppress TNF-α than the unsubstituted drug. Only recently, thalidomide has been suggested as a therapy for chronic heart failure, which frequently leads to cardiac cachexia [121]. In fact, thalidomide has been used to improve restlessness and nausea in patients with advanced cancer, being also useful to improve appetite [122, 123]. In a placebo-controlled study in patients with acute pulmonary tuberculosis, either human immunodeficiency virus positive or negative, thalidomide led to significant weight gain [124].

## Conclusions

Both a dramatic decrease in appetite and an increase in metabolism of fat and lean body mass play a critical role in the development of cachexia. However, a final common pathway has not been established so far, but it appears that TNF-α is part of this pathway. Several therapeutic approaches have been discussed over the past several years. Immunomodulation and immunosuppression seem to be promising techniques to target several aspects of this perturbation. Moreover, the pleiotropic effects of statins comprise immunomodulatory aspects, and some statins have been shown to decrease proinflammatory cytokine activation. Clinical data on the usefulness of statin application in cachexia are not yet available. However, some very early data were disappointing. In this study, hepatoma-bearing cachectic rats were treated with simvastatin, but the drug failed to prevent muscle wasting [125]. The pleiotropic effects of statin treatment are still promising, however, and it might be a matter of choosing the right drug and, of course, the right dose in the right patient. Indeed, very low doses of statins, which do not lower plasma cholesterol, may still confer pleiotropic effects. Future research will hopefully elucidate the impact of statins in cachexia.

## References

1. Levine B, Kalman J, Mayer L et al (1990) Elevated circulating levels of tumor necrosis factor in severe chronic heart failure. N Engl J Med 323:236–241
2. Argiles JM, Lopez-Soriano FJ (1999) The role of cytokines in cancer cachexia. Med Res Rev 19:223–248
3. Roubenoff R, Roubenoff RA, Cannon JG et al (1994) Rheumatoid cachexia: cytokine-driven hypermetabolism accompanying reduced body cell mass in chronic inflammation. J Clin Invest 93:2379–2386
4. Anker SD, Egerer KR, Volk HD et al (1997) Elevated soluble CD14 receptors and altered cytokines in chronic heart failure. Am J Cardiol 79:1426–1430
5. Anker SD, Clark AL, Teixeira MM et al (1999) Loss of bone mineral in patients with cachexia due to chronic heart failure. Am J Cardiol 83:612–615
6. von Haehling S, Genth-Zotz S, Anker SD, Volk HD (2002) Cachexia: a therapeutic approach beyond cytokine antagonism. Int J Cardiol 85:173–183
7. Cerami A, Ikeda Y, Le Trang N et al (1985) Weight loss associated with an endotoxin-induced mediator from peritoneal macrophages: the role of cachectin (tumor necrosis factor). Immunol Lett 11:173–177
8. Anker SD, Volterrani M, Egerer KR et al (1998) Tumour necrosis factor alpha as a predictor of impaired peak leg blood flow in patients with chronic heart failure. QJM 91:199–203
9. Ceconi C, Curello S, Bachetti T et al (1998) Tumor necrosis factor in congestive heart failure: a mechanism of disease for the new millennium? Prog Cardiovasc Dis 41:25–30
10. Anker SD, Ponikowski PP, Clark AL et al (1999) Cytokines and neurohormones relating to body composition alterations in the wasting syndrome of chronic heart failure. Eur Heart J 20:683–693
11. von Haehling S, Jankowska EA, Anker SD (2004) Tumour necrosis factor-alpha and the failing heart – pathophysiology and therapeutic implications. Basic Res Cardiol 99:18–28
12. Anker SD, von Haehling S (2004) Inflammatory mediators in chronic heart failure: an overview. Heart 90:464–470
13. Rauchhaus M, Doehner W, Francis DP et al (2000) Plasma cytokine parameters and mortality in patients with chronic heart failure. Circulation 102:3060–3067
14. Cederholm T, Wretlind B, Hellstrom K et al (1997) Enhanced generation of interleukins 1 beta and 6 may contribute to the cachexia of chronic disease. Am J Clin Nutr 65:876–882
15. Baumann H, Gauldie J (1994) The acute phase response. Immunol Today 15:74–80
16. Kotler DP. Cachexia (2000) Ann Intern Med 133:622–634
17. Llovera M, Garcia-Martinez C, Agell N et al (1998) Ubiquitin and proteasome gene expression is increased in skeletal muscle of slim AIDS patients. Int J Mol Med 2:69–73
18. Garcia-Martinez C, Llovera M, Agell N et al (1995) Ubiquitin gene expression in skeletal muscle is increased during sepsis: involvement of TNF-alpha but not IL-1. Biochem Biophys Res Commun 217:839–944
19. Williams A, Sun X, Fischer JE, Hasselgren PO (1999) The expression of genes in the ubiquitin-proteasome proteolytic pathway is increased in skeletal muscle from patients with cancer. Surgery 126:744–749
20. Bailey JL, Wang X, England BK et al (1996) The acidosis of chronic renal failure activates muscle proteolysis in rats by augmenting transcription of genes encoding proteins of the ATP-dependent ubiquitin-proteasome pathway. J Clin Invest 97:1447–1453
21. Zamir O, Hasselgren PO, Kunkel SL et al (1992) Evidence that tumor necrosis factor participates in

the regulation of muscle proteolysis during sepsis. Arch Surg 127:170–174

22. Zamir O, Hasselgren PO, von Allmen D, Fischer JE (1993) In vivo administration of interleukin-1 alpha induces muscle proteolysis in normal and adrenalectomized rats. Metabolism 42:204–208

23. Goodman MN (1994) Interleukin-6 induces skeletal muscle protein breakdown in rats. Proc Soc Exp Biol Med 205:182–185

24. Hall-Angeras M, Angeras U, Zamir O et al (1990) Interaction between corticosterone and tumor necrosis factor stimulated protein breakdown in rat skeletal muscle, similar to sepsis. Surgery 108:460–466

25. Hasselgren PO, Wray C, Mammen J (2002) Molecular regulation of muscle cachexia: it may be more than the proteasome. Biochem Biophys Res Commun 290:1–10

26. Lee DH, Goldberg AL (1998) Proteasome inhibitors: valuable new tools for cell biologists. Trends Cell Biol 8:397–403

27. Hasselgren PO, Fischer JE (2001) Muscle cachexia: current concepts of intracellular mechanisms and molecular regulation. Ann Surg 233:9–17

28. Fenteany G, Standaert RF, Lane WS et al (1995) Inhibition of proteasome activities and subunit-specific amino-terminal threonine modification by lactacystin. Science 268:726–731

29. Glas R, Bogyo M, McMaster JS et al (1998) A proteolytic system that compensates for loss of proteasome function. Nature 392:618–622

30. Aghajanian C, Soignet S, Dizon DS et al (2002) A phase I trial of the novel proteasome inhibitor PS341 in advanced solid tumor malignancies. Clin Cancer Res 8:2505–2511

31. Orlowski RZ, Stinchcombe TE, Mitchell BS et al (2002) Phase I trial of the proteasome inhibitor PS-341 in patients with refractory hematologic malignancies. J Clin Oncol 20:4420–4427

32. Richardson PG, Barlogie B, Berenson J et al (2003) A phase 2 study of bortezomib in relapsed, refractory myeloma. N Engl J Med 348:2609–2617

33. Ghosh S, May MJ, Kopp EB (1998) NF-kB and Rel proteins: evolutionarily conserved mediators of immune responses. Annu Rev Immunol 16:225–260

34. Adcock IM, Caramori G (2001) Cross-talk between pro-inflammatory transcription factors and glucocorticoids. Immunol Cell Biol 79:376–384

35. Sen R, Baltimore D (1986) Multiple nuclear factors interact with the immunoglobulin enhancer sequences. Cell 46:705–716

36. Baeuerle PA, Baltimore D (1988) I kappa B: a specific inhibitor of the NF-kappa B transcription factor. Science 242:540-546

37. Loewe R, Holnthoner W, Groger M et al (2002) Dimethylfumarate inhibits TNF-induced nuclear entry of NF-kappa B/p65 in human endothelial cells. J Immunol 168:4781–4787

38. Langen RC, Schols AM, Kelders MC et al (2001) Inflammatory cytokines inhibit myogenic differentiation through activation of nuclear factor-kappaB. FASEB J 15:1169–1180

39. Fiorentino DF, Bond MW, Mosmann TR (1989) Two types of mouse T helper cell. IV. Th2 clones secrete a factor that inhibits cytokine production by Th1 clones. J Exp Med 170:2081–2095

40. de Vries JE (1995) Immunosuppressive and anti-inflammatory properties of interleukin 10. Ann Med 27:537–541

41. Riley JK, Takeda K, Akira S, Schreiber RD (1999) Interleukin-10 receptor signaling through the JAK-STAT pathway. Requirement for two distinct receptor-derived signals for anti-inflammatory action. J Biol Chem 274:16513–16521

42. Koj A (1998) Termination of acute-phase response: role of some cytokines and anti-inflammatory drugs. Gen Pharmac 31:9–18

43. Asadullah K, Docke WD, Sabat RV et al (2000) The treatment of psoriasis with IL-10: rationale and review of the first clinical trials. Expert Opin Investig Drugs 9:95–102

44. Moore KW, de Waal Malefyt R, Coffman RL, O'Garra A (2001) Interleukin-10 and the interleukin-10 receptor. Annu Rev Immunol 19:683–765

45. Pestka S, Krause CD, Sarkar D, Walter MR et al (2004) Interleukin-10 and Related Cytokines and Receptors. Annu Rev Immunol 22:929–979

46. Massague J (1998) TGF-b signal transduction. Annu Rev Biochem 67:753–791

47. Karres I, Kremer JP, Steckholzer U et al (1996) Transforming growth factor-beta 1 inhibits synthesis of cytokines in endotoxin-stimulated human whole blood. Arch Surg 131:1310–1316

48. Chuncharunee S, Carter CD, Studtmann KE et al (1993) Chronic administration of transforming growth factor-beta suppresses erythropoietin-dependent erythropoiesis and induces tumour necrosis factor in vivo. Br J Haematol 84:374–380

49. Zugmaier G, Paik S, Wilding G et al (1991) Transforming growth factor beta 1 induces cachexia and systemic fibrosis without an antitumor effect in nude mice. Cancer Res 51:3590–3594

50. Brunet LR, Finkelman FD, Cheever AW et al (1997) IL-4 protects against TNF-alpha-mediated cachexia and death during acute schistosomiasis. J Immunol 159:777–785

51. De Bosscher K, Vanden Berghe W, Haegeman G (2000) Mechanisms of anti-inflammatory action and of immunosuppression by glucocorticoids: negative interference of activated glucocorticoid receptor with transcription factors. J Neuroimmunol 109:16–22

52. Argiles JM, Meijsing SH, Pallares-Trujillo J et al (2001) Cancer cachexia: a therapeutic approach. Med Res Rev 21:83–101

53. Inui A (2002) Cancer anorexia-cachexia syndrome: current issues in research and management. CA Cancer J Clin 52:72–91

54. Mantovani G, Macciò A, Massa E, Madeddu C (2001) Managing cancer-related anorexia/cachexia. Drugs 61:499–514

55. Auphan N, DiDonato JA, Rosette C et al (1995) Immunosuppression by glucocorticoids: inhibition of NF-kappa B activity through induction of I kappa B synthesis. Science 270:286–290

56. Scheinman RI, Cogswell PC, Lofquist AK, Baldwin AS Jr (1995) Role of transcriptional activation of I kappa B alpha in mediation of immunosuppression by glucocorticoids. Science 270:283–286

57. McEwan IJ, Wright AP, Gustafsson JA (1997) Mechanism of gene expression by the glucocorticoid receptor: role of protein-protein interactions. Bioessays 19:153–160

58. Scheinman RI, Gualberto A, Jewell CM et al (1995) Characterization of mechanisms involved in transrepression of NF-kappa B by activated glucocorticoid receptors. Mol Cell Biol 15:943–953

59. Armstrong VW, Oellerich M (2001) New developments in the immunosuppressive drug monitoring of cyclosporine, tacrolimus, and azathioprine. Clin Biochem 34:9–16

60. Buurman WA, Ruers TJ, Daemen IA et al (1986) Cyclosporin A inhibits IL 2-driven proliferation of human alloactivated T cells. J Immunol 136:4035–4039

61. Matsuda S, Koyasu S (2000) Mechanisms of action of cyclosporine. Immunopharmacology 47:119–125

62. Meyer S, Kohler NG, Joly A (1997) Cyclosporine A is an uncompetitive inhibitor of proteasome activity and prevents NF-kappaB activation. FEBS Lett 413:354–358

63. Holschermann H, Durfeld F, Maus U et al (1996) Cyclosporine a inhibits tissue factor expression in monocytes/macrophages. Blood 88:3837–3845

64. Dawson J, Hurtenbach U, MacKenzie A (1996) Cyclosporin A inhibits the in vivo production of interleukin-1b and tumour necrosis factor a, but not interleukin-6, by a T-cell-independent mechanism. Cytokine 8:882–888

65. Garcia JE, de Cabo MR, Rodriguez FM et al (2000) Effect of cyclosporin A on inflammatory cytokine production by U937 monocyte-like cells. Mediators Inflamm 9:169–174

66. Losa Garcia JE, Mateos Rodriguez F et al (1998) Effect of cyclosporin A on inflammatory cytokine production by human alveolar macrophages. Respir Med 92:722–728

67. Rofe AM, Whitehouse MW, Bourgeois CS et al (1990) Prevention of adjuvant-induced cachexia in rats by cyclosporin A. Immunol Cell Biol 68:63–69

68. Dumont FJ (2000) FK506, an immunosuppressant targeting calcineurin function. Curr Med Chem 7:731–748

69. Yard BA, Pancham RR, Paape ME et al (1993) CsA, FK506, corticosteroids and rapamycin inhibit TNF-alpha production by cultured PTEC. Kidney Int 44:352–358

70. Napoli KL, Taylor PJ (2001) From beach to bedside: history of the development of sirolimus. Ther Drug Monit 23:559–586

71. Kay JE, Kromwel L, Doe SE, Denyer M (1991) Inhibition of T and B lymphocyte proliferation by rapamycin. Immunology 72:544–549

72. Jorgensen PF, Wang JE, Almlof M et al (2001) Sirolimus interferes with the innate response to bacterial products in human whole blood by attenuation of IL-10 production. Scand J Immunol 53:184–191

73. Istvan ES, Deisenhofer J (2001) Structural mechanism for statin inhibition of HMG-CoA reductase. Science 292:1160–1164

74. Roberts WC (1997) The rule of 5 and the rule of 7 in lipid-lowering by statin drugs. Am J Cardiol 82:106–107

75. Endo A, Kuroda M, Tsujita Y (1976) ML-236A, ML-236B, and ML-236C, new inhibitors of cholesterogenesis produced by Penicillium citrinium. J Antibiot (Tokyo) 29:1346–1348

76. Rosenson RS (2004) Current overview of statin-induced myopathy. Am J Med 116:408–416

77. Jacobs D, Blackburn H, Higgins M et al (1992) Report of the Conference on Low Blood Cholesterol: Mortality Associations. Circulation 86:1046–1060

78. Newman TB, Hulley SB (1996) Carcinogenicity of lipid-lowering drugs. JAMA 275:55–60

79. Bjerre LM, LeLorier J (2001) Do statins cause cancer? A meta-analysis of large randomized clinical trials. Am J Med 110:716–723

80. Strandberg TE, Pyorala K, Cook TJ et al (2004) for the 4S Group. Mortality and incidence of cancer during 10-year follow-up of the Scandinavian Simvastatin Survival Study (4S). Lancet 364:771–777

81. Liao JK (2002) Isoprenoids as mediators of the biological effects of statins. J Clin Invest 110:285–288

82. Ridker PM, Rifai N, Clearfield M et al (2001) Air Force/Texas Coronary Atherosclerosis Prevention Study Investigators. Measurement of C-reactive protein for the targeting of statin therapy in the primary prevention of acute coronary events. N Engl J Med 344:1959–1965

83. Albert MA, Danielson E, Rifai N, Ridker PM (2001) PRINCE Investigators. Effect of statin therapy on C-reactive protein levels: the pravastatin inflammation/CRP evaluation (PRINCE): a randomized trial and cohort study. JAMA 286:64–70

84. Ridker PM, Cannon CP, Morrow D et al (2005) on behalf of the Pravastatin or Atorvastatin Evaluation and Infection Therapy-Thrombolysis in Myocardial Infarction 22 (PROVE IT-TIMI 22) Investigators. C-reactive protein levels and outcomes after statin therapy. N Engl J Med 352:20–28

85. Rosenson RS, Tangney CC, Casey LC (1999) Inhibition of proinflammatory cytokine production by pravastatin. Lancet 353:983–984

86. Chan DC, Watts GF, Barrett PH et al (2002) Effect of atorvastatin and fish oil on plasma high-sensitivity

C-reactive protein concentrations in individuals with visceral obesity. Clin Chem 48:877–883

87. Koh KK, Son JW, Ahn JY et al (2003) Comparative effects of diet and simvastatin on markers of thrombogenicity in patients with coronary artery disease. Am J Cardiol 91:1231–1234

88. Waehre T, Damas JK, Gullestad L et al (2003) Hydroxymethylglutaryl coenzyme a reductase inhibitors down-regulate chemokines and chemokine receptors in patients with coronary artery disease. J Am Coll Cardiol 41:1460–1467

89. Kinlay S, Schwartz GG, Olsson AG et al; Myocardial Ischemia Reduction with Aggressive Cholesterol Lowering Study Investigators (2003) High-dose atorvastatin enhances the decline in inflammatory markers in patients with acute coronary syndromes in the MIRACL study. Circulation 108:1560–1566

90. Node K, Fujita M, Kitakaze M et al (2003) Short-term statin therapy improves cardiac function and symptoms in patients with idiopathic dilated cardiomyopathy. Circulation 108:839–843

91. Holm T, Andreassen AK, Ueland T et al (2001) Effect of pravastatin on plasma markers of inflammation and peripheral endothelial function in male heart transplant recipients. Am J Cardiol 87:815–818

92. Indolfi C, Cioppa A, Stabile E et al (2000) Effects of hydroxymethylglutaryl coenzyme A reductase inhibitor simvastatin on smooth muscle cell proliferation in vitro and neointimal formation in vivo after vascular injury. J Am Coll Cardiol 35:214–221

93. Bustos C, Hernandez-Presa MA, Ortego M et al (1998) HMG-CoA reductase inhibition by atorvastatin reduces neointimal inflammation in a rabbit model of atherosclerosis. J Am Coll Cardiol 32:2057–2064

94. Walter DH, Schachinger V, Elsner M, Mach S et al (2000) Effect of statin therapy on restenosis after coronary stent implantation. Am J Cardiol 85:962–968

95. Corsini A, Pazzucconi F, Pfister P et al (1996) Inhibitor of proliferation of arterial smooth-muscle cells by fluvastatin. Lancet 348:1584

96. Kureishi Y, Luo Z, Shiojima I et al (2000) The HMG-CoA reductase inhibitor simvastatin activates the protein kinase Akt and promotes angiogenesis in normocholesterolemic animals. Nat Med 6:1004–1010

97. Carmeliet P, Lampugnani MG, Moons L et al (1999) Targeted deficiency or cytosolic truncation of the VE-cadherin gene in mice impairs VEGF-mediated endothelial survival and angiogenesis. Cell 98:147–157

98. Fujio Y, Nguyen T, Wencker D et al (2000) Akt promotes survival of cardiomyocytes in vitro and protects against ischemia-reperfusion injury in mouse heart. Circulation 101:660–667

99. Fulton D, Gratton JP, McCabe TJ et al (1999) Regulation of endothelium-derived nitric oxide production by the protein kinase Akt. Nature 399:597–601

100. Dimmeler S, Fleming I, Fisslthaler B et al (1999) Activation of nitric oxide synthase in endothelial cells by Akt-dependent phosphorylation. Nature 399:601–605

101. Llevadot J, Murasawa S, Kureishi Y et al (2001) HMG-CoA reductase inhibitor mobilizes bone marrow-derived endothelial progenitor cells. J Clin Invest 108:399–405

102. Vasa M, Fichtlscherer S, Adler K et al (2001) Increase in circulating endothelial progenitor cells by statin therapy in patients with stable coronary artery disease. Circulation 103:2885–2890

103. Walter DH, Rittig K, Bahlmann FH et al (2002) Statin therapy accelerates reendothelialization: a novel effect involving mobilization and incorporation of bone marrow-derived endothelial progenitor cells. Circulation 105:3017–3024

104. Kumar B, Andreatta C, Koustas WT et al (2002) Mevastatin induces degeneration and decreases viability of cAMP-induced differentiated neuroblastoma cells in culture by inhibiting proteasome activity, and mevalonic acid lactone prevents these effects. J Neurosci Res 68:627–635

105. Russo G, Leopold JA, Loscalzo J (2002) Vasoactive substances: nitric oxide and endothelial dysfunction in atherosclerosis. Vascul Pharmacol 38:259–269

106. von Haehling S, Anker SD, Bassenge E (2003) Statins and the role of nitric oxide in chronic heart failure. Heart Fail Rev 8:99–106

107. Goldstein JL, Brown MS (1990) Regulation of the mevalonate pathway. Nature 343:425–430

108. Ridley AJ (2001) Rho family proteins: coordinating cell responses. Trends Cell Biol 11:471–477

109. Amano M, Fukata Y, Kaibuchi K (2000) Regulation and functions of Rho-associated kinase. Exp Cell Res 261:44–51

110. Strey A, Janning A, Barth H, Gerke V (2002) Endothelial Rho signaling is required for monocyte transendothelial migration. FEBS Lett 517:261–266

111. Worthylake RA, Lemoine S, Watson JM, Burridge K (2001) RhoA is required for monocyte tail retraction during transendothelial migration. J Cell Biol 154:147–160

112. Wassmann S, Laufs U, Muller K et al (2002) Cellular antioxidant effects of atorvastatin in vitro and in vivo. Arterioscler Thromb Vasc Biol 22:300–305

113. Laufs U, Fata VL, Plutzky J, Liao JK (1998) Upregulation of endothelial nitric oxide synthase by HMG CoA reductase inhibitors. Circulation 97:1129–1135

114. Shaul PW (2002) Regulation of endothelial nitric oxide synthase: location, location, location. Annu Rev Physiol 64:749–774

115. Feron O, Dessy C, Desager JP, Balligand JL (2001) Hydroxy-methylglutaryl-coenzyme A reductase inhibition promotes endothelial nitric oxide synthase activation through a decrease in caveolin abundance. Circulation 103:113–118

116. Pelat M, Dessy C, Massion P et al (2003)

Rosuvastatin decreases caveolin-1 and improves nitric oxide-dependent heart rate and blood pressure variability in apolipoprotein E-/- mice in vivo. Circulation 107:2480–2486

117. Kunz W (1956) N-Phthalyl-glutaminsäure-imid. Arzneimittelforschung 6:426–430

118. Sampaio EP, Kaplan G, Miranda A et al (1993) The influence of thalidomide on the clinical and immunologic manifestation of erythema nodosum leprosum. J Infect Dis 168:408–414

119. Sampaio EP, Sarno EN, Galilly R et al (1991) Thalidomide selectively inhibits tumor necrosis factor a production by stimulated human monocytes. J Exp Med 173:699–703

120. Moreira AL, Sampaio EP, Zmuidzinas A et al (1993) Thalidomide exerts its inhibitory action on tumor necrosis factor a by enhancing mRNA degradation. J Exp Med 177:1675–1680

121. Davey PP, Ashrafian H (2000) New therapies for heart failure: is thalidomide the answer? QJM 93:305–311

122. Bruera E, Neumann CM, Pituskin E et al (1999) Thalidomide in patients with cachexia due to terminal cancer: preliminary report. Ann Oncol 10:857–859

123. Inui A (2002) Cancer anorexia-cachexia syndrome: current issues in research and management. CA Cancer J Clin 52:72–91

124. Tramontana JM, Utaipat U, Molloy A et al (1995) Thalidomide treatment reduces tumor necrosis factor alpha production and enhances weight gain in patients with pulmonary tuberculosis. Mol Med 1:384–397

125. Muscaritoli M, Costelli P, Bossola M et al (2003) Effects of simvastatin administration in an experimental model of cancer cachexia. Nutrition 19:936–939

# Subject Index